Oxford Textbook of
Neurorehabilitation

Oxford Textbooks in Clinical Neurology

PUBLISHED

Oxford Textbook of Epilepsy and Epileptic Seizures
Edited by Simon Shorvon, Renzo Guerrini, Mark Cook, and Samden Lhatoo

Oxford Textbook of Vertigo and Imbalance
Edited by Adolfo Bronstein

Oxford Textbook of Movement Disorders
Edited by David Burn

Oxford Textbook of Stroke and Cerebrovascular Disease
Edited by Bo Norrving

Oxford Textbook of Neuromuscular Disorders
Edited by David Hilton-Jones and Martin Turner

FORTHCOMING

Oxford Textbook of Neuroimaging
Edited by Massimo Filippi

Oxford Textbook of Neuro-oncology
Edited by Tracy Batchelor, Ryo Nishikawa, Nancy Tarbell, and Michael Weller

Oxford Textbook of Cognitive Neurology and Dementia
Edited by Masud Husain and Jonathan Schott

Oxford Textbook of Headache Syndromes
Edited by Michel Ferrari, Joost Haan, Andrew Charles, David Dodick, and Fumihiko Sakai

Oxford Textbook of Clinical Neurophysiology
Edited by Kerry Mills

Free personal online access for 12 months

Individual purchasers of this book are also entitled to free personal access to the online edition for 12 months on *Oxford Medicine Online* (www.oxfordmedicine.com). Please refer to the access token card for instructions on token redemption and access.

Online ancillary materials, where available, are noted at the end of the respective chapters in this book. Additionally, *Oxford Medicine Online* allows you to print, save, cite, email, and share content; download high-resolution figures as Microsoft PowerPoint slides; save often-used books, chapters, or searches; annotate; and quickly jump to other chapters or related material on a mobile-optimised platform.

We encourage you to take advantage of these features. If you are interested in ongoing access after the 12-month gift period, please consider an individual subscription or consult with your librarian.

Oxford Textbook of

Neurorehabilitation

Edited by

Volker Dietz

Professor em. Dr. Spinal Cord Injury Center Balgrist University Hospital, Zurich, Switzerland

Nick S. Ward

Reader in Clinical Neurology & Honorary Consultant Neurologist, UCL Institute of Neurology and The National Hospital for Neurology and Neurosurgery, Queen Square, London, UK

Series Editor

Christopher Kennard

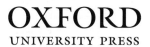

OXFORD

UNIVERSITY PRESS

Great Clarendon Street, Oxford, OX2 6DP,
United Kingdom

Oxford University Press is a department of the University of Oxford.
It furthers the University's objective of excellence in research, scholarship,
and education by publishing worldwide. Oxford is a registered trade mark of
Oxford University Press in the UK and in certain other countries

First Edition published in 2015

Impression: 1

Published in the United States of America by Oxford University Press
198 Madison Avenue, New York, NY 10016, United States of America

British Library Cataloguing in Publication Data

Data available

Library of Congress Control Number: 2014948347

ISBN 978–0–19–967371–1

Printed and bound by
Bell & Bain Ltd, Glasgow

Preface

This volume, Oxford Textbook of Clinical Neurorehabilitation, mainly reflects insights from knowledge gained over the last 25 years. It covers the most relevant aspects of neurorehabilitation approaches as currently applied, most of which are dependent, to a large degree, upon advances made through basic, clinical, therapeutic, social, and technological research during recent decades. We asked the authors-all of whom are acknowledged experts in a specific field of neurorehabilitation-to present their chapters with the current state of the art in their area and, as far as possible, the scientific basis on which contemporary treatment approaches are based. The authors were also asked to make their chapters attractive and accessible for both specialists and non-specialists involved in the neurorehabilitation of patients by including videos, illustrations, and tables to provide a summary of particular aspects of their subject. Where appropriate, different perspectives on a given field are also provided. This volume should serve as a current overview covering all aspects of neurorehabilitation for medical doctors, scientists and therapists working in this diverse and advancing field.

Impressive progress has been made in the field of neurorehabilitation over recent decades. This period of change dawned with an almost exclusively experience-based neurorehabilitation approach, inaugurated by a number of schools and usually practiced in separation from other medical disciplines. Over time, in most subspecialities, evidence-based neurorehabilitation has been gradually established. This move towards a more scientific and integrated paradigm is illustrated by smoother transitions from acute care: for instance, stroke patients into early rehabilitation requiring close multidisciplinary interactions characterized by close cooperation between clinical staff and researchers. This early phase of rehabilitation is followed by longer-term functional training approaches and social integration programmes, which are today being successfully applied for patients with stroke, brain injury, and spinal cord injury (SCI). Such modern rehabilitation approaches have strong theoretical underpinnings, for instance on evidence gained from animal experiments investigating the exploitation potential of neuroplasticity or from well-conducted patient studies concerning the effect of longer training times on the recovery of sensorimotor function during rehabilitation in patient with various forms of central (CNS) and peripheral nervous system damage. However, despite all this recent progress, we must acknowledge the evident limitations of our treatment approaches. After severe CNS damage neurological deficits

remain, and our ongoing aim can only be to achieve more optimal outcomes for individual patients.

Repetitive training of lost functional movements has become established for the recovery of sensorimotor function. This has been associated with an increase in the use and impact of technology in contemporary neurorehabilitation programmes, using assistive devices, feedback information, and virtual reality training conditions. This technology allows standardized training sessions and objective measurement of the trajectory of movement recovery and can motivate the patient through feedback over the course of rehabilitation. Today, the significance of this technology is occasionally considered to be overestimated and its further development is critically discussed. Further progress with technology must be driven by recognition of the physiological requirements for its beneficial application. Nevertheless, there are few doubts that technology will continue to have an increasing impact in neurorehabilitation.

Despite all these promising developments, in several respects there are still hurdles to overcome if we are to achieve optimal neurorehabilitation strategies. Although concepts such as neuroplasticity are well attested in animal experiments, a major problem still concerns the successful translation of basic research into clinical applications. Several causes may perpetuate this problem. Despite promising techniques for inducing neural regeneration in animal models, applying therapies based on these concepts in human patients with SCI has not yet shown convincing results. This failure may be due to the lack of an adequate animal model and a solution will require close cooperation between researchers and clinicians involved in the care of patients with CNS damage.

We are also still at the beginning of building a true understanding of the factors which underlie and influence training effects. For example, which proprioceptive input is required to achieve meaningful limb muscle activation, in turn leading to training effects resulting in improved sensorimotor functional outcomes? How can a treatment programme be optimally adapted to individual abilities and requirements, for example, with respect to movement velocity and complexity? To what extent must training of particular factors, such as equilibrium control during stepping, be challenging?

We must also be aware of the increasing population of elderly people requiring neurorehabilitation. This is having and will continue to have profound medical, therapeutic and social consequences. This situation is frequently neglected and solutions must be identified and developed in the near future. One such solution might be improved transition from an initial, short, focused neurorehabilitation period in specialized centres, prior to early integration into community- or home-based rehabilitation with community-based nursing care and an environment adapted to the individual's needs and access to neurorehabilitation specialists.

Observations indicate that neuroplasticity can still be successfully exploited in elderly patients and lead to a degree of neurological recovery similar to that possible in young patients, although translation in functional gains is usually poor. Elderly people thus require special training approaches focused on a few important daily life activities, something often more successfully achieved in a familiar setting (i.e. at home or in the community) rather than in a specialized centre where elderly people may have difficulty adapting to an unfamiliar setting.

In the future, prediction of outcome will be further improved and will determine the focus of training approaches to be applied.

It might not only allow the optimization of sensorimotor functional rehabilitation but also prevent complications of autonomic dysfunction and the development of pain syndromes. Such early outcome predictions, particularly for sensorimotor functions, are available today, usually using a combination of electrophysiological and imaging assessments in conjunction with clinical examination.

If rehabilitation medicine is to continue its recent progression, close cooperation between basic and clinical research, therapists, and engineers is required to develop and promote useful assessments for an early refined prediction of outcome (sensorimotor and autonomic function and pain syndromes) with the aim of establishing standardized, but individually adapted, treatment programmes.

Volker Dietz
Nick Ward

Contents

Abbreviations

5-HT	5-hydroxytryptamine	CI	confidence interval
AAC	alternative augmentative communication	CIDP	chronic inflammatory demyelinating polyradiculoneuropathy
ABG	arterial blood gas	CIMT	constrained induced movement therapy
Ach	acetylcholine	CISC	clean intermittent self-catheterization
AD	autonomic dysreflexia	CM	centre of mass
AD	Alzheimer's disease	CMA	cingulate motor area
ADH	antidiuretic hormone	CMAd	dorsal cingulate motor area
ADHD	attention deficit hyperactivity disorders	CMT	Charcot–Marie–Tooth
ADL	activities of daily living	CMV	cytomegalovirus
AFO	ankle–foot orthoses	CNP	central neuropathic pain
AIS	American Spinal Injury Association Impairment Scale	CNS	central nervous system
AMA	antimitochondrial antibodies	CONSORT	CONsolidated Standards of Reporting Trials Statement
AMPS	Assessment of Motor and Process Skills	CoP	centre of pressure
ANA	antinuclear antibodies	CPG	central pattern generator
ANS	autonomic nervous system	CRP	C-reactive protein
APBT	active–passive bilateral training	C-SCI	cervical spinal cord injury
ARAT	Action Research Arm Test	CST	corticospinal tract system
ASD	autistic spectrum disorder	CST	corticospinal tract
ASIA	American Spinal Injury Association	CT	combined training
ATC	assistive technology for cognition	CVS	cardiovascular system
AUC	area under the curve	CWRU	Case Western Reserve University
BAT	bilateral arm training	CXR	chest X-ray
BATRAC	Bilateral arm training with rhythmic auditory cueing	DA	dopamine
		DALY	disability adjusted life year
BB	Box and Blocks Test	DCML	dorsal column medial lemniscus
BDNF	brain-derived neurotrophic factor	DDAVP	desmopressin acetate
BI	Barthel Index	DFNS	German Network on Neuropathic Pain
BMSC	bone marrow stromal cells	DG	dentate gyrus
BNAVE	Balance Near Automatic Virtual Environment	DLB	dementia with Lewy bodies
BOLD	blood oxygen level-dependent	DMB	Data Monitoring Board
BP	blood pressure	DO	detrusor overactivity
BrdU	bromodeoxyuridine	DOF	degrees of freedom
BWS	body weight support	DSD	detrusor-sphincter-dyssynergia
BWSTT	body weight-supported treadmill training	DTI	diffusion tensor imaging
CAHAI	Chedoke Arm and Hand Activity Inventory	DWI	Diffusion-weighted imaging
CAT	computer-assisted therapy	EADL	electronic aid for daily living
CBF	cerebral blood flow	EAE	experimental autoimmune encephalomyelitis
CBS	Catherine Bergego Scale	EBV	Epstein–Barr virus
CBT	cognitive-behavioural therapy	EEG	electroencephalography
CCS	central cord syndrome	eEmc	electrical enabling motor control
CF	cystic fibrosis	EFNS	European Federation of Neurological Societies Task Force
CFS	chronic fatigue syndrome		
CHEP	contact heat evoked potential		

EFNS	European Federation of Neurological Societies
EMA	European Medicines Agency
emEmc	electromagnetic stimulation enabling motor control
EMG	electromyography
ENA	extractable nuclear antigens
ES	electrical stimulation
ESC	embryonic stem cells
ESD	early supported discharge
ESR	erythrocyte sedimentation rate
ET	endurance training
EUS	external urethral sphincter
EXCITE	Extremity Constraint Induced Therapy Evaluation
FA	fractional anisotropy
FBC	full blood count
FDA	Food and Drug Administration
FEES	fibreoptic endoscopic evaluation of swallowing
fEmc	Pharmacological enabling motor control
FES	functional electrical stimulation
FIM	Functional Independence Measure
FINE	flat interface nerve electrode
FLAME	Fluoxetine for Motor Recovery after Acute Ischaemic Stroke
FM score	Fugl-Meyer Motor Score
FMA	Fugl-Meyer Arm scale
FMS	Fugl-Meyer Scale
FRA	flexor reflex afferent
FST	functional strength training
GABA	gamma-aminobutyric acid
GABAAR	GABA type A receptor
GABABR	GABA type B receptor
GAPS	Glasgow Augmented Physiotherapy after Stroke
GBA	glucocerebrosidase
GCS	Glasgow Coma Scale
GET	graded exercise therapy
GI	gastrointestinal
GMC	General Medical Council
GMT	goal-management training
GNP	grasping neuroprosthesis
GRADE	Grading of Recommendations Assessment, Development and Evaluation
GRASP	graded repetitive arm supplementary programme
GRASPP	Graded Redefined Assessment of Strength, Sensibility and Prehension
GRF	ground reaction force
GSR	galvanic skin response
HAS	hybrid assistive system
HD	Huntington's disease
HIV	human immunodeficiency virus
HOS	hybrid orthotic system
HPA	hypothalamic-pituitary-adrenal
HR	heart rate
HRG	healthcare resource group
IASP	International Association for the Study of Pain
ICC	intraclass correlation coefficients
ICD 10	International Classification of Diseases 10th edition
ICF	International Classification of Functioning, Disability, and Health

ICF	International Classification of Functioning
ICF model	International Classification of Functioning, Disability and Health Model
ICIDH	International Classification of Impairments, Disabilities and Handicaps
IFN-α	interferon-α
IFN-β	interferon-β
IMMPACT	Initiative on Methods, Measurement, and Pain Assessment in Clinical Trials
iPSC	inducible pluripotent stem cells
IRB	
ISCIBPD	International Spinal Cord Injury Basic Pain Dataset
ISCIP	International Spinal Cord Injury Pain Classification
ISNCSCI	International Standards for Neurological Classification of Spinal Cord Injury
ISRCTN	International Standard Randomized Control Trial Number
ITB	intrathecal baclofen
JTT	Jebsen–Taylor Hand Function Test
L-DOPS	l-threo-3,4-dihydroxyphenylserine
LFT	liver function test
LMR	locomotor mesencephalic region
L-NAME	nitro-l-arginine methyl ester
LOS	length of stay
LTD	long-term depression
LTNC	long-term neurological condition
LTP	long-term potentiation
LTP	long-term potentiation
LUT	lower urinary tract
M1	primary motor cortex
MAL	Motor Activity Log
MCAO	middle cerebral artery occlusion
MCI	mild cognitive impairment
MCID	minimal clinically important difference
MEG	magnetoencephalography
MEP	motor-evoked potential
MeSH	Medical Subject Headings
MHADIE	Measuring Health and Disability in Europe
MI	Motricity Index
MIBG	metaiodobenzylguanidine
MIME	mirror image movement enabling
MPI	Multidimensional Pain Inventory
MRI	magnetic resonance imaging
MS	multiple sclerosis
MSA	multiple system atrophy
MSC	mesenchymal stem cell
MSU	mid-stream urine
mTBI	minor traumatic brain injury
MUST	Malnutrition Universal Screening Tool
MVC	maximal voluntary contraction
NANC	non-adrenergic non-cholinergic
NBD	neurogenic bowel dysfunction
NCS	nerve conduction studies
NDO	neurogenic detrusor overactivity
NE	norepinephrine
NG	nasogastric
NGF	nerve growth factor

NIBS	non-invasive brain stimulation		ROM	range of motion
NICE	National Institute of Health and Care Excellence		RT	resistance training
NIH	National Institutes of Health		rTMS	repetitive transcranial magnetic stimulation
NIHSS	National Institutes of Health Stroke Scale		SARS	sacral anterior root stimulator
NLI	neurological level injury		SC	Schwann cells
NLUTD	neurogenic lower urinary tract dysfunction		SCI	spinal cord injury
NMDAR	NMDA receptor		SCIM	Spinal Cord Independence Measure
NMES	neuromuscular electrical stimulation		SGZ	subgranular zone
NMDA	N-methyl-D-aspartate		SIS	Stroke Impact Scale
NNT	number needed to treat		SLE	systemic lupus erythematosus
NP	neuroprosthesis		SMA	supplementary motor area
NPC	neural precursor cells		SNRI	serotonin-noradrenaline reuptake inhibitors
NPS	Neuropathic Pain Scale		SPECT	single-photon emission computed tomography
NPSI	Neuropathic Pain Symptom Inventory		SR	spinal reflex
NRS	Numerical rating scale		SREBR	Stroke Rehabilitation Evidence-Based Review
NSAID	non-steroidal anti-inflammatory drug		SSEP	somatosensory evoked potential
NSC	Neural stem cells		SSR	sympathetic skin response
NSPC	neural stem/progenitor cells		SSRI	Selective serotonin reuptake inhibitor
OA	osteoarthritis		STROBE	Strengthening the Reporting of Observational Studies in Epidemiology
OB	olfactory bulb			
OEC	olfactory ensheathing cells		STT	spinothalamic tract
OH	orthostatic hypotension		SVZ	subventricular zone
OM	opposing muscle		TBI	traumatic brain injury
OT	other training		TBS	theta burst stimulation
PAF	pure (primary) autonomic failure		TCA	tricyclic antidepressant
PAG	periaqueductal grey		TcMEP	transcranial motor evoked potential
PAS	paired associative stimulation		TCT	trunk control test
pcEmc	transcutaneous electrical stimulation		TDCS	transcranial direct current stimulation
PCS	post-concussion syndrome		tDCS	transcranial direct current stimulation
PD	Parkinson's disease		TENS	transcutaneous electrical nerve stimulation
PEFR	peak expiratory flow rate		TES	therapeutic electrical stimulation
PEG	percutaneous endoscopic gastrostomy		TFT	thyroid function test
PET	positron emission tomography		TIA	transient ischaemic attack
PLIC	posterior limb of the internal capsule		TLE	temporal lobe epilepsy
PLMD	periodic limb movement disorder		TM	target muscle
PLORAS	predicting language outcome and recovery after stroke		TMS	transcranial magnetic stimulation
			tRNS	transcranial random noise stimulation
PMC	pontine micturition centre		tsDCS	transcutaneous spinal direct current stimulation
PMd	dorsolateral premotor cortex			
PMv	ventrolateral premotor cortex		TST	thermoregulatory sweat test
PNF	proprioceptive neuromuscular facilitation		TTZ	training target zone
PNS	peripheral nervous system		U&Es	urea and electrolytes
POTS	postural orthostatic tachycardia syndrome		UDP	use-dependent plasticity
pQCT	peripheral quantitative computed tomography		UTI	urinary tract infection
PREP	Predicting REcovery Potential		VA	Veterans Affairs
PTEN	phosphatase and tensin homologue		VECTORS	Very Early Constraint-Induced Movement during Stroke Rehabilitation
PTSD	post-traumatic stress disorders			
PVS	permanent vegetative state		VI	visual illusion
PWD	persons with disabilities		VM	ventral mesencephalic
QALY	quality-adjusted life year		VR	virtual reality
QDIRT	quantitative direct and indirect test of sudomotor function		VRMT	VR-aided memory training
			WHO	World Health Organization
QSART	quantitative sudomotor axon reflex test		WISC II	Walking Index for Spinal Cord Injury II (WISCI II)
QST	quantitative sensory testing			
RCT	randomized controlled trial		WISCI	Walking Index for Spinal Cord Injury
RLS	restless leg syndrome		WMFT	Wolf Motor Function Test
RMS	rostral migratory stream		WNP	walking neuroprosthesis

Contributors

Roger Barker, Professor of Clinical Neuroscience and Honorary Consultant Neurologist, University of Cambridge and Addenbrooke's Hospital, John van Geest Centre for Brain Repair, Cambridge CB2 0PY, UK

Jo Bayly, Specialist Physiotherapist in Palliative Care, Woodlands Hospice, UHA Campus, Longmoor Lane, Liverpool, UK

Normand Boucher, Center for Interdisciplinary Research in Rehabilitation and Social Integration (CIRRIS) & School of Social Work, Université Laval, Québec, Canada

Jacopo Carpaneto, Biorobotics Institute, Scuola Superiore Sant'Anna, Pisa, Italy

Alan Carson, Department of Clinical Neurosciences, University of Edinburgh, Edinburgh, UK

Mike Craggs, Professor, Royal National Orthopaedic Hospital Trust, Brockley Hill, Stanmore, Middlesex, UK

Jenny Crinion, PhD, Clinical Scientist and Honorary Speech and Language Therapist, UCL Institute of Cognitive Neuroscience, London, UK

Armin Curt, Professor, Balgrist University Hospital, Spinal Cord Injury Center, Zurich, Switzerland

Volker Dietz, Professor, SCI Research, Spinal Cord Injury Centre, Balgrist University Hospital, Zürich, Switzerland

Bruce Dobkin, Professor of Neurology and Neurorehabilitation, UCLA, Los Angeles, CA, USA

Andrew Dorsch, Assistant Professor of Neurology, UCLA, Los Angeles, CA, USA

Jacques Duysens, KU Leuven, Department of Kinesiology, Heverlee, Belgium

V. Reggie Edgerton, Brain Research Institute UCLA, Life Sciences Building Los Angeles, CA, USA

Geoffrey Edwards, Center for Interdisciplinary Research in Rehabilitation and Social Integration (CIRRIS) & Department of Geomatic Sciences, Université Laval, Québec, Canada

Mark Edwards, Sobell Department of Motor Neuroscience and Movement Disorders, Institute of Neurology, University College London, London, UK

Gail Eva, NIHR Postdoctoral Fellow, Brain Repair & Rehabilitation, Institute of Neurology, Faculty of Brain Sciences, UCL, London

Patrick Fougeyrollas, Center for Interdisciplinary Research in Rehabilitation and Social Integration (CIRRIS) & Department of Anthropology, Université Laval, Québec, Canada

Steffen Franz, Spinal Cord Injury Center, Heidelberg University Hospital, Heidelberg, Germany

Angela Gall, Royal National Orthopaedic Hospital Trust, Brockley Hill, Stanmore, Middlesex, UK

Hubert Gascon, Center for Interdisciplinary Research in Rehabilitation and Social Integration (CIRRIS) & Department of Educational Sciences, Université du Québec à Rimouski, Lévis, Canada

Yury Gerasimenko, Brain Research Institute, University of California at Los Angeles, Los Angeles, California, USA

Michèle Hubli, Autonomic Research Lab, International Collaboration on Repair Discoveries (ICORD), University of British Columbia, Vancouver, Canada

Andreas Hug, Spinal Cord Injury Center, Heidelberg University Hospital, Heidelberg, Germany

Tom Hughes, Department of Neurology, University Hospital of Wales, Heath Park, Cardiff, UK

William Huynh, Institute of Neurological Sciences, Prince of Wales Hospital Randwick, NSW, Sydney, Australia; Brain and Mind Research Institute, Level 4, Clinical and Translational Research Building M02F, Camperdown NSW, Sydney, Australia.

Arun Jayaraman, Rehabilitation Institute of Chicago, Chicago, IL, USA

Sebastian Jessberger, Professor, Laboratory of Neural Plasticity, HiFo/Brain Research Institute, University of Zurich, Zurich, Switzerland

Ilse Jonkers, KU Leuven, Department of Kinesiology, Human Movement Biomechanics, Heverlee, Belgium

Matthew Kiernan, Professor, Bushell Chair of Neurology, Brain and Mind Research Institute, Level 4, Clinical and Translational Research Building M02F, Camperdown NSW, Sydney, Australia

Boudewijn Kollen, PhD, Department of General Practice, University of Groningen, University Medical Centre Groningen, AV Groningen, The Netherlands

John W. Krakauer, Professor of Neurology and Neuroscience, The Johns Hopkins University School of Medicine (JHUSOM), Baltimore, Maryland, USA

Gert Kwakkel, Professor, Department of Rehabilitation Medicine, VU University Medical Centre, Amsterdam, The Netherlands

Michael Lee, PhD, Physiotherapist and chiropractor, Neuroscience Research Australia, Randwick NSW, Sydney, Australia. Brain and Mind Research Institute, Level 4, Clinical and Translational Research Building M02F, Camperdown NSW, Sydney, Australia

Alex Leff, Reader in Cognitive Neurology and Honorary Consultant Neurologist, UCL Institute of Cognitive Neuroscience, Queen Square, London, UK

Daniel C. Lu, Ronald Reagan UCLA Medical Center, Department of Neurosurgery, Center for Health Sciences, Los Angeles, CA, USA

Andreas Luft, Neurologische Klinik, Universitätsspital Zürich, Zentrum für ambulante Rehabilitation, ZHW, Zürich, Switzerland

Firas Massaad, KU Leuven, Department of Kinesiology, Research Center for Movement Control and Neuroplasticity, Heverlee, Belgium

Gillian Mead, Professor of Stroke and Elderly Care Medicine, University of Edinburgh, Edinburgh, UK

Ulrich Mehnert, Department of Urology at Ruhruniversität Bochum, Germany

Pieter Meyns, KU Leuven, Department of Kinesiology, Research Center for Movement Control and Neuroplasticity, Tervuursevest 101, B-3001 Heverlee, Belgium

Silvestro Micera, Center for Neuroprosthetics and Institute of Bioengineering, School of Engineering, Ecole Polytechnique Federale de Lausanne (EPFL), Lausanne, Switzerland and Biorobotics Institute, Scuola Superiore Sant'Anna, Pisa, Italy

Luc Noreau, Center for Interdisciplinary Research in Rehabilitation and Social Integration (CIRRIS) & Department of Rehabilitation, Université Laval, Québec, Canada

Rory O'Connor, Senior Lecturer and Honorary Consultant Physician, Academic Department of Rehabilitation Medicine, Leeds, UK

Diane Playford, National Hospital for Neurology & Neurosurgery, Queen Square, London, UK

Arthur Prochazka, Professor, Neuroscience and Mental Health Institute, 507A Heritage Medical Research Centre, University of Alberta, Edmonton, Alberta, Canada

Radek Ptak, Head of Neuropsychology Section, Service de Neurorééducation, Hôpitaux Universitaires de Genève, Genève, Switzerland

Lucia Ricciardi, Sobell Department of Motor Neuroscience and Movement Disorders, Institute of Neurology, University College London, London, UK

Robert Riener, Professor, ETH Zurich, Sensory-Motor Systems Laboratory, University of Zurich, Zurich, Switzerland

John Rothwell, Professor, National Hospital for Neurology & Neurosurgery, Queen Square, London, UK

Francois Routhier, Center for Interdisciplinary Research in Rehabilitation and Social Integration (CIRRIS) & Department of Rehabilitation, Université Laval, Québec, Canada

Roland R. Roy, Brain Research Institute, University of California at Los Angeles, Los Angeles, California, USA

Rüdiger Rupp, Experimental Neurorehabilitation, Spinal Cord Injury Center, University Hospital Heidelberg, Germany

Louise Rutz-LaPitz, Rheinburg Klinik, Walzenhausen, Switzerland

William Rymer, Professor in Physical Medicine and Rehabilitation and Physiology, Northwestern University Feinberg School of Medicine, Chicago, IL, USA

Daniel Schließmann, Experimental Neurorehabilitation, Spinal Cord Injury Center, University Hospital Heidelberg, Germany

Armin Schnider, Professor of Neurorehabilitation, Service de Neurorééducation, Hôpitaux Universitaires de Genève, Genève, Switzerland

Christian Schuld, Experimental Neurorehabilitation, Spinal Cord Injury Center, University Hospital Heidelberg, Germany

Thomas Sinkjaer, Center for Sensory-Motor Interaction (SMI), Aalborg University and The Danish National Research Foundation, Copenhagen, Denmark

Bouwien Smits-Engelsman, KU Leuven, Department of Kinesiology, Heverlee, Belgium; Avans+ University for Professionals, Breda, Netherlands

Orlando Swayne, University College London, London, UK

Geert Verheyden, KU Leuven, Department of Rehabilitation Sciences, Faculty of Kinesiology and Rehabilitation Sciences, Heverlee, Belgium

Claude Vincent, Center for Interdisciplinary Research in Rehabilitation and Social Integration (CIRRIS) & Department of Rehabilitation, Université Laval, Québec, Canada

Derick Wade, Professor, The Oxford Centre for Enablement (OCE), Nuffield Orthopaedic Centre, Windmill Road, Oxford, UK

Nick Ward, National Hospital for Neurology & Neurosurgery, Queen Square, London, UK

Norbert Weidner, Spinal Cord Injury Center, University Hospital Heidelberg, Germany

Killian Welch, Robert Ferguson Unit, Royal Edinburgh Hospital, Edinburgh, UK

Eva Widerström-Noga, Research Professor, Department of Neurological Surgery, Rehabilitation Medicine and Neuroscience Program, and Health Scientist Veterans Affairs, University of Miami, USA

Markus Wirz, Head of Research and Development, Health Departement, Institute of Physiotherapy, ZHAW Zurich University of Applied Sciences, Winterthur, Switzerland

Ulf Ziemann, Department Neurology and Stroke, Hertie Institute for Clinical Brain Research, Eberhard Karls University Tübingen, Tübingen, Germany

General aspects of neurorehabilitation

SECTION 1

General aspects of neurorehabilitation

CHAPTER 1

The International Classification of Functioning, Disability, and Health

Diane Playford

The International Classification of Functioning, Disability, and Health (ICF) provides a framework for the description of health and health-related states and offers a biopsychosocial model of disability. It lists body functions and structure, and activity and participation. The relationship between impairment, activity, and participation is not linear, and can be further moderated by contextual factors, including personal and environmental factors. Each of these components is denoted by a prefix, followed by a numeric code, and then a qualifier, which also has a numeric value. This approach allows clear description of each domain, the extent of any impairment, and the level of performance and capacity at the activity and participation level. There are a wide range of potential applications of the ICF. It has been adopted most widely within rehabilitation services to describe individual functioning, but can also be used at a service and national policy level to describe, monitor, and evaluate different activities. This chapter aims to outline the use of the ICF, consider its strengths, and highlight its function in a range of settings.

The ICF was introduced by the World Health Organization (WHO) in 1999 as a response to the conceptual and practical difficulties posed by its predecessor, the International Classification of Impairment, Disability and Handicap (ICIDH) [1]. For many years there was a tension between medical and social models of disability. In the medical model disability was seen as a problem of the individual's body, whereas the social model identified disability as a consequence of the external environment and societal attitudes [2]. These two views polarize the debate. While it is clearly not acceptable for an individual to be denied their role in society through barriers created by the social, political and physical environment, it is also appropriate for clinicians, if requested, to treat pain, spasticity, weakness and other symptoms.

It is clear that such polarized views were never the only views on this debate. Gzil and colleagues [3] chart clearly the evolution of thinking around disability. However, over the past ten years thinking has shifted as is exemplified by the adoption of the biopsychosocial model of disability described in the WHO ICF. When this was first published adoption was slow, but it is now accepted as a practical model of disability. This chapter will outline the ICF, consider how widely it has been adopted, and identify some of the remaining issues in its widespread adoption and use.

The ICF provides a framework for the description of health and health-related states. It lists body functions and structure, and activity and participation [1]. Functioning refers to all body functions, activities, and participation, while disability is used for impairments, activity limitations, and participation restrictions. The relationship between impairment, activity, and participation is not linear, and can be further moderated by contextual factors, including personal and environmental factors. Body structures and functions, activities, participations, and environmental factors are coded, whereas personal factors are not. For example, the loss of a little finger is an impairment of body structure; in most people this will result in little change in activity or participation, but for an international concert violinist the participation restriction will be considerable and will impact on their ability to maintain paid work. However, whether they are able to accept this participation restriction and go on to find other paid work, say as a cab driver, will depend on personal factors including values and beliefs about paid work, and environmental factors such as their families willingness to support them financially.

The ICF can be drawn out schematically as shown in Figure 1.1.

- **Body functions** are physiological functions of body systems (including psychological functions). Examples of body functions include cognitive and emotional functioning; vision; hearing; and cardiovascular, respiratory, digestive, reproductive, and musculoskeletal functions.

- **Body structures** are anatomical parts of the body such as organs, limbs, and their components. Examples include the oesophagus, stomach, intestine, pancreas, and liver or the brain, spinal cord, and meninges.

- **Impairments** are problems in body function or structure, such as a significant deviation or loss. Examples would include respiratory failure or limb loss.

- **Activity** is the execution of a task or action by an individual, for example, lifting and carrying objects.

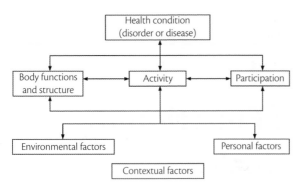

Fig. 1.1 The International Classification of Functioning, Disability and Health (ICF) drawn out schematically.

- **Activity limitations** are difficulties an individual may have in executing activities.
- **Participation** is involvement in a life situation, such as paid employment.
- **Participation restrictions** are problems an individual may experience in involvement in life situations.

Together, activity and participation describes the person's functional status and these are coded together using the following headings: learning and applying knowledge, general tasks and demands, communication, mobility, self care, domestic life, interpersonal interactions and relationships, major life areas and community, and social and civic life.

- **Environmental factors** make up the physical, social, and attitudinal environment in which people live and conduct their lives. They include factors that are not within the person's control, such as work, health, and social care agencies, legislation, and societal norms.
- **Personal factors** include race, gender, age, educational level, coping styles, values, and beliefs. Personal factors are not specifically coded in the ICF because of the wide variability among cultures. They are included in the framework, however, because although they are independent of the health condition they may have an influence on how a person functions.

Each of these components is denoted by a prefix, and is divided into chapters covering different domains:

    b for body function

    s for body structures

    d for activities and participation

    e for environmental factors.

When assigning a code, each prefix is followed by a numeric code that starts with the chapter number (one digit) and followed by second level item (two digits). For example, if we have to code body function for back pain then these are the codes:

b2	Sensory functions and pain	(first-level item)
b280	Sensation of pain	(second-level item)
b2801	Pain in a body part	(third-level item)
b28013	Pain in back	(fourth-level item).

The third and fourth level items are pertinent to some codes and not others.

For example, when coding dysarthria, the code will be as follows:

b3	Voice and speech functions	(first-level item)
b320	Articulation functions	(second-level item).

The domains of ICF become more meaningful when 'qualifiers' are used. Qualifiers are a numerical value and are suffixed after a point (separator) with the ICF code. They record the presence and severity of a problem at the functions, structure and activities, and participation level. The ICF guidelines state that any code should be accompanied by a qualifier, without which the code has no inherent meaning.

For the body structure and function, the qualifiers indicate presence of a problem and, on a five-point scale, the degree of impairment of function and/or structure, that is:

xxx.0 no problem

xxx.1 mild problem

xxx.2 moderate problem

xxx.3 severe problem

xxx.4 complete problem.

For example, b320.3: severe impairment in articulation functions of speech. In this example the (.3) after the main code b320 is the qualifier, and it describes severe impairment.

For activities and participation, there are two qualifiers that are used:

The first is the 'performance qualifier', which describes what individuals do in their current environment. This takes into account the environmental factors, so provides a 'lived experience'.

The second is the 'capacity qualifier', which describes the highest probable level of functioning of an individual in a given domain in a given time. This provides information related to a 'standard' environment.

For example:

d4500.21	In this example, the '2' after the point is the performance qualifier, and the '3' is the capacity qualifier. This will be read as:

d450	walking
d4500	walking short distances
d4500.2–	moderate difficulty in walking short distances in current setting (may include environmental support such as rails, or use of a frame
d4500.–3	severe difficulty in walking in a standard environment.

A further two qualifiers can then be added, including capacity qualifier with assistance and performance qualifier without assistance. This allows one to identify what patients do in their current environment using assistance (first qualifier), what they would do in a standard environment (second qualifier), what they could do in an optimized environment (third qualifier), and what they can do in their current environment without assistance (fourth qualifier).

The qualifier coding for environmental factors helps in indicating whether the environmental factors are facilitating or impeding the person's performance. Thus, they are represented with a plus sign for facilitation, and a minus sign or just a '.' for impediment. For example,

e150.2   design, construction, and building products, and technology of buildings for public use confer a moderate *obstacle*

e150+2   design, construction, and building products, and technology of buildings for public use provide a moderate *facilitating* effect.

This highlights the fact that environment should be assessed according to individual needs, and thus, it cannot be taken as standard. The pavement ramps and slopes can be a facilitator for a wheelchair user, whereas they may provide barrier to a blind person who uses a stick.

The WHO highlights a wide range of potential applications of the ICF. Initially adoption was slow [4]. Reasons highlighted were that activities and participation were categorized together in comparison with the very distinct conceptual differences of disability and handicap found in the earlier ICIDH. It was reported that, as they were conceptually distinct, they should have been categorized separately. However, it was recognized that users could differentiate activity and participation domains in a number of different ways, and this was left up to the user. Many users used to describing disability in terms of loss found the more positive language of the ICF unwieldy. It was felt that the ICF could only be used effectively following training. However, by 2012, Wiegand and colleagues [5] felt that although the adoption of the ICF was widespread in the field of rehabilitation, its implementation in practice was idiosyncratic and had rarely been evaluated properly. A study in 2013 of the implementation of the ICF in Israeli rehabilitation centres among physiotherapists suggested that the majority were familiar with the ICF, and nearly two thirds reported partial implementation in their units [6]. Implementation focused mostly on adopting the biopsychosocial concepts and using ICF terms. The ICF was not used either for evaluating patients or for reporting or encoding patient information, supporting Wiegand's view that evidence that the ICF has lead to real changes is lacking [5].

As suggested by Jacob [6], the place where the ICF has probably been most useful has been in rehabilitation of an individual patient where it provides a shared language within the multidisciplinary teams supporting a comprehensive assessment of an individual with a disability and facilitating treatment planning, which may aim to improve physiological function, maximize activity, alter the environment or support patient adjustment, all with a view to reaching a goal focussed on participation. As the whole data set can be unwieldy a considerable body of work using Delphi methodology has been undertaken, producing comprehensive and brief 'core sets' for different conditions and settings [7, 8]. Examples of such core sets exist for multiple sclerosis (MS) [9, 10], stroke [11], traumatic brain injury [12], and rheumatoid arthritis [13], and also for acute rehabilitation settings [14].

In other domains the ICF has been used less frequently. For example, it is rarely used for the evaluation of treatment and other interventions, or for self-evaluation by patients, although the capacity and performance qualifiers should allow this.

At the institutional level the ICF has potential to be used in planning, developing and evaluating services. Madden and colleagues [15] recently investigated the relationship between the ICF and information in reports published to monitor and evaluate community rehabilitation services. Thirty-six articles were selected for analysis containing 2495 information items. Approximately one third of the 2,495 information items identified in these articles (788 or 32%) related to concepts of functioning, disability and environment, and could be coded to the ICF. These information items were spread across the entire ICF classification with a concentration on activities and participation (49% of the 788 information items) and environmental factors (42%). Based on these findings Madden and colleagues [15] suggest the ICF can be used as a potentially useful framework and classification, providing building blocks for the systematic recording of information related to functioning and disability to inform health professionals and other staff, and to enable national and international comparisons.

The ICF could also be used to guide social policy development, including legislative reviews, model legislation, regulations and guidelines, and definitions for anti-discrimination legislation. For example, at the social level the ICF has potential to be used for eligibility criteria for state entitlements such as social security benefits, disability pensions, workers' compensation, and insurance. A recent study by Anner and colleagues [16] examined the official requirements on medical reporting about disability in social insurance across Europe. They found that four features were demanded: an assessment of work capacity, a socio-medical history, a determination of the feasibility and effectiveness of intervention and the prognosis. Within the reports on working capacity there was an increasing trend for authors to make formal or informal reference to the ICF. However, the formats of reporting on work capacity varied between countries, from free text to semi-structured report forms to fully structured and scaled report forms of working capacity. They suggest the ICF could serve as a reference for describing work capacity, provided the ICF contains all necessary categories. It is of interest that as well as recording the ICF categories the authors recognize the need for a socio-medical history, and a determination of the feasibility and effectiveness of intervention and the prognosis. These features are absent from the ICF and highlight some its potential weaknesses. The Italian Ministry of Health and Ministry of Labor and Social Policies supported a 3-year project for the definition of a common framework and a standardized protocol for disability evaluation based on ICF.

The MHADIE project (Measuring Health and Disability in Europe: Supporting policy development) aimed to develop realistic, evidence-based, and effective national policies for persons with disabilities [17]. A preliminary step towards this goal was the demonstration of the feasibility of employing the ICF in clinical, educational and statistical fields, which corresponds to the recognized need to enhance the European Union's capacity to describe the levels and extent of disability across populations, as highlighted in its Disability Action Plan 2006–2007. The ultimate outcome of the project was the production of 13 policy recommendations, dealing with statistics, clinical, and educational areas, and 4 general policy recommendations focusing on the need to: (a) co-ordinate and integrate disability conceptualization at all policy levels and across sectors; (b) conduct longitudinal cohort studies which include children aged 0–6; (c) review transport policies in light of the requirements of persons with disabilities; (d) review all disability policies to emphasize and support the role of the family, which is a consistent and substantial environmental facilitator in the lives of persons with disabilities.

Similarly the ICF has potential to be used in planning, developing and evaluating education and training for both professionals and patients. Little has been written on the use of the ICF for structuring professional curricula, although Sabariego [18, 19] demonstrated its utility in structuring an educational programme for stroke patients.

In research, the ICF has been used to provide a framework for patient-reported outcomes. Baker et al. described a scale selection strategy for choosing relevant outcomes for a study of robotics to treat the upper limb after stroke [20]. They used the ideas contained in the Food and Drug Administration (FDA) Patient Reported Outcome Measures document and mapped them on to the ICF to select a comprehensive set of measures. A study by Fayed and colleagues [21] used the ICF as a framework to demonstrate how many clinical trials do not capture measures important to children with chronic conditions. In a study of nearly 500 clinical trials less than 8% included an outcome focussed on activity and participation as part of the trial evaluation process.

It seems that, while the ICF has had a profound influence on the thinking of clinicians, it has not been adopted as widely as it could have been at a patient, service, policy, or research level for assessment and evaluation. Some of this may be due to lack of familiarity and it is clear that familiarity is growing. Escorpizo and Stucki [22] argue that disability can be described and measured using the ICF and ICF-related tools such as the Generic Set, ICF Core Sets specific to health conditions or settings, and measurement instruments that have been linked to the ICF. He states that education of those in occupational medicine, work rehabilitation, disability adjudication, policy and legislation, and government agencies about the ICF will lead to greater implementation of the ICF, including determining functional and work capacity and as a reference framework and a language of disability to help facilitate a common ground of understanding.

Some of this may be due to the fact that the full ICF is large and can be seen as unwieldy but the development of core sets mitigates this difficulty. A number of areas where the framework could be strengthened have been identified, many of which were apparent to the authors at first publication

First, the fact that there is lack of clarity in the distinction between activity and participation. Many authors have highlighted the difficulties, including Whiteneck [23]. Typical activities include activities of daily living (ADL) such as bathing, dressing, eating, walking, and talking, various combinations of which may be required to fulfil social roles. Typically, participation includes social roles (such as earning a living, parenting, and leisure activities), fulfilling civic and religious roles (spouse, parent, and citizen), all of which can be fulfilled in a wide variety of ways.

Second, it has been suggested by Wade and Halligan [24] that it needs to be integrated with a model of illnesses. At present, to code

disease the *International Classification of Diseases* 10th edition (ICD 10) has to be used, but there are areas where the ICD 10 and the ICF overlap. Work is currently being undertaken to address these difficulties [25]. However, our understanding of impairment of structure and function continues to develop and can now be considered at molecular, subcellular, cellular, and tissue level. Any categorization of pathology is likely to run the risk of being either simplistic or complex, incomplete and unwieldy. However, within the rehabilitation framework identifying pathology and its treatment is essential to allow rehabilitation physicians and teams to use all the means at their disposal to minimize disability. As recognized by the original authors of the ICF, in addition to failing to recognize pathology, it fails to acknowledge as part of the pathological diagnosis the importance of disease course in managing the treatment of disability; the needs of a person with relapsing remitting MS are quite different than the needs of a patient with a progressive neuropathy, which differ again from someone with a single-incident disorder. The only way to capture this is by recording changes in qualifiers over time.

Third, it does not describe personal factors [24]. Personal factors are not specifically coded in the ICF because of the wide variability among cultures. They are included in the framework, however, because although they are independent of the health condition they may have an influence on how a person functions. However, personal factors are critical to understanding performance; this explains why one patient, ventilated and quadriplegic, might apply to the courts requesting physician-assisted suicide and another similar patient manages with an appropriate care package and technological support to go to work every day for an IT company. It is also personal factors that explain the apparent mismatch between objective and experienced disability.

Closely related to personal factors are values and beliefs [24]. If rehabilitation is concerned with changing behaviour in an adaptive manner, then working with patients to determine their goals demands more than an understanding of the activity limitations and participation restrictions, but also needs an understanding of values and beliefs that lead to the prioritization of one goal over another.

In summary, the ICF represents a significant step forward and has embedded a biopsychosocial approach into rehabilitation thinking. It is used as a framework for considering the disability experienced by individual patients. However, it has not been adopted as widely as envisaged. It has rarely used for evaluating patients, or for reporting or encoding patient information, or for the evaluation of treatment and other interventions. It has potential to be used far more widely, including in education of both professionals and patients, to be used within occupational medicine, vocational rehabilitation, and government policy, allowing a shared language and precise coding of information both within and between services and countries. Some of the reasons for its slow adoption may be that it can feel unwieldy. It is likely that with the increasing use of core sets that the ICF will be used more widely in the future. Other limitations, many of which were highlighted by the authors at outset, include the fact that it does not incorporate any model of illness, or provide descriptors of personal factors, and individual values and beliefs. There is, however, a growing consensus about the use of the ICF and how it should further develop. With time, it is likely to be adopted more widely.

References

1. International Classification of Functioning, Disability and Health: ICF. World Health Organization, Geneva, 2001.
2. Marks D. Models of disability. Disabil Rehabil. 1997;**19**(3):85–91. Review.
3. Gzil F, Lefeve C, Cammelli M, et al. Why is rehabilitation not yet fully person-centred and should it be more person-centred? Disabil Rehabil. 2007;**29**(20–21):1616–1624.
4. Schuntermann MF. The implementation of the International Classification ofFunctioning, Disability and Health in Germany: experiences and problems. Int J Rehabil Res. 2005;**28**(2):93–102.
5. Wiegand NM, Belting J, Fekete C, Gutenbrunner C, Reinhardt JD. All talk, no action?: the global diffusion and clinical implementation of the international classification of functioning, disability, and health. Am J Phys Med Rehabil. 2012;**91**(7):550–560.
6. Jacob T. The implementation of the ICF among Israeli rehabilitation centers—the case of physical therapy. Physiother Theory Pract. 2013;**29**(7):536–546.
7. Grill E, Stucki G. Criteria for validating comprehensive ICF Core Sets anddeveloping brief ICF Core Set versions. J Rehabil Med. 2011;**43**(2):87–91.
8. Yen TH, Liou TH, Chang KH, Wu NN, Chou LC, Chen HC. Systematic review of ICF core set from 2001 to 2012. Disabil Rehabil. 2014;**36**(3):177–184.
9. Coenen M, Cieza A, Freeman J, Khan F, Miller D, Weise A, Kesselring J; Members of the Consensus Conference. The development of ICF Core Sets for multiple sclerosis: results of the International Consensus Conference. J Neurol. 2011;**258**(8):1477–1488.
10. Kesselring J, Coenen M, Cieza A, Thompson A, Kostanjsek N, Stucki G. Developing the ICF Core Sets for multiple sclerosis to specify functioning. Mult Scler. 2008;**14**(2):252–254. Epub 2007 Nov 6. PubMed PMID: 17986511.
11. Geyh S, Cieza A, Schouten J, et al. ICF Core Sets for stroke. J Rehabil Med. 2004;(44 Suppl):135–141.
12. Laxe S, Zasler N, Selb M, Tate R, Tormos JM, Bernabeu M. Development of the International Classification of Functioning, Disability and Health core sets for traumatic brain injury: an International consensus process. Brain Inj. 2013;**27**(4):379–387
13. Stucki G, Cieza A, Geyh S, et al. ICF Core Sets for rheumatoid arthritis. J Rehabil Med. 2004;(44 Suppl):87–93. PubMed PMID: 15370754.
14. Grill E, Ewert T, Chatterji S, Kostanjsek N, Stucki G. ICF Core Sets development for the acute hospital and early post-acute rehabilitation facilities. Disabil Rehabil. 2005 Apr 8–22;**27**(7–8):361–366. Review.
15. Madden RH, Dune T, Lukersmith S, et al. The relevance of the International Classification of Functioning, Disability and Health (ICF) in monitoring and evaluating community-based rehabilitation (CBR). Disabil Rehabil. 2014;**36**(10):826–837.
16. Anner J, Kunz R, Boer WD. Reporting about disability evaluation in European countries. Disabil Rehabil. 2014;**36**(10):848-854
17. Leonardi M, Chatterji S, Ayuso-Mateos JL, et al. Integrating research into policy planning: MHADIE policy recommendations. Disabil Rehabil. 2010;**32**(Suppl 1):S139–147.
18. Sabariego C, Barrera AE, Neubert S, Stier-Jarmer M, Bostan C, Cieza A. Evaluation of an ICF-based patient education programme for stroke patients: a randomized, single-blinded, controlled, multicentre trial of the effects on self-efficacy, life satisfaction and functioning. Br J Health Psychol. 2013 Nov;**18**(4):707–728.
19. Neubert S, Sabariego C, Stier-Jarmer M, Cieza A. Development of an ICF-based patient education program. Patient Educ Couns. 2011;**84**(2):e13–17.
20. Baker K, Cano SJ, Playford ED. Outcome measurement in stroke: a scale selection strategy. Stroke. 2011;**42**(6):1787–1794.
21. Fayed N, de Camargo OK, Elahi I, et al. Patient-important activity and participation outcomes in clinical trials involving children with chronic conditions. Qual Life Res. 2014;**23**(3):751–757.
22. Escorpizo R, Stucki G. Disability evaluation, social security, and theinternational classification of functioning, disability and health: the time is now. J Occup Environ Med. 2013;**55**(6):644–651.
23. Whiteneck G, Dijkers MP. Difficult to measure constructs: conceptual andmethodological issues concerning participation and environmental factors. Arch Phys Med Rehabil. 2009;**90**(11 Suppl):S22–35.
24. Wade DT, Halligan P. New wine in old bottles: the WHO ICF as an explanatory model of human behaviour. Clin Rehabil. 2003;**17**(4):349–354.
25. Escorpizo R, Kostanjsek N, Kennedy C, Nicol MM, Stucki G, Ustün TB; Functioning Topic Advisory Group (fTAG) of the ICD-11 Revision. Harmonizing WHO's International Classification of Diseases (ICD) and International Classificationof Functioning, Disability and Health (ICF): importance and methods to link disease and functioning. BMC Public Health. 2013;**13**:742.

CHAPTER 2

An interdisciplinary approach to neurological rehabilitation

Derick Wade

Introduction

People who have continuing disability often benefit from help to improve their abilities and/or to adapt. Rehabilitation services provide this help. Rehabilitation is a process focused on disability, the functional activities that are limited. It aims to optimize participation in social activities and to minimize distress and discomfort. Neurological and neuromuscular diseases are a common and potent cause of persistent, often progressive disability. Therefore the process of neurological rehabilitation is important to all healthcare.

This chapter discusses the process of rehabilitation, what it is, and how services should be organized. It argues that having access to a specialist team using an interdisciplinary approach is essential for all patients, even people with relatively straightforward problems. It focuses on the benefits that should follow on from using an interdisciplinary approach.

There are many definitions of rehabilitation, but the important core features [1–4] are that:

◆ It is primarily a **process**, not a single or limited set of treatments.

◆ It has as its focus **disability**, not disease.

◆ It necessarily has to take a **holistic view**, actively considering and taking into account all influences on a patient's situation, rather than considering such influences as of interest but to be put to one side as not relevant.

◆ Therefore it necessarily often involves a **wide range of different**:
  • people
  • professions, and also non-professional people
  • agencies and organizations including many outside the healthcare system.

Neurological and neuromuscular disorders pose a particular difficulty for two reasons. The central patient-related processes in rehabilitation are learning and adaptation, and it is the nervous system that is required for these recovery processes. Therefore the process must be adapted to the patient's cognitive ability, which will often be limited by the disease.

At the same time, because the nervous system is central to almost all human skills and activities, the range of losses is great and in particular usually includes a perceived or actual change in a person's identity. Consequently, the knowledge and skills needed cover a very wide range.

Although rehabilitation may appear very different from normal neurological practice, in reality it shares many common features. In particular, success depends upon a full, accurate analysis of the presenting problems (diagnosis) and then undertaking targeted interventions aimed at reversing or ameliorating identified problems (treatment). The primary difference is that the focus of attention in rehabilitation is on disability, the functional activities that are limited, rather than on the underlying damage to or disease of the nervous system, which is the focus of neurological and neurosurgical services.

The main consequence of this different focus—disability, not disease—is that a much wider range of factors is of importance. Even in neurology success requires access to a team covering a wide range of different areas of expertise such as neurophysiology, psychology and neurosurgery. In rehabilitation this is even more important, and the range of expertise needed is much larger.

This chapter outlines, for the non-expert, some more detail on the need for, and benefits of, a multidisciplinary approach, illustrating the very large range of expertise needed. It does so by starting with a short discussion of the analytic framework used within rehabilitation practice. This demonstrates the need for a team approach. It then discusses the rehabilitation process, before considering the membership of the team and how teams should work. One definition of a team is a group of people working towards a common goal, and this emphasizes the central importance of goal setting when faced with complex problems.

The biopsychosocial model of illness

In 1977 Engel wrote a seminal paper that is as relevant and fresh now as it was then [5]. In the paper he drew upon sociological and other research to formalise a much broader approach to analysing and understanding illness. Together with the ideas of Talcott Parsons published in 1952 [6], the biopsychosocial model of illness enabled a fuller understanding of illness. The biopsychosocial model was soon used by the World Health Organization as the basis for the International Classification of Impairments, Disabilities and Handicaps (WHO ICIDH, 1980) [7] and then the improved International Classification of Functioning (WHO ICF, 2001) [8].

The original biopsychosocial model has been developed to make it complete [2–4, 8]. Despite its relevance to all healthcare, it is only now becoming incorporated into wider healthcare systems [9–11]. It will be described briefly here. Many other references in this chapter expand upon it and its use. It is illustrated in Figure 2.1.

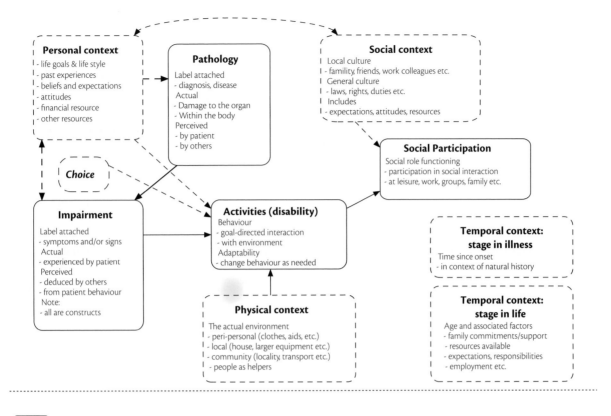

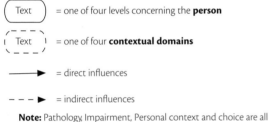

Text = one of four levels concerning the **person**

Text = one of four **contextual domains**

→ = direct influences

- - ► = indirect influences

Note: Pathology, Impairment, Personal context and choice are all **within** the person, and are not directly observable.

Activities and physical context are both directly observable.

Social participation and social context concern meaning and require interpretation or inference of observed actions or situations.

Temporal context is a given, but is often overlooked

Fig. 2.1 Biopsychosocial model of illness: components of importance.

The basic insight is that the complexity of any illness must first be divided into contextual factors and patient-related factors. The patient-related factors come from one of four hierarchical levels: the organ, the body, the person interacting with their physical, observable environment, and the person's interactions with other people. The contextual factors encompass four concepts: the physical environment, the social environment, the person's own pre-existing characteristics and time, which is subdivided to cover both the person's stage in their life and their stage in their illness.

The descriptive framework is also a systems analytic model, and only major interactions are shown in Figure 2.1. As would be predicted from a systems approach, there are multiple and complex interactions between different factors including some that apply in a direction contrary to expectation. One strength of this model, of particular relevance to neurologists is that it predicts the existence of functional illness [3].

Loss, change, and recovery

Recovery following an episode of tissue dysfunction occurs, initially, through restitution of the tissue and thus the functions associated with that tissue. However, when there is residual dysfunction the body and person adapts, a process of learning to achieve goals in a different way. For most internal, physiological functions this is 'automatic' and beyond conscious control. There are exceptions, such as the use of hormone replacement therapy after failure of an organ when the person has to learn to take the replacement appropriately, which is not trivial for insulin (for example).

In conditions where there is a gradual and usually progressive loss of tissue function, such as occurs with muscular dystrophies, multiple sclerosis, Huntington's disease or motor neuron disease, then there is an inevitable process of adaptation than can, in slowly progressive disorders such as Parkinson's disease, be so successful that the patient (to be) may lose significant amounts of tissue without noticing it. In other words, subclinical disease simply reflects very successful adaptation. In some disorders it is other people and not the patient who notice change, so successful is the adaptation. However, eventually most people will notice problems, especially in fluctuating conditions such as multiple sclerosis.

Finally, there are conditions that arise before, at or shortly after birth, when the person is naturally totally dependent anyway. If the damage is fixed, then the person will learn and develop and will incorporate the consequences of their losses (if any) into their normal development which may thus be different from usual. If the person has an additional progressive loss, they will also adapt to their changing abilities.

Rehabilitation

Rehabilitation is no more or less than helping the person to adapt and learn in response to their limited, altered, or changing abilities. Conceptually, it is exactly similar to education, except that it is set in the context of loss or absence of existing or expected abilities arising from a disease or health disorder.

Sometimes, for example when muscles have simply wasted through disuse or after an acute but reversible injury but are still intact, the process is primarily one of encouraging 'natural' recovery and doing so in a safe environment so that, for example, the person does not fall or develop skin pressure ulcers while recovering. More commonly, the process involves identifying and teaching alternative strategies and allowing practice in a safe environment. Also quite commonly, the process involves helping the person recognize that some previous goals or activities are no longer achievable, and helping them and their family adjust to this.

This approach emphasizes that rehabilitation is not only applicable to people with recently acquired losses set in the context of premorbid 'normality'. It is also appropriate for people who have limitations imposed by some congenital or other problem present from birth and for people who have a progressive disorder. In these circumstances the goals may be different and the underlying illness processes may be different, but rehabilitation services can still help the person adapt, set appropriate goals, which may be greater than those expected by the patient, and learn new skills to meet goals.

The **process** of rehabilitation is shown in Figure 2.2 and Figure 2.3. The rehabilitation process depends crucially upon an accurate initial analysis of the situation, identifying:

- Underlying pathology (disease, disorder) if any, because it may:
  - Determine prognostic field and prognostic markers
  - Suggest impairments that should be looked for, or do not need testing for
- Impairments present, nature and severity

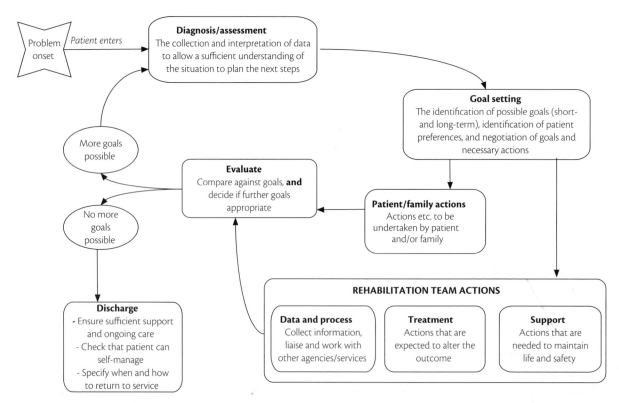

Fig. 2.2 The rehabilitation process—a reiterative cycle.

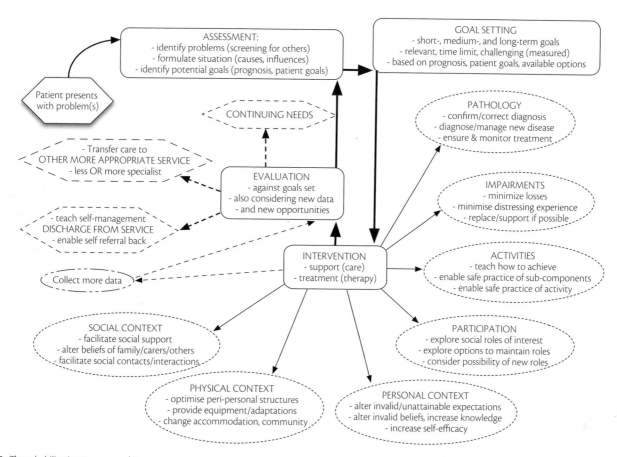

Fig. 2.3 The rehabilitation process and its components.

- Levels of activity and social participation
  - Currently
  - Previously, or in case of life-long illness, anticipated or desired
- Personal contextual factors
  - Expectations of rehabilitation and change
  - Attitudes, strengths, weaknesses, etc.
  - Goals/domains of interest
- Physical contextual factors such as:
  - Accommodation
  - Availability of practical support from people (caring, not social)
  - Equipment and adaptations
- Social contextual factors, such as
  - Attitudes and expectations of family and important others
  - Benefits and other resources available
- Prognosis: likely change and interventions needed and available.

Rehabilitation team

The list given of important components needed to achieve successful (efficient and effective) rehabilitation illustrates why a multidisciplinary team is needed.

For most patients with more complex problems, this detailed and in depth analysis can only be achieved by a group of professionals who have between them appropriate expertise. Without a clear, accurate initial analysis it is probable that the process may be misdirected, attempting to achieve inappropriate goals or not attempting to achieve appropriate goals. Unfortunately, failures in determining and setting expectations early on are still a common cause of both unnecessary disability (people not realizing that they could do more) and of distress, when given unduly optimistic expectations.

Patients with neurological conditions are particularly likely to have complex problems. Complexity is, in fact, difficult to define and in this context it refers to problems that:

- are multifactorial (i.e. are influenced by many different factors such as cognition, mood change, altered sensation)
- have interactions between the different factors that themselves influence the outcome of interest (e.g. combination of blindness and amnesia after posterior cerebral circulation ischaemia makes rehabilitation of both impairments much more difficult)
- have non-linear relationships between the different factors
- usually include also clinical uncertainty about the disease and its prognosis.

This complexity arises particularly in neurological rehabilitation because the nervous system is the central system to being a person, defined in rehabilitation as a social being who learns and adapts to changing circumstances. The brain, in particular, controls almost all conscious and much unconscious behaviour. It analyses situations, plans actions, responds to changes, etc. It also is the basis for personality, emotion and goals. Indeed most people now equate brain damage with a change in their personhood—who they *are*.

There are few if any conditions that affect the central nervous system that do not cause complex problems. Consequently, most patients with continuing problems associated with any neurological disorder may benefit from expert rehabilitation.

Given the wide range of problems that may arise from neurological dysfunction, it should be obvious that no single person or profession is likely to have the very large range of expertise needed to lead to an accurate analysis of a patient's situation. However, without a full understanding both of the deficits and of the areas of preserved or good function, it is likely that each individual professional person involved will not set appropriate goals or undertake appropriate interventions. For example, knowing how much apparent memory loss is actually secondary to depression, or how much apparent motor loss is secondary to a functional disorder may have a major impact on treatments offered.

Teams and teamwork

A team is or should be more than a group of people who simply share factual, analytic information. The word is derived from a team of horses pulling a plough, which illustrates its cardinal feature; a team works towards a common goal, each member contributing according to their expertise and ability.

Teams are themselves complex systems (in a systems analytic sense), and this is or should be manifest in several ways. Team members should:

- have shared knowledge and skills
- share clinical information about patients continuously
- be able to undertake tasks usually undertaken by others within the team; the work is shared and therefore if someone is not available the team can continue to function.

This is **not** to say that the missing person's skills and knowledge are not important, but it does mean that a proper team can continue to function without a member without too much difficulty for a period.

In network terms, teams are resilient and resist degradation, which means that once they are set up, they can continue to function albeit at a reduced level despite loss of a significant proportion of their members. It is worth contrasting how two teams might function in the absence of a particular therapist. One team is a true team, but the other is a 'virtual team', a group of people who just happen to be involved with a particular patient. If a therapist is missing from a true team, it will function quite well for several weeks but in the case of a virtual, single patient 'team' the work will simply not be done.

This feature of teamwork is obvious in many other contexts. For example, a hospital's chief executive will go on holiday, sleep, be away at meetings, etc., but the hospital and the hospital management team continue to function. However, no-one would dispute that organizations need a chief executive and that the absence, or the presence of a poor chief executive leads to organizational failure in the long term.

In rehabilitation there is the potential for endless discussion about:

- the membership of the team
- the type of teamwork used, usually distinguishing between **multi**disciplinary and **inter**disciplinary teams and, more recently **trans**disciplinary practice
- whether or not the patient (and family) are a part of the team (if, like me, you think that this is a meaningless question, then see National Institute of Health and Care Excellence (NICE) guideline on stroke [12])
- who should lead the team.

Some of these issues are best left to one side, but others will be discussed.

It is worth starting by considering what exactly constitutes 'the rehabilitation team', primarily to show that there is no simple single answer.

It is self-evident that no team can include every single expert who might ever be needed by the patients seen by a service. In other words, teams will always need to seek additional knowledge or skills from others in some situations. For example, a small number of patients may need an intrathecal baclofen pump to manage spasticity, but one cannot expect a neurosurgeon to be closely involved with the team.

Moreover, in a team of any significant size the actual group of people involved with a particular patient will be a subset of the whole team in the service. Some patients will have no need for some professions; that patient's team is not the same as the whole team. Even with a highly focused service, every therapist cannot be involved with every patient, and often a person or people or team from elsewhere will be involved to a greater or lesser extent.

Figure 2.4 illustrates the complexity of 'the team' and the difficulty in defining 'the team': the overall group of people who are actively and appropriately involved directly or indirectly can be very large and can come from a wide variety of different organizations or no organization and can come from a wide variety of professions or no profession. Each individual will have his or her own interests, skills, knowledge, experience and expectations. Success depends upon each person acting in concert with all the others, and not against them (usually accidentally).

Figure 2.4 also shows that the potential for miscommunication and misunderstanding is great, and highlights the overwhelming importance of liaison and communication, which is discussed later.

Considering the 'core team'—the group of people who constitute the general 'rehabilitation team'—they may espouse a particular style of teamwork. These are often characterized as one of three types [14]:

- **multidisciplinary**; work undertaken with other disciplines in parallel or sequentially
- **interdisciplinary**; work undertaken jointly with other disciplines
- **transdisciplinary**; work integrated across many disciplines, and undertaken collaboratively.

These are really degrees of integration and sharing, ranging from the incidental group of people who happen to be involved with

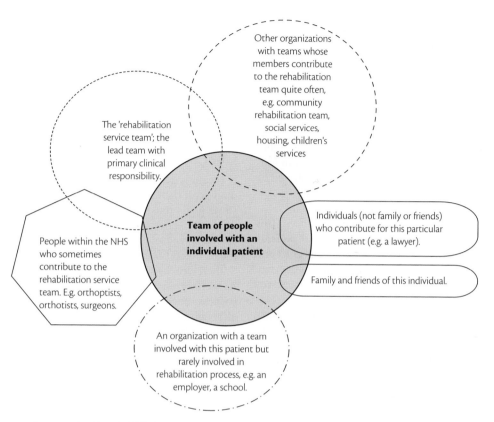

Fig. 2.4 The complex nature of team-work with an individual patient.

one patient but otherwise rarely work together, to a group of people who work together all the time, sharing much knowledge and skills, and working collaboratively.

The ideal is to have a fully integrated team who all work collaboratively, because this is likely to lead to a more efficient and effective team. Evidence in support of this assertion will be reviewed in the next section.

Is teamwork effective?

There is some evidence from healthcare research to support this assertion [13, 14], including some related to rehabilitation [15].

A large observational study [15] on 1688 stroke patients seen by 530 team members from six disciplines in 46 Veteran's Association hospitals showed that three team features were associated with better outcomes in terms of patient functional independence. The team features were:

- task orientation
- order and organization
- utility of quality information.

Teams that scored more highly on effectiveness had shorter lengths of stay.

There is some randomized, controlled trial evidence from neurological rehabilitation. The most convincing comes from stroke rehabilitation where studies show that stroke unit care is more effective that care in general settings [16]. The major differences between stroke unit care and the control intervention have been investigated and many concern teamwork—meeting together

to discuss patients, sharing common processes, team education, and so on. Although the studies were not specified as a contrast between integrated teamwork and either no teamwork, or at best ad hoc multidisciplinary teamwork, they did in fact study that. There is reasonable evidence for other diseases that integrated teams produce better results than 'usual practice', which will generally include therapists working together on a particular patient, but not as a team [17, 18].

Effective team structure and function

Some suggested general principles will be given here, many based on experience, not research. The discussion assumes that:

- it concerns people with an actual or apparent neurological or neuromuscular disorder which includes people with neuromimetic functional disorders
- the service is based with a healthcare system rather than social services (the principles would be the same, but organization names would differ).

The core membership of the team should include sufficient staff with a sufficiently broad range of knowledge and skills to the competent and able to manage at least 80% of the problems posed by the patients seen without needing to seek external help [19]. Teamwork requires individuals to know and trust each other and to have a shared understanding, and this only arises from regular contact and working together. Individuals who have a primary responsibility elsewhere simply cannot be full team members. Therefore most people seeing most patients should work together within the same group, with external people being called in for particular, relatively rare, problems only.

The members of the team should agree and use a single model of illness when analysing or discussing a patient's situation. This will lead to a shared, consistent vocabulary and set of explanations given to others (patient, family, other external teams, etc.). It is manifest by using documentation that has a similar structure.

The management approach to common problems such as patients with amnesia, transferring patients who have poor mobility, and irritability and aggression, should be agreed both in general and for individual patients. To achieve this there should be shared educational activities and training, and agreed protocols (evidence from stroke).

The team must share a single office or group of offices. This facilitates easy communication both about individual patients and about team working practices. It engenders a team spirit and allows meetings to be convened easily and quickly, both when an acute patient problem arises and when team practice needs discussion.

The team must work within a single management and budgetary arrangement. This is essential for several reasons. Different organizations have different priorities, and have organizational meeting and activities that are all likely to differ from other organizations leading to disintegration of the team. Separate budgetary arrangements will also lead to conflicts.

The suggested team membership is listed here. It must be stressed that **all** members of the team are expected to have specific, documented knowledge and skills covering rehabilitation and an appropriate level of experience of neuromuscular disorders. It should also be stressed that every team member needs to be familiar with recognizing and managing emotional problems and behaviour that might pose risk or distress to the patient or others.

The core professional membership must include:

- doctors
- nurses; this is the key group for all in-patient services but is also important for outpatient and domiciliary services
- physiotherapists
- occupational therapists
- speech and language therapists
- clinical neuropsychologists
- social workers; this is a second key group, without which service efficiency and effectiveness is markedly reduced because liaison with social services is so important.

There is a second group of professions where local factors and the patient group seen may need to be considered, but who should often be part of the core team:

- dieticians
- orthotists
- orthoptists.

The team will need ready access to a wide range of other professionals regularly or on an intermittent basis. Generally, it is best to form a particular relationship with one person, so that the specific

person becomes familiar with the rehabilitation team. Professions to consider include:

- clinical engineers and the whole team specializing in equipment, if they are not an integral part of the service
- orthopaedic surgeons
- liaison psychiatrist.

Goal setting

If a team is defined as a group of people working towards a common goal, then the process of identifying, agreeing and setting those goals must be the central, defining process that distinguishes effective teams from less effective teams. If there is no a shared agreed and regularly used process of setting goals used by the members of a team, it cannot be called a team.

Therefore, because goal setting is so central to 'transdisciplinary', integrated team working, this section will expand upon the process especially in the context of neurological rehabilitation, although the evidence comes from a much broader field.

Goal setting increases motivation and engagement [20, 21]. The evidence is very strong that setting goals for individuals and for teams alters behaviour; individuals and teams achieve more when they set appropriate goals. The evidence also suggests that effective goals are:

- considered **relevant** and important by the individual concerned (the patient)
- considered **achievable** by the person concerned (whether or not it is actually achievable)
- considered **challenging** by the person concerned
- supported by **intermediate goals** if the overall goal is set some way in the future
- **specified** rather than general; it needs to be easily known when the goal is reached.

However, it must be recognized that goal setting also carries disadvantages: risks to the patient and the resources used. For example, goal setting can also be demotivating if the goals are too easily achieved or are perceived as impossible or irrelevant. Moreover, achieving goals should not be used to determine any other decision [20], because it decreases engagement. They do not need to be SMART [22] (there is debate about what SMART stands for [22], and one set of terms is Specific, Measureable, Achievable (though originally it was Attributable), Relevant and Time-limited.).

Consequently, when developing rehabilitation goals it is vital to discover what the patient's wishes and expectations are. Furthermore, because the goals set will also be influenced by and have an impact upon others, it is important always to consider the wishes and expectations of others. This applies obviously to family, but less obviously it also applies (for example) to team members and organizations. For example, if a team member disagrees fundamentally with a goal such as returning to live with an abusive partner, or if an organization does not agree with a plan to discharge home with a care package (because they do not want to pay) then they will not work wholeheartedly towards the goals.

At the same time, it is also important to know what change can be expected, both in the absence of any intervention and if there are interventions, and whether theoretically beneficial interventions are actually available to the patient.

All of this information then needs to be used to draw up a plan with long-term and shorter-term goals and a list of specific actions to be undertaken by members of the team. This plan must be compatible with the patient's own wishes and interests.

The plan should always recognize that exact prediction is impossible, and that progress should be reviewed and goals adjusted according to changes that occur in the situation and according to the success or otherwise of interventions tried.

Several specific facts need to be stressed. Although the patient's wishes must be taken into account, it is neither possible nor desirable for team goals simply to repeat a patient's stated wishes. The patient's wishes may be impossible, given the losses or the resources available, the actions needed may not be within the power of the team to execute, or they may be appropriate but only at a later stage.

Second, it is important to explain to the patient how sub-goals are related to their wishes. For example, most patients who lose the ability to walk have regaining that ability has an important goal, but few will express any interest in regaining trunk control (for example). Regaining control over balance may be an essential first stage towards walking but if the patient does not understand and accept this they are unlikely to work towards it as a goal.

Lastly, it is important to accept that changing a patient's beliefs or expectations is a reasonable part of rehabilitation, so that they can expend their effort on achievable goals that are consistent with their overall wishes. For example, after complete spinal cord injury it may be necessary to help the patient accept that they will never walk so that they can learn to use a wheelchair and thereby achieve a greater goal of living independently and working.

Team working

If the goal setting process discussed is followed, the output should be a series of actions that lead towards a set of goals that are relevant to the patient. The goals should all start from the patient's overall wishes, rather than being dominated by what the team members feel that they can do. In other words, the question is 'what do you want us to help you achieve?' rather than 'We can help you achieve these goals; are they useful to you?'.

Within any team there must be an element of shared work, which takes two forms.

First, and by definition, two or more team members will be working together towards a common goal with the patient. This will lead to team members using techniques that are advised by another team member, which reinforces the 'treatment'; for example a speech and language therapist may use specified, agreed techniques for transfer and to manage emotional distress as part of a session aimed at improving speech clarity. This duplication and continuation of a treatment approach within other activities greatly increases the patient's learning.

Second, and more controversially, a team member may at least on occasions, undertake work on behalf of others. The easiest example is when a patient is first assessed. The first team member to see a patient, perhaps in a different setting, can and should collect information that is not important to his or her own profession,

but is relevant to another profession. For example, a therapist might collect information on diagnoses, investigations, and drugs for a doctor, and a speech and language therapist might collect information on transfers (for a physiotherapist) or memory (for a psychologist).

This sharing of roles is of great importance, and although it is sometimes seen as offering a cheap, second-class service it should be something that increases the expertise of team members and also the quality of the service. There are now several examples available in guidelines, the most obvious being the assessment of swallowing in the acute phase after stroke by nursing staff [11]. This has not lead to any diminution in the role of a speech and language therapist.

The risk is that managers may see it as an opportunity to reduce staffing, which then actually greatly reduces team quality. The overall level of team expertise is reduced—it has less depth—and individual professions will avoid or stop supporting each other, and therefore collaborative team-work is destroyed.

An effective collaborative rehabilitation team is likely to have the following characteristics:

- An agreed, shared framework for understanding and analysing and describing a patient's situation. This will now usually be the biopsychosocial model of illness. This is manifest through:
  - A shared terminology and vocabulary
  - A similar lay-out of clinical notes.
- The use of an agreed set of measures for frequently measured domains, such as independence in personal activities of daily living (ADL).
  - The Barthel ADL index is likely to be the measure of personal ADL
  - Measures should be chosen for mobility, dexterity, communication, memory, etc.
- A shared primary clinical record where all professions record all major observations, etc. This is becoming more common. It does not preclude separate professional notes for day-to-day recording and recording specific detailed information.
  - One challenge is that some professions are reluctant to share some data
  - Another challenge is to achieve a comprehensive complete record that can nonetheless be easily searched to find relevant information quickly.
- A single geographic area (office or set of offices) used by all team members.
  - A good team will also have a shared 'social' area for coffee, meals, relaxation.
- Shared treatment spaces, not 'belonging' to any particular profession or department.
- Evidence of actual sharing of roles and responsibilities such as:
  - Chairing or leading multi-disciplinary patient-centred meeting
  - Chairing or leading team and service projects
  - Undertaking clinical work on behalf of other team members.

♦ Multidisciplinary goal-setting meetings on a regular basis for all patients.

- Reviewing all patients under the team on a regular basis, usually weekly
- Reviewing individual patients at a goal-setting meeting or similar, at an appropriate interval.

♦ Shared, agreed protocols for managing common problems (e.g. swallowing problems, aggression).

♦ Shared educational activities.

♦ Be managed as a single unit, including having a single budget shared by the whole team.

Key-workers

One of the recurring areas of discussion within rehabilitation concerns key-workers, with many questions being debated: are they needed or even essential, what are the limits of their responsibility and power, who should be a key-worker?

The idea of a key-worker has arisen in response to quite a wide variety of perceived (not necessarily actual) problems:

♦ Patients and families not knowing who to approach about a particular problem.

♦ Failures in communication within the team, for example about clinical changes and/or changes in the management plan.

♦ Difficulties faced by people from outside the central team (e.g. external social workers) in contacting the team and getting information.

♦ Lack of continuity in care, with an associated lack in consistency in information and advice given.

♦ Failures in goal setting:

- not setting a comprehensive set of goals
- not monitoring progress towards or achievement of goals.

♦ Failures in organizing external management, especially transfers of care.

From this list one can appreciate that a key-worker could easily be overwhelmed! With this list in mind, it is worth considering whether having a key-worker would actually help any of the problems, let alone all.

In all discussions it is assumed that the key-worker is a single, named individual who carries that responsibility for a named patient over a prolonged time (e.g. whole admission, whole episode of out-patient care, one year). It must then also be accepted that key-workers:

♦ may be part-time only

♦ will have periods of leave

♦ will not be on-call every day or all hours

♦ will have other work commitments (i.e. they are not employed primarily as a key-worker)

♦ will have his or her own areas of expertise and therefore other areas where they have limited skills and knowledge.

Consequently, it is quite unrealistic to expect a keyworker to fulfil any of the expectations very well, if at all.

Further reflection shows that the problems identified are really related to team organization, because the team as a whole could easily resolve all of these problems.

Many of the problems concern interaction with other agencies, especially Social Services (as the organization which is, in many countries, responsible for social and domiciliary support, housing, etc.). The primary solution, in the UK at least, would be to insist upon having a social worker as an integral member of the team; this is sadly not the case in many areas within the UK.

Most of the other problems simply require all members of a team to take responsibility for a problem when they are approached. For example, if a patient wants to know about wheelchairs, the key-worker is likely to suggest contacting the appropriate team member, but this could be done by any team member. Indeed, the team member should actually contact the appropriate person directly, rather than delaying the process by asking the key worker to do it.

Thus it is probably better to identify and analyse the problem faced, and to develop a protocol or way for the team to respond to the need, rather than to suggest a key-worker which simply transfers the problem and probably complicates the process still further.

Conclusion

Patients with long-term neurologically based problems present a great challenge to healthcare. The problems for one patient requires the attention of a few to many people delivered over a variable length of time often in a variety of settings. These people constitute that person's team. Other patients will have other problems, some in common and some not. Some of the people involved will help many patients, some only a proportion. Nonetheless, the areas of expertise are similar.

The simplest solution is for there to be a group of people who between them can resolve the majority of problems faced by the majority of people with neurological disease. The evidence suggests, quite strongly, that this leads to a better outcome for the patient at no more cost to the healthcare system. The evidence also suggests that a system focused on the patient's needs and wishes whereby the group of people involved discuss and agree a set of goals which they work towards collaboratively is more effective.

This is a description of an interdisciplinary team. Unfortunately, for practical, political and organizational reasons, the teams are rarely comprehensive and there are still weaknesses. Nonetheless, using a patient-centred goal-setting process based within a biopsychosocial model of illness and an interdisciplinary healthcare rehabilitation team is probably the best achievable method for managing the problems of this group of patients.

References

1. Wade DT, de Jong B. Recent advances in rehabilitation. Br Med J. 2000;**320**:1385–1358.
2. Wade DT, Halligan PW. Do biomedical models of illness make for good healthcare systems? Br Med J. 2004;**329**:1398–1401.
3. Wade DT. (2009) Holistic Health Care. What is it, and how can we achieve it? Available from http://www.ouh.nhs.uk/oce/research-education/documents/HolisticHealthCare09-11-15.pdf (accessed 29 September 2014).
4. Wade DT. Describing rehabilitation interventions. Clin Rehabil. 2005;**19**:811–818.

5. Engel GL. The need for a new medical model: a challenge for bio-medicine Science. 1977;**196**:129–136.

6. Parsons T. The Social System. Free Press. Glencoe, IL, 1951.

7. International Classification of Impairments, Disabilities, and Handicaps. WHO, Geneva, 1980.

8. International Statistical Classification of Diseases and Related Health Problems. 10th Revision. Version for 2007. World Health Organization, Geneva, Switzerland.

9. Multiple Sclerosis. National clinical guideline for diagnosis and management in primary and secondary care. National Institute for Clinical Excellence (NICE). Clinical Guideline 8 Clinical Effectiveness and Evaluation Unit, Royal College of Physicians, London, 2003.

10. Rehabilitation Following Acquired Brain Injury. National Clinical Guidelines. British Society of Rehabilitation Medicine & Royal College of Physicians, London, 2003.

11. National Clinical Guideline for Stroke (Fourth edition) The Intercollegiate Working Party for Stroke. Clinical Effectiveness and Evaluation Unit, Royal College of Physicians, London, 2012.

12. Stroke rehabilitation: Long-term rehabilitation after stroke. NICE Clinical Guideline CG 162. Available from http://www.nice.org.uk/guidance/cg162 (accessed 29 September 2014).

13. Choi BCK, Pak AP. Multidisciplinary, interdisciplinary, and trans-disciplinary in health research, services, education, and policy: 1; Definitions, objectives, and evidence of effectiveness. Clin Invest Med. 2006;**29**:351–364.

14. Zwarenstein M, Reeves S. Knowledge translation and interprofessional collaboration: where the rubber of evidence-based care meets the road of teamwork. J Continuing Educ Health Prof. 2006;**26**:46–54.

15. Strasser DC, Falconer JA, Herrin JS, Bowen SE, Stevens AB, Umoto J. Team functioning and patient outcomes in stroke rehabilitation. Arch Phys Med Rehabil. 2005;**86**:403–409.

16. Stroke Unit Trialists' Collaboration. Organised inpatient (stroke unit) care for stroke. Cochrane Database of Systematic Reviews 2007, Issue 4. Art. No.: CD000197. DOI: 10.1002/14651858.CD000197.pub2.

17. Khan F, Turner-Stokes L, Ng L, Kilpatrick T, Amatya B. Multidisciplinary rehabilitation for adults with multiple sclerosis. Cochrane Database of Systematic Reviews 2007, Issue 2. Art. No.: CD006036. DOI: 10.1002/14651858.CD006036.pub2.

18. Turner-Stokes L, Nair A, Sedki I, Disler PB, Wade DT. Multi-disciplinary rehabilitation for acquired brain injury in adults of working age. Cochrane Database of Systematic Reviews 2005, Issue 3. Art. No.: CD004170. DOI: 10.1002/14651858.CD004170.pub2.

19. Wade DT. Clinical governance and rehabilitation services. Clin Rehabil. 2000;**14**:1–4.

20. Locke EA, Latham GP. Building a practically useful theory of goal setting and task motivation. A 35-year odyssey. Am Psychol. 2002;**57**:705–172.

21. Levack WMM, Taylor K, Siegert RJ, Dean SG. Is goal planning in rehabilitation effective? A systematic review. Clin Rehabil. 2006;**20**:739–755.

22. Wade DT. Goal setting in rehabilitation: an overview of what, why, and how. Clin Rehabil. 2009;**23**:291–295.

CHAPTER 3

The economic benefits of rehabilitation for neurological conditions

Rory O'Connor

Introduction

Rehabilitation produces outcomes that are most apparent at the level of participation [1] or health-related quality of life rather than body function or structure. Measuring outcomes, therefore, requires a greater level of sophistication than simply collecting biochemical or radiological findings and attributing any change to the effect of the treatment [2]. Deriving econometric data from the outcome of rehabilitation interventions relies on using the outcomes generated by rehabilitation programmes combined with the costs of the input.

As rehabilitation is reliant on extensive direct patient contact with healthcare professionals, the apparent cost of interventions can seem high in the early phase. People severely disabled by long-term neurological conditions require considerable medical, nursing and therapy input to maintain and improve their functioning and wellbeing [3]. The initial management of an acute spinal cord injury requires full clinical and radiological examination of the central nervous system, turns to prevent pressure sores by nurses every 2 or 4 hours, active bladder and bowel management, and passive movements of the patient's joints by physiotherapists. The behavioural management of an acquired brain injury often requires 24-hour individual nursing, with intensive neuropsychology and occupational therapy input. The clinicians delivering these therapies are often senior, further increasing the apparent cost.

Rehabilitation environments tend to be enriched and more sophisticated than general hospital wards and departments. Hyperacute rehabilitation following the onset of severe neurological illness or trauma requires considerable space to accommodate the extra staff and equipment to manage the patient's needs. Postacute rehabilitation environments will include adapted bathrooms, kitchens, therapeutic gymnasia, and hydrotherapy pools. These facilities tend to be provided in standalone locations, which tend to have higher overheads per patient than larger institutions. After discharge, community rehabilitation teams will need therapeutic milieu to treat their patients, particularly if patients' home environments are less than suitable [4].

These factors combine to explain the apparent initial high cost of rehabilitation: interventions are extensive, labour intensive, and require expensive facilities. If we accept that rehabilitation is effective [5], can we justify the cost?

Disability is expensive, both for the individuals concerned and for society in general. Costs of equipment and medication, care provision at home or in institutions, welfare payments, lost earnings and consequently reduced tax receipts [6] combine to make disability a major draw on a society's exchequer. If rehabilitation interventions could reduce people's requirements for support in the community, make them more independent and more likely to return to work after illness, then rehabilitation would pay for itself over time. Linking the changes measured by rehabilitation outcome assessments to economic evaluations can demonstrate the financial benefits as well as the functional improvements.

As most of the costs associated with living with a disability in the community are related to the cost of providing personal care (e.g. assistance with washing, dressing, toileting, and meal provision), economic evaluations have focused on recording individual's daily and weekly care requirements and using this information to develop a cost model. Additional expenditure associated with expensive equipment or housing adaptations can be included in this model. Once costs are established for a healthcare economy, then the model can be applied to other patients coming through the system. Once such model is based on the suite of measures developed in Northwick Park Hospital in London, UK [7], which capture the weekly care requirements of people with long-term neurological conditions and translate this into a weekly cost of care. Other models have been developed around the costs associated with a year-of-care, for example, motor neurone disease. But, for many people with a sudden onset neurological condition, improvement can be expected with rehabilitation and costs are loaded towards the initial year after onset [8].

Using this methodology, rehabilitation can be demonstrated to reduce care costs and return the investment of an inpatient multidisciplinary rehabilitation programme within a number of months [9]. However, the upfront costs of rehabilitation can be substantial, particularly if a rehabilitation pathway is not already in existence in a health economy and investment is required for development. Furthermore, most of the potential savings are recouped through reduced social care costs and welfare payments, although health systems benefit through reduced length of stay and fewer secondary complications for patients [10], and improved outcomes for family carers [11]. Therefore, healthcare facilities need to work within integrated health and social care environments to derive full benefit from the cost savings.

History of economic evaluations

Financial assessments of healthcare interventions have always been a topic of interest to communities with medical practitioners. The Code of Hammurabi in ancient Egypt prescribed fiduciary rewards for physicians who successfully treated patients. Unfortunately, adverse outcomes were punished by physical and financial penalties depending on the severity of the mishap [12]. In the 1800s mortality statistics were the primary outcomes reported by healthcare institutions, with no regard for the results of the operations and interventions that were performed within their institutions [13]. These institutions were largely charitable and, apart from ensuring overall financial regularity, no other scrutiny was placed on how their money was spent.

Apart from small experiments in collecting outcome data and relating it to healthcare interventions (14), very few advances were made in the first half of the last Century. A step-change in evaluating health outcomes occurred in the 1960s [15]. Donabedian's work was the first to assess healthcare interventions using the concepts of structure, process and outcomes, with which we are familiar today. In North America in the 1980s and Australia in the 1990s, structure and process were used to develop healthcare resource groups (HRGs)—treatment episodes which are similar in resource use and in clinical response. Only in the last decade are these healthcare economies systematically examining outcomes to justify expenditure.

However, inappropriate outcomes can still be applied to these interventions—this can make it difficult to determine the correct underlying costs if the necessary data are not collected. For instance, survival data are presented for conditions where survival is not at risk. Survival is also often presented in a composite outcome, included with other events, such as recurrence of the index event or additional morbidity, which is inappropriate too, as these outcomes have different impacts on individuals. In some instances prolonging survival may not actually be in a patient's best interests [16]. Therefore, it is essential to choose an outcome that can provide robust patient-level data and adequately register the economic impact of the intervention.

A further consideration formerly under-recognized is that many health status measures ultimately used in economic analyses do not collect information that will completely describe the impact of the rehabilitation input. Many measures used in economic analyses contain impairment or activity level items, such as level of pain or walking, and these may not actually be the relevant outcome for many people—reducing pain or improving walking may only be an antecedent to returning to work or education. There are not many healthcare providers who regularly measure wider, participation outcomes, and yet they are increasingly relevant to

society, particularly in reducing the cost of welfare payments such as incapacity benefits. Therefore, rehabilitation services planning to judge the economic effectiveness of their interventions need to have a measure that is correctly targeted to the population they serve and that population's needs. For example, a rehabilitation unit working with people with severe neurological impairments needing substantial care input would look to reducing the hours and complexity of a package of care on discharge. Similarly, a vocational rehabilitation programme working with clients with traumatic brain injury living in the community would collect data on job return and retention and level of salary achieved in those taking up their first employment.

An illustration of these issues can be seen in the development of the International Classification of Functioning, Disability and Health (ICF) [1]. It was initially proposed that impairments lead in a linear fashion to 'handicap' [17]. However, the limitations of this model were quickly identified as the impact of impairments are modulated by a wide range of factors both internal and external to the individual. So, for example, a heavy goods vehicle driver who developed post-stroke epilepsy would be unable to return to driving as an occupation for up to 10 years, even if he had no other physical manifestations of the his stroke. This is a function of a country's legislation in relation to driver licensing, which would be considered an issue relating to the person's environment in the widest sense. The latest model (Figure 3.1) outlines the complex, bi-directional relationships between each of the factors. The ICF is the currently accepted way to fully describe the impact of a health condition on an individual and complements the International Classification of Diseases.

Methods of economic evaluation

Many of the functional outcome measures that are routinely collected by rehabilitation services will encompass a range of activities of daily living and record the activity limitations that the patients encounter. Whilst this is an important first step in an economic analysis, it is not sufficient to record the full benefit derived by the intervention. Measures such as the Barthel Index [18] and Functional Independence Measure [19] cannot be directly translated into care costs. Only measures which record hours of nursing or care input such as the Northwick Park suite of measures [7] or an health status measure that has been extensively assessed in relation to quality adjusted life years (QALY), such as the EuroQol [20], can be used for economic evaluations.

There is an important difference between these two econometric methods. The first, recording actual care hours, gives a financial cost if the individual is currently in the community receiving care. Whilst care is the most expensive part of community support, due to substantial input from care staff, it is not the only cost and consideration must be given to additional costs such as housing adaptations, welfare and loss of income. It is also a theoretical cost and it assumes that all care will be provided by paid carers. Very many family members take on a carer's role and this is not likely to be recompensed. Indeed, carers may remain out-of-pocket if they choose to give up work to care for their relatives. But for most post-acute rehabilitation services in developed countries it provides a useful overview of the effectiveness, in financial terms, of the rehabilitation programme.

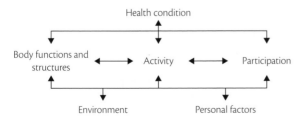

Fig. 3.1 The International Classification of Functioning, Disability and Health.

Translating health-related quality of life into a QALY determines the annual cost that would be required to transform the current quality of life for given individual into full quality of life. This method has been used extensively by statutory bodies, such as the National Institute for Health and Care Excellence, to determine whether to support new health technologies. Whilst many rehabilitation interventions have been judged to be cost-effective [21], others have been judged to be too expensive relative to the change in function produced to be considered for funding.

Trying to convert activity-level data to an economic quantum is fraught with complications. For example, attempts have been made to link the Barthel Index with the EuroQol as there is a commonality in some of the items (mobility, personal care, usual activities). However, the items of the two measures are worded and scored differently, which would result in different responses to the items. More importantly, the Barthel Index is clinician-scored and the EuroQol is self-report, therefore two different and not necessarily equivalent perspectives are recorded [22]. Furthermore, 40% of the items (pain and psychological functioning) in the EuroQol have no correspondence with items on the Barthel Index. This leaves a large, clinically important, component of the QALY unscored, which may result in a floor effect where a potentially important clinical difference is not recorded by the measure [23].

This illustrates a use of the ICF in choosing a suitable measure. Each component of the ICF can be measured (the Barthel Index measures body functions and activity) but this does not directly relate to other components of the ICF. Therefore, to measure participation, one needs to choose a scale that relates directly to the construct that it is intended to measure. This avoids the conceptual discrepancy between collecting data that are expected to change with the proposed rehabilitation intervention and a measure that does not identify that a change has occurred. Examples of measures and how they relate to the ICF constructs are given in Figure 3.2.

Even when using self-report health status measures to gather primary data directly, there are substantial methodological issues with the process that derives the scores. It was initially assumed that health related quality of life was a linear construct from full health through to death. However, most analyses will reveal that many people regard certain health conditions—e.g. the persistent vegetative state—to be much worse than death and these states fall below the floor of the scale and any change through rehabilitation is thus lost. Data also need to be compared to normative groups and as many health status measures are completed by people in full, or near full, health, it can be difficult to benchmark the quality of life of people with long-term conditions. Most people with long-term conditions regard their quality of life as comparable to people without long-term conditions one year after the onset of the condition—the disability paradox [24]. This also reduces the apparent effect of an intervention and consequently it cost effectiveness.

A further limitation of these measures is that they do not produce interval level data, which are critical to allow arithmetic procedures [25]. Money and time are interval-level data and are crucial to calculating the full economic cost of an intervention. However, many health status measures produce, at best, ordinal-level data, which cannot be manipulated arithmetically or correlated to interval-level data, rendering most economic analyses of this type invalid. As an example, one might examine the stairs item of the Barthel index, which records patients' stair climbing abilities into one of three categories: unable (0), needs help (aid, verbal, physical; 1), and independent (2). Independence in stair climbing can make a huge difference to a person's independence when they return home and a great deal of time and rehabilitation staff effort (money) goes into achieving this. Yet, the recording of change by the Barthel Index item (output) will not correlate directly with the input: the effort of generating stair climbing ability at all is very substantial compared to gaining independent stair climbing once this has been achieved [26]. Therefore gaining a Barthel point from 0 to 1 takes far greater resource (and cost) than from 1 to 2, yet would appear to generate the same improvement in the overall Barthel score (a change of 1 point). A better measure for this purpose would be the Assessment of Motor and Process Skills (AMPS), which is based on analyses that produce an interval-level score [27].

An alternative, robust approach will use a functional measure, such as the Northwick Park dependency measures that directly records the care and nursing input that an individual requires. The temporal data generated by these measures can then be costed based on the quantity of input and the pay of those employed to provide this care. Rehabilitation interventions that reduce individual's, dependency will reduce their care needs and therefore the overall cost of their care will be less. As a starting place for an economic evaluation, this provides very robust data, which can be manipulated arithmetically, used in comparisons, and tracked longitudinally.

This approach is straightforward for patients in post-acute inpatient rehabilitation programmes, where the data can be routinely collected as part of the rehabilitation process. Additional data collection must be performed to determine the expenditure associated with hospitalizations and other healthcare-associated costs, social care and welfare, and loss of potential earning and hence exchequer returns. Some of these potential costs are less easy to calculate as future expenditure and earnings can be more difficult to predict. More complicated economic modelling is required to determine these costs.

Case studies of rehabilitation economic evaluations

◆ Liaison rehabilitation in acute and critical care settings

Acute medical and surgical beds in any health economy are a precious and expensive resource and length of stay could be judged to be a reasonable approximation for cost in this

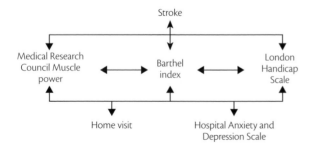

Fig. 3.2 Mapping outcome measures onto the ICF.

setting. Any intervention that reduces length of stay will result in economies. Rehabilitation provided in these settings will not only reduce length of stay, but will also result in avoidable complications such as pressure sores and contractures, which in themselves, will increase length of stay, delay transfer to a definitive rehabilitation facility, and increase the amount of time that the rehabilitation team spends dealing with the complications rather than rehabilitating the underlying condition [10].

At present, there are no economic evaluations of this type of rehabilitation input [28]. Head-to-head studies of different methods of delivering early rehabilitation would be required in order to fully evaluate the economic benefits of these interventions.

◆ Post-acute acquired brain injury rehabilitation

Similarly, there are no published economic assessments on the impact of inpatient rehabilitation for adults in the post-acute phase of their recovery from acquired brain injury. Early work in our own unit (a 19-bed inpatient facility providing goal-orientated rehabilitation to adults with neurological conditions) demonstrates the effectiveness in discharging severely impaired patients to their own homes. From September 2008 to September 2010, 261 patients (174 males; median age 53 years, range 16 to 84) were discharged from inpatient rehabilitation, 85.5% of these patients to their own homes. Discharge destination was not determined by the dependency level, but environmental factors: 93% of patients were discharged home if they lived with a carer and had their own accommodation. Median length of stay was 29 days (interquartile range 32 days). However, only 22% of patients who did not have their own accommodation or live with a carer returned home (length of stay 62 days; IQR 51), illustrating the importance of these factors in promoting a safe and timely discharge relative to the underlying diagnosis or the resultant impairments.

We looked at a subset of these patients using the Northwick Park dependency suite of measures. We included 79 patients (42 males; median age 54 years, range 17–85) who had complete admission and discharge data. All costs were based on direct treatment costs and overheads and are presented in UK pounds sterling at 2010 costs. The median cost of inpatient rehabilitation per patient was £14,026 (interquartile range £8,617 to £23,811). The median weekly cost of care for a patient reduced by £939 from £1,232 to £300. The median time to offset the investment in post-acute rehabilitation was 17 weeks.

◆ Stroke rehabilitation

More data are available for patients in post-acute stroke rehabilitation, much of it originating from the work of the Stroke Trialists in the 1990s who identified that organized stroke rehabilitation does not increase length of stay and produces better outcomes for patients at all levels of disability [29]. Further work illustrated that length of stay could be reduced through the use of community based stroke rehabilitation once patients were initially stabilized and had received early rehabilitation in the stroke unit [30]. Overall costs were not reduced due to the costs of the community service, but inpatient hospital costs were significantly less.

Looking more closely at the reduction in care costs associated with inpatient stroke rehabilitation it has been possible to identify what savings can be achieved [9]. At 2006 costs, median weekly care costs were reduced from £1,900 to £1,100 for 35 inpatients in post-acute stroke rehabilitation.

◆ Spinal cord injury rehabilitation

Prior to the establishment of spinal cord injury rehabilitation units, the life expectancy of a person with tetraplegia was approximately one month. Avoidance of the main complications of spinal cord injury (pressure sores, urinary and respiratory tract infections) and comprehensive rehabilitation has resulted in near normal life expectancy for people living with spinal injury. Returning people to economic activity was one of the main objectives of rehabilitation [31].

Spinal cord injuries tend to occur in a bimodal age distribution with a peak in early adulthood and later life [32]. For the younger cohort, life expectancy approaches that of people with no neurological injury [33], hence comprehensive rehabilitation that facilitates return to, or entry into, work will have an important impact [34]. The initial rehabilitation of people with spinal cord injury is expensive (US $282,000 in 2003) [35], with high annual costs relating to ongoing medical and rehabilitation interventions. Unfortunately, no groups have looked at the comparative effect of rehabilitation interventions in reducing these costs.

◆ Community-based rehabilitation

For many neurological conditions, community-based rehabilitation interventions will be required to maintain individual's functioning in their own environments. This is equally important for people who are discharged from post-acute rehabilitation facilities as well as people with long-term conditions living in the community [4]. Two studies have looked at the costs of supporting individuals in the community. A study of interventions to support people with challenging behaviour after traumatic brain injury identified that while the first year of organized intervention was more costly than usual care, costs decreased substantially in subsequent years [8].

A second study looked at community rehabilitation for people following stroke [36]. With a median input of nine weeks of daily rehabilitation input in 71 people's own homes (45 males; median age 71 years), costs of care reduced from £234 per week (2009 costs) to £102 per week.

Developing an economic evaluation

As a first step in designing an economic evaluation, it is essential to record the costs of the input provided by the rehabilitation programme. For most healthcare economies, approximately three-quarters of costs will be associated with direct staff costs. Premises, medication, equipment and overheads will vary depending on the nature of the programme. Second, an outcome measure is chosen that has good psychometric properties, is linked to a robust economic evaluation, and is targeted to the population participating in the rehabilitation programme (Table 3.1). Then a decision must be made about collecting additional data regarding wider aspects of the population's needs such as welfare benefits, earnings and other costs that need to be offset such as additional childcare for family members who are carers (Box 3.1).

Table 3.1 Requirements for measures suitable for economic analyses

Targeting	The measure has been used in a sample similar to the proposed population. The measure covers the expected range of the construct in the population
Unidimensionality	Only one construct is measured by the scale (or one construct per element of the scale if there are multiple sub-scales)
Scale responses	Each item will be categorical (nominal or ordinal) or continuous (interval or ratio). Only continuous responses can be subjected to arithmetic processes
Reliability	Error is minimized between repeated administrations of the measure (test–retest reliability) and between different clinicians collecting the data (inter-rater reliability)
Validity	The extent to which the scale measures what it purports to measure in relation to an established instrument (concurrent criterion validity) or in terms of predicting an outcome (predictive criterion validity). Content validity is a qualitative assessment of the scale by an expert panel in relation to the items that comprise the scale. Construct validity refers to the relationship between the scale and other scales that purport to measure the same construct
Responsiveness	The ability of the measure to accurately detect change when it has occurred

Box 3.1 Concepts in economic evaluation

Economic evaluations of health status require a transformation from the outcome measure to a utility score. This is a score from 1 to 0 where 1 is full health and 0 is death. This is multiplied by life expectancy and the number of quality adjusted life years (QALY) is obtained.

Another health economic term is the disability adjusted life year (DALY). This is the converse of the QALY and is a construct to be reduced by a health intervention.

To find the value of the utility for an individual, a number of techniques are employed. The most commonly used ones are the standard gamble, time trade-off, magnitude estimation and person trade-off.

The standard gamble is a method of establishing the utility for a health state. A person is asked to state the certainty between being in a certain health state and the probability of being restored to full health (p) or untimely death ($1 - p$). This can be difficult to explain to patients and the time trade-off was developed to overcome this. The person is asked to make a choice between the number of years in their current health state (or other state of disability) and the (fewer) number of years of perfect health. Most reports use either the standard gamble or the time trade-off as the other methods are used much less frequently hence their validity is less well established.

One of the limitations of these techniques in neurological conditions, is that people regularly rate certain outcomes, such as the vegetative state, as a worse than death resulting in a negative health utility. In calculations, this is considered as 0, which underestimates the impact of the condition, reducing the apparent effect of a rehabilitation intervention.

Converting categorical data, such as patient's level of ability, into interval level data, preferably monetary, through the use of measures of recording care, nursing, therapy, and medical input will increase the range of statistical procedures that can be performed on the data. Most data collected through rehabilitation interventions are non-parametric and will require appropriate statistical analyses. If categorical level data cannot be converted, then specialist, less powerful techniques can be applied [37].

Finally, data must be presented in a form that is comprehensible to the commissioners of the rehabilitation service, whether locally or nationally, as many of these will not have a clinical background. The information should also be available to lay people including service users and their families. It is incumbent on us to demonstrate that we are spending money on these services responsibly.

Economic evaluation of rehabilitation and the future

Of course, health and social care provision are not isolated from the wider socio-political environment. Rehabilitation services have always had to respond to wider social and political demands. The two greatest changes to the delivery of rehabilitation in developed countries was the impact of the First and Second World Wars. These catastrophes resulted in the development and expansion of amputee rehabilitation services and neurological rehabilitation services, respectively [38, 39]. Other changes have been more evolutionary rather than revolutionary and have responded to changes in epidemiology [40], technology [41], and service delivery [3]. Cultural changes have also determined that rehabilitation and disability management services are delivered more in the community rather than in institutions [42]. Most of these developments and changes have been positive, resulting in enhanced services and better outcomes for those affected by disabling conditions. More recently, however, global economic pressures have resulted in a contraction of health and social care services, or at least a halt to further investment in new services. Straitened healthcare budgets over the last decade have resulted in a failure to appreciate the benefits of investment-to-save with its upfront budgetary requirements.

It is expected that economic pressures will continue to affect the ability of rehabilitation services to provide the input required to realise the potential savings that can be brought about by appropriate treatments. The longer-term benefits of rehabilitation may be disregarded in favour of the apparent short-term cost-saving measures of disinvestment in rehabilitation services. Therefore, it is important that each rehabilitation service is aware of external socio-political pressures and is proactive in collecting robust information on the full, long-term benefits of rehabilitation input. These efforts will enable rehabilitation services to continue to provide for disabled people into the future.

References

1. World Health Organization. International Classification of Functioning, Disability and Health, 1st edn. WHO, Geneva, 2001.
2. O'Connor RJ, Neumann VC. Payment by results or payment by outcome? The history of measuring medicine. J Roy Soc Med. 2006;**99**(5):226–231.
3. Department of Health Long-term Conditions NSF Team. The national service framework for long-term conditions. Leeds, UK, 2005.

4. O'Connor RJ, Best M, Chamberlain MA. The Community Rehabilitation Unit in Leeds: a resource for people with long-term conditions. Int J Therapy Rehabil. 2006;**13**(3):118–125.

5. Anderson C, Ni Mhurchu C, Brown PM, Carter K. Stroke rehabilitation services to accelerate hospital discharge and provide home-based care: an overview and cost analysis. Pharmacoeconomics. 2002;**20**(8):537–552.

6. Chamberlain MA, Fialka Moser V, Schuldt Ekholm K, O'Connor RJ, Herceg M, Ekholm J. Vocational rehabilitation: an educational review. J Rehabil Med. 2009;**41**(11):856–869.

7. Turner-Stokes L, Tonge P, Nyein K, Hunter M, Nielson S, Robinson I. The Northwick Park Dependency Score (NPDS): a measure of nursing dependency in rehabilitation. Clin Rehabi. 1998;**12**(4):304–318.

8. Feeney TJ, Ylvisaker M, Rosen BH, Greene P. Community supports for individuals with challenging behavior after brain injury: an analysis of the New York state behavioral resource project. J Head Trauma Rehabil. 2001;**16**(1):61–75.

9. O'Connor RJ, Beden R, Pilling A, Chamberlain MA. What reductions in dependency costs result from treatment in an inpatient neurological rehabilitation unit for people with stroke? Clin Med. 2011;**11**(1):40–43.

10. Ross D, Heward K, Salawu Y, Chamberlain MA, Bhakta B. Upfront and enabling: delivering specialist multidisciplinary neurological rehabilitation. Int J Therapy Rehabil. 2009;**16**(2):107–113.

11. Jackson D, McCrone P, Turner-Stokes L. Costs of caring for adults with long-term neurological conditions. J Rehabil Med. 20129;**45**(7):653–661.

12. Schwartz JS, Lurie N. Assessment of medical outcomes. New opportunities for achieving a long sought-after objective. Int J Technol Assess Health Care. 1990;**6**(2):333–339.

13. Cook GC, Webb AJ. Reactions from the medical and nursing professions to Nightingale's 'reform(s)' of nurse training in the late 19th century. Postgrad Med. 2002;**78**(916):118–123.

14. Neuhauser D. Ernest Amory Codman, M.D., and end results of medical care. Int J Technol Assess Health Care. 1990;**6**(2):307–325.

15. Donabedian A. Evaluating the quality of medical care. Milbank Memorial Fund Quarterly. 1966;**44**(3):Suppl:166–206.

16. Voltz R. Palliative therapy in the terminal stage of neurological disease. J Neurol. 1997;**244**(0):S2–S10.

17. World Health Organization. International Classification of Impairments, Disabilities and Handicaps. WHO, Geneva, 1980.

18. Mahoney FI, Barthel DW. Functional evaluation: the Barthel index. Maryland State Med J. 1965;**16**:61–65.

19. Granger CV, Hamilton BB, Keith RA, Zielezny M, Sherwin FS. Advances in functional assessment for medical rehabilitation. Topics Geriatr Rehabil. 1986;**1**(3):59–74.

20. de Haan R, Aaronson N, Limburg M, Hewer RL, van Crevel H. Measuring quality of life in stroke. Stroke. 1993;**24**(2):320–327.

21. National Institute for Health and Care Excellence. Stroke rehabilitation: long-term rehabilitation after stroke. Clinical guidelines, CG162. National Institute for Health and Care Excellence, London, 2013.

22. Andresen EM, Vahle VJ, Lollar D. Proxy reliability: health-related quality of life (HRQoL) measures for people with disability. Qual Life Res. 2001;**10**(7):609–619.

23. O'Connor RJ, Cano SJ, Thompson AJ, Hobart JC. Exploring rating scale responsiveness: does the total score reflect the sum of its parts? Neurology. 2004;**62**(10):1842–1844.

24. Albrecht GL, Devlieger PJ. The disability paradox: high quality of life against all odds. Social Sci Med. 1999;**48**(8):977–988.

25. Cook KF, Ashton CM, Byrne MM, et al. A psychometric analysis of the measurement level of the rating scale, time trade-off, and standard gamble. Social Sci Med. 2001;**53**(10):1275–1285.

26. Teixeira-Salmela LF, Olney SJ, Nadeau S, Brouwer B. Muscle strengthening and physical conditioning to reduce impairment and disability in chronic stroke survivors. Arch Phys Med Rehabil. 1999;**80**(10):1211–1218.

27. Fisher AG. The assessment of IADL motor skills: an application of many-faceted Rasch analysis. Am J Occup Ther. 1993;**47**(4):319–329.

28. Ward AB, Gutenbrunner C, Damjan H, Giustini A, Delarque A. European Union of Medical Specialists (UEMS) section of Physical & Rehabilitation Medicine: a position paper on physical and rehabilitation medicine in acute settings. J Rehabil Med. 2010;**42**(5):417–424.

29. Stroke Unit Trialists' Collaboration. Collaborative systematic review of the randomised trials of organised inpatient (stroke unit) care after stroke. Stroke Unit Trialists' Collaboration. Br Med J. 1997;**314**(7088):1151–1159.

30. Beech R, Rudd AG, Tilling K, Wolfe CD. Economic consequences of early inpatient discharge to community-based rehabilitation for stroke in an inner-London teaching hospital. Stroke. 1999;**30**(4):729–735.

31. Schultke E. Ludwig Guttmann: emerging concept of rehabilitation after spinal cord injury. J Hist Neurosci. 2001;**10**(3):300–307.

32. O'Connor RJ, Murray PC. Review of spinal cord injuries in Ireland. Spinal Cord. 2006;**44**(7):445–448.

33. Ditunno JF, Jr., Formal CS. Chronic spinal cord injury. N Engl J Med. 1994;**330**(8):550–556.

34. Inman C. Effectiveness of spinal cord injury rehabilitation. Clin Rehabi. 1999;**13** Suppl 1:25–31.

35. Priebe MM, Chiodo AE, Scelza WM, Kirshblum SC, Wuermser LA, Ho CH. Economic and societal issues in spinal cord injury. Arch Phys Med Rehabil. 2007;**88**(3 Suppl 1):S84–88.

36. O'Connor RJ, Martyn-Hemphill C, McNicol C, Morrison R. Reduction in care costs with community rehabilitation. Clin Med. 2011;**11**(3):299–300.

37. Svensson E. Guidelines to statistical evaluation of data from rating scales and questionnaires. J Rehabil Med. 2001 Jan;**33**(1):47–48.

38. O'Connor E. 'Fractions of Men': engendering amputation in Victorian culture. Comparative Studies in Society and History. 1997;**39**(4):742–777.

39. Silver JR. The British contribution to the treatment of spinal injuries. J Hist Neurosci. 1993;**2**(2):151–157.

40. Anonymous. Rehabilitation services. Br Med J. 1972;**2**(816):727–728.

41. McColl I, Bunch A, Fanshawe E, et al. Review of artificial limb and appliance centre services. DHSS, London, 1986.

42. Miller EJ, Gwynne GV. A life apart: pilot study of residential institutions for the physically handicapped and young chronic sick. Tavistock Press, London, 1972.

CHAPTER 4

Predicting activities after stroke

Gert Kwakkel and Boudewijn Kollen

Why should we predict activities after stroke?

Stroke recovery is heterogeneous in terms of outcome, and it is estimated that 25 into 25% of the 50 million stroke survivors worldwide require some assistance or are fully dependent on caregivers for activities of daily living (ADL) after their stroke [1]. In addition to medical management after acute stroke to prevent further cerebral damage, early stroke rehabilitation is initiated with the ultimate goal of achieving better recovery in terms of body functions and activities in the first months after stroke, and to reduce disability and handicap during the years that follow [2]. Knowledge about factors that determine the final outcome in terms of activities after stroke is important for early stroke management, in order to set suitable rehabilitation goals, enable early discharge planning, and correctly inform patients and relatives. The current trend to shorten the length of stay in hospital stroke units, as well as the increasing demand for efficiency in the continuity of stroke care, imply that knowledge about the prognosis for the outcome in terms of basic activities such as dressing, mobility, and bathing is crucial to optimize stroke management in the first months post stroke. Knowledge about the prognosis in terms of activities (i.e. functional prognosis) is also important for the effective design of future trials in stroke rehabilitation. In particular, identifying subgroups of patients who may benefit most from a particular intervention [3–5] and stratifying patients into prognostically comparable groups will prevent underpowered studies (i.e. type II errors), keeping in mind that the contribution of stroke rehabilitation services is relatively small (i.e. 5 to 10% of the variance in the outcome) compared to the variability across patients included in trials [6–8]. A number of observational studies suggest that the degree of recovery in terms of impairments and activities after stroke is already largely defined within the first days after stroke onset [9–16]. This finding also suggests that the effectiveness of therapy is not only determined by selecting the most effective therapy but also depends on selecting appropriate patients, who show some potential for recovery of activities after stroke. Moreover, many evidence-based therapies such as constraint-induced movement therapy (CIMT) or modified versions of it, body weight-supported treadmill training (BWSTT), neuromuscular stimulation, and early supported discharge policies by a stroke team are heavily dependent on an appropriate selection of stroke patients [17]. Hence, the establishment of an adequate prognosis by a stroke rehabilitation team will increase the efficiency of stroke services and reduce costs. From a patient's perspective, effective prognostics enable health care professionals to respond to changes that occur over time, to estimate the feasibility of the short- and long-term treatment goals, and to provide correct information to patients and their partners [18].

Despite the above advantages, prognostic research has received little attention in neurology and rehabilitation medicine compared to intervention research, and has not gained much acceptance in clinical practice as a result of: (1) doubts about predictive accuracy due to issues such as bias in observations, (2) problems with the generalization of the results, and (3) the complexity of algorithms, which hampers practical implementation [18–20]. Furthermore, a number of previous systematic reviews of prognostic research have shown that a high proportion of prognostic studies in stroke are of poor methodological quality [18–21]. On the other hand, a favourable trend can be discerned, since the better quality studies were published in the most recent years [18, 20]. This illustrates the growing awareness among investigators of the importance of meeting the methodological criteria for prediction model development.

The present chapter will focus on prediction of activities after stroke. First, we will discuss some methodological shortcomings of prognostic research. Subsequently, based on the most common flaws in prospective cohort studies, we will elucidate the main characteristics about the pattern and hierarchical sequence of recovery of impairments and disability post stroke. Finally, the most important clinical bedside factors will be discussed that independently predict outcome of activities of daily living, dexterity and walking ability post stroke.

What constitutes good quality prognostic research?

In contrast to the CONSORT statements [22], there are no strict methodological criteria for assessing the quality of prognostic research. A number of key factors have been identified in clinical epidemiology that may confound the relationship between the independent variable of interest (i.e. the determinant) and the outcome or dependent variable in the regression model. The methodology of prognostic studies continues to evolve [3, 19, 21, 23–25] and guidelines for reporting observational studies in accordance with the 'strengthening of reporting of observational studies in epidemiology' (STROBE) statement have only recently been established [26].

Table 4.1 summarizes the main factors that affect internal, statistical, and external validity of high-quality prognostic research. This 27-item checklist addresses six major risks of bias: (1) study participation, (2) study attrition, (3) prognostic factor measurement, (4) outcome measurement, (5) statistical analysis, and (6) clinical performance [3, 19, 18, 20, 23, 25, 27, 28]. As shown in Table 4.1, each item can be rated as positive (sufficient information: low risk of bias, 1 point assigned), negative (insufficient information: potential risk of bias, 0 points assigned), or partial/unknown. A total score can be obtained by summing all items that were given a positive rating.

What do we know about the pattern of stroke recovery in terms of body functions and activities?

The development over time of body functions (i.e. impairments) and activities (i.e. disabilities) after stroke is characterized by a large diversity. Some patients show hardly any improvement even in the long term, whereas other patients recover fully within hours or days after their stroke. Even though the outcome of stroke patients is heterogeneous and individual recovery patterns differ, clear mathematical regularities (i.e. logistic and sigmoidal) have been found in these non-linear patterns of recovery, making the outcome in terms of body functions and activities highly predictable [7, 14, 15, 16, 17, 21, 27–31]. Figure 4.1 shows an average common, hypothetical pattern of stroke recovery of patients with a first-ever ischaemic middle cerebral artery (MCA) stroke [32].

As shown in Figure 4.1, the time course after stroke is characterized by larger improvements during the first weeks post stroke than in the post-acute phases beyond 3 months after stroke, reflecting common underlying mechanisms known as 'spontaneous neurological recovery' [17, 30, 33, 34–36]. A number of cohort studies have shown that the initial severity of disability as well as the extent of improvement observed within the first days or weeks post stroke are important indicators of the outcome at 6 months after stroke [20, 33, 34, 37–40]. Another striking feature supporting the existence of a predefined biological pattern in time is the observation that the sequence of progress in activities, as assessed for example with the Barthel Index (BI), is almost fixed in time. Hierarchical scaling procedures of the BI show that in about 80% of all patients with a first-ever MCA stroke, progress of activities follows the same sequence of BI items [41].

As shown in Figure 4.2, skills that allow the use of compensation strategies, such as grooming, recover earlier than more complex skills such as dressing and climbing stairs. The observed sequence in this small sample of patients was recently confirmed by a number of studies using Rasch analysis. Rasch analysis determines the probability of achieving a particular milestone on the basis of 'patient's' ability' and 'item difficulty' [42, 43]. A larger study involving 556 stroke patients [41] found the same hierarchical sequence in terms of BI items. It should be noted, however, that not all items of the BI measure the same underlying concept. Indeed, items that measure body functions (i.e. bladder and bowel control) in the BI [41] and the Functional Independence Measure (FIM) [44, 45] are not suitable for a Rasch analysis, because these items assess different (impairment-related) constructs.

The fact that the recovery of activities after stroke follows a fixed hierarchy is not limited to ADL outcomes measured with instruments like the BI or the FIM [45], but have also been found for the Stroke Impact Scale [46], the National Institutes of Health Stroke Scale (NIHSS) [47], as well as for the recovery of

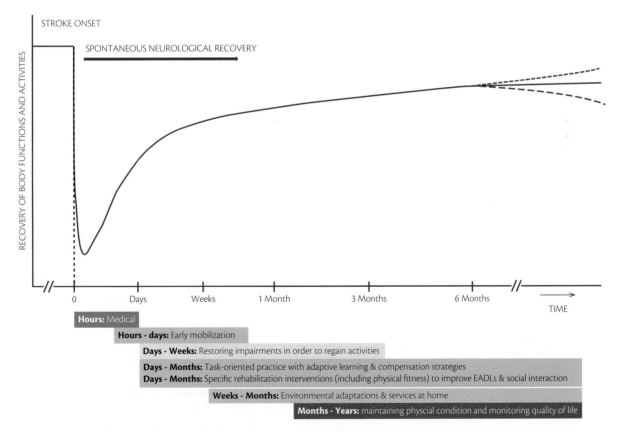

Fig. 4.1 Hypothetical pattern of recovery after stroke with timing of intervention strategies.
Reprinted from Lancet, 14, Langhorne P, Bernhardt J, Kwakkel G, Stroke rehabilitation, 1693–702, Copyright (2011), with permission from Elsevier.

Table 4.1 Quality assessment of reports of prognostic studies

Outcome strategies		Scale	Criteria
Evaluation of study design			
D1	Source population and recruitment	Y/N/?	*Positive* when sampling frame (e.g. hospital based, community based, primary care) *and* recruitment procedure (place and time period, method used to identify sample) are reported.
D2	Inclusion and exclusion criteria	Y/?	*Positive* if both the inclusion and exclusion criteria are explicitly described.
D3	Important baseline key characteristics of study sample	Y/?	*Positive* if the following key characteristics of the sample are described: gender, age, type, localization, number of strokes, stroke severity. Number of strokes is adequate when at least 'a history of stroke' or 'recurrent stroke' is reported.
D4	Prospective design	Y/N/?	*Positive* when a prospective design was used, *or* in case of a historical cohort in which prognostic factors were measured before the outcome was determined.
D5	Inception cohort	Y/N/?	*Positive* if observation started at an uniform time point within 2 weeks after stroke onset.
D6	Information about treatment	Y/N/?	*Positive* if information on treatment during observation period is reported (e.g. medical or paramedical, usual care, randomized, etc.)
Study attrition			
A1	Loss to follow-up	Y/N/?	*Positive* if loss to follow-up during period of observation did not exceed 20%.
A2	Reasons for loss to follow-up	Y/N/?	*Positive* if reasons for loss to follow-up are specified, *or* there was no loss to follow-up.
A3	Methods to deal with missing data	Y/N/?	*Positive* if adequate method of dealing with missing values was used in case of missing values (e.g. multiple imputation), *or* there were no missing values.
A4	Comparison of completers and non-completers	Y/N/?	*Positive* if article reports that there are no significant differences between participants who completed the study and those who did not, concerning key characteristics of gender, age, type and severity *and* candidate predictors and outcome, *or* if there was no loss to follow-up.
Predictor measurement			
P1	Definition of predictors	Y/N/?	*Positive* if the article clearly defines or describes all candidate predictors (concerning *both* clinical and demographic features).
P2	Measurement of predictors reliable and valid	Y/N/?	*Positive* if ≥1 candidate predictor was measured in a valid and reliable way, *or* referral is made to other studies which have established reliability and validity,
P3	Coding scheme and cut-off points	Y/N/?	*Positive* if coding scheme for candidate predictors was defined, including cut-off points *and* rationale for cut-off points; *or* if there was no dichotomization or classification.
P4	Data presentation	Y/N/?	*Positive* if frequencies or percentages or mean (SD/CI), or median (IQR) are reported for all candidate predictors.
Outcome measurement			
O1	Outcome(s) defined	Y/N/?	*Positive* when a clear definition of the outcome(s) of interest is presented.
O2	Measurement of outcome(s) reliable and valid	Y/N/?	*Positive* when outcome was measured in a valid and reliable way, *or* reference is made to other studies which have established reliability and validity.
O3	Coding scheme and cut-off points described	Y/N/?	*Positive* if the coding scheme of the outcome is given, including cut-off points *and* rationale for cut-off points; *or* if there was no dichotomization.
O4	Appropriate end-points of observation	Y/N/?	*Positive* if observation was obtained at a fixed time after stroke onset, *negative* if observation was made at discharge.
O5	Data presentation	Y/N/?	*Positive* if frequencies or percentages or mean (SD/CI) or median (IQR) are reported for the outcome measure.
Statistical analysis			
S1	Strategy for model building described	Y/N/?	*Positive* if the method of the selection process for multivariable analysis is presented (e.g. forward, backward selection, including *p*-value).
S2	Sufficient sample size	Y/N/?	*Positive* if the number of patients with a positive or negative outcome (event) per variable in the logistic regression analysis was adequate, i.e. equal to or exceeding 10 events for each variable in the multivariable model (Events Per Variable), *or* in case of linear regression analysis $N \geq 10$ for each variable.
S3	Presentation of univariate analysis	Y/N/?	*Positive* if univariate crude estimates and confidence intervals (β/SE, OR/CI, RR, HR) are reported. *Negative* when only *p*-values or correlation coefficients are given, *or* if no tests were performed at all.
S4	Presentation of multivariable analysis	Y/N/?	*Positive* if point estimates with confidence intervals (β/SE, OR/CI, RR, HR,) are reported for the multivariable models.
S5	Continuous predictors	Y/N/?	*Positive* if continuous predictors were not dichotomized in the multivariable model.

(continued)

Table 4.1 (Continued)

Outcome strategies		Scale	Criteria
Clinical performance/validity			
C1	Clinical performance	Y/N/?	*Positive* if article provides information concerning at least one of the following performance measures: discrimination (e.g. ROC), calibration (e.g. HL statistic), explained variance, clinical value (e.g. sensitivity, specificity, PPV, NPV)
C2	Internal validation	Y/N/?	*Positive* if appropriate techniques were used to assess internal validity (e.g. cross-validation, bootstrapping), *negative* if split-sample method was used.
C3	External validation	Y/N/?	*Positive* if the prediction model was validated in a second independent group of stroke patients.

Y, Positive, 1 point; N, Negative, 0 points; ?, Partial/unknown.

Veerbeek JM, Kwakkel G, van Wegen EE, et al. Early prediction of outcome of activities of daily living after stroke: a systematic review. Stroke. 42(5):1482–8 © 2011.

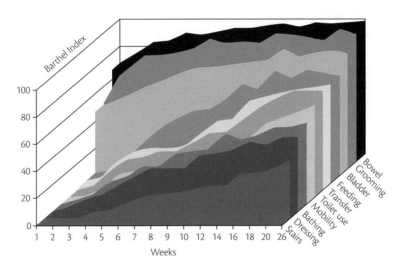

Fig. 4.2 Progress of patients' skills (Barthel Index) in a fixed sequence, with earlier recovery for relatively less complex skills that allow compensation strategies, such as feeding and grooming, and later recovery for more complex skills, such as dressing and climbing stairs. As illustrated in this figure, patients showed an almost consistent sequence of recovery with bowel control restored first, followed by grooming, bladder control, feeding, transfer, toilet use, mobility, bathing, dressing, and finally climbing stairs. The so-called Guttmann scaling procedure yielded a coefficient of scalability ranging from 0.72 for week 26 to 0.85 for week 3 post stroke, suggesting that about 80% of the patients progressed through this fixed sequence in time.

Reprinted from Restor Neurol Neurosci, 22, Kwakkel G, Kollen B, Lindeman E., Understanding the pattern of functional recovery after stroke: facts and theories, 281–99, Copyright (2004), with permission from IOS Press.

the upper limb function measured with the ABILHAND questionnaire [48] or the Action Research Arm Test (ARAT) [49]. These findings support the notion that defining milestones may serve as an important part of multidisciplinary stroke management [50–52] in order to allow the team to focus on realistically attainable treatment goals.

Are we able to predict ADL independence after stroke?

Knowledge about robust and unbiased factors that predict outcome in terms ADL is paramount in early stroke management. A systematic review of 48 studies that aimed to predict ADL outcome showed that the BI and mRS were the two activity level outcome measures most frequently used in prognostic stroke studies. Despite the fact that that only a small proportion of the included studies, i.e. 6 out of 48 (12.5%), was of high quality [20], strong evidence was found that age and scores on scales assessing severity of neurological deficits in the early post-stroke phase, such as the NIHSS and CNS, are strongly associated with the final basic

ADL outcome beyond 3 months post stroke [53]. In a prospective cohort study in 159 stroke victims with a mild to moderate first-ever ischaemic hemispheric stroke, we found that when measured within 72 h post stroke, the NIHSS score was strongly associated with the final outcome in terms of ADL independency as measured with the Barthel Index at 6 months.

The discriminative properties as well as the accuracy of prediction with the NIHSS at baseline seem to be robust and hardly influenced by the timing of assessment in the first 9 days after stroke onset [15]. As shown in Figure 4.3 the area under the curve (AUC) ranged from 0.789 (95%CI, 0.715–0.864) for measurements on day 2 to 0.804 (95%CI, 0.733–0.874) and 0.808 (95%CI, 0.739–0.877) for days 5 and 9, respectively [15].

The systematic review of 48 prognostic studies also showed that gender and the presence of risk factors for stroke, such as atrial fibrillation, did not predict the outcome in terms of basic ADL [20]. Conspicuously, imaging data for the prediction of ADL outcome proved to be of limited value when compared to the contribution

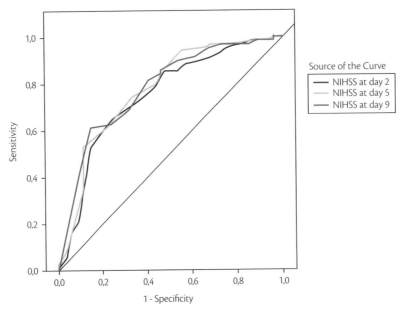

Fig. 4.3 Graphic presentation of ROC analyses of the moment of timing of the assessment of NIHSS scores for the outcome of BI (≥19) at 6 months after stroke. Reprinted from J Neurol Sci, 57– 61, Kwakkel G, Veerbeek J, van Wegen E, et al., Predictive value of the NIHSS for ADL outcome after ischemic hemispheric stroke: does timing of early assessment matter?, 57– 61, Copyright (2010), with permission from Elsevier.

of clinical variables alone [20]. In a previous prospective study in 75 first-ever MCA stroke survivors, we found that age and the initial BI score measured at day 5 post stroke predicted 84% of the AUC for the outcome in terms of ADL independency 1 year post stroke. In this study, patients were classified as ADL-independent if they had a BI score of 19 or 20 points. However, adding magnetic resonance imaging (MRI) findings at 11 days post stroke, such as the presence of white matter lesions, hemisphere of stroke, cortical or subcortical, and lesion and stroke volume, increased the AUC from 0.84 to 0.87 in the surviving patients. [54] In line with other studies in this field that investigated the impact of stroke lesion volumes on the outcome in terms of ADL [55], this prospective cohort study suggests that neuroimaging variables from conventional MRI scans do not increase the accuracy of long-term prediction of ADL [54-56].

In addition to the predictive validity of neurological scales such as NIHSS and CNS, a number of prospective cohort studies have shown that the baseline value of the BI (or FIM) assessed within 2 weeks post stroke is highly associated with the final BI (or FIM) measured at 6 months post stroke [7, 27, 53, 54]. However, the predictive accuracy of the initial BI score seems to be time dependent [53]. For example, a prospective cohort study investigating the diagnostic accuracy of the BI in 206 hemispheric stroke patients [53] showed a significantly higher accuracy in predicting the outcome in terms of the BI at 6 months when assessed at 5 or 9 days post stroke than when assessed at 2 days post stroke. The AUC ranged from 0.785 on day 2 to 0.837 and 0.848 on days 5 and 9, respectively, suggesting that the assessment on day 5 proved to be the earliest post-stroke moment for an optimal prediction of final outcome in terms of ADL (Figure 4.4). This finding suggests that the BI should preferably be measured at the end of the first week in hospital-based stroke units to ensure effective stroke rehabilitation management. This time-dependence of the predictability can be explained by several putative mechanisms. The first is that 2 days post stroke is too early for patients to begin to develop the compensatory strategies that they

will use to carry out ADL. At one week, in contrast, the core compensatory abilities may already be present. The second possibility is that subjects may have a greater tendency to perform below their true maximal capacity early after stroke. The third option is that oedema and metabolic factors, which have their maximal influence in the first 72 hours, could mask the capacity for recovery.

The less than optimal prediction of BI at 6 months for patients assessed within 72 hours in our study may have been caused by the instability of neurological deficits, which is manifested by the neurological worsening observed in approximately 25% of all patients during the first 24 to 48 hours after stroke [53]. However, a parallel study focusing on the timing of an assessment of neurological deficits by the NIHSS in the same population resulted in no significant differences between days 2, 5, and 9 [15], which makes neurological worsening within this period unlikely. A more plausible explanation could be that observers find it difficult to determine the patient's actual performance in terms of basic ADL when the patient is still bedridden. As a consequence, an assessment within 72 h post stroke will underestimate their actual performance. In line with the recommendation by Kasner [57], our findings suggest that even in individuals with a minor stroke who are bedridden during the first few days after stroke, the BI will underestimate outcome scores, making the BI an unsuitable instrument to measure disability within the first 3 days post stroke.

Other determinants reported in valid prospective cohort studies suggest that not only baseline ADL factors such as sitting balance but also urinary incontinence, severity of hemiplegia, cozmorbidity, consciousness at admission, cognitive status, and depression are independent factors that contribute to the outcome in terms of ADL beyond 6 months [18, 19, 20, 27, 58].

Who regains walking ability?

Regaining independent gait is considered a primary goal in stroke rehabilitation. A number of prospective cohort studies have shown that approximately 60% [10, 59] to 80% [21] of stroke patients are able to walk independently at 6 months post stroke. Various prognostic studies suggest that age [60, 61], severity of sensory and motor dysfunction of the paretic leg [62], homonymous hemianopia [61. 62], urinary incontinence [11, 60], sitting balance [11, 13, 21, 63–66], initial disability in ADL and ambulation [10, 11, 13], level of consciousness on admission [60], and the number of days between stroke onset and first assessment [16] are independently associated with gait outcomes 6 months after stroke [21]. For example, the EPOS study, involving 154 first-ever ischaemic stroke patients who were unable to walk independently, used multivariate (or multivariable) logistic modelling to show that accurate prediction within 72 hours is achievable at hospital stroke units by means of two simple bedside tests: namely sitting balance and muscle strength of the paretic leg. Independent gait was defined as 4 points or more on the Functional Ambulation Categories (FAC), suggesting that patients could be classified as safe walkers able to walk independently on flat surfaces [21]. Those non-ambulatory patients who regained their sitting balance as assessed by the trunk control test (TCT) and who developed some voluntary movement of the hip, knee and/or ankle as assessed by the MI–leg score (≥25 points) within the first 72 hours post stroke had about a 98% chance of regaining independent gait within 6 months. In contrast, those patients who were unable to sit independently for 30 seconds and were hardly able to contract the muscles of the paretic lower limb within 72 hours had a probability of about 27% of achieving independent gait [21]. Early reassessment of sitting balance and lower limb strength on days 5 and 9 showed that if sitting ability and lower limb strength failed to recover, the probability of regaining independent gait declined to 23% when assessed on day 5, and 10% when assessed on day 9 post stroke [21].

The increasing accuracy of prediction over time may reflect underlying intrinsic neurological mechanisms of recovery such as elevation of diaschisis after stroke [7, 30]. Comparing these findings with those of other studies is difficult due to the lack of prognostic studies investigating the accuracy of prediction within 72 hours. However, a number of prospective studies have shown that muscle strength of the hemiplegic leg [21, 61, 62] and sitting balance [11, 21, 64], when measured between the second to fourth week after stroke, are significantly associated with improvement of walking ability [13] and achieving independent gait [13, 65, 66] at 6 months. Obviously, the early control of sitting balance as a prerequisite for regaining standing balance and gait is an important factor for the final outcome at 6 months [65]. The importance of balance control for gait is also supported by the study of Kollen and colleagues [13], who showed that improvement in standing balance was the most important variable associated with improvement of gait performance as measured with the FAC [13].

Since the proportion of false positives (≈7%) was clearly smaller than the proportion of false negatives (≈27%) within 2 days post stroke, our study suggests this model is generally somewhat pessimistic, and illustrates that some patients with an initially poor sitting balance and a severe paresis of the hemiplegic limb will nevertheless regain independent gait [13]. This finding is supported by a number of recent longitudinal studies showing that gait recovery is closely related to learning to use compensatory movement strategies [67–69]. For instance, patients learn to keep their balance by shifting their centre of gravity to the non-paretic side [68, 70], despite significant change in motor control on the paretic side is almost lacking [67, 69]. In the same vein, longitudinal studies with repeated measurements over time show that the contribution of the non-paretic side to the increase in comfortable and maximal walking speed is larger than the contribution of the paretic side [71]. To date, all longitudinal studies suggest that patients learn to cope with existing neurological deficits when regaining standing balance [68, 70, 72] and independent gait

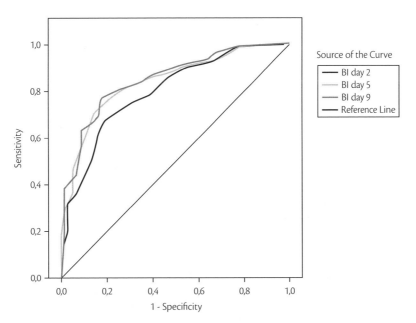

Fig. 4.4 Graphic presentation of ROC analyses of the timing of the assessment of BI on days 2, 5, and 9 for the outcome in terms of dichotomized BI scores (≥19) after 6 months (N = 206).
Kwakkel G, Veerbeek JM, Harmeling-van der Wel BC, van Wegen E, Kollen BJ; Early Prediction of functional Outcome after Stroke (EPOS) Investigators. Diagnostic accuracy of the Barthel Index for measuring activities of daily living outcome after ischemic hemispheric stroke: does early poststroke timing of assessment matter? Stroke. 2011 Feb;42(2):342–6 with permission.

after stroke [67, 69, 73, 74]. Obviously, these adaptation strategies already start as soon as patients learn to accomplish tasks within the first weeks post stroke.

Who regains dexterity after stroke?

Although prospective epidemiological studies are lacking, findings of a number of prospective cohort studies suggest that 33% to 66% of stroke patients with a paretic upper limb do not show any recovery in upper limb function at 6 months after stroke [75, 76]. Depending on the outcome measures used, 5% to 20% achieve full recovery of the upper paretic limb in terms of activities at 6 months [9, 12, 75, 76].

A recent systematic review of 58 studies on prognostic variables relating to upper limb recovery showed that the initial severity of upper limb impairment and function were the most significant predictors of upper limb recovery (i.e. odds ratio 14.84 (95%CI: 9.08–24.25) and 38.62 (95%CI: 8.40–177.53), respectively [28]. With that the most important predictive factor for upper limb recovery following stroke was the initial severity of motor impairment post stroke [28]. However, the interpretation of these results were complicated by methodological factors such as using different upper limb motor outcome scales, timing of baseline and outcome assessments and with that, predictors selected [28].

In order to better understand the functional prognosis of the upper limb, we tested the probability of impairment being reduced and dexterity being regained at 6 months using logistic regression analysis in patients who had an almost flaccid upper limb in the first week post stroke and no dexterity as assessed the FM arm score, as shown in Figure 4.1 [12]. We found that only by those patients with some early reduction of impairment in the upper paretic limb had greater gains later; patients showing some (synergistic) movement in the upper limb within 4 weeks post stroke had a 94% chance of improving their ARAT score, whereas this probability remained below 10% in those who failed to show any return of motor control (Figure 4.5).

This study, with repeated measurements over time, suggests that there is a critical time window in which the final outcome in terms of dexterity is largely determined. In fact, it is the same limited time window that has been found in animal studies for an upregulation of growth-promoting factors, resulting in synapse strengthening and activity-dependent rewiring of neuronal networks to compensate for tissue lost to injury [77].

These findings built on the results of previous prospective studies starting after the first week post stroke [78–81]. For example, Smania et al. [79] showed in a sample of 48 stroke patients that active finger extension at day 7 post stroke is a valid early indicator of a favourable outcome in terms of upper limb function as measured with the nine-hole peg test, the Fugl-Meyer for the arm, and the Motricity Index for the arm. Katrak et al. [80] reported that initial shoulder abduction, measured about 11 days after stroke, is an early predictor of good hand function at 1 and 2 months after stroke. These findings also suggest that the selection of patients in terms of poor or favourable prognosis for upper limb recovery at the impairment level is an important prerequisite for effective stroke rehabilitation. To date, all evidence-based therapies that have proved to be effective for the upper limb, including CIMT, have been based on studies with selected patients with a low level of impairment that allows for superposition of compensatory strategies. In contrast, studies on evidence-based therapies for patients with an unfavourable prognosis at the impairment and function levels are lacking in the literature.

In a more recent prospective study [14] involving 159 stroke victims, we investigated if outcome in terms of upper limb function at 6 months can be predicted within 72 hours after stroke onset. In addition, we reinvestigated the effect of the timing of assessment on the accuracy of prediction by reassessing observed clinical

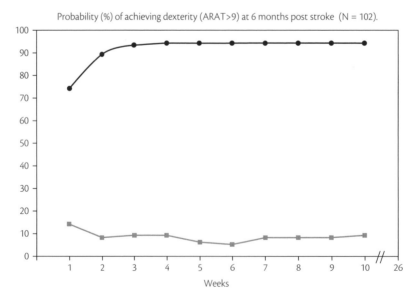

Probability (%) of achieving dexterity (ARAT>9) at 6 months post stroke (N = 102).

Fig. 4.5 Probability of achieving some dexterity at 6 months post stroke. Within the first 3 to 4 months, a critical time window was present in which the outcome in terms of dexterity (dichotomized into ARAT < 10 points or ARAT ≥10) was determined. Optimal prediction was based on the Fugl-Meyer scores of the paretic arm and the motricity index score of the leg (MI-leg).

Kwakkel G, Kollen BJ, van der Grond J, et al. Probability of regaining dexterity in the flaccid upper limb: impact of severity of paresis and time since onset in acute stroke. Stroke. 34:2181–2186 determinants on days 5 and 9 after stroke. The results showed that those patients with some finger extension and some visible shoulder abduction on day 2 after stroke onset had a 98% probability of achieving some upper limb function at 6 months. In contrast, patients who did not show this voluntary motor control had a probability of only 25%. It was also remarkable that 60% of the patients with some finger extension within 72 hours had regained full upper limb function according to the ARAT at 6 months. [14]

This finding confirms the substantial predictive value of finger extension as a positive sign for a favourable outcome for the upper paretic limb in the acute phase after stroke. Retesting the model on days 5 and 9 showed that the probability of regaining function remained 98% for those with some finger extension and shoulder abduction, whereas the probability decreased from 25% to 14% for those without this voluntary control. Obviously, the reservation of some voluntary finger extension reflects the importance of the presence of some intact corticospinal tract fibres of the corticospinal tract system (CST) in the affected hemisphere that can activate distal arm and hand muscles [82], assuming that the forearm and hand lack direct bilateral innervation from both hemispheres [84]. Studies using transcranial magnetic stimulation (TMS) [83–85] and diffusion tensor imaging [86, 87] have further confirmed this hypothesis. For example, Van Kuijk et al. [88] showed that in patients with an initial paralysis of the upper limb, the presence or absence of a motor-evoked potential in the abductor digiti minimi, measured with transcranial magnetic stimulation at the end of the first week after stroke, is highly predictive of the final outcome in terms of dexterity at 6 months. However, the predictive value of the presence or absence of motor-evoked potentials in the abductor digiti minimi is similar to that of clinical assessments alone, suggesting that transcranial magnetic stimulation measurements should focus on the predictive value of motor-evoked potentials of the finger extensors in particular, rather than the finger flexors or the abductor digiti minimi alone [89].

In the same vein, similar to findings from TMS studies, but in contrast to the predictive value of lesion volume of MRI for the outcome in terms of ADL, we found in 75 MCA victims that lesions of the internal capsule detected on MRI were associated with a significantly lower probability of the return of isolated hand motor function than superficial lesions of the cortex, subcortex, and corona radiata [90]. This difference in the relevance of lesion volume in predicting impairment versus ADL was to be expected as the latter largely depends on compensation. The probability of regaining hand function declined from 54% when the corticofugal tract was only partly affected to 13% when both motor cortex and internal capsule were affected. The latter study once again shows that the return of hand function 1 year after stroke largely depends on the preservation of neuroanatomical areas known to represent the corticofugal tract of the upper limb. Obviously, the involvement of structures with a greater density of dysfunctional corticofugal tract fibres, such as the internal capsule, is associated with poor recovery of hand motor function at one year post stroke [90].

Knowledge about the early prediction of final functional outcome for the upper limb function is paramount for the implementation of effective stroke management. In particular, subsequent multidisciplinary rehabilitation services may be optimized based on the probability of regaining function, in view of the fact that many evidence-based therapies for the upper paretic limb, including CIMT, require some return of voluntary wrist and finger extension [91-93]. This finding also suggests that evidence-based practice is not only a matter of applying the most effective therapy for a particular patient but is also about selecting the appropriate patients to be offered this specific therapy.

Are improvements of body functions and cognition predictable post-stroke

Longitudinal regression analyses of change scores have shown that most improvements in motor function, such as in synergism [30, 33], strength of upper [30] and lower paretic limb [59], as well as decline in cognitive impairments, such as neglect [30, 93] and dysphasia [94, 95] are almost entirely defined within the first 10 to 12 weeks post-stroke. Recent kinematic analyses have shown that these improvements, such as in FM-scores, within the first eight post-stroke weeks parallel the restitution of quality of motor control in terms of: (1) the number of degrees of freedom that patients are able to control for in a reaching task [96] and normalization of jerk during, for example, a reaching task [97]. Beyond these first weeks of restitution, often regarded as the period in which true neurological repair takes place, improvements are mainly characterized by substitution and learning to adapt to existing neurological deficits [98]. Furthermore, it has been shown that more severe impairments at stroke onset result in slower patterns of recovery then on average to 3 months post stroke for more severe affected subjects [33].

Interestingly, Prabhakaran and colleagues [16] suggested that the amount of restitution of impairments driven by spontaneous motor recovery is relatively fixed for FM-arm scores, which accounts for approximately 70% of patients' maximal potential recovery. In their study, this maximal potential motor recovery was defined as the difference between initial FM upper limb (FM-UL) measured within 72 hours post stroke and the maximal possible score of 66 points [16: p. 68]. According to this recovery model, patients with an initial severe upper limb impairment (i.e. a low initial FM-UL score) have more room to improve on the FM-UL, and thus have a larger potential for improvent when compared to patients with an initial mild upper limb impairment (i.e. a high initial FM-UL score). This fixed amount of spontaneous neurological change was observed particularly in those with a mild to moderate neurological deficit after a first ever hemispheric stroke, which was the case in the majority (~70%) of ischaemic stroke patients. The reason why patients with more severe initial neurological deficits show less spontaneous neurological improvement remains unknown. One may hypothesize that the reversibility of impaired brain function due to ischemia is influenced by the size of the lesion, and underlying processes involving recovery of neuronal networks including mechanisms of homeostatic neuroplasticity in the first weeks post stroke [7, 77, 98–100] Unfortunately, the study of Prabhakaran et al. [16] does not provide insight in the neurobiological mechanisms responsible for the proportional neurological recovery.

The finding of a fixed proportional recovery after stroke is not unique for motor recovery but is also found for other modalities like speech and inattention. Lazar and colleagues [94] showed that the amount of improvement in aphasia scores following ischaemic stroke was almost fixed; showing an overall relationship of 0.73 between the maximal potential change in aphasia score and the observed change, measured at 3 months post stroke [94]. However, it should be noted that the study was performed in a small sample of 21 stroke patients. Also, neglect after right hemisphere stroke often resolves within 3 months of stroke onset and shows an almost fixed percentage of improvement on for example on the letter cancellation task [30. 93]. Also, neglect after right hemisphere stroke often resolves within 3 months of stroke onset and shows an almost fixed percentage of improvement, on for example a letter cancellation task [93, 101].

The aforementioned preliminary findings suggest that the amount of spontananeous neurological recovery is based on a fixed proportion and is thus highly predictable during the first 3 or 6 months post stroke. Second, one may conclude that the proportional fixed amount of recovery is not specific for motor impairments but rather generic and applies to other impairments such as inattention and dysphasia, obviously reflecting the same underlying biological mechanisms responsible for neurological recovery [77, 98, 99].

The theory behind the maximal proportional recovery of body functions including cognitive impairments, such as inattention and dysphasia, does not support the clinical observation that in many cases patients may improve far beyond the first 3 months of spontaneous neurological recovery post-stroke. For example, Desmond and coauthors performed a battery of neuropsychological tests 3 months and then annually after stroke. Among patients with baseline cognitive impairment, 36% were found to show improved cognitive function beyond the first 3 months after stroke [102]. These results are similar to those that Kotila and colleagues reported [103], and Wade and coworkers found significant recovery in several aspects of memory between 3 and 6 months after stroke [76]. Recovery of constructional apraxia may be seen up to 6 months after stroke. However, it is important to distinguish in these tests between improvements in body function and activities acknowledging that recovery of activities or abilities to perform a clinical test does not per se reflect true neurological repair but rather more optimal using compensation or coping strategies of the patient [99, 104].

Some parts of this Chapter are also written in the Textbook of Neural Repair and Rehabilitation. Predicting activities after stroke. Edited by Michael E. Selzer, Stephanie Clarke, Leonardo G. Cohen, Gert Kwakkel and Robert H. Miller. Volume II, Section 7, Chapter 46, pages 585–601.

References

1. Miller E, Murray L, Richards L, et al, American Heart Association Council on Cardiovascular Nursing and the Stroke Council. Comprehensive overview of nursing and interdisciplinary rehabilitation care of the stroke patient: a scientific statement from the American Heart Association. Stroke. 2010;**41**:2402–2448.
2. Hachinski V, Donnan G, Gorelick P, et al. Stroke: working toward a prioritized world agenda. Stroke. 2010;**41**:1084–1099.
3. Moons KG, Altman DG, Vergouwe Y, Royston P. Prognosis and prognostic research: application and impact of prognostic models in clinical practice. Br Med J. 2009;**338**:b606.
4. Moons K, Royston P, Vergouwe Y, Grobbee D, Altman D. Prognosis and prognostic research: what, why, and how? Br Med J. 2010;**338**:1317–1320.
5. Cramer SC. Stratifying patients with stroke in trials that target brain repair. Stroke. 2010;**41**(10 Suppl):S114–116.
6. Young F, Lees K, Weir C, GAIN International Trial Steering Committee and Investigators. Improving trial power through use of prognosis-adjusted end points. Stroke. 2005;**3**:597–601

7. Veerbeek JM, van Wegen E, van Peppen R, van der Wees PJ, Hendriks E, Rietberg M, Kwakkel G. What is the evidence for physical therapy poststroke? A systematic review and meta-analysis. PLoS One. 2014;**9**(2):e87987.
8. Veerbeek JM, Koolstra M, Ket JC, van Wegen EE, Kwakkel G. Effects of augmented exercise therapy on outcome of gait and gait-related activities in the first 6 months after stroke: a meta-analysis. Stroke. 2011;**42**(11):3311–3315.
9. Nakayama H, Jørgensen HS, Raaschou HO, Olsen TS. Recovery of upper extremity function in stroke patients: the Copenhagen Stroke Study. Arch Phys Med Rehabil. 1994;**75**(4):394–398.
10. Jørgenson H, Nakayama H, Raaschou H, Olsen T. Recovery of walking function in stroke patients: the Copenhagen Stroke Study. Arch Phys Med Rehabil. 1995;**76**:27–32.
11. Wade D, Hewer R. Functional abilities after stroke measurement, natural history and prognosis. J Neurol Neurosurg Psychiatry. 1987;**50**:177–82.
12. Kwakkel G, Kollen BJ, van der Grond J, Prevo AJH. Probability of regaining dexterity in the flaccid upper limb: impact of severity of paresis and time since onset in acute stroke. Stroke. 2003;**34**:2181–2186.
13. Kollen B, Kwakkel G, Lindeman E. Longitudinal robustness of variables predicting independent gait following severe middle cerebral artery stroke: a prospective cohort study. Clin Rehabil. 2006;**20**:262–268.
14. Nijland RH, van Wegen EE, Harmeling-van der Wel BC, Kwakkel G; EPOS Investigators. Presence of finger extension and shoulder abduction within 72 hours after stroke predicts functional recovery: early prediction of functional outcome after stroke: the EPOS cohort study. Stroke. 2010;**41**(4):745–50.
15. Kwakkel G, Veerbeek J, van Wegen E, et al, EPOS Investigators. Predictive value of the NIHSS for ADL outcome after ischemic hemispheric stroke: does timing of early assessment matter? J Neurol Sci. 2010;**294**:57–61.
16. Prabhakaran S, Zarahn E, Riley C, et al. Inter-individual variability in the capacity for motor recovery after ischemic stroke.Neurorehabil Neural Repair. 2008;**22**:64–71.
17. Langhorne P, Bernhardt J, Kwakkel G. Stroke rehabilitation. Lancet. 2011;**377**(9778):1693–702.
18. Kwakkel G, Kollen BJ. Predicting activities after stroke: what is clinically relevant? Int J Stroke. 2013;**8**(1):25–32.
19. Counsell C, Dennis M. Systematic review of prognostic models in patients with acute stroke. Cerebrovasc Dis. 2001;**12**:159–170.
20. Veerbeek JM, Kwakkel G, van Wegen EE, Ket JC, Heymans MW. Early prediction of outcome of activities of daily living after stroke: a systematic review. Stroke. 2011a;**42**(5):1482–8.
21. Veerbeek JM, Van Wegen EE, Harmeling-Van der Wel BC, Kwakkel G; EPOS Investigators. Is accurate prediction of gait in nonambulatory stroke patients possible within 72 hours poststroke?: The EPOS study. Neurorehabil Neural Repair. 2011b;**25**(3):268–74.
22. Moher D, Schulz KF, Altman DG. The CONSORT statement: revised recommendations for improving the quality of reports of parallel-group randomised trials. Lancet. 2001;**357**(9263):1191–1194.
23. Altman D. Systematic reviews of evaluations of prognostic variables. BMJBr Med J. 2001;**323**:224–228.
24. Altman DG, Vergouwe Y, Royston P, Moons KG. Prognosis and prognostic research: validating a prognostic model. Br Med J. 2009;**338**:b605.
25. Hayden J, Côté P, Bombardier C. Evaluation of the quality of prognosis studies in systematic reviews. Ann Intern Med. 2004;**144**:427–437.
26. Von Elm E, Altman D, Egger M, Pocock S, Gøtzsche P, Vandenbroucke J, for the STROBE Initiative. The Strengthening of Reporting of Observational Studies in Epidemiology (STROBE) statement: guidelines for reporting observational studies. Lancet. 2008;**370**:1453–1457.
27. Meijer R, van Limbeek J, Kriek B, Ihnenfeldt D, Vermeulen M, de Haan R. Prognostic social factors in the subacute phase after a stroke for the discharge destination from the hospital stroke-unit. A systematic review of the literature. Disabil Rehabil. 2004;**26**(4):191–197.

28. Coupar F, Pollock A, Rowe P, Weir C, Langhorne P. Predictors of upper limb recovery after stroke: a systematic review and meta-analysis. Clin Rehabil. 2012;26(4):291–313.

29. Koyama T, Matsumoto K, Okuno T, Domen K. A new method for predicting functional recovery of stroke patients with hemiplegia: logarithmic modelling. Clin Rehabil. 2005;19(7):779–789.

30. Kwakkel G, Kollen B, Twisk J. Impact of time on improvement of outcome after stroke. Stroke. 2006;37(9):2348–2353.

31. Zarahn E, Alon L, Ryan SL, Lazar RM, Vry MS, Weiller C, Marshall RS, Krakauer JW. Prediction of motor recovery using initial impairment and fMRI 48 h poststroke. Cereb Cortex. 2011;21(12):2712–2721.

32. Kwakkel G, Wagenaar RC, Twisk JW, Lankhorst GJ, Koetsier JC. Intensity of leg and arm training after primary middle-cerebral-artery stroke: a randomized trial. Lancet. 1999;354(9174):191–196.

33. Duncan PW, Goldstein LB, Matchar D, Divine GW, Feussner J. Measurement of motor recovery after stroke. Outcome assessment and sample size requirements. Stroke. 1992;23:1084–1089.

34. Duncan PW, Goldstein LB, Horner RD, Landsman PB, Samsa GP, Matchar DB. Similar motor recovery of upper and lower extremities after stroke. Stroke. 1994;25:1181–1188.

35. Gresham GE. Stroke outcome research. Stroke. 1986;17(3):358–360.

36. Newman M. The process of recovery after hemiplegia. Stroke. 1972;3(6):702–710.

37. Kwakkel G, Wagenaar RC, Kollen BJ, Lankhorst GJ. Predicting disability in stroke—a critical review of the literature. Age Ageing. 1996;25(6):479–489.

38. Heller A, Wade DT, Wood VA, Sunderland A, Hewer RL, Ward E. Arm function after stroke: measurement and recovery over the first three months. J Neurol Neurosurg Psychiatry. 1987;50(6):714–719.

39. Andrews K, Brocklehurst JC, Richards B, Laycock PJ. The rate of recovery from stroke—and its measurement. Int Rehabil Med. 1981;3(3):155–161.

40. Skilbeck C, Wade D, Hewer R, et al. Recovery after stroke. J Neurol Neurosurg Psychiatry. 1983;46:5–8.

41. Van Hartingsveld F, Lucas C, Kwakkel G, Lindeboom R. Improved interpretation of stroke trial results using empirical Barthel item weights. Stroke. 2006;37(1):162–166.

42. Tennant A, Geddes JM, Fear J, Hillman M, Chamberlain MA. Outcome following stroke. Disabil Rehabil. 1997 Jul;19(7):278–84. PubMed PMID: 9246544.

43. Granger CV, Linn RT. Biologic patterns of disability. J Outcome Meas. 2000;4(2):595–615.

44. Dallmeijer AJ, Dekker J, Roorda LD, et al. Differential item functioning of the Functional Independence Measure in higher performing neurological patients. J Rehabil Med. 2005;37(6):346–352.

45. Nilsson AL, Sunnerhagen KS, Grimby G. Scoring alternatives for FIM in neurological disorders applying Rasch analysis. Acta Neurol Scand. 2005;111(4):264–273.

46. Duncan PW, Bode RK, Min Lai S, Perera S; Glycine Antagonist in Neuroprotection. Rasch analysis of a new stroke-specific outcome scale: the Stroke Impact Scale. Arch Phys Med Rehabil. 2003;84(7):950–963.

47. Heinemann AW, Harvey RL, McGuire JR, et al. Measurement properties of the NIH Stroke Scale during acute rehabilitation. Stroke. 1997;28(6):1174–1180.

48. Simone A, Rota V, Tesio L, Perucca L. Generic ABILHAND questionnaire can measure manual ability across a variety of motor impairments. Int J Rehabil Res. 2011;34(2):131–140.

49. Koh CL, Hsueh IP, Wang WC, Sheu CF, Yu TY, Wang CH, Hsieh CL. Validation of the action research arm test using item response theory in patients after stroke. J Rehabil Med. 2006;38(6):375–380.

50. Daly JJ, Ruff RL. Construction of efficacious gait and upper limb functional interventions based on brain plasticity evidence and model-based measures for stroke patients. Scientific World Journal. 2007 Dec 20;7:2031–2045.

51. Smith MT, Baer GD. Achievement of simple mobility milestones after stroke. Arch Phys Med Rehabil. 1999;80(4):442–447.

52. Wade DT, de Jong BA. Recent advances in rehabilitation. BMJBr Med J. 2000 20;320(7246):1385–1388.

53. Kwakkel G, Veerbeek JM, Harmeling-van der Wel BC, van Wegen E, Kollen BJ; Early Prediction of functional Outcome after Stroke (EPOS) Investigators. Diagnostic accuracy of the Barthel Index for measuring activities of daily living outcome after ischemic hemispheric stroke: does early poststroke timing of assessment matter? Stroke. 2011;42(2):342–346.

54. Schiemanck SK, Kwakkel G, Post MW, Prevo AJ. Predictive value of ischemic lesion volume assessed with magnetic resonance imaging for neurological deficits and functional outcome poststroke: A critical review of the literature. Neurorehabil Neural Repair. 2006b;20(4):492–502.

55. Schiemanck SK, Kwakkel G, Post MW, Kappelle LJ, Prevo AJ. Predicting long-term independency in activities of daily living after middle cerebral artery stroke: does information from MRI have added predictive value compared with clinical information? Stroke. 2006a;37(4):1050–1054.

56. Adams HJ, del Zoppo G, Alberts M, et al, American Heart Association/American Stroke Association Stroke Council, American Heart Association/American Stroke Association Clinical Cardiology Council, American Heart Association/American Stroke Association Cardiovascular Radiology and Intervention Council, Atherosclerotic Peripheral Vascular Disease Working Group, Quality of Care Outcomes in Research Interdisciplinary Working Group. Guidelines for the early management of adults with ischemic stroke: a guideline from the American Heart Association/American Stroke Association Stroke Council, Clinical Cardiology Council, Cardiovascular Radiology and Intervention Council, and the Atherosclerotic Peripheral Vascular Disease and Quality of Care Outcomes in Research Interdisciplinary Working Groups: the American Academy of Neurology affirms the value of this guideline as an educational tool for neurologists. Circulation. 2007;115:e478–e534.

57. Kasner S. Clinical interpretation and use of stroke scales. Lancet Neurol. 2006;5:603–612.

58. Jongbloed L. Prediction of function after stroke: a critical review. Stroke. 1986 Jul-Aug;17(4):765–776. Review.

59. Kollen B, Van de Port I, Lindeman E, Twisk J, Kwakkel G. Predicting improvement in gait after stroke: a longitudinal prospective study. Stroke. 2005;36:2676–2280.

60. Barer DH, Mitchell J. Continence after stroke: useful predictor or goal of therapy? Q J Med. 1989;261:27–39.

61. Sanchez-Blanco I, Ochoa-Sangrador C, Lopez-Munain I, Izquierdo-Sanchez M, Fermoso-Garcia J. Predictive model of functional independence in stroke patients admitted to a rehabilitation programme. Clin Rehabil. 1999;13: 464–475.

62. Patel A, Duncan P, Lai S, Studenski S. The relation between impairments and functional outcomes poststroke. Arch Phys Med Rehabil. 2000;81:1357–1363.

63. Franchignoni F, Tesio L, Ricupero C, et al. Trunk control test as an early predictor of stroke rehabilitation outcome. Stroke. 1997;28:1382–1385.

64. Loewen S, Anderson B. Predictors of stroke outcome using objective measurement scales. Stroke. 1990;21:78–81.

65. Verheyden G, Nieuwboer A, De Wit L, et al. Time course of trunk, arm, leg, and functional recovery after ischemic stroke. Neurorehabil Neural Repair. 2008

66. Verheyden G, Nieuwboer A, De Wit L, Thijs V, Dobbelaere J, Devos H, Severijns D, Vanbeveren S, De Weerdt W. Time course of trunk, arm, leg, and functional recovery after ischemic stroke. Neurorehabil Neural Repair. 2008;22(2):173–179.

67. Buurke J, Nene A, Kwakkel G, Erren-Wolters V, IIzerman M, Hermens H. Recovery of gait after stroke: what changes? Neurorehabil Neural Repair. 2008;22:676–683.

68. De Haart M, Geurts A, Huidekoper S, Fasotti L, van Limbeek J. Recovery of standing balance in postacute stroke patients: a rehabilitation cohort study. Arch Phys Med Rehabil. 2004;85: 886–895.

69. Den Otter AR, Geurts AC, Mulder T, Duysens J. Gait recovery is not associated with changes in the temporal patterning of muscle activity during treadmill walking in patients with post-stroke hemiparesis. Clin Neurophysiol. 2006;117:4–15.

70. Van Asseldonk EHF, Buurke JH, Bloem BR, et al. Disentangling the contribution of the paretic and non-paretic leg to balance control in stroke patients. Exp Neurol. 2006;**201**:441–451.

71. Kwakkel G, Wagenaar RC. Effect of duration of upper- and lower-extremity rehabilitation sessions and walking speed on recovery of interlimb coordination in hemiplegic gait. Phys Ther. 2002;**82**(5):432–448.

72. Kirker SG, Jenner JR, Simpson DS, Wing AM. Changing patterns of postural hip muscle activity during recovery from stroke. Clin Rehabil. 2000;14:618–626.

73. Roerdink M, De Haart M, Daffertshofer A, Donker SF, Geurts AC, Beek PJ. Dynamical structure of center-of-pressure trajectories in patients recovering from stroke. Exp Brain Res. 2006;**174**:256–269.

74. Kollen B, Kwakkel G, Lindeman E. Time dependency of walking classification in stroke. Phys Ther. 2006;**86**(5):618–625.

75. Sunderland A, Fletcher D, Bradley L, Tinson D, Hewer RL, Wade DT. Enhanced physical therapy for arm function after stroke: a one year follow up study. J Neurol Neurosurg Psychiatry. 1994;57:856–858.

76. Wade DT, Langton-Hewer R, Wood VA, Skilbeck CE, Ismail HM. The hemiplegic arm after stroke: measurement and recovery. J Neurol Neurosurg Psychiatry. 1983;**46**:521–524.

77. Murphy TH, Corbett D. Plasticity during stroke recovery: from synapse to behaviour. Nat Rev Neurosci. 2009; **10**(12): 861–872.

78. Smania N, Gambarin M, Tinazzi M, et al. Are indexes of arm recovery related to daily life autonomy in patients with stroke? Eur J Phys Rehabil Med. 2009;**45**: 349–354.

79. Smania N, Paolucci S, Tinazzi M, et al. Active finger extension: a simple movement predicting recovery of arm function in patients with acute stroke. Stroke. 2007;**38**:1088–1090.

80. Katrak P, Bowring G, Conroy P, Chilvers M, Poulos R, McNeil D. Predicting upper limb recovery after stroke: the place of early shoulder and hand movement. Arch Phys Med Rehabil. 1998;**79**:758–761.

81. Beebe JA, Lang CE. Relationships and responsiveness of six upper extremity function tests during the first six months of recovery after stroke. J Neurol Phys Ther. 2009;**33**(2):96–103.

82. Matsui T, Hirano A. An Atlas of the Human Brain for Computerized Tomography. Igaku-Shoin, Tokyo, 1978.

83. Butler AJ, Kahn S, Wolf SL, Weiss P. Finger extensor variability in TMS parameters among chronic stroke patients. J Neuroeng Rehabil. 2005;**2**:10.

84. Fries W, Danek A, Scheidtmann K, Hamburger C. Motor recovery following capsular stroke. Role of descending pathways from multiple motor areas. Brain. 1993; **116**: 369–382.

85. Morecraft RJ, Herrick JL, Stilwell-Morecraft KS, et al. Localization of arm representation in the corona radiata and internal capsule in the non-human primate. Brain. 2002; **125**: 176–198.

86. Newton JM, Ward NS, Parker GJ, et al. Non-invasive mapping of corticofugal fibres from multiple motor areas—relevance to stroke recovery. Brain. 2006;**129**:1844–1858.

87. Stinear CM, Barber PA, Smale PR, Coxon JP, Fleming MK, Byblow WD. Functional potential in chronic stroke patients depends on corticospinal tract integrity. Brain. 2007;**130**(Pt 1):170–180.

88. Van Kuijk AA, Pasman JW, Hendricks HT, Zwarts MJ, Geurts AC. Predicting hand motor recovery in severe stroke: the role of motor evoked potentials in relation to early clinical assessment. Neurorehabil Neural Repair. 2009;**23**:45–51.

89. Pendlebury ST, Blamire AM, Lee MA, Styles P, Matthews PM. Axonal injury in the internal capsule correlates with motor impairment after stroke. Stroke. 1999; **30**: 956–962.

90. Schiemanck SK, Kwakkel G, Post MW, Kappelle LJ, Prevo AJ. Impact of internal capsule lesions on outcome of motor hand function at one year post-stroke. J Rehabil Med. 2008;**40**(2):96–101.

91. Fritz SL, Light KE, Patterson TS, Behrman AL, Davis SB. Active finger extension predicts outcomes after constraint-induced movement therapy for individuals with hemiparesis after stroke. Stroke. 2005;**36**:1172–1177.

92. Wolf SL, Winstein CJ, Miller JP, et al. Effect of constraint-induced movement therapy on upper extremity function 3 to 9 months after stroke: the EXCITE randomized clinical trial. JAMA. 2006;**296**:2095–2104.

93. Nijboer TC, Kollen BJ, Kwakkel G. Time course of visuospatial neglect early after stroke: A longitudinal cohort study. Cortex. 2013;**49**(8):2021–2027.

94. Kwakkel G, Veerbeek JM, van Wegen E.E.H., Wolf SL. Constrained Induced Movement Therapy Post Stroke. Lancet Neurol. 2014 (in press).

95. Lazar RM, Minzer B, Antoniello D, Festa JR, Krakauer JW, Marshall RS. Improvement in aphasia scores after stroke is well predicted by initial severity. Stroke. 2010;**41**(7):1485–1488.

96. van Kordelaar J, van Wegen EE, Nijland RH, Daffertshofer A, Kwakkel G. Understanding adaptive motor control of the paretic upper limb early poststroke: The EXPLICIT-stroke Program. Neurorehabil Neural Repair. 2013a Nov;**27**(9):854–863.

97. van Kordelaar J, van Wegen EE, Kwakkel G. The impact of time on quality of motor control of the paretic upper limb after stroke. Arch Phys Med Rehabil. 2013b;**95**(2):338–344.

98. Buma F, Kwakkel G, Ramsey N. Understanding upper limb recovery after stroke. Restor Neurol Neurosci. 2013;**31**(6):707–722.

99. Krakauer JW. Motor learning: its relevance to stroke recovery and neurorehabilitation. Curr Opin Neurol. 2006;**19**:84–90.

100. Brouns R, De Deyn PP. The complexity of neurobiological processes in acute ischemic stroke. Clin Neurol Neurosurg. 2009;**111**:483–495.

101. Kwakkel G, van Peppen R, Wagenaar RC, et al. Effects of augmented exercise therapy time after stroke: a meta-analysis. Stroke. 2004b;**35**(11):2529–2539.

102. Desmond DW, Moroney JT, Sano M, Stern Y. Recovery of cognitive function after stroke. Stroke. 1996;**27**(10):1798–1803.

103. Kotila M, Waltimo O, Niemi ML, Laaksonen R, Lempinen M. The profile of recovery from stroke and factors influencing outcome. Stroke. 1984;**15**(6):1039–1044.

104. Krakauer JW. Arm function after stroke: from physiology to recovery. Semin Neurol. 2005;**25**:384–395.

CHAPTER 5

Designing a clinical trial for neurorehabilitation

Bruce Dobkin and Andrew Dorsch

Introduction

Clinical research in neurological rehabilitation has at its disposal a wide range of potentially therapeutic techniques, including physical, cognitive, behavioural, pharmacological, neural stimulation, robotic, and perhaps cellular and biological treatments. Determining which of these interventions results in the greatest possible functional improvement requires an evidence base derived from randomized controlled trials (RCT) conducted by investigators with an understanding of the best elements of trial design, implementation, and interpretation. Emerging consensus standards for clinical trials serve as a useful starting point for the investigator planning a clinical trial in neurorehabilitation. In this chapter, we use the recent SPIRIT guidelines [1] as a framework while progressing through the developmental stages of a clinical trial. We emphasize what is most unique about complex interventions to improve motor-related outcomes, since the great majority of RCT, over 500, have been devoted to motor rehabilitation after stroke [2].

Preparing a clinical trial protocol

While formal, large-scale clinical trials are a recent development in neurological rehabilitation, numerous small-population or pilot studies have been reported in the literature for many years. Design and preparation for a clinical trial, regardless of study size, should focus on who will participate, what intervention will be delivered, and how change in function will be measured.

Choice of trial design

When discussing clinical research, the 'gold standard' trial is considered to be a prospective, parallel-group superiority trial that compares a novel intervention to the standard of care in a selected group of participants. Other traditional trial designs such as crossover and factorial designs tend to be used less often in neurological rehabilitation due to concerns about carry-over effects or interactions between interventions, respectively. While the majority of the discussion in this chapter will focus on classical RCT design, it should be emphasized that a RCT is the final step in an iterative preparatory process; alternate trial designs may more efficiently answer questions earlier in an intervention's development.

Descriptive study designs

Different types of descriptive designs utilized in the rehabilitation literature are listed in Table 5.1. These studies can be used to better characterize the natural history of a disease process or to identify clinical trends that bear further investigation. Though the comparison of results from a new intervention to the experience of historical 'controls' is always tempting and drives enthusiasm, descriptive studies offer no strength in terms of causal inferences about interventions and outcomes [3].

n-of-1 designs

This type of trial is most readily comparable to how medicine is practised on a daily basis. In the basic n-of-1 design, measurements are taken to establish the functional baseline of a single person (A), after which an intervention is provided (B) and a re-evaluation (A) is performed to determine if changes in the outcome measure of interest have occurred. More complex permutations including multiple baselines, several repetitions of the AB structure randomized for order of presentation, and combinations of interventions can also be tested. Due to statistical concerns regarding bias in participant selection and the significance of effect size calculated from small sample sizes, the results of these studies should be interpreted with caution; they may not generalize to the population of interest. In contrast, this study type can provide valuable information when attempting to personalize an RCT-evaluated intervention to an individual in a clinical practice setting [4].

Adaptive trial designs

The optimal dose, timing, and intensity of an intervention can be identified from among multiple possible treatment combinations using this study design [5]. Adaptive trial designs involve frequent reassessment of outcomes during the implementation of an intervention and modification of subject assignment or treatment dosage based upon Bayesian statistical methods and computer simulation models [6]. This strategy has been used successfully to assess medication dosing for safety and to get a sense of possible efficacy. Adaptive trial designs can arrive at answers faster than the standard designs in which efficacy is not determined until data have been collected from all study participants. In an adaptive treatment trial, the decision rules for changing assignment or treatment are specified before the trial begins to avoid introducing bias [7].

Table 5.1 Common study designs in neurorehabilitation

Descriptive
case series
cohort
cross-sectional
Small population
n-of-1
adaptive
Randomized
parallel group
crossover
factorial

Participant population

In addition to defining standard detailed inclusion and exclusion criteria, investigators conducting neurorehabilitation clinical trials will have special concerns with regards to the selection and recruitment of study participants.

Selection criteria

When considering the appropriate patient sample for an intervention, investigators should consider whether certain characteristics will alter responsiveness to the treatment strategy or confound an analysis of the response: age, time since injury, lesion location (e.g. cortical vs. subcortical, dominant vs. non-dominant hemisphere, etc.), physical and cognitive impairments, spared function, medical comorbidities, and natural history of the disease (i.e. changes in impairments and disabilities over time). Structural magnetic resonance imaging (MRI) measures of lesion volume and tractography to assess, for example, sparing of the corticospinal tract after stroke [8], may serve as additional study selection criteria.

Most participants recruited to clinical trials in neurological rehabilitation are defined as being in a chronic stage of disease, for example more than 6–12 months after stroke, spinal cord injury, or traumatic brain injury. Though commonly accepted as a means of parsing the recovery process into separate stages, such a classification scheme is overly simplified and ignores the fact that functional improvements, however modest, may occur at varied time scales for each individual. Most important, 'chronic' is not synonymous with clinically stable in the context of neurologic rehabilitation. Trials may one day better classify the stages of recovery using biomarkers or measures of cortical excitability rather than disease chronology, as is starting to be done for acute vascular events [9].

Defining a functional baseline

As recovery of function is the primary goal of most rehabilitation interventions, it is essential that the baseline function of study participants be well characterized. Function is most often defined using the criteria set forth in the International Classification of Functioning, Disability, and Health (ICF), which classifies what an individual can or cannot do based upon personal as well as environmental and contextual factors [10]. *Impairment* is defined

as a problem with body structure or function, for example the inability to voluntarily move the arm after a stroke. Limitations in *activity*, for example buttoning a shirt, occur when a person encounters difficulty in executing a task. *Participation* in life situations can be restricted due to individual limitations in activity or to a lack of accommodation for the disabled person. The assessment of function depends upon the choice of outcome measure, as some measures are specific to one ICF domain while others span several domains.

One must be aware that even for those subjects in the 'chronic' stage of recovery, functional performance can transiently decrease due to medical or psychosocial complications (e.g. depression, pain, urinary tract infection) or increase due to motivational factors (e.g. encouragement from physician or family, participation in a clinical trial). Many persons with neurological disease are relatively inactive when compared to age-matched healthy controls [11] yet retain the latent capacity to rapidly improve when participating in the regular training that forms the key component of many neurorehabilitation interventions. A separate concern regarding the functional capacity of persons participating in rehabilitation trials is the relative frequency with which those who demonstrate mild-to-moderate functional impairments are recruited. Many extant interventions can lead to functional gains in people with mild residual impairment; fewer therapeutic strategies are tested in those suffering from moderate-to-severe loss of physical or cognitive functioning.

Recruitment and consent issues

Persons recovering from neurological diseases are an especially vulnerable population. Special efforts should be made when recruiting and consenting these participants [12]. A standardized assessment should be used to determine decision-making capacity. Obtaining consent from a surrogate decision maker, as is done in dementia research [13], may be appropriate under certain circumstances, given the relative importance of family for post-hospital care. Special care must be taken when recruiting participants from less advantaged socioeconomic groups, whose participation rate in clinical research has been historically low. The difference between standard clinical care and the research intervention should be explicitly stated and the likelihood of individual benefit from the intervention, which is best stated as none, explained in advance. In addition, when designing a clinical trial intervention for disabled persons, one must consider the burden placed upon study participants, especially the time and effort required to return to a study site for repeated assessments.

Intervention

Value of intervention

Given the limited resources available for clinical research, a study must be justified on the basis of the value of information or potential clinical benefit of an experimental intervention [14]. In particular, the novelty of the proposed intervention should be weighed against the ease of its implementation, the prevalence of the condition, the personnel and equipment required, confounders of recruitment, and cost. If it is to be put through a tedious and expensive RCT an intervention ought to hold the realistic possibility that it will have a robust effect that is meaningful to disabled persons. Initial experiments ought to address this possibility.

Intervention components

When describing a trial intervention the essential components (site location, who delivers the intervention and for non-drug trials how the clinicians were trained, timing/duration/intensity of intervention, assessment methods, proposed mechanisms of action, etc.) should be detailed [15]. A growing number of investigators are revealing the details and decision-making of their protocols by publishing them near the beginning of the trial. Two prominent examples in neurologic rehabilitation are the EXCITE [16] and LEAPS [17] trials.

Choice of comparison/control intervention

Defining the intervention delivered to subjects assigned to the comparator arm(s) is of unique importance in neurologic rehabilitation. In general, the concept of clinical equipoise states that there should be genuine uncertainty whether a novel intervention will result in improved outcomes. While pharmaceutical trials can provide a placebo pill to account for participants' attention and motivation (the so-called Hawthorne effect), in neurological rehabilitation, where the intervention of interest is often a variation of existing therapies, providing no intervention to the control group sets up an artificial comparison that does not exist in clinical care as actually practiced. Defining the control intervention to be 'usual care' can also prove troublesome, especially in multicentre studies, where the definition of what constitutes standard therapy (timing, duration, intensity) may be quite different. Indeed, for many people who have suffered a neurological injury, usual care often means no care—that is no practice, no exercise, no additional support.

Now that well-designed trials have shown that many motor rehabilitation therapies improve outcomes if they include a high enough dose of task-related practice and skills learning [18–20], investigators conducting trials in neurologic rehabilitation should drop the notion that no intervention or 'usual care' (if that means no specific intervention) is a proper control for an experimental therapy. Despite the added cost of an active control treatment [21], experimental rehabilitation interventions should be compared to a well-defined control that engages participants, offers a degree of training, and is relevant to the primary outcome measure. The comparison intervention need not target the same presumed neural mechanism for gains.

Randomization and blinding

Randomization aims to ensure that a trial produces unbiased results. Attention should be devoted in the planning stages to formulating a detailed randomization plan [1]. Different randomization methods can be applied to assign study participants to an intervention. Simple randomization uses a constant ratio (1:1, 2:1, etc.) to produce the allocation sequence, whereas 'biased-coin' designs alter the ratio during recruitment to correct for imbalances in assignment. In block randomization, the number of subjects in each intervention group is kept similar by randomly allocating an equal number of participants within each block (i.e. for every ten subjects, five subjects are randomly assigned to the intervention and five to the control). Stratification allocates participants to an intervention based upon a clinical or demographic characteristic, such as age by decade or National Institutes of Health (NIH) Stroke Scale score. Finally, minimization is a technique in which subjects are allocated to an intervention group in such a way as to minimize the difference between groups in prespecified criteria (e.g. age, gender, disability).

The allocation sequence is obtained most often using a random number generator in order to prevent the anticipation of future group assignments based on knowledge of past assignments. Once produced, the sequence should be kept secure until group assignment, a process known as allocation concealment. Use of central telephone or computer databases to implement allocation is rapidly replacing the prior standard of opaque, numbered envelopes to be opened at the time of randomization.

Concealing group assignment to study participants may not always be feasible, but the individuals performing outcome assessments and, if feasible, those providing the intervention must be blinded. An additional benefit of including an active control as opposed to no defined intervention is that subjects in both groups will receive care, which may reduce bias. In place of the use 'single blinded' or 'double blinded' the SPIRIT guidelines suggest specifying whom amongst patients, providers, and assessors is blinded to treatment assignment [1]. As with randomization, the use of a computerized database with separate logins for providers and assessors can assist in maintaining blinding.

Outcome measures

Selecting the optimal outcome measure to quantify the improvement of change of greatest interest requires considerable thought and planning. It is not enough to use a scale that others have employed for similar trials. An increasing number of measurement tools are available, but only a minority has undergone a thorough validation of their psychometric properties in a population of interest. While collections of standardized tests such as those in the NIH Toolbox can be used, if choosing from amongst the multitude of other available tests, the ideal outcome measure would be one that is clinically relevant, reliable, and valid for answering the question at hand for the characteristics of person entered. We would pose the following questions for consideration during the outcome measure selection process:

1. What is being measured?

Quantitative methods such as kinematics and neurophysiological tests (electromyography, cortical excitability) provide objective, if less than perfect measures of the integrity of the motor system and end effector muscles. Functional ability is measured using outcome measures associated with one of the three domains (impairment, activity, participation) of the ICF. Patient self-report about physical functioning can provide valuable supplemental information regarding capabilities, but may not reflect what people actually do. Investigators must be aware that the environment in which testing occurs (i.e. clinic versus home), likely influences behaviour. Indeed, the interpretation of test results obtained while in a controlled setting many not accurately reflect performance in real-world settings.

2. What is the structure of the outcome measure?

Outcome measures can take several forms [22]. Interval scale measurements, such as temperature, have an arbitrary zero point but a consistent magnitude of change for every scale unit. Ratio scale measurements, for example the time elapsed during a 15-metre walk, have an absolute zero value in addition to an interval structure. Measurements on an ordinal scale, by contrast, are assigned to one of several predefined categories that are rank-ordered. Ordinal scales either constitute a single item (e.g. the modified Rankin and Ashworth scales) or a combination of multiple items across categories (e.g. the Barthel Index and Fugl-Meyer (FM) scale). Complex interventions like those employed in neurologic rehabilitation usually require some combination of these types of scales to assess efficacy or express outcomes in ICF or mechanistic terms.

3. How responsive is the measure to change?

Subsumed within this question are issues related to different aspects of the outcome measure's validity. Test–retest validity assesses the variability in responses over repeated test administrations while the degree to which the test measures what it sets out to measure is appraised by its construct validity. A growing number of outcome measures are undergoing formal psychometric evaluation [23] and the results collated in databases such as the StrokEngine based at McGill University.

4. Is the measure appropriate for use in the population under study?

In addition to concerns regarding the cost of study equipment and personnel, the amount of effort, motivation, and time required of a patient to complete tasks should be kept below what may become a burden. Learning and practice effects may need to be accounted for if repeated assessments will be performed in a relatively short time, especially within two weeks of one another. The literature should be reviewed to determine if the measure has been applied previously to patients of similar demographic characteristics and what magnitude of change was reported.

5. How will performance on the measure be analysed?

Ratio scale data are commonly analysed using parametric statistical tests while logistic or non-parametric statistical tests are utilized to analyse ordinal data. A ratio scale outcome measure is not synonymous with collection of normally distributed data; transformation using a logarithmic or other function may be necessary to correct for a skewed distribution. How ordinal data will be analysed, for example as dichotomous versus multi-ordinal outcomes, can affect interpretation of the outcomes [24].

Measures of impairment

The ICF defines impairment as a deficit in body function, whether in consciousness, speech, cognition or physical movement [25]. Commonly used impairment measures, such as the Glasgow Coma Scale and American Spinal Injury Association Impairment Scale, are multiple-item ordinal scales that evaluate a person's neurologic function across multiple domains. Because performance of these measures requires clinician assessment, practical concerns regarding intra- and inter-rater reliability must be addressed through standardized training of assessors [26]. The combination of clinician assessment and anatomic biomarkers, such as integrity of the corticospinal tract, may improve upon the use of a sole metric to measure motor impairment.

Measures of activity

The ICF activity domain encompasses a patient's ability to perform routine tasks, most typically defined as activities of daily living such as bathing, grooming, and feeding. The Barthel Index and Functional Independence Measure (FIM) are the two most commonly used disability scales that measure the amount of assistance a person requires to complete daily tasks. Both scales suffer from floor and ceiling effects, which are especially evident beyond the first 3–6 months after, for example, the onset of a stroke. More global assessments of function such as the modified Rankin Score often include aspects of both impairment and activity.

When evaluating a patient's ability to perform a task, investigators must be aware of how tasks or questions are presented as so not to be confused between functional capacity, what persons can do (or think they can do) in a controlled clinical environment, with functional performance, what a person does in real-world settings [27]. As an example, the function estimated by persons with stroke based upon the Stroke Impact Score does not necessarily correlate well with their actual task performance on objective testing [28].

Measures of participation

How a person interacts with the environment defines participation in the ICF framework. Due to the difficulty in observing people outside of the clinic setting, most evaluation in the participation domain is self-reported and falls under the rubric of 'quality-of-life' or 'patient-derived' outcome measures. Many investigators have moved beyond using one of the first such standardized tools, the SF-36, to validated disease-specific measures such as the Stroke Impact Scale [29] and MS Impact Scale [30]. Despite the potential for bias [31], self-report augments and adds validity to the interpretation of impairment and disability measurements derived from other tools. A growing movement, exemplified by organizations such as the Patient-Centered Outcomes Research Institute (PCORI) in the United States, incorporates input from representative persons with disability throughout the intervention design process in an effort to develop therapies with an impact on daily functioning. Investigators should be aware of the ability of social and electronic media to aggregate and share patient-reported data, which can serve as a testing ground for refining patient-reported outcomes [32].

Quantitative functional assessment

Though technologies such as electromechanical shoe insoles, hard-wired goniometers, video analysis systems, and pedometers have been used for decades to obtain estimates of patient activity, neurological rehabilitation research would optimally measure the type, quantity, and quality of daily activities and skilled motor practice in which patients engage outside of clinical supervision or laboratory testing [33]. Advances in technology have translated into the growing field of wireless health, in which small devices worn on the body or positioned in the home unobtrusively collect quantitative data such as gait speed [34, 35]. It is not unreasonable to assume that, in the near future, clinicians will be able to monitor patient home-based practice or control for practice outside of formal intervention times in a clinical trial using these technologies.

Biomarkers

A range of imaging, biochemical, and neurophysiological tests are reported in the neurologic rehabilitation literature as surrogate biomarkers of plasticity and recovery. Individual genetic polymorphisms, for example in the gene for brain-derived neurotrophic factor (BDNF) [36], or those associated with differential responses to physical exercise [37], may be added to the diagnostic armamentarium in the near future as additional biomarkers for clinical care and research. Especially in early-stage trials of biological interventions, biomarkers may be the only non-invasive means to demonstrate axon growth, remyelination of damaged pathways, and modifications of neural networks in the absence of clinically detectable change. Investigators must be vigilant when using biomarkers so as not to confuse an association between changes in clinical performance and changes in the surrogate as being indicative of causation.

Statistical concerns

It is strongly recommended that investigators preparing a clinical trial consult with a statistician early in the protocol development process. A biostatistician can not only assist with power and sample size calculations, which are key elements of funding proposals, but also suggest appropriate analysis methods for the data to be collected during the clinical trial. By reviewing the intervention, outcomes, and analysis of the trial in detail, potential omissions and errors can be rectified before participants are enrolled. Statisticians, of course, cannot salvage a poorly designed trial.

Sample size and power calculations

The number of participants in each intervention group is dependent upon the statistical test used, the prespecified false error rate (α), the power (1 – β), the expected performance of the control group on the outcome of interest, and the effect size [38]. Potential attrition rates of participants from the trial should be estimated and included in sample size calculations. Sample size calculations are relatively straightforward for the comparison of percentages or means. For more complex statistical analyses, such as mixed effects models, estimates can be provided. It has been stated previously that trials in neurorehabilitation should aim for at least a medium effect size (as defined by Cohen) that corresponds to a fairly robust change in individual patient function [39]. The method used to calculate the effect size should be fully described as it has implications for study design, interpretation of individual participant versus group responses, and comparison of results between studies [40, 41].

Superiority vs. non-inferiority

The prospective, parallel-group RCT is a superiority trial in that the intervention under study is being tested for its ability to provide additional benefit as compared to the standard of care. In contrast, a non-inferiority trial tests the novel intervention for similar efficacy or adverse effects as compared to the standard intervention. A common misconception among clinical trial investigators is that a failure to identify a significant difference between two interventions in a superiority trial means that the interventions are equivalent. Rather, the statistical assumptions and the sample sizes required to validate those assumptions are quite different depending upon the goals of a trial [42].

Primary outcome(s)

The choice of primary outcome is integral to trial design and the interpretation of results. A primary outcome is one that is chosen *a priori* to answer the hypothesis being tested, usually the intervention's possible efficacy. The primary outcome measure must be stated explicitly, preferably when the trial is initially registered. If at all possible only a single primary outcome measure should be defined with the remainder serving as secondary outcome measures. Use of multiple primary outcomes, as is not uncommon [43], requires the use of correction for multiple comparisons to lessen the possibility that one of many outcomes will suggest efficacy when it really does not. Pilot studies using a pre- and post-test without a control group, trials with fewer than 20 subjects in each arm, and even large RCTs that pursue data mining for positive results can be misleading when multiple outcomes are measured and tested for statistical significance. The concern for practicing clinicians is that a repeated testing search for 'significant' *p*-values may hide all the negative results that do not appear in a publication.

Missing data

Prior to conducting a clinical trial the decision must be made as to which participants will be included in the analysis of the primary outcome—all those randomized, subjects meeting a certain level of intervention adherence, only those who completed the trial, etc. The CONSORT statement recommends performing an 'intention to treat' analysis in which all randomized trial participants are analysed in their originally assigned treatment group. As this is not always feasible, detailed reasoning for excluding a subject from analysis should be provided when reporting the study results [44]. Similarly, the method to be used to account for missing data should be specified prior to starting the trial. Frequently employed methods such as last observation carried forward are easy to implement but prone to bias, therefore multiple imputation techniques that make use of the remainder of collected data to estimate missing values are recommended [45].

Common confounders

By highlighting various aspects of this trial design, we hope to have guided the reader past some of the pitfalls that consign neurological rehabilitation trials to equivocal outcomes. Other confounders bear mention.

Conceptual confounding

The term 'plasticity' has perhaps become overused and variably defined in the neurologic rehabilitation literature. It has been established that the adult nervous system is capable of learning, even after neurologic injury. Changes in synaptic efficacy or network connectivity are as likely to occur in a patient after skilled motor practice as in a healthy control. Thus, basing a trial on the capacity of an intervention to produce neural adaptations within the motor network rather than on gains in clinically important motor skills does not make for a sound scientific rationale [46].

In a similar vein, caution should be exercised when attempting to translate the results of preclinical animal studies to interventions in humans. Rodent studies may bear little relationship to the type and timing of injuries and interventions that occur in patients with neurological disease [47]. Behavioural measures in mammals are far less sophisticated and informative than those in humans. The process of rehabilitation involves the use of cues and feedback that have no correlate in animal training. Furthermore, genetic homogeneity and the loss of a natural living environment may alter the responsiveness of animals in ways that are not predictive of changes in function for disabled persons.

Confounding in implementation

As mentioned, the inclusion of chronically impaired persons with seemingly 'stable' functional baselines can be a source of confounding in neurologic rehabilitation trials. To lessen the potential for this effect, one could obtain multiple measures over one month before or after entry, prior to the start of the trial, to look for a stable baseline (see Duncan et al. [17] for an example). An alternate method would be to provide a modest intervention to participants in all trial arms to ensure that each has reached a functional plateau prior to introducing the formal intervention [48]. Either method would be appropriate to remove some of the uncertainty associated with single measurements of function and ensure that any changes after an intervention are most likely a true response and not a clinical-statistical fluctuation [49].

The context, duration, and intensity of an intervention and any concomitant therapies can each affect the interpretation of trial results. People participating in inpatient rehabilitation typically undergo 1–3 hours of formal training from 3–6 days a week, but investigators have little control or knowledge about what they are doing for the remainder of each day during a trial. Study participants may be carrying out practice that further drives gains or inhibits gains, and some may do nothing, which may limit the effects of the formal intervention [50]. Prior efforts to control for subject practice have been limited by available outpatient monitoring technologies [20, 51]. Use of wearable motion-sensing technologies to capture the types and quantity of practice, at least for mobility and upper extremity activities, may help to alleviate this concern.

Finally, variations in how functional outcomes are assessed across sites in a multicentre clinical trial can be an unwanted source of confounding. Even simple tests such as a 10-metre walk can be performed differently, for example starting from a stop versus using a walking lead-in prior to the starting line [52, 53]. It is therefore of utmost importance that assessments be standardized and assessors be properly trained to follow the same procedure [26]. Online training and assessment tools such as video and webinars are increasingly supplanting on-site training and trainer evaluation.

Enrichment

Improving the promise, feasibility, and economy of a clinical trial is possible through the use of enrichment strategies, many of which are aimed at the recruitment and retention of research participants.

The recruitment process can be expedited through the development of a database of patients interested in participating in clinical research. Consent forms approved by the local Institutional Review Board (IRB) can be left in the clinic rooms for patients to fill out and sign. Investigators then search the database looking for matches with regards to the disease, impairment, or disability of interest. Within or across institutions, this becomes a method by which to increase both the rate of recruitment to the study as well as the sample size and therefore power of a trial.

A growing number of formal collaborative networks sponsored by private foundations and government agencies aim to foster more efficient phase II and III clinical trials across (e.g. the NINDS' NeuroNEXT in the United States) as well as within specific neurological diseases. Society websites such as those for the American Society of Neurorehabilitation and the World Federation of NeuroRehabilitation serve as additional sources for potential research collaborations.

The retention of participants in clinical trials can become a concern as the frequency and duration of training time grows, especially in longitudinal [54] or uncontrolled [55] research studies. Reinforcement from family [56] and clinicians [57] can serve to maintain participants' motivation and self-efficacy for change. Personalized feedback or messages delivered to a smartphone could further engage subjects.

Registration

All human clinical research should be registered in a database that is openly accessible to the public. Which database to use varies depending on the type of study and geographic location in which the trial is to be conducted. Commonly utilized databases include clinicaltrials.gov, clinicaltrialsregister.eu, the UK Clinical Research Network Portfolio Database, and the International Standard Randomised Control Trial Number (ISRCTN) Register of Clinical Trials. In addition to meeting regulatory requirements, trial registration serves to increase research transparency, to decrease duplication of research efforts, and to facilitate the identification of trials for potential study participants [1].

Implementing a clinical trial

The overall goal in clinical trial design is to develop a study with high internal validity. The investigator wants to be able to conclude that the intervention produced the observed outcome without interference from potentially confounding variables. As will be discussed, getting to the milestone at which a demonstration of efficacy becomes worthwhile is an iterative process involving several stages of development prior to the RCT [58].

Progression through trial stages

The majority of clinical trials in medicine tend to follow the pattern established for pharmaceutical design and safety testing. *Phase I* involves a relatively high risk or novel intervention given to a small number of healthy or affected people. Establishing safety and examining responsiveness are the primary goals. *Phase II* follows Phase I and builds upon knowledge of risks. More participants are involved. Safety and potential efficacy are studied. The effects of different dosages of a medication or intensity of an intervention are determined, along with the best research methodology and outcome measures, in preparation for Phase III. *Phase III* rigorously assesses the potential for efficacy of the intervention by a randomized trial with blinded outcomes, comparing the new intervention to a standard one or to a placebo. The power for the study may be drawn from *Phase II* studies. *Phase IV* refers to the post-approval phase in which the intervention is approved for use in specified populations of people and provided as a part of routine care. Safety, including interactions with medications, is evaluated in the general population through drug registries and voluntary event reporting to monitoring agencies.

In contrast to this progression, clinical trials in neurorehabilitation may benefit from more strategically planned, consecutive stages. Working with the initial definitions provided by Dobkin [48] we detail the different stages of intervention development using body-weight supported treadmill training (BWSTT) as an example of an intervention of interest for hemiplegic stroke. This perspective aims to address and help correct the cycle of inconclusive pilot studies that suffer from poor design and fail to inform or end up misleading subsequent studies.

Stage 1 (Phase I): feasibility/consideration-of-concept study

In this descriptive stage, an intervention that has been identified from animal experiments, theory, and/or clinical observations is evaluated with regards to its appropriateness for testing in a larger trial. The focus in this stage is on aspects of trial methodology rather than on intervention efficacy [59]. Intervention outcomes under study can include participant willingness to be randomized, recruitment and attrition rates, timing of the intervention, subject responsiveness to different doses of the intervention, and safety [60].

BWSTT was identified as a potential rehabilitative intervention that integrated the concepts of progressive, task-oriented training, and neuroplasticity. It also drew, perhaps inappropriately in the case of stroke and incomplete spinal cord injury (SCI), from feline and rodent models of complete spinal transection at the level of the low thoracic cord that demonstrated evidence for locomotor pattern generation. Initial pilot studies for SCI had reported gains in stepping compared to 'historical' controls. Then reports suggested improvements in selected groups of stroke patients [61]. Though some aspects of BWSTT training were varied to identify the optimal training parameters [62], other aspects such as the most favourable timing after stroke and methods relating practice on the treadmill to aspects of gait and motor control needed for over-ground walking received less attention.

Stage 2 (Phase II): pilot/development-of-concept study

Once the general feasibility of the intervention has been established, the formal trial intervention is optimized through testing in a convenience sample of participants. A series of studies may be needed as new information becomes available from completed work. At this stage an important aim is to pull together the basic components of the proposed larger trial including inclusion/exclusion criteria, randomization method, control group intervention, and blinded assessment. In addition to serving as a test-run for a larger study, this stage can be used to evaluate the variability of potential baseline and outcome measures. Adaptive trial designs, particularly with regards to dose finding, may be useful here; preplanned, periodic assessment of interim data can inform the study and lead to modifications of the design. Though information regarding efficacy can be collected, hypothesis testing should not be the goal at this stage; sample sizes are likely too small to meet criteria for significance [63].

In the case of BWSTT, initial pilot studies and test–retest studies without controls included confounders such as expectation bias on the part of clinicians and participants, impairment severity and amount of residual motor control, Hawthorne effects (the effect of being watched and given feedback), and intensity of practice performed during the formal intervention and outside of the clinic. Issues related to subject selection—including clinical heterogeneity of subjects and a failure to account for relative inactivity of subjects prior to the intervention—and intervention delivery, such as a lack of control for activity performed outside of treadmill walking, likely contributed to bias in the interpretation of outcomes.

Stage 3 (Phase II): pilot/demonstration-of-concept study

This stage presents the opportunity to obtain an estimate of effect size for the formal trial intervention. A pilot might anticipate an effect size of moderate magnitude (defined as 0.4 to 0.6 using Cohen's criteria), which would suggest a meaningful change in function. One potential interpretive flaw at this stage arises from the performance of multiple outcome comparisons to look for statistical significance. At Stage 3, an investigator may not yet be sure about what outcome is most meaningful, so more than one or two may be designated as primary. The raw data for all baseline and outcome measures should be published, showing a histogram of clinically interesting changes so that the number of responders and non-responders can be visualized. The data analysis can be presented with uncorrected p-values, but values corrected for multiple comparisons should also be included if several outcome measures are used.

The first large RCT of BWSTT for stroke was carried out by Visintin and Barbeau [64], who compared walking practice on a treadmill for 6 weeks with versus without support by an overhead harness. In retrospect, this was more of a demonstration of concept, in that treadmill training without weight support is also an experimental intervention and not feasible for many persons with recent stroke. Indeed, the study had a high dropout rate. The results revealed significant gains in walking speed for the BWS group, but the walking speeds achieved (0.34 vs 0.25 m/s) were both quite slow; this should have raised concern about the protocol's intensity, duration, style of training, optimal translation of practice on a moving belt to over-ground walking, and potential for efficacy compared to more conventional training.

Stage 4 (Phase III): RCT/proof-of-concept study

Building upon the results of the previous three stages, the goal of this stage is to test the efficacy of the intervention. This stage of trial development often requires collaboration between multiple study sites to ensure sufficient and timely recruitment of participants. Once initial efficacy has been demonstrated, independent replication of the results by a separate group of investigators is strongly recommended.

The SCILT [65] and LEAPS [20] trials tested BWSTT against more conventional therapies that required over-ground practice or exercise for 12 weeks. The benefits accrued from greater stepping practice and weight support did not exceed those from training of similar intensity. Like other progressive physical therapies, BWSTT achieved good results in mild to moderately impaired participants, who happened to be the focus of most pilot studies. In those with a greater loss of motor control, for whom fewer proven therapies exist, the intervention was not powerful enough to overcome the degree of impairment.

Along with the EXCITE [51] and VA robotics [18] trials, the number of participants in each arm of the LEAPS study necessary to reveal a statistically equivalent or better outcome was no more than 50. With randomization of reasonably homogeneous groups, it seems likely that the efficacy of complex physical interventions can be ascertained for walking and upper extremity function with numbers in this range, in sharp contrast to drug trials that need hundreds of participants in each arm to find an absolute difference in the primary outcome of 1–5%. Drug trials for stroke prevention treatments can afford a high number needed to treat (NNT) to find a clinical benefit that also exceeds the risk of adverse events. Complex rehabilitation studies would seem to require a NNT of <10, at least for the recovery of motor skills. The LEAPS trial found an NNT of 6 for improvement to a higher walking level for both BWSTT and home-based exercise [66].

Stage 5 (Phase IV): translational/implementation-of-concept study

If an intervention is determined to be efficacious across well-designed trials, the final step of its development is to determine its effectiveness—how does the intervention translate into routine clinical care? Barriers to implementation, variations in intervention fidelity, and cost-effectiveness in comparison to other treatments are identified and addressed to optimize patient care and improve functional outcomes [67]. Surveillance studies, registries, and RCTs that examine cost-effectiveness for inpatient or outpatient care can help assure that the new intervention is applicable to real-world settings.

In the case of BWSTT, this translational step was skipped as commercial systems and robotic devices became widespread after initial positive pilot study reports, long before large-scale trials attempted to demonstrate efficacy. With the findings of SCILT, LEAPS, and other BWSTT and robotic-assistive stepping trials to date [68], the initial excitement appears premature, as the costs in time, personnel, and equipment produce no greater improvement in mobility for disabled patients as compared to the same intensity of over-ground training. While robotic and other treadmill-based interventions may yet prove useful for individuals meeting select criteria, the preponderance of evidence at this time suggests that these interventions be used in clinical research but not as a routine therapy.

Data collection, monitoring, and safety

Investigators should give some thought to how they will collect and manage data during the study. A significant proportion of research funds can be expended in designing a homegrown data entry system or purchasing a commercial database product. Common platform endeavours by the NIH and research universities such as REDCap (http://www.project-redcap.org/) may gradually replace the current piecemeal approach by providing a secure, standardized template for data entry and analysis.

While not necessary for every research study, sites such as the DMPTool (https://dmp.cdlib.org/) can assist in preparing a plan for data storage and dissemination. Consideration should be given to data format and how meta-data related to the data of interest, for example a description of how the data were collected, will be organized for efficient search. The collection of data by research collaborations across institutions raises questions of data storage and backup (on-site, cloud, etc.) as well as what limitations will be placed on future use of the data

The SPIRIT guidelines and many governmental funding agencies require the formation of a Data Monitoring Board (DMB) to oversee clinical research studies. In trials where participants are exposed to a greater than minimal risk of harm from the intervention, the DMB will advocate for patient safety by monitoring adverse events and halting the study if predefined stopping rules are triggered. Additionally, the DMB can review incoming data and institute a futility analysis to determine the likely benefit, if any, from the recruitment of additional participants.

Reporting clinical trial results

Standardization

Depending upon the design of the study and type of outcomes being reported, different international consensus standards for trial reporting are recommended (Table 5.2). Results from prospective, randomized clinical trials should follow the Consolidated Standards of Reporting Trials (CONSORT) guidelines [44]. Using clearly understood language, it is expected that subject recruitment, randomization, primary and secondary endpoints, and statistical results will be reported in sufficient detail such that other investigators can replicate the experiment. A growing number of scientific journals require completion of a CONSORT checklist and inclusion of participant flow through the study as the first figure in a manuscript submitted for publication (Figure 5.1).

Positive vs. negative results

Especially in neurologic rehabilitation, where patient recruitment is difficult and the interventions are complicated, it is essential that positive and negative results of important studies be published. With scarce resources, it makes no sense to repeat the same protocol that has not led to better outcomes; serious confounders can be identified from the details of a report.

Determining significance

In contrast to reporting p-values, as has been commonly done in the past, the CONSORT guidelines also recommend the tabulation of confidence intervals for all predefined primary and secondary study outcomes [44]. Confidence intervals (CIs) can contribute to determining the clinical significance of change resulting from an intervention. For example, consider a trial of non-invasive brain stimulation to treat a post-stroke paretic upper extremity that reports a statistically significant improvement of 4 points on the Fugl-Meyer (FM) scale after a course of stimulation. Though the mean change in FM score in this case reached the threshold for significance [69], a large confidence interval could alter the clinical interpretation of the results if the lower bound on the confidence interval is not a meaningful gain in function. Conversely, a mean change with a non-significant p-value could

Table 5.2 Consensus standards for clinical research

Study design
SPIRIT [1]
Test accuracy
STARD [78]
Reporting of study results
EQUATOR [79]
CONSORT [44] (randomized)
STROBE [80] (observational)
PRISMA [81] (meta-analysis)
CONSORT-PRO [82] (patient-reported outcomes)
Level of evidence
GRADE [75]

CONSORT Statement 2010 Flow Diagram

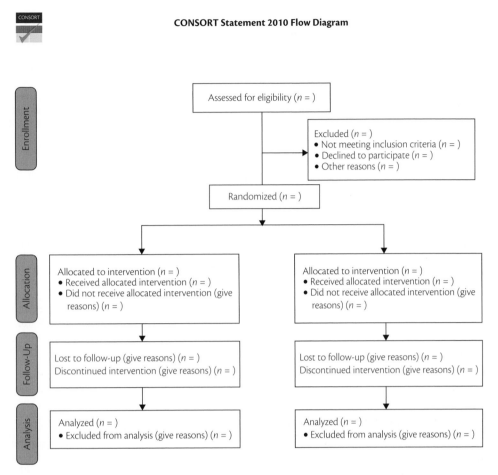

Fig. 5.1 CONSORT flow diagram.

This flow diagram provides a clear, concise method to report the recruitment, randomization, and participation of subjects in a clinical trial. When reporting clinical trial results, it is recommended that this flow diagram be included as the first figure. Copies of this diagram can be obtained from the CONSORT website (http://www.consort-statement.org, accessed 29 September 2014).

have an upper CI bound that includes clinically relevant change, in which case a benefit from the intervention could not be ruled out without recruiting additional study participants [70]. The 4-point change itself may or may not be associated with improved functional use of the arm and hand, raising the concern about clinical meaningfulness.

When results using a multiple-item outcome scale are presented, investigators should tabulate scores on individual scale items to provide the reader a better understanding of where changes are occurring. To continue the aforementioned example, the same total change in upper extremity FM score can result from functional improvements at separate joints, for example the elbow and wrist versus the shoulder. A person would demonstrate improved reach and grasp ability in the former case but not in the latter despite similar overall improvement in the FM score. Failure to differentiate between the two methods of achieving the same change score could lead to highly different interpretations of an intervention's efficacy, which has the potential to affect the direction of future research efforts. Investigators should also be aware that, for many multi-item ordinal scales, the transition from one rank to another is not linear and modern psychometric methods such as IRT or Rasch analysis may need to be applied to ensure scale reliability prior to statistical analysis [71].

The concept of minimal clinically important difference (MCID) is often invoked when ascribing the clinical significance of functional changes due to an intervention. Most typically the MCID links change on the outcome of interest to that on an 'anchor' functional rating scale such as the modified Rankin or Stroke Impact Score [72,73]. Distribution-based methods that make use of the effect size can also be used to calculate the MCID [74]. While the MCID provides an estimate of how much change is required to be clinically significant, investigators should be aware that its magnitude is dependent upon the population being tested and the method of calculation, amongst other factors, and that translation of MCID to another clinical setting or population of different characteristics should be done with caution [41].

Level of evidence

When clinicians consider the results of research studies for their evidence-based practices, they can classify the level of evidence using numerous different rating scales. The Grading of Recommendations Assessment, Development and Evaluation (GRADE) network has produced a rating scale and ongoing discussions of evidence rating based upon quality of evidence [75]. Other classification systems, such as that used by the American Academy of Neurology [76], apply different criteria to arrive at recommendations ranging from strongest (Class I) to least robust (Class IV). Regardless of the classification method used, an intervention does not meet the optimal standard for routine incorporation into clinical practice until a multi-site, Class I trial has shown efficacy for clinically important outcomes and, preferably, has been replicated in another group of similar subjects [77].

References

1. Chan AW, Tetzlaff JM, Gøtzsche PC, et al. SPIRIT 2013 explanation and elaboration: guidance for protocols of clinical trials. Br Med J. 2013;**346**:e7586.
2. Stinear C, Ackerley S, Byblow W. Rehabilitation is initiated early after stroke, but most motor rehabilitation trials are not: a systematic review. Stroke. 2013;**44**:2039–2045.
3. Prasad V, Jorgenson J, Ioannidis JP, Cifu A. Observational studies often make clinical practice recommendations: an empirical evaluation of authors' attitudes. J Clin Epidemiol. 2013;**66**:361–366.
4. Graham JE, Karmarkar AM, Ottenbacher KJ. Small sample research designs for evidence-based rehabilitation: issues and methods. Arch Phys Med Rehabil. 2012;**93**:S111–116.
5. Berry DA. Bayesian clinical trials. Nat Rev Drug Discov. 2006;**5**:27–36.
6. Krams M, Lees KR, Berry DA. The past is the future: innovative designs in acute stroke therapy trials. Stroke. 2005;**36**:1341–1347.
7. Kairalla JA, Coffey CS, Thomann MA, Muller KE. Adaptive trial designs: a review of barriers and opportunities. Trials. 2012;**13**:145.
8. Riley JD, Le V, Der-Yeghiaian L, et al. Anatomy of stroke injury predicts gains from therapy. Stroke. 2011;**42**:421–426.
9. Giles MF, Albers GW, Amarenco P, et al. Early stroke risk and ABCD2 score performance in tissue- vs time-defined TIA: a multicenter study. Neurology. 2011;**77**:1222–1228.
10. World Health Organization. International classification of functioning, disability and health: ICF. World Health Organization, Geneva, 2001.
11. Rand D, Eng JJ, Tang PF, Jeng JS, Hung C. How active are people with stroke?: use of accelerometers to assess physical activity. Stroke. 2009;**40**:163–168.
12. Savage TA. Ethical issues in research with patients who have experienced stroke. Top Stroke Rehabil. 2006;**13**:1–10.
13. Grill JD, Raman R, Ernstrom K, Aisen P, Karlawish J. Effect of study partner on the conduct of Alzheimer disease clinical trials. Neurology. 2013;**80**:282–288.
14. Emanuel EJ, Wendler D, Grady C. What makes clinical research ethical? JAMA. 2000;**283**:2701–2711.
15. Hoffmann TC, Glasziou PP, Boutron I, et al. Better reporting of interventions: template for intervention description and replication (TIDieR) checklist and guide. Br Med J. 2014:**348**:g1687.
16. Winstein CJ, Miller JP, Blanton S, et al. Methods for a multisite randomized trial to investigate the effect of constraint-induced movement therapy in improving upper extremity function among adults recovering from a cerebrovascular stroke. Neurorehabil Neural Repair. 2003;**17**:137–152.
17. Duncan PW, Sullivan KJ, Behrman AL, et al. Protocol for the Locomotor Experience Applied Post-stroke (LEAPS) trial: a randomized controlled trial. BMC Neurol. 2007;**7**:39.
18. Lo A, Guarino P, Richards L, et al. Robot-assisted therapy for long-term upper-limb impairment after stroke. N Engl J Med. 2010;**362**:1772–13.
19. Cumming TB, Thrift AG, Collier JM, et al. Very early mobilization after stroke fast-tracks return to walking: further results from the phase II AVERT randomized controlled trial. Stroke. 2011;**42**:153–158.
20. Duncan PW, Sullivan KJ, Behrman AL, et al. Body-weight-supported treadmill rehabilitation after stroke. N Engl J Med. 2011;**364**:2026–2036.
21. Wolf SL, Winstein CJ, Miller JP, Blanton S, Clark PC, Nichols-Larsen D. Looking in the rear view mirror when conversing with back seat drivers: the EXCITE trial revisited. Neurorehabil Neural Repair. 2007;**21**:379–387.
22. Stevens SS. On the theory of scales of measurement. Science. 1946;**103**:677–680.
23. Edwards DF, Lang CE, Wagner JM, Birkenmeier R, Dromerick AW. An evaluation of the Wolf Motor Function Test in motor trials early after stroke. Arch Phys Med Rehabil. 2012; **93**:660–668.
24. Saver JL. Optimal end points for acute stroke therapy trials: best ways to measure treatment effects of drugs and devices. Stroke. 2011;**42**:2356–2362.
25. Langhorne P, Bernhardt J, Kwakkel G. Stroke rehabilitation. Lancet. 2011;**377**:1693–1702.
26. Sullivan KJ, Tilson JK, Cen SY, et al. Fugl-Meyer assessment of sensorimotor function after stroke: standardized training procedure for clinical practice and clinical trials. Stroke. 2011;**42**:427–432.
27. Lemmens RJ, Timmermans AA, Janssen-Potten YJ, Smeets RJ, Seelen HA. Valid and reliable instruments for arm-hand assessment at ICF activity level in persons with hemiplegia: a systematic review. BMC Neurol. 2012;**12**:21.
28. van Delden AL, Peper CL, Beek PJ, Kwakkel G. Match and mismatch between objective and subjective improvements in upper limb function after stroke. Disabil Rehabil. 2013;**35**:1961–1967.
29. Duncan PW, Bode RK, Min Lai S, et al. Rasch analysis of a new stroke-specific outcome scale: the Stroke Impact Scale. Arch Phys Med Rehabil. 2003;**84**:950–963.
30. Hobart J, Lamping D, Fitzpatrick R, Riazi A, Thompson A. The Multiple Sclerosis Impact Scale (MSIS-29): a new patient-based outcome measure. Brain. 2001;**124**:962–973.
31. Shiffman S, Stone AA, Hufford MR. Ecological momentary assessment. Annu Rev Clin Psychol. 2008;**4**:1–32.
32. Wicks P, Vaughan TE, Massagli MP. The multiple sclerosis rating scale, revised (MSRS-R): development, refinement, and psychometric validation using an online community. Health Qual Life Outcomes. 2012;**10**:70.
33. Dobkin BH, Dorsch A. The promise of mHealth: daily activity monitoring and outcome assessments by wearable sensors. Neurorehabil Neural Repair. 2011;**25**:788–798.
34. Weiss A, Sharifi S, Plotnik M, van Vugt JP, Giladi N, Hausdorff JM. Toward automated, at-home assessment of mobility among patients with Parkinson disease, using a body-worn accelerometer. Neurorehabil Neural Repair. 2011;**25**:810–818.
35. Chumbler NR, Quigley P, Li X, et al. Effects of telerehabilitation on physical function and disability for stroke patients: a randomized, controlled trial. Stroke. 2012;**43**:2168–2174.
36. Cheeran B, Talelli P, Mori F, et al. A common polymorphism in the brain-derived neurotrophic factor gene (BDNF) modulates human cortical plasticity and the response to rTMS. J Physiol. 2008;**586**:5717–5725.
37. Pérusse L, Rankinen T, Hagberg JM, et al. Advances in exercise, fitness, and performance genomics in 2012. Med Sci Sports Exerc. 2013;**45**:824–831.
38. Charles P, Giraudeau B, Dechartres A, Baron G, Ravaud P. Reporting of sample size calculation in randomised controlled trials: review. Br Med J. 2009;**338**:b1732.
39. Dobkin BH. The Clinical Science of Neurologic Rehabilitation. Oxford University Press, New York, 2003.
40. Hobart J, Blight AR, Goodman A, Lynn F, Putzki N. Timed 25-Foot Walk: Direct evidence that improving 20% or greater is clinically meaningful in MS. Neurology. 2013;**80**:1509–1517.
41. Simpson LA, Eng JJ. Functional recovery following stroke: capturing changes in upper-extremity function. Neurorehabil Neural Repair. 2013;**27**:240–250.
42. Christensen E. Methodology of superiority vs. equivalence trials and non-inferiority trials. J Hepatol. 2007;**46**:947–954.

43. Zarin DA, Tse T, Williams RJ, Califf RM, Ide NC. The ClinicalTrials. gov results database—update and key issues. N Engl J Med. 2011;**364**:852–860.

44. Moher D, Hopewell S, Schulz KF, et al. CONSORT 2010 Explanation and Elaboration: Updated guidelines for reporting parallel group randomised trials. J Clin Epidemiol. 2010;**63**:e1–37.

45. Donders AR, van der Heijden GJ, Stijnen T, Moons KG. Review: a gentle introduction to imputation of missing values. J Clin Epidemiol. 2006;**59**:1087–1091.

46. Efrati S, Fishlev G, Bechor Y, et al. Hyperbaric oxygen induces late neuroplasticity in post stroke patients—randomized, prospective trial. PLoS One. 2013;**8**:e53716.

47. Krakauer JW, Carmichael ST, Corbett D, Wittenberg GF. Getting neurorehabilitation right: what can be learned from animal models? Neurorehabil Neural Repair. 2012;**26**:923–931.

48. Dobkin BH. Progressive staging of pilot studies to improve Phase III trials for motor interventions. Neurorehabil Neural Repair. 2009;**23**:197–206.

49. Barnett AG, van der Pols JC, Dobson AJ. Regression to the mean: what it is and how to deal with it. Int J Epidemiol. 2005;**34**:215–220.

50. Chollet F, Tardy J, Albucher JF, et al. Fluoxetine for motor recovery after acute ischaemic stroke (FLAME): a randomised placebo-controlled trial. Lancet Neurol. 2011;**10**:123–130.

51. Wolf SL, Winstein CJ, Miller JP, et al. Effect of constraint-induced movement therapy on upper extremity function 3 to 9 months after stroke: the EXCITE randomized clinical trial. JAMA. 2006;**296**:2095–2104.

52. Guyatt GH, Pugsley SO, Sullivan MJ, et al. Effect of encouragement on walking test performance. Thorax. 1984;**39**:818–822.

53. Graham JE, Ostir GV, Fisher SR, Ottenbacher KJ. Assessing walking speed in clinical research: a systematic review. J Eval Clin Pract. 2008;**14**:552–562.

54. Koski L, Mernar TJ, Dobkin BH. Immediate and long-term changes in corticomotor output in response to rehabilitation: correlation with functional improvements in chronic stroke. Neurorehabil Neural Repair. 2004;**18**:230–249.

55. Harkema S, Gerasimenko Y, Hodes J, et al. Effect of epidural stimulation of the lumbosacral spinal cord on voluntary movement, standing, and assisted stepping after motor complete paraplegia: a case study. Lancet. 2011;**377**:1938–1947.

56. Galvin R, Cusack T, O'Grady E, Murphy TB, Stokes E. Family-mediated exercise intervention (FAME): evaluation of a novel form of exercise delivery after stroke. Stroke. 2011;**42**:681–686.

57. Dobkin BH, Plummer-D'Amato P, Elashoff R, et al. International randomized clinical trial, stroke inpatient rehabilitation with reinforcement of walking speed (SIRROWS), improves outcomes. Neurorehabil Neural Repair. 2010;**24**:235–242.

58. Collins LM, Murphy SA, Nair VN, Strecher VJ. A strategy for optimizing and evaluating behavioral interventions. Ann Behav Med. 2005;**30**:65–73.

59. Arain M, Campbell MJ, Cooper CL, Lancaster GA. What is a pilot or feasibility study? A review of current practice and editorial policy. BMC Med Res Methodol. 2010;**10**:67.

60. Thabane L, Ma J, Chu R, et al. A tutorial on pilot studies: the what, why and how. BMC Med Res Methodol. 2010;**10**:1.

61. Hesse S, Bertelt C, Schaffrin A, Malezic M, Mauritz KH. Restoration of gait in nonambulatory hemiparetic patients by treadmill training with partial body-weight support. Arch Phys Med Rehabil. 1994;**75**:1087–1093.

62. Sullivan KJ, Knowlton BJ, Dobkin BH. Step training with body weight support: effect of treadmill speed and practice paradigms on poststroke locomotor recovery. Arch Phys Med Rehabil. 2002;**83**:683–691.

63. Lancaster GA, Dodd S, Williamson PR. Design and analysis of pilot studies: recommendations for good practice. J Eval Clin Pract. 2004;**10**:307–312.

64. Visintin M, Barbeau H, Korner-Bitensky N, Mayo NE. A new approach to retrain gait in stroke patients through body weight support and treadmill stimulation. Stroke. 1998;**29**:1122–1128.

65. Dobkin B, Apple D, Barbeau H, et al. Weight-supported treadmill vs over-ground training for walking after acute incomplete SCI. Neurology. 2006;**66**:484–493.

66. Nadeau SE, Wu SS, Dobkin BH, et al. Effects of task-specific and impairment-based training compared with usual care on functional walking ability after inpatient stroke rehabilitation: LEAPS Trial. Neurorehabil Neural Repair. 2013;**27**:370–380.

67. Vickrey BG, Hirtz D, Waddy S, Cheng EM, Johnston SC. Comparative effectiveness and implementation research: directions for neurology. Ann Neurol. 2012;**71**:732–742.

68. Dobkin BH, Duncan PW. Should body weight-supported treadmill training and robotic-assistive steppers for locomotor training trot back to the starting gate? Neurorehabil Neural Repair. 2012;**26**:308–317.

69. Hummel FC, Celnik P, Pascual-Leone A, et al. Controversy: Noninvasive and invasive cortical stimulation show efficacy in treating stroke patients. Brain Stimul. 2008;**1**:370–382.

70. Guyatt G, Jaeschke R, Heddle N, Cook D, Shannon H, Walter S. Basic statistics for clinicians: 2. Interpreting study results: confidence intervals. CMAJ. 1995;**152**:169–173.

71. Hobart JC, Cano SJ, Zajicek JP, Thompson AJ. Rating scales as outcome measures for clinical trials in neurology: problems, solutions, and recommendations. Lancet Neurol. 2007;**6**:1094–1105.

72. Lang CE, Edwards DF, Birkenmeier RL, Dromerick AW. Estimating minimal clinically important differences of upper-extremity measures early after stroke. Arch Phys Med Rehabil. 2008;**89**:1693–1700.

73. Tilson JK, Sullivan KJ, Cen SY, et al. Meaningful gait speed improvement during the first 60 days poststroke: minimal clinically important difference. Phys Ther. 2011;**90**:196–208.

74. Revicki D, Hays RD, Cella D, Sloan J. Recommended methods for determining responsiveness and minimally important differences for patient-reported outcomes. J Clin Epidemiol. 2008;**61**:102–109.

75. Guyatt GH, Oxman AD, Vist GE, et al. GRADE: an emerging consensus on rating quality of evidence and strength of recommendations. Br Med J. 2008;**336**:924–926.

76. Gross RA, Johnston KC. Levels of evidence: taking neurology to the next level. Neurology. 2009;**72**:8–10.

77. Ioannidis JP. Why most published research findings are false. PLoS Med. 2005;**2**:e124.

78. Bossuyt PM, Reitsma JB, Bruns DE, et al. Towards complete and accurate reporting of studies of diagnostic accuracy: The STARD Initiative. Ann Intern Med. 2003;**138**:40–44.

79. The EQUATOR Network. www.equator-network.org (accessed 8 September 2014).

80. von Elm E, Altman DG, Egger M, et al. The Strengthening the Reporting of Observational Studies in Epidemiology (STROBE) statement: guidelines for reporting observational studies. Lancet. 2007;**370**:1453–1457.

81. Moher D, Liberati A, Tetzlaff J, et al. Preferred Reporting Items for Systematic Reviews and Meta-Analyses: The PRISMA Statement. PLoS Med. 2009;**6**:e1000097.

82. Calvert M, Blazeby J, Altman DG, et al. Reporting of patient-reported outcomes in randomized trials: the CONSORT PRO extension. JAMA. 2013;**309**:814–822.

CHAPTER 6

The influence of age on neurorehabilitation

Markus Wirz and Louise Rutz-LaPitz

Introduction

General aspects pertaining to age and ageing

The worldwide ageing of the population described later in this section is associated with an expected increase in morbidity and demand for long-term care [1]. There are several important factors to consider regarding the ageing person. Increased age does not necessarily mean inability to work or to be physically fit. International retirement ages are being increased not lowered. Post-retirement people are very active, travel extensively, are politically involved, and believe in continuing personal development (e.g. the Gray Panthers www.graypanthers.org; they participate!). Thus, age should not be the main factor in deciding rehabilitation potential. Stroke is one of the most frequent neurological conditions and is strongly associated with age-related changes of the organism, in particular with the cardiovascular system and typically occurs in older persons. Age is an important, yet not modifiable, risk factor for stroke [2]. Accordingly hemiparesis due to stroke is typically seen in older patients. A marked increase of stroke cases in future decades are predicted based on a combination of estimates regarding the ageing of the population and observed incidence rates [3]. Another neurological condition requiring interdisciplinary neurological rehabilitation is spinal cord injury (SCI). Typical causes for a SCI in young male patients were severe traumas sustained from vehicular or sport accidents. However, the mean age of patients with acquired traumatic SCI has increased in recent years [4]. Beside the traumatic SCI, non-traumatic causes have become more frequent. One of the characteristics of the latter group of patients is an older age compared to those with a traumatic SCI [5]. There is a globally observed trend towards an increase of patients with non-traumatic SCI and correspondingly the number of older patients with an SCI is increasing. Although there are many neurological conditions requiring interdisciplinary rehabilitation this chapter focuses on patients with either stroke or SCI. It can be summarized, that the general principles of neurological rehabilitation are the same in young and old patients. Some aspects, however, need to be considered when an elderly patient is referred to rehabilitation.

Definitions of ageing

Ageing itself can be seen as a process that starts at conception and lasts until death. However, in the context of this chapter, ageing focuses on the period of life following reproductive activity or an age where people are generally considered as aged, elderly, or old. Ageing can not only be defined as a certain period of time an organism exists. The concept of growing old encompasses a variety of additional aspects [6].

Chronological age is commonly used to give a certain age. It refers to the elapsed time, starting from birth. This understanding of the ageing process is, for example, reflected in the Medical Subject Headings (MeSH) where persons are categorized according to their age into different age groups: for example aged 65 through 79 years, or aged 80 and over. The description of a persons' age by using years is useful in numerous ways. However, it can be insufficient for some purposes. Two patients with the same chronological age can exhibit different age-related medical conditions which influence clinical decision making when choosing treatment options. Also for specific research questions matching of an intervention and a control group purely based on chronological age might negatively influence the outcome. A definition of ageing or age-related characteristics, which goes beyond counting years must be adopted.

The concept of *biological age* therefore additionally regards the health and age-associated condition of a person. With increasing age various maintenance mechanisms fail to preserve the normal structure and functions of cells and tissues. Thus, the incidence for cardiovascular diseases, cancer, stroke, and dementia increases with advancing age [7]. In addition, degenerative processes—for example of the musculoskeletal system—limit one's ability to perform activities of daily living. For neurorehabilitation it is important to consider a patient's biological age. Age-related alterations, pain, or accompanying diseases may limit the patient's resources to cope with the new situation.

The society a person lives in has also a concept of ageing. Accordingly, the expectations regarding the role, functions, and tasks of that person within the society change over time. For example, it is considered not normal when a 30-year-old patient with stroke is discharged to a residential care home for the elderly. This aspect of ageing is referred to as *sociological age* [6]. Pertaining to neurorehabilitation sociological age influences the goal-setting process. Incorporating the social background of a patient is important for developing individualized rehabilitation goals.

Demographic changes

General population

According to the World Health Organization's (WHO) health observatory global life expectancy increased from 64 years in

1990 to 70 years in 2011. During the same period the life expectancy grew from 76 years to 80 years in high-income countries [8]. The combination of a decline in fertility rates and increased longevity leads to a shift of the age composition of society. While the relative number of children is decreasing the proportion of older persons (i.e. aged 60 years or over) is growing at an accelerated rate and is reported to amount to 21% in developed countries. It is even expected that the older population will outnumber children by the mid-21st century. Also, within the portion of the older population an increase in age takes place. In 2012 already 14% were aged 80 years and over. It is expected that this figure will further rise to 20% in 2050. This corresponds to approximately 400 million persons worldwide. In more developed regions of the world older persons predominantly live independently, either alone or with their spouses. Among those who live alone there is a discrepancy between men and women. It is reported that almost half of older women, but only a minority of men who live independently alone [9].

Patients with stroke

Worldwide stroke statistics state that stroke is still number three in cause of death. Stroke is the most frequent cause of adult disability and the third cause of reduced quality of life in the elderly [10]. This results in personal and economic encumbrance.

Each year, about 16 million people in the world experience a first-ever stroke. Of these, about 5.7 million die and another 5 million remain disabled [11].

Patients with spinal cord injury

When looking at demographic characteristics of patients with SCI it is important to distinguish between spinal cord lesions due to traumatic and non-traumatic events.

Along with the ageing of the general population the average age at onset of a traumatic SCI has increased over the last decades. In the USA, the average age at injury was 29 years in the 1970s and 41 years in the period 2005–2010 with 2% being 75 years or older [12, 13]. In Europe the corresponding age was 45 years in the latter period [14], (Wirz, unpublished).

With an average age of 60 years and over, patients with non-traumatic SCIs are clearly older at onset than traumatic cases [15–18].

Age adapted neurorehabilitation

The increasing age of patients with stroke, SCI, or other neurological diseases described in the previous sections becomes more and more apparent in rehabilitation settings. It is therefore worthwhile to consider the consequences of the growing number of elderly patients on rehabilitation procedures. Although advancing age is an independent predictor of both short- and long-term survival after stroke [19] it is important to acknowledge that age is not an exclusion criteria or limiting factor for neurorehabilitation of the elderly stroke patient [20]. There are no specific handling methods or concepts for the ageing person. Members of the rehabilitation team working with the ageing adult need to understand typical changes in all systems with advancing age and adapt the principles of rehabilitation accordingly.

International Classification of Functioning, Disability and Health (ICF)

The ultimate goal of neurorehabilitation is to restore function in order to increase quality of life. The challenge for the neurorehabilitation team is in finding the best strategies to access the clients' resources and treat their impairments in order to facilitate reorganization. Neurorehabilitation should therefore be goal directed and requires a structure that is transparent to all members of the rehabilitation team. The variety of professional collaboration requires a common language that is applicable beyond professional barriers, in order to achieve the optimum rehabilitation outcome. The biopsychosocial model of the International Classification of Functioning, Disability and Health (ICF) can serve as such an orientation for many processes of neurorehabilitation. The ICF belongs to the World Health Organization (WHO) family of international classifications [21]. The ICF facilitates the uncovering of impairments, limitations and restrictions as well as resources and capabilities. The ICF comprises two parts, each with two components:

Part 1. Functioning and Disability

    (a) Body Functions and Structures

    (b) Activities and Participation

Part 2. Contextual Factors

    (c) Environmental Factors

    (d) Personal Factors.

When setting rehabilitation goals the whole spectrum of the ICF should be considered. This will influence the choice of therapeutic interventions and assessments. In the following sections we use the ICF to highlight aspects of the aged patient considered to be important for the rehabilitation process.

Age-related conditions

Patients of advanced age exhibit numerous life changes which may interfere with the process of neurorehabilitation. ICF personal context barriers are often not adaptable. This may be a limiting factor in the aged person which will influence therapeutic interventions and outcomes.

Body functions and structures

In older patients numerous physiological body functions and anatomical structures may be altered, the most common changes being in the musculoskeletal system. There are also impairments in other systems, 'age-related alterations in memory, motor activity, mood, sleep pattern, appetite, and neuroendocrine function result from alterations in the structure and function of the brain' (Table 6.1) [22].

With a prevalence of approximately 30% in the general population osteoarthritis (OA) is one of the most frequent diagnoses in general practice. Beside factors like gender or obesity, age is clearly associated with the occurrence of OA. The incidence of OA increases markedly after the age of 50 years [23]. It is clinically characterized by pain, stiffness, functional impairment, and limited movement, as well as deformations in later stages [24]. OA occurs most frequently in the knee, hip, and hand joints with the consequence of walking- and upper extremity-related disabilities.

Table 6.1 Age-related conditions that interfere with neurorehabilitation and have to be regarded for goal setting and assigning patients to treatment programmes—the rehabilitative training has to be adapted according to the current medical condition

- Muscular and cardiovascular deconditioning
- Muscle weakness
- Osteoarthritis
- Artificial joints, usually hip/knee
- Osteoporosis
- Cardiovascular problems
- Pulmonary deficits
- Neuroendocrine function changes
- Diabetes mellitus with possible peripheral sensory deficits
- Increased cholesterol
- Reduced appetite
- Difficulty with eyesight
- Loss of hearing
- Reduced balance with increase in number of falls
- urogenital problems
- Depression
- Reduced memory and general cognition
- Sleep pattern changes

A lack of spinal range of motion may contribute to postural control problems. Due to the expected increase of age (and obesity) of the general population OA related conditions are expected to occur even more frequently [25].

Relating to the musculoskeletal system, other conditions as well as OA become more prevalent with increasing age. Additionally, a loss of muscle mass, and hence voluntary muscle power takes place. It is reported that this age-related sarcopenia starts in the fourth decade with 80% being lost in the eighth decade. This sarcopenia is caused by multiple factors. Inactivity, age-related molecular changes, malnutrition, and other reasons are reported to be associated with the decline in muscle mass. Inactivity can partially be explained by the interference with other diseases that lead to pain and fatigue [26, 27]. The reduction of age-related muscle mass is often associated with an increase in fat mass, resulting in sarcopenic obesity [28].

Age related states like musculoskeletal pain, reduced joint mobility and load capacity, limited muscular strength, obesity, and cardiovascular diseases [29] restrict the ability to train physically, which is an important component of neurorehabilitation. As such, not only the actual neurological condition has to be treated, but also the general status of elderly patients. In turn interventions aiming at improving functions have to be adapted. This issue might also be reflected in clinical evaluation of rehabilitation outcome. For example, the 6-minute walk test might be limited, not primarily because of the neurological disease, but because of pre-existing cardiopulmonary deconditioning or general muscle weakness.

Stroke patients are often tired for weeks post stroke [30]. There are multiple reasons for this phenomenon. Due to incontinence, the client often has a catheter. Bladder Infections are typical and treated with antibiotics, which cause tiredness. Persons who are bedridden lose their capacity for work. Muscles atrophy very fast. Sarcopenia is present in almost all stroke patients, regardless of age [31]. Lack of nutrition, due to loss of appetite or dysphagia, may result in a reduction of energy or deconditioning. These factors, among others, mean that older patients must have more rest periods between therapies which influences quantity and intensity of treatment.

Deficits in cognition, be it memory, planning capabilities, perception, concentration, etc., will affect the success of neurorehabilitation. The elderly person may have had pre-existing problems, which will probably be exacerbated post stroke. These deficits are often the limiting factors for discharge home.

Activities

Activities are tasks or actions conducted by an individual. The performance of activities relate to body functions and structures, but not in a one-to-one relationship. The execution of an activity might be reduced not only due to the actual neurological condition. A history of falls due to balance impairments, for example, can lead to fear of falling with corresponding inactivity in order to prevent future falls. This so called post-fall syndrome leads to a secondary worsening of activity performance [32].

Participation

Participation relates to the involvement in a life situation. This strongly interacts with the concept of sociological aging mentioned earlier in this chapter. According to Swiss statistics, a large percentage of persons aged over 65 rely on walking for mobility, be it for shopping or recreation [33]. The most important first goal for an elderly, or any patient in neurorehabilitation, is usually to be able to walk. The discussion regarding employment, of course, is absent in the elderly, retired population.

Environmental factors

Environmental factors are of special importance in geriatric patients. A majority of persons with advanced age already do not live on their own; in particular, those patients with stroke or SCI may not be able to live independently. The question of where the person will live at discharge from rehabilitation must be considered at an early stage in order to efficiently prepare. However, there are elderly persons who often are capable of doing more in their own home than in a foreign environment. Environment plays a large role in recovery, and must be emphasized. A context factor barrier, which could lead to shorter length of stays in rehabilitation and therefore influence goal setting, could be insurance payment or lack thereof.

Principles of neurorehabilitation

After structuring specific features of the elderly on the basis of the ICF, the following sections look at specific principles of neurorehabilitation and their potential need for adaptation when applied in elderly patients.

Motor learning

A successful rehabilitative training should incorporate task-specific exercises with a high number of repetitions, variations progression, as well as rest periods [34]. It is important to keep in mind that the elderly person has brain plasticity and therefore rehabilitation potential. Mahnke et al. have stated in their research that the ageing person with a stroke does have neuroplasticity and capability to learn. Rehabilitation specialists must be capable of delivering therapies that drive neural reorganization and learning. 'Driving brain plasticity with positive outcomes requires engaging older adults in demanding sensory, cognitive, and motor activities on an intensive basis, in a behavioural context designed to re-engage and strengthen the neuromodulatory systems that control learning in adults' [35]. Recent literature suggests that the principles of motor learning are of importance for relearning motor tasks and to drive neuroplasticity and central nervous system (CNS) reorganization after neurological impairment. One fundamental element is that of repetition. Repetitive exercises should be performed in continual problem solving situations and meaningful goals that drive the patient to practice [36]. Several investigations showed that rehabilitation outcome depends on training intensity (for review see [37, 38]. Older patients may perceive such intense trainings as more challenging than their younger counterparts. Nevertheless, there is evidence that the principle of augmented therapy works in clinical practice. As little as 16 hours of additional training within 6 months after the incident led to small, yet measurable, improvements of outcomes in patients with stroke [39].

Therapeutic tasks, combined with handling skills when necessary, are important for the ageing stroke patient. In order to 'drive' neuroplasticity, the task must be interesting and motivating. The therapist must be able to find tasks that access the client's procedural memory in order to facilitate motor responses. This is a challenge. Tasks can be used to treat impairments such as trunk instability, reduced postural control, balance, hand–eye coordination, upper and lower-extremity impairments, etc. Task-oriented treatment may be used to reduce activity limitations themselves. Intensity of the treatment as well as the progression of the task itself must be developed and monitored by the therapist. An example of task-oriented therapy in appropriate environments, which is of utmost importance for the patient if performed in such a way as to access procedural systems and support/influence motor learning, is transfers in varying everyday situations: from the bed to the wheelchair, toilet, wheelchair, shower, wheelchair, scale, wheelchair, normal chair for breakfast, etc.

Active participation which requires attention and concentration is another important principle [40]. It is essential that the patient be given responsibility for his or her own improvement when possible. Patients tend to be very dependent on rehabilitation staff. Small duties or 'home-exercises' patients are expected to do by themselves are important. A home programme written in a booklet or done in pictures is an example. In the inpatient setting, the patient should always have their booklet with them. It makes an impression when the doctor asks to see their book and requests that the patient show him or her their 'exercises'. Upper extremity range of motion exercises or leg strengthening to be done in sitting are examples.

Verticalization

Inactivity in the elderly causes, as previously stated, muscular and cardiovascular changes. This situation is exacerbated post stroke. In the acute phase, the tendency is to mobilize the patient as soon as possible in order to prevent prolonged bed rest, which adversely affects multiple systems and impedes functional recovery, especially in the elderly. One type of relatively low stress mobilization in the very acute phase is verticalization via a tilt table. The patient must be closely monitored to assess the effect of vertical position [41]. Immediately post stroke there is the danger of increasing the size of the penumbra due to brain hypoperfusion with verticalization. Changes in blood pressure and pulse rates may indicate the angle and amount of time of verticalization the patient can tolerate [42].

The therapist must consider the necessity to bandage the lower extremities in order to prevent hypotension. Standing on the table may have an added effect of positively affecting consciousness via the ascending reticular activating system, will give weight bearing through the lower extremities maintaining dorsal extension in the foot, will affect breathing/lung expansion due to the effect of gravity on the internal organs, and gives vestibular, proprioceptive, and tactile information, as well as body/space perceptual cues.

Robotics

Robots have become increasingly applied in neurorehabilitation. There are devices for the training of the upper and lower extremities. Reaching, grasping, or walking can be trained in a controlled manner. Improvements can be monitored and documented. These devices follow the principles of task-specificity and intensity. They are often equipped with sensors and allow providing feedback to both patients and therapists. Training can be accomplished using motivating games [43]. Some devices are designed for home use under the remote supervision of a rehabilitation specialist. An incompatibility with innovative technology may be present in patients with cognitive impairments. Although the devices possess many sophisticated features (e.g. virtual environment) they still require a certain ability to abstract in order to fully profit from the features of a robotic training. The immersive or non-immersive virtual reality makes the task being completed 'real'. Although there are no conclusive, large-scale studies done on the effect of robotic therapies with virtual reality at the activity or participation levels at this time, the carry-over from the practice situation to real life has been successfully shown in the airline industry with pilots and flight simulators. There is strong evidence that sensorimotor training with robotic devices improves upper extremity functional outcomes, and motor outcomes of the shoulder and elbow, but not the wrist and hand, of stroke patients [44]. The high intensity of training, which is possible by means of robotic training, bears also the risk to overstrain joints or bones of elderly patients. Thus, the dosage must carefully be adapted to the meet the tolerance of the individual. Robotic therapies are excellent for research as they can be standardized and allow for quantification. In conventional therapy trials, standardization and quantification have been very difficult to produce [45].

Cardiovascular training

Heart disease in the elderly is a risk factor for stroke. Premorbid hyperlipidaemia, hypertension, atrial fibrillation, and reduced aerobic capacity is not uncommon. (American Heart Association http://www.heart.org/HEARTORG/). These factors are exacerbated post stroke. Macko has repeatedly shown that patients with strokes have deficient cardiovascular capabilities [46]. He has shown that aerobic training positively influences the patients' cardiac and cerebral blood flow and VO_2. Patients should be encouraged to wheel the wheelchair, walk the treadmill with body support, or to walk short distances, climb stairs, or ride a stationary bike adapted to their physical capabilities. This type of training may also have a positive influence on depression [47].

Novel, translational therapies

Although not specific for ageing patients until now, science has provided new ideas on how to maximize 'traditional/conventional' therapy interventions. Transcranial magnetic stimulation (TMS), transcranial direct current stimulation (TDCS), as well as paired associative stimulation (PAS), are being used to increase recovery of upper extremity function. The results are positive and will be included in future intervention strategies for all stroke patients. 'Noninvasive transcranial brain stimulation combined with motor training did enhance the acquisition of a novel skill with the paretic hand' [48]. Although the mean age of the participants in this study was 58, the positive effects were there for the >70-year-old person [49].

Length of rehabilitation stay

Focused rehabilitation strategies and improved efficiency as well as cost pressure are two reasons for the reduction of rehabilitation length of stay (LOS) [50, 51]. Although somewhat counterintuitive, several investigations show that age is independent from rehabilitation LOS in stroke [52–54] and SCI [55]. Other authors report longer LOS for the very old [56]. It has to be borne in mind that rehabilitation services provision varies widely between countries. However, from a clinical point of view older patients need longer training periods to achieve their goals. This is partially due to the fact that training intensity has to be adapted to the frail body system or that medical instability interferes with the rehabilitative training. Elderly clients also appear to be more tired and recover their general health post stroke more slowly than younger ones. Elderly patients do exhibit difficulties to translate skills and abilities learned within a therapeutic context to everyday life situations. As an example, it has been shown in a cohort of 237 patients with traumatic SCI from different European rehabilitation settings that, although older patients had a favourable recovery of neurological deficits, the improvement in functional tasks was worse compared to younger patients [55].

Early supported discharge

The concept of early supported discharge (ESD) for stroke survivors addresses—among others—the issue of not adequately translating skills learned in the rehabilitation setting to the home environment, by an early discharge from hospital, in combination with continuing multidisciplinary rehabilitation at the home of the patient. According to a systematic review [57] including 11 studies with almost 1,600 patients, such an ESD team typically comprises physiotherapists, occupational therapists, speech- and language therapists, medical doctors, nurses, and social workers. Physio- and occupational therapy are the main components in an ESD team. Family members and spouses or other assistant persons and carer have to be involved from the very beginning. Already established ESD service provided therapy on a daily basis for a period of 3 months. To ensure goal-directed interventions co-ordination meetings on a weekly basis are recommended. The ESD service appeared to be as effective as standard care provided in specialized stroke units. The eligibility for ESD is somewhat limited. Persisting disability, living within a local area and stable medical conditions are prerequisites for the ESD approach. However, patients with a moderate disability (initial Bathel Index of >9) are reported to profit most. In studies for the evaluation of ESD about 41% of patients with stroke were suitable for an early discharge. Pertaining to the outcomes of ESD it has been shown that patients who underwent the ESD procedure had shorter length of hospital stay, a reduced odds of death, dependency for daily life activities, or long-term institutional care [57].

Telerehabilitation

Many elderly patients are either unable physically to go to outpatient therapy or travel is not feasible due to distances, or other context factors. With the novel approach of telerehabilitation it becomes possible to continue rehabilitation at a patient's home without the therapists being physically present. It takes advantage of modern communication technologies in conjunction with home-based robots, which are equipped with sensor technology. Telerehabilitation has been used effectively in Canada and other areas where large distances have made direct contact therapy interventions almost impossible. The therapist has visual contact with the patient and caregivers and can problem solve, change the home programme, etc., via the computer. The use of telerehabilitation has been shown to be an effective strategy of bringing therapists into the home for consultations as well as therapy sessions [58].

Contribution of family members and caregivers to rehabilitation

Ageing patients are often dependent on their children or other caregivers. The spouse is frequently not capable of 24-hour caregiving. The family/caregiver should be included in the rehabilitation process as soon as possible. In the acute phase, the family is also in a situation of shock, and sometimes must be told things repeatedly before they are able to process what is happening.

Family support is very important for the patient. In the perfect situation, the family attends treatment sessions, works with nursing to learn how to help their family member, is in contact with the physicians to understand the medical situation, and will be able to take the family member home or assist them in their own home. After discharge the burden is often on the caregivers. Families are often unable or unwilling to take over the responsibility for the elderly client. This happens less often with the younger person. Even if the elderly client is quite capable, there may be architectural barriers that will make going home a problem.

Discharge destination

A different dilemma with the older person who is able to live in their own home could be isolation. They may be unable to get out into society. Loneliness happens with ageing in any case when the person gradually loses their friends and acquaintances. In this case, a better solution could be specialized nursing facilities with educated rehabilitation staff, appropriate therapies, and contact with others.

If the personal and environmental context factors are such that the patient probably will not be able to go home, social services should be involved soon so there is time to find the best place for the patient to live upon discharge.

Outcome testing

Every patient in therapy should have outcome testing done on a regular basis. The tests used should be reliable and valid, as well as practicable. With elderly patients, different tests or other thresholds or endpoints may be appropriate than with younger patients. The rehabilitation goal might be accomplished when an old patient is able to move around the house independently whereas younger patients also train to go to the community The Functional Independence Measure (FIM) [59] is done routinely in many centres by the nursing staff and gives good information regarding the patient's functional status at the activity level. Physical therapists use different tests for different stages in recovery. At the very low FIM level, one can use the early functional abilities test [60] or the trunk control test [61]. Balance and risk for falling can be tested using the Berg Balance Scale [62] or the Performance Oriented Mobility Assessment [63]. Timed tests are very useful for gait. Upper extremity function can be tested with the nine-hole peg test [64] or the Wolf motor function test [65]. All patients can be tested using the Goal Attainment Scale [66]. The point is that therapists must have objective findings and be able to make clear statements regarding improvement or change.

Evidence

There is no conclusive evidence in neurorehabilitation as to which therapies have the best results for the ageing patient either with stroke or SCI. Most trials have looked at chronic stroke patients with very specific inclusion criteria. The numbers of participants generated for these trials are relatively small. Patients with strokes, especially in the ageing, have very heterogeneous symptoms and are difficult to study in a randomized controlled trial (RCT). Susan D. Horn's ideas for practice-based evidence studies [67] would be more appropriate for this population, but are not yet accepted in the science world as equivalent to RCTs. Single case studies are useful and interesting at the individual level but not for comparing procedures or methods.

Although there are effective treatments that restore brain perfusion and minimize complications and recurrent stroke, there is no treatment proven to facilitate neurological recovery after stroke [35].

It is often seen for research purposes that groups of young and old patients are being compared regarding several outcomes. One has to bear in mind, however, that age might not be the only difference between such groups. Survival, for example, is different in young and old patients. Older patients still alive and referred to rehabilitation may be healthier than their younger counterparts. Depending on the research question such survival effects need to be controlled for. It is also known that pre-existing conditions are sometimes under-reported [68]. There might also be a selection bias in that only patients who have the potential to meet the challenge of rehabilitation are referred to specialized centres [69].

Basic science researchers have shown in animal studies, but also in smaller-scale human studies, the fact of neuroplasticity post stroke, and are attempting to translate this information into neurorehabilitation therapy interventions. There are many reasons why this is difficult. Patients with stroke are a very heterogeneous population. There is not sufficient contact between the researchers and clinicians [70]. Some clinicians are not informed of the restorative neuroscience developments. On the other hand, some scientists are not really aware of the problems clinicians have. Not everything basic science learns in small, very controlled studies is applicable in daily life rehabilitation. Instead of a positive, creative environment to try novel therapies, there may be a situation of antagonism. Evidence, with its translation into the clinic, should be a circular integration of best research evidence, clinical expertise, and patient values [71].

An example of an intervention with good evidence is constraint induced movement therapy (CIMT). CIMT emphasizes task-oriented training, meaningful patient goals, active participation, and repetition. The so called, 'forced-use' of the affected upper extremity with goal-oriented therapy has excellent results for the patients who meet the inclusion criteria. Also, modified CIMT, meaning less hours per day practice over a longer period of time, has also very good outcome results. This therapy, translated from science into practice, can be used in the rehab setting but also at home. The patients who profit the most from this therapy are not cognitively impaired and have some functional recovery in their upper extremities [72].

Patients with SCI

The majority of neurological deficits requiring neurological rehabilitation are hemiparesis due to cerebrovascular stroke. Patients with SCI account to about a tenth of the cases with stroke.

The basis for modern comprehensive SCI rehabilitation was established during World War II when a substantial number of patients with SCI were transferred home [73]. These cases and those who followed after the War were mostly young men who experienced their spinal cord lesion in a traumatic event. Accordingly, assessments and interventions were tailored to the features of this specific patient group. However, there is indication from the literature that the mean age at injury has been increasing in the last decades. More importantly the proportion of cases with non-traumatic SCI is growing and almost exceeds that of traumatic cases [16, 74–76]. One characteristic of the latter group is the markedly older age. So, when considering patients who sustain a SCI with advanced age the cause is most likely of non-traumatic nature.

SCI aetiology

The aetiology of a traumatic SCI varies with the age at injury onset. With approximately 45% a motor vehicle crash is the predominant cause in younger subjects (16–46 years). Falls are the leading aetiology in patients older than 60 years [12].

Non-traumatic SCI is mostly caused by age-related conditions—neoplasms, vascular disease, inflammatory disease, and degenerative spinal stenosis [74, 76].

In summary, older patients are more likely to experience a non-traumatic incomplete SCI, resulting in less severe disability. However, these patients tend to present additional diagnoses, which interfere with the potential good prognosis for recovery.

Clinical presentation

According to registers in the USA [77] and Europe [14], the most frequent condition after a traumatic SCI is incomplete tetraplegia (41% and 33%) followed by complete paraplegia (22% and 27%), incomplete paraplegia (21% and 23%) and complete tetraplegia (16% and 17%). Cases with incomplete SCI at a high cervical level are increasing [13]. A special form of incomplete traumatic tetraplegia is the central cord syndrome (CCS), which is present more frequently in older individuals. It is characterized by a more pronounced paralysis of the upper extremities compared to the lower extremities, which remain less affected. The CCS is caused by a lesion of the central region of the cervical spinal cord involving the grey matter and axons projecting to the upper body. The more laterally located neural structures that project to the lower body are less compromised. CCS frequently occurs during an inadequate minor trauma associated with a trip or a fall. A pre-existing, often clinically non-symptomatic myelopathy due to degenerative processes of the cervical spine in combination with a small trauma, results in CCS. However, CCS is not restricted to elderly people; it can also occur in younger patients following a trauma [78, 79].

There is clear evidence from the literature that patients with a SCI of non-traumatic origin present more often with incomplete paraplegia and higher admission scores on the FIM [15, 16, 74, 76].

Outcome after SCI

When comparing old with young patients one must bear in mind that the two groups differ not only in age but also with respect to other characteristics. For example, such a comparison might be influenced by survival effects. Without the SCI older patients have a more favorable survival rate as compared to the younger group.

Observational studies suggest that neurological and functional outcome after SCI is related to the patients' age at injury (e.g. [80]). However, it is likely that age is not independent from other predictors like severity of injury. As mentioned earlier, older patients experience more incomplete SCI, which is associated with a better outcome. Accordingly, neurological outcome seems not to be negatively influenced by age. It seems, however, that older patients fail to translate their favourable neurological recovery into functional abilities [55, 81].

Age in combination with severity and neurological level of spinal lesion is reported to be associated with mortality after SCI. Old patients with a complete SCI at the cervical level have a substantially increased mortality rate [80–82].

Conclusion

Demographics show that the population of the world is ageing. Risks for strokes and other neurological conditions increase with age. The elderly patient will probably have more comorbidities than the younger patient. In spite of this, the elderly have neurorehabilitation potential. Preserved neuroplasticity, the potential to train muscular strength, cardio-vascular endurance and joint flexibility does not stop at a certain age. Therapy methods and concepts are not particularly age related. They need to be adapted in intensity to the person's capabilities. The rehabilitation period may be longer with the aged, but results in a definite quality of life improvement for the affected person and their family.

References

1. Crocker T, Forster A, Young J, et al. Physical rehabilitation for older people in long-term care. Cochrane Database Syst Rev. 2013;2:CD004294.
2. Panel, Sacco RL, Benjamin EJ, Broderick JP, et al. Risk Factors. Stroke. 1997;28(7):1507–1517.
3. Howard G, Goff DC. Population shifts and the future of stroke: forecasts of the future burden of stroke. Ann N Y Acad Sci. 2012;1268:14–20.
4. Center NSCIS. 2011 NSCISC Annual Statistical Report. National Spinal Cord Injury Statistical Center, Birmingham, AL, 2011.
5. New PW, Sundararajan V. Incidence of non-traumatic spinal cord injury in Victoria, Australia: a population-based study and literature review. Spinal Cord. 2008;46(6):406–411.
6. Balcombe NR, Sinclair A. Ageing: definitions, mechanisms and the magnitude of the problem. Best Practice & Research. 2001;15(6):835–849.
7. Holliday R. Understanding ageing. Philos Trans R Soc Lond B Biol Sci. [Review]. 1997;352(1363):1793–1797.
8. World Health Organization. Global health observatory. WHO, Geneva, 2013. Available from www.who.int/gho (accessed 1 October 2014).
9. Nations U. Population ageing and development: Ten years after Madrid, Department of Economic and Social Affairs PD;2012 December 2012. Report No.: 2012/4.
10. World Health Organization. The global burden of disease: 2004 update. WHO, Geneva, 2008.
11. Strong K, Mathers C, Bonita R. Preventing stroke: saving lives around the world. Lancet Neurol. 2007;6(2):182–187.
12. National Spinal Cord Injury Statistical Center. The 2011 annual statistical report for the spinal cord injury model systems. Birmingham, Alabama 2012. Available from https://www.nscisc.uab.edu/reports.aspx (accessed 1 October 2014).
13. Devivo MJ. Epidemiology of traumatic spinal cord injury: trends and future implications. Spinal Cord. 2012;50(5):365–372.
14. Curt A, Schwab ME, Dietz V. Providing the clinical basis for new interventional therapies: refined diagnosis and assessment of recovery after spinal cord injury. Spinal Cord. 2004;42(1):1–6.
15. McKinley WO, Seel RT, Hardman JT. Nontraumatic spinal cord injury: incidence, epidemiology, and functional outcome. Arch Phys Med Rehabil. 1999;80(6):619–623.
16. New PW, Simmonds F, Stevermuer T. A population-based study comparing traumatic spinal cord injury and non-traumatic spinal cord injury using a national rehabilitation database. Spinal Cord. 2011;49(3):397–403.
17. van den Berg ME, Castellote JM, Mahillo-Fernandez I, de Pedro-Cuesta J. Incidence of spinal cord injury worldwide: a systematic review. Neuroepidemiology. 2010;34(3):184–192; discussion 92.
18. van den Berg ME, Castellote JM, Mahillo-Fernandez I, de Pedro-Cuesta J. Incidence of nontraumatic spinal cord injury: a Spanish cohort study (1972–2008). Arch Phys Med Rehabil. 2012;93(2):325–331.
19. Kammersgaard LP. Survival after stroke. Risk factors and determinants in the Copenhagen Stroke Study. Dan Med Bull. 2010;57(10):B4189.
20. Koch J, Baronti F, Hürlimann U. Neurorehabilitation nach Hirnschlag: Alter ist kein limitierender Faktor. Schweizerische Ärztezeitung. 2007;88(12):531–534
21. World Health Organization. International Classification of Functioning, Disability and Health: ICF. WHO, Geneva, 2001.
22. Sanes JR, Jessell TM. The Aging Brain. Principles of Neural Science, 5th edn. McGraw-Hill, New York, 2013.
23. Neogi T, Zhang Y. Epidemiology of osteoarthritis. Rheum Dis Clin North Am. 2013;39(1):1–19.
24. Sacitharan PK, Snelling SJ, Edwards JR. Aging mechanisms in arthritic disease. Discov Med. 2012;14(78):345–352.
25. Suri P, Morgenroth DC, Hunter DJ. Epidemiology of osteoarthritis and associated comorbidities. PM R. 2012;4(5 Suppl):S10-19.
26. Degens H, Korhonen MT. Factors contributing to the variability in muscle ageing. Maturitas. 2012;73(3):197–201.
27. Walston JD. Sarcopenia in older adults. Curr Opin Rheumatol. 2012;24(6):623–627.
28. Mathus-Vliegen EM. Obesity and the elderly. J Clin Gastroenterol. 2012;46(7):533–544.
29. Seals DR, Walker AE, Pierce GL, Lesniewski LA. Habitual exercise and vascular ageing. J Physiol. 2009;587(Pt 23):5541–5549.
30. van Eijsden HM, van de Port IG, Visser-Meily JM, Kwakkel G. Poststroke fatigue: who is at risk for an increase in fatigue? Stroke Res Treat. 2012;2012:863978.
31. Carda S, Cisari C, Invernizzi M. Sarcopenia or muscle modifications in neurologic diseases: a lexical or patophysiological difference? Eur J Phys Rehabil Med. 2013;49(1):119–130.

32. Murphy J, Isaacs B. The post-fall syndrome. A study of 36 elderly patients. Gerontology. 1982;**28**(4):265–270.

33. Bundesamt für Statistik BfR, editor. Mobilität in der Schweiz, Ergebnisse des Mikrozensus Mobilität und Verkehr 2010. Neuchâtel und Bern, 2012.

34. Bowden MG, Woodbury ML, Duncan PW. Promoting neuroplasticity and recovery after stroke: future directions for rehabilitation clinical trials. Curr Opin Neurol. 2013;**26**(1):37–42.

35. Mahncke HW, Bronstone A, Merzenich MM. Brain plasticity and functional losses in the aged: scientific bases for a novel intervention. Prog Brain Res. 2006;**157**:81–109.

36. Gentile AM. Motor Learning Seminar. Bad Ragaz, 1995.

37. Dobkin BH. Strategies for stroke rehabilitation. Lancet Neurol. 2004;**3**(9):528–536.

38. Krakauer JW. Motor learning: its relevance to stroke recovery and neurorehabilitation. Curr Opin Neurol. 2006;**19**(1):84–90.

39. Kwakkel G, van Peppen R, Wagenaar RC, et al. Effects of augmented exercise therapy time after stroke: a meta-analysis. Stroke. 2004;**35**(11):2529–2539.

40. Winstein CJ, editor. Motor Learning and Motor Control. SeminarRheinburg Clinic, Walzenhausen, 1999.

41. Baltz MJ, Lietz HL, Sausser IT, Kalpakjian C, Brown D. Tolerance of a standing tilt table protocol by patients an inpatient stroke unit setting: a pilot study. J Neurol Phys Ther. 2013;**37**(1):9–13.

42. Heiss WD. The concept of the penumbra: can it be translated to stroke management? Int J Stroke. 2010;**5**(4):290–295.

43. Wirz M, Rupp R. Applications issues for robotics. In: Dietz V, Rymer Z, Nef T, editors. Neurorehabilitation Technology. Springer, Berlin, 2012.

44. Foley N, Teasell R, Jutai J, Bhogal S, Kruger E. Evidence-based review of stroke rehabilitation. Upper extremity interventions. 2012. Available from http://www.ebrsr.com/evidence-review/10-upper-extremity-interventions (accessed 1 October 2014).

45. Cheeran B, Cohen L, Dobkin B, et al. The future of restorative neurosciences in stroke: driving the translational research pipeline from basic science to rehabilitation of people after stroke. Neurorehabil Neural Repair. 2009;**23**(2):97–107.

46. Macko RF, Ivey FM, Forrester LW, et al. Treadmill exercise rehabilitation improves ambulatory function and cardiovascular fitness in patients with chronic stroke: a randomized, controlled trial. Stroke. 2005;**36**(10):2206–2211.

47. Ivey FM, Ryan AS, Hafer-Macko CE, Macko RF. Improved cerebral vasomotor reactivity after exercise training in hemiparetic stroke survivors. Stroke. 2011;**42**(7):1994–2000.

48. Zimerman M, Heise KF, Hoppe J, Cohen LG, Gerloff C, Hummel FC. Modulation of training by single-session transcranial direct current stimulation to the intact motor cortex enhances motor skill acquisition of the paretic hand. Stroke. 2012;**43**(8):2185–2191.

49. Gomez Palacio Schjetnan A, Faraji J, Metz GA, Tatsuno M, Luczak A. Transcranial direct current stimulation in stroke rehabilitation: a review of recent advancements. Stroke Res Treat. 2013;2013:170–256.

50. Meyer M, Britt E, McHale HA, Teasell R. Length of stay benchmarks for inpatient rehabilitation after stroke. Disabil Rehabil. 2012;**34**(13):1077–1081.

51. Tistad M, Ytterberg C, Sjostrand C, Holmqvist LW, von Koch L. Shorter length of stay in the stroke unit: comparison between the 1990s and 2000s. Top Stroke Rehabil. 2012;**19**(2):172–181.

52. Appelros P. Prediction of length of stay for stroke patients. Acta Neurol Scand. 2007;**116**(1):15–19.

53. Ekstrand E, Ringsberg KA, Pessah-Rasmussen H. The physiotherapy clinical outcome variables scale predicts length of hospital stay, discharge destination and future home facility in the acute comprehensive stroke unit. J Rehabil Med. 2008;**40**(7):524–528.

54. Tan WS, Heng BH, Chua KS, Chan KF. Factors predicting inpatient rehabilitation length of stay of acute stroke patients in Singapore. Arch Phys Med Rehabil. 2009;**90**(7):1202–1207.

55. Jakob W, Wirz M, van Hedel HJ, Dietz V. Difficulty of elderly SCI subjects to translate motor recovery—'body function'—into daily living activities. J Neurotrauma. 2009;**26**(11):2037–2044.

56. Saposnik G, Cote R, Phillips S, et al. Stroke outcome in those over 80: a multicenter cohort study across Canada. Stroke. 2008;**39**(8):2310–2317.

57. Langhorne P, Taylor G, Murray G, et al. Early supported discharge services for stroke patients: a meta-analysis of individual patients' data. Lancet. 2005;**365**(9458):501–506.

58. Linder SM, Reiss A, Buchanan S, et al. Incorporating robotic-assisted telerehabilitation in a home program to improve arm function following stroke. J Neurol Phys Ther. 2013;**37**(3):125–132.

59. Keith RA, Granger CV, Hamilton BB, Sherwin FS. The functional independence measure: a new tool for rehabilitation. Adv Clin Rehabil. 1987;**1**:6–18.

60. Alvsaker K, Walther SM, Kleffelgard I, Mongs M, Draegebo RA, Keller A. Inter-rater reliability of the early functional abilities scale. J Rehabil Med. 2011;**43**(10):892–899.

61. Sheikh K, Smith DS, Meade TW, Brennan PJ, Ide L. Assessment of motor function in studies of chronic disability. Rheumatol Rehabil. 1980;**19**(2):83–90.

62. Berg K. Measuring balance in the elderly: preliminary development of an instrument. Physiotherapy Canada. 1989;**41**(6):304–311.

63. Tinetti ME. Performance-oriented assessment of mobility problems in elderly patients. J Am Geriatr Soc. 1986;**34**(2):119–126.

64. Kellor M, Frost J, Silberberg N, Iversen I, Cummings R. Hand strength and dexterity. Am J Occup Ther. 1971;**25**(2):77–83.

65. Wolf SL, Lecraw DE, Barton LA, Jann BB. Forced use of hemiplegic upper extremities to reverse the effect of learned nonuse among chronic stroke and head-injured patients. Exp Neurol. 1989;**104**(2):125–132.

66. Malec JF, Smigielski JS, DePompolo RW. Goal attainment scaling and outcome measurement in postacute brain injury rehabilitation. Arch Phys Med Rehabil. 1991;**72**(2):138–143.

67. Horn SD, DeJong G, Deutscher D. Practice-based evidence research in rehabilitation: an alternative to randomized controlled trials and traditional observational studies. Arch Phys Med Rehabil. 2012;**93**(8 Suppl):S127–137.

68. van Middendorp JJ, Albert TJ, Veth RP, Hosman AJ. Methodological systematic review: mortality in elderly patients with cervical spine injury: a critical appraisal of the reporting of baseline characteristics, follow-up, cause of death, and analysis of risk factors. Spine. 2010;**35**(10):1079–1087.

69. McKinley W, Cifu D, Seel R, et al. Age-related outcomes in persons with spinal cord injury: a summary paper. NeuroRehabilitation. 2003;**18**(1):83–90.

70. Cumberland Consensus Working Group. Cheeran B, Cohen L, Dobkin B, et al. The future of restorative neurosciences in stroke: driving the translational research pipeline from basic science to rehabilitation of people after stroke. Neurorehabil Neural Repair. 2009;**23**(2):97–107.

71. Isaac CA, Franceschi A. EBM: evidence to practice and practice to evidence. J Eval Clin Pract. 2008;**14**(5):656–659.

72. Wolf SL, Winstein CJ, Miller JP, et al. Effect of constraint-induced movement therapy on upper extremity function 3 to 9 months after stroke: the EXCITE randomized clinical trial. JAMA. 2006;**296**(17):2095–2104.

73. Donovan WH. Donald Munro Lecture. Spinal cord injury—past, present, and future. J Spinal Cord Med. 2007;**30**(2):85–100.

74. Catz A, Goldin D, Fishel B, Ronen J, Bluvshtein V, Gelernter I. Recovery of neurologic function following nontraumatic spinal cord lesions in Israel. Spine. 2004 Oct 15;**29**(20):2278–2282; discussion 83.

75. Guilcher SJ, Munce SE, Couris CM, et al. Health care utilization in non-traumatic and traumatic spinal cord injury: a population-based study. Spinal Cord.2010;**48**(1):45–50.

76. Ho CH, Wuermser LA, Priebe MM, Chiodo AE, Scelza WM, Kirshblum SC. Spinal cord injury medicine. 1. Epidemiology and classification. Arch Phys Med Rehabil. 2007;**88**(3 Suppl 1):S49–54.

77. Spinal cord injury facts and figures at a glance. J Spinal Cord Med. 2012;**35**(1):68–69.

78. McKinley W, Santos K, Meade M, Brooke K. Incidence and outcomes of spinal cord injury clinical syndromes. J Spinal Cord Med. 2007;**30**(3):215–224.

79. Aito S, D'Andrea M, Werhagen L, et al. Neurological and functional outcome in traumatic central cord syndrome. Spinal Cord. 2007;**45**(4):292–297.

80. Wilson JR, Cadotte DW, Fehlings MG. Clinical predictors of neurological outcome, functional status, and survival after traumatic spinal cord injury: a systematic review. J Neurosurg Spine. 2012;**17**(1 Suppl):11–26.

81. Furlan JC, Fehlings MG. The impact of age on mortality, impairment, and disability among adults with acute traumatic spinal cord injury. J Neurotrauma. 2009;**26**(10):1707–1717.

82. DeVivo MJ, Stover SL, Black KJ. Prognostic factors for 12-year survival after spinal cord injury. Arch Phys Med Rehabil. 1992;**73**(2):156–162.

CHAPTER 7

The applicability of motor learning to neurorehabilitation

John W. Krakauer

Introduction

Statements to the effect that recovery is a form of learning or relearning are commonplace in the field of neurorehabilitation. In this chapter, motor training will refer to what is done to the patient and motor learning will refer to what the patient may do in response. This distinction is important—just because training is happening does not mean that anything is being learned. The relearning premise for neurorehabilitation is based on three other a priori assumptions. First, that the nature of the deficit to be rehabilitated through learning is known. Second, that the kind of motor learning that should be targeted by training is known. Third, that patients after stroke have an intact learning capacity despite impaired performance. In this chapter the focus will be mainly on rehabilitation of arm paresis after stroke, which results from damage to motor cortical areas and/or their descending pathways. This narrower focus is essential if the topic of learning and neurorehabilitation is to remain within the bounds of a single chapter. That said it is hoped that the general principles introduced here, which will be emphasized over details, are broadly applicable across the range of post-stroke impairments and to other neurological conditions.

Arm paresis after stroke refers to loss of strength and motor control, along with changes in phasic and tonic muscle tone [1]. Non-neural peripheral changes in muscle, joint and tendon properties can also contribute to the paresis phenotype. In this chapter it will be assumed that treatments for strength, tone (spasticity) and contractures are not based on motor learning principles and so will not be addressed further. Note again that one can *train* for strength but this is not motor *learning*. Thus, the starting point for this chapter is that when learning is invoked it implies either improving motor control or finding alternative compensatory strategies with effectors/joints/muscles in which motor control remains relatively intact; in either case, response to training is assumed to have mechanistic commonalities with motor learning in healthy subjects. It will become apparent after reading this chapter that the assumption that one can equate recovery and motor learning is subject to several fundamental caveats.

A taxonomy for motor learning

The fundamental problem for motor learning is to find the appropriate motor commands that will bring about a desired task outcome. Motor learning is a fuzzy category that encompasses action selection guided by instruction, reward, or error, and subsequent improved execution of the selected actions. Skill is a very popular term but is hard to define. Here, it will suffice to say that one is skilled at a task when practice has led to it being performed better than baseline because of selection of optimal mean actions that are then executed with high speed and precision. We will briefly describe the motor learning components in the following section. A question that should always be kept in mind is whether these components of motor learning are relevant or effective in reversing identified motor deficits after stroke or any other neurological condition.

The role of *instruction* in selecting task-appropriate actions has been surprisingly under-emphasized in the motor learning literature despite the ubiquity of coaching and teaching in sport, music and dance; all quintessential motor skill-requiring activities. Similarly, the existence of physical and occupational therapists attests to the crucial role of instruction in rehabilitation. We have recently posited [2] that neglect of the crucial roles of knowledge and instruction for motor learning originates in part from an over-emphasis on simple implicit adaptation tasks due to the classic result in the patient H.M., who retained memory of mirror-drawing ability across days despite no explicit memory of ever having performed the task [3]. This led, in our view, to over-generalization of the notion of procedural learning/memory from this simple task to all motor skills. We have recently argued instead that everyday motor skills such as cooking or driving cannot be extrapolated from motor adaptation tasks and cannot be learned without knowledge and instruction [2]. In agreement with our position, a recent paper has shown that a motor task with redundant structure cannot be learned without explicit awareness of this structure [4]. We, and others, have recently shown that even adaptation tasks have a crucial explicit component [5, 6].

In *reinforcement learning*, actions are selected with increased or decreased frequency based on rewards and punishments, respectively. Reward can be intrinsic, based on self-perceived success or failure, or it can be based on extrinsically provided loss or gain in points or praise. Rewards can be short-term or long-term, and the balance between these is of central computational importance in the field of reinforcement learning. A local action solution can be found based on short-term rewards that is 'just good enough', which then becomes habitual, even though with more time and exploration, a more optimal action could have been found. For example, if a person is given a pair of skis and told to get down a mountain, they may well find a way to do so on their own but they are very unlikely to discover the best technique, which would require instruction and more extended practice. Later in the chapter we will argue that compensatory strategies after stroke often represent precisely this kind of premature adoption of habitual 'just good enough' actions. Constraint-induced therapy is an attempt to prevent adoption of the bad habit of choosing the unaffected arm to perform tasks rather than doing the harder work of improving the affected side [7].

Sensorimotor adaptation refers to reduction of errors in response to a perturbation. Sensorimotor adaptation tasks have been extensively studied experimentally and modeled computationally [8–11]. The prevailing idea is that adaptation occurs through cerebellar-dependent reduction of errors through updating of a forward model via sensory prediction errors [12, 13]. The relevance of adaptation to rehabilitation remains unclear, however, because although imposed errors can lead to fast and large changes in behaviour, these changes do not seem to last once the perturbation is removed. For example, the paretic arm can be made adapt to a viscous force field set to amplify baseline directional reaching biases. When the force field is switched off, aftereffects are now in a direction that negates the biases [14]. A similar 'error augmentation' approach has been used using a split-belt treadmill to reduce step asymmetry in hemiparetic gait [15]. In both cases, however, the desirable aftereffects are very short lived. In the case of force-field adaptation of the arm, after effects lasted for only 30–60 movements after 600 training movements [14]. More recently it has been shown that repeated exposure over multiple sessions prolongs split-belt treadmill over-ground after-effects in patients with stroke [16]. Interestingly, repeated exposure is also required for prism adaptation in the treatment of neglect after stroke [17]. One explanation for the short-lived nature of adaptation is that newly adapted behaviours are out-competed by baseline behaviours that have been reinforced over much longer periods of time and have become habits. In support of this idea is the recent finding that if a newly adapted behaviour, once it has reached asymptote, is reinforced by switching from error to binary feedback, the adapted behaviour is retained for longer [18]. Thus, if adaptation paradigms are going to be used to have patients quickly converge on desired behaviours, then error-based and reinforcement-based learning mechanisms will likely need to be combined. A potential way to do this would be to adapt a patient first and then reinforce the after-effect.

We have recently introduced the term 'motor acuity', drawing a direct parallel with perceptual acuity, for the component of motor skill by which movement variability and smoothness improve with practice [19]. This kind of learning probably occurs in the same motor cortical areas that are responsible for the motor commands themselves [20]. Motor acuity increases with repeated practice and could potentially be modelled as a form of statistical learning.

Finally, there has been a great deal of recent interest in *use-dependent plasticity* (UDP). It will be argued here that the assumption that UDP is a form of motor learning or motor memory relevant to neurorehabilitation is likely incorrect. The core problem is the tendency to blur the distinction between plasticity and learning. Plasticity refers to the capacity of the nervous system to change its input–output characteristics with various forms of training. These input–output relationships can be assayed in a variety of ways, which include single-unit recording in animal models and non-invasive brain stimulation in humans. Learning does imply that a plastic change has occurred but a plastic change does not imply that learning of a new behaviour has occurred. Thinking otherwise is to commit the classic logical fallacy called 'affirming the consequent': (1) If P, then Q. (2) Q. (3) Therefore, P. Unfortunately, a sizable literature appears to consider UDP important to neurorehabilitation, based largely on this logical fallacy. To appreciate the misunderstanding, consider the classic paper in this area by Classen and colleagues [21]. Transcranial magnetic stimulation (TMS) of the motor cortex was used to evoke isolated and directionally consistent thumb movements through activation of the abductor pollicis brevis muscle. Subjects were then required to practice thumb movements for 30 minutes in the direction approximately opposite to that elicited by TMS. The critical finding was that subsequent TMS was found to evoke movements in or near the direction practiced rather than in the pre-training baseline direction. This is a very interesting result with regard to how movement repetition (it is not really training in so much as the goal is not to improve performance in any way) can lead to changes in cortical representation. Indeed, a very similar mechanism is likely at play in the series of controversial papers published by Graziano and colleagues showing that long duration trains of intracortical microstimulation of monkey motor cortical areas elicit movements that look like natural movements performed at high frequency in everyday life [22]. More recently, it has been shown that TMS in piano players elicits different finger postures than in non-piano players [23].

The crucial point when considering all these UDP-like results is that it is not at all clear what they mean for *voluntary* movements. To appreciate this objection, consider the thumb experiment; although TMS after training causes the thumb to move in a direction roughly similar to the one practised, if a subject is asked to move their thumb in the original pretrained direction they do not suddenly find themselves going in reverse! That is to say, the plastic changes assayed with TMS have not changed voluntary behaviour. Now it is true that when looked for, movement repetitions in one direction can lead to small biases in other directions [24–26] but these biases are only a fraction of the trained direction and can be easily over-ridden in a few trials. Thus at the current time, experiments that induce UDP are informative about how the brain changes with repetition but these changes do not lead to learning of new task-relevant behaviours. Further support for this conclusion comes from the many reported failures of haptic and robotic guidance to benefit training [27, 28]. It appears that the interest in these cortical epiphenomena is out of proportion to their practical usefulness for neurorehabilitation.

To learn complex everyday tasks almost certainly requires that instruction and knowledge combine with adaptation, reinforcement, and acuity mechanisms. For example, instruction and imitation can help select the mean movement that then becomes more precise and reinforced with repeated practice. All these normal learning mechanisms, if intact after stroke, could be used to increase the acuity and accuracy of compensatory movements without any recovery per se.

Table 7.1 Types of motor learning

Type	Anatomy	Example	Relevance
Instruction	Prefrontal cortex	Transfer from bed-to-chair	High
Error-based adaptation	Cerebellum and parietal cortex	Split-belt treadmill for gait	Medium
Reward- and failure-based reinforcement	Motor cortex and basal ganglia	Constraint-induced therapy of arm	High
Motor acuity	Motor cortex	None as of yet	Unclear
Use-dependent plasticity	Motor cortex	None as of yet	Low

Thus far, we have spoken about the different ways that new actions can be acquired and improved. As has already been alluded to for the case of adaptation, acquisition is not of great use if what is learned is not retained across sessions. In addition to retention, it is hoped that training the limb on a task in the rehabilitation clinic will generalize to other activities of daily living. It is surprising how little investigation there has been of retention and generalization of motor learning in the context of neurorehabilitation. One possible reason is that, as we argue here, rehabilitation is mainly compensatory and does not generalize because learning to compensate suffers from the same 'curse of task specificity' as normal motor learning [29]. A notable exception, as already mentioned, is work performed by Bastian and colleagues looking at retention of split-belt treadmill adaptation and its generalization to over-ground walking [16].

All the kinds of motor learning described here (see Table 7.1) for healthy subjects are predicated on the existence of normal neural substrate for the expression of learning, that is, that the motor system can execute the chosen motor commands. It should be immediately apparent that if the neural substrate that generates motor commands is damaged, for example the corticospinal tract (CST) after a capsular infarct, then learning might not be expressible, even if normal [30]. This example should already make it clear that learning is not, on the face of it, an obvious mechanism for reversal of a stroke's effect on performance. It will be argued here that motor learning in response to rehabilitative training after stroke can only operate within the residual performance envelope that the remaining nervous system is capable of after spontaneous biological recovery is complete. That is to say, based on reasoning and current empirical data, the null position taken in this chapter is that motor learning in response to training in the period after spontaneous biological recovery is complete cannot reverse the loss of motor control but is only relevant to learning of compensatory strategies.

Motor learning in the sensitive period after stroke: interaction with spontaneous biological recovery

There is now extensive evidence in both humans and in non-human animal models that almost all recovery of motor control (impairment) occurs in a time-limited window or sensitive period post-stroke; such training-independent recovery is often referred to as spontaneous biological recovery [31]. The sensitive period lasts about 3 months in humans [32, 33] and 1 month in rodents [34]. Evidence suggests that most recovery occurs within the sensitive period because of a unique plasticity environment that is initiated by ischaemia and falls off as a function of time and distance from the infarct. This post-ischaemic environment can be characterized by unique changes in gene expression, in the structure and physiology of synapses, and in excitatory/inhibitory balance [31, 35–37]. The crucial point to be made here is that spontaneous biological recovery in the sensitive period is not motor learning per se but an endogenous repair process that presumably relies on residual intact neural architecture as a template for reorganization. That the repair process may interact with and be augmented by training is of great importance, but task-specific training is not necessary for spontaneous biological recovery [38] and training alone cannot reproduce spontaneous biological recovery outside of the sensitive period. A clear demonstration that recovery can occur in the absence of directed training is the predictable change in the Fugl-Meyer Scale (FMS) between the first week after stroke and 3 months later [33, 39]. The FMS tests the ability to isolate joints and to make multi-joint movements in and out of synergy. As the FMS does not have functional components it is never used for training, nevertheless the FMS can dramatically improve in the sensitive period (Figure 7.1).

The obvious question is how to combine the task specificity of training with the general recovery allowed by spontaneous biological recovery in the sensitive period? Experiments in animal models suggest that the response of the brain to training in the sensitive period is uniquely enhanced and that this responsiveness diminishes as the interval between the stroke and training is increased. In one influential experiment in rats, it was demonstrated that starting re-training 5 days after stroke was much more effective than waiting 2 weeks. By one month the efficacy of task-specific training was not greater than social housing alone. These results, and others, strongly suggest that motor learning in the sensitive period is qualitatively different from motor learning in the chronic state and in healthy animals, and bears similarities to conditions early in development [31, 40]. In primates, a partial ischaemic lesion in motor cortex leads to loss of hand dexterity that recovers fully if training is initially early but is lost completely if delayed [41]. As of this writing, two crucial questions remain unanswered in the case of humans: (1) Does any form of rehabilitation in the sensitive period enhance the generalizing effects of spontaneous biological recovery? (2) Is the response to any given amount of task-specific training greater inside versus outside the sensitive period? These questions are a challenge to address and so it is not so surprising that we do not yet know the answers to them. One problem is that studies need to be adequately powered to detect additional changes riding on top of spontaneous biological recovery. Another is that it is almost certainly necessary to provide high intensity and dosage of training to exploit enhanced plasticity mechanisms, levels that current practice does not come close to achieving in the relevant time window.

A recent study determined that patients were active only 13% of the time and were alone 60% of the time during inpatient rehabilitation [42]. Lang and colleagues, in a study of how much movement practice is provided during rehabilitation (inpatient

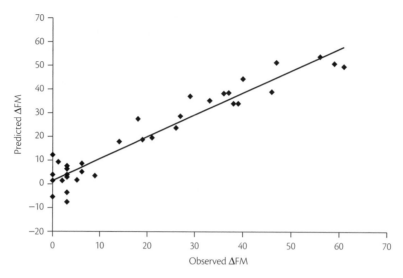

Fig. 7.1 The observed change in Fugl-Meyer Scale (ΔFM) from the first 72 hours after stroke to 3 months is very predictable in most patients using a regression model with initial FMS as a predictor.

and outpatient), found that practice of task-specific, functional upper-extremity movements occurred in only 51% of the rehabilitation sessions that were meant to address upper-limb rehabilitation and that even then the average number of repetitions per session was only 32 [43]. Data from the animal literature suggest that this dosage of repetitions is too low; changes in synaptic density in the primary motor cortex occur after 400 but not 60 reaches [44, 45]. In most rodent stroke recovery studies that use reaching as part of the rehabilitation protocol, there is often no limit imposed on the amount of reaching allowed; rats will typically reach 300 times in a training session. In a recent experiment, the amount of reaching rats were permitted was varied, and it was found that there was a threshold for the amount below which recovery did not occur [46].

Thus current rehabilitation in humans does not come close to reproducing either the dosages or intensities achieved in rodent and primate studies. Further support for the idea that current therapy early after stroke is too under-dosed to have an impact on impairment is the predictability of recovery at 3 months in the FMS after just 48 h: subsequent intervening therapy does not seem to be changing the trajectory of spontaneous biological recovery. On a more hopeful note, a recent feasibility study found that it is possible to deliver a similar number of upper-limb repetitions to stroke patients in a 1-hour therapy session as occurs in typical animal rehabilitation studies [47].

Whenever discussion turns to early intense rehabilitation after stroke, the objection of a possible adverse effect is raised both with respect to exacerbation of lesion volume and a worse behavioural outcome in the affected limb. This objection originates from a series of well-cited studies by Schallert and colleagues in the rat, in which they reported that immobilization of the unaffected forelimb with a hard cast for 15 days post-lesion induction led to less use of the affected side once the cast was removed from the unaffected side compared to when the affected side itself had been immobilized for the same duration. Immobilization of the unaffected limb not only had an adverse effect on behaviour but was also accompanied by expansion in lesion volume [48, 49]. What is less well appreciated is

that in these early studies, the lesions were electrolytic rather than ischaemic, making their relevance to stroke questionable. Subsequently, however, the same group of investigators asked the same question for ischaemic lesions using a middle cerebral artery occlusion (MCAO) model in the rat. Here the results are more equivocal. In the case when 45 minutes of MCAO caused moderate cortical ischaemia, 10 days of casting of the unaffected limb did not lead to exaggeration of infarct volume but did lead to worse behavioural performance [50]. For more severe cortical ischaemia, induced by 90 minutes of three-vessel occlusion, there was no deleterious effect on lesion volume or outcome. In a distal MCAO model that caused subcortical (striatal) infarction, forced non-use but not over-use of the affected forelimb led to detrimental behavioural outcomes but without exaggeration of lesion size [50]. More recently, the same investigators failed to show a behavioural consequence of casting the unaffected limb despite exaggerations of cortical lesion volume [51]. Indeed in this study, as in the earlier subcortical study, it was *disuse* of the affected forelimb that had detrimental effects. Importantly, in these later experiments the cast was smaller and lighter and the rats were housed in larger cages with littermates. Carmichael and colleagues have revisited the effects of overuse. They induced overuse of the affected forelimb one day after the stroke by using Botox in the unaffected limb; there was no increase in infarct size with this approach [52] but the same authors have demonstrated that there is instability in cortical excitability for about 3 to 5 days post-stroke [36, 53].

All the studies cited thus far with respect to deleterious effects of early over-use of the affected limb have been in rodents. Support for a similar effect in humans came from the VECTORS study, in which 52 patients with stroke were randomized at about 10 days post-stroke to two levels of intensity of constraint-induced movement therapy (CIMT) or standard upper-extremity therapy [54]. It should be stated that intense here meant 3 hours versus 2 hours of shaping therapy per day. The surprising result was that at 90 days, affected upper-extremity functional outcome measured with the Arm Research Action Test was worse for the more intensive CIMT group. An impairment measure was not reported in VECTORS. Interestingly, over 60% of the high intensity group had involvement of the dominant limb versus only 30% for the low intensity group. There have been reports of asymmetries in degree of bilateral and non-affected limb use with right and left hemispheric strokes [55], so other factors could have played a role in the results. Finally, longitudinal magnetic resonance imaging (MRI) in a subset of the patients did not show any enlargement of the brain lesion that could be related to intensity of treatment, so there was no evidence for infarct expansion, which was the putative explanation for intensity-related worsening in the early rodent models [48]. A study similar to VECTORS enrolled 23 patients within one week after stroke onset but with only one CIMT intensity level. In this case, the trend favored CIMT, although in the control group, therapy was more intensive than usual in order to match the CIMT group [56].

It is hard not to conclude that as rodent experiments have become more sophisticated, the purported detrimental effects of early affected limb use have become less convincing. In addition, the more recent experiments raise the possibility that immobilizing the unaffected limb can *reduce* practice with the affected limb; in none of these studies was actual frequency or total use of the affected side ever documented, it was just inferred indirectly. Thus it cannot be ruled out that it is immobilization of the unaffected side that is the problem rather than overuse of the affected side. A conservative approach, to allay lingering fears about early exacerbation, might be to ramp up the dose and intensity over the first 5 days post-stroke in the case of large cortical infarcts. It should also be emphasized that CIMT is not the only way to instigate early use of the affected side. For example, increased dosage and intensity of training could be accomplished by robotic therapy of the affected side without any need to immobilize the unaffected side but there have been very few studies of robotics in the first 3 months after stroke to date.

To summarize this section, evidence in humans and in animal models demonstrates that there is a sensitive period after stroke in which most recovery from impairment occurs and in which there is heightened responsiveness to motor training. Future advances in reduction in impairment will almost certainly exploit this sensitive period.

Motor learning in chronic stroke: it's all about compensation

This section is predicated on the assumption that in chronic stroke—that is when patients are 6 months or more post-stroke—brain plasticity and the response to training are no different to what is seen in healthy subjects, with the consequence that treatment effects on impairment are minimal and only compensatory responses can be expected to lead to meaningful improvements in function. Significant decreases in impairment occur almost exclusively in the first 3 months after stroke as a result of an interaction between spontaneous biological recovery and training in this sensitive period. As already outlined, conventional neurorehabilitation in the sensitive period is so low in dose and intensity that it fails to exploit the unique potential for motor learning. Instead, patients are prematurely made to learn compensatory strategies when they should be focusing on reducing impairment in the short time available.

There is undeniable irony in the course taken in neurorehabilitation research thus far—training at the doses and intensities that would potentially be highly beneficial in the sensitive period have instead been attempted almost exclusively outside of it, when it is too late for such training to have an effect on impairment and so only compensation is possible. Here, the term compensation will be restricted to changes in effector, joints and muscles, and not to use of external aids such as walkers, canes, or orthoses. In this framework, motor learning in patients with chronic hemiparesis is in no way different to a healthy person learning to write with their non-dominant arm after breaking their dominant arm, or learning to lean forward and shuffle when walking on a slippery surface. The failure to distinguish between the unique learning conditions that pertain to the sensitive period and the ordinary motor learning that occurs during the rehabilitation of patients with chronic stroke, has led, in our view, to significant conceptual confusion and the design of ill-conceived trials.

The two major forms of neurorehabilitation of the paretic arm in chronic stroke based on motor-learning principles are CIMT, and robotics. There are other learning-based approaches, which include action observation [57, 58], bilateral priming [59], Arm Ability Training [60], electromyography (EMG)-triggered neuromuscular stimulation [61], and virtual reality [62]. We will not cover these other approaches here in any detail because they have received less experimental attention and because the principles that will be discussed here, in our view, apply to them to a large degree.

Constraint-induced movement therapy

CIMT was the focus of the first multicentre randomized trial in neurorehabilitation, EXCITE [7]. The technique has two components: (1) Restraint of the less affected arm and/or hand with a sling or mitten for 90% of waking hours. (2) Task-oriented practice with the affected side using a form of training called *shaping*. The weightings for the two components and the length of the overall treatment have varied considerably in studies since the original trial. It is perhaps under-appreciated that EXCITE was based on some well-thought-out principles first established in de-afferented monkeys by Taub and colleagues. A chapter on motor learning and rehabilitation is a good place to consider the learning principles underlying CIMT in more detail and ask whether they were well suited to application to hemiparesis after stroke in humans.

Taub and colleagues wrote an influential paper in 1994 titled: 'An operant approach to rehabilitation medicine overcoming learned non-use by shaping' [63]. In this paper, the authors presented their new rehabilitation framework based on experiments in monkeys that had been deafferented in one forelimb via dorsal rhizotomy. The key observation was that the monkeys did not resume use of the de-afferented limb even after spinal shock had resolved and use of the limb was again possible. The explanation was that early on when the limb was severely impaired, the monkeys learned that it was useless through negative reinforcement. This learning became a habit despite return of a latent capacity that was not explored. The authors discovered that the habit of non-use could be overcome if the good limb was restrained over days. In addition to use of the restraint, the authors also re-trained the limb in two different ways. In conditioned response training, the monkeys were made to make isolated repetitive movements across single joints and resist against loads. It was noted that these exercises did not generalize to functional tasks (the relevance of this finding to much conventional human neuro-rehabilitation cannot go unnoted). A second, more effective training method, which they called shaping, was to incrementally reward successive approximations to a functional behaviour. In essence, shaping attempted through reward to reverse the non-use that had developed through failure. In the same paper, some promising preliminary data were presented in three patients with stroke. We can now fast forward to EXCITE, a clinical trial predicated on the ideas of restraint and shaping developed in these early studies by Taub and colleagues.

EXCITE showed that patients who received CIMT for 2 weeks had greater responses in a test of motor function and in self-report of performance quality in common daily activities. There was no assessment of motor impairment [7]. What is CIMT accomplishing? Evidence suggests that it is not leading to either significant reductions in impairment or a return to closer to normal levels of motor control [64]. Instead patients seem to be learning to compensate better for their deficit by practising particular tasks using intact residual capacities. The subtle but critical point is that, unlike in the case of a monkey's recovery from spinal shock, patients are not discovering a capacity that they lost and then latently regained. Instead compensatory strategies in the chronic state are performed with capacities that were present from the time of the stroke or were recovered in the sensitive period; they just had not been incorporated into functional tasks through practice. Thus while it seems that an operant approach, as in de-afferented monkeys, does teach useful compensatory strategies in patients after stroke, the mechanistic parallels between CIMT after stroke and after de-afferentation are limited. Learned non-use has never been documented in humans, nor is there evidence of a latent return of capacity in the chronic state. Mention of plasticity and reorganization in the setting of CIMT is misleading unless these terms are thought to apply equally to healthy subjects. For example, to also occur when a healthy person's elbow is splinted into flexion so that within a few attempts they flex their trunk to make a reaching movement. To summarize, CIMT is a rehabilitation approach based on reinforcement through verbal instruction. It relies on the existence of residual actions that can be selected through rewarded practice and incorporated into functional tasks. CIMT has not been shown to lead to the recovery of lost motor control.

Robotic therapy

It is of historical interest that the most popular robotic device for therapy of the upper limb after stroke evolved from the same planar robot used in initial ground-breaking studies of a form of motor learning, force-field adaptation [8]. Two distinct approaches have since been used with robots in the setting of therapy. One approach has been to have the robot guide or constrain the arm to more normal straight trajectories (i.e. shaping). Alternatively, robot-applied force fields may be used to make patients' trajectory errors even larger than their baseline errors (error augmentation [14]). Here, the idea is that when the force field is switched off, immediate after-effects will be more similar to normal movements. Thus two very different kinds of motor learning have been used with the same robotic device: incremental reinforcement (shaping) versus fast error-based learning (adaptation). Interestingly, the data suggest that the former approach has small but lasting effects [65], whereas the latter has impressive but short-lived effects [14]. Similarly, an increasingly investigated split-belt treadmill

paradigm used for gait rehabilitation has shown rapid improvements in gait symmetry in patients with hemiparesis after stroke, presumably through cerebellar-dependent error-based learning but these improvements revert back to baseline asymmetry fairly rapidly (25 strides) when patients return to over-ground ambulation [15]. Planar movements have a unique solution in joint space if the trunk is restrained, which means that it is not compensatory movements that are being trained but instead an attempt is being made to have subjects regain more normal motor control. Thus, robotics is quite different from CIMT. It is important to be clear on what kind of motor learning is being targeted by an approach and whether the goal is impairment reduction or compensation. It is of interest that although not intentional, both CIMT and robotics have reinforcement as their core learning mechanism but ended up having differential efficacy on function and impairment, respectively.

There have been 67 robotic stroke trials between 1997 and 2011. The learning principles underlying the trials are rarely overtly described. The largest robotics trial to date treated patients with chronic stroke (> 6 months) using the MIT-Manus device [66] with results that were essentially negative: patients who received robotic therapy gained only 2 Fugl-Meyer points over the usual care group. A minimum meaningful effect size for the FMS is a change of 7 [67]. A meta-analysis of robotic therapy has also reported a very small FMS change overall [65]. Despite unimpressive results, there are very important lessons to be learned from the Veterans Association ROBOTICS study. First, the study showed that standard of care has no effect at all on impairment, disability or quality of life. This observation alone cries out for the need for new treatments. Second, therapists outside of a research setting would not be able to consistently provide doses of assisted arm movements of around 1,000 per session (the average in real-world settings is 20–45). Third, there were no serious adverse events in 49 patients who performed 1,024 movements per session with the robot, three times a week for 12 weeks.

The reason why the effect sizes on impairment for robotic studies have been so disappointing is that, as previously stated, almost all recovery from impairment occurs in the sensitive period. This window had closed by the time patients were enrolled in almost all the robotic studies to date. Only five robotic trials have been conducted in the first 3 months after stroke, with only one of these showing a FMS change of 5 or more (68). It is not enough, however, to provide robotic therapy in the first 3 months; the kinds of movement will also almost certainly matter. The MIT-Manus robot trains patients to make non-ecological horizontal planar movements; the shoulder and elbow are level with each other. In a very interesting study, six healthy subjects were given a wearable motion-tracking system to record their arm movements as they went about their daily life [69]. Despite the large range of possible movements, the investigators found that during most normal everyday tasks the arms are confined to a small volume of space around the body and movements are predominantly in the vertical, not the horizontal, plane across a variety of tasks. Thus it could be objected that trials with the MIT-Manus and other single joint or planar devices may have failed not because they were outside the sensitive period, but because patients were not trained on functional movements. This possibility has now been addressed in a recently published trial in chronic stroke that used a 3D exoskeletal robot with 7 degrees of freedom [70]. Patients in the study (77 randomized) had fairly severe impairment with a mean FMS of 20/66. Patients received 45 minutes of robotic or standard therapy, three times a week for 8 weeks. Not much detail is provided about either the robotic protocol used or of the motor learning framework it was embedded in. It should be said that it is fairly typical for rehabilitation studies to provide little in the way of methodological detail or conceptual justification with respect to theories of learning. The change in FMS was 4.7 in the case of robotic assistance and 3.1 points after conventional therapy. The difference of 0.78 reached significance but unfortunately this is clinically trivial.

At the current time the most parsimonious conclusion is that no amount of training alone, no matter what motor learning mechanism is recruited, is going to reverse impairment in the chronic state after stroke. It is a biological not a technological limit. It is to be hoped that there will not be a loss of faith in robotic therapy just because it has for the most part been deployed in the wrong time frame after stroke.

Does stroke have an effect on motor learning?

The question of whether learning and not just motor control is impaired after stroke is asked surprisingly infrequently [71]. The question itself can be misunderstood and is also very difficult to answer for methodological reasons. First of all, the relevant question is not whether or not certain strategically localized strokes can cause learning deficits, because the answer is clearly yes. For example, we know that cerebellar and parietal infarcts can have detrimental effects on visuomotor adaptation [72–74]. The critical question is whether the infarcts in motor cortical areas and/or their output pathways that cause hemiparesis also cause a learning deficit. At the time of writing, it has not been convincingly demonstrated that there is a learning deficit in the paretic arm after stroke [71]. One reason that the question is very difficult to answer is that there is a no assumption-free way to compare learning rate, retention or generalization between patients and controls when the levels of initial performance are not matched, as is the obviously case in the setting of hemiparesis. Any attempt to match through normalization, either additive or multiplicative, makes unproven assumptions and can lead to contradictory results [75]. The only way forward is to either have a good justifiable a priori learning model that is predicated on either additive or multiplicative effects, or to try and stratify patients who overlap performance-wise with controls. Such stratification is treacherous because of regression to the mean—one may be conditioning on noise rather than comparing true overlapping high values from one group and low values from another, and therefore requires good estimates of the measurement noise in the learning task chosen. Alternatively one can ask what the degree of retention or generalization is for patients based on what is considered desirable for them rather than making any comparison to controls.

Conclusions and future approaches

Here the case has been made that training has a unique effect on learning and repair in the first 3 months after stroke. In this time window, true reductions in impairment occur both through spontaneous biological recovery and interactions between post-ischaemic plasticity and training. In the chronic phase, motor learning is normal and only leads to task-specific compensatory effects rather than any true reversal of the paretic deficit. It is to be hoped that in the future, pharmacological agents (e.g. selective serotonin receptor inhibitors [76]), trophic support from stem cells, and brain stimulation techniques will augment [77], extend and even re-open the sensitive period in the chronic period [78, 79]. Most clinicians can provide anecdotes about patients who made true progress at the impairment level way beyond the 3-month sensitive period; such patients are also to be found in reported clinical trials. Whether these late responding patients comprise a special subset remains to be investigated but several possibilities suggest themselves. One is that these patients are outliers with respect to the sensitive period. Another is that their main deficit is not classic CST hemiparesis—for example, they have proprioceptive loss, dystonia, or apraxia. Another may be biomechanical or peripheral, for example, fixing one part of the system (e.g. painful or stiff shoulder) allows apparent reduction in impairment elsewhere (distally). Finally, perhaps something has allowed them to reopen their sensitive period to training. In the mean time, the best hope for patients with hemiparesis after stroke is to greatly increase the dose and intensity of impairment-focused therapy for the first 3 months after stroke based on the new findings with regard to learning, plasticity, and neural repair in this sensitive period.

References

1. Krakauer JW. Arm function after stroke: from physiology to recovery. Semin Neurol. 2005;**25**(4):384–395.
2. Stanley J, Krakauer JW. Motor skill depends on knowledge of facts. Front Hum Neurosci. 2013;**7**:503.
3. Milner B. Les troubles de la memoire accompagnant des lesions hippocampiques bilaterales. Physiologie de l'Hippocampe. Centre National de la Recherche, Paris, 1962,, p. 257–272.
4. H Manley, Dayan, P, Diedrichsen J. When Money is Not Enough: Awareness, Success, and Variability in Motor Learning. PLoS One. 2014;**9**(1):e86580
5. Benson BL, Anguera JA, Seidler RD. A spatial explicit strategy reduces error but interferes with sensorimotor adaptation. J Neurophysiol. 2011;**105**(6):2843–2851.
6. Taylor J, Krakauer J, Ivry R. Explict and implicit contributions to learning in a sensorimotor adaptation task. J Neurosci. 2014;**34**(8):3023–3032.
7. Wolf SL, Winstein CJ, Miller JP, et al. Effect of constraint-induced movement therapy on upper extremity function 3 to 9 months after stroke: the EXCITE randomized clinical trial. JAMA. 2006;**296**(17):2095–2104.
8. Shadmehr R, Mussa-Ivaldi FA. Adaptive representation of dynamics during learning of a motor task. J Neurosci. 1994;**14**(5 Pt 2):3208–3224.
9. Krakauer JW, Pine ZM, Ghilardi MF, Ghez C. Learning of visuomotor transformations for vectorial planning of reaching trajectories. J Neurosci. 2000;**20**(23):8916–8924.
10. Thoroughman KA, Shadmehr R. Learning of action through adaptive combination of motor primitives. Nature. 2000;**407**(6805):742–747.
11. Smith MA, Ghazizadeh A, Shadmehr R. Interacting adaptive processes with different timescales underlie short-term motor learning. PLoS Biol. 2006;**4**(6):e179.
12. Mazzoni P, Krakauer JW. An implicit plan overrides an explicit strategy during visuomotor adaptation. J Neurosci. 2006;**26**(14):3642–3645.
13. Tseng Y-W, Diedrichsen J, Krakauer JW, Shadmehr R, Bastian AJ. Sensory prediction errors drive cerebellum-dependent adaptation of reaching. J Neurophysiol. 2007;**98**(1):54–62.

14. Patton JL, Stoykov ME, Kovic M, Mussa-Ivaldi FA. Evaluation of robotic training forces that either enhance or reduce error in chronic hemiparetic stroke survivors. Exp Brain Res. 2006;**168**(3):368–383.

15. Reisman DS, Wityk R, Silver K, Bastian AJ. Split-belt treadmill adaptation transfers to overground walking in persons poststroke. Neurorehabil Neural Repair. 2009;**23**(7):735–744.

16. Reisman DS, McLean H, Keller J, Danks KA, Bastian AJ. Repeated split-belt treadmill training improves poststroke step length asymmetry. Neurorehabil Neural Repair. 2013;**27**(5):460–468.

17. Newport R, Schenk T. Prisms and neglect: what have we learned? Neuropsychologia. 2012;**50**(6):1080–1091.

18. Shmuelof L, Huang VS, Haith AM, Delnicki RJ, Mazzoni P, Krakauer JW. Overcoming motor 'forgetting' through reinforcement of learned actions. J Neurosci. 2012;**32**(42):14617–14621.

19. Shmuelof L, Krakauer JW, Mazzoni P. How is a motor skill learned? Change and invariance at the levels of task success and trajectory control. J Neurophysiol. 2012;**108**(2):578–594.

20. Shmuelof L, Krakauer JW. Are we ready for a natural history of motor learning? Neuron. 2011;**72**(3):469–476.

21. Classen J, Liepert J, Wise SP, Hallett M, Cohen LG. Rapid plasticity of human cortical movement representation induced by practice. J Neurophysiol. 1998;**79**(2):1117–1123.

22. Graziano MSA, Taylor CSR, Moore T. Complex movements evoked by microstimulation of precentral cortex. Neuron. 2002 May 30;**34**(5):841–851.

23. Gentner R, Gorges S, Weise D, aufm Kampe K, Buttmann M, Classen J. Encoding of motor skill in the corticomuscular system of musicians.. 2010;**20**(20):1869–1874.

24. Diedrichsen J, White O, Newman D, Lally N. Use-dependent and error-based learning of motor behaviors. J Neurosci. 2010;**30**(15):5159–5166.

25. Huang VS, Haith A, Mazzoni P, Krakauer JW. Rethinking motor learning and savings in adaptation paradigms: model-free memory for successful actions combines with internal models. Neuron. 2011;**70**(4):787–801.

26. Verstynen T, Sabes PN. How each movement changes the next: an experimental and theoretical study of fast adaptive priors in reaching. J Neurosci. 2011;**31**(27):10050–10059.

27. Winstein CJ, Pohl PS, Lewthwaite R. Effects of physical guidance and knowledge of results on motor learning: support for the guidance hypothesis. Res Q Exerc Sport. 1994;**65**(4):316–323.

28. Liu J, Cramer SC, Reinkensmeyer DJ. Learning to perform a new movement with robotic assistance: comparison of haptic guidance and visual demonstration. J Neuroengineering Rehabil. 2006;**3**:20.

29. Bavelier D, Green CS, Pouget A, Schrater P. Brain plasticity through the life span: learning to learn and action video games. Annu Rev Neurosci. 2012;**35**:391–416.

30. Takahashi CD, Reinkensmeyer DJ. Hemiparetic stroke impairs anticipatory control of arm movement. Exp Brain Res. 2003;**149**(2):131–140.

31. Zeiler SR, Krakauer JW. The interaction between training and plasticity in the poststroke brain. Curr Opin Neurol. 2013;**26**(6):609–616.

32. Duncan PW, Goldstein LB, Matchar D, Divine GW, Feussner J. Measurement of motor recovery after stroke. Outcome assessment and sample size requirements. Stroke J Cereb Circ. 1992;**23**(8):1084–1089.

33. Prabhakaran S, Zarahn E, Riley C, et al. Inter-individual variability in the capacity for motor recovery after ischemic stroke. Neurorehabil Neural Repair. 2008;**22**(1):64–71.

34. Biernaskie J, Chernenko G, Corbett D. Efficacy of rehabilitative experience declines with time after focal ischemic brain injury. J Neurosci. 2004;**24**(5):1245–1254.

35. Murphy TH, Corbett D. Plasticity during stroke recovery: from synapse to behaviour. Nat Rev Neurosci. 2009;**10**(12):861–872.

36. Clarkson AN, Huang BS, Macisaac SE, Mody I, Carmichael ST. Reducing excessive GABA-mediated tonic inhibition promotes functional recovery after stroke. Nature. 2010;**468**(7321):305–309.

37. Carmichael ST. Brain excitability in stroke: the yin and yang of stroke progression. Arch Neurol. 2012;**69**(2):161–167.

38. Biernaskie J, Corbett D. Enriched rehabilitative training promotes improved forelimb motor function and enhanced dendritic growth after focal ischemic injury. J Neurosci. 2001;**21**(14):5272–5280.

39. Zarahn E, Alon L, Ryan SL, Lazar RM, Vry M-S, Weiller C, et al. Prediction of motor recovery using initial impairment and fMRI 48 h poststroke. Cereb Cortex.. 2011;**21**(12):2712–2721.

40. Cramer SC, Chopp M. Recovery recapitulates ontogeny. Trends Neurosci. 2000;**23**(6):265–271.

41. Nudo RJ, Wise BM, SiFuentes F, Milliken GW. Neural substrates for the effects of rehabilitative training on motor recovery after ischemic infarct. Science. 1996;**272**(5269):1791–1794.

42. Bernhardt J, Dewey H, Thrift A, Donnan G. Inactive and alone: physical activity within the first 14 days of acute stroke unit care. Stroke J Cereb Circ. 2004;**35**(4):1005–1009.

43. Lang CE, Macdonald JR, Reisman DS, et al. Observation of amounts of movement practice provided during stroke rehabilitation. Arch Phys Med Rehabil. 2009;**90**(10):1692–1698.

44. Remple MS, Bruneau RM, VandenBerg PM, Goertzen C, Kleim JA. Sensitivity of cortical movement representations to motor experience: evidence that skill learning but not strength training induces cortical reorganization. Behav Brain Res. 2001;**123**(2):133–141.

45. Luke LM, Allred RP, Jones TA. Unilateral ischemic sensorimotor cortical damage induces contralesional synaptogenesis and enhances skilled reaching with the ipsilateral forelimb in adult male rats. Synapse. 2004;**54**(4):187–199.

46. MacLellan CL, Keough MB, Granter-Button S, Chernenko GA, Butt S, Corbett D. A critical threshold of rehabilitation involving brain-derived neurotrophic factor is required for poststroke recovery. Neurorehabil Neural Repair. 2011;**25**(8):740–748.

47. Birkenmeier RL, Prager EM, Lang CE. Translating animal doses of task-specific training to people with chronic stroke in 1-hour therapy sessions: a proof-of-concept study. Neurorehabil Neural Repair. 2010;**24**(7):620–635.

48. Kozlowski DA, James DC, Schallert T. Use-dependent exaggeration of neuronal injury after unilateral sensorimotor cortex lesions. J Neurosci. 1996;**16**(15):4776–4786.

49. Humm JL, Kozlowski DA, James DC, Gotts JE, Schallert T. Use-dependent exacerbation of brain damage occurs during an early post-lesion vulnerable period. Brain Res. 1998;**783**(2):286–292.

50. Bland ST, Pillai RN, Aronowski J, Grotta JC, Schallert T. Early overuse and disuse of the affected forelimb after moderately severe intraluminal suture occlusion of the middle cerebral artery in rats. Behav Brain Res. 200129;**126**(1–2):33–41.

51. Bland ST, Schallert T, Strong R, Aronowski J, Grotta JC, Feeney DM. Early exclusive use of the affected forelimb after moderate transient focal ischemia in rats: functional and anatomic outcome. Stroke J Cereb Circ. 2000;**31**(5):1144–1152.

52. Overman JJ, Clarkson AN, Wanner IB, et al. A role for ephrin-A5 in axonal sprouting, recovery, and activity-dependent plasticity after stroke. Proc Natl Acad Sci U S A. 2012;**109**(33):E2230–2239.

53. Clarkson AN, Overman JJ, Zhong S, Mueller R, Lynch G, Carmichael ST. AMPA receptor-induced local brain-derived neurotrophic factor signaling mediates motor recovery after stroke. J Neurosci. 2011;**31**(10):3766–3775.

54. Dromerick AW, Lang CE, Birkenmeier RL, et al. Very Early Constraint-Induced Movement during Stroke Rehabilitation (VECTORS): A single-center RCT. Neurology. 2009;**73**(3):195–201.

55. Harris JE, Eng JJ. Individuals with the dominant hand affected following stroke demonstrate less impairment than those with the nondominant hand affected. Neurorehabil Neural Repair. 2006;**20**(3):380–389.

56. Boake C, Noser EA, Ro T, Baraniuk S, Gaber M, Johnson R, et al. Constraint-induced movement therapy during early stroke rehabilitation. Neurorehabil Neural Repair. 2007;**21**(1):14–24.

57. Ertelt D, Hemmelmann C, Dettmers C, Ziegler A, Binkofski F. Observation and execution of upper-limb movements as a tool for rehabilitation of motor deficits in paretic stroke patients: protocol of a randomized clinical trial. BMC Neurol. 2012;**12**:42.

58. Cowles T, Clark A, Mares K, Peryer G, Stuck R, Pomeroy V. Observation-to-imitate plus practice could add little to physical therapy benefits within 31 days of stroke: translational randomized controlled trial. Neurorehabil Neural Repair. 2013;**27**(2):173–182.

59. Stinear CM, Petoe MA, Anwar S, Barber PA, Byblow WD. Bilateral priming accelerates recovery of upper limb function after stroke: a randomized controlled trial. Stroke J Cereb Circ. 2014;**45**(1):205–210.

60. Plautz EJ, Milliken GW, Nudo RJ. Effects of repetitive motor training on movement representations in adult squirrel monkeys: role of use versus learning. Neurobiol Learn Mem. 2000;**74**(1):27–55.

61. Cauraugh J, Light K, Kim S, Thigpen M, Behrman A. Chronic motor dysfunction after stroke: recovering wrist and finger extension by electromyography-triggered neuromuscular stimulation. Stroke J Cereb Circ. 2000;**31**(6):1360–1364.

62. Turolla A, Dam M, Ventura L, et al. Virtual reality for the rehabilitation of the upper limb motor function after stroke: a prospective controlled trial. J Neuroengineering Rehabil. 2013;**10**:85.

63. Taub E, Crago JE, Burgio LD, et al. An operant approach to rehabilitation medicine: overcoming learned nonuse by shaping. J Exp Anal Behav. 1994;**61**(2):281–293.

64. Kitago T, Liang J, Huang VS, et al. Improvement after constraint-induced movement therapy: recovery of normal motor control or task-specific compensation? Neurorehabil Neural Repair. 2013;**27**(2):99–109.

65. Kwakkel G, Kollen BJ, Krebs HI. Effects of robot-assisted therapy on upper limb recovery after stroke: a systematic review. Neurorehabil Neural Repair. 2008;**22**(2):111–121.

66. Lo AC, Guarino PD, Richards LG, Haselkorn JK, Wittenberg GF, Federman DG, et al. Robot-assisted therapy for long-term upper-limb impairment after stroke. N Engl J Med. 2010;**362**(19):1772–1783.

67. Gladstone DJ, Danells CJ, Black SE. The Fugl-Meyer assessment of motor recovery after stroke: a critical review of its measurement properties. Neurorehabil Neural Repair. 2002;**16**(3):232–240.

68. Hesse S, Werner C, Pohl M, Rueckriem S, Mehrholz J, Lingnau ML. Computerized arm training improves the motor control of the severely affected arm after stroke: a single-blinded randomized trial in two centers. Stroke J Cereb Circ. 2005;**36**(9):1960–1966.

69. Howard IS, Ingram JN, Körding KP, Wolpert DM. Statistics of natural movements are reflected in motor errors. J Neurophysiol. 2009;**102**(3):1902–1910.

70. Klamroth-Marganska V, Blanco J, Campen K, et al. Three-dimensional, task-specific robot therapy of the arm after stroke: a multicentre, parallel-group randomised trial. Lancet Neurol. 2013;**13**(2):159–66;

71. Kitago T, Krakauer JW. Motor learning principles for neurorehabilitation. Handb Clin Neurol. 2013;**110**:93–103.

72. Mutha PK, Sainburg RL, Haaland KY. Left parietal regions are critical for adaptive visuomotor control. J Neurosci. 2011;**31**(19):6972–6981.

73. Martin TA, Keating JG, Goodkin HP, Bastian AJ, Thach WT. Throwing while looking through prisms. I. Focal olivocerebellar lesions impair adaptation. Brain J Neurol. 1996;**119** (Pt 4):1183–1198.

74. Donchin O, Rabe K, Diedrichsen J, Lally N, Schoch B, Gizewski ER, et al. Cerebellar regions involved in adaptation to force field and visuomotor perturbation. J Neurophysiol. 2012;**107**(1):134–147.

75. Kitago T, Krakauer JW. Losing control: brain vs spinal cord. Neurology. 2010;**74**(16):1250–1251.

76. Chollet F, Tardy J, Albucher J-F, et al. Fluoxetine for motor recovery after acute ischaemic stroke (FLAME): a randomised placebo-controlled trial. Lancet Neurol. 2011;**10**(2):123–130.

77. Reis J, Schambra HM, Cohen LG, et al. Noninvasive cortical stimulation enhances motor skill acquisition over multiple days through an effect on consolidation. Proc Natl Acad Sci U S A. 2009;**106**(5):1590–1595.

78. Takesian AE, Hensch TK. Balancing plasticity/stability across brain development. Prog Brain Res. 2013;**207**:3–34.

79. Gervain J, Vines BW, Chen LM, et al. Valproate reopens critical-period learning of absolute pitch. Front Syst Neurosci. 2013;**7**:102.

Physiological consequences of CNS damage

CHAPTER 8

Spinal neuronal dysfunction after deprivation of supraspinal input

Michèle Hubli and Volker Dietz

Introduction

In the last two decades, the field of spinal cord injury (SCI) research has achieved a number of discoveries that help to understand the processes of degeneration, inflammation and recovery of function after this devastating condition. Several experimental approaches in animal models indicate promising findings concerning a partial repair of damaged neuronal tracts even after a severe SCI in humans. The main experimental strategies for repair include: (i) neuroprotective and anti-inflammatory treatments; (ii) enhancement of axonal fibre regeneration and compensatory axonal sprouting; and (iii) transplantation of bridges or stem cells [1]. Most of these treatment strategies show some improvement in animal models on the anatomical and/or the functional level [2, 3]. However, the current situation with regard to translate these experimental treatments to human SCI is less convincing.

Several clinical trials failed or were aborted since the promising achievements in animal experiments often could not be replicated in human SCI [2–4]. For example, one of the most promising treatments was the application of the neuroprotective steroid methylprednisolone that showed beneficial neuroanatomical and functional changes in rodent SCI [5, 6] as well as partial efficacy in human SCI [7, 8]. Although methylprednisolone was accepted as a neuroprotective treatment for acute human SCI today in most countries its application in clinical practice has been given up due to low efficacy and significant side effects in human SCI [9].

A successful translation of promising experimental treatments of SCI into a clinical trial in humans relies on specific features pertaining to human SCI condition [10]. Several factors could explain the discrepancy in results between animal models and clinical studies, such as differences in the level and type of lesion, or the treatment onset. For example, treatments in rodents are usually administered directly after the injury, while treatment effects in the subacute and chronic stage of rodent SCI are less usual and little understood [11]. In humans, however, repair treatments are frequently delayed until a chronic stage (ca. 1 year post-lesion) because at this time the clinical condition is more stable and no spontaneous neurological recovery is expected [12].

Interestingly, the only effective therapy for functional recovery following SCI and stroke up to now are rehabilitative training approaches. Well-established rehabilitation approaches focus on the facilitation of neuroplasticity by training to improve muscle activation and function. This positive neuroplasticity is opposed by negative neuroplasticity (for review see [13]). During the past decade, a focus of research was to investigate the change of neuronal activity below the level of lesion in non-trained, that is, immobilized SCI [14–16] and severely affected hemiparetic stroke subjects [17]. Evidence arose from studies in subjects with chronic motor-complete SCI that the function of spinal neuronal circuits below the level of lesion is impaired [14, 15]—that is when signs of a 'negative' neuroplasticity become apparent. The preservation of spinal neuronal function below the level of lesion is an important prerequisite for the success of any kind of future regeneration-inducing therapies. Therefore, the purpose of this chapter is to summarize the alterations of spinal neuronal circuits that lack supraspinal input after an SCI and stroke, and to discuss potential countermeasures to prevent neuronal dysfunction in the chronic stage of the injury.

Electrophysiological assessment of spinal neuronal function

Information about changes of spinal neuronal function after a severe lesion to the spinal cord can be gained by non-invasive electrophysiological assessments, such as lower leg muscle electromyography (EMG) recordings of locomotor activity during assisted locomotion of subjects, and spinal reflex (SR) recordings (see Figure 8.1). Within the last 10 years such assessments, mainly performed in subjects with motor-complete SCI and hemiparetic stroke revealed significant alterations in spinal neuronal function several months after injury [14, 15, 17]. This might affect rehabilitation outcome of subjects suffering from a severe SCI or stroke in the future. In this section of the chapter we describe two different techniques acting as neuronal windows into spinal neuronal circuitries underlying locomotion and their changes after deprivation of supraspinal drive.

Neuronal basis of locomotor activity

A century of research into the organization of the neuronal processes underlying the control of locomotion in invertebrates and vertebrates has demonstrated that the basic neuronal circuitries responsible for generating efficient stepping patterns are embedded within the lumbosacral spinal cord [18]. At the beginning of the last century Graham-Brown postulated his 'half-centre' hypothesis which demonstrated the intrinsic capacity of the mammalian spinal neuronal circuitries to generate rhythmic motor patterns without descending or sensory input [19]. For example,

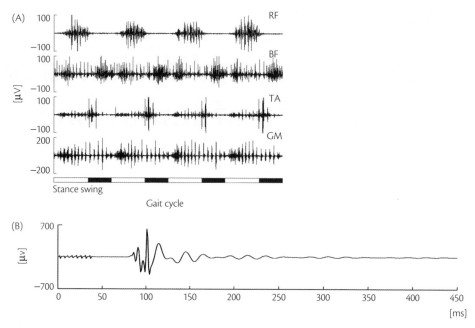

Fig. 8.1 Electrophysiological assessments of spinal neuronal function. (A) Example of locomotor EMG activity during assisted walking in the driven gait orthosis Lokomat in an acute (3 months after SCI) paraplegic subject. This subject suffered a motor-complete SCI and leg muscle activity was recorded in rectus femoris (RF), biceps femoris (BF), tibialis anterior (TA), and gastrocnemius medialis (GM). (B) Polysynaptic SR response (early component, latency ~80 ms) in a healthy subject (25 years old). Reflex response is recorded in the ipsilateral tibialis anterior muscle (ankle flexor) evoked by tibial nerve stimulation at the dorsal aspect of the medial malleolus. The stimulus artefact of the electrical pulse (eight bipolar rectancular pulses, 2 ms pulse width, 200 Hz) is present at the onset of the EMG recording.
Modified from [15] and [42], with permission.

cats with a complete spinal cord transection at thoracic segments gradually improve hindlimb locomotion on a treadmill following 2–3 weeks of daily locomotor training [20, 21]. The spinal cat can relearn walking with alternating steps in the hindlimbs, body weight support, and plantar foot placement. Under such circumstances the EMG activity of the hindlimbs was remarkably similar before and after the spinal cord transection. It has been shown that, with ongoing training, the body support can be decreased associated with improved locomotor capacity until no more support of body weight is required and well-coordinated hindlimb stepping movements can be performed [22]. Also, in non-human primates with complete spinal cord lesions the isolated spinal cord has the capacity to produce stepping patterns [23].

In contrast to cats and non-human primates, stepping-like leg movements are more difficult to induce after a complete SCI in humans. However, when an appropriate afferent input is provided during assisted stepping, a well-organized rhythmic locomotor EMG pattern can be induced even in subjects with complete SCI (see Figure 8.1A) [24–27]. The analysis of such locomotor EMG patterns produced in the absence of descending supraspinal control, as for example in complete SCI subjects, provides important information regarding the role of spinal neuronal circuits and their interaction with afferent input to generate locomotor activity.

Spinal reflex behaviour

The simplest and best understood SR is the monosynaptic H-reflex, where the stimulated muscle/nerve site is also target of the reflex response. On the other hand, polysynaptic reflexes have several interneurons intercalated in the mediating reflex pathway. The most known examples of such polysynaptic reflexes are the

flexor (or withdrawal) reflex and the cutaneous reflex [28]. These reflexes are evoked either by a short train of electrical noxious stimuli (flexor reflex) or non-noxious stimuli (cutaneous reflex) that are applied to a leg nerve. A true withdrawal response of the ipsilateral leg can only be obtained by applying a strong, that is, noxious nerve stimulation. In contrast to monosynaptic reflexes, polysynaptic reflexes can consist of two reflex responses: an early and a late component which appear in synergistic muscle groups—predominantly in the flexor muscles of the stimulated leg. Figure 8.1B shows a typical example of a polysynaptic reflex response (early reflex component) in the ankle flexor of a healthy subject to non-noxious nerve stimulation.

This chapter will only focus on the alterations of polysynaptic SR behaviour evoked by non-noxious nerve stimulation after SCI and stroke. It is assumed that polysynaptic SR closely interact with spinal neuronal centres that control locomotion (central pattern generators), and might even form a part of them [15]. Therefore, the analysis of polysynaptic SR can provide complementary insights into the behaviour of spinal neuronal circuitries. Information about the changes in organization of propriospinal neurons and the interaction of proprioceptive input to spinal locomotor circuitries can be provided by SR recording evoked by electrical stimulation of a leg nerve in subjects with deprived supraspinal input.

Time course of spinal neuronal dysfunction

The longitudinal examination of changes in spinal neuronal function after SCI has only been recently addressed. It represents an important step towards the understanding of changes in spinal neuronal function below the level of a spinal cord lesion. So far, the relationship between polysynaptic SR and muscle spasms [29, 30] or the influence of force-related input on these reflex responses [31, 32] have been the focus of research in SCI subjects.

In general, spinal neuronal dysfunctions after a severe SCI can be divided in three different stages (see Figure 8.2). The next section will give an insight into longitudinal changes of SR behaviour and locomotor EMG activity in SCI subjects in relation to clinical signs of a severe SCI.

Acute, transition, and chronic stages of SCI

The very acute phase of a severe SCI classified according to the American Spinal Injury Association Impairment Scale (AIS) as AIS A and B (motor-complete) is followed by a spinal shock. During this phase locomotor ability is lost, and no polysynaptic SR can be evoked, but H-reflex is still present [33]. Approximately 6 weeks after the injury, when spinal shock vanishes, an early SR component (latency ~80 ms) which is normally present in neurologically intact healthy subjects (see Figure 8.1B), reappears following tibial nerve stimulation [15, 33]. A comparable phenomenon of SR behaviour can be observed in rats with complete spinal cord transection [34, 35]. The reappearance of SR activity is accompanied by the capability to induce a locomotor EMG activity in both rats [34] and humans [15, 36] when an appropriate proprioceptive input (loading, hip extension) is provided during assisted leg movements with body weight support, for example, by a driven gait orthosis. Over the subsequent weeks the amplitude of locomotor EMG pattern and SR activity increases. However, compared to healthy subjects, the locomotor EMG amplitude stays on a low level.

A steady state of spinal neuronal activity that underlies both locomotor and SR function is reached after about 6 months [33]. Recordings of SR show successively smaller amplitudes of the early reflex component, while H-reflex remains unchanged [33].

In the transition phase (between 6 and 12 months after SCI) a shift from dominant early to dominant late SR components occurs [15]. Clinically, a complete SCI at this stage is characterized by the development of spasticity including increased muscle tone, spasms, and exaggerated tendon tap reflexes. Several studies have indicated that long-latency (or polysynaptic) reflexes are reduced in amplitude after SCI or stroke and that the increased muscle tone at this and later stages of the central neural lesion cannot be explained by a neuronal hyperactivity but, rather by secondarily occurring non-neuronal changes, such as altered muscle mechanics [37, 38]. Changes in mechanical muscle properties can involve loss of sarcomeres, changes in muscle–joint relationship [39], and the properties of collagen tissue and tendons. These changes can partly compensate for paresis and allow support of body weight during walking in incomplete SCI and stroke subjects, as seen in the condition of spastic movement disorder (for review see [40]).

The most profound changes in spinal neuronal function occur about 1 year after a severe SCI. At this chronic stage spinal neuronal dysfunction is fully developed (for review see [41, 42]) and is reflected in two major phenomena: (i) a shift from a dominant early to a dominant late SR component and (ii) a locomotor EMG exhaustion. These two important alterations in spinal neuronal function after a severe SCI occur simultaneously (Figure 8.3).

The late (latency ~ 250 ms) SR component following tibial nerve stimulation appears around 6 to 12 months after a severe SCI and fully dominates about 2 years post-injury while no more early component appears. This alteration in SR pattern is accompanied by changes in spinal locomotor circuitries producing a locomotor EMG pattern during assisted locomotion of SCI subjects. Also, the locomotor EMG exhaustion phenomenon starts around 6 to 12 months post-injury and is characterized by a drop of EMG amplitude to near noise level within the first 5 to 10 min of assisted locomotion [14]. The EMG exhaustion is more pronounced in the

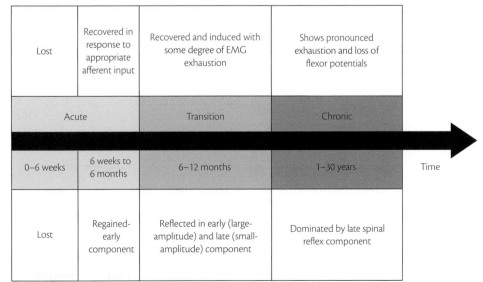

Fig. 8.2 Time course of electrophysiological changes after severe SCI in humans. EMG, electromyographic.

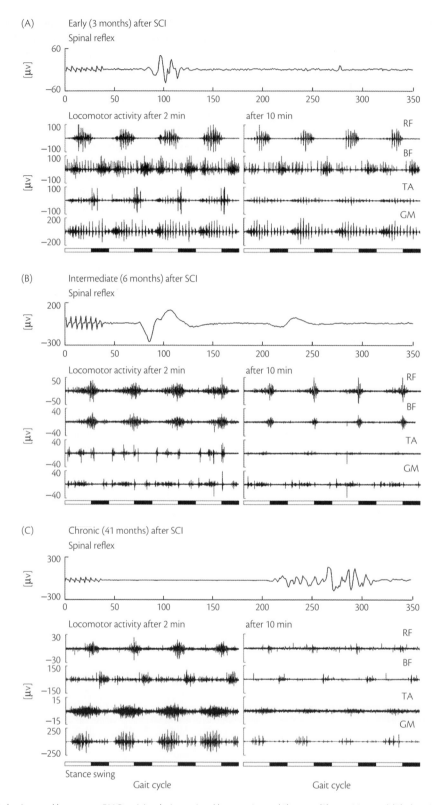

Fig. 8.3 Time course of SR behaviour and locomotor EMG activity during assisted locomotion at (A) acute, (B) transition and (C) chronic stage following a complete SCI. SR was evoked at the tibial nerve and recorded in the ipsilateral tibialis anterior muscle. Locomotor activity of four leg muscles is shown at the beginning and 10 min after assisted locomotion.

Modified from [15] and [42], with permission.

leg flexor than extensor muscles. In addition, a partial loss of EMG activity (see Figure 8.3A–C) occurs at this stage, independently of the EMG exhaustion. The initially partial, and later almost complete, loss of EMG potentials mainly concerns the tibialis anterior muscle. This might be attributed to a transsynaptic degeneration of motoneurons after SCI [43, 44].

The exhaustion phenomenon itself is assumed to take part at premotoneuronal, that is, spinal interneuronal level [14]. Two observations support this assumption: first, repetitive nerve stimulation does not change the amplitudes of muscle action potentials and of H-reflexes [45]; second, despite EMG exhaustion of locomotor activity, leg muscle activity can suddenly increase due to muscle cramps/spasms induced by stumbling.

Earlier studies have investigated the development of neuronal dysfunction only in severe (AIS A and B) SCI. However, studies in the last few years have shown that long-lasting immobility and the concurrent reduced proprioceptive input to spinal neuronal circuitries rather than the completeness of an SCI contributes to the development of the EMG exhaustion phenomenon and change in SR pattern. Also immobilized, motor-incomplete (AIS C) show a neuronal dysfunction [16]. Although in most motor-complete SCI subjects (AIS A and B) an EMG exhaustion occurs during assisted locomotion, subjects with motor-incomplete SCI (AIS C and D) who regularly perform stepping movements show no EMG exhaustion, and the early SR component remains dominant. In contrast, incomplete SCI subjects who are wheelchair-bound show the same exhaustion of EMG activity associated with a dominant late SR component as do AIS A and B SCI subjects [16].

Comparisons with chronic stroke

Stroke and SCI are both central nervous system (CNS) lesions and affected subjects share several clinical and functional similarities, such as paresis, increased muscle tone, and exaggerated tendon tap reflexes, leading to a spastic movement disorder. In contrast to SCI subjects, hemiparetic stroke subjects have partially preserved neuronal interactions between the unaffected and the affected leg [46, 47], which might lead to different alterations in spinal neuronal circuitries compared to SCI. It has been shown that also in stroke subjects polysynaptic SR undergo changes in the chronic stage, such as the development of a dominant late SR component [17]. However, in contrast to SCI subjects, this late component was only present in the affected leg of severely disabled chronic stroke subjects [17]. Another difference to SCI subjects was that in stroke subjects the dominant late SR component was not associated with an EMG exhaustion of leg muscle activity during assisted locomotion, even when stepping movements were performed solely by the affected leg [17]. Explanations for these differences between chronic hemiparetic stroke and SCI subjects might be the compensatory function of the unaffected leg and the interlimb interactions in stroke subjects. This would be in line with the neuronal coupling between the affected and unaffected legs during locomotion [46, 48]. Another explanation could be the observation that an improvement in walking ability is not associated with a change in leg muscle activation and the small, little modulated EMG amplitude in the affected leg during walking after stroke [49, 50]. This might prevent a locomotor EMG exhaustion in hemiparetic stroke subjects.

Despite common clinical characteristics of stroke and SCI, there are specific effects on spinal neuronal circuits underlying locomotion. The unilateral deprivation of supraspinal drive (stroke) leads to a dysfunction of spinal neuronal circuits over time which differs to some extent from the bilateral one (SCI): for example, no change in the leg muscle activation pattern occurs in the affected leg after stroke [50]. Consequently, neurorehabilitation in hemiparetic stroke subjects should focus on the affected leg, in a similar way to constraint-induced movement therapy of the affected arm in stroke subjects [51]. Using such an approach of a specific training of the affected leg, compensation by the unaffected leg could be diminished and a spinal neuronal dysfunction (i.e. a shift to dominant late SR components), might be avoided.

Pathophysiological basis of neuronal dysfunction

The pathophysiology underlying the EMG exhaustion phenomenon and the development of a dominant late SR component in SCI subjects is not yet fully understood. It is assumed that the neuronal changes occur on a premotoneuronal, that is, interneuronal level [41]. Two potential mechanisms have been considered to contribute to spinal neuronal dysfunction after severe SCI: first, a neuronal degradation and second, a phenomenon ascribed to a synaptic 'fatigue' resulting from a dominant inhibitory drive of synaptic transmission following the lack of use of neural pathways in immobilized subjects with chronic stroke/SCI. Recent studies in subjects with motor-complete and incomplete SCI subjects favour the latter idea. The following section elaborates pro and contra arguments for the mechanisms underlying a spinal neuronal dysfunction after SCI.

Dysbalance of excitatory and inhibitory drive

The observation that locomotor training in motor-complete SCI subjects can neither reverse the EMG exhaustion nor the dominance of the late SR component would be in line with the assumption of a degradation of spinal neuronal function [14, 16]. In contrast, the persistent possibility to induce a locomotor pattern by assisted walking in motor-complete SCI subjects even more than 25 years after the injury favours the assumption that the changes in locomotor and SR function in chronic SCI origin from a shift towards the dominance of inhibitory drive within neuronal circuits leading to a neuronal dysfunction, rather than from a degradation of neuronal function. Another argument that strengthens the latter assumption is the finding that locomotor EMG exhaustion and development of a dominant late SR component can be reversed by intensive locomotor training in motor-incomplete SCI subjects [16]. Thus, the functional state of spinal neuronal circuitries is not fixed, but rather plastic and it can be altered by an appropriate training [16] (see section 'Countermeasures and clinical impact').

The lack of use of neuronal pathways underlying locomotion in chronic SCI due to loss of supraspinal and appropriate proprioceptive input is suggested to cause a dominance of inhibitory drive within locomotor circuitries (see Figure 8.4). This suggestion is based on the knowledge that the locomotor pattern in vertebrates is shaped by a close interaction of excitatory and inhibitory drive within interneuronal circuitries [18, 52]. An SCI leads to a deprivation of input to excitatory interneurons from supraspinal and appropriate proprioceptive input (Figure 8.4B and C). As a consequence, this deprivation leads to a dominance of inhibitory drive and weakening of excitatory

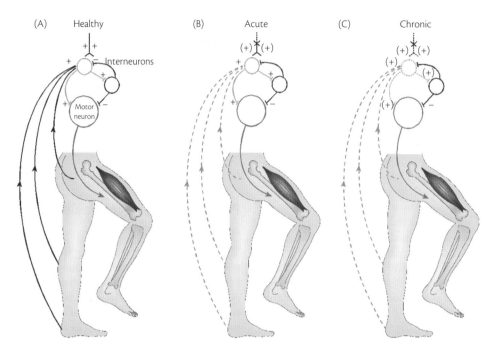

Fig. 8.4 Alterations of spinal neuronal function controlling locomotion and spinal reflexes after SCI. In healthy subjects (A) and SCI subjects in the acute stage (<1 year post-lesion) (B), excitatory and inhibitory spinal neuronal circuits shape the locomotor pattern. After an SCI, the supraspinal and appropriate sensory input that normally activates excitatory neuronal pathways (A) becomes lost (B). Over the subsequent months, this loss leads to impaired function of excitatory spinal neuronal circuits, while the function of the inhibitory neurons remains intact (C). Thus, in the chronic stage of an SCI, the balance between excitatory and inhibitory spinal neuronal circuits shaping the locomotor output shifts towards a predominance of inhibitory signalling.
Modified from [14], with permission.

interneuronal activity. Such a bias to neuronal inhibition could explain the decrease of EMG amplitude during assisted locomotion and the dominance of a late SR component (for review see [41, 42]). The proposed mechanism is still a hypothesis and has to be proven in the future. Comparable changes in balance between excitatory and inhibitory drive within spinal neuronal circuitries have been described in cats with SCI [53, 54]. As a consequence weakening the inhibitory glycinergic drive by a locomotor training could improve walking capacity in spinal cats [55, 56].

Countermeasures and clinical impact

The success of any regeneration inducing therapy to partially repair an SCI and to induce functional recovery will heavily depend on the preserved function of spinal neuronal circuitries below the level of lesion. It is expected that presently such therapies applied in chronic SCI subjects could hardly be beneficial due to spinal neuronal dysfunction, until appropriate countermeasures are developed. The next section provides some insights into possible countermeasures to prevent the development of neuronal dysfunction after SCI. Especially functional locomotor training has an important role in this regard.

Locomotor training—appropriate sensory cues

Although the EMG exhaustion phenomenon and the dominant late SR component could not yet be reversed in the chronic stage of a motor-complete SCI [14, 16], in the last few years evidence came up that spinal neuronal dysfunction can be, at least partially, reversed by an intensive locomotor training in severely affected incomplete SCI subjects (AIS C) [16]. The crucial aspect for a successful functional training seems to be the provision of appropriate sensory cues to strengthen

the activity in excitatory neuronal circuitries underlying the generation of a locomotor pattern. Afferent input from muscles, joints, and skin receptors interact dynamically with spinal neuronal circuitries and this interaction shapes the locomotor activity (for review see [57]). The most relevant proprioceptive input to activate spinal locomotor circuitries in subject with SCI originates from load and hip joint receptors [25, 58]. Load information is provided from leg extensor muscles (namely Ib afferent signals from Golgi tendon organs), and probably also from mechanoreceptors in the foot sole [59]. In addition, the following observations highlight the significance of hip joint receptors in the activation of spinal neuronal circuits underlying the generation of a locomotor pattern [27]. Robotic assisted locomotion with blocked knee and/or ankle joint movements induces a 'normal' locomotor EMG activity in motor-complete SCI subjects. However, when the hip joint becomes blocked, only focal stretch reflexes are present.

One month of intense locomotor training with the appropriate load and hip joint related afferent input and additional functional electrical stimulation of the peroneal nerve at the onset of the swing phase has shown to reverse spinal neuronal dysfunction in a severely affected, non-ambulatory, but motor-incomplete SCI subject [16]. Such a combination of afferent input provided during locomotor training might attenuate inhibitory activity and re-establish a balance between inhibitory and excitatory drive within spinal neuronal circuitries. Corresponding observations were made earlier in a cat model after hindlimb locomotor training [55] or in spinal rats in which 'non-functional' neuronal circuits were transformed into a 'functional' state using epidural stimulation and pharmacological interventions together with locomotor training [60].

Neuromodulatory approaches

The importance of appropriate afferent information from peripheral receptors as a source of activating spinal neuronal circuitries became obvious from experiments in completely transected animals and motor-complete SCI subjects during the last decades. Reduced proprioceptive feedback after an SCI has a negative impact on spinal neuronal function as well as on the concurrent recovery of locomotor function. Therefore, besides an intensive functional training, tools to artificially activate spinal neuronal circuits are needed. Several neuromodulatory strategies aim to increase excitability of spinal neuronal circuitries in order to tune their physiological state to a level that leads to a locomotor facilitation and might even counteract the development of spinal neuronal dysfunction in chronic SCI subjects. Examples of such potential strategies include continuous vibration of the quadriceps and hamstring muscle groups [61], continuous electrical stimulation of the peroneal or sural nerves [62], and magnetic stimulation of the spinal cord [63]. The latter approach, applied repetitively over the thoracolumbar spine, was able to activate spinal locomotor circuitries in healthy subjects. However, so far there is no evidence that this kind of non-noxious magnetic stimulation is able to enhance spinal neuronal activity and, consequently evoke a locomotor activity also in SCI subjects. Electrical epidural stimulation at the thoracolumbar level of the spinal cord in complete SCI subjects could induce locomotor EMG activity [64–66]. Besides electrical or magnetic stimulation approaches, various pharmacological agents, such as serotonergic and noradrenergic agonists, can increase spinal neuronal activity in animals [60]. Following human SCI, there is so far only limited evidence available for a pharmacological facilitation of spinal neuronal circuits underlying locomotion (for review see [67]).

Recently, two novel promising, non-invasive techniques, called paired associative stimulation [68–70] and transcutaneous spinal direct current stimulation (tsDCS) [71–74], have been applied in humans to modulate spinal neuronal excitability. The latter technique is derived from transcranial direct current stimulation and influences spinal neuronal excitability by anodal or cathodal polarization of the cord tissue [75]. So far, tsDCS has been mainly applied in healthy subjects as a tool to modulate transsynaptic efficacy in monosynaptic [72, 74] and polysynaptic reflex pathways [71]. Only one study has applied this technique in subjects with SCI. Increased amplitudes of polysynaptic SR after 20 min of anodal tsDCS were described [73]. This leads to the assumption that tsDCS can modulate spinal neuronal excitability in chronic SCI subjects. It remains to be determined whether anodal tsDCS can be used to counteract the development of spinal neuronal dysfunction after severe SCI.

Conclusion

Facilitation of neuroplasticity plays a major role in the rehabilitation of subjects with SCI and stroke. The development of a 'negative' plasticity occurring in patients deprived of supraspinal input after damage of CNS structures was recognized only a few years ago. This 'negative' plasticity is reflected in the development of a neuronal dysfunction within spinal neuronal circuits in severely affected subjects with stroke/SCI who do not undergo a functional training. This phenomenon is important insofar as a neuronal dysfunction could prevent a successful application of future regeneration inducing therapies. A severe CNS damage leads to dysfunction of spinal neuronal circuitries involved in the generation of locomotor (only SCI) and SR activity. This spinal neuronal dysfunction becomes fully established around 1 year post-lesion and is represented in an exhaustion of locomotor EMG activity during assisted locomotion and a shift from dominant early to dominant late SR components. The proposed cause of this 'negative' neuroplasticity is a bias to inhibitory signalling within spinal neuronal circuitries. It is assumed that immobility with its associated loss of appropriate proprioceptive feedback to spinal neuronal circuitries weakens the excitatory drive within spinal neuronal networks and leads to the bias of an inhibitory drive in interneuronal activity. Countermeasures to prevent or to reverse the development of neuronal dysfunction include intensive training approaches in combination with stimulation techniques. Promising non-invasive neuromodulatory techniques, which increase spinal neuronal excitability, might justify future investigations to counteract the development of spinal neuronal dysfunction in chronic CNS damage.

References

1. Filli L, Schwab ME. The rocky road to translation in spinal cord repair. Ann Neurol. 2012;**72**(4):491–501.
2. Tator CH. Review of treatment trials in human spinal cord injury: issues, difficulties, and recommendations. Neurosurgery. 2006;**59**(5):957–982; discussion 82–7.
3. Hawryluk GW, Rowland J, Kwon BK, Fehlings MG. Protection and repair of the injured spinal cord: a review of completed, ongoing, and planned clinical trials for acute spinal cord injury. Neurosurg Focus. 2008;**25**(5):E14.
4. Baptiste DC, Fehlings MG. Update on the treatment of spinal cord injury. Prog Brain Res. 2007;**161**:217–233.
5. Oudega M, Vargas CG, Weber AB, Kleitman N, Bunge MB. Long-term effects of methylprednisolone following transection of adult rat spinal cord. Eur J Neurosci. 1999;**11**(7):2453–2464.
6. Holtz A, Nystrom B, Gerdin B. Effect of methylprednisolone on motor function and spinal cord blood flow after spinal cord compression in rats. Acta Neurol Scand. 1990;**82**(1):68–73.
7. Bracken MB, Shepard MJ, Collins WF, et al. A randomized, controlled trial of methylprednisolone or naloxone in the treatment of acute spinal-cord injury. Results of the Second National Acute Spinal Cord Injury Study. N Engl J Med. 1990;**322**(20):1405–1411.
8. Bracken MB, Shepard MJ, Holford TR, et al. Administration of methylprednisolone for 24 or 48 hours or tirilazad mesylate for 48 hours in the treatment of acute spinal cord injury. Results of the Third National Acute Spinal Cord Injury Randomized Controlled Trial. National Acute Spinal Cord Injury Study. JAMA. 1997;**277**(20):1597–1604.
9. Hurlbert RJ, Hamilton MG. Methylprednisolone for acute spinal cord injury: 5-year practice reversal. Can J Neurol Sci. 2008;**35**(1):41–45.
10. Dietz V, Curt A. Neurological aspects of spinal-cord repair: promises and challenges. Lancet Neurol. 2006;**5**(8):688–694.
11. Houle JD, Tessler A. Repair of chronic spinal cord injury. Exp Neurol. 2003;**182**(2):247–260.
12. Mackay-Sim A, Feron F, Cochrane J, et al. Autologous olfactory ensheathing cell transplantation in human paraplegia: a 3-year clinical trial. Brain. 2008;**131**(9):2376–2386.
13. Dietz V. Neuronal plasticity after a human spinal cord injury: positive and negative effects. Exp Neurol. 2012;**235**(1):110–115.
14. Dietz V, Muller R. Degradation of neuronal function following a spinal cord injury: mechanisms and countermeasures. Brain. 2004;**127**(10):2221–2231.

15. Dietz V, Grillner S, Trepp A, Hubli M, Bolliger M. Changes in spinal reflex and locomotor activity after a complete spinal cord injury: a common mechanism? Brain. 2009;**132**(8):2196–2205.

16. Hubli M, Dietz V, Bolliger M. Spinal reflex activity: a marker for neuronal functionality after spinal cord injury. Neurorehabil Neural Repair. 2012;**26**(2):188–196.

17. Hubli M, Bolliger M, Limacher E, A.R. L, Dietz V. Spinal neuronal dysfunction after stroke. Exp Neurol. 2012;**234**(1):153–160.

18. Grillner S. Neurobiological bases of rhythmic motor acts in vertebrates. Science. 1985;**228**(4696):143–149.

19. Graham-Brown T. The intrinsic factors in the act of progression in the mammal. Proc R Soc Lond B Biol Sci. 1911:308–319.

20. Barbeau H, Rossignol S. Recovery of locomotion after chronic spinalization in the adult cat. Brain Res. 1987;**412**(1):84–95.

21. De Leon RD, Hodgson JA, Roy RR, Edgerton VR. Full weight-bearing hindlimb standing following stand training in the adult spinal cat. J Neurophysiol. 1998;**80**(1):83–91.

22. Barbeau H, Rossignol S. Enhancement of locomotor recovery following spinal cord injury. Curr Opin Neurol. 1994;**7**(6):517–524.

23. Vilensky JA, O'Connor BL. Stepping in nonhuman primates with a complete spinal cord transection: old and new data, and implications for humans. Ann N Y Acad Sci. 1998;**860**:528–530.

24. Dietz V, Colombo G, Jensen L. Locomotor activity in spinal man. Lancet. 1994;**344**(8932):1260–1263.

25. Harkema SJ, Hurley SL, Patel UK, Requejo PS, Dobkin BH, Edgerton VR. Human lumbosacral spinal cord interprets loading during stepping. J Neurophysiol. 1997;**77**(2):797–811.

26. Dobkin BH, Harkema S, Requejo P, Edgerton VR. Modulation of locomotor-like EMG activity in subjects with complete and incomplete spinal cord injury. J Neurol Rehabil. 1995;**9**(4):183–190.

27. Dietz V, Muller R, Colombo G. Locomotor activity in spinal man: significance of afferent input from joint and load receptors. Brain. 2002;**125**(12):2626–2634.

28. Pierrot-Deseilligny E, Burke D. Cutaneomuscular, withdrawal and flexor reflex afferent responses. In: Bachmann V, editor. The circuitry of the human spinal cord. Cambridge University Press, New York, 2005. pp. 384–451.

29. Andersen OK, Finnerup NB, Spaich EG, Jensen TS, Arendt-Nielsen L. Expansion of nociceptive withdrawal reflex receptive fields in spinal cord injured humans. Clin Neurophysiol. 2004;**115**(12):2798–2810.

30. Hornby TG, Rymer WZ, Benz EN, Schmit BD. Windup of flexion reflexes in chronic human spinal cord injury: a marker for neuronal plateau potentials? J Neurophysiol. 2003;**89**(1):416–426.

31. Conway BA, Knikou M. The action of plantar pressure on flexion reflex pathways in the isolated human spinal cord. Clin Neurophysiol. 2008;**119**(4):892–896.

32. Schmit BD, McKenna-Cole A, Rymer WZ. Flexor reflexes in chronic spinal cord injury triggered by imposed ankle rotation. Muscle Nerve. 2000;**23**(5):793–803.

33. Hiersemenzel LP, Curt A, Dietz V. From spinal shock to spasticity: neuronal adaptations to a spinal cord injury. Neurology. 2000;**54**(8):1574–1582.

34. Lavrov I, Gerasimenko YP, Ichiyama RM, et al. Plasticity of spinal cord reflexes after a complete transection in adult rats: relationship to stepping ability. J Neurophysiol. 2006;**96**(4):1699–1710.

35. Valero-Cabre A, Fores J, Navarro X. Reorganization of reflex responses mediated by different afferent sensory fibers after spinal cord transection. J Neurophysiol. 2004;**91**(6):2838–2848.

36. Dietz V, Colombo G, Jensen L, Baumgartner L. Locomotor capacity of spinal cord in paraplegic patients. Ann Neurol. 1995;**37**(5):574–582.

37. Dietz V, Quintern J, Berger W. Electrophysiological studies of gait in spasticity and rigidity. Evidence that altered mechanical properties of muscle contribute to hypertonia. Brain. 1981;**104**(3):431–449.

38. O'Dwyer NJ, Ada L, Neilson PD. Spasticity and muscle contracture following stroke. Brain. 1996;**119**:1737–1749.

39. Lieber RL, Friden J. Spasticity causes a fundamental rearrangement of muscle-joint interaction. Muscle Nerve. 2002;**25**(2):265–270.

40. Dietz V, Sinkjaer T. Spastic movement disorder: impaired reflex function and altered muscle mechanics. Lancet Neurol. 2007;**6**(8):725–733.

41. Dietz V. Behavior of spinal neurons deprived of supraspinal input. Nat Rev Neurol. 2010;**6**(3):167–174.

42. Hubli M, Bolliger M, Dietz V. Neuronal dysfunction in chronic spinal cord injury. Spinal Cord. 2011;**49**(5):582–587.

43. Chang CW. Evident transsynaptic degeneration of motor neurons after spinal cord injury: a study of neuromuscular jitter by axonal microstimulation. Am J Phys Med Rehabil. 1998;**77**(2):118–121.

44. Lin CS, Macefield VG, Elam M, Wallin BG, Engel S, Kiernan MC. Axonal changes in spinal cord injured patients distal to the site of injury. Brain. 2007;**130**(4):985–994.

45. Muller R, Dietz V. Neuronal function in chronic spinal cord injury: divergence between locomotor and flexion- and H-reflex activity. Clin Neurophysiol. 2006;**117**(7):1499–1507.

46. Kloter E, Wirz M, Dietz V. Locomotion in stroke subjects: interactions between unaffected and affected sides. Brain. 2011;**134**(3):721–731.

47. Reisman DS, Wityk R, Silver K, Bastian AJ. Locomotor adaptation on a split-belt treadmill can improve walking symmetry post-stroke. Brain. 2007;**130**(7):1861–1872.

48. Zehr EP, Loadman PM. Persistence of locomotor-related interlimb reflex networks during walking after stroke. Clin Neurophysiol. 2012;**123**(4):796–807.

49. Buurke JH, Nene AV, Kwakkel G, Erren-Wolters V, Ijzerman MJ, Hermens HJ. Recovery of gait after stroke: what changes? Neurorehabil Neural Repair. 2008;**22**(6):676–683.

50. Den Otter AR, Geurts AC, Mulder T, Duysens J. Gait recovery is not associated with changes in the temporal patterning of muscle activity during treadmill walking in patients with post-stroke hemiparesis. Clin Neurophysiol. 2006;**117**(1):4–15.

51. Taub E, Uswatte G, Pidikiti R. Constraint-induced movement therapy: a new family of techniques with broad application to physical rehabilitation—a clinical review. J Rehabil Res Dev. 1999;**36**(3):237–251.

52. Grillner S, Deliagina T, Ekeberg O, et al. Neural networks that co-ordinate locomotion and body orientation in lamprey. Trends Neurosci. 1995;**18**(6):270–279.

53. Tillakaratne NJ, de Leon RD, Hoang TX, Roy RR, Edgerton VR, Tobin AJ. Use-dependent modulation of inhibitory capacity in the feline lumbar spinal cord. J Neurosci. 2002;**22**(8):3130–3143.

54. Ichiyama RM, Broman J, Edgerton VR, Havton LA. Ultrastructural synaptic features differ between alpha- and gamma-motoneurons innervating the tibialis anterior muscle in the rat. J Comp Neurol. 2006;**499**(2):306–315.

55. de Leon RD, Tamaki H, Hodgson JA, Roy RR, Edgerton VR. Hindlimb locomotor and postural training modulates glycinergic inhibition in the spinal cord of the adult spinal cat. J Neurophysiol. 1999;**82**(1):359–369.

56. Ichiyama RM, Broman J, Roy RR, Zhong H, Edgerton VR, Havton LA. Locomotor training maintains normal inhibitory influence on both alpha- and gamma-motoneurons after neonatal spinal cord transection. J Neurosci. 2011;**31**(1):26–33.

57. Rossignol S, Dubuc R, Gossard JP. Dynamic sensorimotor interactions in locomotion. Physiol Rev. 2006;**86**(1):89–154.

58. Dietz V, Colombo G. Effects of body immersion on postural adjustments to voluntary arm movements in humans: role of load receptor input. J Physiol. 1996;**497**:849–856.

59. Bastiaanse CM, Duysens J, Dietz V. Modulation of cutaneous reflexes by load receptor input during human walking. Exp Brain Res. 2000;**135**(2):189–198.

60. Courtine G, Gerasimenko Y, van den Brand R, et al. Transformation of nonfunctional spinal circuits into functional states after the loss of brain input. Nat Neurosci. 2009;**12**(10):1333–1342.

61. Gurfinkel VS, Levik YS, Kazennikov OV, Selionov VA. Locomotor-like movements evoked by leg muscle vibration in humans. Eur J Neurosci. 1998;10(5):1608–1612.

62. Selionov VA, Ivanenko YP, Solopova IA, Gurfinkel VS. Tonic central and sensory stimuli facilitate involuntary air-stepping in humans. J Neurophysiol. 2009;101(6):2847–2858.

63. Gerasimenko Y, Gorodnichev R, Machueva E, et al. Novel and direct access to the human locomotor spinal circuitry. J Neurosci. 2010;30(10):3700–3708.

64. Dimitrijevic MR, Gerasimenko Y, Pinter MM. Evidence for a spinal central pattern generator in humans. Ann N Y Acad Sci. 1998;860:360–376.

65. Minassian K, Jilge B, Rattay F, al. Stepping-like movements in humans with complete spinal cord injury induced by epidural stimulation of the lumbar cord: electromyographic study of compound muscle action potentials. Spinal Cord. 2004;42(7):401–416.

66. Harkema S, Gerasimenko Y, Hodes J, et al. Effect of epidural stimulation of the lumbosacral spinal cord on voluntary movement, standing, and assisted stepping after motor complete paraplegia: a case study. Lancet. 2011;377(9781):1938–1947.

67. Domingo A, Al-Yahya AA, Asiri Y, Eng JJ, Lam T. A systematic review of the effects of pharmacological agents on walking function in people with spinal cord injury. J Neurotrauma. 2012;29(5):865–879.

68. Cortes M, Thickbroom GW, Valls-Sole J, Pascual-Leone A, Edwards DJ. Spinal associative stimulation: a non-invasive stimulation paradigm to modulate spinal excitability. Clin Neurophysiol. 2011;122(11):2254–2259.

69. Meunier S, Russmann H, Simonetta-Moreau M, Hallett M. Changes in spinal excitability after PAS. J Neurophysiol. 2007;97(4):3131–3135.

70. Leukel C, Taube W, Beck S, Schubert M. Pathway-specific plasticity in the human spinal cord. Eur J Neurosci. 2012;35(10):1622–1629.

71. Cogiamanian F, Vergari M, Schiaffi E, et al. Transcutaneous spinal cord direct current stimulation inhibits the lower limb nociceptive flexion reflex in human beings. Pain. 2010;152(2):370–375.

72. Winkler T, Hering P, Straube A. Spinal DC stimulation in humans modulates post-activation depression of the H-reflex depending on current polarity. Clin Neurophysiol. 2010;121(6):957–961.

73. Hubli M, Dietz V, Schrafl-Altermatt M, Bolliger M. Modulation of spinal neuronal excitability by spinal direct currents and locomotion after spinal cord injury. Clin Neurophysiol. 2013;124(6):1187–1195.

74. Lamy JC, Ho C, Badel A, Arrigo RT, Boakye M. Modulation of Soleus H-reflex by spinal DC stimulation in humans. J Neurophysiol. 2012;108(3):906–914.

75. Nitsche MA, Cohen LG, Wassermann EM, et al. Transcranial direct current stimulation: State of the art 2008. Brain Stimul. 2008;1(3):206–223.

CHAPTER 9

Secondary changes after damage of the central nervous system: significance of spastic muscle tone in rehabilitation

Volker Dietz and Thomas Sinkjaer

Introduction

Spasticity is a well-known syndrome, most commonly arising after stroke, multiple sclerosis, spinal cord injury (SCI), traumatic brain injuries, and other central nervous system (CNS) lesions. These patients suffer a spastic movement disorder, with slowing of stepping and impaired voluntary limb movements. Clinical diagnosis of spasticity is based on the combination of physical signs in the passive patient—exaggerated tendon reflexes and muscle hypertonia defined as a velocity-dependent resistance of a muscle to stretching [1]. Spastic muscle tone can differently be distributed in flexor and extensor muscles as well as a focal or generalized increase in muscle tone can be experienced depending on the cause of the spastic symptoms [2].

One problem in the clinic when diagnosing spasticity is that it is not easy with the current applied methods, such as the Ashworth and the Tardieu scales, to distinguish between reflex and passive muscle-mediated changes [3, 4]. Also the term spasticity is inconsistently defined and the measures used do not correspond to the clinical features of spasticity [5].

In this chapter, we relate the definition of spasticity by Lance [1] to the knowledge of the mechanisms underlying the associated movement disorder. On the basis of the clinical signs it was assumed in the past that neural overactivity, causing exaggerated reflexes, might be responsible for muscle hypertonia, which then leads to spastic movement disorder [6–10]. This view was supported by experiments on decerebrate cats [[11], which showed that muscle tone during stretching is substantially reduced after severing the nerves involved in the stretch-reflex loop. Therefore, it became established that most treatment approaches should be directed to attenuate or abolish reflex activity and thereby to reduce muscle tone [6, 12].

This view did not take into account several points. First, the decerebrate cat is not an adequate model for human spasticity as rigid muscle tone develops immediately after decerebration, whereas human spasticity develops over weeks after acute lesions.

Correspondingly, human tendon tap reflexes are enhanced on the affected side already early after stroke without increase in muscle tone. Second, exaggerated tendon reflexes are only a small part of the mechanisms that contribute to the control of functional movement, such as walking. Third, most studies on the effect of antispastic drugs are focused on isolated clinical signs, such as reflex activity, and not on the spastic movement disorder that hampers patients. Fourth, without the development of spastic muscle tone (e.g. after stroke/SCI), most patients would be unable to walk because of the paresis. Fifth, clinical examination of spasticity is done in the relaxed/passive patient and does not reflect the state of neuronal circuits within the CNS underlying natural movements such as walking.

No convincing animal model exists for human spasticity (see [13]), perhaps because the pathophysiology of spasticity is multifactorial. Any changes in the neuronal or biomechanical systems, for example differences in the site and duration of a central lesion, are of importance in determining which neural control mechanisms are deficient and contribute to the movement disorder [14]. Furthermore, such changes might already be secondary and compensatory to the primary dysfunction of sensorimotor systems. There are some differences in the appearance of spasticity between spinal and supraspinal lesions and lesions of different origin (e.g. inflammatory or traumatic). However, these factors have little influence on the impairment of function which essentially depends on the severity of CNS damage.

Research on functional movement in recent years indicates that the clinical signs of spasticity are little related to the spastic movement disorder, which hampers patients and should be the focus of any treatment. For example, exaggerated reflexes, a dominant sign in clinical assessments, have little effect on the movement disorder. In this chapter, we describe the role of reflex and muscle activity and muscle mechanics in patients with spasticity and the resulting muscle tone in two conditions (cf. [15]): passive (clinical) and active (functional). This serves as a basis for an appropriate treatment which will be presented and discussed in a third section.

Clinical signs of spasticity

In a clinical setting, muscle tone and tendon tap reflexes are routinely examined in relaxed patients. Exaggerated tendon tap reflexes of the affected limb muscles and an increased resistance of a muscle to stretching indicate the presence of spasticity caused by a central motor lesion.

Exaggerated reflexes: short-latency reflex activity

The nature and mechanisms underlying exaggerated tendon reflex activity (monosynaptic or oligosynaptic segmental reflexes) have been the focus of many studies in patients with spasticity. The short-latency reflex activity is mediated by fast conducting group Ia nerve fibres from the muscle spindles to the spinal cord. A severe acute central lesion is associated with a loss of tendon tap reflexes followed by hyperreflexia which is suggested to be due to a neuronal reorganization in both cats [16] and humans [17, 18].

Exaggerated reflexes were thought to result from hyperactivity of fusimotoneurons [19, 20] (also called gamma motoneurons), which correspond to the alpha motoneurons innervating normal muscle fibres, although only indirect approaches have been applied, and this has not been proven convincingly [21–23]. Furthermore, increased reflex activity is not likely to be caused by either reduced recurrent inhibition of motoneurons via Renshaw cell activity [24, 25] or intraspinal nerve sprouting [26].

There is evidence for reduced presynaptic inhibition of Ia afferent fibres in leg muscles after SCI, but not in hemiplegic stroke subjects [27, 28], as a possible mechanism underlying exaggerated tendon tap reflexes. However, there is no association between decreased presynaptic inhibition of Ia afferents and the degree of muscle hypertonia as assessed by the Ashworth scale [28].

In addition, deficient disynaptic reciprocal inhibition [29], increased excitability of reciprocal Ia inhibitory [29] pathways [30–32], changed postactivation depression [33] and disinhibition of group II pathways [34–36] were suggested to contribute to hyper-reflexia after SCI or stroke and other mechanisms might also be involved [28, 37].

A severe central motor lesion is followed by flaccid paresis with a loss of tendon tap reflexes. In contrast, the H-reflex (an electrically elicited short-latency reflex excluding muscle spindles) is already present during spinal shock when tendon reflexes cannot yet be elicited [18]. After 1–2 weeks, tendon reflexes and muscle tone reappear. At later stages (4–6 weeks) clinical signs of spasticity (i.e. exaggerated reflexes and increased muscle tone), become established. The loss of reflexes is usually attributed to a reduced excitability of alpha- and gamma motoneurons due to the sudden loss of input from supraspinal centres [18]. When spasticity has developed, the threshold of the soleus stretch reflex is decreased in patients with spasticity [38, 39], possibly due to an increase in alpha and gamma motoneuron excitability [40]. Repetitive clonic muscle contractions are more likely to be due to an impaired interaction of central and peripheral mechanisms than to a recurrent stretch reflex activity [41].

Exaggerated reflexes: flexor reflex activity

The flexor reflex is a polysynaptic spinal reflex that might be connected with spinal locomotor centres [42]. While a great variability of flexion reflex responses exists in patients with a SCI [43], the dominant view is that flexor reflexes are exaggerated after a

central nervous lesion and might cause muscle spasms after spinal cord injury [44]. Furthermore, it seems that the sites where flexor reflexes can be elicited become expanded in patients with a spinal or supraspinal lesion as compared to healthy humans [45, 46].

Several mechanisms are suggested to underlie flexor reflex activity after a CNS lesion. For example, spontaneous firing of motoneurons during rest was suggested to lead to muscle spasms [47, 48], initially caused by receptor upregulation and later on by neuronal sprouting [49, 50]. Flexor reflexes in patients with chronic SCI are also believed to reflect neuronal plateau potentials [37, 51].

After an acute, complete SCI, flexor reflex excitability and spastic muscle tone develop in parallel [18]. However, after a few months, there is a divergent course in which the severity and occurrence of muscle spasms increase, whereas flexor reflex amplitude decreases [18]. In line with this, patients with complete chronic SCI compared to healthy people show a lower incidence of the early flexor reflex component [43, 52] and they produce smaller leg joint torques [53]. These observations suggest that the activity of flexor reflexes is little or only indirectly related to the occurrence of muscle spasms in spasticity of spinal origin.

Spastic muscle tone

Muscle hypertonia is clinically assessed in the passive muscle using the Ashworth scale and is clinically defined as a velocity-dependent resistance to stretch [54]. This is particularly true for the leg extensor [55, 56] and arm flexor—the antigravity muscles [40, 57]. Spastic muscle hypertonia is associated with muscle activity measured by electromyography, which exceeds that seen in healthy subjects [58, 59].

In addition to the extra-electromyographic activity (EMG) passive stiffness (eg, muscle contracture) at the ankle joint is also increased and contributes to the clinically defined spastic muscle hypertonia [4, 60–62]. Consequently, it becomes evident that the abnormal stretch reflex activity is insufficient to explain increased muscle tone in people with spasticity [59, 63–65]. Reflex-mediated stiffness in the active ankle extensors [65] and elbow flexor muscles [40, 58, 66] in patients with spasticity can even be within the range of healthy controls and seems to be only slightly increased in patients with SCI [67]. From investigating the ankle joint stiffness in stroke, multiple sclerosis, and SCI participants Lorentzen et al [4] concluded that the clinical diagnosis of spasticity includes changes in both active and passive muscle properties, and the two can hardly be distinguished based on routine clinical examination. The truth is still in the eye of the beholder [68]. Today, it is believed that a combination of mechanisms contributes to clinical spasticity, that is an increase in passive stiffness of a muscle to stretch due to changes in collagen tissue and tendons [59, 61, 65], an enhancement of intrinsic stiffness of muscle fibres (Gracies, 2005), and a loss of sarcomeres [69], leading to subclinical contractures (for review see [70]). In addition, morphometric and histochemical investigations changes take place in muscle-fibre properties [71–73] that might contribute to spastic muscle tone. Consequently, clinical muscle hypertonia seems to be more associated with subclinical muscle contracture rather than with reflex hyperexcitability [64, 69, 74]. Conversely, changes in biomechanical conditions of a muscle (i.e. loss of sarcomeres) might again have an effect on the stretch reflex behaviour (possibly via group III/IV muscle afferents) in people with spasticity [75, 76].

In conclusion, exaggerated reflexes elicited in passive spastic muscles, as seen in clinical bedside examination, are not solely responsible for the increased resistance of a spastic muscle to stretch. Secondary changes in intrinsic and extrinsic muscle properties contribute to spastic muscle tone (e.g. [70]). This assumption is based on observations made in patients with central motor lesions of different origin (e.g. traumatic SCI, stroke, and multiple sclerosis [12]).

Spastic movement disorder

After central motor lesions, patients suffer a movement disorder. To achieve adequate treatment, it is crucial to address the mechanisms underlying the impaired function. Actual studies indicate that the clinical signs of spasticity are little related to the movement disorder. The most relevant aspect concerns the fact that an 'extra-activity' contributes to muscle tone in the passive, clinical condition, but during functional movements a reduced muscle activation becomes partially compensated for by secondary changes in muscle mechanics. In this section, we discuss some of the mechanisms underlying impaired functional movements after a CNS lesion.

Pattern of leg muscle activity during locomotion

During a functional movement, such as locomotion, patients with spastic paraparesis have typical patterns of leg muscle activation recorded with electromyography. Spastic gait is associated with a low level of leg muscle activity compared with that in healthy people [77–79]. The reduction depends on the severity of paresis. In line with this, the fast regulation of motoneuron discharge, which

characterizes functional muscle activation, is absent in spasticity [71, 80]. However, the timing of the pattern (i.e. the reciprocal activation of antagonistic leg muscles) is largely preserved [78, 81, 82]. Only rarely does some coactivation of antagonistic leg muscles occur during the stance phase of walking [83–85]. Premature leg extensor activation in the early stance phase of gait [83–85] is associated with the plantar-flexed position of the spastic-paretic foot and is not spasticity-specific. Premature leg extensor activation in the early stance phase, or even before impact, also occurs when healthy people walk by voluntarily tip-toeing (i.e. the extensor activation depends on the foot position before impact). Furthermore, also co-activation of antagonistic leg muscles can be recorded in healthy people when they are walking with slightly flexed knees. In a few patients with spasticity, the impact of the forefoot is associated with the appearance of isolated stretch-reflex potentials [83–85].

The leg extensor EMG amplitude modulation, which in healthy people typically occurs during the stance phase, is reduced or lacking in people with spasticity [86] due to the attenuated integration of afferent input (long-latency reflex) activity to the ongoing locomotor leg extensor activity (Figure 9.1) [86, 87].

Reflex behaviour during locomotion

In healthy people, group Ia afferent input to the spinal cord becomes suppressed during the stance phase of gait [88, 89]. Because of reduced Ia suppression in spasticity, short-latency stretch reflexes commonly appear in the leg extensor muscles during the transition from the swing to the stance phase of gait, which is rarely the case in healthy people. Furthermore, the inability to

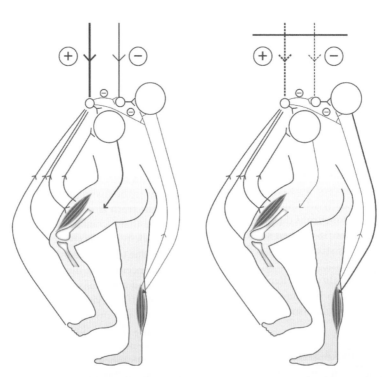

Fig. 9.1 Reflex behaviour during human gait. Left: In the healthy physiological condition, afferent feedback from long-latency reflex activity is facilitated by supraspinal drive and becomes significantly involved in leg muscle activation to adapt the locomotor pattern to the ground conditions. Ia afferent-mediated inputs are inhibited. Right: after a spinal or supraspinal lesion, the functionally essential activity of long-latency reflexes is impaired owing to the loss of supraspinal input.
Reprinted from Lancet Neurol, 6, Dietz V, Sinkjaer T, Spastic movement disorder: impaired reflex function and altered muscle mechanics, 725–733 © 2007, with permission from Elsevier.

suppress stretch reflex excitability during the swing phase of gait might contribute to impaired walking [89–95].

During walking in healthy subjects, the H- reflex and short-latency stretch reflex (both mediated by group Ia afferents) in leg muscles become modulated in a specific way [90, 91]. In subjects suffering spastic paresis, this physiological reflex modulation is impaired [91–95]. Also, the modulation of cutaneous reflexes is reduced during gait [93]. Furthermore, the quadriceps-tendon jerk-reflex depression, which is present in healthy people, is absent in patients with spinal lesions and is associated with a loss of modulation during the step cycle [91]. In general there are no qualitative differences in reflex behaviour between spasticity of cerebral origin and that of spinal origin [91], although direct comparisons are rare.

During perturbations of gait in people with stroke (e.g. short acceleration impulses of the treadmill during the stance phase of stepping) in the unaffected leg, short-latency stretch reflex components are followed by large compensatory long-latency reflexes in leg extensor [89, 96, 97] and dorsiflexor muscles [98]. By contrast, in the spastic leg, short-latency reflexes are isolated without out the presence of a significant long-latency EMG component [77, 99]. The consequence is reduced adaptation of muscle activity to the ground conditions [86], which, together with the reduced capacity to modulate reflex activity over the normal range, might contribute to the spastic movement disorder [96, 100].

Reflex behaviour in the active muscle: controlled conditions

The observations made during locomotion are in agreement with the results obtained when the voluntarily activated muscle becomes investigated in well-controlled lab conditions. Studies that apply joint displacements in voluntarily activated limb muscles show similar results as during functional movements and, therefore, differ from those obtained in the passive muscle. These studies show a uniform pattern of compensatory electromyographic responses in arm and leg muscles to the displacements. When background EMG levels are matched to normal levels in patients with spasticity, little evidence exists for exaggerated reflex activity [65, 100–102]. In unaffected muscles, the short-latency reflex is followed by longer latencies reflexes [78, 88]. In spasticity of spinal and cerebral origin this long-latency reflex activity is reduced or absent in arm and leg muscles [58, 66, 103]. Nevertheless, the automatic resistance to the joint displacement is of similar amplitude on the affected and unaffected sides.

During muscle contractions of healthy people, some inhibitory mechanisms on reflexes are removed [14]. By contrast, in spasticity, presynaptic inhibition, postactivation depression, and reciprocal inhibition do not further decrease during contraction Figure 9.2). Therefore, short-latency stretch reflexes in patients with spasticity differ less in size between the relaxed (clinical) and active (functional) conditions compared with those in healthy subjects [14, 58]. These short-latency reflexes are prominent but not functional and they show no task-dependent modulation in the spastic paretic condition as seen in healthy subjects. During isotonic leg muscle contractions, modulation and inhibition of Ib afferents (innervating the force-sensitive Golgi tendon organs) is reduced [104] and some co-contraction of antagonistic arm muscles can occur [105, 106].

In conclusion, there is similar reflex behaviour during displacements applied to activated limb muscles in both non-functional and functional conditions. These findings might result from impaired use of afferent input by spinal neuronal circuits after central lesions. In spastic limb muscles, stretch evoked EMG-activity and the resulting torque is near normal in the active condition but is increased in the passive (i.e. clinical) condition. Spastic subjects have difficulties to switch off limb muscle/reflex activity in a passive condition [66]. Thus, modulation of stretch-reflex-induced EMG-activity is restricted to a smaller range between passive and active conditions compared to healthy subjects.

Tension development

Muscle tone, as defined clinically, cannot be examined during movement. However, tension development at the Achilles tendon, resulting from a combination of muscle stiffness and EMG activity, can be recorded during locomotion. Tension development differs between the affected and unaffected legs in patients with spastic hemiparesis [77]. On the unaffected side, changes in tension at the Achilles tendon parallel the amplitude of triceps surae electromyographic activity. On the spastic side, the tension development is associated with a stretching of the triceps surae during the stance phase of gait. During this period, the leg extensor muscles are tonically activated with low electromyographic amplitude [77]. This is interpreted as tension development on a simpler level of organization on the spastic side due to changes in mechanical properties of the leg extensor muscles [15]. The possible mechanisms underlying these changes have been previously outlined. Thus, secondary to a spinal/cerebral lesion, there is a major alteration in motor unit properties [107] and in the normal muscle–joint relationships [69, 108, 109] that allow for support of the body during stepping movements.

In subjects suffering a spinal damage at the caudal level, the flaccid leg muscle paresis does usually not allow to perform stepping without prostheses to stabilize knee and ankle joints. With regard to this aspect, spastic muscle tone is beneficial to regain the capacity to support the body and to perform stepping movements.

Cerebral versus spinal spasticity

In this review, mechanisms of spasticity of cerebral and spinal origin are discussed. Although spasticity due to spinal or cerebral lesions has rarely been compared, no qualitative difference in the clinical appearance seems to exist. This is also true for the contribution of spasticity to the movement disorder in cerebral palsy [110]. A recent study [111] suggests failure of normal development of central drive to ankle dorsiflexors relates to gait deficits in children with cerebral palsy. These differences between the least and most affected tibialis anterior muscles were unrelated to differences in the magnitude of EMG in the two muscles but positively correlated with ankle dorsiflexion velocity and joint angle during gait,

Alterations between the different forms of spasticity existed, for example, in the degree of presynaptic inhibition which is greater in spinal cord injured subjects [28], are not reflected in any clinical or functional difference. Nevertheless, there are some quantitative differences in the clinical manifestation of spinal and cerebral spasticity. First, compared to a spinal lesion, complete plegia of a limb rarely occurs in stroke patients and, second, the recovery of function is usually stronger in cerebral compared to spinal lesions. Consequently also, spastic signs, which are related to the degree of paresis, are usually less pronounced in cerebral compared to

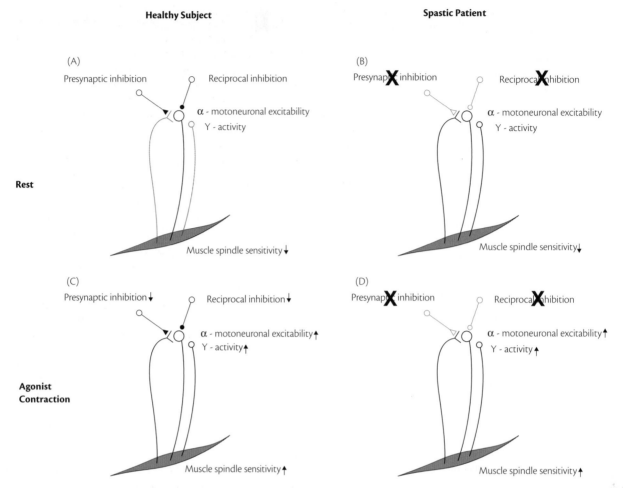

Fig. 9.2 Short-latency reflex behaviour in passive and active muscle. In healthy people, the stretch reflex activity is low at rest (A), which is explained by low excitability of spinal motor neurons, low muscle-spindle sensitivity, low discharge rate of Ia afferents, and pronounced presynaptic inhibition (Ib and Ia afferent discharge increase, whereas presynaptic inhibition (Ib inhibition and Ia inhibition) decreases. stretch reflex activity is consequently high. In spasticity, presynaptic Ib and Ia inhibition is already decreased at rest (C) and stretch reflex activity is high already. During voluntary contraction (D) there is little change in these parameters and the stretch reflex activity is not very different from that at rest. The arrows designate whether the mechanism is decreased or increased during contraction compared with rest.
Nielsen J, Petersen N, Crone C, Sinkjaer T, Stretch reflex regulation in healthy subjects and patients with spasticity, Neuromodulation, John Wiley & Sons © 2005.

spinal lesions. This is suggested to be due to the fact that in a unilateral brain damage some non-crossing corticospinal tract fibres supply the affected side.

Conclusion

Studies on spastic movement disorder provide evidence that the central pattern of leg muscle activation is largely preserved after a central lesion and the clinically dominant hyperreflexia play a minor role in leg muscle activation during gait. Attenuated integration of afferent feedback and a reduction of supraspinal drive lead to a tonic mode of leg muscle activity with a small EMG amplitude with the consequence of hampered walking. Secondary to a central lesion, changes in muscle, ligament, and tendon properties occur that compensate at part for the loss of supraspinal drive. The obvious consequence is the regulation of muscle tone on a simpler level (Figure 9.3). This behaviour of the spastic muscle allows for the support of the body during walking. This is also reflected in the fact that the level of spastic tone depends on the severity of paresis [112]. Therefore, such changes should be considered as adaptive to a primary disorder.

They may even be viewed as optimum for a given state of the system of movement production [113]. Knowledge about the nature of the changes in muscle mechanics is still rudimentary.

Therapeutic consequences

Any treatment of spasticity should focus on the movement disorder of individual patients. The physical signs obtained during the clinical examination such as exaggerated tendon tap reflexes are little related to the functional condition, as natural movements involve reflex mechanisms that are not assessed by the clinical examination (Figure 9.3). Impaired walking is mainly caused by disabling paresis and impaired use of afferent input by spinal neuronal circuits [114] and not by spastic muscle tone [69]. As a result, antispastic medications that are directed to reduce clinical signs of spasticity, such as exaggerated reflexes and muscle tone, do not improve movement disorder [115–119]. Medication can even increase weakness [117, 120, 121], which might interfere with functional movements, such as walking.

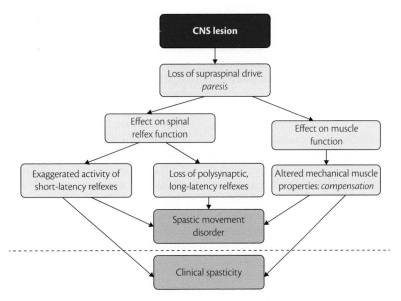

Fig. 9.3 Mechanisms involved in spastic movement disorder. A central motor lesion leads to changes in the integration of afferent feedback and consequently, excitability of spinal reflexes as well as a loss of supraspinal drive. As a consequence, changes in muscle function occur and lead to altered mechanical muscle properties. The combination of all sequels of the primary lesion leads to the spastic movement disorder.
Reprinted from Lancet Neurol, 6, Dietz V, Sinkjaer T, Spastic movement disorder: impaired reflex function and altered muscle mechanics, 725–733 © 2007, with permission from Elsevier.

Similarly, Botulinum toxin type A is assumed to frequently result in a cosmetic effect on spastic signs without functional improvement [121, 122], although this toxin might reduce the dominance of forearm flexor muscle tone, which can impede grasp movements [123, 124]. Also, intrathecal baclofen is reported to reduce hyperactive reflexes without producing significant weakness [125–127].

In conclusion, therapeutic interventions in patients with spastic paresis due to an incomplete SCI or stroke should consist primarily in physiotherapy. It should be focused on the training, relearning and activation of residual motor function [128, 129]. A focus of rehabilitation concerns the locomotor training of spastic para- and hemiparetic subjects [13, 130]. Such a training can be adapted in duration and intensity to the individual needs by robotic devices [131]. In addition, secondary complications, such as muscle contractures can be prevented by functional training [132].

Antispastic drug therapy might predominantly of benefit in non-ambulatory patients by reducing muscle tone and relieving muscle spasms [133], which might in turn improve nursing care for these patients.

Specific treatment approaches

Practical management

Pharmacological management of spasticity is usually focused on the reduction of reflex activity and muscle tone under clinical conditions. In fact, only a few reports exist about the effects of antispastic drugs on functional movement (see [15]). These usually fail to show any significant improvement in function. Similar conclusions can be drawn for other non-drug treatments of spasticity. Adequately controlled trials have rarely been performed, and some studies were empirically, not objectively, conducted (see

[12]). For an overview of methods for treating spasticity, see the reviews: [12, 134].

Non-specific procedures

Painful flexor spasms and increased muscle tone frequently result from an increase in cutaneous reflex activity induced by noxious or potentially painful afferent activity such as is associated with infections of the urinary tract, other infections combined with fever, and skin ulcerations, as well as by clothes irritating the skin. Consequently, worsening of spastic symptoms can frequently be alleviated by appropriate treatment of bladder function and skin care in paraplegic patients, as well as by early detection and management of the responsible factors (e.g. appropriate shoes or clothes) [12].

Physiotherapy

Physiotherapy represents a most definitive mode of treatment for mobile and non-ambulatory spastic patients, although this statement is not based on hard data. Active and passive manipulative forms of physiotherapeutic treatment are of importance for both groups of patients. On the one hand, in non-ambulatory patients residual motor functions can be improved by training. On the other hand, contractures of muscles and joints that are difficult to treat when established can be prevented at an early stage by frequent muscle stretching. Exercise therapy should be directed toward defined functions for which training is specifically indicated and required for daily living tasks. Benefits have been shown to depend on the intensity of rehabilitative training [135, 136].

Based on divergent empirical evidence, different physiotherapeutic procedures are being applied. Proprioceptive neuromuscular facilitation (PNF) and myofeedback techniques are believed to activate reflexively spinal neuronal circuits. The techniques of Bobath and Vojta are primarily used to treat children with cerebral palsy [88]. Stereotyped movements become activated by such stimulation techniques when they are applied to specific dermatomes and joints. The Vojta method tries to activate complex movements that are believed to be programmed in the central nervous system. In contrast, the Bobath method tries to inhibit spastic symptoms in flexor muscles of the upper extremity and extensors of the lower limbs.

All these physiotherapeutic techniques are directed to achieve the following goals: (1) to avoid secondary complications (i.e. pneumonia, skin ulcerations, and deep vein thrombosis); (2) to prevent and treat muscle contractures; (3) to reduce muscle hypertonia; (4) to train posture and automatically performed movements by the induction of voluntarily initiated and controlled complex movements; (5) to learn and train coordinated movements by the involvement of tactile, auditory, vestibular, and visual cues; and (6) to apply appropriate supportive aids, such as rollator, wheelchair, crutches, orthoses, and technical equipment (e.g. special shoes).

Each of these techniques is based on empirical observations and not well funded theories. Controlled studies documenting positive effects of the treatment exist for none of them. Therefore, it is not yet possible to perform an appropriate evaluation and to arrive at a recommendation based on the objective superiority of one of these techniques compared with another in the treatment of a given spastic patient.

Nevertheless, physiotherapy must be part of a multidisciplinary integrated approach to patients. It also includes occupational therapy and nursing assistance. These all are means to achieve greater mobility and, as far as possible, independence for the patient.

Locomotor training

The locomotor training can improve both spasticity and locomotor function. It is based on observations made in cats with complete spinal lesions [137]. Such animal experiments have shown that repetitive afferent input is essential for such a motor learning task [138].

Interactive locomotor training is performed on a treadmill with various percentages of the subjects' body weight (about 30–70%) mechanically supported by an overhead harness using a strain-gauge transducer. In such a condition rudimentary coordinated stepping movements associated with a proper muscle activation can be facilitated. In severely affected people with stroke or SCI this training is associated with a great expenditure—two physiotherapists are required to assist leg movements. Recent developments of driven gait orthoses can compensate for this drawback (e.g. [131, 139]).

During the course of training, a progressively 'normal' locomotor EMG pattern with stronger leg muscle activation is developed: that is patients can take over more body weight [140, 141]. Reduction of spastic symptoms and improvement of locomotor function by such an activation of spinal locomotor centres is also influenced by the repetitive elements of the training approach. Also upper limb spasticity can be reduced and function be improved by active training approaches [142]. In line with this, functional training combined with electrical muscle stimulation can improve function in upper [143] and lower [144] limbs, associated with a reduction in muscle tone. Even severely impaired chronic incomplete paraplegic patients, this training can successfully be applied [13, 130, 145–147]. It should be considered, however, that the effect of body weight supported treadmill training

in walking rehabilitation of post-stroke patients have been inconclusive. Some studies favour body weight supported treadmill training to other forms of walking rehabilitation such as conventional physiotherapy and over ground walking exercise, whereas others have found there to be little difference [147]. At present, evidence suggests that body weight supported treadmill training is equally effective but not a superior method of rehabilitation when compared to other means of walking therapy [148]. This is not surprising, as any form of functional training should be expected to improve locomotor ability in people with stroke and SCI [149]. An overground walking therapy, however, in severely affected patients requires the assistance of two physiotherapists and therefore limits training time. In less severely affected patients it should be recognized that body weight supported treadmill training is a good supplement to over ground walking rehabilitation for enabling a higher intensity of task-orientated training [147].

Drug therapy of spasticity

The presumed actions of the best established antispastic drugs are illustrated in Figure 9.4. As a rule, the use of only one substance of these substances at a time is recommended, at least to begin with. There are patients who do best with modest doses of two medications that have different target of action (baclofen and tizanidine, for example), so combination of drugs may eventually be necessary. Because relief of spasms and muscle hypertonia may only be achieved at the cost of reduced muscle power, doses should be kept to minimum, especially in mobile patients. In addition, drug therapy should always be combined with physiotherapy. Almost all antispastic drugs may induce side effects, often consisting of drowsiness and nausea (see [12]).

Best antispastic effects are reported for baclofen, tizanidine, and benzodiazepines (e.g. clonazepam). Therefore, these are the drugs of first choice for spastic patients. They are more effective in spasticity of spinal than of cerebral origin such as with multiple sclerosis and traumatic or neoplastic spinal cord lesions ([134, 150]).

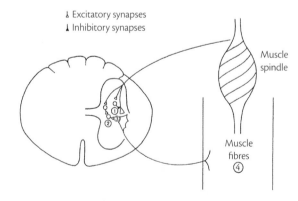

Fig. 9.4 Presumed site of action of drugs with antispastic effects. (1) Clonazepam/diazepam facilitate GABA-A mediated presynaptic inhibition; (2) baclofen inhibits activity of polysynaptic reflexes by GABA-B-receptor activation; (3) tizanidine acts on alpha$_2$-adrenergic receptors; (4) dantrolene reduces the sensitivity of peripheral intra-muscular receptors and reduces release of calcium ions from the sarcoplasmic reticulum, which thus weakens muscle contraction.
Reprinted from Neurological Disorders Course and Treatment (Second Edition), Dietz V, Young R, The Syndrome of Spastic Paresis, 1247–1257, Copyright (2003), with permission from Elsevier.

Baclofen acts as a gamma-aminobutyric acid (GABA)-B ago-nist on a spinal level presynaptically and (less) postsynaptically. Monosynaptic stretch reflexes are depressed more effectively than polysynaptic reflexes. Baclofen can alleviate spasms and muscle hypertonia, especially in non-ambulatory patients with spastic-ity [151, 152]. A long-term side-effect of baclofen concerns the mechanical properties of motor units: that is a reduced force development and an increased fatiguability [153].

Gabapentin, a GABA-related drug, is effective particularly for the treatment of painful muscle spasms [154]. Tizanidine is an imidazoline derivative closely related to clonidine. Both are thought to act on alpha-2-adrenergic receptors, especially in spas-ticity of supraspinal origin. It is suggested that these substances reduce the activity of polysynaptic reflexes, in ways similar to the action of baclofen [116, 119].

Clonidine and tizanidine also have effects on spinal cord neural curcuits that are generally inhibitory.In part at least, they reduce the release of glutamate. Clonidine and presumably also tizani-dine produce marked inhibition of spinal reflex responses in alpha motoneurons to group II activity in the spinal cat [155]. Tizanidine also results in non-opiate analgesia by action on alpha-2-receptors in the spinal dorsal horn, which inhibit release of substance P. This is assumed to diminish flexor reflex afferent (FRA)-mediated actions with the consequence that clonidine reduces the frequency and severity of spasms particularly in patients with spinal cord injury [25].

Benzodiazepines (e.g. clonazepam) amplify the inhibitory action of GABA-A at presynaptic and postsynaptic levels and thereby, excitatory actions become dampened with a negative rebound. It is believed that increasing presynaptic inhibition of afferent fibres in the spinal cord of patients with spasticity should reduce the release of excitatory transmitters from afferent fibres and, consequently, reduce the gain of spinal stretch- and flexor-reflexes. One can assume that these compounds act directly within the spinal cord [156]. For diazepam, serious side effects such as development of tolerance, dependency, and drowsiness are reported [134].

Small doses (5 mg) of cannabinoids have already been reported to be beneficial for the mobility of patients suffering multiple scle-rosis without having an effect on spastic muscle tone assessed by the Ashworth test [157].

Intrathecal infusion of baclofen

In immobilized patients with severe spastic symptoms, oral anti-spastic drugs are frequently not well tolerated in the long term because of their adverse effects. In these cases intrathecal baclofen application can efficiently reduce painful symptoms and has toler-able side effects [158–161].

The intrathecal dose is minute (100–400 μg/day), but the antispastic effects, especially on muscle tone and spasms, are powerful. In non-ambulatory patients severe spasticity can be transformed into flaccid paresis, which usually makes nurs-ing easier. During the first month, some tolerance develops, which often makes an increase in dosage necessary [162]. In patients with severe spasticity caused by lesions at any level of the CNS, but most frequently in non-ambulatory patients with (in-) complete SCI at a thoracic level, continuous intrath-ecal baclofen infusion is a safe and effective adjunct to physi-cal therapy [163]. After termination of chronic treatment with

intrathecal baclofen, lasting reduction in spasticity has been reported [164].

The main side effects of intrathecal baclofen consist of drow-siness and somnolence, perhaps associated with depression of respiration. These side effects are usually due to an overdose of baclofen reaching the lower brainstem. The catheter system must eventually be repaired; its failure is the main cause of interruption of drug delivery [165].

Local antispastic therapy

For the treatment of circumscribed muscle hypertonia, local injection of botulinum toxin, which acts to reduce release of acetylcholine from motor nerve endings, has become an estab-lished therapy [166, 167]. Its application is commonly based on electromyographic recordings made during muscle contractions. Injections of botulinum toxin A reduce moderate spasticity (for review see [168–170]) and especially focal spasticity (e.g. domi-nance of forearm flexor tone [171]) by the reversible induction of peripheral paresis (chemical denervation). This usually lasts 3 to 5 months [122]. The combination of botulinum toxin type A with constraint movement therapy has a beneficial effect on upper limb function and spasticty [172]. It also represents a tech-nique for the improvement of bladder function in patients with incomplete voiding caused by hypertonia of the sphincter exter-nus muscle [173].

Less established treatments

There is a long history of neurosurgical alleviation of spasticity, specifically concerning localized treatment of spastic symptoms by interruption of the peripheral reflex arc. Selective dorsal rhizot-omy [174, 175] or dorsal longitudinal myelotomy [176] was applied in children with spasticity. These procedures reduce afferent input that is assumed to be responsible for increased muscle tone. Abnormal movement patterns, however, persist although spastic muscle tone is somewhat reduced [177–179]). Consequently some clinical signs become improved, while impairment of functional movements is little changed [122].

Similarly, infiltration of ventral roots or muscle nerves by phe-nol or alcohol can transform a spastic into a flaccid paresis [180]. These treatments are rarely used (most frequently in complete SCI), because spasticity usually reappears after some months and unwelcome sequels, such as skin ulcerations caused by sensory loss in the corresponding dermatomes, are not uncommon.

Beneficial effects on spasticity are also reported with functional electrical stimulation (FES) [181, 182] and by transcutaneous elec-trical stimulation of muscles [183]. A combined use of intensive vol-untary exercise and electrical stimulation of spastic arm muscles can have a beneficial effect on arm function in post-stroke hemiple-gic patients [184]. Also repetitive transcranical magnetic stimula-tion was reported to ameliorate spasticity [128]. For most patients with moderate spasticity such a treatment is too awkward to be used regularly and negative results have also been reported [185].

Conclusion

This chapter describes the differential roles of limb muscle acti-vation and reflex function in the passive, clinical condition and during functional movements after a stroke, multiple sclerosis or SCI. According to actual research studies, the assessment of exaggerated tendon reflexes is important for the clinical diagnosis but has a minor impact in spastic movement disorder. Following a CNS lesion, changes in mechanical muscle fibre properties lead to a regulation of muscle tone on a simpler level of organization. Thus, during functional movements, spastic muscle tone compensates for the loss of supraspinal neuronal drive. Therefore, in ambulatory people with a CNS damage, antispastic drugs should be kept to a minimum as they can accentuate paresis. Further studies are needed to understand the details of the intracellular and extracellular modifications of skeletal muscle that occur secondary to a spinal or supraspinal lesion. This might help in the development of novel therapeutic interventions to improve antispastic treatments in patients with overshooting spasticity.

References

1. Lance J. Symposium synopsis. In: RG Feldman, RR Young, WP Koella (Eds.). Spasticity: disordered motor control. Year Book Medical Publishers, Chicago, 1980, pp. 485–495.
2. Wissel J, Ward AB, Erztgaard P, et al. European consensus table on the use of botulinum toxin type A in adult spasticity. J Rehabil Med. 2009;**41**:13–25.
3. Malhotra S, Cousins E, Ward A, et al. An investigation into the agreement between clinical, biomechanical and neurophysiological measures of spasticity. Clin Rehabil. 2008; **22**:1105–1115.
4. Lorentzen J, Grey MJ, Crone C, Mazevet D, Biering-Sørensen F, Nielsen JB. Distinguishing active from passive components of ankle plantar flexor stiffness in stroke, spinal cord injury and multiple sclerosis. Clin Neurophysiol. 2010;**121**:1939–1951.
5. Malhotra S, Pandyan AD, Day CR, Jones PW, Hermens H. Spasticity, an impairment that is poorly defined and poorly measured. Clin Rehabil. 2009;**23**:651–658.
6. Abbruzzese G. The medical management of spasticity. Eur J Neurol. 2002;**9** Suppl 1:30–34; discussion 53–61.
7. Denny-Brown D. Historical aspects of the relation of spasticity to movements. In: RG Feldmann, RR Young, WP Koella (Eds.). Spasticity: disordered motor control. Year Book Medical Publishers, Chicago, 1980, pp. 1–15.
8. Gracies JM. Pathophysiology of impairment in patients with spasticity and use of stretch as a treatment of spastic hypertonia. Phys Med Rehabil Clin N Am. 2001;**12**:747–768.
9. Sheean G. The pathophysiology of spasticity. Eur J Neurol. 2002;**9** Suppl 1:3–9; dicussion 53–61.
10. Wiesendanger M. Neurobiology of spasticity. In: M Emre, R Benecke (Eds.). Spasticity. The current status of research and treatment. New Trends in Clinical Neurology Series, Parthenon, Carnforth, 1989, pp. 45–61.
11. Lidell E, Sherrington C. Reflexes in response to stretch (myotatic reflexes). Proc R Soc. 1924;**96**:212–242.
12. Dietz V, Young R. The syndrome of spastic paresis. In: T Brandt, L Caplan, J Dichgans, C Diener and C Kennard (Eds.). Neurological Disorders. Course and treatment. Academic Press, Amsterdam, 2003, pp 1247–1257.
13. Dietz V. Studies on the spastic rat: an adequate model for human spastic movement disorder? J Neurophysiol. 2008;**99**:1039–1040; author reply 1041.
14. Nielsen J, Petersen N, Crone C, Sinkjaer T. Stretch reflex regulation in healthy subjects and patients with spasticity. Neuromodulation. 2005;**8**:49–57.
15. Dietz V, Sinkjaer T. Spastic movement disorder: impaired reflex function and altered muscle mechanics. Lancet Neurol. 2007;**6**:725–733.
16. Mendell LM. Modifiability of spinal synapses. Physiol Rev. 1984;**64**:260–324.
17. Carr LJ, Harrison LM, Evans AL, Stephens JA. Patterns of central motor reorganization in hemiplegic cerebral palsy. Brain. 1993;**116** (Pt 5):1223–1247.
18. Hiersemenzel LP, Curt A, Dietz V. From spinal shock to spasticity: neuronal adaptations to a spinal cord injury. Neurology. 2000;**54**:1574–1582.
19. Dietrichson P. The fusimotor system in relation to spasticity and parkinsonian rigidity. Scand J Rehabil Med. 1973;**5**:174–178.
20. Rushworth G. Spasticity and rigidity: an experimental study and review. J Neurol Neurosurg Psychiatry. 1960;**23**:99–118.
21. Hagbarth KE, Wallin G, Lofstedt L. Muscle spindle responses to stretch in normal and spastic subjects. Scand J Rehabil Med. 1973;**5**:156–159.
22. Vallbo AB, Hagbarth KE, Torebjork HE, Wallin BG. Somatosensory, proprioceptive, and sympathetic activity in human peripheral nerves. Physiol Rev. 1979;**59**:919–957.
23. Wilson LR, Gandevia SC, Inglis JT, Gracies J, Burke D. Muscle spindle activity in the affected upper limb after a unilateral stroke. Brain. 1999;**122** (Pt 11):2079–2088.
24. Mazzocchio R, Rossi A. Involvement of spinal recurrent inhibition in spasticity. Further insight into the regulation of Renshaw cell activity. Brain. 1997;**120** (Pt 6):991–1003.
25. Shefner JM, Berman SA, Sarkarati M, Young RR. Recurrent inhibition is increased in patients with spinal cord injury. Neurology. 1992;**42**:2162–2168.
26. Nacimiento W, Mautes A, Topper R, et al. B-50 (GAP-43) in the spinal cord caudal to hemisection: indication for lack of intraspinal sprouting in dorsal root axons. J Neurosci Res. 1993;**35**:603–617.
27. Burke D, Ashby P. Are spinal 'presynaptic' inhibitory mechanisms suppressed in spasticity? J Neurol Sci. 1972;**15**:321–326.
28. Faist M, Mazevet D, Dietz V, Pierrot-Deseilligny E. A quantitative assessment of presynaptic inhibition of Ia afferents in spastics. Differences in hemiplegics and paraplegics. Brain. 1994;**117** (Pt 6):1449–1455.
29. Crone C, Nielsen J, Petersen N, Ballegaard M, Hultborn H. Disynaptic reciprocal inhibition of ankle extensors in spastic patients. Brain. 1994;**117** (Pt 5):1161–1168.
30. Boorman G, Hulliger M, Lee RG, Tako K, Tanaka R. Reciprocal Ia inhibition in patients with spinal spasticity. Neurosci Lett. 1991;**127**:57–60.
31. Knutsson E, Martensson A, Gransberg L. Influences of muscle stretch reflexes on voluntary, velocity-controlled movements in spastic paraparesis. Brain. 1997;**120** (Pt 9):1621–1633.
32. Okuma Y, Lee RG. Reciprocal inhibition in hemiplegia: correlation with clinical features and recovery. Can J Neurol Sci. 1996;**23**:15–23.
33. Nielsen J, Petersen N, Crone C. Changes in transmission across synapses of Ia afferents in spastic patients. Brain. 1995;**118** (Pt 4):995–1004.
34. Marque P, Simonetta-Moreau M, Maupas E, Roques CF. Facilitation of transmission in heteronymous group II pathways in spastic hemiplegic patients. J Neurol Neurosurg Psychiatry. 2001;**70**:36–42.
35. Nardone A, Schieppati M. Reflex contribution of spindle group Ia and II afferent input to leg muscle spasticity as revealed by tendon vibration in hemiparesis. Clin Neurophysiol. 2005;**116**:1370–1381.
36. Remy-Neris O, Denys P, Daniel O, Barbeau H, Bussel B. Effect of intrathecal clonidine on group I and group II oligosynaptic excitation in paraplegics. Exp Brain Res. 2003;**148**:509–514.
37. Nielsen JB, Crone C, Hultborn H. The spinal pathophysiology of spasticity—from a basic science point of view. Acta Physiol (Oxf). 2007;**189**:171–180.
38. Levin MF, Feldman AG. The role of stretch reflex threshold regulation in normal and impaired motor control. Brain Res. 1994;**657**:23–30.
39. Nielsen JF, Sinkjaer T. A comparison of clinical and laboratory measures of spasticity. Mult Scler. 1996;**1**:296–301.

40. Powers RK, Marder-Meyer J, Rymer WZ. Quantitative relations between hypertonia and stretch reflex threshold in spastic hemiparesis. Ann Neurol. 1988;**23**:115–124.

41. Beres-Jones JA, Johnson TD, Harkema SJ. Clonus after human spinal cord injury cannot be attributed solely to recurrent muscle-tendon stretch. Exp Brain Res. 2003;**149**:222–236.

42. Bussel B, Roby-Brami A, Azouvi P, Biraben A, Yakovleff A, Held JP. Myoclonus in a patient with spinal cord transection. Possible involvement of the spinal stepping generator. Brain. 1988;**111** (Pt 5):1235–1245.

43. Muller R, Dietz V. Neuronal function in chronic spinal cord injury: divergence between locomotor and flexion- and H-reflex activity. Clin Neurophysiol. 2006;**117**:1499–1507.

44. Ditunno JF, Little JW, Tessler A, Burns AS. Spinal shock revisited: a four-phase model. Spinal Cord. 2004;**42**:383–395.

45. Andersen OK, Finnerup NB, Spaich EG, Jensen TS, Arendt-Nielsen L. Expansion of nociceptive withdrawal reflex receptive fields in spinal cord injured humans. Clin Neurophysiol. 2004;**115**:2798–2810.

46. Schmit BD, McKenna-Cole A, Rymer WZ. Flexor reflexes in chronic spinal cord injury triggered by imposed ankle rotation. Muscle Nerve. 2000;**23**:793–803.

47. Bennett DJ, Sanelli L, Cooke CL, Harvey PJ, Gorassini MA. Spastic long-lasting reflexes in the awake rat after sacral spinal cord injury. J Neurophysiol. 2004;**91**:2247–2258.

48. Gorassini MA, Knash ME, Harvey PJ, Bennett DJ, Yang JF. Role of motoneurons in the generation of muscle spasms after spinal cord injury. Brain. 2004;**127**:2247–2258.

49. Goldberger ME, Murray M. Patterns of sprouting and implications for recovery of function. Adv Neurol. 1988;**47**:361–385.

50. Little JW, Ditunno JF, Jr., Stiens SA, Harris RM. Incomplete spinal cord injury: neuronal mechanisms of motor recovery and hyperreflexia. Arch Phys Med Rehabil. 1999;**80**:587–599.

51. Hornby TG, Rymer WZ, Benz EN, Schmit BD. Windup of flexion reflexes in chronic human spinal cord injury: a marker for neuronal plateau potentials? J Neurophysiol. 2003;**89**:416–426.

52. Knikou M, Conway BA. Effects of electrically induced muscle contraction on flexion reflex in human spinal cord injury. Spinal Cord. 2005;**43**:640–648.

53. Deutsch KM, Hornby TG, Schmit BD. The intralimb coordination of the flexor reflex response is altered in chronic human spinal cord injury. Neurosci Lett. 2005;**380**:305–310.

54. Ashworth B. Preliminary trial of cardioprodal in multiple sclerosos. Practitioner. 1964;**192**:540–542.

55. Sinkjaer T, Toft E, Andreassen S, Hornemann BC. Muscle stiffness in human ankle dorsiflexors: intrinsic and reflex components. J Neurophysiol. 1988;**60**:1110–1121.

56. Toft E, Sinkjaer T, Andreassen S, Larsen K. Mechanical and electromyographic responses to stretch of the human ankle extensors. J Neurophysiol. 1991;**65**:1402–1410.

57. Condliffe EG, Clark DJ, Patten C. Reliability of elbow stretch reflex assessment in chronic post-stroke hemiparesis. Clin Neurophysiol. 2005;**116**:1870–1878.

58. Dietz V, Trippel M, Berger W. Reflex activity and muscle tone during elbow movements in patients with spastic paresis. Ann Neurol. 1991;**30**:767–779.

59. Hufschmidt A, Mauritz KH. Chronic transformation of muscle in spasticity: a peripheral contribution to increased tone. J Neurol Neurosurg Psychiatry. 1985;**48**:676–685.

60. Malouin F, Bonneau C, Pichard L, Corriveau D. Non-reflex mediated changes in plantarflexor muscles early after stroke. Scand J Rehabil Med. 1997;**29**:147–153.

61. Sinkjaer T, Magnussen I. Passive, intrinsic and reflex-mediated stiffness in the ankle extensors of hemiparetic patients. Brain. 1994;**117** (Pt 2):355–363.

62. Thilmann AF, Fellows SJ, Ross HF. Biomechanical changes at the ankle joint after stroke. J Neurol Neurosurg Psychiatry. 1991;**54**: 134–139.

63. Galiana L, Fung J, Kearney R. Identification of intrinsic and reflex ankle stiffness components in stroke patients. Exp Brain Res. 2005;**165**:422–434.

64. O'Dwyer NJ, Ada L. Reflex hyperexcitability and muscle contracture in relation to spastic hypertonia. Curr Opin Neurol. 1996;**9**:451–455.

65. Sinkjaer T, Toft E, Larsen K, Andreassen S, Hansen HJ. Non-reflex and reflex mediated ankle joint stiffness in multiple sclerosis patients with spasticity. Muscle Nerve. 1993;**16**:69–76.

66. Ibrahim IK, Berger W, Trippel M, Dietz V. Stretch-induced electromyographic activity and torque in spastic elbow muscles. Differential modulation of reflex activity in passive and active motor tasks. Brain. 1993;**116** (Pt 4):971–989.

67. Mirbagheri MM, Barbeau H, Ladouceur M, Kearney RE. Intrinsic and reflex stiffness in normal and spastic, spinal cord injured subjects. Exp Brain Res. 2001;**141**:446–459.

68. Stokic DS. Spasticity 30 years later: The truth is still in the eye of the beholder. Clin Neurophysiol. 2010;**121**:1789–1791.

69. O'Dwyer NJ, Ada L, Neilson PD. Spasticity and muscle contracture following stroke. Brain. 1996;**119** (Pt 5):1737–1749.

70. Chung SG, van Rey E, Bai Z, Rymer WZ, Roth EJ, Zhang LQ. Separate quantification of reflex and nonreflex components of spastic hypertonia in chronic hemiparesis. Arch Phys Med Rehabil. 2008;**89**:700–710.

71. Dietz V, Ketelsen UP, Berger W, Quintern J. Motor unit involvement in spastic paresis. Relationship between leg muscle activation and histochemistry. J Neurol Sci. 1986;**75**:89–103.

72. Edstrom L. Selective changes in the sizes of red and white muscle fibres in upper motor lesions and Parkinsonism. J Neurol Sci. 1970;**11**:537–550.

73. Lieber RL, Steinman S, Barash IA, Chambers H. Structural and functional changes in spastic skeletal muscle. Muscle Nerve. 2004;**29**:615–627.

74. Vattanasilp W, Ada L, Crosbie J. Contribution of thixotropy, spasticity, and contracture to ankle stiffness after stroke. J Neurol Neurosurg Psychiatry. 2000;**69**:34–39.

75. Kamper DG, Schmit BD, Rymer WZ. Effect of muscle biomechanics on the quantification of spasticity. Ann Biomed Eng. 2001;**29**:1122–1134.

76. Schmit BD, Benz EN, Rymer WZ. Afferent mechanisms for the reflex response to imposed ankle movement in chronic spinal cord injury. Exp Brain Res. 2002;**145**:40–49.

77. Berger W, Horstmann G, Dietz V. Tension development and muscle activation in the leg during gait in spastic hemiparesis: independence of muscle hypertonia and exaggerated stretch reflexes. J Neurol Neurosurg Psychiatry. 1984;**47**:1029–1033.

78. Dietz V. Spinal cord pattern generators for locomotion. Clin Neurophysiol. 2003b;**114**:1379–1389.

79. Dietz V, Berger W. Normal and impaired regulation of muscle stiffness in gait: a new hypothesis about muscle hypertonia. Exp Neurol. 1983;**79**:680–687.

80. Rosenfalck A, Andreassen S. Impaired regulation of force and firing pattern of single motor units in patients with spasticity. J Neurol Neurosurg Psychiatry. 1980;**43**:907–916.

81. Kautz SA, Patten C, Neptune RR. Does unilateral pedaling activate a rhythmic locomotor pattern in the nonpedaling leg in post-stroke hemiparesis? J Neurophysiol. 2006;**95**:3154–3163.

82. Maegele M, Muller S, Wernig A, Edgerton VR, Harkema SJ. Recruitment of spinal motor pools during voluntary movements versus stepping after human spinal cord injury. J Neurotrauma. 2002;**19**:1217–1229.

83. Dietz V, Quintern J, Berger W. Electrophysiological studies of gait in spasticity and rigidity. Evidence that altered mechanical properties of muscle contribute to hypertonia. Brain. 1981;**104**:431–449.

84. Knutsson E, Richards C. Different types of disturbed motor control in gait of hemiparetic patients. Brain. 1979;**102**:405–430.

85. Levin MF, Selles RW, Verheul MH, Meijer OG. Deficits in the coordination of agonist and antagonist muscles in stroke patients: implications for normal motor control. Brain Res. 2000;853:352–369.

86. Mazzaro N, Nielsen JF, Grey MJ, Sinkjaer T. Decreased contribution from afferent feedback to the soleus muscle during walking in patients with spastic stroke. J Stroke Cerebrovasc Dis. 2007;16:135–144.

87. Nardone A, Galante M, Lucas B, Schieppati M. Stance control is not affected by paresis and reflex hyperexcitability: the case of spastic patients. J Neurol Neurosurg Psychiatry. 2001;70:635–643.

88. Dietz V. Neurophysiology of gait disorders: present and future applications. Electroencephalogr Clin Neurophysiol. 1997;103:333–355.

89. Dietz V. Proprioception and locomotor disorders. Nat Rev Neurosci. 2002;3:781–790.

90. Faist M, Dietz V, Pierrot-Deseilligny E. Modulation, probably presynaptic in origin, of monosynaptic Ia excitation during human gait. Exp Brain Res. 1996;109:441–449.

91. Faist M, Ertel M, Berger W, Dietz V. Impaired modulation of quadriceps tendon jerk reflex during spastic gait: differences between spinal and cerebral lesions. Brain. 1999;122 (Pt 3):567–579.

92. Fung J, Barbeau H. Effects of conditioning cutaneomuscular stimulation on the soleus H-reflex in normal and spastic paretic subjects during walking and standing. J Neurophysiol. 1994;72:2090–2104.

93. Jones CA, Yang JF. Reflex behavior during walking in incomplete spinal-cord-injured subjects. Exp Neurol. 1994;128:239–248.

94. Sinkjaer T, Andersen JB, Nielsen JF. Impaired stretch reflex and joint torque modulation during spastic gait in multiple sclerosis patients. J Neurol. 1996;243:566–574.

95. Sinkjaer T, Toft E, Hansen HJ. H-reflex modulation during gait in multiple sclerosis patients with spasticity. Acta Neurol Scand. 1995;91:239–246.

96. Dietz V. Human neuronal control of automatic functional movements: interaction between central programs and afferent input. Physiol Rev. 1992;72:33–69.

97. Dietz V. Spastic movement disorder: what is the impact of research on clinical practice? J Neurol Neurosurg Psychiatry. 2003a;74:820–821.

98. Christensen LO, Andersen JB, Sinkjaer T, Nielsen J. Transcranial magnetic stimulation and stretch reflexes in the tibialis anterior muscle during human walking. J Physiol. 2001;531:545–557.

99. Sinkjaer T, Andersen JB, Nielsen JF, Hansen HJ. Soleus long-latency stretch reflexes during walking in healthy and spastic humans. Clin Neurophysiol. 1999;110:951–959.

100. Burne JA, Carleton VL, O'Dwyer NJ. The spasticity paradox: movement disorder or disorder of resting limbs? J Neurol Neurosurg Psychiatry. 2005;76:47–54.

101. Gracies JM. Pathophysiology of spastic paresis. I: Paresis and soft tissue changes. Muscle Nerve. 2005;31:535–551.

102. Lum PS, Patten C, Kothari D, Yap R. Effects of velocity on maximal torque production in poststroke hemiparesis. Muscle Nerve. 2004;30:732–742.

103. Toft E, Sinkjaer T, Andreassen S, Hansen HJ. Stretch responses to ankle rotation in multiple sclerosis patients with spasticity. Electroencephalogr Clin Neurophysiol. 1993;89:311–318.

104. Marita H, Shinds M, Momoi H, Yanagawa S, Yanagisawa N. Lack of modulation of Ib inhibition during antagonist contraction in spasticity. Neurology. 2006;67:52–56.

105. Dewald JP, Pope PS, Given JD, Buchanan TS, Rymer WZ. Abnormal muscle coactivation patterns during isometric torque generation at the elbow and shoulder in hemiparetic subjects. Brain. 1995;118 (Pt 2):495–510.

106. Kamper DG, Harvey RL, Suresh S, Rymer WZ. Relative contributions of neural mechanisms versus muscle mechanics in promoting finger extension deficits following stroke. Muscle Nerve. 2003;28:309–318.

107. Kallenberg LA, Hermens HJ. Motor unit peroperties of biceps brachii during dynamic contractions in chronic stroke patients. Muscle Nerve. 2011;43:112–119.

108. Foran JR, Steinman S, Barash I, Chambers HG, Lieber RL. Structural and mechanical alterations in spastic skeletal muscle. Dev Med Child Neurol. 2005;47:713–717.

109. Lieber RL, Friden J. Spasticity causes a fundamental rearrangement of muscle-joint interaction. Muscle Nerve. 2002;25:265–270.

110. Lin JP. The contribution of spasticity to the movement disorder of cerebral palsy using pathway analysis: Does spasticity matter? Dev Med Child Neurol. 2011;53:7–9

111. Petersen TH, Farmer SF, Kliim-Due M, Nielsen JB. Failure of normal development of central drive to ankle dorsiflexors relates to gait deficits in children with cerebral palsy. J Neurophysiol. 2013;109: 625–639.

112. Urban PP, Wolf T, Uebele M, et al. Occurence and clinical predictors of spasticity after ischemic stroke. Stroke. 2010;41:2016–2020.

113. Latash M, Anson J. What are 'normal movements' in atypic populations? Behav Brain Sci. 1996;19: 55–106.

114. Kloter E, Wirz M, Dietz V. Locomotion in stroke subjects: Interactions between unaffected and affected sides. Brain. 2011;134:721–731.

115. Bass B, Weinshenker B, Rice GP, et al. Tizanidine versus baclofen in the treatment of spasticity in patients with multiple sclerosis. Can J Neurol Sci. 1988;15:15–19.

116. Bes A, Eyssette M, Pierrot-Deseilligny E, Rohmer F, Warter JM. A multi-centre, double-blind trial of tizanidine, a new antispastic agent, in spasticity associated with hemiplegia. Curr Med Res Opin. 1988;10:709–718.

117. Hoogstraten MC, van der Ploeg RJ, vd Burg W, Vreeling A, van Marle S, Minderhoud JM. Tizanidine versus baclofen in the treatment of spasticity in multiple sclerosis patients. Acta Neurol Scand. 1988;77:224–230.

118. Lapierre Y, Bouchard S, Tansey C, Gendron D, Barkas WJ, Francis GS. Treatment of spasticity with tizanidine in multiple sclerosis. Can J Neurol Sci. 1987;14:513–517.

119. Stien R, Nordal HJ, Oftedal SI, Slettebo M. The treatment of spasticity in multiple sclerosis: a double-blind clinical trial of a new anti-spastic drug tizanidine compared with baclofen. Acta Neurol Scand. 1987;75:190–194.

120. Latash ML, Penn RD. Changes in voluntary motor control induced by intrathecal baclofen in patients with spasticity of different etiology. Physiother Res Int. 1996;1:229–246.

121. Thach W, Montgomery E. Motor systems. In: Pearlman A and Collins R, eds. Neurobiology Disease. Oxford University Press, Oxford, 1990, pp. 168–196.

122. Corry IS, Cosgrove AP, Walsh EG, McClean D, Graham HK. Botulinum toxin A in the hemiplegic upper limb: a double-blind trial. Dev Med Child Neurol. 1997;39:185–193.

123. Miscio G, Del Conte C, Pianca D, et al. Botulinum toxin in post-stroke patients: stiffness modifications and clinical implications. J Neurol. 2004;251:189–196.

124. Trompetto C, Curra A, Buccolieri A, Suppa A, Abbruzzese G, Berardelli A. Botulinum toxin changes intrafusal feedback in dystonia: a study with the tonic vibration reflex. Mov Disord. 2006;21:777–782.

125. Boviatsis EJ, Kouyialis AT, Korfias S, Sakas DE. Functional outcome of intrathecal baclofen administration for severe spasticity. Clin Neurol Neurosurg. 2005;107:289–295.

126. Meythaler JM, Guin-Renfroe S, Hadley MN. Continuously infused intrathecal baclofen for spastic/dystonic hemiplegia: a preliminary report. Am J Phys Med Rehabil. 1999;78:247–254.

127. Sadiq SA, Wang GC. Long-term intrathecal baclofen therapy in ambulatory patients with spasticity. J Neurol. 2006;253:563–569.

128. Centonze D, Koch G, Versace V, et al. Repetitive transcranial magnetic stimulation of the motor cortex ameliorates spasticity in multiple sclerosis. Neurology. 2007;68:1045–1050.

129. Diserens K, Perret N, Chatelain S, et al. The effect of repetitive arm cycling on post stroke spasticity and motor control: repetitive arm cycling and spasticity. J Neurol Sci. 2007;253:18–24.

130. Dietz, V, Harkema SJ. Locomotor activity in spinal cord injured persons. J Appl Physiol. 2004;**96**:1954–1960.

131. Riener R, Lueneburger L, Jezernik S, Anderschitz M, Colombo G, Dietz V. Locomotor training in subjects with sensori-motor deficits: An overview of the robotic gait orthosis lokomat. J Healthc Eng. 2010;**1**:197–216.

132. Pin T, Dyke P, Chan M. The effectiveness of passive stretching in children with cerebral palsy. Dev Med Child Neurol. 2006;**48**:855–862.

133. Barnes MP, Kent RM, Semlyen JK, McMullen KM. Spasticity in multiple sclerosis. Neurorehabil Neural Repair. 2003;**17**:66–70.

134. Glenn MB, Whyte J. The Practical Management of Spasticity in Children and Adults. Lea &Febiger, Philadelphia, London, 1990.

135. Kwakkel G, Wagenaar RC, Twisk JW, Lankhorst GJ, Koetsier JC. Intensity of leg and arm training after primary middle-cerebral-artery stroke: a randomised trial. Lancet. 1999;**354**:191–196.

136. Ansari NN, Adelmanesh F, Naghdi S, et al. The effect of physiotherapeutic ultrasound on muscle spasticity in patients with hemiplegia: A pilot study. Electromygr Clin Neurophysiol. 2006;**46**:247–252.

137. Barbeau H, Fung J. New experimental approaches in the treatment of spastic gait disorders. In: Fossberg H and Hirschfeld H, editors. Movement Disorders in Children, **Vol 36**. Karger, Basel, 1992, pp. 234–246.

138. Sakamato T, Porte LL, Asanuma H. Functional rote of the sensory cortex in learning motor skills in cats. Brain Res. 1989;**503**:258–264.

139. Lam T, Wirz M, Lunenburger L, Dietz V. Swing phase resistance enhances flexor muscle activity during treadmill locomotion in incomplete spinal cord injury. Neurorehabil Neural Repair. 2008;**22**:438–446.

140. Dietz V, Colombo G, Jensen L. Locomotor activity in spinal man. Lancet. 1994;**344**:1260–1263.

141. Visintin M, Barbeau H. The effects of body weight support on the locomotor pattern of spastic paretic patients. Can J Neurol Sci. 1989;**16**: 315–325.

142. Posteraro F, Mazzoleni S, Aliboni S, et al. Upper limb spasticty reduction following active training: A robot-mediated study in patients with chronic hemiparesis. J Rehabil Med. 2010;**42**:279–281.

144. Alon G, Sunnerhagen KS, Geurts A, et al. A home-based, self-administered stimulation program to improve selected hand functions of chronic stroke. NeuroRehabilitation. 2003;**18**:215–225.

144. Yan T, Hui-Chan CWY, Li LSW. Functional electrical stimulation improves motor recovery of the lower extremity and walking ability of subjects with first acute stroke: A randomized placebo-controlled trial. Stroke. 2005;**36**:80–85.

145. Wernig A, Muller S, Nanassy A, Cagol E. Laufband therapy based on 'rules of spinal locomotion' is effective in spinal cord injured persons. Eur J Neurosci. 1995;**7**:823–829.

146. Wirz M, van Hedel HJ, Rupp R, Curt A, Dietz V. Muscle force and gait performance: relationships after spinal cord injury. Arch Phys Med Rehabil. 2006;**87**:1218–1222.

147. Aaslund MK, Helbostad JL, Moe-Nilssen R. Walking during body-weight-supported treadmill training and acute responses to varying walking speed and body-weight support in ambulatory patients post-stroke. Physiother Theory Pract 2013;**29**: 278–289.

148. Dobkin, B.H., Duncan PW. Should body weight supported treadmill training and robotic-assistive steppers for locomotor training trot back to the starting gate? Neurorehabil Neural Repair. 2012;**26**:308–17.

149. Dietz V. Neuronal plasticity after human spinal cord injury: Positive and negative effects. Exp Neurol. 2012;**235**:110–115.

150. Montané E, Vallano A, Laporte JR. Oral antispastic drugs in nonprogressive neurologic diseases: A systematic review. Neurology. 2004;**63**:1357–1363.

151. Duncan GW, Shahani BT, Young RR. An evaluation of baclofen treatment for certain symptoms in patients with spinal cord lesions. A double-blind, cross-over study. Neurology. 1976;**26**:441–446.

152. Hattab JR. Review of European clinical trials with baclofen. In: RG Feldman, RR Young, WP Koella (Eds.), Spasticity: Disordered Motor Control. Year Book, Chicago, 1980, pp. 71–85.

153. Thomas CK, Hager-Ross CK, Klein CS Effects of baclofen on motor units paralysed by chronic cervical spinal cord injury. Brain. 2010;**133**:117–125.

154. Cutter NC, Scott DD, Johnson JC, Whiteneck G. Gabapentin effect on spasticity in multiple sclerosis: a placebo-controlled, randomized trial. Arch Phys Med Rehabil. 2000;**81**:164–169.

155. Schomburg ED, Steffens H. The effect of DOPA and clonidine on reflex pathways from group II muscle afferents to alpha-motoneurones in the cat. Exp Brain Res. 1988;**71**:442–446.

156. Davidoff RA. Antispasticity drugs: mechanisms of action. Ann Neurol. 1985;**17**:107–116.

157. Zajicek J, Fox P, Sanders H, et al, UK MS-Reseach Group. Cannabinoids for treatment of spasticity and other symptoms related to multiple sclerosis (CAMS study): Multicenter randomised placebo-controlled trial. Lancet. 2003;**362**:1517–1526.

158. Latash ML, Penn RD, Corcos DM, Gottlieb GL. Short-term effects of intrathecal baclofen in spasticity. Exp Neurol. 1989;**103**:165–172.

159. Ochs G, Struppler A, Meyerson BA, et al. Intrathecal baclofen for long-term treatment of spasticity: a multi-centre study. J Neurol Neurosurg Psychiatry. 1989;**52**:933–939.

160. Penn RD, Savoy SM, Corcos D, et al. Intrathecal baclofen for severe spinal spasticity. N Engl J Med. 1989;**320**:1517–1521.

161. Zdolsek HA, Olesch C, Antolovich G, et al. Intrathecal baclofen therapy: Benefits and complications. J Intellect Dev Disabil. 2011;**36**:B207–213.

162. Coffey JR, Cahill D, Steers W, et al. Intrathecal baclofen for intractable spasticity of spinal origin: results of a long-term multicenter study. J Neurosurg. 1993;**78**:226–232.

163. Stewart-Wynne EG, Silbert PL, Buffery S, Perlman D, Tan E. Intrathecal baclofen for severe spasticity: five years experience. Clin Exp Neurol. 1991;**28**:244–255.

164. Dressnandt J, Conrad B. Lasting reduction of severe spasticity after ending chronic treatment with intrathecal baclofen. J Neurol Neurosurg Psychiatry. 1996;**60**:168–173.

165. Schurch B. Errors and limitations of the multimodality checking methods of defective spinal intrathecal pump systems. Case report. Paraplegia. 1993;**31**:611–615.

166. Davis D, Jabbari B. Significant improvement of stiff-person syndrome after paraspinal injection of botulinum toxin A. Mov Disord. 1993;**8**:371–373.

167. Al-Khodairy AT, Gobelet C, Rossier AB. Has botulinum toxin type A a place in the treatment of spasticity in spinal cord injury patients? Spinal Cord. 1998;**36**:854–548.

168. Hecht MJ, Stolze H, Auf dem Brinke M, et al. Botulinum neurotoxin type A injections reduce spasticity in mild to moderate hereditary spastic paraplegia—report of 19 cases. Mov Disord. 2008;**23**:228–233.

169. Ozcakir S, Sivrioglu K. Botulinum toxin in poststroke spasticity. Clin Med Res. 2007;**5**:132–138.

170. Simpson DM, Gracies JM, Graham HK, et al. Assessment: Botulinum neurotoxin for the treatment of spasticity (an evidence-based review): report of the Therapeutics and Technology Assessment Subcommittee of the American Academy of Neurology. Neurology. 2008;**70**:1691–1698.

171. Marciniak C, Rader L, Gagnon C. The use of botulinum toxin for spasticity after spinal cord injury. Am J Phys Med Rehabil. 2008;**87**:312–317; quiz 318–320, 329.

172. Sun SF, Hsu CW, Sun HP, et al. Combined botulinum toxin type A with modified constraint-induced movement therpy for chronic stroke patients with upper extremity spasticity: A randomized controlled study. Neurorehabil Neural Repair. 2010;**24**:34–41.

173. Schurch B, Hauri D, Rodic B, Curt A, Meyer M, Rossier AB. Botulinum-A toxin as a treatment of detrusor-sphincter dyssynergia: a prospective study in 24 spinal cord injury patients. J Urol. 1996;**155**:1023–1029.

174. Laitinen LV, Nilsson S, Fugl-Meyer AR. Selective posterior rhizotomy for treatment of spasticity. J Neurosurg. 1983;**58**: 895–899.

175. Peacock WJ, Staudt LA. Functional outcomes following selective posterior rhizotomy in children with cerebral palsy. J Neurosurg. 1991;**74**:380–385.

176. Putty TK, Shapiro SA. Efficacy of dorsal longitudinal myelotomy in treating spinal spasticity: a review of 20 cases. J Neurosurg. 1991;**75**:397–401.

177. Giuliani CA. Dorsal rhizotomy for children with cerebral palsy: support for concepts of motor control. Phys Ther. 1991;**71**:248–259.

178. McLaughlin JF, Bjornson KF, Astley SJ, et al. Selective dorsal rhizotomy: efficacy and safety in an investigator-masked randomized clinical trial. Dev Med Child Neurol. 1998;**40**:220–232.

179. Wright FV, Sheil EM, Drake JM, Wedge JH, Naumann S. Evaluation of selective dorsal rhizotomy for the reduction of spasticity in cerebral palsy: a randomized controlled tria. Dev Med Child Neurol. 1998;**40**:239–247.

180. Scott BA, Weinstein Z, Chiteman R, Pulliam MW. Intrathecal phenol and glycerin in metrizamide for treatment of intractable spasms in paraplegia. Case report. J Neurosurg. 1985;**63**:125–127.

181. Pease WS. Therapeutic electrical stimulation for spasticity: quantitative gait analysis. Am J Phys Med Rehabil. 1998;**77**:351–355.

182. Weingarden HP, Zeilig G, Heruti R, et al. Hybrid functional electrical stimulation orthosis system for the upper limb: effects on spasticity in chronic stable hemiplegia. Am J Phys Med Rehabil. 1998;**77**:276–281.

183. Seib TP, Price R, Reyes MR, Lehmann JF. The quantitative measurement of spasticity: effect of cutaneous electrical stimulation. Arch Phys Med Rehabil. 1994;**75**:746–750.

184. Popovic MR, Keller T, Pappas IP, Dietz V, Morari M. Surface-stimulation technology for grasping and walking neuroprosthesis. IEEE Eng Med Biol Mag. 2001;**20**:82–93.

185. Sonde L, Kalimo H, Fernaeus SE, Viitanen M. Low TENS treatment on post-stroke paretic arm: a three-year follow-up. Clin Rehabil. 2000;**14**:14–19.

CHAPTER 10

Autonomic nervous system dysfunction

Angela Gall and Mike Craggs

Introduction

The autonomic nervous system (ANS) regulates, adjusts, and coordinates visceral functions of the body. An understanding of its normal functions and pathophysiology is essential to improve diagnosis, investigation, and management in autonomic neurorehabilitation [1].

The ANS, which is divided into the sympathetic and parasympathetic systems, is primarily an efferent system. It receives its afferent input from many visceral afferent neurons, sometimes interacting with somatic reflexes. The ANS has both central nervous system (CNS) and peripheral nervous system (PNS) components. The outflow of both the sympathetic and the parasympathetic nervous system follows a two-neuron pathway, which consists of a preganglionic neuron located within the CNS and a postganglionic neuron located outside the CNS. Sympathetic fibres leave the CNS at the thoracolumbar level, and the parasympathetic fibres leave at the craniosacral level. In general, the sympathetic and parasympathetic nervous systems have opposing effects on visceral function. The hypothalamus serves as the major control centre for most ANS functions; local reflex circuits that interrelate visceral afferent and autonomic efferent activity are an integrated control system in the spinal cord and brainstem.

It is the sympathetic division of the ANS, which is primarily activated in response to stressors such as exercise, temperature fluctuations, low blood glucose, and other environmental challenges. The sympathetic nervous system is critical for maintaining blood pressure as we move from the horizontal to the vertical and for this control it is an automatic reflex that constricts the blood vessels in the legs and abdomen to prevent blood rushing from our head to pool in these regions. During exercise, sympathetic activity increases the frequency and strength of heartbeats whilst also controlling sweating and blood flow to the skin to maintain a physiologically appropriate body temperature. Sympathetic influences also help to maintain continence.

The parasympathetic division provides an important counterbalance, or opposition, to sympathetic activity in many organs of the body, for example by slowing the heart during sleep, emptying the bladder and bowel, and constricting the pupils. However, there are some end organs, for example peripheral blood vessels, which have only a sympathetic supply.

It is not surprising, knowing the extent of ANS control of the visceral organs, that problems can arise both globally and regionally, and show up in many different ways. For example, lesions in the hypothalamus, spinal cord, or the sympathetic nerves controlling sweat glands could seriously impair perspiration leading to poor temperature control; likewise diseases or trauma in the brain stem, spinal cord, or parasympathetic nerves could lead to urinary retention and erectile dysfunction in men.

Interestingly, autonomic failure is often associated with the side effects of drugs being taken for treating other disorders, particularly those pharmacological agents that interfere with normal chemical neurotransmission within autonomic pathways. So, for example, treating recumbent hypertension in the elderly using antihypertensive drugs, which interfere with adrenergic mechanisms in the sympathetic nervous system, may result in more serious complications of hypotension and dizziness when the person stands up. Another common example is the experience of dry-mouth and urinary retention associated with antidepressant medication.

In the context of understanding ANS dysfunction for advancing neurorehabilitation practice, this chapter aims to deliver the following aspects: an overview of autonomic functions, their central control and pathophysiology; a review of the most important and specific autonomic system disorders, their causes, management and assessment; and finally, future directions for neurorehabilitation following autonomic failure.

Peripheral autonomic function and its central control

The peripheral ANS, comprising sympathetic and parasympathetic neural pathways, is primarily an efferent system innervating smooth muscle of the target visceral end organs to provide specific functions (Figure 10.1). Most organs are supplied by both of these pathways that are said to have opposing efferent and regulatory controls such as dilating or constricting the pupils or accelerating or slowing heart rate, in each case by sympathetic or parasympathetic activity, respectively. However, there are four end organs that have only sympathetic supply: these are peripheral blood vessels, sweat glands, apocrine glands, and the erector pili muscles, one exception to this being the cavernosus tissue in the penis and clitoris, which have both sympathetic and parasympathetic fibres.

Autonomic efferent pathways

Preganglionic pathways of autonomic peripheral efferent systems have their origins in either the midbrain, the brainstem or spinal

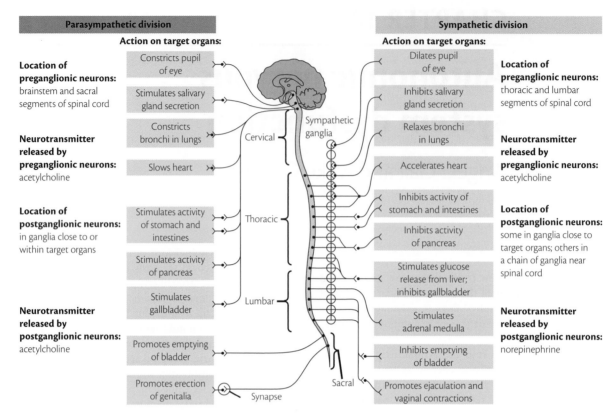

Fig. 10.1 Autonomic innervation and functional effects on visceral organs.

cord. The sympathetic division has its peripheral origins at the level of the thoracolumbar spinal cord whereas the parasympathetic division has two origins, one in the cranial nerves of the brainstem and the other in the sacral spinal cord. For both divisions those preganglionic nerves originating in the spinal cord have their cell bodies in the intermediolateral part of the grey matter. Postganglionic pathways of both divisions originate in peripheral ganglia, but whereas parasympathetic ganglia are always located at or close to the effector organs, those of the sympathetic pathways synapse mainly in the paravertebral sympathetic chain of ganglia or one of four more peripheral ganglia, superior cervical,

coeliac, superior mesenteric, or inferior mesenteric (Figure 10.2). This description is overly simplistic as it does not reflect the extensive neuronal convergence and divergence characteristic of the ANS. That is, each postganglionic cell receives information from multiple preganglionic cells and each preganglionic cell communicates with multiple postganglionic cells. Futhermore, nerves from individual spinal segments can have widespread effects on multiple organs.

Both sympathetic and parasympathetic preganganglionic nerves have a common neurotransmitter, acetylcholine, which acts via nicotinic receptors (i.e. not blocked by atropine.) It is the

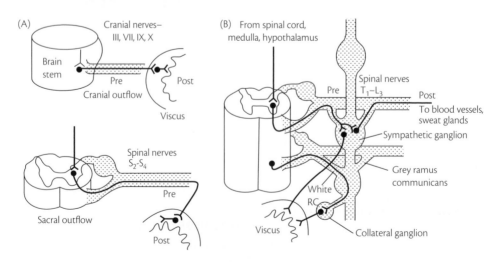

Fig. 10.2 Pre- and postganglionic peripheral efferent autonomic pathways. (A) Parasympathetic (B) Sympathetic.

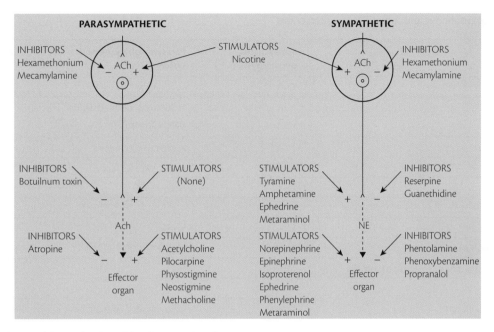

Fig. 10.3 Neurotransmitters and drug actions in peripheral autonomic pathways.

postganglionic neurons through their specific neurotransmitters, noradrenaline for sympathetic pathways and acetylcholine (via muscarinic receptors of which there are a number of different types, e.g M2, M3, M4) for parasympathetic pathways, which determines the final functional effects on the different effector organs. Although norepinephrine (noradrenaline) is the principal neurotransmitter for postganglionic sympathetic nerves there are a few exceptions where there is cholinergic neurotransmission (for example sudomotor nerves, vasodilator nerves of skeletal muscle, and the adrenal medulla.) Interestingly, the adrenal medulla secretes both norepinephrine (noradrenaline) and epinephrine (adrenaline), which respectively mediate vasoconstriction through actions on α_1 (postsynaptic) or α_2 (presynaptic) adrenoceptors. In the case of skeletal muscle vasodilatation is effected through β_2 adrenoceptors. It should also be mentioned here that both the rate and force of heart contractions is mediated through β_1 adrenoceptors.

Interestingly, it is at both the ganglia and end organ sites that many therapeutic exogenous pharmacological agents act (Figure 10.3) and can alter autonomic function [2], but in some cases these can unintendedly compromise function in non-targeted pathways.

It is also interesting to note that the concept of simple antagonism between catecholaminergic (noradrenergic) and cholinergic neurotransmission is now believed to be simplistic. For example, it is known from recent histochemistry, unlike the originally proposed principle by Dale of one neurotransmitter for one synapse [3], that sympathetic ganglia have nearly 50% acetylcholine containing neurons in which non-adrenergic non-cholinergic (NANC) purinergic neurotransmission is now accepted [4]. Evidence for this can be seen in some ganglion cells, such as those in the posterior root ganglia, where there can be as many as ten neuropeptides acting as neurotransmitters at the same synapse [5]. However, we still know little about the full purpose of such

multitransmitter actions. Finally, and as a further complication, studies have shown that presynaptic cholinergic receptors may affect noradrenergic sympathetic neurotransmission and this influence could indirectly neuromodulate the effects of acetylcholine to produce both inhibitory and excitatory phenomena in the same ganglion [6].

Autonomic afferent pathways, somatic interaction, and spinal reflexes

Autonomic afferents carry deep, and often poorly localizable, sensations like pain. Since they provide pain sensation for the viscera, or internal organs, they are also called visceral afferents. The afferent pathways of autonomic reflexes can originate in individual organs but ordinarily they can have their origins anywhere, so that direct reflex interactions can take place between different organs (for example, the urinary bladder and bowel) [7]. Also, somatic and autonomic afferent pathways can interact (Table 10.1) at the segmental level to give necessary coordinated effects on the one hand or unusual referred sensations on the other. Coordinated effects, for example, are particularly important for proper function of the lower urinary tract whereby if the bladder and the striated urethral sphincter are not coordinated (detrusor–sphincter dyssynergia) then continence and efficient emptying can be seriously compromised, as in the neurogenic bladder [8].

Another common example of interaction between somatic and visceral afferents is in referred pain, where for example, a myocardial infarction can manifest itself as pain in the shoulder and down the left arm. Such a phenomenon gives support for the 'convergence-projection' theory of referred visceral pain where these converging viscerosomatic pathways in the spinal cord, mediated via long supraspinal loops, including the spinoreticular and spinothalamic tracts, to elicit appropriate CNS sensory and motor responses [9].

Table 10.1 Peripheral autonomic and somatic reflex interactions

Organ or system	Sympathetic nervous system	Parasympathetic nervous system	Somatic system
Heart	T1–T5	Vagus nerve (Cranial X)	None
Blood vessels		In salivary & gastro-intestinal glands (Cranial X)	
Upper body	T1–T5		None
Lower body	T5–L2	In genital erectile tissue	None
Bronchopulmonary	T1–T5	Vagus nerve (Cranial X)	C3–C8 T1–T12
Sweat glands	T1–L2	None	None
Lower urinary tract			
Bladder detrusor muscle	T10–L1	S2–S4	None
Bladder neck, proximal urethra	T10–L2	S2–S4?	None
External (striated) urethral sphincter (+smooth muscle?)	T10–L2?	None	S2–S4
Gastrointestinal tract			
Oesophagus to splenic flexure	T1–L2	Vagus nerve (Cranial X)	None
Splenic flexure to internal anal sphincter	T1–L2	S2–S4	None
External (striated) anal sphincter (+smooth muscle?)	T10–L2	S2–S4	S2-S4
Genitals			
Penis and testicles	T10–L2	S2–S4	None
Vagina and uterus	T10–L2	S2–S4	None

Central control of autonomic function

It is said that the 'highest' level of integration for autonomic function resides in the hypothalamus although it is very much under the influence of the cerebral cortex and relies on extrahypothalamic structures, such as the 'limbic system,' essential to its operation [10]. The hypothalamus takes a central role in processing those aspects of sensory input important for instinctive drives such as hunger, thirst, and sexual needs. In other words, the hypothalamus functions to determine the choice of behaviours, based on sensory information from a changing environment, and to maintain homeostasis. A good example of such functions concerns temperature regulation, by the redistribution of blood in the circulation, to maintain a constant core temperature through peripheral dilatation in the presence of stressful environmental temperature changes.

Local reflex circuits that interrelate visceral afferent and autonomic efferent activity are integrated into a hierarchic control system in the spinal cord and brain stem. Progressively greater complexity in the responses and greater precision in their control occur at each higher level of the nervous system. As mentioned earlier, most visceral reflexes contain contributions from the lower motoneurons that innervate skeletal muscles as part of their response patterns. The distinction between purely visceral and somatic reflex hierarchies becomes less and less meaningful at the higher levels of hierarchic control and behavioural integration.

For most autonomic-mediated functions, the hypothalamus serves as the major control centre. The hypothalamus, which

has connections with the cerebral cortex, limbic system, and pituitary gland, is in a prime position to receive, integrate, and transmit information to other areas of the nervous system. The neurons concerned with thermoregulation, thirst, and feeding behaviours are found in the hypothalamus. The hypothalamus is also the site for integrating neuroendocrine function. Hypothalamic releasing and inhibiting hormones control the secretion of anterior pituitary hormones (thyroid-stimulating hormone, adrenocorticotropic hormone, growth hormone, luteinizing hormone, follicle-stimulating hormone, and prolactin). The supraoptic nuclei of the hypothalamus are involved in water metabolism through synthesis of antidiuretic hormone (ADH) and its release from the posterior pituitary gland. Oxytocin, which causes contraction of the pregnant uterus and milk let-down during breastfeeding, is synthesized in the hypothalamus and released from the posterior pituitary gland in a manner similar to that of ADH.

The organization of many life-support reflexes occurs in the reticular formation of the medulla and pons. These areas of reflex circuitry, often called *centres*, produce complex combinations of autonomic and somatic efferent functions required for the respiration, gag, cough, sneeze, swallow, and vomit reflexes, as well as the more purely autonomic control of the cardiovascular system. At the hypothalamic level, these reflexes are integrated into more general response patterns, such as rage, defensive behaviour, eating, drinking, voiding, and sexual function. Forebrain, and especially limbic system control of these behaviours, involves inhibiting or facilitating release of the response patterns according to social pressures during general emotion-provoking situations.

Reflex adjustments of cardiovascular and respiratory function occur at the level of the brainstem. A prominent example is the carotid sinus baroreflex. Increased blood pressure in the carotid sinus increases the discharge from afferent fibres that travel by way of the ninth cranial nerve to cardiovascular centres in the brainstem. These centres increase the activity of descending efferent vagal fibres that slow heart rate, while inhibiting sympathetic fibres that increase heart rate and blood vessel tone. One of the striking features of ANS function is the rapidity and intensity with which it can change visceral function. Within 3 to 5 seconds, it can increase heart rate to about twice its resting level. Bronchial smooth muscle tone is largely controlled by way of parasympathetic fibres carried in the vagus nerve. These nerves produce mild to moderate constriction of the bronchioles.

Important ANS reflexes are located at the level of the spinal cord. As with other spinal reflexes, these reflexes are modulated by input from higher centres (Figure 10.4). When there is loss of communication between the higher centres and the spinal reflexes, as occurs in spinal cord injury, these reflexes function in an unregulated manner. There is uncontrolled sweating, vasomotor instability, and reflex bowel and bladder function.

Much of our more recent knowledge of autonomic control has been achieved through the use of functional imaging of the brain in both healthy individuals and people with a variety of disorders [11]. Although complementary anatomical and neurophysiological studies in both animals and humans continue to be essential for investigating the finer mechanisms of autonomic control we can expect that with improved resolution of brain and spinal cord imaging our insight into functional changes associated with disease and trauma will greatly assist our understanding of mechanisms, improve our diagnostics, and hence lead to better treatment and management of autonomic failures.

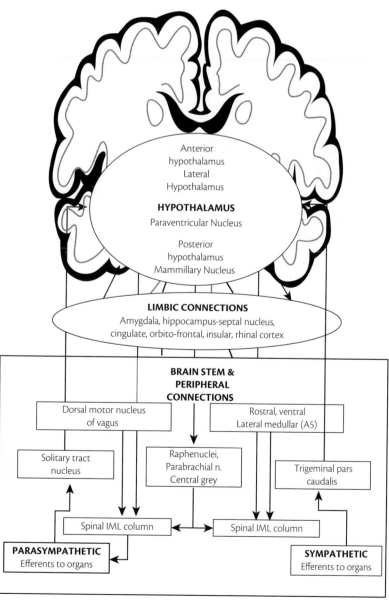

Fig. 10.4 Central control of autonomic function.

Exemplars of specific autonomic functions and failures

Control of normal cardiovascular function

The cardiovascular system (CVS) has a pivotal role in homeostasis, controlling blood flow to specific vascular beds, depending on metabolic need. It is the control of blood flow that is most important, arterial pressure being simply a means to drive flow [12]. Adequate perfusion of organs is controlled by the CNS through a combination of both cardiac output and arterial vascular resistance to meet the demands of the CVS accompanying different behavioural states such as sleep, digestion, exercise, and emotional responses.

Circulation to the brain, spinal cord, and other vital centres is largely controlled by autonomically mediated circulatory reflexes that match pressure and flow to the needs of the individual tissue beds (Figure 10.5). When going from the supine to the standing position, for example, cerebral blood flow is protected by the baroreceptor reflex. This reflex incorporates pressure-sensitive receptors in the carotid sinus and aorta, cardiovascular regulatory centres in the brainstem, and autonomic effector responses that alter heart rate and total peripheral resistance to meet the changing demands of the circulatory system and to maintain blood flow to vital centres. Volume receptors control total blood volume and are the circulatory system's protection against inadequate filling of the vascular compartment. Disorders of circulatory function occur when the autonomic reflexes controlling cardiovascular function are exaggerated, deficient, or inappropriate. They include such disorders as cardiac dysrhythmias and abnormal blood pressure responses to normal activities of daily living.

Orthostatic hypotension represents an abnormal drop in blood pressure that occurs sometimes when resuming an upright position. It may result from an impaired vasoconstrictor response and peripheral pooling of blood with a temporary lack of blood flow to the brain.

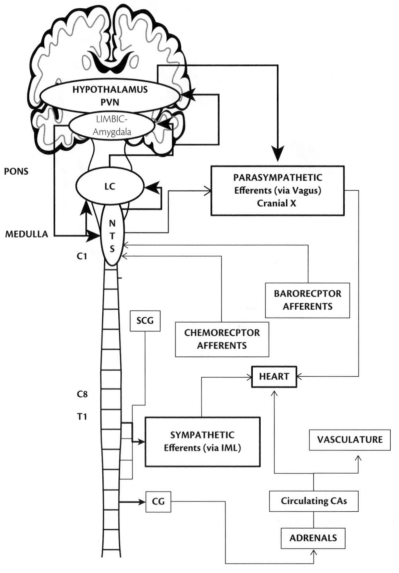

Fig. 10.5 Control of the cardiovascular system.

Fainting or syncope refers to a transient loss of consciousness resulting from inadequate cerebral blood flow. It usually is preceded by sweating, pallor, blurred vision, dizziness, and nausea. Fainting may have an abrupt onset, with an initial increase in sympathetic activity leading to increased heart rate and vascular resistance. The initial sympathetic response is brief and followed by a sudden drop in heart rate, a decrease in vascular resistance, a profound fall in blood pressure and cerebral blood flow, and loss of consciousness. Fainting is more common in people who are in the upright position, and resumption of the supine position during a faint usually results in a return of consciousness. Factors that predispose to fainting include a reduction in venous return to the heart resulting from orthostatic or postural stress, blood loss, or an increased intrathoracic pressure because of performance of the Valsalva manoeuvre. The risk of syncope is increased in a hot environment because of vasodilatation and loss of extracellular fluid volume caused by sweating. Emotional fainting can occur as the result of reduced vasoconstrictor outflow and increased vasodilator outflow from CNS centres that influence blood vessel tone. Most healthy people can precipitate presyncopal conditions, particularly in hot weather, when they hyperventilate and produce cerebral vasoconstriction secondary to decreased cerebral carbon dioxide levels. Assumption of the standing position or standing without moving the legs to promote venous return contributes to the presyncopal condition. Immobility and prolonged bed rest lead to a decrease in vascular volume and deconditioning of vascular smooth muscle and the skeletal muscle pumps that return blood to the heart. Thus, dizziness and the potential for fainting are common after immobility or bed rest. Micturition syncope can occur immediately after bladder emptying. Loss of consciousness is abrupt, and recovery is rapid and complete. A full bladder causes vasoconstriction, a condition that does not usually produce hypertension because it is counteracted by the baroreceptor reflex. It has been suggested that syncope occurs when the constricted vessels suddenly dilate. It is more common in males than in females, probably because the standing position contributes to pooling of blood in the extremities. The reflex effects of bladder distention on circulation are much more pronounced in paraplegic people with cord injuries above T6.

The baroreceptor reflex is less efficient in many elderly people, and this may contribute to syncope and falls. This is particularly true when multiple stresses are placed on the circulation. These stresses include sudden assumption of the standing position from either the seated or supine position, vasodilatation caused by a warm room or bed, a full bladder, use of medications that impair autonomic function, and decreased vascular volume because of inadequate fluid intake or the use of diuretics.

Postprandial hypotension is a decrease in blood pressure that occurs after a meal. Insulin release has a depressant effect on baroreflex function. Consequently, the consumption of a meal that is high in carbohydrate content, with the subsequent release of insulin, has the potential for producing a postprandial decrease in blood pressure. This aspect of autonomic function has many practical implications for people who already have disorders of ANS function, such as elderly people and people who have had a stroke. Several studies have shown a significant reduction of postprandial blood pressure in elderly people. In people who have had a stroke, autoregulation of the cerebral vessels in the affected area is lost; slight orthostatic falls in blood pressure after carbohydrate ingestion have the potential of further compromising blood flow to the area. Therefore, ingestion of small, low-carbohydrate meals and afterward avoidance of positions that produce orthostatic hypotension are suggested as a means of minimizing brain ischaemia. These cardiovascular consequences of autonomic failure and their management and assessment are covered in more detail later in this chapter.

Control of the lower urinary tract

Coordinated function of the urinary bladder and its sphincters depends on the complete integrity of central and peripheral nervous pathways in a complex neural control system located in the brain, spinal cord and somato-visceral nerves [13] involving sympathetic, parasympathetic and somatic interactions (Figure 10.6).

Micturition, or 'urination', occurs involuntarily in infants and young children until the age of 3 to 5 years, after which it is regulated voluntarily. The neural circuitry that controls this process is complex and highly distributed: it involves pathways at many levels of the brain, spinal cord, and peripheral nervous system and is mediated by multiple neurotransmitter systems. Diseases or injuries of the nervous system in adults can cause the re-emergence of involuntary or reflex micturition, leading to urinary incontinence. This is a major health problem, especially in those with neurological impairment. The neural control of micturition and how disruption of this control leads to abnormal storage and release of urine is essential to address the issues of diagnosis and treatment [14].

The control system for micturition is believed to act like a switching circuit in the pontine region of the brain to maintain a reciprocal and coordinated relationship between the reservoir function of the bladder and sphincteric outlet function of the urethra [15]. As the bladder slowly fills, any tendency for spontaneous contractions of the detrusor smooth muscle in the bladder wall are inhibited, while urethral smooth and striated muscle sphincters are contracted to prevent leakage. Furthermore, voluntary control of the striated urethral sphincter and pelvic floor muscles are also an essential part of the continence mechanism. Voiding requires a complete relaxation of the sphincters, coupled with a coordinated sustained detrusor contraction so that urine is expelled quickly and efficiently from the bladder. This synergistic relationship between the smooth muscle of the bladder wall and the sphincters around the urethra is essential for maintaining continence on the one hand and unobstructed voiding on the other [16] (Figure 10.7A).

Damage or disease in any of the nervous pathways controlling the lower urinary tract can have serious consequences for this relationship, leading to uncoordinated somatovisceral reflexes, impairment of normal vesicourethral function, voiding dysfunction, and incontinence. For example, in the event of an upper motor neuron lesion, as in a suprasacral spinal cord injury, there is damage to the spinobulbar pathways (i.e. connecting the lumbosacral segments with the brainstem) and, whether complete or incomplete, causes serious disruption to coordination of the bladder and sphincters leading to un-inhibited pelvic (parasympathetic) reflexes [17] (Figure 10.7B).

The main aim for the treatment and management in rehabilitation of the neurogenic bladder is to establish a low-pressure high-capacity bladder that does not compromise renal function [18].

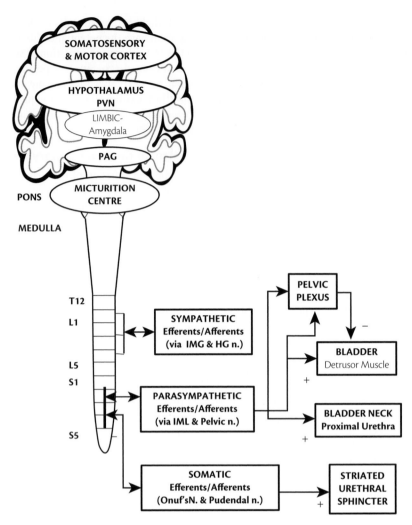

Fig. 10.6 Principal central and peripheral pathways controlling the bladder and sphincters.

As a postscript it should not be forgotten that urine is formed in the kidneys and that their function in body sodium regulation is extremely important for body fluid volume homeostasis. This regulation is now believed to be dependant on sympathetic control of the three renal neuroeffectors in the blood vessels, the tubules, and the juxtaglomerular granular cells. Abnormalities of these autonomic control mechanisms can be a significant contributor to the pathophysiology of clinically important disease states such as hypertension and sodium-retaining oedema-forming conditions (e.g. congestive heart failure) gives promise of future therapeutic interventions [19].

A more comprehensive guide to management and neurorehabilitation of the bladder (and bowel) can be found in Chapter 24.

Autonomic system disorders

Autonomic failure can be global or regional. When global, the impairment can affect all aspects of function. Less commonly ANS failure is confined to sympathetic or parasympathetic systems. The autonomic nervous system pathways are also interrupted in other CNS disorders such as multiple sclerosis and also particularly after spinal cord injury (SCI), resulting in regional impairments. Depending on the level of cord injury, the ANS

innervation to various structures will be affected, resulting in important clinical sequelae. Autonomic failure may be primary or secondary, depending on whether an underlying cause from outside the autonomic system can be demonstrated.

Causes of autonomic failure

Primary autonomic failures includes those which are presumably neurodegenerative, including multiple system atrophy (MSA), pure autonomic failure, Parkinson's disease (PD) with autonomic failure, and dementia with Lewy bodies (DLB). There are links between these conditions at a pathological level with the presence of alpha synuclein inclusion bodies. These inclusion bodies are neuronal in the CNS in PD with autonomic failure and diffuse Lewy body disease, neuronal within the peripheral nervous system in pure autonomic failure, and glial in the CNS in MSA. These primary forms of autonomic failure are now referred to as autonomic alpha synucleinopathies.

MSA can be thought of as a spectrum of clinical disorders in which there are shared pyramidal features and a variable degrees of autonomic failure, cerebellar and Parkinsonian involvement. Where cerebellar features dominate the term MSA-C is used. Where Parkinsonian features are the more prominent the term

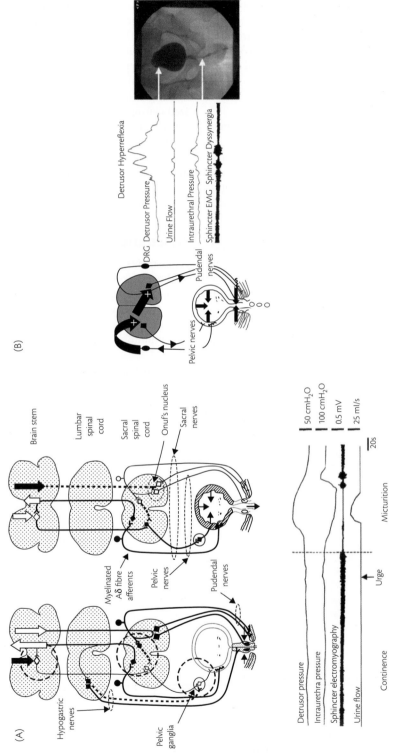

Fig. 10.7 Normal control of bladder–sphincter coordination (A) and aberrant sacral reflexes resulting in detrusor hyperreflexia (neurogenic detrusor overactivity (NDO)) with sphincter dyssynergia in spinal cord injury (B).

used is MSA-P. MSA is a distinctive clinical entity with many characteristic features including anterocollis, laryngeal spasm, rapid eye movement sleep disorder and a tendency to take deep sighing breaths. Patients are typically younger than in other primary forms of autonomic failure and progression can be relatively rapid.

Pure (or primary) autonomic failure (PAF) can present in a similar way to MSA but patients are likely to be older, there may be a longer clinical history and evidence of more widespread degeneration will be absent. PAF has a relatively good prognosis and although symptoms may become limiting in time there is, in contrast to MSA, little effect on overall life expectancy.

Autonomic failure is an important non-motor complication of PD and in some cases can become a dominant clinical feature. The prognosis will be better than in MSA. Autonomic failure can also occur in DLB.

A summary of central nervous system disorders resulting in autonomic dysfunctions is shown in Figure 10.8. As can be seen from the figure, the autonomic sequelae vary according to the anatomy and pathology of the disorder.

Secondary causes of autonomic failure are much more varied. There are acute and chronic causes and they include treatable conditions and conditions where autonomic failure is a feature of a serious associated illness that needs disease specific management.

Secondary autonomic failure may present acutely or chronically. Causes of acute autonomic failure include paraneoplasia,

porphyria, Guillain–Barré syndrome, botulism, drugs, and auto-immune ganglionic neuropathy. A more chronic form of secondary autonomic failure occurs with peripheral neuropathies. Although some of autonomic involvement is present in many neuropathies it is more pronounced in diabetic neuropathy, amyloidosis, and hereditary sensory and autonomic neuropathy type III (Riley–Day syndrome). Table 10.2 summarizes the principal causes of autonomic neuropathy.

Secondary causes of autonomic failure can present in similar ways to primary causes. Clinical pointers might include a younger age at presentation, a family history, clinical features of generalized neuropathy, impaired heart rate control where there is vagal involvement, and impaired sweating of the extremities.

Our understanding of autonomic failures, whether through primary or secondary causes, and their clinical features and management, have advanced significantly during the last 30 years and have become the subject of many excellent textbooks on this very important aspect of medicine [20].

Assessment of autonomic function

Assessments of autonomic function include both quantitative and qualitative testing. First line assessments include checking lying, sitting, standing and postprandial heart rate (HR) and blood pressures (BP). Other uncommon bedside stimuli that can be used to assess for a rise in blood pressure during continuous blood pressure monitoring include isometric exercise (sustained hand grip

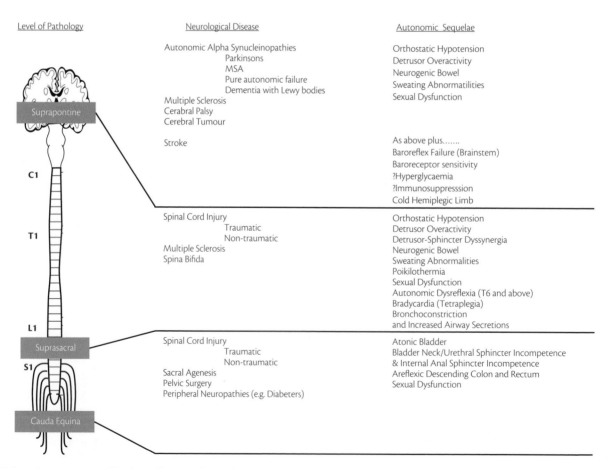

Fig. 10.8 Central nervous system disorders and autonomic sequelae.

Table 10.2 Causes of autonomic neuropathy

Ageing (postural hypotension and disordered thermoregulation are common in the elderly)

Causes linked with systemic diseases:

    Diabetic autonomic neuropathies

    Alcoholic neuropathy

    Subacute combined degeneration

    Hepatic disease

    Uraemic neuropathy

    Amyloid neuropathies

Infectious causes:

    Human immunodeficiency virus (HIV)

    Lyme disease

    Leprosy

    Chagas' disease

Toxic causes:

    Vincristine

    Cisplatin

    Amiodarone

    Pyridoxine overdose

    Thallium poisoning

Immune-mediated causes:

    Rheumatoid arthritis

    SLE

    Sjögren's syndrome

    Systemic sclerosis

    Autoimmune thyroiditis

    Neuropathy related to inflammatory bowel disease

    Postural orthostatic tachycardia syndrome (POTS)

    Guillain–Barré syndrome

    Chronic inflammatory demyelinating neuropathy

    Acute pandysautonomia

    Acute cholinergic pandysautonomia

    Eaton–Lambert syndrome

    Holmes–Adie syndrome

    Paraneoplastic autonomic neuropathy

Hereditary causes:

    Anderson–Fabry disease

    Hereditary types (I to V)

    Tangier disease

    Multiple endocrine neoplasia (type 2b)

SLE, systemic lupus erythematosus.

for 3 min), a cold pressor test (immersion of a hand in ice water for 90 s), and mental arithmetic (with serial-7 or serial-17 subtraction), all of which stimulate sympathetic outflow and elevate blood pressure in healthy patients. Multiple daily blood pressures or 24–48-hour ambulatory blood pressure monitoring examine for diurnal fluctuation: A difference of >15 mmHg with either systolic or diastolic blood pressure between daytime (awake) values and night-time (sleeping) values could indicate presence of autonomic neuropathy.

More standardized autonomic testing may be performed to assess the severity of the impairment and to help localize the parts of the autonomic nervous system that are involved [21].

Assessment of cardiovagal (parasympathetic) innervation

Heart rate (HR) response to deep breathing—this test approaches the optimal test for cardiovagal function. Both the afferent and efferent pathways are vagal. The end point is the maximal HR variability obtained under laboratory conditions.

Valsalva ratio—this ratio is derived from the maximal HR generated by the Valsalva manoeuvre divided by the lowest HR following the manoeuvre.

HR response to standing or tilt table (30:15 ratio)—the initial HR responses to standing consist of a tachycardia at 3 then 12 seconds followed by a bradycardia at 20 seconds. The initial cardioacceleration is an exercise reflex, while the subsequent tachycardia and bradycardia are baroreflex mediated. The 30:15 ratio (R-R interval at beat 30)/(R-R interval at beat 15), has been recommended as an index of cardiovagal function.

These three tests evaluate cardiovagal function. They have a high sensitivity and specificity and are simple, safe and cost-effective. The tests are well standardized and reproducible, with a coefficient of variation of 20%. The confounding variables are well known for response to deep breathing and the Valsalva manoeuvre but less well known for the standing test.

Laboratory indices of adrenergic function—beat-to-beat blood pressure (BP) responses to the Valsalva manoeuvre. The availability of a well-validated photoplethysmographic volume clamp technique to measure beat-to-beat BP30–35 has permitted the application of the well-known properties of the phases of the Valsalva manoeuvre to the clinical laboratory. The test greatly enhances the sensitivity and specificity of the laboratory evaluation of adrenergic function. The test should be classified as an established test.

BP response to sustained hand grip—sustained muscle contraction causes a rise in systolic and diastolic BP and HR. The stimulus derives from exercising muscle and central command. Efferent fibres travel to the muscle and heart, resulting in increased cardiac output, BP, and HR. This autonomic maneouvre has been adapted as a clinical test of sympathetic autonomic function. BP is measured using a sphygmomanometer cuff. The test is of limited sensitivity and specificity. Confounding variables are not well known. It should be regarded as an investigational test.

BP and HR responses to tilt-up or active standing—blood pressure and heart rate response to standing. Supine and tilted BP recordings, especially when supplemented with beat-to-beat BP and HR recordings, can be used as an established test.

Assessment of sudomotor function

Quantitative sudomotor axon reflex test (QSART)—measures axon reflex-mediated sudomotor responses quantitatively and evaluates postganglionic sudomotor function. Four regions are tested: forearm, proximal leg, distal leg, and dorsum of the foot. Electrical stimulation (iontophoresis) is applied to the skin, and the volume of sweat produced can be measured. The test has a high sensitivity, specificity, and reproducibility, with a coefficient of variation of 20%. Confounding variables are well known. The test is straightforward and is an established test.

Thermoregulatory sweat test (TST)—is used to evaluate both preganglionic and postganglionic thermoregulatory pathways and function over the entire anterior body surface. It evaluates the distribution of sweating by a change in color of an indicator powder. The TST is now well standardized and has recently been rendered semiquantitative and expressed as a percentage of anterior body anhidrosis. The test has a high sensitivity. As a stand-alone test, it has a low specificity, and limited information is available on its reproducibility and confounding variables. Combined with QSART, its specificity for delineating the site of the lesion is greatly enhanced. The test has been in clinical use for at least four decades. It is an established test. When evaluated together in the same patient, TST and QSART can differentiate preganglionic from postganglionic lesions

Sympathetic skin response (SSR)—this test can be used to identify indirect evidence of sweat production via measurement of changes in skin conductance on the palm/sole in response to an electrical stimulus. Brief electrical stimuli are administered at intermittent intervals and a response is measured from the hands or the feet, representing a change in skin resistance due to sweating. The test is of relatively low sensitivity and uncertain specificity and habituates. Its greatest advantage is its relative ease of performance. The test is of some value as part of an autonomic battery. It is a commonly used test that will likely be replaced by better tests such as the QSART or sweat imprint as these become more conveniently available.

Quantitative direct and indirect test of sudomotor function (QDIRT)/ silastic sweat imprint—involves making a silicone impression of a patient's skin while sweating is induced by acetylcholine iontophoresis. The presence of sweat droplets can be quantified in the silicone cast, providing a marker of sudomotor function. The test seems to be sensitive and quantitative. It is an established test.

Assessment of gastrointestinal function

Video-fluoroscopy—is useful in assessment of swallowing in the presence of oropharyngeal dysphagia. A barium swallow study, meal, and follow-through study are helpful in suspected upper gastrointestinal disorders, though endoscopic assessment provides the opportunity for biopsy in particular situations, as well as better visualization.

Oesophageal manometry—may be of value in disorders of motility and oesophagogastric function and gastric motility may be assessed by using radioisotope methods and scintigraphic scanning. Diabetic patients with symptoms of oesophageal dysmotility have insufficient lower oesophageal sphincter relaxation and a higher percentage of simultaneous waves detected, while diabetic patients with cardiovascular autonomic neuropathy have greater pathological simultaneous contractions. In cases of small-bowel disorders suspected to be neurological in nature, manometry may be of value in discriminating myopathic from

neuropathic disorders. Large-bowel dysfunction can be assessed via measurement of transit time.

Anorectal manometry—is the most well established and widely available tool for investigating anorectal function. Anal sphincter tone can be quantified by anorectal manometry. The anorectal sensory response, anorectal reflexes, rectal compliance, and defecatory function are also assessed by anorectalmanometry. Anal sphincter function is assessed by measurement of resting sphincter pressure, squeeze sphincter pressure, and the functional length of the anal canal. Changes in anal and rectal pressures during attempted defecation are also assessed, particularly useful in the diagnosis of dyssynergic or obstructive defecation, a common cause of constipation. Assessment of rectal sensation is useful in patients with faecal incontinence or rectal hyposensitivity. The presence or absence of the rectoanal contractile reflex and the rectoanal inhibitory reflex is also documented. Rectal compliance is calculated and reflects the capacity and distensibility of the rectum. Rectal compliance is calculated by plotting the relationship between balloon volume (dV) and steady state intrarectal pressure (dP). The balloon expulsion test is used to assess rectoanal co-ordination during defecatory manoeuvres. The test evaluates a patient's ability to expel a filled balloon from the rectum, providing a simple and more physiologic assessment of defecation dynamics [22].

A guide to management and neurorehabilitation of the bowel (and bladder) can be found in Chapter 24.

Assessment of urinary tract function

The urinary bladder has two functions, to store at low-pressure urine from the kidneys and empty efficiently, that is leave no residual that could lead to urinary tract infection. The neurogenic bladder is optimally assessed for detrusor hyper-reflexia (neurogenic detrusor overactivity—NDO) and detrusor–sphincter dyssynergia by urodynamics with sphincter electromyography or more usefully, videourodynamics [13] (see Figure 10.7B).

A guide to management and neurorehabilitation of the bladder (and bowel) can be found in Chapter 24.

Assessment of sexual function

Erectile and ejaculatory dysfunction are clinical complaints and confirmed through history taking. Specific tests are not usually indicated if diagnosis and aetiology are clear. Semen samples for World Health Organization (WHO) analysis will be required if male fertility is uncertain, and in patients with neurological compromise [23] (e.g. spinal cord lesions) these can be obtained usually by penile vibro-ejaculation or more invasively by ano-rectal electrical ejaculation or aspiration.

Assessment of pupillary responses

Pupillometry measure changes in papillary response and is being investigated at some institutions as a potential marker for autonomic neuropathy [24].

Other specialized assessments

Neurophysiological tests of nerve conduction, spinal reflexes, and electromyography can sometimes be very helpful to determine the extent of preservation or damage to central and peripheral

Table 10.3 A summary of assessments of autonomic function

Assessment of cardiovagal innervation	Heart rate response to: Breathing Valsalva manoeuvre Standing or tilt table
Assessment of adrenergic function	BP response to: Valsalva manoeuvre Sustained hand grip Standing or tilt table
Assessment of sudomotor function	Quantitative sudomotor axon reflex test (QSART) Thermoregulatory sweat test (TST) Sympathetic skin response (SSR) Quantitative direct and indirect test of sudomotor function (QDIRT)
Assessment of gastrointestinal function	Videofluoroscopy, barium swallow Oesophogeal manometry Gastric scintigraphy Small bowel manometry Transit time Anorectal manometry
Assessment of urinary tract function	Flowmetry, MSU, Standard urodynamics with sphincter EMG or more ideally video-urodynamics. Post void residual urine.
Asessment of sexual function	Specific lab assessment not usually necessary. Semen analysis required for fertility assessment.
Assessment of pupillary responses	Pupillometry
Nerve conductions studies and electromyography	Including quantitative sensory testing
Imaging	MIBG cardicac scintigraphy Cardiac PET and SPECT scanning
Specific diagnostic tests for underlying disorder	Ganglionic Ach receptor antibody Imaging and other Ix to confirm MSA/PD etc Shirmer test Skin biopsy

MSU, mid-stream urine; MIBG, metaiodobenzylguanidine; PET, positron emission tomography; SPECT, single-photon emission computerized tomography.

nerous pathways. Findings on nerve conduction studies (NCS) and electromyography (EMG) can be normal in pure autonomic neuropathies because the involved fibres are small myelinated and unmyelinated fibres, which cannot be assessed with NCS or EMG. However in autonomic neuropathies with concomitant sensory neuropathy, absence of sensory potentials may occur. In autonomic neuropathies with concomitant sensorimotor neuropathy, marked loss of motor and sensory potentials is noted.

Quantitative sensory testing (QST) can be helpful in autonomic disorders with sensory neuropathy. QST permits comparison of sensory thresholds by using vibration and temperature perception to assess both large and small-fibre modalities. These patients typically have impaired thresholds for heat and pain, but vibration and cool sensitivity may be normal.

Imaging by postitron emission tomography (PET), functional magnetic resonance imaging (MRI) and types of computerized tomography (e.g. peripheral quantitative computed tomography pQCT) are becoming recognized not only for their benefit in understanding neural mechanisms in the central nervous system but also for the development of potentially useful diagnostic techniques in autonomic disorders [25]. Improvements in resolution (e.g. 4 Tesla MRI) may enable much more functional detail and, together with sophisticated methods of analysis, the identification of specific pathways in the CNS (e.g. tractography).

Specialist investigations are occasionally indicated in the assessment of the cardiac effects of autonomic disorders. Reduced sympathetic noradrenergic innervation has been seen in the left myocardium by single-photon emission computerized tomography (SPECT) and ^{123}I or thoracic 6-(^{18}F) fluorodopamine PET scanning in patients with PD and postural hypotension. SPECT and PET scanning may identify cardiac sympathetic dysfunction in both type I and type II diabetes mellitus. MIBG (metaiodobenzylguanidine) cardiac-scintigraphy may also be helpful. Table 10.3 summarizes the assessment of autonomic function.

Clinical features and management

The clinical sequelae of autonomic dysfunction depends on the extent of the dysfunction and whether the dysfunction is global or regional. The following sections look at the specific effects of autonomic dysfunction on different systems and discuss assessment and management strategies [26]. Table 10.4 summarizes the clinical features of autonomic dysfunction generally and outlines the autonomic problems, assessment, and management specifically after spinal cord injury are outlined later in Table 10.8.

The management of primary chronic autonomic failure is symptomatic, supportive and targeted to the particular pattern of failure present in an individual. In secondary causes there may also be treatment of the underlying disease process. For example, if an autoimmune neuropathy is present, attempted management with immunomodulatory therapies should be considered. If diabetes mellitus is the underlying cause, strict control of blood glucose to prevent further worsening is essential. Following spinal cord injury the management may be either supportive (in complete stable SCI) or may involve optimizing functional recovery.

Specific system disorders and their management

Cardiovascular system

Bradycardia

Bradycardia, along with hypertension, may occur in cerebral tumours and during autonomic dysreflexia in high SCI. In the latter, the afferent and vagal efferent components of the baroreflex arc are intact, and the heart slows in an attempt to control the rise in blood pressure. In phaeochromocytoma, bradycardia with escape rhythms and atrioventricular dissociation may occur in response to a rapid rise in pressure. In diabetes mellitus, the presence of a cardiac vagal neuropathy may increase the likelihood

Table 10.4 Clinical Features of principal autonomic disorders

Primary autonomic failure	Suggested if pyramidal features, cerebellar involvement, parkinsonian features
Secondary autonomic failure	Suggested if younger age, family history, features of generalized neuropathy
Cardiovascular symptoms and signs	Postural hypotension
	Impaired heart rate control, particularly bradycardia
	Baroreflex failure
	Autonomic dysreflexia
	Long-term cardiovascular disease
	Paroxysmal sympathetic and motor overactivity ('storming' after acquired brain injury)
Respiratory symptom & signs	Relative bronchoconstriction
	Increased secretions
	Laryngeal spasm
	Tendancy to deep sighing breathes
Sweating abnormalities	Increased sweating
	Reduced ability to sweat (may result in hyperpyrexia)
Bladder dysfunction	Voiding dysfunction
	Urinary retention
	Detrusor overactivity
	Urinary incontinence
	Detrusor sphincter dyssynergia
Gastrointestinal dysfunction	Reflux oesophagitis, delayed gastric emptying
	Constipation
	Impaired control of evacuation
	Incomplete evacuation
	Incontinence
Sexual dysfunction	Erectile dysfunction
	Ejaculatory dysfunction
	Impaired vaginal lubrication in females
	Impaired orgasm
	Impaired male fertility

of cardio-respiratory arrest during anaesthesia. Disorders of cardiac conduction are common in Chagas' disease and occur in amyloidosis.

Severe bradycardia can occur in cervical cord injuries. The inability to increase sympathetic activity is likely to contribute. Cardiac dysrhythmias and cardiac arrest can occur leading to baseline bradycardia. Disrupted sympathetic innervation after SCI results in unopposed parasympathetic activity. The intact vagi are sensitive to hypoxia and stimuli such as tracheal suction which can induce bradycardia and cardiac arrest.

Bradycardia is more frequently encountered in the acute phase, and is more severe in the first 2–6 weeks after trauma.

Management of bradycardia after SCI

There is limited data available regarding the optimal and best treatment available for symptomatic bradycardia after SCI. All data is based on case reports, case series and observational studies. Atropine is generally recommended as the first-line agent for bradycardia after cervical spinal cord injury. Atropine

should be kept readily available at the bedside at all times. Other medications used include sympathomimetic agents such as dopamine or epinephrine. The methylxanthine agents, including aminophylline and theophylline, have been used effectively for the management of refractory symptomatic bradycardia when other agents have failed. In addition, there are reports of methylxanthines used specifically as a successful first line treatment for bradycardia associated with cervical spinal cord injury.

Prevention of further episodes of bradycardia in patients with frequent episodes is important. Strategies include optimizing oxygenation, and prophylactic atropine for precipitating procedures such as rolling or tracheal suction. There are reports on the benefits of xanthine derivates as prophylaxis, although this is not standard management.

Currently, there are no established guidelines regarding permanent pacemaker placement in this population. Permanent pacemakers may still be considered in patients with refractory or recurrent bradycardia however their implantation will have implications for future imaging (by MRI) and management as currently functional electrical stimulation treatments are contraindicated in individuals with implanted pacemakers [27].

Tachycardia

Rarely, autonomic disorders are associated with tachyarrythmias; In postural orthostatic tachycardic syndrome (POTS), the tachycardia usually is associated with head-up postural change and exertion. Tachycardia caused by increased sympathetic discharge may occur along with hypertension in Guillain–Barré syndrome and in tetanus. In phaeochromocytoma, it results from autonomous catecholamine release and β adrenoceptor stimulation [28].

Orthostatic hypotension (OH)

The management of orthostatic hypotension has both non pharmacological and pharmacological aspects [29–31]. Non-pharmacological aspects include maintaining a good fluid intake and ensuring adequate dietary salt. The action of drinking an extra one to two glasses of water can have a significant beneficial effect on systolic blood pressure. In patients with severe neurogenic OH, intake of this volume led to an increase in systolic blood pressure of more than 30 mmHg—plasma norepinephrine (noradrenaline) in this patient group increased, and this vasopressor response was almost completely abolished by intravenous ganglion blockade. Therefore, simply drinking water increases blood pressure not only by increasing volume status, but also by increasing sympathetic activity.

Education to understand factors likely to be associated with lower blood pressures is also important. These include warm environments, following large meals (known as 'dumping'), following alcohol, exercise, and medications with hypotensive effects. Blood pressure can also be lowered by factors associated with elevations in intrathoracic (e.g. coughing) and intra-abdominal (micturition/defaecation) pressures. Slow cautious movements between different body postures should be emphasized. Encourage patients to sit or lie down upon the initiation of orthostatic symptoms. The head of the bed can be elevated so the patient sleeps at a 15–20° angle to stimulate nocturnal mineralocorticoid release. Physical counter-manoeuvres should also be attempted. The manoeuvres

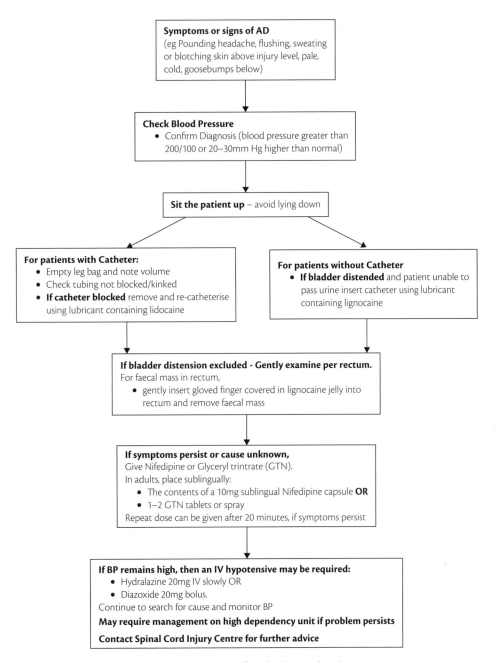

Symptoms or signs of AD
(eg Pounding headache, flushing, sweating or blotching skin above injury level, pale, cold, goosebumps below)

Check Blood Pressure
- Confirm Diagnosis (blood pressure greater than 200/100 or 20–30mm Hg higher than normal)

Sit the patient up – avoid lying down

For patients with Catheter:
- Empty leg bag and note volume
- Check tubing not blocked/kinked
- **If catheter blocked** remove and re-catheterise using lubricant containing lidocaine

For patients without Catheter
- **If bladder distended** and patient unable to pass urine insert catheter using lubricant containing lignocaine

If bladder distension excluded - Gently examine per rectum.
For faecal mass in rectum,
- gently insert gloved finger covered in lignocaine jelly into rectum and remove faecal mass

If symptoms persist or cause unknown,
Give Nifedipine or Glyceryl trintrate (GTN).
In adults, place sublingually:
- The contents of a 10mg sublingual Nifedipine capsule **OR**
- 1–2 GTN tablets or spray
Repeat dose can be given after 20 minutes, if symptoms persist

If BP remains high, then an IV hypotensive may be required:
- Hydralazine 20mg IV slowly **OR**
- Diazoxide 20mg bolus.
Continue to search for cause and monitor BP
May require management on high dependency unit if problem persists
Contact Spinal Cord Injury Centre for further advice

Fig. 10.9 Algorithm for the clinical features and management of autonomic dysreflexia (AD) in spinal cord injury.

include crossing the legs, squatting, and tensing the leg muscles, abdominal muscle, buttocks, or whole body.

Compressive stockings should be used. The thigh-high moderate compression stockings give the most benefit, although they are difficult to put on and can be uncomfortable. Patients should be strongly encouraged to use these as much as possible. Gentle isometric exercises to help build up muscle tone is essential for patients with orthostatic hypotension. Water aerobics, water jogging, or gentle aerobic exercises may help or use of a recumbent bicycle, to avoid putting them in a position where they may experience loss of consciousness or fall.

Pharmacological therapy of orthostatic intolerance should be attempted in more difficult cases or when conservative therapy is unsuccessful. Several medications are effective in controlling orthostatic hypotension and include mineralocorticoids such as

fludrocortisone (50 to 400 μg daily) and adrenergic agonists such as ephedrine (15–30 mg tds) and Midodrine (2.5–10 mg tds). Care has to be taken with the use of sympathetomimetic agents in patients where there is baroreceptor failure as extreme hypertension can occur. Both of these medications may lead to supine hypertension and a balance may be difficult to strike. Other medications used, with some success include selective serotonin reuptake inhibitors, phenobarbitone, erythropoietin (particularly patients with diabetes who have anaemia and orthostatic hypotension) and desmopressin acetate DDAVP (vasopressin). Subcutaneous doses of octreotide 25 to 150 μg 30 minutes before a meal may be used to reduce postprandial orthostatic hypotension.

A systematic review looking specifically at SCI patients [32] has concluded there is no evidence on the effect of salt or fluid regulation alone for OH management in SCI. Salt and fluid regulation was evaluated in combination with other pharmacological interventions and thus, the effects of salt and fluid regulation cannot be determined. There is conflicting evidence that elastic stockings/abdominal binders have any effect on cardiovascular responses in individuals with SCI, although there is level 2 evidence that pressure from elastic stockings and abdominal binders may improve cardiovascular physiological responses during submaximal upper-extremity exercises. Nevertheless most clinicians continue to recommend these for initial management of postural hypotension.

Functional electrical stimulation (FES) has been shown to be an important adjunct treatment to minimize cardiovascular changes during postural orthostatic stress and there is level 4 evidence that 80 sessions of active stand training improves cardiovascular control such as response to orthostatic stress after tetraplegia. Further evidence for the role of physical interventions is likely to emerge.

Nitro-L-arginine methyl ester (L-NAME), in 2 studies, L-threo-3,4-ihydroxyphenylserine (L-DOPS) in a case report and ergotamine with fludrocortisone in a case report have been shown to be of benefit. Further evidence for the role and effectiveness of these, and other drugs, is required.

Autonomic dysreflexia (AD)

AD is a clinical emergency in individuals particularly with spinal cord injury at or above the level of T6. An episode of AD is usually characterized by acute elevation of arterial blood pressure (BP) with bradycardia (occasionally tachycardia) [33]. Other clinical features of AD are shown in Table 10.5 [34].

AD usually occurs as a result of noxious or potentially noxious peripheral or visceral stimulation below the injury level and affects individuals with lesions above the outflow to the splanchnic and renal vascular beds (T5–T6). AD is found in individuals with both complete and incomplete injury. The incidence of AD in individuals with SCI varies from 20 to 70% of the at risk SCI population, regardless of age at injury.

Several factors that could trigger AD have been described in the literature. Urinary retention from missed or blocked catheter is the most common cause. Catheterization and manipulation of an indwelling catheter, urinary tract infection, detrusor sphincter dyssynergia, and bladder percussion are also precipitating factors. Faecal impaction and constipation may also trigger AD. Stimuli that would be noxious if pain sensation was preserved, such as bone fractures or abdominal emergencies, may also be triggering factors. Sexual activity may induce AD in both sexes, and the risk of AD during pregnancy and delivery is also increased. Iatrogenic causes also occur such as cystoscopy, urodynamics, vibro- or electroejaculation, as well as electrical stimulation of muscles [35].

The stimulation below the lesion level can induce a widespread activation of the sympathetic nervous system demonstrated by an increase in noradrenaline release. This induces vasoconstriction in the muscle, skin, kidneys, and splanchnic vascular beds below the level of injury. Baroreceptors are then activated by the resultant increase in arterial blood pressure and, as part of homeostasis, act to reduce the effects of the vasoconstriction by reducing sympathetic activity and increasing parasympathetic activity. This results in dilation of vascular beds above the lesion level (with intact central control) and a reduction in HR (vagal innervation to the heart is unaffected by SCI).

Objectively, an increase in systolic BP greater than 20–30 mmHg is considered a dysreflexic episode. Individuals with cervical and high thoracic SCI have resting arterial BPs that are lower than able-bodied individuals. As such, acute elevation of BP to normal or slightly elevated ranges could indicate AD in this population. Intensity of AD can vary from asymptomatic, mild discomfort and headache to a life threatening emergency when systolic blood pressure can reach 300 mmHg, and symptoms can be severe.

Untreated episodes of autonomic dysreflexia may have serious consequences, including intracranial hemorrhage, cardiac complications, retinal detachments, seizures, and death. During an episode of AD, a significant increase in visceral sympathetic activity with coronary artery constriction can result in myocardial ischaemia, even in the absence of coronary artery disease [36–39].

The identification of the possible trigger and decrease of afferent stimulation to the spinal cord is the most effective prevention strategy in clinical practice. Where this is not immediately possible then medication can be used to control the blood pressure [40]. Nifedipine, nitrates, or captopril are most commonly used. See Figure 10.9 for a management algorithm [26].

For further discussion on these aspects of autonomic dysfunction following, for example, spinal cord injury see the rationale for additions to the International Standards for Neurological Assessment [41, 42].

Sweating abnormalities

Hypohidrosis is usually seen below the level of lesion after SCI, whereas hyperhidrosis may be present above as well as below the level of lesion, and may be a sign of an ongoing pathological process such as syringomyelia or autonomic dysreflexia, or may accompany micturition and defecation. Hyperhidrosis may also be present without any known cause. Patients who have lack of sweat output need to be educated about the risk of heat intolerance. They should be encouraged to avoid excessive and prolonged heat exposure as they may have poor thermoregulation and be at risk of hyperthermia.

For patients who have increased sweat output, several medications have been used, with varying effects. Botulinum toxin has been used for focal hyperhidrosis. If patient's symptoms are

Table 10.5 Typical clinical features of autonomic dysreflexia

Sudden uncontrolled rise in blood pressure with other signs of sympathetic overactivity:

- ◆ systolic pressures reaching up to 250–300 mmHg
- ◆ diastolic pressures reaching up to 200–220 mmHg.

Other features of autonomic imbalance vary, but may include:

- ◆ pounding headache
- ◆ sweating or silvering
- ◆ feelings of anxiety
- ◆ chest tightness
- ◆ blurred vision
- ◆ nasal congestion
- ◆ blotchy skin rash or flushed above the level of their spinal injury (due to parasympathetic activity
- ◆ cold with goosebumps (cutis anserina) below the level of injury (due to the sympathetic activity).

more generalized, medications with anticholinergic action or side effects may be tried. Clonidine has been used to treat hyperhydrosis after SCI [43–52].

Temperature dysregulations

Temperature dysregulation after SCI includes poikilothermia (adopting the environmental temperature, e.g. becoming hypothermic in cold conditions) and exercise-induced fever. Body temperature is under direct autonomic control via hypothalamic regulation. Peripheral cold and warm receptors project to the hypothalamus via the spinal cord, although deep temperature sensors are also present. When core temperature decreases, sympathetic (noradrenergic) mechanisms induce piloerection, shivering, and vasoconstriction to produce body heat and shunt blood away from the cool surface. Areas lacking connection between the hypothalamus and the sympathetic system do not mount this response. Given a large enough surface area lacking these mechanisms, core temperature will decline. In practical terms, individuals with lesions at T6 and above exhibit the problem, since a loss of descending sympathetic control of more than half of the body is present [41]. Management relies on awareness, prevention then correcting the temperature as much as possible. One of the best ways for a person with a SCI to cool down is to have a cold wet towel wrapped around the back of the neck. The skin could also be damped down or sprayed with cool water to allow water to evaporate from the skin, and cool the body. If a person gets too cold, then layers of clothing and warm fluids can bring the core temperature back up to normal. Occasionally warmed, humidified oxygen, heated intravenous saline, warmed blankets or heat lamps will be required although care must be taken on insensate skin.

Respiratory system

The respiratory system, including the lung, respiratory muscles, and neural control system, is a complex integrated physiological system that is not yet fully understood. The respiratory system is unique in that it must operate in a cyclical and highly coordinated fashion for 24 hours per day in order to sustain life. Respiratory complications continue to be one of the leading causes of morbidity and mortality in people with SCI, especially among cervical and higher thoracic injuries. The effects on lung mechanics are outwith the scope of this chapter; however, SCI affects the autonomic supply to the repiratory system, which has important clinical consequences.

Interruption of the sympathetic innervation and unopposed vagal activity results in increased secretions and heightened airway tone, with a reduction in baseline airway calibre i.e. relative bronchoconstriction. This, in combination with the mechanical difficulties of secretion clearance, results in the high incidence of respiratory complications seen.

In studies, the majority of tetraplegics manifest non-specific airway hyperreactivity following pretreatment with histamine, methacholine, and ultrasonically nebulized distilled water. There are several potential mechanisms for hyperresponsiveness in tetraplegia including loss of sympathetic autonomic input with relatively unopposed parasympathetic input, altered mechanical lung properties with decreased deep breathing and 'stretching' of airways, and non-specific airway hyperresponsiveness similar to subjects with asthma.

Schlero et al. [53] demonstrated a significant increase in airway calibre following inhalation of ipratropium bromide, an anticholinergic agent, suggesting that reduction in airway calibre is not due to acquired airway fibrosis stemming from repeated infections or to abnormal hysteresis secondary to chronic inability of subjects to inhale to predicted total lung capacity.

There is some evidence to show that use of bronchodilators (beta 2 agonists and anticholinergics) can elicit a positive response in pulmonary function with bronchodilatation and normalizing of airway calibre. Bronchodilators can be recommended for short-term use in patients with obstructive impairment. Further research is required to understand the effects of brocnhodilators on respiratory symptoms and complications [53–58].

The lower urinary tract and bowel

A guide to management and neurorehabilitation of the bladder (and bowel) can be found in Chapter 24.

The gastrointestinal (GI) system

Reflux oesophagitis, delayed gastric emptying, constipation, impaired control of evacuation, and incomplete evacuation can all occur as a result of autonomic dysfunction. Incontinence, oesophageal dysmotility and delayed gastric emptying may occur in up to 50% of diabetic patients. In particular, reports of abdominal fullness predicted delayed gastric emptying [59]. Oesophageal dysmotility, delayed gastric emptying, and autonomic neuropathy correlate to disturbed glucose homeostasis [59]. Possible management for gastrointestinal autonomic neuropathy in patients with diabetes may include aminoguanidine, which can prevent diabetes-induced changes in nitric oxide synthase-related changes in animal models of ileum autonomic neuropathy.

Damage to the nervous system has a large impact on function of the large bowel and maintenance of faecal continence. Stool transit through the bowel may be slowed placing the individual at high risk of constipation. Sensory and motor control of the ano-rectum may be impaired leaving the individual with reduced or absent voluntarily control of the process of defaecation. Most evidence for managing these problems is found in the literature around spinal cord injury. With appropriate assessment and evaluation, this knowledge can be applied to helping individuals with bowel dysfunction due to other neurological conditions.

A guide to management and neurorehabilitation of the bowel (and bladder) can be found in Chapter 24.

Exemplar of specific conditions: stroke— autonomic sequelae and management

Autonomic dysfunction is a common complication after acute stroke [60] (see Table 10.6). The exact incidence and prevalence is unknown. The dysfunction may be cardiovascular, thermoregulatory, or be of bowel, bladder, or sexual function.

Cardiovascular dysfunction after stroke

In terms of cardiovascular dysfunction, in one-study abnormal scores on autonomic symptoms questionnaire were present in 72.7% of patients with ischaemic stroke [61]. It has been identified in 69.0% patients without carotid stenosis and 88.9% with carotid stenosis [62] and cardiovascular autonomic dysfunction

Table 10.6 A summary of autonomic sequelae in stroke

Cardiovascular regulation
Myocardial infarction
Cardiac arrhythmias
ECG-abnormalities
Hypo- and hypertonia
Decreased heart rate and blood pressure variability
Thermoregulation
Asymmetric sweating
Cold hemiplegic limbs
Urogenital regulation
Urinary incontinence and retention
Impotence and orgasmic disability
Gastrointestinal regulation
Gastroparesis
Stress ulcers

has been diagnosed in 31.8% of patients with abnormal sympathetic skin responses in 81.8% of patients [62].

Some studies' results point to gradual recovery of autonomic dysfunction within the first months following the acute phase [63, 64]. However in other study impairments persisted at 6 months after stroke [65] and another suggests cardiovascular autonomic function is persistently deranged after stroke in older people [66].

The pathophysiology of the impairments is not fully understood. Brainstem stroke, damaging the baroreflex relay nuclei, is typically associated with baroreflex failure and blood pressure instability [67], but acute ischaemic stroke also causes significant damage to the cardiovascular autonomic system, manifesting as abnormalities of heart rate variability [68], although interestingly, patients with carotid stenosis show more severely impaired parasympathetic and sympathetic functions [62].

Baroreflex impairment has been demonstrated in acute ischaemic and haemorrhagic stroke [69–72]. The level of baroreflex dysfunction does not appear to differ between ischaemic and haemorrhagic stroke, although different pathophysiological mechanisms may exist [73] and the associations between autonomic function and early stroke outcome in different subtypes of cerebral infarct have shown different autonomic function properties between acute large artery atherosclerotic infarction and lacunar infarction groups [74].

There is increasing evidence that the central autonomic network, including a hemispheric network, is involved [69] and, in particular, the insular cortex seems to play a principal role in modulating baroreceptor sensitivity [75–78].

In summary, several consequences of autonomic dysfunction may impact on the pathophysiology and outcome following stroke and Sykora et al. [79] hypothesize that autonomic dysfunction in acute stroke, as expressed by decreased baroreceptor sensitivity, may have effects on outcome via inadequate cerebral perfusion due to the increased blood pressure variability and impaired cerebral autoregulation, increased cardiovascular complications, and secondary brain injury due to inflammation, hyperglycaemia, and blood–brain barrier disruption.

Autonomic dysfunction in patients with stroke worsens their health status and can induce life-threatening complications [61].

Disease manifestations that may indicate baroreceptor reflex dysfunction, such as hypertensive crises or high blood pressure variability, often accompany the acute phase of ischaemic or haemorrhagic stroke [80]. Poor outcomes may be related to secondary brain injury, hyperglycaemia, immunosuppression, and cardiovascular complications.

A significant and independent association has been demonstrated between impaired baroreceptor sensitivity, blood pressure variability, and short-term outcome in patients with intracerebral haemorrhage [12]. Because cerebrovascular autoregulation seems to be impaired in both acute ischaemic and haemorrhagic stroke, fluctuations in blood pressure may significantly alter cerebral perfusion [81–83].

Autonomic impairment also potentially plays an important role in non-haemodynamically mediated secondary brain injury after stroke. A shift to sympathetic predominance has previously been shown to be associated with proinflammatory cytokine production, hyperglycaemia, and increased blood–brain barrier permeability. In turn, these mechanisms have been proposed to be involved in secondary brain injury after stroke [79].

Autonomic shift to sympathetic overactivity has been repeatedly observed in acute stroke. Sykora et al. [84] again hypothesize that hyperglycemia in acute stroke relates to autonomic imbalance and that the adverse effects on stroke outcome may be cross-linked. They observed an association between hyperglycaemia and decreased baroreceptor sensitivity in non-diabetic patients, suggesting that hyperglycaemic reaction in acute stroke may reflect stroke-related autonomic changes and suggest outcome effects of autonomic changes and hyperglycaemia are interdependent, having the sympathovagal imbalance as a common underlying mechanism. The possible therapeutic relevance of this warrants further studies.

Autonomic abnormalities may predispose to infection and a study [85] on the influence of lesion location within middle cerebral artery (MCA) territory on parameters related to activation of sympathetic adrenomedullar pathway, immunodepression, and associated infection suggests a specific role of the insular lesion in the pathogenesis of stroke-induced sympathetic hyperactivation and immunodepression.

Baroreflex impairment has been independently related to less favourable long- and short-term outcomes after acute ischaemic stroke or after intracerebral haemorrhage [72] and may be relevant to the risk of all-cause and cardiovascular mortality in stroke survivors at increased risk for developing cardiac complications, and demonstrate a significantly higher cardiovascular morbidity and mortality [79].

Existing knowledge about baroreflex dysfunction in acute stroke raises questions regarding therapeutic implications. Baroreflex sensitivity can be influenced by drugs, especially beta blockers [86, 87], although several other drugs have been proposed to enhance baroreflex sensitivity, including ketanserin [88] clonidine, moxonidine, and mecobalamin [89, 90]. There is no good clinical evidence yet that these medications will have a role in management but further studies seem justified.

New devices to stimulate baroreceptors are emerging in the treatment of chronic refractory hypertension. By stimulating the carotid baroreceptors electrically, these devices ameliorate baroreflex sensitivity and reduce hypertension [91], however, there is no evidence as yet for their role after stroke.

The effects of body weight supported treadmill training (BWSTT) [92] and Repetitive transcranial magnetic stimulation (rTMS) of the sensorimotor cortex on autonomic dysfunction have started to be explored and may in the future have a role in promoting autonomic function and managing autonomic dysfunction after stroke.

Bowel and bladder dysfunction after stroke [93]

Urinary and faecal incontinence are both common in the early stages post-stroke; 40–60% of people admitted to hospital after a stroke can have problems with urinary incontinence, with 25% still having problems on discharge and 15% remaining incontinent after 1 year. Increased age, stroke severity, the presence of diabetes, prostatic hypertrophy, pre-existing impairment in urinary function, and the occurrence of other disabling diseases, increase the risk of urinary incontinence after stroke.

Incontinence is a major burden on patients and carers. Management of both bladder and bowel problems should be seen as an essential part of rehabilitation. Acute use of an indwelling catheter may facilitate management of fluids, prevent urinary retention, and reduce skin breakdown in patients with stroke; however, use of an indwelling urinary catheter greater than 48 hours post-stroke increases the risk of urinary tract infection.

Faecal incontinence occurs in a substantial proportion of patients after a stroke, but clears within two weeks in the majority of patients. Continued faecal incontinence is a poor prognostic factor.

Constipation and faecal impaction are more common after stroke than faecal incontinence. Immobility and inactivity,

Table 10.7 Stroke—bladder and bowel management [94]

Management of bladder and bowel after stroke: Recommendations from the Royal College of Physicians (UK) National Guidelines 2012.

- All wards and stroke units should have established assessment and management protocols for both urinary and faecal incontinence, and for constipation in stroke patients.
- Patients with stroke who have continued loss of bladder control 2 weeks after diagnosis should be reassessed to identify the cause of incontinence, and have an ongoing treatment plan involving both patients and carers.
- The patient should:
  - have any identified causes of incontinence treated
  - have an active plan of management documented
  - be offered simple treatments such as bladder retraining, pelvic floor exercises, and external equipment first
  - only be discharged with continuing incontinence after the carer (family member) or patient has been fully trained in its management and adequate arrangements fora continuing supply of continence aids and services are confirmed and in place.
- All stroke patients with a persistent loss of control over their bowels should:
  - be assessed for other causes of incontinence, which should be treated if identified
  - have a documented, active plan of management
  - be referred for specialist treatments if the patient is able to participate in treatments
  - only be discharged with continuing incontinence after the carer (family member) or patient has been fully trained in its management and adequate arrangements for a continuing supply of continence aids and services are confirmed and in place.
- Stroke patients with troublesome constipation should:
  - have a prescribed drug review to minimize use of constipating drugs
  - be given advice on diet, fluid intake and exercise
  - be offered oral laxatives
  - be offered rectal laxatives only if severe problems remain.

Table 10.8 Summary of autonomic problems, their assessments and management after SCI

Clinical problem	Assessment	Management
Bradycardia	ECG cardiac monitor	Optimize oxygenation Atropine for acute episodes Consider prophylactic atropine for vagal stimulating procedures ? Methylxanthine agents Pacemaker only if refractory or recurrent
Orthostatic hypotension	Lying/sitting/standing BP measurement	Education on exacerbating factors and prevention Compressive stockings Abdominal binder Trial medications either ephedrine, midodrine, or fludrocortisone
Autonomic dysreflexia	In patients with injuries at/above T6 BP measurement Assess for cause	See Figure 10.9
Sweating abnormalities—hyper or hypohydrosis	Exclude other pathology, e.g. syrinx, autonomic dysreflexia	Education on effects and preventative strategies Consider medication, e.g. clonidine Consider botulinum toxin if focal
Temperature dysregulation	Temperature measurement	Education/awareness/prevention strategies Cold towels/cool spray if hyperthermic Clothing, warm fluids if hypothermic Occasionally humidified oxygen, heated intravenous saline, warmed blankets if more severe hypothermia
Impaired respiratory function	Chest examination, Vital capacity, PEFR if able, SaO$_2$, ABGs/CXR if indicated	Oxygen/humidification beta-2-agonists and anticholinergics Manual therapy techniques to promote sputum clearance, increase ventilation and reduce work of breathing
Urinary incontinence	See Chapter 24	See Chapter 24
Constipation	See Chapter 24	See Chapter 24
Faecal incontinence	See Chapter 24	See Chapter 24
Impaired sexual function	See Chapter 24	See Chapter 24

ABG, arterial blood gas; BP, blood pressure; CXR, chest X-ray; PEFR, peak expiratory flow rate.

inadequate fluid or food intake, depression or anxiety, a neurogenic bowel, constipating side effects of medications, impaired sensation, lack of transfer ability, and cognitive impairments may each contribute to this problem. Goals of management are to ensure adequate intake of fluid and fibre and to help the patient establish a regular toileting routine. Bowel training is more effective if the routine is consistent with the patient's previous bowel habits. Stool softeners and laxatives may be helpful. Trans-anal irrigation may be considered if conservative management is unsuccessful [94]. Table 10.7 summarizes the bowel and bladder management after stroke and Table 10.8 summarizes autonomic imparments and management after SCI.

Conclusions and future directions for neurorehabilitation

Autonomic failures are a feature of many neurological conditions, which can last a lifetime and be exacerbated by further medical complications in the ageing process. There is a need for improving the detection and diagnoses of these failures as well as finding new and inventive therapies to overcome them for better neurorehabilitation. Conservative approaches and minimally invasive therapies are gaining favour in practice, but surgical interventions continue to be necessary in some cases.

In diagnostics there have been many significant advances of which neuroimaging is perhaps the one that will take us well into the future. Recent functional imaging studies have, for example, helped us to identify brain and spinal cord structures that are concerned with particular vegatative functions including the control of cardiovascular arousal mechanisms [95] and more recently, central control of the bladder [96].

CNS areas that exert particular autonomic control, including central as well as peripheral pathways may then become the targets for various interventions including smart drugs and devices. An example of the latter is the use of conditional neuro-stimulators which only apply their stimulation when abnormal activity such as neurogenic bladder overactivity (detrusor hyper-reflexia) is detected and then suppressed (conditional neuromodulation) [97].

In medical therapies there are bound to be much further advances in pharmacological agents that can more precisely target specific organs and their autonomic nervous control to effect benefit. Medical device delivery of drugs that are now widely used in spasticity control (e.g. baclofen pumps) are now being adapted to deliver drugs for long-term pain management [98] and the potential for targeted delivery in other areas of the central nervous system are possible, including those controlling autonomic function. Furthermore, these types of drugs may work better in combination with other therapies involving implantable neuro-stimulators which could be used to promote drug action by stimulating the autonomic pathways in the targeted areas.

Neurophysiological approaches using devices to promote restoration of autonomic function are gaining prominence in neurorehabilitation. There is deep brain stimulation for various conditions and some of these techniques are having considerable success including benefits for autonomic function; for example, in PD deep brain stimulation has also been shown to have a beneficial effect in suppressing associated urinary bladder overactivity [99]. During recent years the emphasis in neurophysiological approaches has been to develop non-invasive therapeutic interventions such as brain and spinal cord stimulation using transcranial magnetic and direct current stimulation (TMS and TDS respectively). The techniques of repetitive forms of TMS (rTMS) are believed to have an impact on influencing neuroplasticity such that it could have therapeutic benefits in the future [100].

Unlike the expected potential of TMS as a therapy, physiotherapy techniques, such as pelvic floor muscle training for improved bladder and bowel control are already demonstrating tangible benefits in conditions such as multiple sclerosis [101] and stroke [102]. Again, these therapies probably result from being able to tap into the neuroplasticity within the pathways of the ANS. Along with physiotherapeutic approaches there has been much research into psychosocial or behavioural therapies for ANS conditions such as those involving the cardiovascular system. However, it appears that such therapies are more concerned with preventative measures rather than addressing cardiovascular failures per se [103], but for those patients with an established cardiovascular disease then a multifactorial lifestyle intervention is recommended [104].

Finally, there is the exciting development of possible biological solutions to neuroprotection, neural repair and neuroregeneration of central and peripheral pathways following disease or trauma. In spinal cord injury, for instance, the biological approach to restoring lost function is often termed 'the cure' and although there have been significant experimental advances made over approximately the last three decades, mainly in the field of restoring locomotor function, the so-called 'cure' remains elusive. This is especially true for autonomic dysfunction where only recently have scientists begun to take a broader interest in these aspects of experimental scientific research in spinal cord injury [105]. It remains to be seen how much of this translates generally into developing newer techniques in neurorehabilitation.

References

1. Mathias CJ, Iodice V, Low D. Autonomic dysfunction: recognition, diagnosis, investigation, management, and autonomic neurorehabilitation. Handb Clin Neurol. 2013;**110**:239–253.
2. Tonkin AL, Frewin DB. Drugs, chemicals and toxins that alter autonomic function. In: Mathias CJ, Bannister R (eds) Autonomic Failure, 5th edn. Oxford University Press, Oxford, 2013, pp. 860–867.
3. Dale HH. Pharmacology and nerve-endings. Proc Roy Soc Med. 1934;**28** (3):319–330.
4. Burnstock G. Physiology and pathophysiology of purinergic neurotransmission. Physiol Rev.2007;**87**:659–797.
5. Burnstock G. Purinergic co-transmission. Exp Physiol. 2008;**94** (1):20–24.
6. de Groat WC, Booth AM. Inhibition and facilitation in parasympathetic ganglia of the urinary bladder. Fed Proc. 1980;**39**(12):2990–2996.
7. Kaplan SA, Dmochowski R, Cash BD, Kopp ZS, Berriman SJ, Khullar V. Systematic review of the relationship between bladder and bowel function: implications for patient management. Int J Clin Pract. 2013;**67**(3):205–216.
8. Blok BFM. Pathophysiology of detrusor-sphincter dyssynergia. In Corcos J and Schick E (eds) Neurogenic Bladder. Taylor & Francis, London, 2004, pp. 163–168.
9. Cervero F. Visceral nociception: peripheral and central aspects of visceral nociceptive systems. Philos Trans R SocLond B Biol Sci. 1985;**308**(1136):325–337.
10. Benarroch EE. The central autonomic network: functional organization, dysfunction, and perspective. Mayo Clin Proc. 1993;**68** (10):988–1001.
11. Critchley HD, Mathias CJ. Functional neuroimaging of autonomic control. In: Mathias CJ, Bannister R (eds) Autonomic Failure, 5th edn. Oxford University Press, Oxford, 2013, pp. 143–168.

12. Paton JFR, Spyer KM. Central nervous control of the cardiovascular system. In: Mathias CJ, Bannister R (eds) Autonomic Failure, 5th edn. Oxford University Press, Oxford, 2013, pp. 35–51.

13. Drake MJ, Fowler CJ, Griffiths D, Mayer E, Paton JFR, Birder L. Neural control of the lower urinary and gastrointestinal tracts: supraspinal CNS mechanisms. Neurourol Urodynam. 2010;29:119–127.

14. Fowler CJ, Griffiths D, deGroat WC. The neural control of micturition. Nature. 2008;9:453–466

15. De Groat WC, Booth AM, Yoshimura N. Neurophysiology of micturition and its modifications in animal models of human disease. In: Maggi CA (ed.) Nervous Control of the Urogenital System. The Autonomic Nervous System; vol 3. Harwood, London, 1993. pp 227–290

16. Craggs MD, Vaizey CJ. Neurophysiology of the bladder and bowel. In Fowler CJ (ed.) Neurology of Bladder, Bowel and Sexual Dysfunction. Blue Books of Practical Neurology; vol 23. Butterworth-Heinemann, Boston, 1999, pp. 19–32.

17. Craggs MD. Pelvic somato-visceral reflexes after spinal cord injury: measures of functional loss and partial preservation. Progr Brain Res. 2006;152:205–219.

18. Panicker JN, de Sèze M, Fowler CJ. Rehabilitation in practice: neurogenic lower urinary tract dysfunction and its management. Clin Rehabil. 2010;24(7):579–589.

19. DiBona GF. Neural control of the kidney: past, present, and future. Hypertension. 2003;41:621–624.

20. Mathias CJ, Bannister R (eds). Autonomic failure. In: A Textbook of Clinical Disorders of the Autonomic Nervous System, 5th edn. Oxford University Press, Oxford, 2013.

21. England JD, Gronseth GS, Franklin G, et al. Practice Parameter: evaluation of distal symmetric polyneuropathy: role of autonomic testing, nerve biopsy, and skin biopsy (an evidence-based review). Report of the American Academy of Neurology, American Association of Neuromuscular and Electrodiagnostic Medicine, and American Academy of Physical Medicine and Rehabilitation. Neurology. 2009;72(2):177–184

22. Jie-Hyun Kim. How to interpret conventional anorectal manometry. J Neurogastroenterol. Motil. 2010;16(4):437–439.

23. Patki P, Woodhouse J, Hamid R, Craggs M, Shah J. Effects of spinal cord injury on semen parameters. J Spinal Cord Med. 2008;31(1): 27–32.

24. Davies DR, Smith SE. Pupil abnormality in amyloidosis with autonomic neuropathy. J Neurol Neurosurg Psychiatry. 1999;67(6):819–822.

25. Critchley HD, Josephs O, O'Doherty J. Human cingulate cortex and autonomic cardiovascular control: converging neuroimaging and clinical evidence. Brain. 2003;216:2139–2156.

26. Mathias CJ. Disorders of the autonomic nervous system. In: Bradley WG, Daroff RB, Fenichel GM, Marsden CD (eds) Neurology in Clinical Practice, vols I and II, 2nd edn. Butterworth-Heinemann, Boston, MA, 1996, pp. 1953–1981.

27. Sadaka F, Veremakis C. Bradycardia secondary to cervical spinal cord injury. In: Breijo-Marquez FR (ed.) Cardiac Arrhythmias—New Considerations) InTech China, Shanghai, 2012, pp. 395–402.

28. Mathias CJ. Autonomic diseases: clinical features and laboratory evaluation. J Neurol Neurosurg Psychiatry. 2003;74:31–41.

29. Freeman R. Clinical practice.Neurogenic orthostatic hypotension. N Engl J Med. 2008;358(6):615–624.

30. Lahrmann H, Cortelli P, Hilz M, Mathias CJ, Struhal W, Tassinari M. Orthostatic hypotension. In: Gilhus NE, Barnes MP, Brainin M (eds) European Handbook of Neurological Management, 2nd edn, Vol. 1. Wiley-Blackwell, Oxford, 2011, pp. 469–475.

31. Consensus statement on the definition of orthostatic hypotension, pure autonomic failure, and multiple system atrophy. The Consensus Committee of the American Autonomic Society and the American Academy of Neurology. Neurology. 1996;46(5):1470.

32. Krassioukov A, Wecht JM, Teasell RW, Eng JJ. Orthostatic hypotension following spinal cord injury. In: Eng JJ, Teasell RW, Miller WC, et al. (eds) Spinal Cord Injury Rehabilitation Evidence (SCIRE). Version 4.0. Vancouver, 2012, pp. 1–21.

33. Krassioukov A, Blackmer J, Teasell RW, Eng JJ. (012). Autonomic Dysreflexia Following Spinal Cord Injury. In: Eng JJ, Teasell RW, Miller WC, et al. (eds) Spinal Cord Injury Rehabilitation Evidence (SCIRE). Version 4.0. Vancouver, 2012, pp. 1–34.

34. Gall A, Turner-Stokes L. Chronic spinal cord injury: management of patients in acute hospital settings. Clin Med. 2008;8(1):70–74.

35. Teasell RW, Arnold JM, Krassioukov A, Delaney GA. Cardiovascular consequences of loss of supraspinal control of the sympathetic nervous system following spinal cord injuries. Arch Phys Med Rehabil. 2000;81:506–516

36. Yarkony GM, Katz RT, Wu Y. Seizures secondary to autonomic dysreflexia. Arch Phys Med Rehabil. 1986;67:834–835

37. Pine ZM, Miller SD, Alonsa JA. Atrial fibrillation associated with autonomic dysreflexia. Am J Phys Med Rehabil. 1991;70:271–273.

38. Eltorai I, Kim R, Vulpe M, Kasravi H, Ho W. Fatal cerebral hemorrhage due to autonomic dysreflexia in a tetraplegic patient: case report and review. Paraplegia. 1992;30:355–360

39. Valles M, Benito J, Portell E, Vidal J. Cerebral hemorrhage due to autonomic dysreflexia in a spinal cord injury patient. Spinal Cord. 2005;43:738–740.

40. Krassioukov A, Warburton DER, Teasell R, Eng JJ. A systematic review of the management of autonomic dysreflexia following spinal cord injury. On behalf of the SCIRE Team. Arch Phys Med Rehabil. 2009;90(4):682–695.

41. Krassioukov AV, Karlsson A-K, Wecht JM, Wuermser L-A, Mathias CJ, Marino RJ, Joint Committee of American Spinal Injury Association and International Spinal Cord Society. J Rehabil Res Dev. 2007;44:103–112.

42. Consortium for Spinal Cord Medicine.Acute management of autonomic dysreflexia: individuals with spinal cord injury presenting to health-care facilities, 2nd edn. Paralyzed Veterans of America, Washington, 2001.

43. Freedberg IM (ed.). Fitzpatrick's Dermatology in General Medicine, 5th edn. McGraw-Hill, Health Professions Division, New York (NY): 1999.

44. Stolman LP. Treatment of hyperhidrosis. Dermatol Clin. 1998;16(4):863–869.

45. Canaday BR, Stanford RH. Propantheline bromide in the management of hyperhidrosis associated with spinal cord injury. Ann Pharmacother. 1995;29(5):489–492.

46. Tashjian EA, Richter KJ. The value of propoxyphene hydrochloride (Darvon) for the treatment of hyperhidrosis in the spinal cord injured patient: an anecdotal experience and case reports. Paraplegia. 1985;23(6):349–353.

47. Torch EM. Remission of facial and scalp hyperhidrosis with clonidine hydrochloride and topical aluminum chloride. South Med J. 2000;93(1):68–69.

48. Birch JF, Varma SK, Narula AA. Botulinum toxoid in the management of gustatory sweating (Frey's syndrome) after superficial parotidectomy. Br J Plast Surg. 1999;52(3):230–231.

49. Laccourreye O, Akl E, Gutierrez-Fonseca R, Garcia D, Brasnu D, Bonan B. Recurrent gustatory sweating (Frey syndrome) after intra- cutaneous injection of botulinum toxin type A: incidence, manage- ment, and outcome. Arch Otolaryngol Head Neck Surg. 1999;125(3):283–286.

50. Glogau RG. Treatment of palmar hyperhidrosis with botulinum toxin. Semin Cutan Med Surg.2001;20(2):101–108.

51. Heckmann M, Ceballos-Baumann AO, Plewig G. Botulinum toxin A for axillary hyperhidrosis (excessive sweating). N Engl J Med. 2001;344(7):488–493.

52. Heckmann M, Breit S, Ceballos-Baumann A, Schaller M, Plewig G. Side-controlled intradermal injection of botulinum toxin A in recal- citrant axillary hyperhidrosis. J Am Acad Dermatol. 1999;41(6):987–990

53. Schilero GJ, Spungen AM, Bauman WA, Radulovic M, Lesser M. Pulmonary function and spinal cord injury. Respir Physiol Neurobiol. 2009;166(3):129–141

54. Dicpinigaitis PV, Spungen AM, Bauman WA, AbsgartenA, Almenoff PL. Bronchial hyper-responsiveness after cervical spinal cord injury. Chest. 1994;**105**:1073–1076.

55. Fein ED, Grimm M, Lesser M, Bauman WA, Almenoff PL. The effects of ipratopium bromide on histamine- induced bronchoconstriction in subjects with cervical spinal cord injury. J Asthma. 1998;**35**:49–55.

56. Grimm DR, Arias E, Lesser M, Bauman WA, Almenoff PL. Airway hyper-responsiveness to ultrasonically nebulized distilled water in subjects with tetraplegia. J Appl Physiol. 1999;**86**:1165–1169

57. Singas E, Grimm DR, Almenoff PL, Lesser M. Inhibition of airway hyperreactivity by oxybutynin chloride in subjects with cervical spinal cord injury. Spinal Cord. 1999;**37**(4):279–283.

58. Grimm DR, Chandy D, Almenoff PL, Schilero G, Lesser M. Airway hyperreactivity in with tetraplegia is associated with reduced baseline airway caliber. Chest. 2000;**118**:1397–1404.

59. Ohlsson B, Melander O, Thorsson O, Olsson R, Ekberg O, Sundkvist G. Oesophageal dysmotility, delayed gastric emptying and autonomic neuropathy correlate to disturbed glucose homeostasis. Diabetologia. 2006;**49**(9):2010–2014.

60. Korpelainen JT, Sotaniemi KA, Myllylä VV. Autonomic nervous system disorders in stroke. Clin Auton Res. 1999;**9**:325–333.

61. Xiong L, Leung HW, Chen XY, et al. Acta Neurol Scand. Autonomic dysfunction in ischemic stroke with carotid stenosis.2012;**126**(2):122–128.

62. Labuz-Roszak B. Pierzchala K. Stroke induces disturbances of autonomic system function. Neurologia i Neurochirurgia Polska. 2007;**41**(6):495–503.

63. Barron SA, Rogovski Z, Hemli J. Autonomic consequences of cerebral hemisphere infarction. Stroke. 1994;**25**:113–116.

64. Korpelainen JT, Sotaniemi KA, Suominen K, Tolonen U, Myllyla VV. Cardiovascular autonomic reflexes in brain infarction. Stroke. 1994;**25**: 787–792.

65. Korpelainen JT, Sotaniemi KA, Huikuri HV, Myllya VV. Abnormal heart rate variability as a manifestation of autonomic dysfunction in hemispheric brain infarction. Stroke. 1996;**27**:2059–2063.

66. McLaren A, Kerr S, Allan L, et al. Autonomic function is impaired in elderly stroke survivors. Stroke. 2005;**36**(5):1026–1030,

67. Phillips AM, Jardine DL, Parkin PJ, Hughes T, Ikram H. Brain stem stroke causing baroreflex failure and paroxysmal hypertension. Stroke. 2000;**31**:1997–2001.

68. Chen CF. Lin HF. Lin RT. Yang YH. Lai CL. Relationship between ischemic stroke location and autonomic cardiac function. J Clin Neurosci. 2013;**20**(3):406–409,

69. Robinson TG, James M, Youde J, Panerai R, Potter J. Cardiac baroreceptor sensitivity is impaired after acute stroke. Stroke. 1997;**28**: 1671–1676.

70. Eames PJ, Blake MJ, Dawson SL, Panerai RB, Potter JF. Dynamic cerebral autoregulation and beat to beat blood pressure control are impaired in acute ischaemic stroke. J Neurol Neurosurg Psychiatry. 2002;**72**:467–472.

71. Eveson DJ, Robinson TG, Shah NS, Panerai RB, Paul SK, Potter JF. Abnormalities in cardiac baroreceptor sensitivity in acute ischaemic stroke patients are related to aortic stiffness. Clin Sci Lond. 2005;**108**:441–447.

72. Sykora M, Diedler J, Rupp A, Turcani P, Rocco A, Steiner T. Impaired baroreflex sensitivity predicts outcome of acute intracerebral hemorrhage. Crit Care Med. 2008;**36**:3074–3079.

73. Sykora M, Diedler J, Rupp A, Turcani P, Steiner T. Impaired baroreceptor reflex sensitivity in acute stroke is associated with insular involvement, but not with carotid atherosclerosis. Stroke. 2009;**40**:737–742.

74. Chen PL. Kuo TB. Yang CC. Parasympathetic activity correlates with early outcome in patients with large artery atherosclerotic stroke. J Neurol Sci. 2012;**314**(1–2):57–61.

75. Oppenheimer SM, Gelb A, Girvin JP, Hachinski VC. Cardiovascular effects of human insular cortex stimulation. Neurology. 1992;**42**:1727–1732.

76. Zhang ZH, Rashba S, Oppenheimer SM. Insular cortex lesions alter baroreceptor sensitivity in the urethane-anesthetized rat. Brain Res. 1998; **813**:73–81.

77. Saleh TM, Connell BJ. Role of the insular cortex in the modulation of baroreflex sensitivity. Am J Physiol. 1998;**274**:R1417–R1424.

78. Zhang ZH, Dougherty PM, Oppenheimer SM. Characterization of baroreceptor-related neurons in the monkey insular cortex. Brain Res. 1998;**796**:303–306.

79. Sykora M. Diedler J. Turcani P. Hacke W. Steiner T. Baroreflex: a new therapeutic target in human stroke. Stroke. 2009;**40**(12):678–682.

80. Ketch T, Biaggioni I, Robertson R, Robertson D. Four faces of baroreflex failure: hypertensive crisis, volatile hypertension, orthostatic tachycardia, and malignant vagotonia. Circulation. 2002;**105**:2518–2523.

81. Immink RV, van Montfrans GA, Stam J, Karemaker JM, Diamant M, van Lieshout JJ. Dynamic cerebral autoregulation in acute lacunar and middle cerebral artery territory ischemic stroke. Stroke. 2005;**36**: 2595–2600.

82. Kuwata N, Kuroda K, Funayama M, Sato N, Kubo N, Ogawa A. Dysautoregulation in patients with hypertensive intracerebral hemorrhage: a SPECT study. Neurosurg Rev. 1995;**18**:237–245.

83. Diedler J, Sykora M, Rupp A, et al. Impaired cerebral vasomotor activity in spontaneous intracerebral hemorrhage. Stroke. 2009;**40**:815–919.

84. Sykora M, Diedler J, Poli S, et al. Association of non-diabetic hyperglycemia with autonomic shift in acute ischaemic stroke. Eur J Neurol. 2012;**19**(1):84–90.

85. Walter U, Kolbaske S, Patejdl R, et al. Insular stroke is associated with acute sympathetic hyperactivation and immunodepression. Eur J Neurol. 2013;**20**(1):153–159.

86. Elghozi JL, Julien C. Sympathetic control of short-term heart rate variability and its harmacological modulation. Fundam Clin Pharmacol.2007;**21**:337–347.

87. Mortara A, La Rovere MT, Pinna GD, Maestri R, Capomolla S, Cobelli F. Nonselective adrenergic blocking agent, carvedilol, improves arterial baroflex gain and heart rate variability in patients with stable chronic heart failure. J Am Coll Cardiol. 2000;**36**: 1612–1618.

88. Liu AJ, Ma XJ, Shen FM, Liu JG, Chen H, Su DF. Arterial baroreflex: a novel target for preventing stroke in rat hypertension. Stroke. 2007;**38**: 1916–1923.

89. Ma XJ, Shen FM, Liu AJ, Shi KY, Wu YL, Su DF. Clonidine, moxonidine, folic acid, and mecobalamin improve baroreflex function in stroke-prone, spontaneously hypertensive rats. Acta Pharmacol Sin. 2007;**28**:1550–1558.

90. Turcani M. Biphasic dose-dependent modulation of cardiac parasympathetic activity by moxonidine, an imidazoline IL-receptor agonist. J Cardiovasc Pharmacol. 2008;**52**:524–535.

91. Uppuluri SC, Storozynsky E, Bisognano JD. Baroreflex device therapy in the treatment of hypertension. Curr Hypertens Rep. 2009; **11**:69–75.

92. Magagnin V, Bo I, Turiel M, Fornari M, Caiani EG, Porta A. Effects of robot-driven gait orthosis treadmill training on the autonomic response in rehabilitation-responsive stroke and cervical spondylotic myelopathy patients. Gait & Posture. 2010;**32**(2):199–204.

93. Stroke Guideline for the Management of Stroke Rehabilitation. Department of Veterans Affairs Department of Defense And The American Heart Association/American Stroke Association Prepared by: THE MANAGEMENT OF STROKE REHABILITATION Working Group With support from: The Office of Quality and Performance, VA, Washington, DC & Quality Management Division, United States Army MEDCOM, Version 2.0 2010.

94. Royal College of Physicians (UK). Management of bladder and bowel after stroke: Recommendations. National Guidelines. Royal College of Physicians, London, 2012.

95. Critchley HD, Corfield DR, Chandler MP, Mathias CJ, Dolan RJ. Cerebral correlates of autonomic cardiovascular arousal: A functional neuroimaging investigation. J Physiol. Lond. 2000;**523**:259–270.

96. Kavia RB, Dasgupta R, Fowler CJ. Functional imaging and the central control of the bladder. J Comp Neurol. 2005;**493**:27–32.

97. Craggs M. Restoration of complete bladder function by neurostimulation. In Corcos J and Schick E (eds) Neurogenic Bladder. 2nd edn. Taylor & Francis, London, 2008, pp. 625–635.

98. Ghafoor VL, Epshteyn M, Carlson GH, Terhaar DM, Charry O, Phelps PK. Intrathecal drug therapy for long-term pain management. Am J Health Syst Pharm. 2007;**64**(23):2447–2461.

99. Seif C, Herzog J, van der Horst C, et al. Effect of subthalamic deep brain stimulation on the function of the urinary bladder. Ann Neurol. 2004;**55**(1):118–120.

100. Ridding MC, Rothwell JC. Is there a future for therapeutic use of transcranial magnetic stimulation? Nat Rev Neurosci. 2007;**8**(7):559–567.

101. McClurg D, Ashe RG, Marshall K, Lowe-Strong AS. Comparison of pelvic floor muscle training, electromyography biofeedback, and neuromuscular electrical stimulation for bladder dysfunction in people with multiple sclerosis: a randomized pilot study. Neurourol Urodyn. 2006;**25**(4):337–348.

102. Tibaek S, Gard G, Jensen R. Pelvic floor muscle training is effective in women with urinary incontinence after stroke: a randomised, controlled and blinded study. Neurourol Urodyn. 2005;**24**(4):348–357.

103. De Backer G Ambrosioni E, Borch-Johnsen, et al. European guidelines on cardiovascular disease prevention in clinical practice: Third Joint Task Force of European and other Societies on Cardiovascular Disease Prevention in Clinical Practice (constituted by representatives of eight societies and by invited experts). Eur J Cardiovasc Prevent Rehabil. 2003;**10**:S1–S78.

104. Blokstra A, van Dis I, Verschuren WM. Efficacy of multifactorial lifestyle interventions in patients with established cardiovascular diseases and high risk groups. Eur J Cardiovasc Nurs. 2012;**11**(1):97–104.

105. Weaver LC, Polosa C (eds). Autonomic dysfunction after spinal cord injury. Progress in Brain Research. Volume 152. Elsevier, Amsterdam, 2006.

CHAPTER 11

Functional recovery in CNS disease: impact of animal models

Steffen Franz, Andreas Hug, and Norbert Weidner

Introduction

Animal models are crucial for the understanding of elementary mechanisms and the natural/interventional course of disease. Moreover, regulatory authorities like the Food and Drug Administration (FDA) or the European Medicines Agency (EMA) demand safety analyses of potential therapeutics in animal models. Despite extensive preclinical research efforts in the field of central nervous system (CNS) diseases, a large translational gap still remains between 'effective' preclinical and actual clinical treatment interventions.

In the clinical setting, functional recovery after CNS damage is conceptualized by the interplay of multidimensional factors in order to restitute/compensate disability by intra-individual (neurological recovery, psychological status/coping strategies) as well as extra-individual (supporting aids, human resources, financial resources, health care system infrastructure) means [1]. With respect to clinical translation, this multidimensional conceptualization of functional recovery discloses the difficulties and limitations of animal research. While animal models are certainly suitable to investigate elementary concepts of pathophysiological recovery mechanisms at the somatic level (cellular/subcellular, basic behavioural analyses), other intra- and extra-individual dimensions, as previously described, can hardly be mimicked. For example, the level of somatic functions by applying the National Institutes of Health Stroke Scale (NIHSS) or the assessment of activities of daily living (ADL) and mobility, reflected by the Barthel ADL Index in the stroke setting cannot be replicated in small animals.

Traumatic spinal cord injury (SCI) and ischaemic stroke are acute onset CNS disorders with a high ratio of long-term disability [2, 3]. SCI and stroke have in common that they have an acute onset of the primary injury followed by distinct mechanisms of secondary damage [4, 5]. Both conditions are routinely treated with a defined standard of care.

With respect to novel treatments there are fundamental differences. In ischaemic stroke the main focus is currently on the development of so called neuroprotective therapeutic interventions, which aim at the restriction of injury to the brain by preventing neuronal cell death. The region of interest in this context is represented by the so called penumbra, an area surrounding the core of the lesion. Over the years more than 1,000 preclinical studies have been completed. The majority of them indeed showed functional benefits in relevant animal models of ischaemic stroke.

Nevertheless, until today, albeit the conduction of almost 200 clinical trials, not a single neuroprotective therapy has shown superior outcome [6].

In contrast, in SCI the most promising focus has been on neuroregenerative strategies. These approaches aim at the stimulation of injured axon pathways to reconnect CNS regions rostral and caudal to the injury site. Destroyed CNS tissue is replaced by factor-, cell- or biomaterial-based interventions [7, 8]. In SCI this approach was spurred by early studies showing that the failure of injured mammalian CNS axons to regrow in the adult can be overcome by introducing an axon growth conducive environment into the injured spinal cord [9]. In subsequent years many preclinical strategies were developed, which were reported to promote structural and functional recovery mostly in spinal cord injured small animals. Paralleling translational efforts in ischaemic stroke, all of those studies, be it factor- or cell-based, failed to demonstrate efficacy in human SCI (for review see [10, 11]).

The fact that SCI and stroke are different in many aspects—affection of spinal cord versus brain, mainly traumatic versus solely cardiovascular aetiology or mainly axonal versus combined cell body and axonal damage—allows us to investigate whether the failure to identify effective therapies represents a disease-specific or a higher-order error. In other words, we want to identify either individual factors of the respective disease responsible for the poor translational success or more general problems of similar neurological disease entities, which prevent prediction of therapeutic efficacy in human individuals. To achieve this, aspects influencing the predictive value of preclinical models in stroke and SCI will be analysed in this chapter: (1) the choice of animal species including preferred gender and age; (2) the disease mimicking intervention, (3) the consideration of standard therapies within preclinical models; (3) the accurary in translating preclinically assessed therapies into the clinical trial; and (4) the coherence of structural and functional outcome parameters in preclinical models and disease.

Factors related to the animal model
Choice of experimental animal

Animal size

Preclinical stroke and SCI research is almost exclusively performed in small animals such as rats and mice [12, 13]. Recent guidelines for stroke therapy trials recommend that in case a given treatment is effective in rodents, the effectiveness still needs to be replicated in gyrencephalic models like cats, pigs or non-human primates prior to the start of the clinical trials [14]. In stroke, which affects in particular the cortex and thus higher cognitive functions, a gyrencephalic model is important. In SCI, spinal cord dimensions (human spinal cord including the lesion area is at least 10 times larger than rat spinal cord) demand the use of an animal species, which at least approaches the dimensions of the human spinal cord. Until now there are only very few examples of large animal studies, which were translated into a clinical trial. The neuroprotective agent NXY-059 was investigated in a primate middle cerebral artery occlusion (MCAO) model [15] and was investigated in a clinical trial, which again failed to demonstrate efficacy of the drug [16, 17]. An antibody against the myelin component Nogo was reported to be effective in a monkey lateral cervical spinal cord hemisection model [18], which eventually served as the basis for a first in man open-label multicentre clinical study. The publication of the results of this study is still pending.

Taken together, official recommendations in stroke and SCI research [19, 20] strongly recommend the use of large animals based on theoretical considerations, which have yet to demonstrate their usefulness on the way to successful clinical translation. In particular, species-specific ethical issues such as appropriate animal husbandry and financial resources required to set up an apporpriate infrastructure for large animal reseach have to be considered [21, 22].

Animal age
Stroke is a disease of the elderly population. Cofactors pronounced in the elderly population such as multimorbidity and impaired translation of neurological recovery into function tremendously influence the outcome [23]. In contrast, most experimental stroke models do not sufficiently account for age. Even more, mainly young inbred healthy male animals without comorbidities are preferably investigated (Table 11.1). Rodent models for aged animals or animals with other relevant cardiovascular risk factors like hypertension exist, however, they did not provide the preclinical basis for translation into the clinic so far [24].

In traumatic SCI—paralleling findings in stroke—the recovery of sensorimotor function correlates inversely with increasing age with regard to recovery of function (e.g. locomotor function) [25]. However, considering the average age at traumatic SCI onset

(between 30 to 38 years of age; [26]), the typical animal age in preclinical studies reflects the clinical situation better. Widely used inbred female rodents are typically 10 to 12 weeks of age, which corresponds to 16–18 years of age in humans [27] (Table 11.1).

Animal gender
Gender preferences exist in both stroke and SCI animal models. While epidemiological data suggest that stroke is a relatively balanced disorder in terms of gender distribution (28), male animal models are usually employed in preclinical studies (Table 11.1). It is known that important pathophysiological processes vary depending on the gender. For example, the infarct size in female mice is smaller than in males [29], which additionally illustrates potential gender biases.

In SCI, the predominant gender is the complete opposite preclinically and clinically. In animal models female rodents are preferred, since manual bladder emptying in females is facilitated due to obvious neuroanatomical advantages (Table 11.1). Clinically, many more male individuals suffer from traumatic SCI with a male to female ratio of up to 6.7:1 [26]. The female rodent preference might lead to false positive functional outcome assessments, since female rats have been shown superior spontaneous recovery following spinal cord contusion compared to male rats [30].

Strain/species
Depending on the species and strain, vascular variations (anomalies in the circle of Willis) have been described, which differentially affect the susceptibility to a given stroke model. Hence, different neurological/functional deficits might arise despite the application of the same stroke model [31–33]. Therefore, the comparability of interventional effects between identical stroke models but different small animal strains is limited (Table 11.1).

In small animal SCI models substantial differences have been reported in terms of morphological changes at the lesion site. Mice lack cystic cavity formation at the lesion site [34, 35], whereas rats—paralleling pathological findings in primates and human subjects—develop typical cystic lesion defects. Such species differences can have profound implications. As an example, PTEN (phosphatase and tensin homolog) inactivation in mice, which activates the intrinsic axon regrowth capacity, promotes axon regrowth across the non-cystic lesion site [36]. In the clinical setting such an approach would not yield structural and

Table 11.1 Lesion models versus human disease characteristics

	Stroke		SCI	
	Small animal	Human	Small animal	Human
Age	8–16 weeks, corresponds to 16–18 years of human age	Mean age 69	10–12 weeks, corresponds to 16–18 years of human age	mean age 45*
Gender	Predominantly male	Female: male ≈ 1:1	Predominantly female	Female: male ≈ 1:3.5*
Lesion type	LOCAL vessel occlusion	Thromboembolic occlusion	Knife transection or contusion	Contusion or long-term compression
Lesion Level/region	Middle cerebral artery	Multifocal	Thoracic level**	Cervical: thoracic level ≈ 1:1*
Severity	Extensive	variable, mostly circumscribed	Predominantly incomplete	Complete: incomplete ≈ 1:1.2*

*Based on 'European Multicenter Study about Spinal Cord Injury (EMSCI)' data set (2001–2012) (Rupp, unpublished data).

**Related to contusion injury/only few models use cervical contusion injury.

consecutive functional improvement without combinatorial treatment approaches aiming for cyst replacement. Furthermore, the choice of the animal strain can influence the observed functional outcome (Table 11.1). Sprague–Dawley rats for instance regain quicker and superior locomotor function following contusional SCI, compared to Long–Evans rats [37].

Other strain/species dependent differences have to be considered in respect to neuroanatomy, neuroplasticity and neuroimmunological diversity, which may differentially affect functional outcome after SCI [38–43].

Lesion model and severity

Lesion model

In stroke and SCI, two principal types of lesion models are typically applied. First, more artificial lesion models, which do not really represent the pathophysiology of the respective disease entity. However, they are justified since they allow to address specific basic scientific questions. For instance, can target reinnervation—as a prerequisite for functional recovery in complete SCI—be achieved at all in a wire knife partial spinal cord transection model? Second, lesion models do exist that mimic the human disease as close as possible. Such a lesion model, for example embolic artery occlusion in stroke, is employed to get as much confidence as possible that an experimental paradigm is likely to work after translation into the clinical setting [33].

Ischaemic stroke is a heterogeneous disease with respect to aetiology. Typically, a brain-supplying vessel is occluded by either thrombotic or embolic mechanisms causing focal cerebral ischaemia to the brain. Several experimental procedures have been established to mimic the different clinical stroke aetiologies in animals [44]. Those range from highly artificial photothrombotic stroke in rodents over selective thermocoagulation of blood vessels in squirrels to clinically relevant models such as embolic artery occlusion models using homologous clots [44–46]. Since most of these preclinical studies failed in terms of clinical translation, the question arises, whether the applied stroke models do sufficiently resemble the clinical situation [47, 48] (Table 11.1).

Compared to the human situation, CNS lesions in animal models are considered to be rather uniform and homogeneous. However, a hypothetical power calculation for the widely applied intraluminal MCAO filament (suture) model in mice with an occlusion time of 60 minutes [49] gives a different impression. Due to collateral blood vessels from the anterior and posterior circulation, infarct volumes are highly dependent on the concomitant occlusion or patency of these collaterals. In the setting of collateral vessel patency the mean infarct volume was 49.2 mm^3 with a standard deviation of 17.2 (Leach correction). Assuming that a new therapy would lead to an infarct volume reduction of 10%, a sample size of 205 animals per group would be necessary (double-sided alpha error rate of 0.05, statistical power of 0.8, t-test for independent groups).

In the clinical setting, most spinal cord injuries occur via a blunt trauma to the spinal cord, leading to the combination of a contusion/compression injury [50, 51]. Preclinically, partial to complete knife/scissor transection as well as contusion/compression are in use (Table 11.1).

Transection SCI models do only reflect human pathology in very few instances [52, 53]. However, these models allow analysing fundamental pathophysiological mechanisms and generate very limited interindividual lesion size variability. Transection models are well suited to investigate axonal regrowth and sprouting [54]. Over many years, it was proposed but never demonstrated that regenerative approaches aim for reinnervation of target neurons, which requires both long-distance axon regeneration and proper target recognition. Therefore, a highly artificial rat cervical lesion model was established, where the dorsal columns containing the ascending proprioceptive projections were transected close to the target neuron area in the medulla oblongata—the nucleus cuneatus. Indeed, combined cellular transplantation and neurotrophin overexpression promoted axon regrowth across the lesion site and proper target reinnervation [55], including recovery of function [56]. These studies provided for the first time the proof of principle that target reinnervation can be achieved after experimental SCI.

Overall, rat thoracic weight drop contusion injury models closely mimic morphological, neurophysiological, and functional changes described in the human situation [57]. Even though contusion/compression injuries to the spinal cord are induced by means of a clip, forceps or an inflated balloon with a defined force [58–63], the heterogeneity between lesioned animals is much higher compared to transection SCI, since they are very sensitive to differences in velocities of impact [59, 64].

The choice of the lesion model also affects the incidence of typical SCI-related complications. For example, a hemisection model, as opposed to a contusion spinal cord injury, has been shown to promote the occurrence of neuropathic-pain related parameters (allodynia). This needs to be considered, when side effects, such as neuropathic pain, are evaluated after an experimental therapy administration [37].

Lesion severity

The clinical heterogeneity of stroke, especially with respect to infarct size is not only relevant for the lesion and neurological deficit itself, but also for ensuing complications (immunodepression, infectious complications) [65]. With respect to the clinical translation of immunological consequences however, rodent models are only of limited usefulness due to phylogenetically different immunological responses [66]. Moreover, other prognosis relevant complications like hypertension, hyperglycemia or fever are only incompletely modeled by most experimental stroke studies [33].

While in clinical stroke infarcts are usually small in size (4.5–14% of the ipsilateral hemisphere), most experimental rodent stroke models generate rather large infarcts with sizes up to 55% of the hemisphere [67] (Table 11.1). These models might be of value for the analysis of fundamental disease mechanisms. For an analysis of interventional treatment effects others than decompressive surgery, these large infarcts are unsuitable. In the clinical setting comparable infarct volumes would lead to space-occupying malignant infarcts with mortality rates up to 80% [68], unless a life-saving decompressive hemicraniectomy is performed [69].

Unlike stroke models, rat contusion SCI creates lesion dimensions, which are in relation to the size of the spinal cord comparable to human SCI. Paralleling pathological findings in the human injured spinal cord, the gray matter is severely affected with a variable degree of white matter sparing. In contrast to human SCI, which affects ventral and dorsal white matter equally, rat contusion SCI primarily lesions the dorsal white matter [53] (Table 11.1).

In SCI, the degree of disability and secondary complications are critically influenced by the neurological level of injury. In humans the majority of injuries occur at cervical level [26, 70], which are accompanied by many potentially disease-modifying complications (respiratory failure, infections, pressure sores). In contrast, the majority of preclinical studies prefer thoracic SCI, since due to severe immobility and respiratory problems complete cervical SCI cannot be handled in the preclinical setting (Table 11.1). Incomplete cervical contusion SCI models with clinically observable functional deficits, such as forelimb/hand motor deficits or autonomic dysfunction, have been established, but only to a limited extent [71, 72].

Factors related to therapy

Standard of care therapy

The only available FDA-approved treatment of acute ischaemic stroke, which improves functional outcome, both on the level of body function and the level of activities, is intravenous thrombolysis with alteplase (tissue type plasminogen activator) within 4.5 hours after stroke onset [73–75]. Why other preclinically promising intravenous thrombolytics failed, remains a matter of debate [76–78]. With respect to functional recovery, the start of an early on and ongoing neurorehabilitation programme remains the mainstay of treatment after ischaemic stroke [79–81].

Given these two proven strategies to improve functional recovery in ischaemic stroke (reperfusion therapy and neurorehabilitation) (Table 11.2), there is a need for their implementation in preclinical work. Novel treatment strategies need to demonstrate additional benefit before implementation in the clinical setting, where established therapies will be administered.

In the rodent experimental setting, rehabilitation strategies might exhibit a couple of dissimilarities compared to the clinical situation. While formal forelimb training in rodents improves skilled reaching [82–84], forced use paradigms established for upper limb rehabilitation in chronic clinical stroke [85–87], might lead to the exacerbation of infarct size and worsening of behavioural tests if initiated too early [88–90]. Vice versa, when started too late, beneficial effects might be missed due to the rapid spontaneous recovery or reduced efficacy of a delayed rehabilitative intervention, respectively [91–93].

After spinal cord trauma, an effective causal treatment like vessel recanalization in ischaemic stroke is not available. Operative and non-operative interventions for spine stabilization are widely accepted among clinicians albeit missing scientific evidence [94, 95] (Table 11.2). The main goals of spinal surgical interventions (decompression, stabilization) are to reduce pressure and/or improve perfusion of the injured cord and to allow rehabilitation in patients as soon as possible [96]. It has yet to be confirmed whether spine stabilization or timely surgical spine decompression improves the outcome after traumatic spinal cord injury [97]. Preclinical studies dedicated to investigate beneficial effects of early decompression suggest an improved outcome [98]. Almost all SCI models—except for the ballon compression model—require laminectomy before the actual SCI lesion, which can be considered as a potential outcome influencing prophylactic neuroprotective measure. Therefore, decompression as it is applied to human subjects is not reflected properly as standard care treatment in small animals. Only few animal studies investigating regeneration promoting tools included spine stabilization into their standard therapeutic regimen [30, 45, 99].

Uncertainty also exists with respect to early and high dose methylprednisolone treatment after traumatic spinal cord injury, leading to ambiguity in current clinical guidelines [100–102]. According to a recently published survey around 50% of acute SCI patients still receive high-dose steroid treatment in Germany

Table 11.2 Standard of care and experimental therapy

	Stroke		SCI	
	Animal	Human	Animal	Human
Standard of care	◆ None	◆ Thrombolysis ◆ Decompressive hemicraniectomy in malignant cerebral infarction ◆ Management of risk factors/complications ◆ Rehabilitation	◆ Laminectomy before contusion ◆ Postoperative manual bladder evacuation and prophylactic antibiotic treatment	◆ Laminectomy subsequent to contusion/compression ◆ Spinal fixation ◆ Management of risk factor/complications ◆ Permanent/intermittent catheterization ◆ Rehabilitation
Experimental therapy				
Timing of therapeutic intervention	◆ Drug administration frequently immediately after induction of ischaemia	◆ Drug administration frequently delayed between 4–6 h post ischaemia onset	◆ Drug administration/cell transplantation usually within few days after injury	◆ Prolonged interval between injury and administration of drug/cells
Route of administration	◆ Frequently systemic i.v./i.p. administration	◆ Frequently systemic i.v. administration	◆ Frequently drug administration locally at injury site ◆ Cell transplantation without imaging guidance into lesion centre	◆ Drug frequently administered not locally ◆ Cell grafting under ultrasound guidance around lesion centre

[103]. While there might be a slight treatment effect for improved sensory-motor function in the very acute phase of up to 8 hours after injury, adverse events like infectious complications are doubtlessly increased with methylprednisolone treatment [100].

Standard procedures during the post-acute stage of SCI are based on rehabilitative concepts to restore independence to a maximum level. Depending on the lesion level and severity, existing sensorimotor dysfunction will be restored or compensated. Albeit missing evidence for individual rehabilitative concepts, lesions of the autonomic nervous system, in particular neurogenic bowel and bladder dysfunction, require significant therapeutical attention. Regulation of bowel evacuation and handling of voiding dysfunction thus represent standard therapeutical targets in clinical routine, which are yet rarely introduced into preclinical studies evaluating regenerative approaches [104, 105]. Preclinical evidence emphasizes that the combination of a regenerative therapy with specific rehabilitative measures may impair functional outcome, if not synchronized properly [105]. Accordingly, regenerative strategies considered for clinical translation should be evaluated in combination with rehabilitative interventions.

Experimental therapies

In order to allow optimal predictability of a targeted neuroprotective/-regenerative therapy, respective modes of drug/cell administration have to be harmonized as close as possible. Timing of therapeutic intervention in relation to the lesion time point represents a highly relevant issue in the translation of a given therapeutic intervention.

Timing of therapeutic intervention

Neuroprotective therapies in ischaemic stroke target early pathophysiological events (excitotoxicity, inflammatory changes, neural apoptosis, free radicals, calcium influx). Therefore, short intervals between disease onset and drug administration are considered to be critical in neuroprotective therapies following the theme 'time is brain'. In preclinical studies, this prerequisite has been met (Table 11.2). However, clinical studies investigating the efficacy of neuroprotective agents following cerebral ischaemia, frequently struggle with the timely drug administration. For example, the free radical scavenging drug NXY-059 was applied within 4 hours after stroke onset [106], whereas respective clinical trials allowed to administer the drug within a 6 hour time frame [16, 17]. Preclinical and clinical assessment of another free radical scavenger—Tirilazid—yielded even more pronounced differences with respect to treatment delay (10 minutes in preclinical experiments versus 5 hours in the clinical trial) [107].

Cell-/biomaterial-, soluble drug- or gene therapy- based neuroregenerative therapies should ideally be applied within a narrow time frame after SCI. Depending on the particular therapeutic intervention, the time frame compared to neuroprotective strategies is not as critical in respect to the time post injury. Nevertheless, in order to increase the predictability of clinical efficacy, preclinical and clinical treatment windows should be matched as close as possible (Table 11.2). Looking at soluble factor based regenerative therapies, which were translated into clinical trials, significant discrepancies between preclinical and clinical drug administration are apparent. A dura-permeable formulation of C3-transferase—BA-210—aiming

for Rho-inactivation was applied locally immediately after injury, whereas in the clinical trial a treatment delay between 7.83 and 146.1 hours was reported [108]. In case of specific antibodies aiming to eliminate axon growth inhibitory effects of the myelin-associated protein Nogo, the differential treatment delay in preclinical versus clinical studies was even more pronounced. Preclinical studies investigated structural and functional effects of respective antibodies only resulting from drug administration immediately post SCI [109]. In the clinical trial, antibodies were then applied in a time frame up to 28 days post injury [110]. Looking at logistically challenging cell-based regenerative studies the maintainance of a proper treatment interval is even more difficult. An ongoing clinical trial investigates allogenic fetal derived neural stem cells in the subacute phase of SCI between 3 months and 1 year after injury [111]. In contrast, respective preclinical studies administered the cells 9 days after contusion SCI in mice [112]. Applying autologous cell transplantation based therapies represents the most difficult strategy in terms of timely therapeutic intervention. Cells need to be harvested from patients' tissue samples, isolated and propagated in culture to be transplanted back into the patient. Most preclinical studies aiming at autologous transplantation mimic this rather complex cell preparation procedure by substituting syngenic cells. A study in spinal cord injured rats has provided proof of principle that within an 8-week time frame autologous neural progenitor cells can be isolated and propagated in sufficient quantities from small subventricular zone biopsies and transplanted into the spinal cord lesion site eliciting substantial structural repair [113]. Whether a comparable time frame is feasible for autologous transplants in the clinical setting remains to be demonstrated.

Therapy administration route

In experimental and clinical stroke neuroprotective treatment administration routes are rather homogenous. The majority of clinical trials follow the preclinical administration strategy—usually systemic i.v., i.p. or s.c. treatment. For example, the neuroprotective drugs Tirilazad and NXY-059 were both investigated primarily after i.v. infusion in rats [107, 114]. Correspondingly, in respective clinical trials the study medication was also administered i.v. [16, 115].

In contrast, in SCI, relevant differences do exist with respect to the therapy administration route. Preclinical studies investigating the regenerative capacity of anti-Nogo antibodies applied the drug continuously either intrathecally remote from the lesion site (respective antibody secretion by hybridoma cells implanted intracerebral [116]) or at the lesion site [18, 117]. In contrast, in the respective clinical trial anti-Nogo antibodies were applied either continuously intrathecally via a lumbar catheter or as repetitive bolus injection also via lumbar intrathecal injection. Indeed, the pharmacokinetics in terms of drug distribution after intrathecal or intracerebral and local spinal versus lumbar infusion (in human subjects) have yet to be determined. Lumbar intrathecal bolus injections have not been evaluated in small animal studies investigating anti-Nogo administration after SCI (Table 11.2). Regarding cell-based local transplantation strategies, cells are frequently transplanted into the area of the spinal cord lesion without exact non-invasive identification (magnetic resonance imaging

(MRI), ultrasound) of the lesion boundaries in preclinical studies (Table 11.2). Clinical trials aiming at translation of respective cell-based therapies, increasingly employ ultrasound guided injection of cell grafts into the rostral and caudal boundaries of the lesion cyst [118–120].

Factors related to outcome parameters

Outcome in CNS disease is determined by both, true recovery (axonal regrowth and sprouting) as well as compensation mechanisms (e.g. compensatory movements in order to improve skilled reaching). Standard behavioural tests in the clinical as well as in the preclinical setting are usually not suited to discriminate between true recovery and compensation (Table 11.3). Depending on the mode of action of new treatment interventions, correct outcome parameters need to be chosen.

Ideally, relevant animal models should not only reflect neuronanatomical and physiological changes (level of somatic functions), but in addition further aspects such as ADL in order to serve as useful predictors of therapeutic efficacy in CNS disease. Outcome parameters for small animals, which correlate with ADL, have yet to be developed. Meaningful outcome parameters in animal models need to reflect the expected mode of action by the treatment under investigation as close as possible.

For example, treatments with potential effects on upper extremity sensorimotor function including fine motor control in humans are not properly reflected by BBB locomotor assessment. Assessment of fine motor skills in rodents is quite challenging, considering the fact that corticospinal projections in lysencephalic rodents are different from those in gyrencephalic humans [40, 121]. Therefore, species-specific neuroanatomical/-physiological differences represent a major obstacle in the translation of potential treatments.

Assessment of structural changes

In ischaemic stroke, the final infarct size or reduction of final infarct size, which can be analyzed postmortem by histology or non-invasively in the living animal by MRI, represent the most frequently applied structural outcome measures in preclincal models, targeting the effects of neuroprotective therapies (Table 11.3). The infarct size can easily be quantified by the given methods in any species and it correlates moderately to strong with short- and long-term clinical outcome [122–126]. The gold standard for this rather crude morphological analysis in animal models is still postmortem histopathology [127] (Table 11.3). But recently, MR stroke imaging has become a robust tool for the intravital measurement of infarct size, even in small animals [128, 129]. Hence, serial correlations with behavioural outcome measures

Table 11.3 Outcome measures in animal models and humans

	Stroke		SCI	
	Small animal	**Human**	**Small animal**	**Human**
Neurological impairment	◆ None	◆ Standardized neurological examination (NIHSS)	◆ None	◆ Standardized neurological examination (ISNCSCI)
Functional impairment				
Locomotion	◆ Rotarod ◆ Foot-fault test ◆ Step test	◆ Repetitive task training ◆ Several walking tests	◆ BBB ◆ Footprint analysis ◆ Beam walking ◆ Kinematics	◆ Walking Index for Spinal Cord Injury (WISCI) ◆ Spinal Cord Independence Measure (SCIM)*
Hand/Arm Function	◆ Cylinder rearing test ◆ Montoya Staircase test	◆ Repetitive task training	◆ Forelimb reaching	◆ Graded Redefined Assessment of Strength, Sensibility and Prehension (GRASPP)
Independence	◆ Morris Watermaze test (examining spatial memory/learning)	◆ Barthel Index ◆ mRankin	◆ None	◆ SCIM**
Patient-reported outcome				
Quality of Life	◆ None	◆ Several assessments available	◆ None	◆ Several assessments available
Neurophysiology	◆ None	◆ None	◆ Somatosensory evoked potential (SSEP) ◆ Transcranial motor evoked potential (TcMEP)	◆ Somatosensory evoked potential (SSEP) ◆ Transcranial motor evoked potential (TcMEP)
Imaging	◆ Histology ◆ Small animal MRI	◆ MRI	◆ Histology	◆ MRI

* Domain 'Mobility'.
** Domain 'Self-Care' and 'Respiration and Sphincter Management'.

are possible in rodents and non-human primates [130, 131]. The advantage of infarct size assessment is that non-invasive MRI can easily be translated from the animal study to the clinical trial. However, can it really be expected that a given neuroprotective treatment saves brain tissue as whole or would such a treatment rather protect defined neuronal populations, which are most likely not visible by just measuring the infarct size? Or in other words, is MRI infarct size assessment just not sensitive enough to detect neuroprotective therapy related changes?

Mere infarct size measurement does not specify the underlying mechanisms with respect to true neurological recovery versus behavioural compensation. In the animal setting for example, treatment with an enriched environment leads to a better functional outcome despite the induction of approximately 8 % larger cerebral infarcts [132]. Underlying mechanisms of these at first sight inconsistent effects remain obscure.

In SCI structural outcome assessment following a therapy aiming for neuroregeneration is more diverse. Several histopathological methods exist to analyse axonal regrowth and sprouting after experimental SCI. Axons can be visualized and quantified via immunohistochemistry, anterograde and retrograde tracing of motor, sensory and autonomic pathways [133–136]. However, as already mentioned, axon regrowth does not necessarily mean re-establishment of neuronal connections, which have been interrupted. Few studies actually show reinnervation of previous neuronal targets [55, 56]. Furthermore, myelination and the status of oligodendroglial survival/replacement can be assessed ultrastructurally [137–139]. Of course, such a structural post mortem assessement is not applicable to clinical trials. Here, non-invasive visualization of the human spinal cord is exclusively based on MRI, which can also be employed for *in vivo* small animal imaging [140, 141]. MRI technology has advanced tremendously within the last decade and it is in principle capable of detecting changes related to axon integrity (diffusion tensor imaging) and myelination status (magnetization transfer ratio). However, these sequences cannot yet be applied to the spinal cord, where surrounding bone structures, metal artefacts resulting from spine stabilization and respiration associated motion artefacts impede specific structural analysis. As in ischaemic stroke, MRI can visualize the lesion size in both experimental and human SCI. In general, the correlation between the lesion size detected with MRI and functional outcome is rather poor [142, 143]. But, as already mentioned, metal artefacts due to spine stabilization in most instances heavily restrict the analysis of the lesion area.

Assessment of functional changes

In clinical reality, it is not a structural surrogate readout parameter that is essential for the patients. Instead, it is a clinically meaningful functional improvement. Several preconditions are essential for an accurate measurement of functional outcome in the clinical as well as in the preclinical setting. (1) Test validity: does the test measure what it is alleged to measure? (2) Test reliability: does the test produce similar results under consistent conditions? (3) statistical methodology: selection of a correct statistical model.

For the clinical setting of acute ischaemic stroke, validated test instruments exist to measure functional outcome on the body level (NIHSS) as well as on the activity level (modified Rankin Scale [mRS], Barthel Index) (Table 11.3). As a surrogate marker for functional outcome in the clinical setting, stroke volume is a reliable and major predictor for both the body function level and activity level [144–146]. For estimation of the functional outcome, the time course of spontaneous recovery, which takes a period of 3 to 4 months in humans, needs to be taken in to account [147, 148]. For details on spontaneous recovery, its mechanisms and restorative therapies see: [149, 150]. In addition, compensatory movements in the animal model (rat) improve functional activity scores for forelimb function without true neurological improvement [151, 152]. Thus, understanding recovery and compensatory mechanisms might be relevant for future designs of treatment interventions [153].

Outcome scores/analyses should be applied according to the anticipated mode of action of the new treatment. While for an 'all or nothing' treatment like thrombolysis a dichotomized outcome scale (favorable versus unfavorable according to the mRS) might be appropriate, this approach appears to be rather inappropriate for a supposed neuroprotective agent [154, 155]. In other cases again, it might be wise to choose an activity-level based or a body-level based outcome test, respectively.

In the clinical setting robust baseline scores are available for SCI. These are reliable predictors for final outcome [156–159]. However, in the experimental setting similar behavioural scores, indicating the completeness of the lesion at baseline are missing (Table 11.3). Such scores would not only be helpful in the experimental setting to improve baseline risk stratification, but might also be beneficial with respect to clinical translation (functional versus structural completeness).

The most important clinical assessments in SCI are the 'International Standards for Neurological Classification in Spinal Cord Injury (ISNCSCI)' of the 'American Spinal Injury Association (ASIA)' and the 'Walking Index for Spinal Cord Injury (WISCI)', as well as the 'Spinal Cord Independence Measure (SCIM)', respectively [160–162] (Table 11.3).

For the most commonly used animal experiments (rodent models) mainly open-field behavioural assessments like BBB and BMS scores are applied [163, 164]. These scores were developed and validated for the analysis of hindlimb locomotor function in rats and mice. Main problems of the tests are the lacking rater-objectivity and the nonlinear/discrete distribution of the test results. Moreover, there is no clear consensus on how much difference in the BBB score from baseline is a meaningful change with respect to clinical translation. Thus, there is a need for more objective functional tests with transferability or rather comparability to the clinical setting [165–167]. Even more differentiated tests with improved inter-rater reliability, more detailed covering of changes in functional performance and more objective evaluation of different locomotion parameters, such as the 'Ladder Beam Walking Task' in mice [168] or the 'CatWalk-Assisted Gait Analysis' in rats [169], do eventually represent poor surrogates for the actual used clinical outcome parameters. Recently, sophisticated treadmill approaches were added to the repertoire of functional outcome/gait analysis assessments in rodents [170, 171]. Notwithstanding the fact that the latter assessments concern quadrupeds, one might draw a parallel to clinically used gait analysis concepts [172, 173]. Even though, a systematic transitional evaluation of these tests as surrogate markers has not yet taken place.

Since the majority of clinical spinal cord injuries are located at cervical level with consecutive upper extremity dysfunction, corresponding functional assessment of forelimb function in respective animal models represents a challenging task. Effects on fine motor skills are modest and hard to assess in rodents and therefore of limited sensitivity regarding the translation into the clinical setting [142, 174]. Generally used assessments in animals are gross sensorimotor skill tests like the 'forelimb reaching task', meanwhile refined by differentiated video motion analysis to identify compensatory movements of spinal cord injured rat [175–179]. Skilled forelimb reaching is also reflected by the 'Montoya Staircase Test' and the 'Cylinder Rearing Test', which have been used in several models of CNS diseases including SCI [72, 180, 181]. Whether non-human primate models suffice to close the translational gap remains to be evaluated [22].

In the clinical context, the Graded Redefined Assessment of Strength Sensibility and Prehension (GRASSP) has been established to assess upper limb function in tetraplegic patients in a standardized fashion [182, 183].

Reliable assessment tools for autonomic dysfunction (bladder, bowel, cardiovascular and sexual function), which substantially affects quality of life in SCI subjects, receive increasing attention both in the preclinical and clinical setting in recent years [184, 185]. However, the predictive value of such assessments still needs to be investigated.

Neurophysiological measurements, in particular somatosensory-evoked potentials (SSEP) and motor-evoked potentials (MEP) allow objective assessment of long distance neural connectivity in animals as well as in patients [186, 187] (Table 11.3). Even so, the translatability of preclinical neurophysiological findings into the clinical setting has not been demonstrated yet.

Summary and conclusion

With the use of preclinical models, substantial knowledge about fundamental CNS disease mechanisms (degeneration, regeneration, inflammation) and potential modes of action of treatments has been gathered for spinal cord injury and ischaemic stroke over the past decades. Nevertheless, the output in terms of successful clinical translation of promising preclinical research results is poor [4, 11,188–193]. And this is despite joined efforts in both diseases to define the most important criteria, which have to be considered in order to substantially increase the likelihood that a given preclinical therapy will successfully translate into a clinically approved treatment. Already 10 years ago, first recommendations based on meta-analysis of existing preclinical studies—so called Stroke Treatment Academic Industry Roundtable (STAIR)—were presented in ischaemic stroke. [14, 19]. In SCI, guidelines for the conduct of clinical trials have also been established [159, 186, 194, 195]. In terms of preclinical studies, a survey in the scientific community investigating the most relevant factors of preclinical studies and recommendations for the optimal conduct of preclinical experiments has recently been published [196].

In the following, we summarize pitfalls of stroke and SCI disease models, which can be considered as either disease-specific or systematic.

Disease-specific pitfalls in stroke

1. Regarding the investigation of neuroprotective therapies in ischaemic stroke, particular concerns are focusing on the choice of structural outcome parameters. Most preclinical studies report successful neuroprotection as soon as a reduction of the infarct volume (determined by histology or MRI) is detected. However, this approach is rather crude, since neuroprotective interventions primarily aim to protect neurons and not the entire neuropil. Moreover, in due consideration of neuroanatomic aspects, it cannot be translated one to one into a corresponding structural analysis in human subjects. In SCI, in recent years more and more efforts have been made to detect mechanisms of given neuroregenerative approaches such as reinnervation, which are likely to account for functional recovery [55, 56].

2. Compared to SCI, the discrepancy in terms of average animal age and average age of patients is much more apparent in stroke.

3. The ischaemic territory (middle cerebral territory) is rather uniform throughout the majority of preclinical studies. In SCI, a wider variety of lesion levels (cervical or thoracic) and severity (incomplete versus complete) are available in the experimental setting.

Disease-specific pitfalls in SCI

1. Potential pitfalls particularly relevant for SCI concern the animal size in the context of axon regeneration. Axons have to regrow over much longer distances in humans to promote reinnervation compared to small animals. In neuroprotective therapies in stroke the issue of animal size is less relevant.

2. Another issue in SCI relates to the timing of the therapeutic intervention. Neuroprotective therapies in stroke models are applied immediately after induction of the ischaemia. Likewise in humans, the goal is to initiate the respective therapy within an early time window after the ischaemia. In neuroregenerative approaches for SCI, timing is still less stringent in both animal models and clinical trials. In most regenerative therapy approaches, the application of the drug, cell or biomaterial frequently needs time (surgery required, cells need to be delivered/prepared). Furthermore, it is not precisely known, which time point of intervention in animal studies translates into corresponding time points in humans.

3. The route of therapy administration (soluble factors and cell transplantation) in preclinical SCI studies is frequently not properly translated into respective clinical trials. In ischaemic stroke, both preclinical and clinical therapies are consistently applied systemically (mostly i.v.)

Unspecific pitfalls

1. In SCI, functional outcome assessments almost completely neglect the field of autonomic dysfunction (neurogenic bowel and bladder or sexual dysfunction), since respective functional outcome tools are rather complex to implement or have not yet been developed. In ischaemic stroke, assessments investigating higher cognitive function—frequently contributing substantially to disability—are missing.

2. In terms of the predictive value, both stroke and SCI employ highly controlled, homogenous, mostly inbred-strain based animal populations, which do not reflect the clinical situation.

3. Comorbidities are not properly addressed in both animal models. In stroke, diabetes and hypertension that could influence the outcome of stroke significantly, do not play a role in respective animal models. In SCI, additional polytrauma associated lesions such as fractures, organ damage (e.g. lung contusion) and secondary complications in the acute situation (e.g. pressure sores, pneumonia) are not considered in animal models. Undoubtedly, these aspects can hardly be introduced into preclinical models.

4. Both SCI and stroke models employ uniform lesion mechanisms, which do not adequately reflect the aetiology of these diseases in humans. In stroke, primary large and small vessel occlusions as well as arterial embolisms cause ischaemic events. However, only vessel occlusion models are used as reliable stroke model. Traumatic SCI, both in humans and in the animal model, is characterized by mostly blunt forces. In humans, there is a mixture of longer lasting compression (bone fragments are dislocated into the spinal canal) and short lasting contusion (e.g. in elderly patients with spinal stenosis). In the majority of the animal models, reflecting the clinical situation as close as possible, the spinal cord is contused without longer-lasting cord compression.

5. Gender preferences, which can be observed in both diseases (male in stroke, female in SCI), can easily be adjusted in future preclinical trials. Standard of care, which can positively and negatively influence the outcome, is mostly neglected or at least not controlled for in stroke and SCI models. Vessel recanalization and all other measures applied in stroke units and rehabilitation centres are in most instances not part of preclinical stroke models. Properly timed decompression, spine stabilization, bladder/bowel management and rehabilitation measures are in most instances not part of preclinical SCI models.

6. Large animal models are desirable for both disease entities. However, to date only few published studies exist in this context. This is understandable considering ethical issues, financial restrictions and large animal numbers that are needed to get statistically relevant results.

Taken together, issues inherent to disease models, as well as higher-level pitfalls independent from the disease model, support the notion that animals fail to closely reflect the respective human disease entities stroke and SCI. Even if these factors were identified, they could not always be addressed in the preclinical setting. Therefore, preclinical models can at best provide proof of principle that a neuroprotective or neuroregenerative therapy will be effective. Specific attention should be paid to the detection of underlying structural mechanisms of recovery and robust and reproducible functional improvement in respective animal models. A provocative conclusion would be to proceed from the culture dish straight to the patient, employing animal models only for safety and pharmacokinetic analysis. However, this is not a realistic approach, which would find acceptance within the basic and clinical science community. As mentioned, there is still significant room for improvement. Current and future preclinical neuroprotective and neuroregenerative therapy cnvestigations

need to demonstrate whether published requirements [14, 19, 52, 109, 197–199] will help to substantially enhance the predicitive value of preclinical experiments.

References

1. World Health Organization. International Classification of Functioning, Disability and Health (ICF). WHO, Geneva, 2001.
2. Appelros P, Nydevik I, Viitanen M. Poor outcome after first-ever stroke: predictors for death, dependency, and recurrent stroke within the first year. Stroke. 2003;**34**(1):122–126.
3. Steeves JD, Kramer JK, Fawcett JW, Cragg J, Lammertse DP, Blight AR, et al. Extent of spontaneous motor recovery after traumatic cervical sensorimotor complete spinal cord injury. Spinal Cord. 2011;**49**(2):257–265.
4. Moskowitz MA, Lo EH, Iadecola C. The science of stroke: mechanisms in search of treatments. Neuron. 2010;**67**(2):181–198.
5. David S, Lopez-Vales R, Wee Yong V. Harmful and beneficial effects of inflammation after spinal cord injury: potential therapeutic implications. Handbook of Clinical Neurology. 2012;**109**:485–502. Epub 2012/10/27.
6. Sutherland BA, Minnerup J, Balami JS, Arba F, Buchan AM, Kleinschnitz C. Neuroprotection for ischaemic stroke: translation from the bench to the bedside. Int J Stroke. 2012;**7**(5):407–418. Epub 2012/03/08.
7. Franz S, Weidner N, Blesch A. Gene therapy approaches to enhancing plasticity and regeneration after spinal cord injury. Exp Neurol. 2012;**235**(1):62–69. Epub 2011/02/02.
8. Blesch A, Fischer I, Tuszynski MH. Gene therapy, neurotrophic factors and spinal cord regeneration. Handbook of Clinical Neurology. 2012;**109**:563–574. Epub 2012/10/27.
9. Richardson PM, McGuinness UM, Aguayo AJ. Axons from CNS neurons regenerate into PNS grafts. Nature. 1980;**284**(5753):264–265. Epub 1980/03/20.
10. Hug A, Weidner N. From bench to beside to cure spinal cord injury: lost in translation? Int Rev Neurobiol. 2012;**106**:173–196.
11. Filli L, Schwab ME. The rocky road to translation in spinal cord repair. Ann Neurol. 2012;**72**(4):491–501.
12. Kwon BK, Okon E, Hillyer J, et al. A systematic review of non-invasive pharmacologic neuroprotective treatments for acute spinal cord injury. J Neurotrauma. 2011;**28**(8):1545–1588. Epub 2010/02/12.
13. Rosenzweig ES, McDonald JW. Rodent models for treatment of spinal cord injury: research trends and progress toward useful repair. Curr Opin Neurol. 2004;**17**(2):121–131. Epub 2004/03/17.
14. Saver JL, Albers GW, Dunn B, Johnston KC, Fisher M, Consortium SV. Stroke Therapy Academic Industry Roundtable (STAIR) recommendations for extended window acute stroke therapy trials. Stroke. 2009;**40**(7):2594–2600.
15. Marshall JW, Cummings RM, Bowes LJ, Ridley RM, Green AR. Functional and histological evidence for the protective effect of NXY-059 in a primate model of stroke when given 4 hours after occlusion. Stroke. 2003;**34**(9):2228–2233. Epub 2003/08/16.
16. Lees KR, Zivin JA, Ashwood T, et al. NXY-059 for acute ischemic stroke. N Engl J Med. 2006;**354**(6):588–600. Epub 2006/02/10.
17. Shuaib A, Lees KR, Lyden P, et al. NXY-059 for the treatment of acute ischemic stroke. N Engl J Med. 2007;**357**(6):562–571. Epub 2007/08/10.
18. Freund P, Schmidlin E, Wannier T, et al. Nogo-A-specific antibody treatment enhances sprouting and functional recovery after cervical lesion in adult primates. Nat Med. 2006;**12**(7):790–792. Epub 2006/07/05.
19. Fisher M. Recommendations for standards regarding preclinical neuroprotective and restorative drug development. Stroke. 1999;**30**(12):2752–2758.
20. Fisher M, Feuerstein G, Howells DW, et al. Update of the stroke therapy academic industry roundtable preclinical recommendations. Stroke. 2009;**40**(6):2244–2250.

21. Blesch A, Tuszynski MH. Spinal cord injury: plasticity, regeneration and the challenge of translational drug development. Trends Neurosci. 2009;32(1):41–47. Epub 2008/11/04.

22. Courtine G, Bunge MB, Fawcett JW, et al. Can experiments in nonhuman primates expedite the translation of treatments for spinal cord injury in humans? Nat Med. 2007;13(5):561–566. Epub 2007/05/05.

23. Ones K, Yalcinkaya EY, Toklu BC, Caglar N. Effects of age, gender, and cognitive, functional and motor status on functional outcomes of stroke rehabilitation. NeuroRehabilitation. 2009;25(4):241–249. Epub 2009/12/29.

24. Liu F, McCullough LD. Interactions between age, sex, and hormones in experimental ischemic stroke. Neurochem Int. 2012;61(8):1255–1265. Epub 2012/10/17.

25. Jakob W, Wirz M, van Hedel HJ, Dietz V. Difficulty of elderly SCI subjects to translate motor recovery—'body function'—into daily living activities. J Neurotrauma. 2009;26(11):2037–2044. Epub 2009/07/17.

26. van den Berg ME, Castellote JM, Mahillo-Fernandez I, de Pedro-Cuesta J. Incidence of spinal cord injury worldwide: a systematic review. Neuroepidemiology. 2010;34(3):184–192; discussion 92.

27. Andreollo NA, Santos EF, Araujo MR, Lopes LR. Rat's age versus human's age: what is the relationship? Arquivos brasileiros de cirurgia digestiva: ABCD = Brazilian Archives of Digestive Surgery. 2012;25(1):49–51. Epub 2012/05/10.

28. Roger VL, Go AS, Lloyd-Jones DM, et al. Heart disease and stroke statistics—2011 update: a report from the American Heart Association. Circulation. 2011;123(4):e18-e209. Epub 2010/12/17.

29. Liu F, McCullough LD. Middle cerebral artery occlusion model in rodents: methods and potential pitfalls. J Biomed Biotechnol. 2011;2011:464701.

30. Silva NA, Sousa RA, Fraga JS, et al. Benefits of spine stabilization with biodegradable scaffolds in spinal cord injured rats. Tissue Eng C Methods. 2013;19(2):101–108. Epub 2012/07/12.

31. Bardutzky J, Shen Q, Henninger N, Bouley J, Duong TQ, Fisher M. Differences in ischemic lesion evolution in different rat strains using diffusion and perfusion imaging. Stroke. 2005;36(9):2000–2005.

32. Cheng MH, Lin LL, Liu JY, Liu AJ. The outcomes of stroke induced by middle cerebral artery occlusion in different strains of mice. CNS Neurosci Therapeutics. 2012;18(9):794–795.

33. Howells DW, Porritt MJ, Rewell SSJ, et al. Different strokes for different folks: the rich diversity of animal models of focal cerebral ischemia. J Cerebr Blood Met. 2010;30(8):1412–1431.

34. Ma M, Basso DM, Walters P, Stokes BT, Jakeman LB. Behavioral and histological outcomes following graded spinal cord contusion injury in the C57Bl/6 mouse. Exp Neurol. 2001;169(2):239–254. Epub 2001/05/19.

35. Inman DM, Steward O. Physical size does not determine the unique histopathological response seen in the injured mouse spinal cord. J Neurotrauma. 2003;20(1):33–42. Epub 2003/03/05.

36. Liu K, Lu Y, Lee JK, Samara R, et al. PTEN deletion enhances the regenerative ability of adult corticospinal neurons. Nature Neurosci. 2010;13(9):1075–1081. Epub 2010/08/10.

37. Mills CD, Hains BC, Johnson KM, Hulsebosch CE. Strain and model differences in behavioral outcomes after spinal cord injury in rat. J Neurotrauma. 2001;18(8):743–756.

38. Joosten EA, Gribnau AA, Dederen PJ. An anterograde tracer study of the developing corticospinal tract in the rat: three components. Brain Res. 1987;433(1):121–130.

39. Lawrence DG, Kuypers HG. The functional organization of the motor system in the monkey. II. The effects of lesions of the descending brain-stem pathways. Brain. 1968;91(1):15–36.

40. Lemon RN, Griffiths J. Comparing the function of the corticospinal system in different species: organizational differences for motor specialization? Muscle Nerve. 2005;32(3):261–279. Epub 2005/04/05.

41. Oudega M, Perez MA. Corticospinal reorganization after spinal cord injury. The J Physiol. 2012;590(Pt 16):3647–3663.

42. Sasaki S, Isa T, Pettersson LG, et al. Dexterous finger movements in primate without monosynaptic corticomotoneuronal excitation. J Neurophysiol. 2004;92(5):3142–3147.

43. Weidner N, Ner A, Salimi N, Tuszynski MH. Spontaneous corticospinal axonal plasticity and functional recovery after adult central nervous system injury. Proc Natl Acad Sci U S A. 2001;98(6):3513–3518. Epub 2001/03/15.

44. Bacigaluppi M, Comi G, Hermann DM. Animal models of ischemic stroke. Part two: modeling cerebral ischemia. Open Neurol J. 2010;4:34–38.

45. Liu F, Luo ZJ, You SW, et al. Significance of fixation of the vertebral column for spinal cord injury experiments. Spine. 2003;28(15):1666–1671. Epub 2003/08/05.

46. Nudo RJ, Larson D, Plautz EJ, Friel KM, Barbay S, Frost SB. A squirrel monkey model of poststroke motor recovery. ILAR journal/National Research Council, Institute of Laboratory Animal Resources. 2003;44(2):161–174.

47. Mergenthaler P, Meisel A. Do stroke models model stroke? Dis Model Mech. 2012;5(6):718–725.

48. Endres M, Engelhardt B, Koistinaho J, et al. Improving outcome after stroke: overcoming the translational roadblock. Cerebrovasc Dis. 2008;25(3):268–278.

49. Chen Y, Ito A, Takai K, Saito N. Blocking pterygopalatine arterial blood flow decreases infarct volume variability in a mouse model of intraluminal suture middle cerebral artery occlusion. J Neurosci Methods. 2008;174(1):18–24.

50. Sekhon LH, Fehlings MG. Epidemiology, demographics, and pathophysiology of acute spinal cord injury. Spine. 2001;26(24 Suppl):S2–12. Epub 2002/01/24.

51. Rowland JW, Hawryluk GW, Kwon B, Fehlings MG. Current status of acute spinal cord injury pathophysiology and emerging therapies: promise on the horizon. Neurosurg Focus. 2008;25(5):E2. Epub 2008/11/05.

52. Kwon BK, Okon EB, Tsai E, et al. A grading system to evaluate objectively the strength of pre-clinical data of acute neuroprotective therapies for clinical translation in spinal cord injury. J Neurotrauma. 2011;28(8):1525–1543. Epub 2010/05/29.

53. Metz GAS, Curt A, van de Meent H, Klusman I, Schwab ME, Dietz V. Validation of the weight-drop contusion model in rats: A comparative study of human spinal cord injury. J Neurotrauma. 2000;17(1):1–17.

54. Raineteau O, Schwab ME. Plasticity of motor systems after incomplete spinal cord injury. Nat Rev Neurosci. 2001;2(4):263–273.

55. Alto LT, Havton LA, Conner JM, Hollis ER, 2nd, Blesch A, Tuszynski MH. Chemotropic guidance facilitates axonal regeneration and synapse formation after spinal cord injury. Nat Neurosci. 2009;12(9):1106–1113. Epub 2009/08/04.

56. Bonner JF, Connors TM, Silverman WF, Kowalski DP, Lemay MA, Fischer I. Grafted neural progenitors integrate and restore synaptic connectivity across the injured spinal cord. J Neurosci. 2011;31(12):4675–4686. Epub 2011/03/25.

57. Metz GA, Curt A, van de Meent H, Klusman I, Schwab ME, Dietz V. Validation of the weight-drop contusion model in rats: a comparative study of human spinal cord injury. J Neurotrauma. 2000;17(1):1–17. Epub 2000/02/16.

58. Young W. Spinal cord contusion models. Progr Brain Res. 2002;137:231–255.

59. Scheff SW, Rabchevsky AG, Fugaccia I, Main JA, Lumpp JE, Jr. Experimental modeling of spinal cord injury: characterization of a force-defined injury device. J Neurotrauma. 2003;20(2):179–193.

60. Fehlings MG, Tator CH. The relationships among the severity of spinal cord injury, residual neurological function, axon counts, and counts of retrogradely labeled neurons after experimental spinal cord injury. Exp Neurol. 1995;132(2):220–228.

61. Rivlin AS, Tator CH. Effect of duration of acute spinal cord compression in a new acute cord injury model in the rat. Surg Neurol. 1978;**10**(1):38–43.

62. Holtz A, Nystrom B, Gerdin B. Spinal cord blood flow measured by 14C-iodoantipyrine autoradiography during and after graded spinal cord compression in rats. Surg Neurol. 1989;**31**(5):350–360.

63. Martin D, Schoenen J, Delree P, et al. Experimental acute traumatic injury of the adult rat spinal cord by a subdural inflatable balloon: methodology, behavioral analysis, and histopathology. J Neurosci Res. 1992;**32**(4):539–550.

64. Sparrey CJ, Choo AM, Liu J, Tetzlaff W, Oxland TR. The distribution of tissue damage in the spinal cord is influenced by the contusion velocity. Spine. 2008;**33**(22):E812–E9.

65. Chamorro A, Meisel A, Planas AM, Urra X, van de Beek D, Veltkamp R. The immunology of acute stroke. Nat Rev Neurol. 2012;**8**(7):401–410.

66. Seok J, Warren HS, Cuenca AG, et al. Genomic responses in mouse models poorly mimic human inflammatory diseases. Proc Natl Acad Sci U S A. 2013;**110**(9):3507–3512.

67. Carmichael ST. Rodent models of focal stroke: size, mechanism, and purpose. NeuroRx. 2005;**2**(3):396–409.

68. Hacke W, Schwab S, Horn M, Spranger M, DeGeorgia M, von-Kummer R. 'Malignant' middle cerebral artery territory infarction—Clinical course and prognostic signs. Arch Neurol-Chicago. 1996;**53**(4):309–315.

69. Vahedi K, Hofmeijer J, Juettler E, et al. Early decompressive surgery in malignant infarction of the middle cerebral artery: a pooled analysis of three randomised controlled trials. Lancet Neurol. 2007;**6**(3):215–222.

70. McKinley W, Santos K, Meade M, Brooke K. Incidence and outcomes of spinal cord injury clinical syndromes. J Spinal Cord Med. 2007;**30**(3):215–224.

71. Anderson KD, Sharp KG, Steward O. Bilateral cervical contusion spinal cord injury in rats. Exp Neurol. 2009;**220**(1):9–22. Epub 2009/06/30.

72. Streijger F, Beernink TM, Lee JH, et al. Characterization of a cervical spinal cord hemicontusion injury in mice using the infinite horizon impactor. J Neurotrauma. 2013;**30**(10):869–883. Epub 2013/01/31.

73. Jauch EC, Saver JL, Adams HP, Jr., et al. Guidelines for the early management of patients with acute ischemic stroke: a guideline for healthcare professionals from the American Heart Association/ American Stroke Association. Stroke. 2013;**44**(3):870–947.

74. Hacke W, Kaste M, Bluhmki E, et al. Thrombolysis with alteplase 3 to 4.5 hours after acute ischemic stroke. N Engl J Med. 2008;**359**(13):1317–1329.

75. Marler JR, Brott T, Broderick J, et al. Tissue-plasminogen activator for acute ischemic stroke. N Engl J Med. 1995;**333**(24):1581–1587.

76. Hacke W, Furlan AJ, Al-Rawi Y, et al. Intravenous desmoteplase in patients with acute ischaemic stroke selected by MRI perfusion-diffusion weighted imaging or perfusion CT (DIAS-2): a prospective, randomised, double-blind, placebo-controlled study. Lancet Neurol. 2009;**8**(2):141–150.

77. Medcalf RL, Davis SM. Plasminogen activation and thrombolysis for ischemic stroke. Int J Stroke. 2012;**7**(5):419–425.

78. Saver JL. Improving reperfusion therapy for acute ischaemic stroke. J Thromb Haemost. 2011;**9**:333–343.

79. Langhorne P, Bernhardt J, Kwakkel G. Stroke rehabilitation. Lancet. 2011;**377**(9778):1693–1702.

80. Stroke Unit Trialists C. Organised inpatient (stroke unit) care for stroke. Cochrane Database Syst Rev. 2007(4):CD000197.

81. Dobkin BH. Strategies for stroke rehabilitation. Lancet Neurol. 2004;**3**(9):528–536.

82. Maldonado MA, Allred RP, Felthauser EL, Jones TA. Motor skill training, but not voluntary exercise, improves skilled reaching after unilateral ischemic lesions of the sensorimotor cortex in rats. Neurorehabil Neural Repair. 2008;**22**(3):250–261.

83. Will B, Galani R, Kelche C, Rosenzweig MR. Recovery from brain injury in animals: relative efficacy of environmental enrichment, physical exercise or formal training (1990–2002). Progr Neurobiol. 2004;**72**(3):167–182.

84. Biernaskie J, Corbett D. Enriched rehabilitative training promotes improved forelimb motor function and enhanced dendritic growth after focal ischemic injury. J Neurosci. 2001;**21**(14):5272–5280.

85. Taub E, Uswatte G, King DK, Morris D, Crago JE, Chatterjee A. A placebo-controlled trial of constraint-induced movement therapy for upper extremity after stroke. Stroke. 2006;**37**(4):1045–1049.

86. Sterr A, Elbert T, Berthold I, Kolbel S, Rockstroh B, Taub E. Longer versus shorter daily constraint-induced movement therapy of chronic hemiparesis: An exploratory study. Arch Phys Med ad Rehabil. 2002;**83**(10):1374–1377.

87. Wolf SL, Winstein CJ, Miller JP, et al. Effect of constraint-induced movement therapy on upper extremity function 3 to 9 months after stroke—The EXCITE randomized clinical trial. JAMA. 2006;**296**(17):2095–2104.

88. Humm JL, Kozlowski DA, James DC, Gotts JE, Schallert T. Use-dependent exacerbation of brain damage occurs during an early post-lesion vulnerable period. Brain research. 1998;**783**(2):286–292.

89. DeBow SB, McKenna JE, Kolb B, Colbourne F. Immediate constraint-induced movement therapy causes local hyperthermia that exacerbates cerebral cortical injury in rats. Can J Physiol Pharm. 2004;**82**(4):231–237.

90. Kozlowski DA, James DC, Schallert T. Use-dependent exaggeration of neuronal injury after unilateral sensorimotor cortex lesions. J Neurosci. 1996;**16**(15):4776–4786.

91. Biernaskie J, Chernenko G, Corbett D. Efficacy of rehabilitative experience declines with time after focal ischemic brain injury. J Neurosci. 2004;**24**(5):1245–1254.

92. Livingston-Thomas JM, Tasker RA. Animal models of post-ischemic forced use rehabilitation: methods, considerations, and limitations. Exp Transl Stroke Med. 2013;**5**(1):2.

93. Krakauer JW, Carmichael ST, Corbett D, Wittenberg GF. Getting neurorehabilitation right: what can be learned from animal models? Neurorehabil Neural Repair. 2012;**26**(8):923–931.

94. Bagnall AM, Jones L, Duffy S, Riemsma RP. Spinal fixation surgery for acute traumatic spinal cord injury. Cochrane Database Syste Rev. 2008(1):CD004725. Epub 2008/02/07.

95. Wilson JR, Singh A, Craven C, Verrier MC, Drew B, Ahn H, et al. Early versus late surgery for traumatic spinal cord injury: the results of a prospective Canadian cohort study. Spinal Cord. 2012;**50**(11):840–843.

96. McDonald JW, Sadowsky C. Spinal-cord injury. Lancet. 2002;**359**(9304):417–425. Epub 2002/02/15.

97. van Middendorp JJ, Hosman AJ, Doi SA. The effects of the timing of spinal surgery after traumatic spinal cord injury: a systematic review and meta-analysis. J Neurotrauma. 2013. Epub 2013/07/03.

98. Dimar JR, Glassman SD, Raque GH, Zhang YP, Shields CB. The influence of spinal canal narrowing and timing of decompression on neurologic recovery after spinal cord contusion in a rat model. Spine. 1999;**24**(16):1623–1633.

99. Rooney GE, Vaishya S, Ameenuddin S, et al. Rigid fixation of the spinal column improves scaffold alignment and prevents scoliosis in the transected rat spinal cord. Spine. 2008;**33**(24):E914–919. Epub 2008/11/18.

100. Bracken MB. Steroids for acute spinal cord injury. Cochrane Database Syst Rev. 2012;**1**:CD001046. Epub 2012/01/20.

101. Hurlbert RJ. Methylprednisolone for acute spinal cord injury: an inappropriate standard of care. J Neurosurg. 2000;**93**(1 Suppl):1–7. Epub 2000/07/06.

102. Short DJ, El Masry WS, Jones PW. High dose methylprednisolone in the management of acute spinal cord injury—a systematic review from a clinical perspective. Spinal Cord. 2000;**38**(5):273–286. Epub 2000/05/24.

103. Druschel C, Schaser KD, Schwab JM. Current practice of methylprednisolone administration for acute spinal cord injury in Germany: a national survey. Spine. 2013;**38**(11):E669–677. Epub 2013/03/01.

104. Garcia-Alias G, Fawcett JW. Training and anti-CSPG combination therapy for spinal cord injury. Exp Neurol. 2012;**235**(1):26–32. Epub 2011/09/29.

105. Maier IC, Ichiyama RM, Courtine G, et al. Differential effects of anti-Nogo-A antibody treatment and treadmill training in rats with incomplete spinal cord injury. Brain. 2009;**132**(Pt 6):1426–1440. Epub 2009/04/18.

106. Savitz SI. A critical appraisal of the NXY-059 neuroprotection studies for acute stroke: a need for more rigorous testing of neuroprotective agents in animal models of stroke. Exp Neurol. 2007;**205**(1):20–25. Epub 2007/04/06.

107. Sena E, Wheble P, Sandercock P, Macleod M. Systematic review and meta-analysis of the efficacy of tirilazad in experimental stroke. Stroke. 2007;**38**(2):388–394. Epub 2007/01/06.

108. Fehlings MG, Theodore N, Harrop J, et al. A phase I/IIa clinical trial of a recombinant Rho protein antagonist in acute spinal cord injury. J Neurotrauma. 2011;**28**(5):787–796. Epub 2011/03/09.

109. Reier PJ, Lane MA, Hall ED, Teng YD, Howland DR. Translational spinal cord injury research: preclinical guidelines and challenges. Handbook of Clinical Neurology. 2012;**109**:411–433. Epub 2012/10/27.

110. Abel R, Baron H, Casha S. Therapeutic Anti-Nogo-A Antibodies in acute spinal cord injury: safety and pharmacokinetic data from an ongoing first-in-human trial. ISCOS annual scientific meeting; Washington, DC, USA, 2011.

111. Sandner B, Prang P, Rivera FJ, Aigner L, Blesch A, Weidner N. Neural stem cells for spinal cord repair. Cell Tiss 2012;**349**(1):349–362. Epub 2012/03/06.

112. Cummings BJ, Uchida N, Tamaki SJ, et al. Human neural stem cells differentiate and promote locomotor recovery in spinal cord-injured mice. Proc Natl Acad Sci U S A. 2005;**102**(39):14069–14074. Epub 2005/09/21.

113. Pfeifer K, Vroemen M, Caioni M, Aigner L, Bogdahn U, Weidner N. Autologous adult rodent neural progenitor cell transplantation represents a feasible strategy to promote structural repair in the chronically injured spinal cord. Regen Med. 2006;**1**(2):255–266. Epub 2007/05/01.

114. Bath PMW, Gray LJ, Bath AJG, et al. Effects of NXY-059 in experimental stroke: an individual animal meta-analysis. Br J pharmacol. 2009;**157**(7):1157–1171.

115. Haley EC, Jr. High-dose tirilazad for acute stroke (RANTTAS II). RANTTAS II Investigators. Stroke. 1998;**29**(6):1256–1257. Epub 1998/06/17.

116. Merkler D, Metz GA, Raineteau O, Dietz V, Schwab ME, Fouad K. Locomotor recovery in spinal cord-injured rats treated with an antibody neutralizing the myelin-associated neurite growth inhibitor Nogo-A. J Neurosci. 2001;**21**(10):3665–3673. Epub 2001/05/23.

117. Liebscher T, Schnell L, Schnell D, et al. Nogo-A antibody improves regeneration and locomotion of spinal cord-injured rats. Ann Neurol. 2005;**58**(5):706–719. Epub 2005/09/21.

118. Rapalino O, Lazarov-Spiegler O, Agranov E, et al. Implantation of stimulated homologous macrophages results in partial recovery of paraplegic rats. Nat Med. 1998;**4**(7):814–821. Epub 1998/07/14.

119. Knoller N, Auerbach G, Fulga V, et al. Clinical experience using incubated autologous macrophages as a treatment for complete spinal cord injury: phase I study results. J Neurosurg Spine. 2005;**3**(3):173–181. Epub 2005/10/21.

120. Lammertse DP, Jones LA, Charlifue SB, et al. Autologous incubated macrophage therapy in acute, complete spinal cord injury: results of the phase 2 randomized controlled multicenter trial. Spinal Cord. 2012;**50**(9):661–671. Epub 2012/04/25.

121. Lemon RN. Descending pathways in motor control. Annu Rev Neurosci. 2008;**31**:195–218.

122. Saver JL, Johnston KC, Homer D, et al. Infarct volume as a surrogate or auxiliary outcome measure in ischemic stroke clinical trials. Stroke. 1999;**30**(2):293–298.

123. Zaidi SF, Aghaebrahim A, Urra X, et al. Final infarct volume is a stronger predictor of outcome than recanalization in patients with proximal middle cerebral artery occlusion treated with endovascular therapy. Stroke. 2012;**43**(12):3238–3244.

124. Yoo AJ, Chaudhry ZA, Nogueira RG, et al. Infarct volume is a pivotal biomarker after intra-arterial stroke therapy. Stroke. 2012;**43**(5):1323–1330.

125. Schiemanck SK, Post MWM, Kwakkel G, Witkamp TD, Kappelle LJ, Prevo AJH. Ischemic lesion volume correlates with long-term functional outcome and quality of life of middle cerebral artery stroke survivors. Restor Neurol Neurosci. 2005;**23**(3–4):257–263.

126. Thijs VN, Lansberg MG, Beaulieu C, Marks MP, Moseley ME, Albers GW. Is early ischemic lesion volume on diffusion-weighted imaging an independent predictor of stroke outcome? A multivariable analysis. Stroke. 2000;**31**(11):2597–2602.

127. Bederson JB, Pitts LH, Germano SM, Nishimura MC, Davis RL, Bartkowski HM. Evaluation of 2,3,5-triphenyltetrazolium chloride as a stain for detection and quantification of experimental cerebral infarction in rats. Stroke. 1986;**17**(6):1304–1308.

128. Duong TQ. MRI in experimental stroke. Methods Mol Biol. 2011;**711**:473–485.

129. Weber R, Ramos-Cabrer P, Hoehn M. Present status of magnetic resonance imaging and spectroscopy in animal stroke models. J Cerebr Blood Flow Metab. 2006;**26**(5):591–604.

130. Karki K, Knight RA, Shen LH, et al. Chronic brain tissue remodeling after stroke in rat: a 1-year multiparametric magnetic resonance imaging study. Brain Res. 2010;1360:168–176.

131. Liu Y, D'Arceuil HE, Westmoreland S, et al. Serial diffusion tensor MRI after transient and permanent cerebral ischemia in nonhuman primates. Stroke. 2007;**38**(1):138–145.

132. Janssen H, Bernhardt J, Collier JM, et al. An Enriched environment improves sensorimotor function post-ischemic stroke. Neurorehabil Neural Repair. 2010;**24**(9):802–813.

133. Bareyre FM, Kerschensteiner M, Raineteau O, Mettenleiter TC, Weinmann O, Schwab ME. The injured spinal cord spontaneously forms a new intraspinal circuit in adult rats. Nat Neurosci. 2004;**7**(3):269–277.

134. McKenna JE, Prusky GT, Whishaw IQ. Cervical motoneuron topography reflects the proximodistal organization of muscles and movements of the rat forelimb: a retrograde carbocyanine dye analysis. J Comp Neurol. 2000;**419**(3):286–296. Epub 2000/03/21.

135. Lane MA, White TE, Coutts MA, et al. Cervical prephrenic interneurons in the normal and lesioned spinal cord of the adult rat. J Comp Neurol. 2008;**511**(5):692–709. Epub 2008/10/17.

136. Lane MA, Lee KZ, Fuller DD, Reier PJ. Spinal circuitry and respiratory recovery following spinal cord injury. Respir Physiol Neurobiol. 2009;**169**(2):123–132. Epub 2009/08/25.

137. Biernaskie J, Sparling JS, Liu J, al. Skin-derived precursors generate myelinating Schwann cells that promote remyelination and functional recovery after contusion spinal cord injury. The J Neurosci. 2007;**27**(36):9545–9559. Epub 2007/09/07.

138. Ruff CA, Wilcox JT, Fehlings MG. Cell-based transplantation strategies to promote plasticity following spinal cord injury. Exp Neurol. 2012;**235**(1):78–90. Epub 2011/02/22.

139. Fouad K, Schnell L, Bunge MB, Schwab ME, Liebscher T, Pearse DD. Combining Schwann cell bridges and olfactory-ensheathing glia grafts with chondroitinase promotes locomotor recovery after complete transection of the spinal cord. J Neurosci. 2005;**25**(5):1169–1178. Epub 2005/02/04.

140. Sandner B, Pillai DR, Heidemann RM, et al. In vivo high-resolution imaging of the injured rat spinal cord using a 3.0T clinical MR scanner. JMRI. 2009;**29**(3):725–730. Epub 2009/02/27.

141. Weber T, Vroemen M, Behr V, et al. In vivo high-resolution MR imaging of neuropathologic changes in the injured rat spinal cord. Am J Neuroradiol. 2006;27(3):598–604. Epub 2006/03/23.

142. Hurd C, Weishaupt N, Fouad K. Anatomical correlates of recovery in single pellet reaching in spinal cord injured rats. Exp Neurol. 2013;247:605–614.

143. Naismith RT, Xu J, Klawiter EC, et al. 2013. Spinal cord tract diffusion tensor imaging reveals disability substrate in demyelinating disease. Neurology. 2013;80:2201–2209.

144. Vogt G, Laage R, Shuaib A, Schneider A, Collaboration V. Initial lesion volume is an independent predictor of clinical stroke outcome at day 90: an analysis of the Virtual International Stroke Trials Archive (VISTA) database. Stroke. 2012;43(5):1266–1272.

145. Schiemanck SK, Kwakkel G, Post MW, Prevo AJ. Predictive value of ischemic lesion volume assessed with magnetic resonance imaging for neurological deficits and functional outcome post-stroke: A critical review of the literature. Neurorehabil Neural Repair. 2006;20(4):492–502.

146. Weimar C, Konig IR, Kraywinkel K, Ziegler A, Diener HC, German Stroke Study C. Age and National Institutes of Health Stroke Scale Score within 6 hours after onset are accurate predictors of outcome after cerebral ischemia: development and external validation of prognostic models. Stroke. 2004;35(1):158–162.

147. Jorgensen HS, Nakayama H, Raaschou HO, Vivelarsen J, Stoier M, Olsen TS. Outcome and time-course of recovery in stroke.1. Outcome—the Copenhagen Stroke Study. Arch Phys Med Rehabil. 1995;76(5):399–405.

148. Jorgensen HS, Nakayama H, Raaschou HO, Vivelarsen J, Stoier M, Olsen TS. Outcome and time-course of recovery in stroke.2. Time-course of recovery—the Copenhagen Stroke Study. Archives of physical medicine and rehabilitation. 1995;76(5):406–412.

149. Cramer SC. Repairing the human brain after stroke. II. Restorative therapies. Ann Neurol. 2008;63(5):549–560.

150. Cramer SC. Repairing the human brain after stroke: I. Mechanisms of spontaneous recovery. Ann Neurol. 2008;63(3):272–287.

151. Alaverdashvili M, Whishaw IQ. Compensation aids skilled reaching in aging and in recovery from forelimb motor cortex stroke in the rat. Neuroscience. 2010;167(1):21–30.

152. Moon SK, Alaverdashvili M, Cross AR, Whishaw IQ. Both compensation and recovery of skilled reaching following small photothrombotic stroke to motor cortex in the rat. Exp Neurol. 2009;218(1):145–153.

153. Murphy TH, Corbett D. Plasticity during stroke recovery: from synapse to behaviour. Nat Rev Neurosci. 2009;10(12):861–872.

154. Bath PMW, Lees KR, Schellinger PD, et al. Statistical analysis of the primary outcome in acute stroke trials. Stroke. 2012;43(4):1171–1178.

155. Lees KR, Bath PMW, Schellinger PD, et al. Contemporary outcome measures in acute stroke research choice of primary outcome measure. Stroke. 2012;43(4):1163–U451.

156. Kirshblum SC, O'Connor KC. Predicting neurologic recovery in traumatic cervical spinal cord injury. Arch Phys Med Rehabil. 1998;79(11):1456–1466.

157. Spiess MR, Muller RM, Rupp R, Schuld C, van Hedel HJ. Conversion in ASIA impairment scale during the first year after traumatic spinal cord injury. J Neurotrauma. 2009;26(11):2027–2036. Epub 2009/05/22.

158. Wilson JR, Cadotte DW, Fehlings MG. Clinical predictors of neurological outcome, functional status, and survival after traumatic spinal cord injury: a systematic review. J Neurosurg Spine. 2012;17(1 Suppl):11–26.

159. Fawcett JW, Curt A, Steeves JD, et al. Guidelines for the conduct of clinical trials for spinal cord injury as developed by the ICCP panel: spontaneous recovery after spinal cord injury and statistical power needed for therapeutic clinical trials. Spinal Cord. 2007;45(3):190–205. Epub 2006/12/21.

160. Kirshblum SC, Burns SP, Biering-Sorensen F, et al. International standards for neurological classification of spinal cord injury (revised 2011). J Spinal Cord Med. 2011;34(6):535–546. Epub 2012/02/15.

161. Ditunno JF, Jr., Ditunno PL, Scivoletto G, et al. The Walking Index for spinal cord injury (WISCI/WISCI II): nature, metric properties, use and misuse. Spinal Cord. 2013;51(5):346–355. Epub 2013/03/06.

162. Furlan JC, Noonan V, Singh A, Fehlings MG. Assessment of disability in patients with acute traumatic spinal cord injury: a systematic review of the literature. J Neurotrauma. 2011;28(8):1413–1430. Epub 2010/04/07.

163. Basso DM, Beattie MS, Bresnahan JC. A sensitive and reliable locomotor rating scale for open field testing in rats. J Neurotrauma. 1995;12(1):1–21. Epub 1995/02/01.

164. Basso DM, Fisher LC, Anderson AJ, Jakeman LB, McTigue DM, Popovich PG. Basso Mouse Scale for locomotion detects differences in recovery after spinal cord injury in five common mouse strains. J Neurotrauma. 2006;23(5):635–659. Epub 2006/05/13.

165. Zorner B, Filli L, Starkey ML, et al. Profiling locomotor recovery: comprehensive quantification of impairments after CNS damage in rodents. Nat Methods. 2010;7(9):701–708.

166. Muir GD, Prosser-Loose EJ. Assessing spinal cord injury. Neuromethods. 2011;62(Ii):401–418.

167. Sedy J, Urdzikova L, Jendelova P, Sykova E. Methods for behavioral testing of spinal cord injured rats. Neurosci Biobehav Rev. 2008;32(3):550–580.

168. Cummings BJ, Engesser-Cesar C, Cadena G, Anderson AJ. Adaptation of a ladder beam walking task to assess locomotor recovery in mice following spinal cord injury. Behav Brain Res. 2007;177(2):232–241. Epub 2007/01/02.

169. Hamers FP, Koopmans GC, Joosten EA. CatWalk-assisted gait analysis in the assessment of spinal cord injury. J Neurotrauma. 2006;23(3–4):537–548. Epub 2006/04/25.

170. Redondo-Castro E, Torres-Espin A, Garcia-Alias G, Navarro X. Quantitative assessment of locomotion and interlimb coordination in rats after different spinal cord injuries. J Neurosci Methods. 2013;213(2):165–178. Epub 2013/01/08.

171. Couto PA, Filipe VM, Magalhaes LG, et al. A comparison of two-dimensional and three-dimensional techniques for the determination of hindlimb kinematics during treadmill locomotion in rats following spinal cord injury. J Neurosci Methods. 2008;173(2):193–200. Epub 2008/07/09.

172. Wirz M, Zemon DH, Rupp R, et al. Effectiveness of automated locomotor training in patients with chronic incomplete spinal cord injury: a multicenter trial. Arch Phys Med Rehabil. 2005;86(4):672–680. Epub 2005/04/14.

173. Norman KE, Pepin A, Ladouceur M, Barbeau H. A treadmill apparatus and harness support for evaluation and rehabilitation of gait. Arch Phys MedRehabil. 1995;76(8):772–778. Epub 1995/08/01.

174. Anderson KD, Gunawan A, Steward O. Spinal pathways involved in the control of forelimb motor function in rats. Exp Neurol. 2007;206(2):318–331.

175. Whishaw IQ, Pellis SM, Gorny BP, Pellis VC. The impairments in reaching and the movements of compensation in rats with motor cortex lesions: an endpoint, videorecording, and movement notation analysis. Behav Brain Res. 1991;42(1):77–91. Epub 1991/01/31.

176. Metz GA, Antonow-Schlorke I, Witte OW. Motor improvements after focal cortical ischemia in adult rats are mediated by compensatory mechanisms. Behav Brain Res. 2005;162(1):71–82. Epub 2005/06/01.

177. Whishaw IQ, Pellis SM, Gorny B, Kolb B, Tetzlaff W. Proximal and distal impairments in rat forelimb use in reaching follow unilateral pyramidal tract lesions. Behav Brain Res. 1993;56(1):59–76. Epub 1993/07/30.

178. Metz GA, Whishaw IQ. Skilled reaching an action pattern: stability in rat (Rattus norvegicus) grasping movements as a function of

changing food pellet size. Behav Brain Res. 2000;**116**(2):111–122. Epub 2000/11/18.

179. Girgis J, Merrett D, Kirkland S, Metz GA, Verge V, Fouad K. Reaching training in rats with spinal cord injury promotes plasticity and task specific recovery. Brain. 2007;**130**(Pt 11):2993–3003. Epub 2007/10/12.

180. Montoya CP, Campbell-Hope LJ, Pemberton KD, Dunnett SB. The 'staircase test': a measure of independent forelimb reaching and grasping abilities in rats. J Neurosci Methods. 1991;**36**(2–3):219–228. Epub 1991/02/01.

181. Clarke J, Ploughman M, Corbett D. A qualitative and quantitative analysis of skilled forelimb reaching impairment following intracerebral hemorrhage in rats. Brain Res. 2007;1145:204–212. Epub 2007/03/10.

182. Kalsi-Ryan S, Curt A, Verrier MC, Fehlings MG. Development of the Graded Redefined Assessment of Strength, Sensibility and Prehension (GRASSP): reviewing measurement specific to the upper limb in tetraplegia. Journal of neurosurgery Spine. 2012;**17**(1 Suppl):65–76. Epub 2012/09/19.

183. Kalsi-Ryan S, Beaton D, Curt A, et al. The Graded Redefined Assessment of Strength Sensibility and Prehension: reliability and validity. J Neurotrauma. 2012;**29**(5):905–914. Epub 2011/05/17.

184. Krassioukov AV, Karlsson AK, Wecht JM, Wuermser LA, Mathias CJ, Marino RJ. Assessment of autonomic dysfunction following spinal cord injury: rationale for additions to International Standards for Neurological Assessment. J Rehabil Res Dev. 2007;**44**(1):103–112. Epub 2007/06/07.

185. Inskip JA, Ramer LM, Ramer MS, Krassioukov AV. Autonomic assessment of animals with spinal cord injury: tools, techniques and translation. Spinal Cord. 2009;**47**(1):2–35. Epub 2008/06/11.

186. Steeves JD, Lammertse D, Curt A, et al. Guidelines for the conduct of clinical trials for spinal cord injury (SCI) as developed by the ICCP panel: clinical trial outcome measures. Spinal Cord. 2007;**45**(3):206–221. Epub 2006/12/21.

187. Blight AR. Spinal cord injury models: neurophysiology. J Neurotrauma. 1992;**9**(2):147–149; discussion 9–50. Epub 1992/01/01.

188. Schwab JM, Brechtel K, Mueller CA, et al. Experimental strategies to promote spinal cord regeneration—an integrative perspective. Progr Neurobiol. 2006;**78**(2):91–116.

189. Sun F, He Z. Neuronal intrinsic barriers for axon regeneration in the adult CNS. Curr Opin Neurobiol. 2010;**20**(4):510–518. Epub 2010/04/27.

190. Benowitz LI, Popovich PG. Inflammation and axon regeneration. Curr Opin Neurol. 2011;**24**(6):577–583. Epub 2011/10/05.

191. O'Collins VE, Macleod MR, Donnan GA, Horky LL, van der Worp BH, Howells DW. 1,026 experimental treatments in acute stroke. Ann Neurol. 2006;**59**(3):467–477.

192. Priestley JV, Michael-Titus AT, Tetzlaff W. Limiting spinal cord injury by pharmacological intervention. Handbook of Clinical Neurology. 2012;**109**:463–484. Epub 2012/10/27.

193. Dietz V, Fouad K. Restoration of sensorimotor functions after spinal cord injury. Brain. 2013. Epub 2013/10/10.

194. Tuszynski MH, Steeves JD, Fawcett JW, et al. Guidelines for the conduct of clinical trials for spinal cord injury as developed by the ICCP Panel: clinical trial inclusion/exclusion criteria and ethics. Spinal Cord. 2007;**45**(3):222–231. Epub 2006/12/21.

195. Lammertse D, Tuszynski MH, Steeves JD, et al. Guidelines for the conduct of clinical trials for spinal cord injury as developed by the ICCP panel: clinical trial design. Spinal Cord. 2007;**45**(3):232–242. Epub 2006/12/21.

196. Kwon BK, Hillyer J, Tetzlaff W. Translational research in spinal cord injury: a survey of opinion from the SCI community. J Neurotrauma. 2010;**27**(1):21–33. Epub 2009/09/16.

197. Macleod MR, Fisher M, O'Collins V, et al. Good laboratory practice preventing introduction of bias at the bench. Stroke. 2009;**40**(3):E50–E2.

198. Kwon BK, Soril LJ, Bacon M, et al. Demonstrating efficacy in preclinical studies of cellular therapies for spinal cord injury—How much is enough? Exp Neurol. 2013;**248C**:30–44. Epub 2013/06/04.

199. Steeves J, Blight A. Spinal cord injury clinical trials translational process, review of past and proposed acute trials with reference to recommended trial guidelines. Handbook of Clinical Neurology. 2012;**109**:386–397. Epub 2012/10/27.

Neuroplasticity and repair

SECTION 3

Neuroplasticity and repair

CHAPTER 12

Animal models of damage, repair, and plasticity in the brain

Andreas Luft

Introduction

Successful therapies in medicine are based on a thorough understanding of their (patho-) physiological mechanisms. In neurorehabilitation, mechanistic insights were achieved through the advancement of the neurosciences and have provided mechanistic explanations for some therapeutic approaches that originated from experience—'post-hoc' so to say. Still, much is unknown.

Animal models complement the study of human physiology because they allow for the use of methodologies that cannot be used in humans. Differences in anatomy and physiology between humans and animals, however, limit the interpretability and applicability for human medicine. Since most of these methods are invasive, ethical questions need to be looked at carefully. Knowledge gains must potentially be substantial to justify the use of animals. In rehabilitation and recovery sciences, so little is known about the brain's potential for recovery and the best ways to exploit this potential that animal experiments are necessary.

Why animal models

In the past, experience and observation served as a basis for the development of neurorehabilitation therapies. While this is certainly a valuable strategy, it falls short of the translational approach in which a physiological mechanism provides the idea of a therapeutic intervention and serves as a surrogate marker for its optimization. Constraint-induced movement therapy was developed based on monkey experiments showing that the non-use of a deafferentiated limb can be reversed by restricting the movement of, that is, immobilizing, the intact limb [1]. Deeper insights into the neurophysiology can only be reached by using animal models.

Animal models are also needed to test invasive interventions such as drugs [e.g. 2] or brain stimulation especially invasive brain stimulation [e.g. 3]. Such methods have not yet entered the clinical routine of stroke rehabilitation but are effective treatment approaches in extrapyramidal movement disorders such as Parkinson's disease or tremor. Without the evidence from animal experimentation would human use be difficult to ethically justify.

Animal models carry a decisive advantage, that is, their homogeneity. The optimal model has the least interindividual variability that is related to methodology, for example, to the size of the brain lesion or the genetic background of the animals. This homogeneity allows to detect effects of interventions that are rather small and that would require large human samples and lengthy and costly clinical studies. This methodological advantage of animal models may help to identify drug side effects on neuroplasticity—that is drugs that reduce or interfere with learning and recovery processes. Stroke patients receive a multitude of medications against seizures, depression, hypertension, agitation etc. Some of these drugs—based on their pharmacological action—potentially reduce neural plasticity, as it may be the case for the antiepileptic levetiracetam [4]. If these drugs had dramatic effects of recovery, their detrimental action would probably have been noticed clinically. More likely, however, these effects are small and may add up to explain why some patients recover better then others. Such small effect sizes are easier to detect in animal models of neuroplasticity that use a surrogate marker instead of behavioural recovery as their outcome measure.

Whether animal models are also apt to investigate mechanisms or efficiency of motor training methods is questionable. The neuroanatomy of the rodent motor system and the movement patterns used by rats are substantially different from humans, which limits comparability. Non-human primate model may be required to explore, for example, the neurophysiology of robot-assisted motor training. Non-human primates are able to be trained in a task-related manner after experimental stroke similar to humans [5].

Why not—limitations of animal models

While we argued above that homogeneity is an advantage of animal models as compared with human studies, it is also their most significant disadvantage. Human stroke is largely variable—factors contributing to this variability are the site of the brain lesion, stroke aetiology, deficit severity, comorbidity, social factors, cognition, and likely other unknown factors. Many of these factors interact with each other, for example the presence of aphasia with the relationship to the caregiver/spouse and depression. An influence of these factors on recovery is likely [6]. Animal models cannot simulate such complex situations, which limits their comparability to humans.

Because most models of post stroke recovery use rats, differences in neuroanatomy need to be considered. The rat's motor system is substantially different from the human motor system: It is unclear whether the separation between primary motor, premotor cortex, and supplementary motor area also exists in the rat [7]. In the rat, primary motor and somatosensory cortex overlap, whereas in humans they are separated [8]. In rats subcortical regions play a bigger role in motor control. This is why behavioural deficits after

Table 12.1 Ischaemic stroke models

Model	Pro	Con
Middle cerebral artery occlusion (MCAO) ◆ suture/thread reversible occlusion ◆ distal MCAO via craniotomy ◆ thromboembolic occlusion with microspheres or thrombotic emboli	Pathophysiology comparable to human stroke, technically simple (except distal MCAO)	◆ Variable lesion size (especially in thromboembolic models) ◆ Subarachnoid haemorrhage in 10–20% of cases ◆ Permanent ligation of ECA for suture insertion produces mastication deficits with subsequent weight loss ◆ Involvement of hypothalamus (except distal MCAO) produces hyperthermia exacerbating cell death.
Multiple vessel occlusion (both carotid arteries, cortical MCA)	Similar to MCAO but produces smaller lesions	Craniotomy with increased preparation time, injury and surgery related morbidity/mortality
Focal interruption of cortical blood supply	Small cortical lesions	Variable lesion size depending on individual vascular anatomy
Endothelin-1 injection (vasoconstrictor)	◆ Focal well-defined lesions ◆ Deep (lacunar) lesions possible	Side effects of endothelin include facilitation of axonal sprouting and astrocytosis Questionable comparability to human with respect to (especially) early course/recovery
Photothrombosis	◆ Focal, well-defined lesions ◆ Technically simple and noninvasive	Microvascular occlusion with lack of penumbra and concomitant formation of vasogenic and cytotoxic oedema Questionable comparability to human with respect to (especially) early course/recovery

a cortical lesion are often small and only detectable in sensitive motor tests [9, 10].

The interpretation of movement deficits related to a brain lesion also has to consider the innate movement patterns of the animal. Rats are quadripedal and typically utilize their forelimbs in a bilaterally symmetrical fashion. Humans, in contrast, are bipedal and therefore require a more sophisticated motor control of balance. Upper extremity movement in humans are mostly unilateral and if they are bilateral then both arms/hands are used in a cooperative manner, for example while opening a bottle [11]. Rats can perform unilateral movements but they have to

slowly acquire and train these movements [12]. Considering that pre-existing knowledge of a task influences its recovery [13], the fact that most movements that serve as a measure for recovery are new to the rat while humans aim to recover motor tasks that they had performed thousands of times before, can limit rat-to-human comparability.

One more difficulty in rodent models of stroke recovery is related to the ischaemia model itself.

Models of experimental brain injury

Several methods exist for inducing ischaemia in the brain of mice or rats and each has its own advantages and disadvantages [14] (Table 12.1). Most models involve cortical or cortical+subcortical strokes. Occlusion of the middle cerebral artery (MCAO) by using a filament inserted through the internal carotid artery, ligating the artery or injecting embolic materials is commonly used. MCAO-induced lesions vary in size [14]. Other models like photothrombosis (Figure 12.1) or intra- or epicortical injections of endothelin-1, a vasoconstrictor that produces reversible ischaemia for up to 3 hours, produce more homogeneous lesions, but are pathophysiologically distinct from human stroke. A substantial proportion of strokes in human affect solely subcortical white matter and/or basal ganglia—the typical lacunar strokes. Rodent models of subcortical stroke use stereotactic injections of endothelin-1 into the internal capsule [15] or into the subcortical white matter [16].

Apart from brain ischaemia models, recovery has also been studied in models of traumatic brain injury [17, 18]. The typical model involves a controlled cortical impact performed by cylinder that is driven by a linear velocity transducer [19].

Comparing learning and recovery

Studies on learning and memory have revealed many processes involving lasting reorganization of neural networks, termed plasticity. In particular, paradigms of motor learning were found to be associated with synaptic [20] and structural plasticity in motor cortices [21]. Because neural reorganization has been found during recovery [22] and learning, it is assumed that both processes share similar mechanisms. Behaviourally, learning and recovery share a dependency on training and training intensity [23].

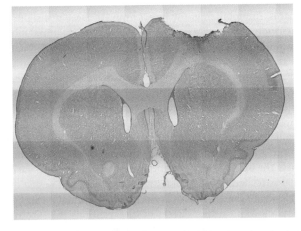

Fig. 12.1 Example of a cortical lesion in rat produced by photothrombosis.

Despite these similarities, a convincing proof that learning and recovery share a common mechanism is still lacking.

Animal models of learning

Learning and memory have been extensively investigated in animal models. While in humans, the distinction between explicit and implicit learning is well established—'explicit' referring to hippocampus dependent memorization of contents of conscious experience, 'implicit' referring to the unconscious learning of procedures or movements—it is less clear in animals. Spatial learning in a maze depends on the hippocampus [24, 25]. Motor learning such as the learning of a skilled forelimb task depends on motor cortex and striatum [26–28], but not on hippocampus [29].

Because brain ischaemia models in rat mainly injure cortex and basal ganglia, recovery research has focused mainly on motor tasks. Complex movements are sensitive measures of functional deficits induced by cortical lesions. Recovery of motor performance has been compared to the healthy learning of these tasks. Skilled forelimb reaching is the motor skill learning model most often used. The rat learns to reach for a food pellet that is placed outside the cage through a slit in the cage's wall. The animals usually require several training days to reach a performance plateau. This task depends on protein synthesis in motor cortex [27] and—to a lesser extent—in basal ganglia [26]. It involves synaptic plasticity in motor-to-sensory cortex transcortical projections [20]. During learning of the reaching movement motor cortex representation maps are transiently modified [30, 31]. Learning is also associated with synaptogenesis (structural plasticity) in motor cortex [32]. Learning to reach depends on acetylcholine [33] and dopamine [34, 35] to be released in motor cortex during training. The reaching task is sufficiently complex to induce learning over several days which is an advantage when trying to augment/reduce learning by certain interventions.

Alternative motor skill learning paradigms are pasta reaching [36], rotarod [37], acrobatic walking tasks [37–39], staircase reaching, in which rats reach for food pellets from different distances—the greater the distance reached from, the better is the performance in this task [40]. The sticky tape test, in which an animal has to remove a piece of tape attached to the forelimb, is sensitive to somatosensory deficits [41]. For a summary of motor paradigms see Table 12.2.

Animal models of plasticity

The term 'plasticity' has been used for a variety of phenomena that represent lasting modifications to neural structure or function. 'Lasting' in this context can refer to several minutes or to a lifetime. Functional plasticity typically means the change of synaptic strength between neurons. Changes in synaptic strength can be mediated by different cellular modifications, such as receptor trafficking, changes in dendritic spines, or synaptogenesis. The latter two may also be regarded as structural plasticity. The term structural plasticity also refers to processes that involve architectural modifications of neuronal circuits especially the growth of new fibres as measured, for example, by increased dendritic branching.

Animal models offer the opportunity to directly investigate the processes of functional or structural plasticity. Long-term potentiation (LTP) of synapses is often used as a measure of functional plasticity. LTP can be induced by costimulation of two input projections to a neuron or by high-frequency stimulation of one projection. The responses of this neuron are then amplified and this amplification persists for several hours or days.

In motor cortex slices, LTP can be observed on the population level—that is in field potentials recorded from motor cortex during sensory cortex stimulation. LTP can be induced by a high frequency burst of stimuli [42]. This form of LTP is used during motor skill learning [20, 43]. LTP in motor cortex can also be observed by recording single neurons [44, 45].

Dendritic spine formation [46] and dendritic branching [21] in motor cortex in response to motor training can be seen as evidence for structural plasticity.

Animal models of recovery

Animal studies investigating interventions in the acute phase of stroke usually determine lesion volume and parameters of behavioural recovery as their measures of outcome [14]. Examples are the cylinder test, in which the symmetry of forelimb use is measured while the rat is exploring a cylindric cage from inside, or the sticky tape test in which the time required to remove a sticky tape from the forepaw is recorded. Complex walking tasks like the rotarod test, beam, or ladder walking are used to assess gait.

Tasks like the cylinder test are highly dependent on motivation, fear, and novelty of the environment, hence assessing compound deficits going beyond the motor domain. The motor assessments

Table 12.2 Motor test (learning) paradigms

Model	Pro	Con
Pellet or pasta reaching task, including staircase reaching	Sensitive to deficits induced by small cortical strokes affecting the motor system	◆ Requires pre-learning over several days to learn to task ◆ A change in movement strategy is not recognized
Skilled walking tests (beam, ladder, rotarod, rotating pole)	Simple set up involving short learning to plateau performance	◆ Involves whole body movement programme, including balance, locomotion under subcortical/extrapyramidal and brainstem control ◆ Quick learning to plateau performance renders studies on learning processess difficult
Forelimb adhesive tape removal test	◆ Requires no special equipment ◆ Good quantification via time attending to stimulus (=tape)	A change in movement strategy is not recognized
Robotic manipulandum	Precise quantification via several parameters that are sensitive to learning	◆ Complex setup ◆ Long pre-training times

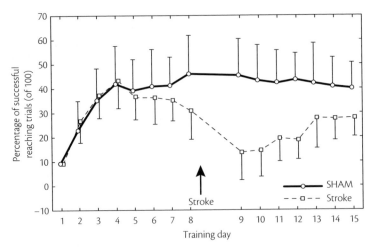

Fig. 12.2 Typical learning and recovery curve of a skilled forelimb reaching task. The rat learns over a period of 8 days to reach for a food pellet with the forepaw. The photothrombotic lesion to the forelimb area of the caudal motor cortex induces a decline in reaching performance. Performance then recovers over the course of 7–14 days (with permission from [13]).

are composed of movement patterns that are novel and not derived from the rat's daily life. The tasks are complex and are learned over several training sessions (days). As a consequence, repeated exposure will induce learning that confounds the assessment of recovery—that is, one cannot discern whether an improvement after a brain lesion is related to recovery of motor function or it is a consequence of the learning of the task.

Because recovery processes that are often non-linear, it is mandatory to use several (more than two) repetitions of an assessment of motor function. Repeated testing assumes high test–retest reliability of the assessment. Task learning reduces reliability. The solution is to over-train the task before lesioning the brain—that is, to train for a sufficient amount of time so that performance reaches a plateau. Based on this plateau one can then determine the lesion-related deficit and subsequent recovery identified by an improvement in performance.

The task that is most often used for assessing recovery of motor function after stroke is the skilled forelimb reaching task [12]. A lesion to the forelimb area of the caudal motor cortex (e.g. induced by photothrombosis) produces a decline in performance which subsequently recovers over a period of 10–14 days to reach nearly pre-stroke levels (Figure 12.2) [13]. Alternative tasks are the opening of sunflower seeds [47] or the staircase reaching task [40, reviewed in 48].

One general problem exists with all these paradigms of post-stroke recovery. They cannot differentiate between the assessment of motor function and training. If the animal is exposed to a task several times to assess a deficit at different time points during recovery, repeated testing itself is a form of rehabilitative training. Hence, one cannot separate spontaneous from therapy-induced recovery. This differentiation may be irrelevant for testing drugs or supportive interventions such as brain stimulation, but, a comparison of different training methods will be difficult. Testing the latter hypothesis would require that assessments do not interfere with the training and that the effectiveness of the training methods to be tested is substantially larger than the training effects mediated by the assessment. Otherwise, the assessment-induced training will occlude the effect of the training methods in focus and no difference will be found.

Another difficulty relates to the limited sensitivity and the large variability of motor tasks such as skilled reaching. A rat can successfully reach for a food pellet by using different motor strategies. Hence, the outcome criterion 'pellet successfully reached' can be achieved in different ways. Some animals simply alter their motor strategy after a stroke coping with a deficit to reach as many pellets as before. Only a video-based movement analysis can then discern different motor strategies, but is difficult to analyse [10]. Alternatively, a robotic sensorized manipulandum can be used [49, 50]. This manipulandum records the kinematics and forces during reaching and pulling to allow for an improved evaluation of the changes occurring during recovery (see Video 12.1 in the online material).

In humans, implementing and integrating improvements in motor function into daily life is often a problem. This problem cannot be addressed in animal models as long as motor tasks that are irrelevant for the rat's daily life are used. The problem occurs already before: a small cortical lesion does not induce a noticeable deficit in the rat's home-cage behaviour. Larger lesions, however, lead to major disability and discomfort. Many animals die or are not motivated for training or behavioural assessment.

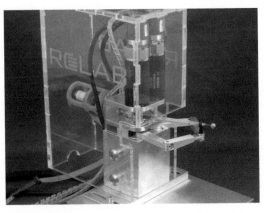

Video 12.1 Rodent robotic manipulandum ETH Pattus.

Conclusions and outlook

Animal models offer the only possibility to reach a deeper understanding of the neuronal processes that underly recovery and rehabilitation, but, they have clear limitations in the comparability to humans.

Animal models allow the direct exploration of functional and structural plasticity processes during recovery. Novel therapies to improve plasticity and recovery can (should) only be developed and be mechanistically explained by using animal models. Whether interventions that successfully improve recovery in animals also work in humans, however, is unpredictable.

To date, most interventions in neurorehabilitation are insufficiently understood. To move the field forward, answers need to be found as to why certain interventions work in some patients better than in others, as to why certain elements of therapy are more effective than others, and what prerequisites a patient must have to benefit from an intervention. To resolve these questions, more basic science in animals and humans is necessary.

References

1. Taub E, Uswatte G, Elbert T. New treatments in neurorehabilitation founded on basic research. Nat Rev Neurosci. 2002;**3**:228–236.
2. Long D, Young J. Dexamphetamine treatment in stroke. Q J Med. 2003;**96**:673–685.
3. Kleim JA, Bruneau R, VandenBerg P, MacDonald E, Mulrooney R, Pocock D. Motor cortex stimulation enhances motor recovery and reduces peri-infarct dysfunction following ischemic insult. Neurol Res. 2003;**25**:789–793.
4. Heidegger T, Krakow K, Ziemann U. Effects of antiepileptic drugs on associative LTP-like plasticity in human motor cortex. Eur J Neurosci. 2010;**32**:1215–1222.
5. Nudo RJ, Friel KM. Cortical plasticity after stroke: implications for rehabilitation. Rev Neurol (Paris). 1999;**155**:713–717.
6. Carod-Artal FJ, Egido JA. Quality of life after stroke: the importance of a good recovery. Cerebrovasc Dis. 2009;**27** Suppl 1:204–214.
7. Passingham RE, Myers C, Rawlins N, Lightfoot V, Fearn S. Premotor cortex in the rat. Behav Neurosci. 1988;**102**:101–109.
8. Hall RD, Lindholm EP. Organization of motor and somatosensory cortex in the albino rat. Brain Res. 1974;**66**:23–38.
9. Napieralski JA, Banks RJ, Chesselet MF. Motor and somatosensory deficits following uni- and bilateral lesions of the cortex induced by aspiration or thermocoagulation in the adult rat. Exp Neurol. 1998;**154**:80–88.
10. Gharbawie OA, Gonzalez CL, Whishaw IQ. Skilled reaching impairments from the lateral frontal cortex component of middle cerebral artery stroke: a qualitative and quantitative comparison to focal motor cortex lesions in rats. Behav Brain Res. 2005;**156**:125–137.
11. Dietz V, Macauda G, Schrafl-Altermatt M, Wirz M, Kloter E, Michels L. Neural Coupling of cooperative hand movements: a reflex and fMRI study. Cerebral Cortex. 2013 Oct 11. [Epub ahead of print].
12. Buitrago MM, Ringer T, Schulz JB, Dichgans J, Luft AR. Characterization of motor skill and instrumental learning time scales in a skilled reaching task in rat. Behav Brain Res. 2004;**155**:249–256.
13. Schubring-Giese M, Molina-Luna K, Hertler B, Buitrago MM, Hanley DF, Luft AR. Speed of motor re-learning after experimental stroke depends on prior skill. Exp Brain Res (Experimentelle Hirnforschung Expérimentation cérébrale). 2007;**181**:359–365.
14. Carmichael ST. Rodent models of focal stroke: size, mechanism, and purpose. NeuroRx. 2005;**2**:396–409.
15. Frost SB, Barbay S, Mumert ML, Stowe AM, Nudo RJ. An animal model of capsular infarct: endothelin-1 injections in the rat. Behav Brain Res. 2006;**169**:206–211.
16. Sozmen EG, Kolekar A, Havton LA, Carmichael ST. A white matter stroke model in the mouse: axonal damage, progenitor responses and MRI correlates. J Neurosci Methods. 2009;**180**:261–272.
17. Darrah SD, Darrah SH, Chuang J, et al. Dilantin therapy in an experimental model of traumatic brain injury: effects of limited versus daily treatment on neurological and behavioral recovery. J Neurotrauma. 2011;**28**:43–55.
18. Soblosky JS, Colgin LL, Chorney-Lane D, Davidson JF, Carey ME. Some functional recovery and behavioral sparing occurs independent of task-specific practice after injury to the rat's sensorimotor cortex. Behav Brain Res. 1997;**89**:51–59.
19. Dixon CE, Clifton GL, Lighthall JW, Yaghmai AA, Hayes RL. A controlled cortical impact model of traumatic brain injury in the rat. J Neurosci Methods. 1991;**39**:253–262.
20. Rioult-Pedotti MS, Friedman D, Donoghue JP. Learning-induced LTP in neocortex. Science. 2000;**290**:533–536.
21. Wang L, Conner JM, Rickert J, Tuszynski MH. Structural plasticity within highly specific neuronal populations identifies a unique parcellation of motor learning in the adult brain. Proc Natl Acad Sci U S A. 2011;**108**:2545–2550.
22. Nudo RJ. Postinfarct cortical plasticity and behavioral recovery. Stroke. 2007;**38**:840–845.
23. Kwakkel G, Wagenaar RC, Twisk JW, Lankhorst GJ, Koetsier JC. Intensity of leg and arm training after primary middle-cerebral-artery stroke: a randomised trial. Lancet. 1999;**354**:191–196.
24. Naghdi N, Majlessi N, Bozorgmehr T. The effects of anisomycin (a protein synthesis inhibitor) on spatial learning and memory in CA1 region of rat hippocampus. Behav Brain Res. 2003;**139**:69–73.
25. Guzowski JF, Lyford GL, Stevenson GD, et al. Inhibition of activity-dependent arc protein expression in the rat hippocampus impairs the maintenance of long-term potentiation and the consolidation of long-term memory. J Neurosci. 2000;**20**:3993–4001.
26. Wächter T, Röhrich S, Frank A, et al. Motor skill learning depends on protein synthesis in the dorsal striatum after training. Exp Brain Res Experimentelle Hirnforschung Expérimentation cérébrale. 2010;**200**:319–323.
27. Luft AR, Buitrago MM, Ringer T, Dichgans J, Schulz JB. Motor skill learning depends on protein synthesis in motor cortex after training. J Neurosci. 2004;**24**:6515–6520.
28. Luft AR, Buitrago MM, Kaelin-Lang A, Dichgans J, Schulz JB. Protein synthesis inhibition blocks consolidation of an acrobatic motor skill. Learning Memory. 2004;**11**:379–382.
29. Gould TJ, Rowe WB, Heman KL, et al. Effects of hippocampal lesions on patterned motor learning in the rat. Brain Res Bull. 2002;**58**:581–586.
30. Kleim JA, Barbay S, Nudo RJ. Functional reorganization of the rat motor cortex following motor skill learning. J Neurophysiol. 1998;**80**:3321–3325.
31. Molina-Luna K, Hertler B, Buitrago MM, Luft AR. Motor learning transiently changes cortical somatotopy. Neuroimage. 2008;**40**:1748–1754.
32. Kleim JA, Barbay S, Cooper NR, et al. Motor learning-dependent synaptogenesis is localized to functionally reorganized motor cortex. Neurobiol Learn Mem. 2002;**77**:63–77.
33. Conner JM, Culberson A, Packowski C, Chiba AA, Tuszynski MH. Lesions of the Basal forebrain cholinergic system impair task acquisition and abolish cortical plasticity associated with motor skill learning. Neuron. 2003;**38**:819–829.
34. Molina-Luna K, Pekanovic A, Rohrich S, et al. Dopamine in motor cortex is necessary for skill learning and synaptic plasticity. PloS ONE. 2009;**4**:e7082.
35. Hosp JA, Pekanovic A, Rioult-Pedotti MS, Luft AR. Dopaminergic projections from midbrain to primary motor cortex mediate motor skill learning. J Neurosci. 2011;**31**:2481–2487.
36. Ballermann M, Metz GA, McKenna JE, Klassen F, Whishaw IQ. The pasta matrix reaching task: a simple test for measuring skilled reaching distance, direction, and dexterity in rats. J Neurosci Methods. 2001;**106**:39–45.

37. Buitrago MM, Schulz JB, Dichgans J, Luft AR. Short and long-term motor skill learning in an accelerated rotarod training paradigm. Neurobiol Learning Memory. 2004;**81**:211–216.

38. Kleim JA, Lussnig E, Schwarz ER, Comery TA, Greenough WT. Synaptogenesis and Fos expression in the motor cortex of the adult rat after motor skill learning. J Neurosci. 1996;**16**:4529–4535.

39. Mattiasson GJ, Philips MF, Tomasevic G, Johansson BB, Wieloch T, McIntosh TK. The rotating pole test: evaluation of its effectiveness in assessing functional motor deficits following experimental head injury in the rat. J Neurosci Methods. 2000;**95**:75–82.

40. Montoya CP, Campbell-Hope LJ, Pemberton KD, Dunnett SB. The 'staircase test': a measure of independent forelimb reaching and grasping abilities in rats. J Neurosci Methods. 1991;**36**:219–228.

41. Andersen CS, Andersen AB, Finger S. Neurological correlates of unilateral and bilateral 'strokes' of the middle cerebral artery in the rat. Physiol Behav. 1991;**50**:263–269.

42. Rioult-Pedotti MS, Friedman D, Hess G, Donoghue JP. Strengthening of horizontal cortical connections following skill learning. Nat Neurosci. 1998;**1**:230–234.

43. Rioult-Pedotti MS, Donoghue JP, Dunaevsky A. Plasticity of the synaptic modification range. J Neurophysiol. 2007;**98**:3688–3695.

44. Castro-Alamancos MA, Donoghue JP, Connors BW. Different forms of synaptic plasticity in somatosensory and motor areas of the neocortex. J Neurosci. 1995;**15**:5324–5333.

45. Aroniadou VA, Keller A. Mechanisms of LTP induction in rat motor cortex in vitro. Cereb Cortex. 1995;**5**:353–362.

46. Harms KJ, Rioult-Pedotti MS, Carter DR, Dunaevsky A. Transient spine expansion and learning-induced plasticity in layer 1 primary motor cortex. J Neurosci. 2008;**28**:5686–5690.

47. Gonzalez CL, Kolb B. A comparison of different models of stroke on behaviour and brain morphology. Eur J Neurosci. 2003;**18**:1950–1962.

48. Kleim JA, Boychuk JA, Adkins DL. Rat models of upper extremity impairment in stroke. ILAR J. 2007;**48**:374–384.

49. Vigaru B, Lambercy O, Graber L, et al. A small-scale robotic manipulandum for motor training in stroke rats. IEEE Int Conf Rehabil Robot. 2011;**2011**:5975349.

50. Vigaru B, Lambercy O, Schubring-Giese M, Hosp J, Schneider M, Osei-Atiemo C, et al. A robotic platform to assess, guide and perturb rat forelimb movements. IEEE Trans Neural Syst Rehabil Eng 2013;**21**(5):796–805.

CHAPTER 13

Animal models of damage, repair, and plasticity in the spinal cord

V. Reggie Edgerton, Roland R. Roy, Daniel C. Lu, and Yury Gerasimenko

Enabling motor control via neuromodulation of the spinal cord networks

A series of experiments conducted over the last several decades have revealed important physiological principles of the neural networks in mice [1, 2], rats [3–12], cats [13–16], and humans [17–20] that control posture, locomotion, and even voluntary control. Some rather subtle adjustments in how different network properties can be modulated to dramatically improve motor function after paralysis have been identified when these principles are merged into a comprehensive synergistic strategy. These principles also suggest that a paradigm shift in present-day concepts regarding the neural control of movement should be considered. More specifically, those properties that are of fundamental importance in achieving functional recovery as demonstrated in several animal models of spinal cord injury include the following: (1) extensive plasticity among the spinal networks can persist for prolonged periods after an injury; (2) an important component of this plasticity is that the spinal networks can learn a motor task and it learns what is practiced—a clear example of activity-dependent plasticity; (3) relatively non-specific signals projecting into the spinal networks can trigger very complex motor behaviours, including postural regulation and stepping at different loads, speeds, and even directions; (4) those signals triggering such complex behaviours can be generated or facilitated by different modes of electrical stimulation and by pharmacological modulation; and (5) sensory information (e.g. proprioceptive and cutaneous inputs), can serve as the controller in generating relatively fine and complex motor tasks in the absence of any supraspinal input.

While the properties listed have emerged over a period of several decades, there have been two seemingly relatively subtle differences not previously fully recognized that have resulted in what might be considered a paradigm shift in thinking about the mechanisms that control motor function. First, it only has been recently fully recognized that the spinal circuitry itself, without any assistance from input from the brain, has the capability to serve as the sole source of control of a wide variety of motor tasks that can be performed by the hindlimbs when the spinal cord circuitry is sufficiently neuromodulated to an appropriate level of excitability. Recognition of this capability has clear implications to how the nervous system controls movement normally, that is, in the non-injured state. Second, we have identified multiple strategies to neuromodulate the spinal circuitry within the relatively narrow range of excitability necessary to enable the spinal circuitry to process complex ensembles of motor-task specific proprioceptive and cutaneous information, as well as enabling residual descending networks that traverse a 'complete' spinal cord injury to serve as a source of volitional control of movement. For example, the application of electrical, pharmacological, and/or sensory stimulation can induce locomotor-like movements, even after a severe spinal cord injury. It is within this critical window of net excitability of the spinal cord that the sensory input can function as the source of movement control without any supraspinal input.

The importance of the sensory system in modulating postural or locomotor movements has been known from the early studies focused on the neural control of movement [16, 21, 22]. Only recently, however, has it been clearly demonstrated that the pattern of dynamic sensory input can provide an ensemble of information from multiple sensory receptors to inform the spinal networks of what mechanical events have just occurred ('feedback') and what is expected to occur subsequently ('feedforward'). Thus the key concept underlying the ability to realize significant improvement in motor function after paralysis is that the spinal networks can be neuromodulated using a range of interventions such that the spinal circuitry becomes enabled to generate complex movements using intrinsic control mechanisms as long as the physiological state of the spinal networks remain within a critical range of excitability [23, 24].

Electrical enabling motor control (eEmc)

The experiments performed by Shik and colleagues [25] more than four decades ago provided data that formed a substantial part of the foundation for the concept of automaticity in the neural control of posture and locomotion. They demonstrated that tonic stimulation of selected areas of the brainstem, now known as the mesencephalic locomotor region (MLR), in an acutely decerebrated cat could induce stepping on a treadmill belt over a range of speeds. Details of the characteristics of the stepping were a function of the precise site of stimulation, the intensity of stimulation, and the sensory information from the hindlimbs. One of the major points from these studies is that a simple tonic stimulus can induce a complex motor behaviour (stepping). These data also provided an important clue as to the degree to which details of posture and locomotion are defined by the spinal circuitry. Subsequently, Grillner and Zangger [26] demonstrated that the functionally isolated lumbosacral circuitry of a mammal could generate rhythmic, coordinated output of flexor and extensor motor nerves for hours. This was shown in adult, acutely spinalized cats with the hindlimbs functionally deafferented (curarized) and by providing a pharmacological stimulus (L-dopa and nialimide) presented systemically. Immediately following these experiments Edgerton and colleagues [27] performed the first series of experiments designed to begin to determine the interneuronal basis of this complex locomotor rhythmicity. These experiments demonstrated that interneurons throughout the dorsal, middle, and ventral laminae of the grey matter of the lumbosacral spinal cord were active in a precise and consistent rhythmic pattern, with each interneuron having a unique on/off and frequency modulation. The main result from these experiments was that there was an expansive network of neurons that participate in 'fictive locomotion' in a large mammal even in the absence of any sensory input. Since that time hundreds of experiments have been performed in attempts to determine the mechanisms of the underlying motor rhythms generated by the spinal cord in mammals commonly known as central pattern generation [16, 28–33].

While our understanding of some of the basic mechanisms of central pattern generation has advanced considerably, there has been relatively little progress in understanding how this network of neurons that can generate this motor rhythmicity also can process infinite complex patterns of sensory information associated with posture and locomotion [20, 34, 35]. Furthermore, the ability to translate important observations derived from central pattern generation experiments to humans has been relatively slow. This limitation largely has been associated with the inability to perform the necessary critical experiments under *in vivo* conditions in adult mammals. An objective of the present chapter is to summarize some of the new approaches that have made it possible to partially overcome some of these limitations from the perspective of studying adult systems *in vivo* with the possibility of translating the findings to human subjects with severe paralysis due to spinal cord injury. To give some insight as to the progress to date we are presenting examples of several types of experimental interventions that show promise toward translation in developing rehabilitative procedures to facilitate recovery of motor and autonomic function after a spinal cord injury in human subjects.

eEmc of the lumbosacral spinal cord

eEmc of the lumbosacral spinal cord is one intervention that has been shown to have considerable potential in facilitating recovery of significant levels of motor, and to some extent autonomic, function. For example, highly coordinated locomotor patterns can be generated in decerebrated cats by tonically electrically stimulating the dorsum of the lumbosacral spinal cord as demonstrated initially by Iwahara and colleagues [36]. Since that study this preparation has been examined more extensively using electromagnetic as well as electrical stimulation [37] showing that highly coordinated, full weight-bearing stepping over a range of speeds and loads can be performed with epidural stimulation at any of several locations along the spinal cord, for example stimulation at a cervical level (Figure 13.1A). A further important observation is that epidural stimulation can have the same effect after an acute

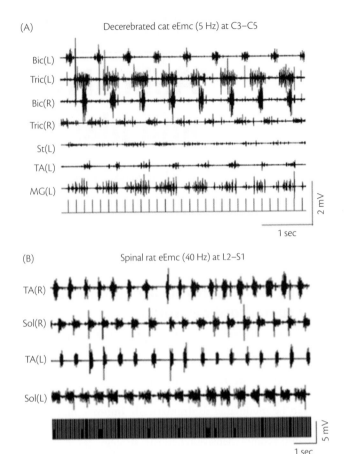

Fig. 13.1 Locomotor-like EMG patterns induced by epidural stimulation (eEmc) in a decerebrated cat (A) and in an adult complete spinal cord transected rat (~T8) 6 weeks after injury (B) are shown. In the decerebrated cat eEmc (5 Hz, pulse duration of 0.5 ms, and 20–100 μA) at a cervical level (spinal cord level C3–C5) induced and facilitated quadrupedal stepping movements in the forelimbs and hindlimbs (A). Rhythmic alternating EMG activity in selected hindlimb muscles induced by eEmc (40 Hz) at spinal cord levels L2 and S1 is shown for a complete spinal cord transected rat (B). The bottom trace in each panel indicates the stimulation frequency. Abbreviations: Bic, biceps; Tric, triceps; St, semitedinosus; TA, tibialis anterior; MG, medial gastrocnemius; Sol, soleus; (R), right; (L), left.
Modified from Bogacheva et al. [37] and from Gad et al. [96].

or chronic mid-thoracic complete spinal cord transection in cats and rats when stimulation was applied at the lumbosacral region of the spinal cord (Figure 13.1B). These figures illustrate how modulation of the cervical and lumbosacral circuitry by stimulating electrically can facilitate highly coordinated locomotor patterns in spinal cord injured mammals.

Pharmacological neuromodulation (fEmc)

It is very clear that monoaminergic neurotransmitter systems play an important role in the control of posture and locomotion. Some examples of how the modulation of different monoaminergic receptors impact locomotor function is shown in Figure 13.2. eEmc applied at L4–L5 (5 Hz, 80–100 μA) in decerebrated cats routinely elicits coordinated hindlimb stepping on the moving treadmill belt with robust alternating flexor–extensor electromyography (EMG) bursts (Figure 13.2A) and weight-bearing stepping with plantar foot placement. After ketanserin (a blocker of

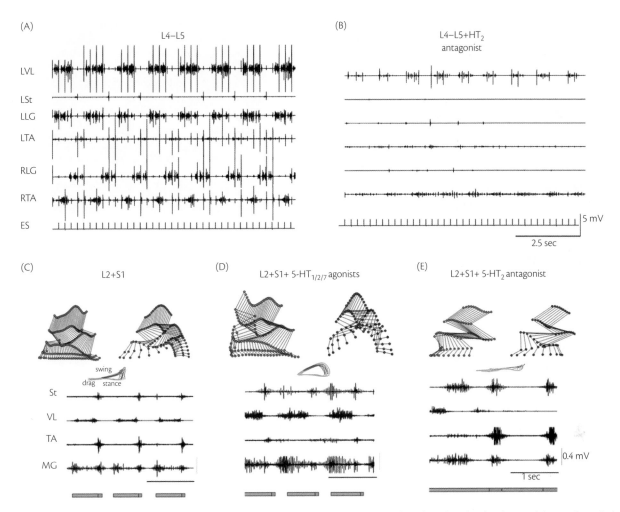

Fig. 13.2 The effects of monoamine drug administration on the stepping pattern induced by eEmc in a decerebrated cat (A, B) and in an adult complete spinal cord transected rat (C, D, E) are shown. EMG recordings from selected hindlimb muscles of a decerebrated cat are shown during quadrupedal stepping at 0.3–0.4 m/s induced by eEmc alone (A) or by eEmc plus ketanserin (a blocker of 5-HT$_2$ receptors) administration (B). Note that administration of ketanserin markedly reduces the EMG bursting in all muscles. The effects of eEmc alone (C), eEmc in the presence of 5-HT$_{1/2/7}$ agonists (8-OHDPAT and quipazine) (D), and eEmc in the presence of a 5-HT$_2$ antagonist (ketanserin) (E) on the kinematics and EMG activity in selected hindlimb muscles of a spinal rat are shown. The stick figures in C, D, and E illustrate a single stance and swing phase for each of the three experimental conditions. Below these stick figures the x–y trajectories of the paw for multiple cycles are shown. VL, vastus lateralis; LG, lateral gastrocnemius; ES, electrical stimulation. All other abbreviations are the same as in Figure 13.1. Horizontal bars show the stance (including drag) phase of each step cycle (in C, D, E).
Modified from Gerasimenko et al. [97] and Musienko et al. [42].

5-HT$_2$ receptors) administration, the EMG activity is depressed (Figure 13.2B) and only weak rhythmic movements without plantar foot placement are observed. eEmc (40 Hz) at L2 and S1 in spinal cord transected rats initiates EMG bursting patterns in the hindlimb muscles with partial, but limited, body weight support (Figure 13.2C). Simultaneous activation of 5-HT$_{1/7}$ (8-OHDPAT) and 5-HT$_2$ (quipazine) receptors results in a significant increase in proximal extensor and flexor muscle EMG activity compared with stepping enabled by eEmc alone (compare Figure 13.2C and D). Administration of ketanserin significantly reduces extensor activity and consequently severely impairs stepping (Figure 13.2E). These results demonstrate how the spinal circuitry output can be modulated pharmacologically and how these pharmacological effects interact with eEmc.

The efficacy of fEmc also has been shown in spinal animals. Adult cats were spinally transected at the T12–T13 junction and then trained to stand for 30 minutes per day for 12 weeks [38].

These spinal cats that were trained to stand could support their body weight using their hindlimbs for prolonged periods, but stepped very poorly (Video 13.1). The administration of strychnine (a glycinergic receptor antagonist) induced full-weight bearing stepping in the hindlimbs within 30–45 minutes (Video 13.2).

Electromagnetic stimulation (emEmc)

The cervical and lumbosacral circuitry of decerebrated cats (Figure 13.3A, B) and the lumbosacral circuitry in non-disabled human subjects (Figure 13.3C, D) are highly responsive to electromagnetic stimulation. One of the more unique features of emEmc is that cyclic activity can be initiated within the first stimulation pulse. This immediate response contrasts with that shown with application of mechanical vibration of muscles and tendons in humans [38]. This immediate response demonstrates that a single electromagnetically generated pulse can result in a critical level of excitatory input to the interneuronal networks that

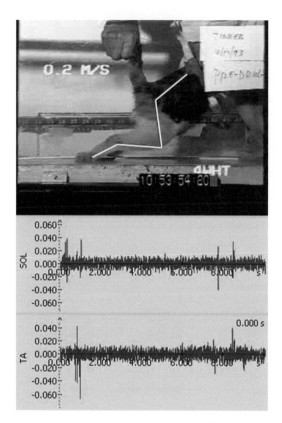

Video 13.1 After a complete transection of the spinal cord at a mid-thoracic level, the animal was trained to stand for 30 minute a day over a period of three months. At that point the animal had learned to successfully stand, but it was unable to generate any load-bearing stepping movements.

From the Edgerton Neuromuscular Research Laboratory (UCLA, USA) and courtesy of Ray de Leon and Roland R. Roy.

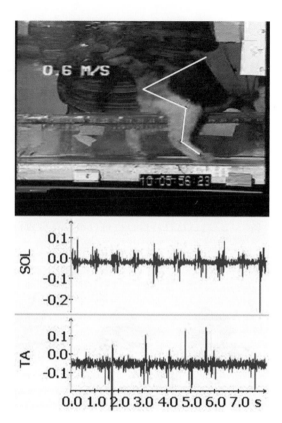

Video 13.2 Thirty minutes after being administered a modest dose of strychnine, which blocks inhibition and thereby facilitates activation, the animal was able to generate full weight-bearing stepping over a range of speeds when the hindlimbs were placed on a moving treadmill belt. This video demonstrates the potential of the spinal circuitry controlling the lower limbs to be activated using a pharmacological intervention (strychnine) from a totally non-functional state for stepping to a fully functional circuitry. This effect lasts for 30 to 60 minutes.

From the Edgerton Neuromuscular Research Laboratory (UCLA, USA) and courtesy of Ray de Leon and Roland R. Roy.

excites multiple motor pools in a highly coordinated fashion. An example of the effects of emEmc in an uninjured subject without (Video 13.3) and with (Video 13.4) mechanical vibration is shown in Videos 13.3 and 13.4.

The observations of facilitating stepping pharmacologically via neuromodulation of the lumbosacral spinal circuitry in the cat and by electromagnetic and sensory stimulation in humans and cats provide examples of how animal models can provide the rationale and experimental strategy for examining similar approaches that could be successfully developed for the clinic.

Transcutaneous electrical stimulation (pcEmc)

Application of electrical pulses generated with electrodes placed cutaneously over selected cervical, thoracic, and lumbosacral spinal segments, depending on the motor function of interest, is another intervention that shows considerable potential as a means of neuromodulating spinal networks. This technique appears to be capable of generating and facilitating motor responses similar to those elicited via epidurally placed electrodes. Although the amount of current that is necessary to generate motor effects is greater with pcEmc than eEmc, it is highly significant that at least some of the motor effects can be realized using a completely non-invasive strategy. Examples of how pcEmc can affect lower limb

movement in an uninjured subject and in a completely paralysed spinal cord injured subject are shown in Figure 13.4.

While each of these interventions shows considerable promise as a tool that could be used to facilitate recovery of motor function after a spinal cord injury, all of them are in the early stages of development technically and in understanding the new physiology that is emerging from these neuromodulatory techniques. Some of the more notable observations from experiments studying the neuromodulation of sensorimotor spinal circuits using electrical stimulation and/or pharmacological neuromodulation are:

1. At the higher levels of excitation via neuromodulatory interventions the end result tends very strongly to be a locomotor-like pattern characterized by alternating flexion and extension of the ipsilateral and contralateral limbs.

2. On the other hand, and more importantly from a clinical translation point of view, when more modest levels of neuromodulation are imposed in severely paralysed animals and humans the networks intrinsic to the spinal circuitry and minimal residual brain–spinal cord connectivity that may remain can serve to control functionally useful movements. This has led to the 'enabling' concept, which means that the spinal circuitry can be neuromodulated in a way that enables the individual to

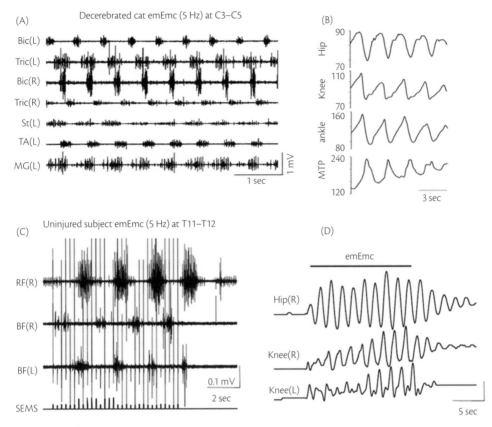

Fig. 13.3 Locomotor-like EMG patterns (A, C) and lower limb kinematics (B, D) induced by electromagnetic stimulation (emEmc) in a decerebrated cat (A, B) and a non-injured human subject (C, D) are shown. emEmc (5 Hz, 0.3–0.5 tesla) at C3–C5 in a decerebrated cat induces stepping-like EMG patterns in selected forelimb and hindlimb muscles (A) and coordinated joint movements (B) during quadrupedal stepping. The y-axis units are in degrees. emEmc (5 Hz, 70% maximum, i.e. ~1.8 tesla) at T11–T12 in a non-injured human subject induces stepping-like EMG patterns in selected lower limb muscles (C) and coordinated joint movements (D) under gravity-neutral conditions. RF, rectus femoris; BF, biceps femoris; MTP, metatarsophalangeal. All other abbreviations are the same as in Figure 13.1 and Figure 13.2.
Modified from Bogacheva et al. [37] and Gorodnichev et al. [98].

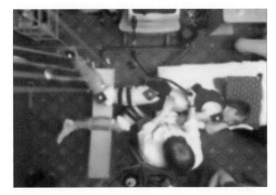

Video 13.3 Activation of the lumbosacral spinal cord of an uninjured individual when placed in a gravity-neutral apparatus enables the lower limbs to move in a step-like manner. The subject is asked to relax and to not move his legs. Step-like movements were initiated by stimulating directly (electromagnetic stimulation) at 5 Hz at vertebral level T12.
This work was conducted in collaboration with Y. Gerasimenko, (Pavlov Institute of Physiology, Russia) and R. Gorodnichev (Velikie Luky State Academy of Physical Education and Sport, Russia).

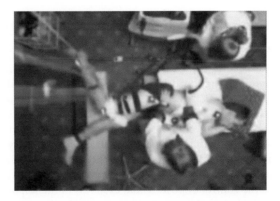

Video 13.4 A combination of vibration (60 Hz) of the quadriceps muscles and electromagnetic stimulation at 5 Hz at vertebral level T12 is imposed on the subject showing an additive effect of sensory and spinal stimulation. Involuntary locomotor-like movements were generated, suggesting that coordinated bilateral oscillatory movement of the lower limbs can be induced when the lumbosacral spinal circuitry is activated sufficiently.
This work was conducted in collaboration with Y. Gerasimenko (Pavlov Institute of Physiology, Russia) and R. Gorodnichev (Velikie Luky State Academy of Physical Education and Sport, Russia).

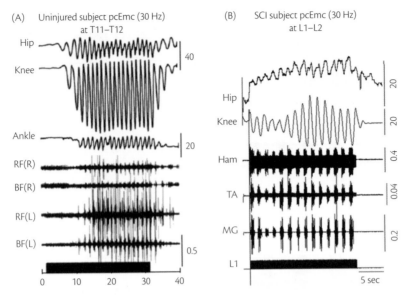

Fig. 13.4 Kinematics and EMG features reflecting locomotor-like patterns induced by transcutaneous electrical stimulation (pcEmc) in a non-injured subject (A) and a motor complete spinal cord injured subject (B) are shown. Angular movements at the hip, knee, and ankle joints and representative EMG activity in selected lower limb muscles bilaterally during involuntary locomotor-like activity induced by pcEmc (30 Hz) applied at the T11–T12 vertebral level (A) or at the L1–L2 vertebral level (B). The lower limbs of these subjects were suspended in a gravity-neutral position as in Figure 13.3C. Amplitude calibration values in (B) are expressed in mV. Modified from Gorodnichev et al. [99] and data from the spinal cord injured subject is unpublished.

initiate and generate a motor task as desired, and not as defined by a specific stimulation pattern that imposes a specific motor response at a specific time. This new source of control can be from peripheral sensory input to the spinal cord or from newly emerged voluntarily controlled descending pathways.

3. The success of enabling spinal circuits electrically is highly dependent on the fine-tuning of the levels of current, frequency and shape of the electrical pulses, and the spinal segment sites.

4. There appears to be a considerable 'enabling' potential when stimulating at levels considerably below motor threshold.

Synergism of Emc and sensorimotor training

Concepts of Emc

As a first general principle in rehabilitative efforts to recover sensorimotor function it is important to engage the relevant spinal cord circuits. To re-engage these circuits after prolonged periods of paralysis one or more neuromodulatory interventions are needed to achieve an enabling physiological state. As noted earlier the ability to use stimulation (electrically and/or pharmacologically) of the spinal cord circuitry to induce stepping has been known for decades. Less attention has been given to the control of posture and even less to the importance of the spinal cord circuitry in the control of voluntary movement. Initial evidence for enabling was reflected in experiments where sensory input was observed to vary the motor response to brainstem stimulation [25]. This idea, however, remained submerged for decades with a primary focus on inducing stepping via spinal cord epidural stimulation and stimulation of the mesencephalic locomotor region. Several changes in this focus were necessary to reach the current state of the concept of Emc of the spinal cord, with the idea of neuromodulation coming to the forefront. Via mechanisms still not fully understood the

physiological state of the spinal circuitry can be modulated to a state that falls within a relatively narrow window of excitability. Sensory input can reach the crucial interneurons that actually control posture and locomotion dynamically from millisecond to millisecond. The higher the level of stimulation above the motor threshold, the greater the motor response is. The consequences of a larger motor response is that it is inversely related to the ability to capitalize on the potential for sensory control—that is the ability to have an enabling or facilitating effect as opposed to an inducing effect leaving the sensory system with no 'say-so' as to what the motor response will be. Although the difference in the source and level of stimulation is a nonfactor by design in studies of central pattern generation, experiments that integrate sensory input into a central pattern generation similar to that occurring under *in vivo* conditions seems almost necessary to effectively translate these basic biological concepts to enabling motor control of multiple motor tasks after a severe spinal cord injury in animal models and now in humans. Inducing activity to enable or facilitate movement by engaging the multiple mechanical receptors associated with limb movement, as well as engaging the seemingly little residual descending motor projections below the lesion that may be greater than generally recognized, provides a newly realized strategy for successful rehabilitation [19, 39–43].

For performance of a motor task to improve first there must be engagement of the neural networks necessary to perform that task—the residual networks after prolonged dysfunction must be re-engaged. This can be accomplished using a number of neuromodulatory strategies. An additional physiological component of successful rehabilitation must be that the networks that generate a motor task can learn to perform that motor task when they are engaged repetitively over a period of minutes, days, or months. In effect, the appropriate spinal networks must be able to adapt and, more specifically, learn. It is clear from decades of experiments that the spinal networks can learn to perform specific motor tasks without any supraspinal input [13, 14, 44–50].

The power of proprioception and sensory input

The importance of sensorimotor spinal networks in the control of movement has been viewed as a reflex phenomenon. This oversimplified concept was modified to some degree with the realization of central pattern generation. As the concept of central pattern generation became so dominant the other capabilities of this circuitry has largely been unexplored. It is gradually becoming clearer that it is not only, or even primarily, the ability of the central pattern generator to induce alternating flexion and extension in a rhythmic manner that is important, but its ability to interpret complex sensory ensembles from multiple receptors located throughout the hindlimbs in real time [43, 51]. This interpretation includes the ability to make appropriate decisions to activate and inhibit those networks within the spinal cord that generate well-coordinated movements and correct responses to perturbations.

Can the spinal cord interpret load bearing-related sensory input to balance and maintain equilibrium during postural and locomotor tasks?

Until recently there was no strong evidence that the lumbosacral circuitry had any ability to sustain equilibrium and balance during posture or locomotion. We have performed a series of experiments over the last few years that demonstrate very clearly that decerebrated cats have the ability to generate useful corrective responses that help to maintain posture and to maintain the position of the hindquarters in a state of equilibrium during full weight-bearing locomotion when the lumbosacral spinal cord is receiving eEmc at the segments (Figure 13.5). Even when the hindlimbs collapse when stepping on a treadmill belt (Figure 13.5A), the hindquarters can regain full weight-bearing stepping and sustain sufficient equilibrium of the hindquarters so that stepping can be sustained over a period of minutes [52]. Although these data cannot exclude sources of control involving the brainstem given that the animals were decerebrated and not spinalized, more recent data demonstrate qualitatively similar but less robust responses in chronic spinal cats (Musienko et al., unpublished observations). In addition it has been reported that chronic spinal cats can learn to stand without assistance for up to 20 minutes [13].

Potential effects of neuromodulatory interventions and training regimens in regaining 'autonomic' function after a spinal cord injury: An integrative physiological response

The level of automaticity within the autonomic nervous system is more evident than in the somatic motor system. Therefore, hypothetically, these autonomically controlled functions would seem to be a viable target for neuromodulation post-injury. In some ways, however, it may be more complicated because of the extensive functional interconnections of multiple autonomic as well as motor systems. The neurotransmitter systems for autonomic control differ from those of the motor system and mainly involve sympathetic and parasympathetic networks. Common medical complications secondary to spinal cord injury are orthostatic hypotension, autonomic dysreflexia, and bladder dysfunction (i.e., detrusor sphincter dyssynergia) due to interruption of the balance between the sympathetic and parasympathetic outflow of the spinal cord. Interestingly, improvements in autonomic function, particularly in bladder function, after eEmc and motor training have been observed [19, 53, 54]. Therefore, we will focus the discussion on bladder function to serve as an example of how some autonomic function may be regained after a spinal cord injury using neuromodulatory strategies.

Because a component of micturition is normally under voluntary control, the lower urinary tract requires complex efferent pathway interactions via the autonomic (mediated by sympathetic and parasympathetic nerves) and somatic (mediated by pudendal nerves) systems [55, 56] (Figure 13.6). The thoracolumbar cord produces sympathetic innervation, while the sacral cord produces parasympathetic and somatic innervation. A spinal cord injury above the lumbosacral cord disrupts control of voiding via central, volitional inputs. It also alters the status of micturition centres in the cord that initially produce an areflexic bladder with urinary retention. After a period of recovery, there is development of automatic/reflexive micturition and neurogenic detrusor overactivity mediated by spinal micturition circuits [57]. The volume and rate of urine flow is poor because of the often coincident contractions of the bladder and the urethral sphincter (detrusor–sphincter dyssynergia).

The sacral spinal micturition circuitry has been studied in cats with complete paralysis. In this model, neurogenic detrusor overactivity mediated by heightened C-fibre activity has been observed. Clinical evidence suggests this mechanism also may exist in humans. Therapies to improve bladder function may have to re-set C-fibre tone to a pre-injury level. In rats, post-injury neuroplasticity has been associated with nerve growth factor (NGF) in the bladder and spinal cord [58–60]. Additional neuromodulatory factors TRPV1 [61], P2X3 [61] and/or the sensory neuropeptides substance P and calcitonin-gene-related peptide [62], may play a role in the transition from areflexia and retention shortly after injury to automatic/reflexive voiding in chronic injury. An understanding of how these established signaling systems could be used to mediate improvements in bladder function with neuromodulatory interventions may be a productive approach in regaining some bladder control [19, 53, 63]. Although there are a variety of stimulation techniques that are in current use to regain some improvement in bladder function, they almost all involve some surgical procedures, such as denervation of selected nerves and/or dorsal roots. The existing devices produce a subset of the micturition behaviour but do not result in enduring plastic changes to the circuitry that allow patients to become device independent. Peripheral nerve stimulators have been used with variable success. For example, the Finetech–Brindley posterior/anterior stimulator often is accompanied by dorsal root rhizotomy. These surgical interventions in themselves have permanent effects on other autonomic functions such as the loss of sexual function. Recent development of a closed-loop neuroprosthesis interface that bypasses the volitional or supraspinal input measures bladder fullness through implanted afferent dorsal roots into microchannel

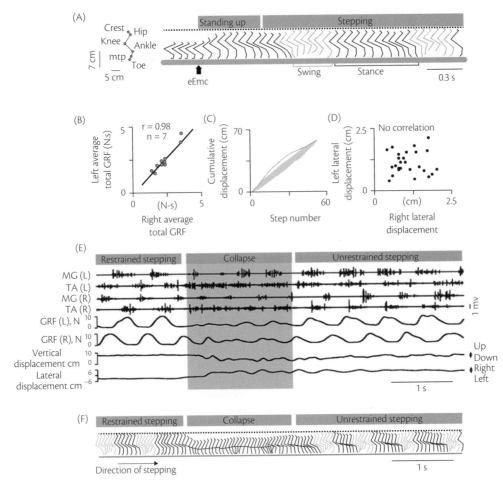

Fig. 13.5 Weight-bearing hindlimb stepping facilitated by eEmc at L4–L5 (5 Hz) in a decerebrated cat and the adaptive postural responses when initiated from a collapsed position. Stick diagrams (60 ms between sticks) of joint movements after the initiation of eEmc during the transition from sitting to standing and for the initial step cycle swing (light green) and stance (grey) phases. crest, iliac crest; mtp, metatarsophalangeal (A). Correlation for the average left vs. right total ground reaction force (GRF) within the entire duration of the stepping trial for ten experiments in seven cats (P < 0.01) (B). Cumulative right and left pelvis displacements plotted in order of occurrence (grey line) or randomized (Monte Carlo 500 times, light green line) (C). No correlation exists when all right and left lateral displacements are randomized with respect to their order of occurrence (D). EMG recordings from the MG and TA muscles bilaterally, GRFs bilaterally, and vertical and lateral pelvis displacements during stepping with the pelvis restrained by clamps (restrained stepping), collapse due to the release of the clamps (shaded area), and stepping during recovery from collapse (unrestrained stepping) (E). Stick diagrams (50 ms between sticks; swing (**light green**), stance (black), and collapse (dark green)) for the same step sequences shown in (E) (F).
Modified from Musienko et al. [52].

electrodes that interpret sensory activity related to bladder fullness. Continence was established with a high-frequency depolarizing block to the ventral roots in spinal rats, while bladder emptying was accomplished by low-frequency stimulation of ventral nerve roots [64]. While promising, the viability of this chronically implanted dorsal root–microchannel electrode system in humans has yet to be established. Furthermore, the above strategies focus on modulating and controlling the peripheral nerve activity rather than restoring the normal bladder spinal and supraspinal circuitry. In contrast, rats subjected to epidural stimulation and motor training have restored micturition function without the need for bladder expression (54) and subjects implanted with an epidural stimulator demonstrated improved volitional control of bladder function without catheterization after daily repetitive stimulation over a period of months [19, 65]. Such a phenomenon may be occurring by activating dormant residual pathways or reorganization of existing supraspinal pathways, such that the coordinated events responsible for micturition

are restored. Another possibility is that the stimulation lowers the threshold of activation of the interneuronal networks necessary for bladder control. Further studies are necessary to elucidate the mechanism of eEmc enabled micturition function after a spinal cord injury. Given the interest in the last few years of the potential of eletroceutical interventions and the importance of recovery of bladder control in a variety of neural disorders, it is almost certain that new and probably successful strategies will be developed to address this important problem.

Reorganization of supraspinal and spinal networks and sensory motor learning after a spinal cord injury

Numerous studies have demonstrated extensive reorganization of supraspinal and spinal circuits in response to a spinal cord injury, progressive neuromotor diseases, and during the process

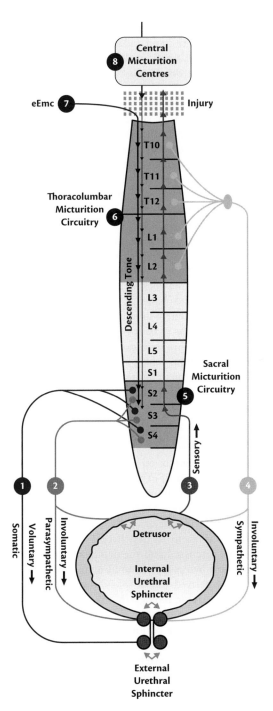

Fig. 13.6 Elements of micturition control: (1) Voluntary control of the external urethral sphincter is via the pudendal nerve. (2) Involuntary control of micturition requires that the internal urethral sphincter be relaxed via pelvic nerve parasympathetic tone. (3) The state of the bladder is modulated by sensory projections that synapse locally and project centrally. (4) Involuntary control also requires hypogastric nerve sympathetic activity for increasing the bladder wall (detrusor) and decreasing the internal urethral sphincter tone. Local circuits (highlighted in dark green) that can modulate micturition are found at the sacral (5) and thoracolumbar (6) levels. Both interact in a coordinated fashion to receive supraspinal input (black line, 8) to maintain continence or control of micturition. Injury can affect descending input or tone to render it to a subthreshold level. Electrical stimulation (eEmc, 7) can be used to activate the local spinal circuits and unmask descending spared axons and to activate micturition volitionally.

of recovery, whether it be spontaneous or driven by some specific intervention. These network reorganizations have been documented with behavioural, pharmacological, anatomical, and biochemical evidence [16, 31, 32, 39, 66–76]. A challenge that is increasingly obvious is how to coordinate supraspinal and spinal reorganization to regain some level of integration of consciously and the more automatically performed motor tasks largely generated by the spinal circuitry [77]. For example we know that the spinal circuits below a complete spinal cord lesion can undergo changes sufficient to generate very effective loadbearing stepping forward, backwards and sidewards [4, 12] and to adjust the activation patterns of motor pools to accommodate varying loads [78–80]. We also know that the spinal circuits can balance the hindquarters during standing and even during stepping without input from the brain [13, 14]. On the other hand it is not known whether supraspinal networks can reorganize without some concomitant plasticity occurring in the spinal networks.

Intuitively, it would seem likely that use-dependent engagement of supraspinal and spinal networks simultaneously, as might occur when a severely injured individual is consciously attempting a movement such as stepping, would be necessary for the two networks to function as a larger, single functionally synergistic network. In this case it seems that the subject's volitional effort is more likely to become integrated with the more automatic aspects of the control of movement. It is difficult to comprehend the combination of biological events that must occur for the reorganization of the supraspinal and spinal networks related to motor control, and the reintegration of these two networks to reach a functionally useful state. The fact that this level of reorganization seems to occur in laboratory animals [5, 11, 81] and in humans [19, 82] seems even more overwhelming considering that the combinations of pathways and circuits involved are not the same as they were before the injury or even after the injury and before any adaptive processes have been initiated [83].

Mechanisms of supraspinal–spinal functional reconnectivity after a spinal cord injury

There are multiple repair strategies possible to regain recovery of motor function. One presumed and commonly viewed strategy is that descending and ascending pathways can be reestablished with an emphasis on the corticospinal tract. For this reparative process to be functionally successful several events must occur. In humans, axons would have to project for long distances in most cases (i.e., 5 to 20 cm in adults). These axons then must functionally reconnect to those interneurons and motoneurons that control the coordination among those motor pools, performing an infinite number of movements differing from millisecond to millisecond kinetically and kinematically. This process seems highly improbable given the number of newly formed connections that must occur directly or indirectly over multiple spinal segments. It appears, however, that this kind of growth and reorganization may not be necessary to regain significant levels of function [5, 19, 84]. It seems that the descending supraspinal pathways can eventually find novel input to propriospinal networks that can carry out the functions necessary for recruitment and coordination of motor pools required for successfully generating volitional motor commands [19]. Whatever the mechanistic strategy, it is almost certain that some degree of formation of new control circuits occurs over time with one of the underlying means of network reorganization being the strengthening and weakening of specific sets of synapses within a network via some activity-dependent phenomenon.

The fineness of the control is likely to become functionally more meaningful when some critical level of new supraspinal–spinal connectivity has occurred. There is considerable experimental evidence consistent with an alternative reparative strategy that seems to be more feasible. This repair strategy consists of establishing new interconnections in the region of the injury when some supraspinal–spinal connectivity remains. This condition seems to exist in many human patients, even when clinical assessments indicate complete paralysis [85–87]. If a critical level of new functional interconnections at the point of injury persists even when there is a severe impairment, perhaps this residual connectivity combined with the formation of new functional synaptic connections can provide a greater level of intrasegmental and intersegmental connectivity to the more or less intact residual networks distal to the lesion. It seems that supraspinal input can trigger highly functional motor tasks if proprioception and cutaneous sensory input from the limbs can be engaged to control the details necessary to achieve meaningful movements. Experimental models supporting this conceptual framework have been derived from the insight gained from central pattern generation experiments [28], and *in vivo* experiments in which animals regain significant locomotor function after transection of some corticospinal pathways that reach a functional target directly or indirectly via the brainstem [5, 88].

This segmental reorganization strategy has gained further support from recent experiments in which individuals with motor complete paralysis have recovered volitional control of movements of all joints of the lower limbs in the presence of eEmc [19]. Within a matter of days or weeks of training for a specific motor task with eEmc for about 1 hour per day these individuals have recovered significant levels of control of movement with regard to the timing of the effort, rate of force developed, and the level of force that can be generated at individual joints. When individuals with motor incomplete, but severe, paralysis are given instructions to move a specific joint, there often is a mass action simultaneous response of flexor and extensors of both legs, indicating a significant loss of the ability to activate and coordinate the desired motor pools needed to generate the intended motor event [89, 90]. The most probable explanation for the newly realized volitional function is that most of the details of the neural pathways generating the volitional demands are in the spinal circuitry. Thus, perhaps the supraspinal signals can be general as long as there is access to the fine control potential intrinsic to the spinal circuitry—that is the combination of proprioceptive and cutaneous input is a central component of the networks underlying fine motor control.

Spinal circuitry reorganization

The potential for reorganization of spinal circuits completely independent of supraspinal influence has been shown in numerous experimental models. This learning-related phenomenon reflects the reorganization potential for performing behaviours ranging from a spinal rat learning to control paw position to avoid shock to spinal cats learning to stand and step and to avoid obstacles and other mechanical perturbations during stepping [13, 14, 44–50]. Biochemical adaptive events associated with spinal cord injury and subsequent network reorganization associated with inhibitory processes after the loss of supraspinal input and its return to near normal levels after stand and step training have been reported [3, 69, 75, 91–93]. Several experiments have shown that the number and kind of interneurons activated during stepping are reduced in spinal animals that have been trained to step and the number of interneurons activated is indirectly related to the skill level regained in stepping after a complete spinal cord transection (i.e., fewer neurons are activated in the animals having the greatest skill in stepping [4, 8]).

Hypothetically, after a severe spinal cord injury and after newly acquired supraspinal input to the spinal circuitry, there will have been significant and permanent changes in the way the two networks interact. Each network will have experienced extensive reorganization [94]. The challenge is to provide a mechanism for these two sources of control to find new solutions, that is to activate novel combinations of neurons to generate movements that may not have been within their domain in the non-injured nervous system. After an injury there is a 'new' nervous system. Novel combinations of neurons can be engaged to generate a motor task that normally would not have occurred in the absence of an injury.

Outlook

The content of this chapter on models of spinal cord injury has focused on a wide range of experimental strategies using principally mice, rats, cats, and humans. This focus is primarily because these are the animal models that have most recently contributed to the evolution of the concepts associated with spinal cord neuromodulation. It is fair to say that virtually all of the neuromodulatory concepts discussed and the demonstrations of how these concepts are now being applied to humans with a severe spinal cord injury were derived almost solely from this range of animal models. The underlying biology that has led to these concepts, however, is based on studies using even a wider range of different animal models over a period of decades. Although we have not discussed any of the basic findings from the lamprey model [95], this particular early vertebrate model has served as the core of much of the ideas discussed in this chapter. Obviously locomotion in the lamprey and humans differs substantially at the 'systems' level, but there are remarkable similarities at the synaptic, cellular, and subcellular levels, and even to some degree at the systems level that have provided the basic biological core of the more complex integrative systems in humans and other mammals. The concept of automaticity at its most basic level certainly can be attributed to the concept of central pattern generation, a phenomenon that occurs in multiple physiological systems and in virtually all multi-cellular organisms. As we learn more about the basic principles controlling the multiple and highly integrated systems in mammals under *in vivo* conditions there undoubtedly will be the emergence of experimental models focusing on species other than those that might be popular at that particular time. An example of this has been the recent emergence in the use of the miniature pig model, the principal reason being the need for an intermediate-sized mammal in developing new technologies that can be applied in efforts to translate basic findings from, for example, the mouse-to-human. The use of any of these animal models does not imply that the experimental results will be identical in the laboratory animal being tested compared to that in human subjects. In fact, in some cases these results can be very misleading if improperly interpreted as being comparable. The view of the present authors is that progress in the development of new strategies to enhance recovery from paralysis using humans as the only experimental subjects is a far less effective strategy than using a wide range of species for testing specific basic neural control mechanisms, some of which are highly likely to result in effective translation from animal models to the human. The success of this approach is likely to become even more effective as our technology improves so that more fundamental questions can be addressed with little or minimal adverse or disruptive effects on human subjects.

Conclusion

This chapter summarizes some of the basic experiments related to neuromodulation of the spinal circuitry using techniques that can generate immediate and/or long-term effects on multiple physiological systems. This neuromodulation can be generated using several different techniques to modulate the spinal circuits electrically (e.g., applying AC currents, electromagnetic), pharmacologically (e.g., using monaminergic agonists), and using specific sources of artificially imposed sensory input to the spinal cord or the sensory input generated by proprioceptive and cutaneous receptors when movements are being generated. In effect, under normal conditions supraspinal centres, including all of the sensory systems being processed by the supraspinal centres, also are continuously modulating the spinal circuitry. This modulation of the spinal circuitry essentially determines how and when it will respond to a particular stimulus or ensemble of stimuli. It appears that the spinal circuitry can be effectively neuromodulated to improve motor function in large part because of the intrinsic automaticity of the spinal circuitry. This automaticity provides the spinal circuitries with the ability to make decisions related to the appropriate activation of selected spinal networks based on the processing of proprioceptive and cutaneous information in real time in an animal or human injured to the extent that there is no remaining supraspinal input. The challenge continues to be to determine the extent to which it is possible to take advantage of this automaticity to regain motor and autonomic function after a severe injury or progressive dysfunction of the nervous system. The results reported herein provide examples suggesting that perhaps this potential has been generally underestimated.

Acknowledgements

This research was supported by the National Institute of Biomedical Imaging and Bioengineering (NIBIB) R01EB007615, the National Institute of Health (NIH) R01NS062009, Christopher and Dana Reeve Foundation, the Walkabout Foundation, and the RFBR grant №13-04-12030 ofi-m as well as by a grant from the Russian Scientific Fund project № 14-45-00024. The work is performed according to the Russian Government Program of Competitive Growth of Kazan Federal University. DISCLOSURE OF INTEREST: V.R.E, D.C.L., R.R.R. and Y.G. hold shareholder interest in NeuroRecovery Technologies. V.R.E is also President and Chair of the company's Board of Directors. V.R.E, D.L., R.R.R. and Y.G. hold certain inventorship rights on intellectual property licensed by The Regents of the University of California to NeuroRecovery Technologies and it's subsidiaries.

References

1. Fong AJ, Cai LL, Otoshi CK, et al. Spinal cord-transected mice learn to step in response to quipazine treatment and robotic training. J Neurosci. 2005;**25**(50):11738–11747.
2. Steuer I, Guertin PA. Spinal cord injury research in mice: 2008 review. Sci World J. 2009;**9**:490–498.
3. Bose PK, Hou J, Parmer R, Reier PJ, Thompson FJ. Altered patterns of reflex excitability, balance, and locomotion following spinal cord injury and locomotor training. Frontiers Physiol. 2012;**3**:258.
4. Courtine G, Gerasimenko Y, van den Brand R, et al. Transformation of nonfunctional spinal circuits into functional states after the loss of brain input. Nat Neurosci. 2009;**12**(10):1333–1342.
5. Courtine G, Song B, Roy RR, et al. Recovery of supraspinal control of stepping via indirect propriospinal relay connections after spinal cord injury. Nat Med. 2008;**14**(1):69–74.
6. Giszter SF, Hockensmith G, Ramakrishnan A, Udoekwere UI. How spinalized rats can walk: biomechanics, cortex, and hindlimb muscle scaling—implications for rehabilitation. Ann NY Acad Sci. 2010;**1198**:279–293.
7. Hillen BK, Abbas JJ, Jung R. Accelerating locomotor recovery after incomplete spinal injury. Ann NY Acad Sci. 2013;**1279**:164–174.
8. Ichiyama RM, Courtine G, Gerasimenko YP, et al. Step training reinforces specific spinal locomotor circuitry in adult spinal rats. J Neurosci. 2008;**28**(29):7370–7375.
9. Ichiyama RM, Gerasimenko YP, Zhong H, Roy RR, Edgerton VR. Hindlimb stepping movements in complete spinal rats induced by epidural spinal cord stimulation. Neurosci Lett. 2005;**383**(3):339–344.
10. See PA, de Leon RD. Robotic loading during treadmill training enhances locomotor recovery in rats spinally transected as neonates. J Neurophysiol. 2013;**110**(3):760–767.
11. Shah PK, Garcia-Alias G, Choe J, et al. Use of quadrupedal step training to re-engage spinal interneuronal networks and improve locomotor function after spinal cord injury. Brain. 2013;**136**(Pt 11):3362–3377.
12. Shah PK, Gerasimenko Y, Shyu A, et al. Variability in step training enhances locomotor recovery after a spinal cord injury. Eur J Neurosci. 2012;**36**(1):2054–2062.
13. de Leon RD, Hodgson JA, Roy RR, Edgerton VR. Full weight-bearing hindlimb standing following stand training in the adult spinal cat. J Neurophysiol. 1998;**80**(1):83–91.
14. de Leon RD, Hodgson JA, Roy RR, Edgerton VR. Locomotor capacity attributable to step training versus spontaneous recovery after spinalization in adult cats. J Neurophysiol. 1998;**79**(3):1329–1340.
15. Murray M, Goldberger ME. Restitution of function and collateral sprouting in the cat spinal cord: the partially hemisected animal. J Comp Neurol. 1974;**158**(1):19–36.
16. Rossignol S, Frigon A. Recovery of locomotion after spinal cord injury: some facts and mechanisms. Ann Rev Neurosci. 2011;**34**:413–440.
17. Dietz V. Spinal cord pattern generators for locomotion. Clin Neurophysiol. 2003;**114**(8):1379–1389.
18. Dietz V. Neuronal plasticity after a human spinal cord injury: positive and negative effects. Exp Neurol. 2012;**235**(1):110–115.
19. Harkema S, Gerasimenko Y, Hodes J, et al. Effect of epidural stimulation of the lumbosacral spinal cord on voluntary movement,

standing, and assisted stepping after motor complete paraplegia: a case study. Lancet. 2011;**377**(9781):1938–1947.

20. Jilge B, Minassian K, Rattay F, et al. Initiating extension of the lower limbs in subjects with complete spinal cord injury by epidural lumbar cord stimulation. Exp Brain Res. 2004;**154**(3):308–326.

21. Grillner S. Control of locomotion in bipeds, tetrapods, and fish. In: Brookhart, JM and Mountcastle VB (eds.) Handbook of Physiology, Section 1, The Nervous System, Volume II, Motor Control, Part 1. American Physiological Society, Bethesda, MD, 1981, pp. 1179–1236.

22. Gurfinkel VS, Levik YS, Kazennikov OV, Selionov VA. Locomotor-like movements evoked by leg muscle vibration in humans. Eur J Neurosci. 1998;**10**(5):1608–1612.

23. Gerasimenko Y, Gorodnichev R, Machueva E, et al. Novel and direct access to the human locomotor spinal circuitry. J Neurosci. 2010;**30**(10):3700–3708.

24. Gerasimenko Y, Roy RR, Edgerton VR. Epidural stimulation: comparison of the spinal circuits that generate and control locomotion in rats, cats and humans. Exp Neurol. 2008;**209**(2):417–425.

25. Shik ML, Severin FV, Orlovskii GN. [Control of walking and running by means of electric stimulation of the midbrain]. Biofizika. 1966;**11**(4):659–666.

26. Grillner S, Zangger P. On the central generation of locomotion in the low spinal cat. Exp Brain Res. 1979;**34**(2):241–261.

27. Edgerton VR, Grillner S, Sjostrom A, Zangger P. Central generation of locomotion in vertebrates. In: Herman R, Grillner S, Stein PSG, Stuart DG (eds) Neural Control of Locomotion. Plenum Publishing Corporation, New York, 1976, pp. 439–464.

28. Grillner S, Jessell TM. Measured motion: searching for simplicity in spinal locomotor networks. Curr Opin Neurobiol. 2009;**19**(6):572–586.

29. Grillner S, Wallen P, Saitoh K, Kozlov A, Robertson B. Neural bases of goal-directed locomotion in vertebrates—an overview. Brain Res Rev. 2008;**57**(1):2–12.

30. Jordan LM, Slawinska U. Chapter 12—modulation of rhythmic movement: control of coordination. Progr Brain Res. 2011;**188**:181–195.

31. Kiehn O. Locomotor circuits in the mammalian spinal cord. Ann Rev Neurosci. 2006;**29**:279–306.

32. Kiehn O. Development and functional organization of spinal locomotor circuits. Curr Opin Neurobiol. 2011;**21**(1):100–109.

33. Lavrov I, Courtine G, Dy CJ, et al. Facilitation of stepping with epidural stimulation in spinal rats: role of sensory input. J Neurosci. 2008;**28**(31):7774–7780.

34. Minassian K, Jilge B, Rattay F, et al. Stepping-like movements in humans with complete spinal cord injury induced by epidural stimulation of the lumbar cord: electromyographic study of compound muscle action potentials. Spinal Cord. 2004;**42**(7):401–416.

35. Shapkova E. Spinal locomotor capability revealed by electrical stimulation of the lumbar enlargement in paraplegic patients. In: Latash MLM (ed.) Progress in Motor Control. Human Kinetics, Champaign, Illinois. 2004, p. 253–289.

36. Iwahara T, Atsuta Y, Garcia-Rill E, Skinner RD. Spinal cord stimulation-induced locomotion in the adult cat. Brain Res Bull. 1992;**28**(1):99–105.

37. Bogacheva IN, Musienko PE, Shcherbakova NA, Moshonkina TR, Savokhin AA, Gerasimenko Iu P. [Analysis of locomotor activity in decerebrated cats during electromagnetic and epidural electrical spinal cord stimulation]. Rossiiskii fiziologicheskii zhurnal imeni IM Sechenova/Rossiiskaia akademiia nauk. 2012;**98**(9):1079–1093.

38. Selionov VA, Ivanenko YP, Solopova IA, Gurfinkel VS. Tonic central and sensory stimuli facilitate involuntary air-stepping in humans. J. Neurophysiol. 2009;**101**(6):2847–2858.

39. Courtine G, van den Brand R, Roy RR, Edgerton VR. Multi-system neurorehabilitation in rodents with spinal cord injury. In: Dietz V, Nef T, Rymer Z (eds) *Neurorehabilitation Technology.* Springer-Verlag, London, 2012, pp. 3–21.

40. Herman R, He J, D'Luzansky S, Willis W, Dilli S. Spinal cord stimulation facilitates functional walking in a chronic, incomplete spinal cord injured. Spinal Cord. 2002;**40**(2):65–68.

41. Musienko P, Heutschi J, Friedli L, van den Brand R, Courtine G. Multi-system neurorehabilitative strategies to restore motor functions following severe spinal cord injury. Exp Neurol. 2012;**235**(1):100–109.

42. Musienko P, van den Brand R, Marzendorfer O, et al. Controlling specific locomotor behaviors through multidimensional monoaminergic modulation of spinal circuitries. J Neurosci. 2011;**31**(25):9264–9278.

43. Musienko PE, Zelenin PV, Lyalka VF, Gerasimenko YP, Orlovsky GN, Deliagina TG. Spinal and supraspinal control of the direction of stepping during locomotion. J Neurosci. 2012;**32**(48):17442–17453.

44. Barbeau H, Rossignol S. Recovery of locomotion after chronic spinalization in the adult cat. Brain Res. 1987;**412**(1):84–95.

45. Grau JW, Crown ED, Ferguson AR, Washburn SN, Hook MA, Miranda RC. Instrumental learning within the spinal cord: underlying mechanisms and implications for recovery after injury. Behav Cogn Neurosci Rev. 2006;**5**(4):191–239.

46. Hodgson JA, Roy RR, de Leon R, Dobkin B, Edgerton VR. Can the mammalian lumbar spinal cord learn a motor task? Med Sci Sports Exerc. 1994;**26**(12):1491–1497.

47. Jindrich DL, Joseph MS, Otoshi CK, et al. Spinal learning in the adult mouse using the Horridge paradigm. J Neurosci Methods. 2009;**182**(2):250–254.

48. Lovely RG, Gregor RJ, Roy RR, Edgerton VR. Effects of training on the recovery of full-weight-bearing stepping in the adult spinal cat. Exp Neurol. 1986;**92**(2):421–435.

49. Lovely RG, Gregor RJ, Roy RR, Edgerton VR. Weight-bearing hindlimb stepping in treadmill-exercised adult spinal cats. Brain Res. 1990;**514**(2):206–218.

50. Zhong H, Roy RR, Nakada KK, et al. Accommodation of the spinal cat to a tripping perturbation. Frontiers Physiol. 2012;**3**:112.

51. Roy RR, Harkema SJ, Edgerton VR. Basic concepts of activity-based interventions for improved recovery of motor function after spinal cord injury. Arch Phys Med Rehabil. 2012;**93**(9):1487–1497.

52. Musienko P, Courtine G, Tibbs JE, et al. Somatosensory control of balance during locomotion in decerebrated cat. J Neurophysiol. 2012;**107**(8):2072–2082.

53. Horst M, Heutschi J, van den Brand R, et al. Multisystem neuroprosthetic training improves bladder function after severe spinal cord injury. J Urol. 2013;**189**(2):747–753.

54. Gad PN, Roy RR, Zhong H, Lu DC, Gerasimenko YP, Edgerton VR. Initiation of bladder voiding with epidural stimulation in paralyzed, step trained rats. PLoS One. 2014;**9**(9):e108184.

55. Fowler CJ, Griffiths D, de Groat WC. The neural control of micturition. Nat Rev Neurosci. 2008;**9**(6):453–466.

56. Sakakibara R, Kishi M, Tsuyusaki Y, Tateno F, Uchiyama T, Yamamoto T. Neurology and the bladder: how to assess and manage neurogenic bladder dysfunction. With particular references to neural control of micturition. Rinsho Shinkeigaku [Clinical Neurology]. 2013;**53**(3):181–190.

57. de Groat WC, Yoshimura N. Mechanisms underlying the recovery of lower urinary tract function following spinal cord injury. Progr Brain Res. 2006;**152**:59–84.

58. Seki S, Sasaki K, Fraser MO, et al. Immunoneutralization of nerve growth factor in lumbosacral spinal cord reduces bladder hyperreflexia in spinal cord injured rats. J Urol. 2002;**168**(5):2269–2274.

59. Seki S, Sasaki K, Igawa Y, et al. Suppression of detrusor-sphincter dyssynergia by immunoneutralization of nerve growth factor in lumbosacral spinal cord in spinal cord injured rats. J Urol. 2004;**171**(1):478–482.

60. Vizzard MA. Neurochemical plasticity and the role of neurotrophic factors in bladder reflex pathways after spinal cord injury. Progr Brain Res. 2006;**152**:97–115.

61. Brady CM, Apostolidis A, Yiangou Y, et al. P2X3-immunoreactive nerve fibres in neurogenic detrusor overactivity and the effect of intravesical resiniferatoxin. Eur Urol. 2004;46(2):247–253.

62. Smet PJ, Moore KH, Jonavicius J. Distribution and colocalization of calcitonin gene-related peptide, tachykinins, and vasoactive intestinal peptide in normal and idiopathic unstable human urinary bladder. Lab Invest. 1997;77(1):37–49.

63. Ward P, Herrity A, Smith R, et al. Novel multi-system functional gains via task specific training in spinal cord injured male rats. J Neurotrauma. 2013;31(9):819–833.

64. Chew DJ, Zhu L, Delivopoulos E, et al. A microchannel neuroprosthesis for bladder control after spinal cord injury in rat. Sci Transl Med. 2013;5(210):210ra155.

65. Angeli CA, Edgerton VR, Gerasimenko YP, Harkema SJ. Altering spinal cord excitability enables voluntary movements after chronic complete paralysis in humans. Brain. 137; 1394-1409.

66. Edgerton R, Roy RR, de Leon R, Tillakaratne N, Hodgson JA. Does motor learing occur in the spinal cord? The Neuroscientist. 1997;3:287–294.

67. Edgerton VR, Courtine G, Gerasimenko YP, et al. Training locomotor networks. Brain Res Rev. 2008;57(1):241–254.

68. Edgerton VR, de Leon RD, Tillakaratne N, Recktenwald MR, Hodgson JA, Roy RR. Use-dependent plasticity in spinal stepping and standing. Adv Neurol. 1997;72:233–247.

69. Edgerton VR, Leon RD, Harkema SJ, Hodgson JA, London N, Reinkensmeyer DJ, et al. Retraining the injured spinal cord. J Physiol. 2001;533(Pt 1):15–22.

70. Edgerton VR, Tillakaratne NJ, Bigbee AJ, de Leon RD, Roy RR. Plasticity of the spinal neural circuitry after injury. Annu Rev Neurosci. 2004;27:145–167.

71. Fong AJ, Roy RR, Ichiyama RM, et al. Recovery of control of posture and locomotion after a spinal cord injury: solutions staring us in the face. Progr Brain Res. 2009;175:393–418.

72. Hultborn H, Nielsen JB. Spinal control of locomotion—from cat to man. Acta Physiol. 2007;189(2):111–121.

73. Ichiyama RM, Gerasimenko Y, Jindrich DL, Zhong H, Roy RR, Edgerton VR. Dose dependence of the 5-HT agonist quipazine in facilitating spinal stepping in the rat with epidural stimulation. Neurosci Lett. 2008;438(3):281–285.

74. Maier IC, Schwab ME. Sprouting, regeneration and circuit formation in the injured spinal cord: factors and activity. Philos Trans Roy Soc Lond B, Biol Sci. 2006;361(1473):1611–1634.

75. Rossignol S, Barriere G, Frigon A, et al. Plasticity of locomotor sensorimotor interactions after peripheral and/or spinal lesions. Brain Res Rev. 2008;57(1):228–240.

76. Rossignol S, Frigon A, Barriere G, et al. Chapter 16—spinal plasticity in the recovery of locomotion. Progr Brain Res. 2011;188:229–241.

77. Shik ML. Recognizing propriospinal and reticulospinal systems of initiation of stepping. Motor Control. 1997;1:310–313.

78. de Leon RD, Reinkensmeyer DJ, Timoszyk WK, London NJ, Roy RR, Edgerton VR. Use of robotics in assessing the adaptive capacity of the rat lumbar spinal cord. Progr Brain Res. 2002;137:141–149.

79. Harkema SJ, Hurley SL, Patel UK, Requejo PS, Dobkin BH, Edgerton VR. Human lumbosacral spinal cord interprets loading during stepping. J Neurophysiol. 1997;77(2):797–811.

80. Timoszyk WK, Nessler JA, Acosta C, et al. Hindlimb loading determines stepping quantity and quality following spinal cord transection. Brain Res. 2005;1050(1–2):180–189.

81. Bareyre FM, Kerschensteiner M, Raineteau O, Mettenleiter TC, Weinmann O, Schwab ME. The injured spinal cord spontaneously forms a new intraspinal circuit in adult rats. Nat Neurosci. 2004;7(3):269–277.

82. Jarosiewicz B, Masse NY, Bacher D, et al. Advantages of closed-loop calibration in intracortical brain-computer interfaces for people with tetraplegia. J Neural Eng. 2013;10(4):046012.

83. Jankowska E, Maxwell DJ, Bannatyne BA. On coupling and decoupling of spinal interneuronal networks. Arch Ital Biol. 2007;145(3–4):235–250.

84. Zaporozhets E, Cowley KC, Schmidt BJ. Neurochemical excitation of propriospinal neurons facilitates locomotor command signal transmission in the lesioned spinal cord. J Neurophysiol. 2011;105(6):2818–2829.

85. Dimitrijevic MR. Residual motor functions in spinal cord injury. Adv Neurol. 1988;47:138–155.

86. Kakulas BA. Neuropathology: the foundation for new treatments in spinal cord injury. Spinal Cord. 2004;42(10):549–563.

87. Sherwood AM, Dimitrijevic MR, McKay WB. Evidence of subclinical brain influence in clinically complete spinal cord injury: discomplete SCI. J Neurol Sci. 1992;110(1–2):90–98.

88. van den Brand R, Heutschi J, Barraud Q, et al. Restoring voluntary control of locomotion after paralyzing spinal cord injury. Science. 2012;336(6085):1182–1185.

89. Alexeeva N, Sames C, Jacobs PL, et al. Comparison of training methods to improve walking in persons with chronic spinal cord injury: a randomized clinical trial. J Spinal Cord Med. 2011;34(4):362–379.

90. Maegele M, Muller S, Wernig A, Edgerton VR, Harkema SJ. Recruitment of spinal motor pools during voluntary movements versus stepping after human spinal cord injury. J Neurotrauma. 2002;19(10):1217–1229.

91. de Leon RD, Tamaki H, Hodgson JA, Roy RR, Edgerton VR. Hindlimb locomotor and postural training modulates glycinergic inhibition in the spinal cord of the adult spinal cat. J Neurophysiol. 1999;82(1):359–369.

92. Tillakaratne NJ, de Leon RD, Hoang TX, Roy RR, Edgerton VR, Tobin AJ. Use-dependent modulation of inhibitory capacity in the feline lumbar spinal cord. J Neurosci. 2002;22(8):3130–3143.

93. Tillakaratne NJ, Mouria M, Ziv NB, Roy RR, Edgerton VR, Tobin AJ. Increased expression of glutamate decarboxylase (GAD(67)) in feline lumbar spinal cord after complete thoracic spinal cord transection. J Neurosci Res. 2000;60(2):219–230.

94. Beauparlant J, van den Brand R, Barraud Q, Friedli L, Musienko P, Dietz V, et al. Undirected compensatory plasticity contributes to neuronal dysfunction after severe spinal cord injury. Brain. 2013;136(Pt 11):3347–3361.

95. Grillner S, Kozlov A, Dario P, et al. Modeling a vertebrate motor system: pattern generation, steering and control of body orientation. Progr Brain Res. 2007;165:221–234.

96. Gad P, Woodbridge J, Lavrov I, et al. Forelimb EMG-based trigger to control an electronic spinal bridge to enable hindlimb stepping after a complete spinal cord lesion in rats. J Neuroeng Rehabil. 2012;9:38.

97. Gerasimenko Y, Musienko P, Bogacheva I, et al. Propriospinal bypass of the serotonergic system that can facilitate stepping. J Neurosci. 2009;29(17):5681–5689.

98. Gorodnichev RM, Machueva EN, Pivovarova EA, et al. [Novel method for activation of the locomotor circuitry in human]. Fiziologiia Cheloveka. 2010;36(6):95–103.

99. Gorodnichev RM, Pivovarova EA, Pukhov A, et al. [Transcutaneous electrical stimulation of the spinal cord: non-invasive tool for activation of locomotor circuitry in human]. Fiziologiia Cheloveka. 2012;38(2):46–56.

CHAPTER 14

Stem cell application in neurorehabilitation

Sebastian Jessberger, Armin Curt, and Roger Barker

Introduction

Over the last 30 years major advances have been made in the field of neural restoration and this includes not only better strategies for endogenous repair but also the ability to actively intervene through neural grafting, for example (see Table 14.1). This revolution stems from a better understanding of the processes underlying intrinsic repair, the realisation that endogenous processes such as neurogenesis still occur in the adult mammalian brain [1], and that neurotrophic factors can be used to encourage cell survival and fibre outgrowth in diseased cells within the central nervous system (CNS). In addition, we now recognise that some cellular transplants can survive in the adult CNS and make and receive connections with functional benefits to the grafted animal. In this chapter we explore various aspects of these processes including the role of adult neurogenesis in health and disease as well as the cell-based approaches that have been used to treat a whole variety of CNS disorders but especially Parkinson's disease (PD) Huntington's disease (HD) and spinal cord injury (see Table 14.2).

Basic biology of stem cells

Endogenous neurogenesis in the adult mammalian brain

It has been a long-held concept in the neurosciences that the generation of neurons tapers off with the end of embryonic development. For decades the leading opinion in the field was that the adult mammalian brain is not capable of generating new neurons throughout life due to the absence of any neurogenic, dividing cells—neural stem cells (NSCs). It was assumed that the neuronal networks and circuitries in the mature CNS are too complex to allow for the maturation and integration of newborn neuronal cells. Thus, the most common strategy to ameliorate disease symptoms and promote rehabilitation in the context of neuropsychiatric disease was to pharmacologically treat abnormalities in transmitter networks and enhance functional plasticity within the surviving networks and brain areas. However, the concept that the adult brain loses its capacity to regenerate was challenged in the mid 1960s, when the first experiments suggested that there may be proliferating cells in the restricted areas of the adult brain that appeared to have the potential to generate new neurons [2, 3]. In these pioneering studies by Altman, Kaplan, and others, radioactively labelled thymidine was used to visualize proliferating cells doubling their DNA content prior to cytokinesis. However, at this time it was technically extremely difficult to truly confirm that: (i) a cell is newborn and (ii) differentiates into a neuron. However, the idea that the adult brain may even be capable of generating new neurons was fuelled by the findings that cells could be isolated and propagated in vitro that showed NSC properties meaning that these cells were able to self-renew and to generate neurons in the culture dish [4]. This technical breakthrough, leading to the acceptance that neurogenesis occurs in the mammalian brain throughout life, came with the use of thymidine-analogues (such as bromodeoxyuridine; BrdU) that could be visualized using antibodies in combination with techniques to label neuronal cells using confocal microscopy (e.g. [5]).

With this strategy—that was later complemented using specific retroviruses that selectively label dividing cells and their progeny and transgenesis-based approaches—two main neurogenic regions in the adult mammalian brain could be identified: the subventricular zone (SVZ) lining the lateral ventricles out of which newborn cells migrate along the rostral migratory stream (RMS) towards the olfactory bulb (OB) where they differentiate into several types of mostly gamma-aminobutyric acid (GABA) ergic olfactory neurons, and the subgranular zone (SGZ) of the hippocampal dentate gyrus (DG) where exclusively glutamatergic, excitatory granule cells are generated [6]. In these two neurogenic areas, NSCs (with certain astrocytic properties) that are largely quiescent (i.e. do rarely divide) under normal conditions, give rise to more proliferative progenitors that generate new, immature neurons [7]. These new neurons mature structurally and functionally over the course of several weeks before they integrate into the pre-existing neural circuitries in the OB and DG. Interestingly, the functional properties of young, immature neurons substantially differ from their older progeny that are generated during embryonic development. These newborn cells are much more excitable and display a higher degree of plasticity which is believed to be the reason why the adult brain invests in the energetically demanding exercise of supporting these two neurogenic (and highly plastic) regions [7].

Notably, the number of neurons generated is not static but rather is dynamically regulated. Positive stimuli, such as physical exercise and environmental enrichment, strongly enhance the number of newborn neurons, whereas negative regulators such as stress and aging substantially decrease neurogenesis [7]. Initially, based on these correlative data, it was hypothesized that adult

Table 14.1 Approaches to cell-based repair of the CNS

Approach	Advantages	Disadvantages	Example
Promotion of intrinsic repair through increased neurogenesis	Uses an innate system so is more physiological No tumourigenic potential	Neurogenesis is only found at a few restricted sites in the adult CNS Limited capacity to upregulate this process	Depression
Exogenous transplants of cells	Many choices in terms of cell that can be used each with their own merits Unlimited supply in theory Many different cell types can be generated to treat multiple different conditions	Ethical concerns with some cell sources Tumourigenic and cell proliferation/migration concerns with some cell types Immunogenic problems with using non-autologous cells; Risk of infection with cultured cells Limited ability to get cells to truly adopt phenotype needed Often need to be delivered by invasive neurosurgical procedure with all the risks associated with it	Parkinson's disease Huntington's disease Spinal cord injury
Direct transdifferentiation of cells in situ	No cell injections needed	Ability to do this effectively and therapeutically is unproven May damage or kill cells	Parkinson's disease

neurogenesis may be not only important for physiological brain function but may also contribute to certain disease processes—for example, in the context of affective disorders such as major depression, as well as neurodegenerative disorders [8]. Indeed, in mouse models of stress and depression it could be shown that certain antidepressants strongly enhanced neurogenesis and that their behavioural effects depend on this pharmacologically enhanced neurogenesis [9]. Besides, a contribution of altered or failing neurogenesis to certain disease processes, the identification of endogenous NSCs also opened up the possibility of activating and recruiting NSCs or their neuronal progeny to lesioned or injured brain areas to replace lost neurons: for example, in the

context of ischaemic stroke. Thus, targeting endogenous NSCs that generate new neurons throughout life presented a novel treatment option to improve or restore brain function in a number of CNS diseases and disorders.

Exogenous stem cells for neural repair

There have been numerous experimental attempts, as well as in the clinic, over the last decades to replace lost neurons not only by mobilizing endogenous NSCs but also by transplanting exogenous cells with the capacity to produce new neurons into the diseased or injured brain. For example, fetal progenitors have been used to replace lost dopaminergic neurons in the context of PD (see later). However, it became evident soon on that heterogeneity of clinical response and difficulties in standardizing cell isolation and cell quality made it extremely challenging to use fetal human progenitors as a standard treatment option to replace dopamine-based pharmacotherapy. Thus, new cellular sources had to be identified and developed that could restore and replace specific neural structures lost to brain injury/degeneration.

Much hope to find a reliable source for neuronal cell replacement was invested in human embryonic stem cells (ESCs). ESCs are derived from the inner cell mass early during embryonic development, and represent a cell type that shows pluripotency—which means that these cells are capable of generating all tissues of the organism besides the trophoblast—along with the capacity for almost indefinite self-renewal. Notably, there has been substantial progress over the last decades to develop protocols to direct ESCs toward specific neuronal lineages, such as dopaminergic neurons (e.g. [10]). Furthermore, the protocols have been substantially improved to reduce the risk of transplanting undifferentiated, and thus dividing, ESCs that have the potential to form tumours within the transplanted tissue, so called teratomas. Nevertheless, the clinical use of ESCs is still challenged by ethical concerns (given that human ESCs are derived from the progeny of in vitro fertilized oocytes) and the fact that transplanted ESCs are non-autologous transplants, requiring at least a certain degree of

Table 14.2 Disorders of the CNS being considered for neural repair

Inborn errors of metabolism/myelination
- Battens' diseases; Perlizeus Merzbacher

Neurodegenerative disorders
- Parkinson's disease; multiple system atrophy; Huntington's disease; motorneuron disease

Neuroimmunological disorders
- Multiple sclerosis

Vascular diseases/disorders
- Stroke

Traumatic injuries
- Spinal cord injury

Neuropsychiatric conditions
- Depression

Other
- Epilepsy
- Retinal disease/macular degeneration

immunosuppression to prevent rejection of the transplanted tissue by the host.

Given these limitations, the discovery that virtually every somatic cell can be reprogrammed to adopt a pluripotent state by introducing defined transcription factors opened novel possibilities for patient-specific cell replacement strategies. These cells, called induced pluripotent stem cells (iPSCs), can be easily generated from each individual (e.g. by a simple skin biopsy and isolating fibroblasts that are then subjected to reprogramming) yielding an isogenic and patient-selective source for therapeutic cell replacement strategies [11].

In the following sections we will briefly review the evidence that altered neurogenesis in the adult brain contributes to neuropsychiatric disease processes and how the mobilization of endogenous or the use of exogenous, transplanted stem cells may provide novel treatment options in the context of neurodegeneration, specifically in PD and HD, as well as other CNS disorders such as spinal cord injury.

Therapeutic targeting of neural stem cells in neuropsychiatric disease

Adult hippocampal neurogenesis and affective disorders

Affective disorders such as major depression represent a major social and financial burden to Western societies, given their high prevalence. Even though a number of classes of antidepressant drugs have been in clinical use for decades, there remains a substantial fraction of patients with therapy-resistant disease, indicating the need to (i) better understand the aetiology and neural consequences of affective disorders and (ii) develop novel treatment strategies. One of the key risk factors (besides age, see 'Age-associated cognitive decline') to develop affective disorders is stress, which was found to dramatically reduce neurogenesis [12]. In combination with the findings that a structural hallmark of patients suffering from depression is a reduction of hippocampal volume as measured by non-invasive imaging approaches, this initiated a large number of studies aiming at understanding a potential link between the onset or maintenance of affective disorders and adult hippocampal neurogenesis [9]. Strikingly, a number of antidepressants such as selective serotonin re-uptake inhibitors (SSRIs) enhance the number of neurons generated and depend at least partially on neurogenesis for their efficacy (e.g., [13]. Supporting the potential contribution of failing neurogenesis to the depressive disease process has been the fact that many antidepressants show a latency of 2 to 4 weeks between being taken and having a therapeutic effect—a time that may reflect the antidepressant-induced generation, maturation, and functional integration of newborn neurons [9].

However, genetic enhancement of hippocampal neurogenesis turned out to not be sufficient for theirdirect mood-regulating effects, even though this needs to be studied in more detail [14]. Furthermore, more studies are required that investigate if new neurons directly affect mood or are only indirectly contributing to affect through modulation of hippocampus-dependent cognition. In summary, it seems reasonable to speculate that neurogenesis in the adult hippocampus represents a novel therapeutic target to ameliorate disease symptoms in major depressive disorders. On the other hand, it is unlikely that hippocampal neurogenesis is the major and sole cause whose alterations may lead to or, if pharmacologically targeted, cure depression. Most importantly, more evidence needs to be produced that neurogenesis may indeed be affected in patients suffering from affective disorders.

Age-associated cognitive decline and reduced neurogenesis

Ageing is associated with a substantial decline in several cognitive domains that may eventually lead to impairments in activities in daily living [15, 16]. Interestingly, the number of neurons that are generated in the adult hippocampus (and SVZ/OB system) dramatically decreases with advancing age (without coming to a complete stop) [1, 7]. Furthermore, the number of neurons born in older age does correlate with the performance of rodents on hippocampus-dependent learning tasks [17]. Thus, it has been speculated that hippocampal neurogenesis may be a critical mediator of cognition with aging. This idea has been supported for example by imaging-based findings in humans that the first structure showing functional and structural alterations in cognitively challenged, aged individuals is indeed the hippocampal dentate gyrus [18]. In addition, known regulators of neurogenesis, such as running and environmental enrichment, have turned out to be effective in enhancing neurogenesis in aged rodents, which was again associated with improved performance in hippocampus-dependent learning tasks [19, 20].

Current projects aim to elucidate the cellular and molecular mechanisms that are responsible for the age-dependent drop of neurogenesis. Furthermore, it remains unclear if enhancing neurogenesis is sufficient to ameliorate cognition in advanced age. Be that as it may, the observed association between cognitive decline and decreased neurogenesis suggests a mechanism at least partially explaining the drop in hippocampus-dependent cognition with old age.

Altered neurogenesis in epilepsy

Besides the aforementioned diseases that reduce the amount of neurons, there are also disease states that at least transiently enhance the number of neurons generated. For example it has been shown that neurogenesis is dramatically enhanced in rodent models of temporal lobe epilepsy (TLE) [21]. Notably, not only the number of neurons generated is enhanced: epileptic activity also leads to ectopic migration of newborn granule cells into the hilar region of the dentate gyrus and the aberrant formation of hilar basal dendrites that form ectopic synapses and potentially impair proper synaptic transmission and connectivity within the dentate circuitry [22, 23]. Strikingly, it has also been shown that ectopic neurogenesis is sufficient to drive epileptogenesis, further supporting the findings that enhanced, but massively altered neurogenesis in the context of TLE, is potentially a contributing disease factor [24]. However, neurogenesis may not only be involved in the establishment of epileptogenic circuitries as it has also been shown that in more advanced or chronic disease stages, neurogenesis is strongly downregulated and may represent one factor responsible for cognitive decline that is commonly observed in patients affected by chronic or therapy refractory forms of TLE [25]. Thus, drugs aiming to enhance neurogenesis in the context of affective disorders or ageing may also turn out to be effective in ameliorating cognitive symptoms in advanced stages of TLE by increasing the number of newborn granule cells.

This has been also aimed for in animal models of TLE, through the transplantation of exogenous NSCs into the epileptic hippocampus. First results are promising, even though the invasiveness and associated risks when considering the next steps in taking such a strategy into the clinical setting are substantial [26].

Stem cell-based therapeutic approaches in Parkinson's disease

PD is a common neurodegenerative disorder of the CNS that affects about 1 in 800 people and typically presents around 70 years of age. It has as part of its core pathology the loss of the nigrostriatal dopaminergic neurons and the formation of alpha synuclein-positive Lewy bodies. However, in recent years a number of fundamental new concepts have emerged with respect to PD:

(1) The disease process is not restricted to dopaminergic nigrostriatal neurons but involves many sites within the brain and even neurons outside of the CNS (e.g. in the enteric nervous system) [27].

(2) PD is not simply a disorder affecting motor control but embraces a range of non-motor features, some of which may even precede the onset of the movement disorder (so-called prodromal or promotor PD) [28].

(3) The disease process may even begin in the periphery and then spread into the CNS with alpha synuclein behaving in a prion-like fashion [29].

(4) Whilst the pathogenesis of the disease process may involve protein spread, it is still unknown why people develop PD in the first place although there is now substantial evidence to show that there are major genetic risk factors for getting it [30]. This includes heterozygote mutations in genes coding for glucocerebrosidase (GBA), the gene that leads to the autosomal recessive condition Gaucher's disease [31].

(5) There are now a large number of Mendelian forms of PD described, some of which resemble idiopathic PD both clinically and pathologically [30].

(6) Idiopathic PD is heterogeneous and the basis for this may relate to common genetic variants that are also linked to the risk of getting it in the first place [32, 33].

All of this has had implications for the use of stem cells in the study and treatment of PD in two main ways;

(i) Disease modelling using iPSCs, typically from patients with Mendelian forms of PD or stem cell lines transfected by the gene of interest [34].

(ii) The fact that neural grafting with dopaminergic cell transplants will only help some patients with PD and then only some of their symptoms and signs—in other words it will never be a treatment for all patients with PD but will only deal with their dopaminergic responsive clinical features [35].

PD disease modelling

iPSCs derived from patients offer a powerful in vitro disease model as these should carry the identical cellular pathological features of the disease in that patient [36]. However, there are a number of key assumptions with this approach. First, that any pathology seen in neurons so derived after a few days or weeks in culture is disease relevant and speaks to the pathology seen in the CNS of the patient that has taken decades to develop. Second, it assumes that the disease process is cell autonomous, as the only cells being studied are the neurons so generated, and it does not, and cannot, interrogate how different cellular players may talk to each other in the disease process (e.g. the role of inflammation). Third, the reprogramming of the cells may remove some of the age-related factors that are critical in the development of PD, given this is the biggest risk factor for PD. Finally, it has to be shown that the neurons so produced are truly authentic neurons of the type wanted. This is especially true for dopaminergic neurons as there are at least 10 subtypes of dopaminergic neurons in the adult brain (A8–A17) [37], all of which show specific electrophysiological, neurochemical, and transcriptional profiles and only some of which are lost in PD [38].

Despite a number of obstacles, several groups have produced PD patient-specific inducible dopaminergic neurons [iDA] derived from iPSCs and early studies found that the differentiated cells did not show any disease-related phenotype [39]. In addition it was noted that residual transgene expression in virus-carrying iPSCs influenced their molecular properties, which has led to the use of derivation methods free of reprogramming factors in the modeling of human disease. Subsequently, it has been shown that iDA derived from iPSCs do display specific PD pathology using cell lines from patients with sporadic and LRRK2-associated PD [40]. As with the earlier study [39], no difference was observed between the iDA from PD patients and controls in the differentiation efficiency, morphology and phenotype after 30 days in culture. However, long-term culture (<75 days) of iDA derived from sporadic PD cases revealed altered morphology, with a decrease in the number and length of neurites and an increased susceptibility to degeneration. iDA from PD patients also exhibit defective autophagosome clearance [39].

While the vast majority of PD cases are idiopathic (>95 %), several causative genes have been identified in families harbouring mendelian forms of the disease [41]. So far, five PD-related genes have been studied using iPS cell technology including neurons derived from patients carrying mutations in the SNCA, *glucocerebrosidase, Leucine-Rich Repeat Kinase-2* (LRRK2), phosphatase and tensin homolog (*PTEN*)-induced putative kinase 1 (*PINK1*), and *Parkin* genes. All of these have shown some pathological changes, although they are often subtle and their relevance to the disease process in the affected patient is unclear.

In recent years, neurons differentiated from iPSCs whilst providing new insights into the cellular mechanisms involved in the pathophysiology of PD, have also been considered for transplantation. However, concerns remain with respect to their safety, mainly due to their proliferative, tumorigenic potential [42]. To overcome this issue, several groups have developed methods that allow direct conversion of human differentiated somatic cells, such as fibroblasts, into functional neurons avoiding any intermediate pluripotent state. The first study to do this converted mouse embryonic and postnatal fibroblasts into functional neurons by the overexpression of three transcription factors (Ascl1, Brn2, and Mytl1) [43]. Subsequently, human fibroblasts have also been successfully converted into functional neurons by overexpressing the same transcription factors [44] and this has now also been done in disease conditions (e.g. Alzheimer's disease patients [45]). For PD, obviously making dopaminergic neurons would be of interest and it has been shown that the addition of two transcription factors specific to the dopaminergic lineage (Lmx1a and FoxA2), along with the three original factors, is sufficient to generate dopaminergic-like neurons [44, 46]. However, the gene expression profiles of these reprogrammed DA neurons differed significantly from primary midbrain DA neurons in these studies and so more recent attempts to generate iDA-like midbrain dopaminergic neurons have used six reprogramming factors (Ascl1, Pitx3, Nurr1, Lmx1a, Foxa2, and En1), as well as the patterning factors Shh and FGF8 [47]. While these iDA expressed many of the relevant markers of dopaminergic neurons, the cells only partially restored dopamine function *in vivo*, and have failed to exhibit similar levels of midbrain transcription levels to those found in embryonic or adult midbrain dopamine neurons [47]. More recently, a combination of five transcription factors (Ascl1, Pitx3, Nurr1, Sox2, and Ngn2) generated iDA that further provided benefit when grafted in the 6-hydroxydopamine [6-OHDA] rat model of PD, suggesting that these reprogrammed cells display functional midbrain dopaminergic neuronal properties [48].

Because the direct conversion does not go through a proliferative state, the quantity of neurons that can be obtained is limited by the accessible number of fibroblasts used as starting material for conversion. Nevertheless, direct conversion of the patient's fibroblasts into relevant neuronal subtypes is very promising for disease modelling and may even ultimately have a role in neural grafting.

Neural transplantation

The core loss of the dopaminergic neurons in PD coupled to the response of patients to dopaminergic drugs led in the 1980s to the idea that this condition could be treated through the transplantation of dopaminergic cells into the diseased basal ganglia. This initially involved autografts of the catecholamine-rich adrenal medulla, although the results were generally disappointing both experimentally and in patients. It was therefore not long before this approach was superseded by transplants of fetal ventral mesencephalic (VM) tissue [49]. This approach involves harvesting the dopaminergic neurons from the developing ventral midbrain and then grafting them into the site where dopamine normally works, namely the striatum. Experimentally, it was shown that this approach worked well when the cells were harvested at the time they normally develop (E13–14 in rats and mice; 6–8 weeks post conception in humans) as the grafted cells could survive, make, and receive connections from the host brain and release dopamine in a regulated manner with functional benefits to the grafted animal. It was on this background that open label studies were undertaken in patients with PD both in Europe and the US. These studies showed that some patients could derive long-term benefit from these grafts and that these clinical improvements correlated with F-dopa-positron emission tomography (PET) imaging showing evidence of dopamine cell survival at the site of implantation. A correlation that was confirmed in a few post mortem studies [50]. The success of this approach gave confidence in some quarters to push on and undertake more rigorous double blind placebo controlled trials even though the results from the open-label studies had been variable and the optimal way of giving the therapy not resolved [51].

These two double-blind placebo-controlled trials that were published in 2001 and 2003 showed that the therapies were ineffective in so much as they failed to deliver on their primary end point [52, 53]. Furthermore, significant numbers of patients developed involuntary movements in the absence of L-dopa but in the presence of the graft; so-called graft-induced dyskinesias. Thus, in many eyes it was shown that this approach did not work, produced side effects, and subsequently it was also shown that the transplants even develop the pathology they are designed to treat [54].

However, a more critical review of the trial data leads one to a rather different conclusion, which is that the fetal VM grafts can work very well in some patients and that understanding why this is the case, will determine whether this whole approach has a future (reviewed in [55]). However, the use of human fetal tissue as the source of cells for grafting is clearly not possible in the long term, for a range of ethical and practical reasons, and as such there is a need to find a more ethically acceptable, readily available source of dopaminergic neurons for grafting [56] (see Table 14.3).

One such cell source is ESCs [57]. However, the use of these cells has been hampered by problems of cell overgrowth; immune rejection, and the ability to truly direct them into authentic nigral dopaminergic neurons. Of late though advances have been made in this area with the production of large numbers of A9-looking nigral neurons, which can survive grafting in animal models of PD with functional benefits and no tumour formation [10]. However, even these cells whilst looking very promising fail to grow axons to the extent that fetal dopaminergic neuroblasts do, and they are also, of course, not free of ethical concerns. As an alternative iDA generated from iPSCs derived from patients' skin fibroblasts are very appealing candidates [58], not only because they circumvent ethical issues but exclude the risk of immune rejection. One other benefit in using iPS cells is the possibility of rejuvenating the cells from an aged patient and thus eliminating the pathologies associated with ageing to restore tissue proliferation and function. The potential of iDA derived from iPS cells for cell replacement therapy has been assessed [59], and whilst encouraging the data is less robust than that seen in ESC-derived dopaminergic neurons. More recently, it has been shown that differentiated inducible neurons [iN] and iDA can have effects in the 6-OHDA lesioned rat, but the effects are modest at best with the cells not looking like mature nigral neurons [46].

Stem cell-based therapeutic approaches in Huntington's Disease (HD)

HD is an autosomal dominant disorder in which the abnormal gene codes for a mutant huntingtin protein that is expressed in every cell of the body. The disease typically presents in mid-life with a combination of motor, cognitive, and psychiatric problems, and it then progresses over a 20–25 year period to death [60]. The pathological changes become more widespread with disease progression, and whilst it was initially thought that the striatum was the main site of pathology in early HD, this view is in need of qualification based on the results of recent studies in early and premanifest HD [61]. These studies have shown that whilst the striatum is an early site of pathology, many other areas are affected, which is important given that the transplant approach to HD has only concentrated on repairing the medium spiny output neurons of the striatum.

Table 14.3 Types of stem cells being considered for neural repair

Type of stem cell	Advantages	Disadvantages
Embryonic stem (ES) cells	Easy to grow Easy to manipulate Unlimited supply	Ethical concerns with their derivation Tumour formation Ability to truly differentiate them into appropriate progeny Immunogenicity
Inducible pluripotent stem (iPS) cells	Allows for autologous grafting Relatively easy to grow to large numbers Capacity to correct genetic defects in them	Tumour formation Problems due to reprogramming Ability to truly differentiate them into appropriate progeny Immunogenicity
Neural precursor cells (NPC)	Allows for autologous grafting if using adult NPC in brain No tumour risk	Ethical concerns with their derivation if derived from fetal or ES source Limited expansion and manipulation compared to ES/iPS cells Ability to truly differentiate them into appropriate progeny Immunogenicity
Bone marrow derived stem cells	Allows for autologous grafting No tumour risk No ethical concerns No immunogenic concerns	Limited expansion possible Ability to truly differentiate them into appropriate neural cells is debatable

In the 1980s–1990s (before the gene for HD was discovered and thus the advent of HD transgenic mice) it was shown experimentally that grafts of fetal striatal tissue placed in the excitotoxic lesioned striatum could survive, differentiate, receive, and make synaptic connections with the host brain and restore behaviour (reviewed in [62])—results which have been less impressive in transgenic animal models of disease [63].

Thus based on the work in the non-transgenic models of HD, early clinical trials were done using human fetal striatal allografts in patients with mild to moderate disease. This was most notably done in the US and Europe and showed mixed results [64].

In the first major study to report, the French group found that three of their five grafted patients showed some transient benefits and that these were linked to evidence of metabolic activity at the site of transplantation [65]. This was followed by a negative study from the group based in South Florida where they found no benefit in any of their patients [66]. This transplant trial used a different approach with respect to the tissue dissection and this could help explain why they did not find any benefits. Interesting of late though, there has been work showing that the grafts in these patients have pathology resembling that seen in the host HD brain [67]. Other studies, most notably one in the UK, have tended to show that the approach using the current protocols are largely unsuccessful [68], although occasional successes have been seen in individual cases [69]. This variability is now being further explored in a large clinical study in France.

Whilst it is unclear whether fetal striatal allografting is useful and even sensible in HD, it has nevertheless led many to look at making striatal output neurons from stem cell sources for possible use in this way. Whilst to date the number of studies doing this have been limited, it is encouraging that the ability to make these cells is possible and that they do have some benefits in animal models of HD [70, 71].

An alternative use of these cells is to study disease pathogenesis in much the same way as has been done in PD. Thus, work has

been done using stem cells transfected with part of the mutant *huntingtin* gene and more recently neurons derived from iPS cells from HD patients have been produced [72]. This has helped confirm some of the key steps in the disease process, and whilst these cells have not as yet been thought of as being useful in autografting therapies, this may evolve if the technologies for correcting gene defects can be perfected.

Finally, the ability to use stem cells to repair the brain from within has always held great attraction since it was first shown that adult neurogenesis occurs in the mammalian brain. In the case of animal models of HD it has been shown that abnormalities exist in hippocampal neurogenesis and this may account for some of the cognitive and affective aspects of the disease [73, 74]. Whilst the basis of this and its relevance to human disease is unknown, it does suggest that intrinsic repair strategies around this system may offer some potential therapeutic avenues worth exploring. In addition there have some reports of increased neurogenesis in the SVZ in HD [75], although again the relevance and significance of this is unknown as are changes in this same system seen in PD and mediated through a midbrain dopaminergic projection and ciliary neurotrophic factor [CNTF] and epidermal growth factor [EGF] signalling pathways (see for example [76]).

Stem cell-based therapeutic approaches in stroke

Stroke is a common disorder that affects many people and encompasses a range of different pathologies from large vessel occlusions with hemispheric loss of tissue to small vessel events causing lacunar infarcts. As a result, there has been much interest in using cells to repair the brain in stroke, although exactly how these cells might do this is debatable. Indeed, the idea has been pursued that they could be used for cell replacement, although this seems unlikely to work given the complexity and diversity of cells lost as part of the original insult. Nevertheless, there has been great interest in developing therapies that either recruit endogenous stem cells for repair or the implantation of exogenous grafts of stem cell derived progenitors that work to enhance repair through some form of paracrine effect.

After experimental stroke in rodents (e.g. occlusion of the middle cerebral artery; MCAO) proliferation of NSCs in the SVZ is strongly enhanced and a small fraction of these newborn cells can migrate away from the SVZ towards the striatum where they differentiate into neuronal cells (e.g. [77]). Similar observations have been made in human samples [78]. However, at this time it remains unclear if stroke-induced endogenous neurogenesis functionally contributes to recovery [79]. Furthermore, it appears that the number of neurons generated is very low. Thus, strategies need to be developed that either enhance the survival or increase the recruitment of newborn cells generated from endogenous NSCs towards the ischaemic lesion.

In the case of neural grafting, this has now evolved to the level of early clinical trials, even though their experimental basis is often not that convincing. The most recent of these is a small open-label study by ReNeuron, in which implants of their immortalized human cortical cell line have been delivered to patients with well-established infarcts. Whilst the data from this study has yet to be published, the preliminary data presented at meetings suggests this approach is safe with some small signal of effect (Muir K, personal communication). This is not the first trial using this approach as various other small open-label studies have been undertaken. However, none have produced robust enough effects to be confident that these cells have a future in the treatment of this common condition (see Bhasin et al [80]).

Stem cell-based therapeutic approaches in multiple sclerosis

Multiple sclerosis (MS) is an autoimmune disease that leads to chronic demyelination followed by axonal loss and a loss of neuronal function. Stem cell-based strategies to ameliorate disease progression and/or clinical symptoms have been trialled (e.g. [81, 82]) and may work through modulation of the autoimmune response and stem cell-mediated regeneration [83, 84].

Interestingly, peripheral administration of neural stem cells (NSCs) and mesenchymal stem cells (MSCs) seems to attenuate the immune reaction in animal models of MS such as experimental autoimmune encephalomyelitis (EAE), most probably by interfering with B-cell proliferation and promoting T-cell anergy. This leads to fewer inflammatory infiltrates and slowed disease progression in EAE. How stem cells exactly mediate these effects remains largely unknown, but given that they can be easily delivered into the periphery this approach could translate into the clinical setting rather rapidly if proven preclinically to be of value [84].

However, a large problem in MS is the degeneration of axons followed by neuronal dysfunction that eventually occurs even in the absence of a strong inflammatory state. Thus, strategies aiming to enhance remyelination are urgently required to truly advance regeneration in MS brains. Again in preclinical EAE models, the transplantation of stem cells with the ability to differentiate into oligodendrocytes reduced disease features. Furthermore, the targeted differentiation into myelinating oligodendrocytes derived from endogenous NSCs in the murine SVZ turned out also to be beneficial in EAE (e.g. Rafalski et al [85]). Thus, current experiments aim to identify small molecules that may enhance the endogenous generation of functional oligodendrocytes to ameliorate disease features in chronic demyelinating disease [86].

Stem approaches in multiple system atrophy and motorneuron disease

Stem cells have also been used in other neurological conditions, including multiple system atrophy (MSA). In this disease MSCs from the bone marrow have been used and in all cases the benefits seem marginal and need confirming in other studies [97]. The rationale for this approach is that these cells can have immune modulating effects as well as releasing trophic factors, all of which can help repair the brain. The same is also true for the adoption of similar strategies in motor neuron disease [88].

Stem cell-based approaches in traumatic spinal cord injury

Spinal cord injury (SCI) is a rare disorder (incidence ranges from 15–30/million of the population) [89] and in many countries regulatory offices grant an orphan disorder designation to it. Due to an increased level of life expectancy achieved over the last three decades (overall normal life expectancy depending on the level of lesion is about 90% compared to age-matched controls) the prevalence of people living with SCI is steadily increasing (in US an estimated incidence of about 12,000 new cases per year and a prevalence of patients living with SCI is about 1 million of the population) [90]. In about 50% of patients the spinal cord injury is due to a traumatic event and for this specific population of patients, rehabilitation standards and outcome assessments have been continuously developed since the first conception and installation of a dedicated SCI rehabilitation programme (in Stoke Mandeville UK, 1942) [91, 92]. Traumatic SCI typically affects healthy and younger subjects (although in the recent decades a shift towards elderly subjects is observed with an increase of the mean age from 30 to 45 years), and compared to other neurological disorders of the brain (like MS, stroke, etc.) constitutes a non-degenerative and non-progressive disorder [93–95]. Furthermore, SCI represents a very distinct disorder within the central nervous system due to a rather localized lesion within the cord. Although the spinal cord is embedded in the CNS compartment (sealed by the blood–brain barrier) the SCI also clinically affects important neural structures that project and form part of the peripheral nervous system—alpha motoneurons. This is clinically evident in the assessment of motor function where typically motor weakness of an upper motorneuron (increased tone, spasticity, increased reflexes) and lower motoneuron (reduced muscle tone, muscle atrophy, loss of reflexes) origin can be seen in the same patient. In these motor segments (myotomes) originating from areas with cord damage, there is always some alpha motoneuron damage, while below the level of lesion motor weakness is due to loss of the descending central motor fibre tracts (i.e. pyramidal spinal tract) [96]. As for the brain, the cord contains neural networks (integration and modulation of in/outputs that affect the facilitation or inhibition of neural inputs) and conductive pathways (longitudinal ascending/descending fibre tracts). Accordingly, the cord is not only involved in conveying afferent–efferent signals but also has a capacity to influence even rather complex sensorimotor functions (like walking) in a sub-hierarchical capacity relative to the brain. The aforementioned findings indicate that the potential use of stem cells to improve the outcome of human SCI can potentially affect many different aspects of the spinal cord.

So far there is no approved or established treatment of the injured spinal cord itself and all the success achieved to date is through rehabilitation and the better outcome of patients with SCI is based on improved management of secondary medical problems (like bowel and bladder function). Although patients undergoing conventional rehabilitation programmes achieve advanced levels of functional outcome they still have a strong desire to improve their medical condition (patients acknowledge that they learned to live with SCI but they want to go beyond this). Due to these strong emotional desires many patients seek any potential treatment and they may even circumvent regulated (i.e. controlled) health care provisions (many will travel abroad to receive unproven treatments with any kind of cells). They even accept to pay at their own expense, enormous amounts of money (20,000–30,000 USD) to receive these cell applications even though none of the provided interventions have been proven to be effective.

Concepts and preclinical models of cell-based therapies in SCI follow in principal the same considerations as in stroke and other CNS disorders (Figure 14.1). Most commonly applied are preclinical models applying olfactory ensheathing cells (OEC) [97, 98], Schwann cells (SC) [99, 100], bone marrow stromal cells (BMSC) [101], and neural stem/progenitor cells (NSPC) [102, 103]. While the latter approaches have transferred to a degree to clinical trials, embryonic (ESC) and induced pluripotent stem cells (iPSC), although also intensively tested in animal models, have not yet reached a required level of safety and confidence for their application in humans, outside of a small trial funded by Geron.

The improvement of locomotor recovery and surgical feasibility of cell transplantation has been shown in several experimental paradigms and includes: adult mice neural precursor cells [104]; combined SC, OEC [105], and chondroitinase ABC [106]; human Schwann cells [107]: OEC [108]; homologous macrophages [109]; human ESC oligo-progenitors [110]; human umbilical cord cells [111]; human neurons from an embryonal teratocarcinoma cell line [112]; human neural precursor cells [113]; and human adult neural stem cells-described herein [114–117].

So far in preclinical models the three most likely mechanisms for using stem cells on the damaged cord include: (1) de-novo remyelination, (2) neurotrophic effects increasing neural plasticity, and (3) replacement of lost cells [118]. These occur to differing extents and the functional readouts in the animal mainly disclose minimal to moderate effects on locomotion. To enhance treatment effects combinatorial interventions are becoming increasingly tested and hold some promise [119, 120].

While in principle, the application of stem cells in animal SCI models appears feasible and reasonably safe, many important aspects for translating these application into human treatments are unresolved: (i) What is the most reasonable animal model (is there a need for non-human primate studies)?; (ii) What injury model (contusion versus cut lesions) and extent (completeness of cord damage) of cord injury is most relevant?; (iii) What kind of cell line may be superior and are there any reliable dose dependencies on outcomes?(iv) What is the most sensitive timing after injury (what constitutes acute and how is that established in animals and humans) for cell transplantation [121]?

Furthermore, the estimation of potential effects sizes as observed in the animal models to those involving patients is unclear [122].

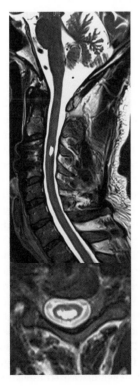
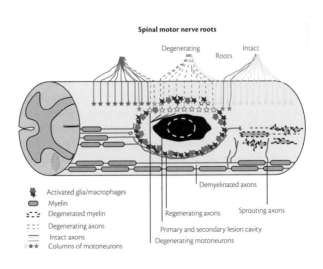

Fig. 14.1 Spinal cord injury.

While in human studies the stratification of patients is typically based on clinical phenotypes (level and completeness of lesion, time after injury, and accompanying medical complications), animal studies often apply a post hoc analysis with a stratification based on performance and biological markers that eventually allows one to find differences in outcomes. Clinical phase I/II trials concentrate on safety and feasibility (route of application, interactions of cells with host, interference of cell transplantation on recovery profiles, etc.) and so far animal models are of limited predictive value in terms of safety concerns [123]. One of the serious anxieties relates to the induction or increase of neuropathic pain, which is frequently an on-going challenge for patients following SCI (in about 60–70% of patients) [124, 125]. The induction of pain has not only been reported in animal models [126] but also in a case control series of intrathecal autologous bone marrow transplantations in humans with chronic SCI [127].

All the aforementioned issues need to be carefully considered when thinking about the translation of preclinical findings into a clinical trial [128].

In humans the procedural (surgical) and biological (cell integration, immunogeneicity) safety of cell transplantation into the spinal cord has been revealed in three recently completed cell-based trials applying intramedullary injections of cells [129–131]. Although the applied cells were of various types of non-CNS autografts, the overall findings revealed the general feasibility of the approach and the surgical risk of cell implantation into the injured spinal cord was considered favourable. The first trial was a Phase I study performed in Israel and assessed the safety of implanting incubated autologous macrophages within 14 days of injury [130]. The premise for this study was based on the concept of 'protective autoimmunity' in which endogenous activated macrophages and T cells are assumed to help augment spinal cord repair in the subacute inflammatory phase (1–2 weeks post injury). The study enrolled eight patients with complete injury between C5 and T11 and the intervention consisted of four microinjections (60 μl) of autologous harvested macrophages (total 4 million cells) at the caudal border of the cord injury. No adverse events were attributed to the experimental therapy, and no acute or delayed morbidity associated with the volume or cell dose injected into the spinal cord was observed. This study resulted in a Phase II study that enrolled 50 subjects before study cancellation for financial reasons. The safety and efficacy data from this study will be analysed and eventually published [132].

The second cell-based study involved implantation of autologous bone marrow cells in combination with systemic granulocyte macrophage colony-stimulating factor - administration in a Phase I/II trial [131]. In this study a series of 35 patients with complete cervical or thoracic injuries were implanted with autologous bone marrow cells at various stages after injury (acute, subacute, and chronic). The premise of the study was based on the possibility of bone marrow derived cells producing neuroprotective cytokines or differentiating into neural cells helpful for repair. The surgical procedure involved exposing the injured cord and injecting 200 million cells in a total suspension volume of 1.8 ml (six 300 μl aliquots) 'surrounding the lesion site.' One patient reported a transient postoperative reduction in hand strength and three patients had increased incisional muscle rigidity (presumably related to the surgical exposure). The authors reported that neuropathic pain was observed in a higher proportion (20%) of the patients who underwent transplantation, as opposed to the parallel 'control' (non-transplanted) patient group (7.7%). The increased neuropathic pain was predominantly noted in those patients transplanted in the subacute and chronic stage. The quality and nature of the neuropathic pain was not fully characterized in the report and pretransplant pain assessments were not quantified. In addition, the confounding variable of the second surgery necessary for the bone marrow cell transplantation as compared to the single stabilization surgery performed in the control group was not accounted for in the analysis of the neuropathic pain. The third study using a cell-based strategy for spinal cord injury involved the injection of autologous OES in three patients with a complete thoracic cord injury [129]. The cell doses in this limited series ranged between 12 and 28 million cells and were injected into the area of injury and adjacent cord using a pattern between 270 to 630 spinal cord injections. No deterioration in function or neuropathic pain was reported for the three subjects in this limited trial.

In 2009, the US Food and Drug Administration approved a Phase 1 clinical trial (Geron company) to evaluate the safety of a human embryonic stem cell-based product candidate, GRNOPC1, in patients with acute thoracic spinal cord injuries. The study was open to patients with a neurologically complete (ASIA Impairment Scale A) traumatic spinal cord injury limited to the thoracic region between T3 and T11. The administration of GRNOPC1 was supposed to occur between 7 and 14 days after the injury. In total about five patients were enrolled in this study, until in November 2011 the company, due to strategic considerations, abandoned the study. There have been no serious adverse events reported so far.

The findings summarised in this section (the list of studies is by no means considered to be complete) reveal that, although there have been a limited number of studies in humans, the application of stem cells for human SCI appears to be feasible. So far, however, there have been no findings in humans that reveal major or clinically obvious improvements in motor or sensory function.

Conclusion

The current possibilities for the structural and functional repair of the injured and diseased CNS are still extremely limited and lesions to the adult brain or spinal cord often result in a detrimental and disabling failure of CNS function. Thus, novel therapeutic avenues are needed. The identification of somatic stem cells within the adult nervous tissue and the improved handling and generation of various multipotent and pluripotent human stem cells, has raised hopes that these cells, whether endogenous or transplanted, will be useful for tissue repair. Even though stem cells are today not routinely used in the clinics to treat CNS diseases, a growing number of clinical studies have identified their potential for functional repair or support of injured tissue. Ongoing studies of stem cell-based treatments at this time are starting to explore their tolerability and to some extent efficacy. It seems plausible that diseases with a relatively well- defined pathology—that is the loss of distinct cell populations such as dopaminergic cells in the substantia nigra in PD, represent more promising targets compared to those with more diffuse neural tissue damage occurring for example after stroke. Further, disease stratification, based on the identification of patient subgroups that may benefit more than others from such interventions, will be important to ultimately judge the potential of stem cell therapies for treating a number of neuropsychiatric diseases. Clearly, future preclinical and clinical studies will have to identify the appropriate source for transplanted cells, be they patient-derived such as iPSCs, or derived from other human tissue representing allografts. Safety, comparability, and large-scale availability of cells are certainly a prerequisite for the routine clinical use of stem cells or their derivatives. Important for the field and subsequently the clinical success of stem cell-based therapies will be the need to avoid premature and over-optimistic expectations of their efficacy as we move towards patients in the clinic.

References

1. Spalding KL, Bergmann O, Alkass K, et al.Dynamics of hippocampal neurogenesis in adult humans. Cell. 2013;**153**(6):1219–1212

2. Altman J, Das GD. Post-natal origin of microneurons in the rat brain. Nature. 1965;**207**:953–956.

3. Kaplan MS, Hinds JW. Neurogenesis in the adult rat: electron microscopic analysis of light radioautographs. Science. 1977;**197**:1092–1094.

4. Reynolds BA, Weiss S. Generation of neurons and astrocytes from isolated cells of the adult mammalian central nervous system. Science. 1992;**255**:1707–1710.

5. Kuhn HG, Dickinson-Anson H, Gage FH. Neurogenesis in the dentate gyrus of the adult rat: age-related decrease of neuronal progenitor proliferation. J Neurosci. 1996;**16**:2027–2033.

6. Gage F. Mammalian neural stem cells. Science. 2000;**287**:1433–1438.

7. Zhao C, Deng W, Gage FH. Mechanisms and functional implications of adult neurogenesis. Cell. 2008;**132**:645–660.

8. Armstrong RJ, Barker RA. Neurodegeneration: a failure of neuroregeneration? Lancet. 2001;**358**:1174–1176.

9. Sahay A, Hen R. Adult hippocampal neurogenesis in depression. Nat Neurosci. 2007;**10**:1110–1115.

10. Kriks S, Shim JW, Piao J, et al. Dopamine neurons derived from human ES cells efficiently engraft in animal models of Parkinson's disease. Nature. 2011;**480**:547–551.

11. Takahashi K, Tanabe K, Ohnuki M, et al. Induction of pluripotent stem cells from adult human fibroblasts by defined factors. Cell. 2007;**131**:861–872.

12. Gould E, Tanapat P. Stress and hippocampal neurogenesis. Biol Psychiatry. 1999;**46**:1472–1479.

13. Santarelli L, Saxe M, Gross C, et al. Requirement of hippocampal neurogenesis for the behavioral effects of antidepressants. Science. 2003;**301**:805–809.

14. Sahay A, Scobie KN, Hill AS, et al. Increasing adult hippocampal neurogenesis is sufficient to improve pattern separation. Nature. 2011;**472**:466–470.

15. Barnes CA. Memory deficits associated with senescence: a neurophysiological and behavioral study in the rat. J Comp Physiol Psychol. 1979;**93**:74–104.

16. Burke SN, Barnes CA. Neural plasticity in the ageing brain. Nat Rev. 2006;**7**:30–40.

17. Drapeau E, Mayo W, Aurousseau C, Le Moal M, Piazza PV, Abrous DN. Spatial memory performances of aged rats in the water maze predict levels of hippocampal neurogenesis. Proc Natl Acad Sci U S A. 2003;**100**:14385–14390.

18. Small SA, Schobel SA, Buxton RB, Witter MP, Barnes CA. A pathophysiological framework of hippocampal dysfunction in ageing and disease. Nat Rev Neurosci. 2011;**12**:585–601.

19. Kempermann G, Gast D, Gage FH. Neuroplasticity in old age: sustained fivefold induction of hippocampal neurogenesis by long-term environmental enrichment. Ann Neurol. 2002;**52**:135–143.

20. van Praag H, Shubert T, Zhao C, Gage FH. Exercise enhances learning and hippocampal neurogenesis in aged mice. J Neurosci. 2005;**25**:8680–8685.

21. Parent JM, Yu TW, Leibowitz RT, Geschwind DH, Sloviter RS, Lowenstein DH. Dentate granule cell neurogenesis is increased by seizures and contributes to aberrant network reorganization in the adult rat hippocampus. J Neurosci. 1997;**17**:3727–3738.

22. Jessberger S, Zhao C, Toni N, Clemenson GD, Jr., Li Y, Gage FH. Seizure-associated, aberrant neurogenesis in adult rats characterized with retrovirus-mediated cell labeling. J Neurosci. 2007;**27**:9400–9407.

23. Walter C, Murphy BL, Pun RY, Spieles-Engemann AL, Danzer SC. Pilocarpine-induced seizures cause selective time-dependent changes to adult-generated hippocampal dentate granule cells. J Neurosci. 2007;**27**:7541–7552.

24. Pun RY, Rolle IJ, Lasarge CL, et al. Excessive activation of mTOR in postnatally generated granule cells is sufficient to cause epilepsy. Neuron. 2012;**75**:1022–1034.

25. Scharfman HE, Hen R. Neuroscience. Is more neurogenesis always better? Science. 2007;**315**:336–338.

26. Shetty AK. Progress in cell grafting therapy for temporal lobe epilepsy. Neurotherapeutics. 2011;**8**:721–735.

27. Braak H, Del Tredici K, Bratzke H, Hamm-Clement J, Sandmann-Keil D, Rub U. Staging of the intracerebral inclusion body pathology associated with idiopathic Parkinson's disease (preclinical and clinical stages). J Neurol. 2002;**249** Suppl 3:III/1–5.

28. Chaudhuri KR, Odin P. The challenge of non-motor symptoms in Parkinson's disease. Progr Brain Res. 2010;**184**:325–341.

29. Brundin P, Kordower JH. Neuropathology in transplants in Parkinson's disease: implications for disease pathogenesis and the future of cell therapy. Progr Brain Res. 2012;**200**:221–241.

30. Lubbe S, Morris HR. Recent advances in Parkinson's disease genetics. J Neurol. 2013;**261**(2):259–266

31. Winder-Rhodes SE, Evans JR, et al. Glucocerebrosidase mutations influence the natural history of Parkinson's disease in a community-based incident cohort. Brain. 2013;**136**:392–399.

32. Williams-Gray CH, Evans JR, Goris A, et al. The distinct cognitive syndromes of Parkinson's disease: 5 year follow-up of the CamPaIGN cohort. Brain. 2009;**132**:2958–2969.

33. Kehagia AA, Barker RA, Robbins TW. Neuropsychological and clinical heterogeneity of cognitive impairment and dementia in patients with Parkinson's disease. Lancet Neurol. 2010;**9**:1200–1213.

34. Drouin-Ouellet J, Barker RA. Parkinson's disease in a dish: what patient specific-reprogrammed somatic cells can tell us about Parkinson's disease, if anything? Stem Cells Int. 2012;**926**:147.

35. Dyson SC, Barker RA. Cell-based therapies for Parkinson's disease. Expert Rev Neurother. 2011;**11**:831–844.

36. Daley GQ. The promise and perils of stem cell therapeutics. Cell Stem Cell. 2012;**10**:740–749.

37. Prakash N, Wurst W. Development of dopaminergic neurons in the mammalian brain. Cell Mol Life Sci. 2006;**63**:187–206.

38. Damier P, Hirsch EC, Agid Y, Graybiel AM. The substantia nigra of the human brain. II. Patterns of loss of dopamine-containing neurons in Parkinson's disease. Brain. 1999;**122** (Pt 8):1437–1448.

39. Soldner F, Hockemeyer D, Beard C, et al. Parkinson's disease patient-derived induced pluripotent stem cells free of viral reprogramming factors. Cell. 2009;**136**:964–977.

40. Sanchez-Danes A, Richaud-Patin Y, Carballo-Carbajal I, et al. Disease-specific phenotypes in dopamine neurons from human iPS-based models of genetic and sporadic Parkinson's disease. EMBO Mol Med. 2012;**4**:380–395.

41. Lesage S, Brice A. Parkinson's disease: from monogenic forms to genetic susceptibility factors. Hum Mol Genet. 2009;**18**:R48–59.

42. Miura K, Okada Y, Aoi T, et al. Variation in the safety of induced pluripotent stem cell lines. Nat Biotechnol. (2009) **27**:743–745.

43. Vierbuchen T, Ostermeier A, Pang ZP, Kokubu Y, Sudhof TC, Wernig M. Direct conversion of fibroblasts to functional neurons by defined factors. Nature. 2010;**463**:1035–1041.

44. Pfisterer U, Kirkeby A, Torper O, et al. Direct conversion of human fibroblasts to dopaminergic neurons. Proc Natl Acad Sci U S A. 2011;**108**:10343–10348.

45. Qiang L, Fujita R, Yamashita T, et al. Directed conversion of Alzheimer's disease patient skin fibroblasts into functional neurons. Cell. 2011;**146**(3): p. 359–371.

46. Caiazzo M, Dell'Anno MT, Dvoretskova E, et al. Direct generation of functional dopaminergic neurons from mouse and human fibroblasts. Nature. 2011;**476**:224–227.

47. Kim J, Su SC, Wang H, et al. Functional integration of dopaminergic neurons directly converted from mouse fibroblasts. Cell Stem Cell. 2011;**9**:413–419.

48. Liu X, Li F, Stubblefield EA, Blanchard B, et al. Direct reprogramming of human fibroblasts into dopaminergic neuron-like cells. Cell Res. 2012;**22**:321–332.

49. Brundin P, Barker RA, Parmar M. Neural grafting in Parkinson's disease Problems and possibilities. Progr Brain Res. 2010;**184**:265–294.

50. Kordower JH, Rosenstein JM, Collier TJ, et al. Functional fetal nigral grafts in a patient with Parkinson's disease: chemoanatomic, ultrastructural, and metabolic studies. J Comp Neurol. 1996;**370**:203–230.

51. Galpern WR, Corrigan-Curay J, Lang AE, et al. Sham neurosurgical procedures in clinical trials for neurodegenerative diseases: scientific and ethical considerations. Lancet Neurol. 2012;**11**:643–650.

52. Freed CR, Greene PE, Breeze RE, et al. Transplantation of embryonic dopamine neurons for severe Parkinson's disease. N Engl J Med. 2001;**344**:710–719.

53. Olanow CW, Goetz CG, Kordower JH, et al. A double-blind controlled trial of bilateral fetal nigral transplantation in Parkinson's disease. Ann Neurol. 2003;**54**:403–414.

54. Olanow CW, Kordower JH, Lang AE, Obeso JA. Dopaminergic transplantation for Parkinson's disease: current status and future prospects. Ann Neurol. 2009;**66**:591–596.

55. Barker RA, Barrett J, Mason SL, Bjorklund A. Fetal dopaminergic transplantation trials and the future of neural grafting in Parkinson's disease. Lancet Neurol. 2013;**12**:84–91.

56. Barker RA, de Beaufort I. Scientific and ethical issues related to stem cell research and interventions in neurodegenerative disorders of the brain. Progr Neurobiol 2013;**110**:63–73

57. Lerou PH, Daley GQ. Therapeutic potential of embryonic stem cells. Blood Rev. 2005;**19**:321–331.

58. Cai J, Yang M, Poremsky E, Kidd S, Schneider JS, Iacovitti L. Dopaminergic neurons derived from human induced pluripotent stem cells survive and integrate into 6-OHDA-lesioned rats. Stem Cells Dev. 2010;**19**:1017–1023.

59. Wernig M, Zhao JP, Pruszak J, et al. Neurons derived from reprogrammed fibroblasts functionally integrate into the fetal brain and improve symptoms of rats with Parkinson's disease. Proc Natl Acad Sci U S A. 2008;**105**:5856–5861.

60. Phillips W, Shannon KM, Barker RA. The current clinical management of Huntington's disease. Mov Disord. 2008;**23**:1491–1504.

61. Tabrizi SJ, Scahill RI, Owen G, et al. Predictors of phenotypic progression and disease onset in premanifest and early-stage Huntington's disease in the TRACK-HD study: analysis of 36-month observational data. Lancet Neurol. 2013;**12**(7): 637–649.

62. Clelland CD, Barker RA, Watts C. Cell therapy in Huntington disease. Neurosurg Focus. 2008;**24**:E9.

63. Cisbani G, St. Pierre M, Cicchetti F. Single cell suspension methodology favours survival and vascularization of fetal striatal grafts in the YAC128 mouse model of Huntington's disease. Cell Transplant. 2013; Jun 17. doi: 10.3727/096368913X668636

64. Wijeyekoon R, Barker RA. The current status of neural grafting in the treatment of Huntington's disease. A review. Front Integr Neurosci. 2011;**5**:78.

65. Bachoud-Levi AC, Deglon N, Nguyen JP, et al. Neuroprotective gene therapy for Huntington's disease using a polymer encapsulated BHK cell line engineered to secrete human CNTF. Hum Gene Ther. 2000;**11**:1723–1729.

66. Hauser RA, Sandberg PR, Freeman TB, Stoessl AJ. Bilateral human fetal striatal transplantation in Huntington's disease. Neurology. 2002;**58**:1704; author reply 1704.

67. Cicchetti F, Soulet D, Freeman TB. Neuronal degeneration in striatal transplants and Huntington's disease: potential mechanisms and clinical implications. Brain. 2011;**134**(Pt 3):641–652.

68. Barker RA, Barrett J, Mason SL, Bjorklund A. The long-term safety and efficacy of bilateral transplantation of human fetal striatal tissue in patients with mild to moderate Huntington's disease. J Neurol Neurosurg Psychiatry. 2013;**84**(6):657–665.

69. Reuter I, Tai YF, Pavese N, et al. Long-term clinical and positron emission tomography outcome of fetal striatal transplantation in Huntington's disease. J Neurol Neurosurg Psychiatry. 2008;**79**:948–951.

70. Ma L, Hu B, Liu Y, et al. Human embryonic stem cell-derived GABA neurons correct locomotion deficits in quinolinic acid-lesioned mice. Cell Stem Cell. 2012;**10**:455–464.

71. Carri AD, Onorati M, Lelos MJ, et al. Developmentally coordinated extrinsic signals drive human pluripotent stem cell differentiation toward authentic DARPP-32+ medium-sized spiny neurons. Development. 2013;**140**:301–312.

72. The HD iPSC Consortium. Induced pluripotent stem cells from patients with Huntington's disease show CAG-repeat-expansion-associated phenotypes. Cell Stem Cell. 2012;**11**:264–278.

73. Phillips W, Morton AJ, Barker RA. Abnormalities of neurogenesis in the R6/2 mouse model of Huntington's disease are attributable to the in vivo microenvironment. J Neurosci. 2005;**25**:11564–11576.

74. Clelland CD, Choi M, Romberg C, et al. A functional role for adult hippocampal neurogenesis in spatial pattern separation. Science. 2009;**325**:210–213.

75. Curtis MA, Penney EB, Pearson AG, et al. Increased cell proliferation and neurogenesis in the adult human Huntington's disease brain. Proc Natl Acad Sci U S A. 2003;**100**:9023–9027.

76. O'Keeffe GC, Tyers P, Aarsland D, Dalley JW, Barker RA, Caldwell MA. Dopamine-induced proliferation of adult neural precursor cells in the mammalian subventricular zone is mediated through EGF. Proc Natl Acad Sci U S A. 2009;**106**:8754–8759.

77. Arvidsson A, Collin T, Kirik D, Kokaia Z, Lindvall O. Neuronal replacement from endogenous precursors in the adult brain after stroke. Nat Med. 2002;**5**:5.

78. Jin K, Wang X, Xie L, et al. Evidence for stroke-induced neurogenesis in the human brain. Proc Natl Acad Sci U S A. 2006;**103**:13198–13202.

79. Lindvall O, Kokaia Z. Stem cells in human neurodegenerative disorders—time for clinical translation? J Clin Invest. 2010;**120**:29–40.

80. Bhasin A, Srivastava MV, Kumaran SS, et al. Autologous mesenchymal stem cells in chronic stroke. Cerebrovasc Dis Extra. 2011;**1**:93–104.

81. Connick P, Kolappan M, Crawley C, et al. Autologous mesenchymal stem cells for the treatment of secondary progressive multiple sclerosis: an open-label phase 2a proof-of-concept study. Lancet Neurol. 2012;**11**(2):150–156.

82. Rice CM, Mallam EA, Whone AL, et al. Safety and feasibility of autologous bone marrow cellular therapy in relapsing-progressive multiple sclerosis. Clin Pharmacol Ther. 2010;**87**(6):679–685.

83. Martino G, Pluchino S. The therapeutic potential of neural stem cells. Nat Rev Neurosci. 2006;**7**:395–406.

84. Jadasz JJ, Aigner L, Rivera FJ, Kury P. The remyelination Philosopher's Stone: stem and progenitor cell therapies for multiple sclerosis. Cell Tiss Res. 2012;**349**:331–347.

85. Rafalski VA, Ho PP, Brett JO, et al. Expansion of oligodendrocyte progenitor cells following SIRT1 inactivation in the adult brain. Nate Cell Biol. 2013;**15**(6):614–624.

86. Huang JK, Fancy SP, Zhao C, Rowitch DH, French-Constant C, Franklin RJ. Myelin regeneration in multiple sclerosis: targeting endogenous stem cells. Neurotherapeutics. 2011;**8**:650–658.

87. Lee PH, Lee JE, Kim HS, et al. A randomized trial of mesenchymal stem cells in multiple system atrophy. Ann Neurol. 2012;72:32–40.

88. Mazzini L, Vercelli A, Ferrero I, Boido M, Cantello R, Fagioli F. Transplantation of mesenchymal stem cells in ALS. Progr Brain Res. 2012;201:333–359.

89. Cripps RA, Lee BB, Wing P, Weerts E, Mackay J, Brown D. A global map for traumatic spinal cord injury epidemiology: towards a living data repository for injury prevention. Spinal Cord. 2011;49(4):49

90. Middleton JW, Hontecillas R, Horne WT, et al. Life expectancy after spinal cord injury: a 50-year study. Spinal Cord. 2012;250(11):803–811

91. Meinecke FW, Exner G. Treatment of patients with spinal cord lesions in Germany 1996-state of the art. Spinal Cord. 1997;35(7):411

92. Schultke E, Guttmann G. Emerging concept of rehabilitation after spinal cord injury. J Hist Neurosci. 2001;10(3):300–307.

93. Furlan JC, Hitzig SL, Craven BD. The influence of age on functional recovery of adults with spinal cord injury or disease after inpatient rehabilitative care: a pilot study. Aging Clin Exp Res. 2013;25(4):463–471.

94. Shin JC, Kim DH, Yu SJ, Yang HE, Yoon SY. Epidemiologic change of patients with spinal cord injury. Ann Rehabil Med. 2013;37(1):50–56.

95. Wirz M, Dietz V. Concepts of aging with paralysis: implications for recovery and treatment. Handb Clin Neurol. 2012;109:77–84.

96. Dietz V, Curt A. Neurological aspects of spinal-cord repair: promises and challenges. Lancet Neurol. 2006;5(8):688–694. Review.

97. Kalincik T, Jozefcikova K, Sutharsan R, Mackay-Sim A, Carrive P, Waite PM. Selected changes in spinal cord morphology after T4 transection and olfactory ensheathing cell transplantation. Auton Neurosci. 2010;158(1–2):31–38.

98. Zhang J, Wang B, Xiao Z, et al. Olfactory ensheathing cells promote proliferation and inhibit neuronal differentiation of neural progenitor cells through activation of Notch signaling. Neuroscience. 2008;153(2):406–413.

99. Wills TE, E. Batchelor EP, Kerr NF, et al. Corticospinal tract sprouting in the injured rat spinal cord stimulated by Schwann cell preconditioning of the motor cortex. Neurol Res. 2013;35(7):763–772.

100. Guest JD, Hiester ED, Bunge RP. Demyelination and Schwann cell responses adjacent to injury epicenter cavities following chronic human spinal cord injury. Exp Neurol. 2005;192(2):384–393.

101. Alexanian AR, Fehlings MG, Zhang Z, Maiman DJ. Transplanted neurally modified bone marrow-derived mesenchymal stem cells promote tissue protection and locomotor recovery in spinal cord injured rats. Neurorehabil Neural Repair. 2011;25(9):873–880.

102. Harrop JS, Hashimoto R, Norvell D, et al. Evaluation of clinical experience using cell-based therapies in patients with spinal cord injury: a systematic review. J Neurosurg Spine. 2012;17(1 Suppl):230–246.

103. Kumamaru H, Ohkawa Y, Saiwai H, et al. Direct isolation and RNA-seq reveal environment-dependent properties of engrafted neural stem/progenitor cells. Nat Commun. 2012;3:1140.

104. Eftekharpour ES, Karimi-Abdolrezaee S, Fehlings MG. Current status of experimental cell replacement approaches to spinal cord injury. Neurosurg Focus. 2008;24(3–4): p. E19.

105. Mackay-Sim A, St John JA. Olfactory ensheathing cells from the nose: clinical application in human spinal cord injuries. Exp Neurol. 2011;229(1):174–180.

106. Fouad K, Pearse DD, Tetzlaff W, Vavrek R. Transplantation and repair: combined cell implantation and chondroitinase delivery prevents deterioration of bladder function in rats with complete spinal cord injury. Spinal Cord. 2009;47(10):727–732.

107. Bunge RP. Schwann cells in central regeneration. Ann N Y Acad Sci 1991;633:229–233.

108. Ramon-Cueto A, Hontecillas R, Horne WT, et al. Functional recovery of paraplegic rats and motor axon regeneration in their spinal cords by olfactory ensheathing glia. Neuron. 2000;25(2):425–435.

109. Rapalino O, Lazarov-Spiegler O, Agranov E, et al. Implantation of stimulated homologous macrophages results in partial recovery of paraplegic rats. Nat Med. 1998;4(7):814–821.

110. Keirstead HS, Nistor G, Bernal G, et al. Human embryonic stem cell-derived oligodendrocyte progenitor cell transplants remyelinate and restore locomotion after spinal cord injury. J Neurosci. 2005;25(19):4694–4705.

111. Saporta S, Kim JJ, Willing AE, Fu ES, Davis CD, Sanberg PR. Human umbilical cord blood stem cells infusion in spinal cord injury: engraftment and beneficial influence on behavior. J Hematother Stem Cell Res. 2003;12(3):271–278.

112. Saporta S, Makoui AS, Willing AE, et al., Functional recovery after complete contusion injury to the spinal cord and transplantation of human neuroteratocarcinoma neurons in rats. J Neurosurg. 2002;97(1 Suppl):63–68.

113. Iwanami A, Kaneko S, Nakamura M, et al. Transplantation of human neural stem cells for spinal cord injury in primates. J Neurosci Res. 2005;80(2):182–190.

114. Cummings BJ, Uchida N, Tamaki SJ, et al. Human neural stem cells differentiate and promote locomotor recovery in spinal cord-injured mice. Proc Natl Acad Sci U S A. 2005;102(39):14069–14074.

115. Cummings BJ, Uchida N, Tamaki SJ, Anderson AJ. Human neural stem cell differentiation following transplantation into spinal cord injured mice: association with recovery of locomotor function. Neurol Res. 2006;28(5):474–481.

116. Hooshmand MJ, Sontag CJ, Uchida N, Tamaki S, Anderson AJ, Cummings BJ. Analysis of host-mediated repair mechanisms after human CNS-stem cell transplantation for spinal cord injury: correlation of engraftment with recovery. PLoS One. 2011;4(6):e5871.

117. Salazar DL, Uchida N, Hamers FP, Cummings BJ, Anderson AJ. Human neural stem cells differentiate and promote locomotor recovery in an early chronic spinal cord injury NOD-scid mouse model. PLoS One. 2010;5(8):e12272

118. Ruff CA, Wilcox JT, Fehlings MG. Cell-based transplantation strategies to promote plasticity following spinal cord injury. Exp Neurol. 2012;235(1):78–90.

119. Lu P, Hontecillas R, Horne WT, et al. Computational modeling-based discovery of novel classes of anti-inflammatory drugs that target lanthionine synthetase C-like protein 2. PLoS One. 2012;7(4):e34643.

120. Karimi-Abdolrezaee S, Schut D, Wang J, Fehlings MG. Chondroitinase and growth factors enhance activation and oligodendrocyte differentiation of endogenous neural precursor cells after spinal cord injury. PLoS One. 2012;7(5):e37589.

121. Curt A. Human neural stem cells in chronic spinal cord injury. Expert Opin Biol Ther. 2012;12(3):271–273.

122. Dietz V, Curt A. Translating preclinical approaches into human application. Handb Clin Neurol. 2012;109:399–409.

123. Fehlings MG, Vawda R. Cellular treatments for spinal cord injury: the time is right for clinical trials. Neurotherapeutics. 2011;8(4):704–720.

124. Taylor J, Huelbes S, Albu S, Gomez-Soriano J, Penacoba C, Poole HM. Neuropathic pain intensity, unpleasantness, coping strategies, and psychosocial factors after spinal cord injury: an exploratory longitudinal study during the first year. Pain Med. 2012;13(11):1457–1468.

125. Zanca JM, Dijkers MP, Hammond FM, Horn SD. Pain and its impact on inpatient rehabilitation for acute traumatic spinal cord injury: analysis of observational data collected in the SCIRehab study. Arch Phys Med Rehabil. 2013;94(4 Suppl):S137–144.

126. Hofstetter CP, Holmstrom NA, Lilja JA, et al. Allodynia limits the usefulness of intraspinal neural stem cell grafts; directed differentiation improves outcome. Nat Neurosci. 2005;8(3):346–353.

127. Kishk NA, Gabr H, Hamdy S, et al. Case control series of intrathecal autologous bone marrow mesenchymal stem cell therapy for chronic spinal cord injury. Neurorehabil Neural Repair. 2010;24(8):702–708.

128. Curt A. The translational dialogue in spinal cord injury research. Spinal Cord. 2012;**50**(5):352–357.

129. Feron F, Perry C, Cochrane J, et al. Autologous olfactory ensheathing cell transplantation in human spinal cord injury. Brain. 2005;**128**(Pt 12):2951–2960.

130. Knoller N, Auerbach G, Fulga V, et al. Clinical experience using incubated autologous macrophages as a treatment for complete spinal cord injury: phase I study results. J Neurosurg Spine. 2005;**3**(3):173–181.

131. Yoon SH. Shim YS, Park YH, et al. Complete spinal cord injury treatment using autologous bone marrow cell transplantation and bone marrow stimulation with granulocyte macrophage-colony stimulating factor: Phase I/II clinical trial. Stem Cells. 2007;**25**(8):2066–2073.

132. Lammertse DP, Jones LA, Charlifue SB, et al. Autologous incubated macrophage therapy in acute, complete spinal cord injury: results of the phase 2 randomized controlled multicenter trial. Spinal Cord. 2012;**50**(9):661–671.

CHAPTER 15

The role of neuroimaging in understanding the impact of neuroplasticity after CNS damage

Nick Ward

Introduction

Acute injury to the central nervous system (CNS) is often followed by some degree of recovery. Scientists and clinicians have been interested in the mechanisms of this recovery for years. Based on observations in animal models of focal CNS injury it is often assumed that a number of processes jointly referred to as neuroplasticity make a major contribution (see Chapters 13 and 14). Experiments in animal models have demonstrated alterations in cerebral organization that occur after injury are related to recovery [1]. Specifically, focal cortical damage in adult brains renders widespread surviving cortical regions more able to change structure and function in response to afferent signals in a way normally only seen in the developing brain]2]. An increased potential for neuroplasticity will in itself not enhance recovery, but it may increase the impact of training strategies since training works through mechanisms of experience-dependent plasticity [1].

The management of patients with incomplete recovery following CNS injury often draws on specific rehabilitation interventions aimed at assisting adaptation to impairment. However, partly because of a growing awareness of the role of neuroplasticity there is an interest in designing therapeutic strategies to promote cerebral reorganisation as a way of reducing rather than compensating for impairment. These include incorporating ideas about learning into neurorehabilitation (see Chapter 7) as well as strategies to enhance the potential for neuroplastic change, such as neuropharmacological (see Chapter 17) and non-invasive brain stimulation (see Chapter 16).

These developments are clearly very exciting for clinicians. A key part of developing future strategies will involve building an empirical understanding of how the brain responds to injury and how such changes may be manipulated in a way that promotes functional recovery. The investigation of cerebral reorganization after focal brain injury in humans is less well advanced than similar work in animal models. There are clearly greater limitations in studying the human brain, but structural and functional imaging provide opportunities to do so. This chapter will explore how neuroimaging has contributed to understanding the impact of neuroplasticity after CNS injury, and how it might contribute in the future. It will largely concentrate on motor recovery after stroke to illustrate how neuroimaging provides a window onto neuroplasticity after CNS damage, but examples from the study of different types of patients (spinal cord injury) and different domains (language) will be referred to in order to examine how much it is possible to generalize these ideas.

Imaging techniques
Functional imaging

Functional neuroimaging techniques allow examination of human brain function *in vivo*. In the context of CNS injury, functional brain imaging provides a way of assessing how focal damage to cortical or subcortical regions alters the way surviving neural networks operate, and how these changes are related to impairment and recovery. Functional imaging of the brain has been carried out with four main techniques: positron emission tomography (PET), functional magnetic resonance imaging (fMRI), electroencephalography (EEG) and magnetoencephalography (MEG). A detailed theoretical background to the techniques is beyond the scope of this chapter. In brief however, both PET and fMRI rely on the assumption that neuronal activity is closely coupled to a local increase in cerebral blood flow (CBF) secondary to an increase in metabolism. PET relies on mapping the distribution of inert, freely diffusible radioactive tracers deposited in tissue as a function of regional perfusion (rCBF). fMRI comprises different methods, but the studies described in the next section use blood oxygen level-dependent (BOLD) imaging techniques. During an increase in neuronal activation there is an increase in local CBF, but only a small proportion of the greater amount of oxygen delivered locally to the tissue is used. There is a resultant net increase in the tissue concentration of oxyhaemoglobin and a net reduction in paramagnetic deoxyhaemoglobin in the local capillary bed and draining venules. The magnetic properties of haemoglobin depend on its level of oxygenation so that this change results in an increase in local tissue derived signal intensity on T_2*-weighted MR images. EEG and MEG on the other hand are techniques that measure the magnetic fields emanating from the scalp, which are created perpendicular to the electrical current (according to Maxwell's equation) that is created by neuronal activity. EEG systems are cheaper and more readily available than MEG, but MEG has some advantages. EEG signals are strongly degraded by heterogeneity in conductivity within head tissues, but this is far less of a problem in MEG. MEG directly measures neuronal activity and has a temporal resolution in the scale of milliseconds. Studies measuring rCBF with PET are less common now but MEG studies are on the increase.

Structural imaging techniques

Ideally, changes in CNS functional organization should be viewed in the context of the anatomy of the structural damage. However, structural imaging in stroke for example, has generally been used to examine the vascular territory involved, without too much consideration of the important functions subserved by the grey and white matter structures that are damaged. This is probably because there has been no good way to quantify damage to key structures using computerized tomography (CT) or T_1- and T_2-weighted MRI. This opened the way for diffusion-weighted imaging (DWI), which is sensitive to the diffusion of water molecules within tissue. Diffusion tensor imaging (DTI) is based on DWI and allows evaluation of the integrity of the white matter by calculation of fractional anisotropy (FA). Probabilistic DTI tractography uses voxel-wise FA values to map probable fibre trajectories by following the estimated fibre orientation of successive voxels to generate streamlines connected to chosen start points. These tractography algorithms then provide quantitative information about the integrity and orientation of white matter tracts in the brain. Its accuracy has been validated using post-mortem specimens [3].

Imaging motor recovery after stroke

Cross-sectional studies in chronic stroke

The first functional imaging studies to examine cortical reorganization of the motor system were performed in recovered chronic subcortical stroke patients. These patients were found to have relative overactivation in a number of motor-related brain regions during the performance of a simple motor task compared to control subjects. In particular, overactivations were seen in brain regions such as dorsolateral premotor cortex (PMd), ventrolateral premotor cortex (PMv), supplementary motor area (SMA), cingulate motor areas (CMA), parietal cortex, and insula cortex [4–7]. A recent meta-analysis on activation data derived from over 50 neuroimaging experiments confirmed that enhanced activity in

contralesional primary motor cortex (M1), bilateral ventral premotor cortex and supplementary motor area (SMA) are a highly consistent findings after motor stroke compared to healthy controls for a wide range of hand motor tasks [8]. These findings were initially interpreted as indicating that recruitment of these brain regions, particularly those in the unaffected hemisphere, might be responsible for recovery.

However, stroke patients are variable and if one studies patients with a range of late post-stroke outcome, results suggest that those with the best outcome have a 'normal' activation pattern when compared to normal controls, whereas those with poorer outcome show significant differences. Although care needs to be taken in conducting and interpreting 'task-related' studies, the differences between stroke patients and healthy controls generally take the form of: (i) overactivations in non-primary motor areas, particularly in the contralesional hemisphere; and (ii) shifts in somatotopic representation in primary and possibly non-primary motor areas [9]. In fact, when the relationship between impairment and regional brain activation was examined for the first time, a negative correlation was found between the magnitude of brain activation in secondary motor areas and outcome [10] (Figure 15.1). In other words, this result confirmed that those with more impairment were the ones with overactivations previously described.

A subsequent study used TMS to quantify the 'functional integrity' of the corticospinal system to test whether this may be the key variable leading to alterations in patterns of task-related activity after stroke. Patients with more corticospinal system damage exhibited less task-related activity in ipsilesional M1 (hand area) and greater activity in secondary motor areas in both hemispheres [11]. A similar result was observed in a group of patients with different levels of impairment studied at approximately 10 days post stroke illustrating that lesion induced reorganization occurs quickly [12]. These results point to a shift away from primary to secondary motor areas with increasing disruption to corticospinal system, presumably because in some patients ipsilesional M1 is less able to influence motor output. However, this is highly likely to depend on the exact pattern of disruption to the descending pathways.

The results from similar studies performed in patients with injury occurring to the CNS at a much earlier age (e.g. cerebral palsy) provide similar results. Prominent contralesional activity

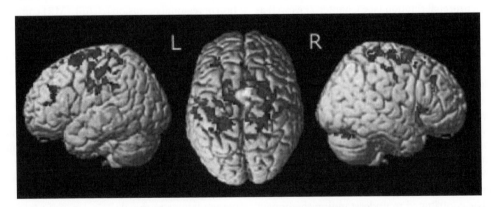

Fig. 15.1 Brain regions in which activity during affected hand grip correlates with impairment. Greater upper limb impairment was associated with greater activity during affected hand grip in these regions. Results are surface-rendered onto a canonical brain. The brain is shown (from left to right) from the left side, from above (left hemisphere on the left) and from the right.

Ward NS, Brown MM, Thompson AJ, Frackowiak RSJ, Neural correlates of outcome after stroke: a cross-sectional fMRI study, Brain, 2003, 126, 1430–48, by permission of Oxford University Press.

has been observed, both in premotor and primary motor cortex, with the latter more likely to be recruited in those with larger lesions [13]. As in those with adult stroke, there is variability in motor system organization related to lesion extent and level of impairment.

The evolution of cerebral reorganization after stroke

Cross-sectional studies are simpler to perform, but do not tell us is how this reorganized state evolved from the earliest time after infarction. Two early longitudinal studies with early and late time points demonstrated initial task-related overactivations in motor-related brain regions followed by a reduction over time in patients said to recover fully [14, 15]. A detailed multisession longitudinal fMRI study of patients with infarcts not involving M1 looked at changes in motor-related brain activity as a function of recovery (rather than time). At approximately 10–14 days after stroke, an initial overactivation was seen in many primary and non-primary motor regions [16]. As in the chronic setting, this was more extensive when the clinical deficit was greatest (i.e. early after stroke). Improvement in motor performance was associated with a steady decrease in task-related activity in these areas (Figure 15.2) suggesting that successful recovery is associated with a normalization of pathologically enhanced brain activity over time, which has been confirmed by a number of subsequent studies [17–19]. Even earlier changes were examined by a serial fMRI study, in which stroke patients with motor impairment were scanned several times in the first 2 weeks post-stroke starting within 3 days after symptom onset [18]. In those with only mild impairment, task-related activation (movement of the affected hand) was not different from healthy controls. However, in those with more marked impairment, there was a general reduction of cerebral activity in the first 1–3 days after stroke, which increased in both hemispheres over and above that seen in healthy controls over the next 10 days. Four months later, cortical overactivity had returned to levels observed in healthy controls in those with recovery of hand function, similar to earlier longitudinal studies.

The early absence of activity is an interesting finding that might represent a real decrease in neural activity or possibly merely reduced BOLD due to neurovascular uncoupling. Intriguingly, however, reduced BOLD reactivity has been linked with increased levels of gamma-aminobutyric acid (GABA) [20]. This is of particular interest as, the balance between inhibition and excitation in the cortex is thought to be a key mediator of neural plasticity. The temporal pattern of reduced then elevated BOLD might point towards the kinds of alterations in lesion induced plasticity that evolve over time that are seen in animal models of focal brain injury [1].

Brain reorganization in response to therapeutic interventions

The studies described so far have examined alterations in organization of cortical motor areas in response to damage (to the corticospinal pathways). There are a number of studies that have looked at the effects of physical therapies (for review see [21]). The standard design is to use functional imaging before and after a particular treatment protocol. Most found treatment-associated increases in ipsilesional hemisphere activity in keeping with the previous longitudinal studies, but others saw a shift in the balance of activation in the opposite direction. The evidence suggests that the contribution of contralesional motor regions varies, but it is not clear what baseline characteristics might predict such shifts. In other words, it is likely individual differences in the anatomy of the damage and time since stroke will determine what topography of therapeutic change is observed.

These results are likely to represent the consequences of functional improvement rather than the mechanism of action of the treatment itself. Only one study has looked at the differential longitudinal changes in brain reorganization for one form of therapy compared to another [22]. Bilateral arm training with rhythmic auditory cueing (BATRAC) led to significantly higher increases in activation in some ipsilesional motor-related areas including PMd and SMA than after matched intensity 'standard' physiotherapy. From a clinical perspective it was disappointing that there were no overall differences in clinical gains for either group. Although a negative clinical trial, it means that the functional imaging differences are not confounded by different therapeutic gains. In other words, the results here do suggest a possible cerebral mechanism for BATRAC compared to intense 'standard' physiotherapy.

In general, functional imaging is unlikely to be useful purely as a marker of clinical improvement, something that is measurable with simple outcome scores. Functional imaging may become a useful marker of the *potential* for change in damaged brain, and this will be discussed later in the chapter.

Is this reorganization functionally relevant?

Most longitudinal studies have been performed in those who end up with reasonable recovery and support the importance of regaining normal patterns of brain activity. However, the cross-sectional studies tell us that not all patients achieve this normalization and those with incomplete recovery can be left with prominent task-related activity in secondary motor areas, particularly in contralesional hemisphere. What is the evidence that this pattern of cortical activity during attempted movement is either contributing to or hindering recovery of motor function?

Do these distributed cortical motor regions have any direct influence over muscles in recovering limbs? One way to look at this is to measure the coherence between oscillatory signals from both the brain (measured with MEG) and the affected muscles (measured with electromyography, EMG) simultaneously during a simple movement. Corticomuscular coherence here implies some kind of functional coupling between the cortical region and the recovering muscle. In a group of chronic stroke patients, the cortical source of the peak corticomuscular coherence was widely distributed compared to controls [23]. In particular, peak corticomuscular coherence was seen in contralesional hemisphere in a number of patients (Figure 15.3), implying direct influence over affected muscle activity.

Transiently disrupting cortical activity in either ipsilesional or contralesional PMd with transcranial magnetic stimulation (TMS) usually does not affect healthy volunteers, but can lead to worsening of recovered motor behaviours in some chronic subcortical stroke patients [24–26]. The effect is usually dependent on residual impairment. For example, TMS to contralesional PMd is

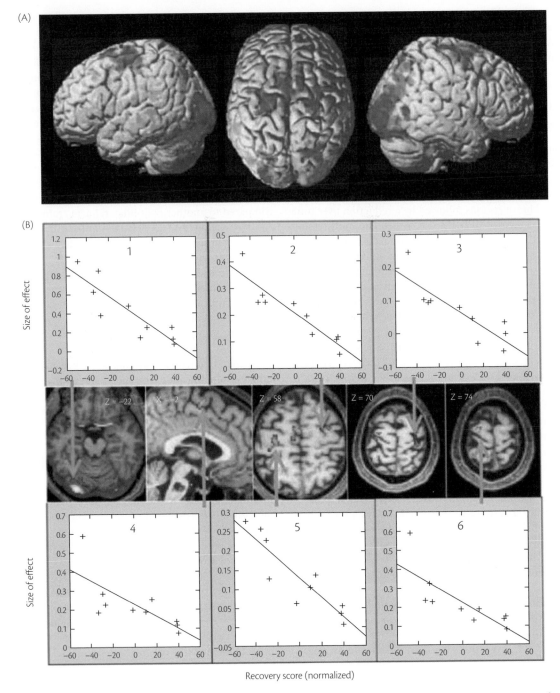

Fig. 15.2 Results of single subject longitudinal analysis examining for changes in brain activations during affected (right) hand grip over sessions as a function of recovery. The patient suffered from a left-sided pontine infarct resulting in right hemiparesis. (A) Results are surface rendered onto a canonical brain; red areas represent recovery-related decreases in task-related activation across sessions, and green areas represent the equivalent recovery-related increases. The brain is shown (from left to right) from the left (ipsilesional, IL) side, from above (left hemisphere on the left), and from the right (contralesional, CL). (B) Results are displayed on patient's own normalized T₁-weighted anatomical images with corresponding plots of magnitude of task-related activation against recovery score (higher number = less impairment), for selected brain regions.
Ward NS, Brown MM, Thompson AJ, Frackowiak RSJ, Neural correlates of motor recovery after stroke: a longitudinal fMRI study, Brain, 2003, 126, 2476–96, by permission of Oxford University Press.

more disruptive in patients with greater impairment [25], whereas TMS to ipsilesional PMd is more disruptive in less impaired patients [24], implying a contralesional shift in balance of functionally relevant activity in those patients with greater impairment. These findings are in keeping with the functional imaging findings previously discussed.

Another approach is based on the assumption that activity in brain areas that are functionally involved in producing a specific behaviour, co-vary with modulation of the task parameters. For example, activity in contralesional sensorimotor and premotor cortices might increase in proportion to the frequency of finger movements in well recovered stroke patients in contrast to control

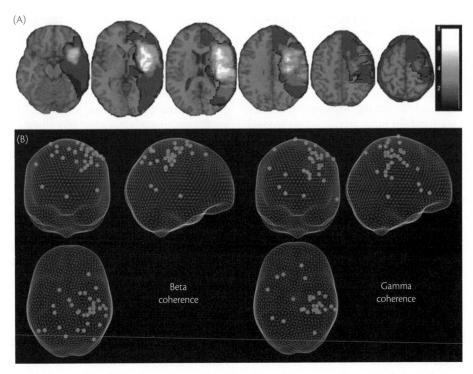

Fig. 15.3 Altered location of peak corticomuscular coherence after stroke. (A) Lesion overlap of stroke patients from axial slices on a template brain demonstrating the variety in cortical and subcortical damage across the group. Scale indicates number of patients overlapping. (B) 3D plot of peak coherence coordinates for beta (left) and gamma (right) (grip performed with left hand). Control subjects are shown in blue and patients are shown in red. Results are displayed on a 'glass brain' and shown from behind (top left), from the right side (top right) and from above (bottom left). Reproduced from Rossiter et al (2012) [23].

subjects [27]. Another study asked subjects to vary force output, rather than movement rate, and then examined for regional changes in the control of force modulation [28]. In healthy humans increasing force production is associated with linear increases in BOLD signal in contralateral M1 and medial motor regions, implying that they have a functional role in force production [29]. In stroke patients with minimal corticospinal system damage and excellent recovery, the cortical motor system behaved in a way that was similar to younger healthy controls. However, in patients with greater corticospinal system damage, force-related signal changes were seen mainly in contralesional dorsolateral premotor cortex, bilateral ventrolateral premotor cortices and contralesional cerebellum, but not ipsilesional primary motor cortex [28]. A qualitatively similar result was found in healthy volunteers with increasing age suggesting that this 'reorganization' might be a generic property of the cortical motor system in response to a variety of insults [30]. In relation to lesion-induced reorganization, not only do premotor cortices become increasingly active during movement as corticospinal system integrity diminishes [11], but also take on a new 'M1-like' role during modulation of force output, which implies a new and functionally relevant role in motor control.

The timing of the task-related activity might also be useful in determining function in relation to action. For example, using event-related fMRI contralesional M1 activity peaks seconds before ipsilesional M1 in stroke patients, in comparison to controls in whom the opposite relationship is observed [31]. On the other hand, in a different study using the fine temporal resolution of EEG, contralesional hemisphere activity was detected after the motor response had been made, suggesting that it was not

related to movement initiation in these patients [32]. Despite its temporal resolution, EEG lacks fine spatial resolution, and so it is not certain which contralesional brain region this result related to: M1 or premotor cortex for example. Others have used directed EEG coherence to investigate whether there is increased the flow of information from the ipsilateral motor cortex following motor stroke [33]. This approach suggested that in stroke patients with residual impairment, the contralesional hemisphere was the main 'driver' (at least in the beta band activity) for task-related flow of information during grip with the affected hand, whereas in recovered patients and controls cortical activity was driven from the ipsilesional (contralateral in controls) sensorimotor cortex.

The results described so far indicate that there is some novel contribution to motor control from the contralesional hemisphere after stroke. Some studies have moved their attention to the premotor cortex. At rest, it seems that the influence of contralesional PMd on ipsilesional motor cortex is inhibitory in well recovered patients, but becomes more facilitatory in those with greater clinical impairment [34]. By using concurrent TMS-fMRI, it was also possible to examine which brain regions contralesional PMd was influencing. During affected hand movement there was a stronger influence of contralesional PMd on two posterior parts of the ipsilesional sensorimotor cortex [34]. This provides a possible mechanism by which contralesional PMd might exert its state-dependent influence over the surviving cortical motor system, since ipsilesional sensorimotor cortex is most likely to be able to generate descending motor signals to the spinal cord to support recovered motor function.

The results presented so far suggest that activity in contralesional hemisphere contributes to motor control after stroke, particularly in more impaired patients. However, an alternative view is that motor areas in the contralesional hemisphere, in particular M1, are pathologically overactive after stroke. There are both TMS [35] and fMRI [36] studies which suggest that in some subcortical stroke patents, contralesional M1 although 'active', may exert an abnormally high degree of interhemispheric inhibitory drive towards ipsilesional M1 during attempted voluntary movement of the affected hand. In other words, contralesional M1 overactivity somehow suppresses ipsilesional M1 activity and consequently motor performance and recovery. Others have used this concept to suppress excitability in contralesional M1 using non-invasive brain stimulation, in an attempt to enhance the effect of motor training. There are now many small studies [37]. Although initially positive, the publication bias is gradually being corrected and negative studies are being published [38]. What is likely to emerge is that the anatomical and neurophysiological characteristics of the individual patient will determine if and how it is possible to prime the motor system so that training regimes have more effect. This will allow stratification of approaches based on mechanistic understanding [39].

The anatomical substrates of motor recovery

Reorganization of cortical motor systems is most prominent in patients with greatest clinical deficit and presumably with the most significant damage to the descending motor pathways. Clearly, recruitment of secondary motor areas does not get patients back to normal, but the evidence is that in many it is at least supporting what recovered function they have. If so, what are the possible anatomical substrates of this effect? A key determinant of motor recovery is sparing of the fast direct motor pathways from ipsilesional M1 to spinal cord motor neurons [40, 41]. There is little evidence that ipsilateral projections from motor cortex to forelimbs exist in primates [42], although this does not rule out such a possibility in humans. This makes ipsilateral projections from contralesional M1 a less likely substrate, but what about those from secondary motor areas? In primates, projections from secondary motor areas to spinal cord motor neurons are usually less numerous and less efficient at exciting spinal cord motoneurons than those from M1 [43, 44]. Studies in primates in which layer V (the 'output' layer) cortical neurons were stimulated and stimulus-triggered averages of electromyographic activity measured from forelimb muscles during a reach-to-grasp task [45, 46]. The onset latency and magnitude of facilitation effects from premotor areas PMd, PMv, SMA, and dorsal cingulate motor area (CMAd) were significantly longer and weaker than those from M1. Although there was evidence for the first time of a small number of direct projections to spinal cord motoneurons at least as fast as those from M1, from each of the secondary motor areas, the majority are unlikely to have a direct influence. Alternative pathways to spinal cord motoneurons would include via corticocortical connections with ipsilesional M1 or via interneurons in the spinal cord. Finally, it is often cited that secondary motor areas only have meaningful projections to proximal rather than distal muscles. In these studies, proximal muscles were predominantly represented in PMd and PMv but for both SMA and CMAd, facilitation effects were more common in distal compared to proximal

muscles. These medial motor areas are almost always 'overactive' in stroke patients compared to control subjects.

Another possibility is that premotor areas are able to send descending motor signals via alternative pathways such as reticulospinal projections to cervical propriospinal premotoneurons [47–49]. These pathways have divergent projections to muscle groups operating at multiple joints [50, 51], which might account for the multijoint 'associated' movements such as the synergistic flexion seen when patients with only poor and moderate recovery attempt isolated hand movements [47]. Although some see these synergistic movements as a barrier to further improvements in motor control (towards 'normal' patterns of movement), it is likely that these patients do not in fact have enough of the appropriate anatomical substrate (fast direct contralateral projections from ipsilesional M1) to support 'normal' movement. In this context, synergistic movements can contribute to functional improvement. Overall, it is feasible that a number of motor networks acting in parallel could generate an output to the spinal cord necessary for movement, and that damage in one of these networks could be at least partially compensated for by activity in another [52, 53].

Imaging language recovery after stroke

In the language domain, functional imaging studies of brain reorganization after stroke have focused largely on patients with anomia, a symptom present in almost all types of aphasia. Many of the functional imaging studies have demonstrated post-stroke activity in a right hemisphere homologue of either Broca's (BA 44/45) or Wernicke's (BA 22) area [54]. Attempts to find a correlation between the magnitude of right hemisphere activation and recovery of language function were unsuccessful, unlike the equivalent studies in the motor domain [10], suggesting that the story is most likely more complicated than simply switching a function from one hemisphere to the other.

This is illustrated by a longitudinal study in which early (within 12 days of stroke) overactivity in right Broca's area compared to controls correlated with better naming ability. After this early phase the relationship between right Broca's area activity and naming performance altered with declining activity occurring at a time of continued clinical improvement [55]. In the same study, there was little task-related BOLD signal very early after stroke (2 days), but it is not clear whether this was neural in origin or due to neurovascular uncoupling. Interestingly, the same early post-stroke reduction in task-related BOLD signal has been reported in the motor domain [56]. In keeping with this apparent alteration in the relationship between naming performance and right Broca's activity, attempted disruption of naming with transcranial magnetic stimulation was more successful in the first 2 weeks after stroke compared to 2 months later [57]. So, as in the motor domain, the role of surviving cortical regions changes with time after stroke.

Looking beyond Broca's, early recovery of naming ability is dependent on restoration of perfusion to at least one of three key areas in the dominant hemisphere—BA37 (posterior middle and inferior temporal/fusiform gyrus) and BA 22 (Wernicke's area) as well as Broca's area (BA 44/45) [58]. The most important of these for naming is BA 37, with perfusion-diffusion mismatch (i.e. salvageable tissue) in this area predicting good recovery [59]. Recovery of single word auditory comprehension however is most likely seen with reperfusion in BA22. One possibility is that damage to more posterior temporal structures (such as BA 22) can disrupt activity in more anterior superior temporal regions that are usually spared in middle cerebral artery territory strokes [60].

As in the motor domain, there have been studies examining treatment related alterations in activation pattern. The results are rather conflicting, possibly because of variations in patients (lesion anatomy, clinical phenotype) and the task used during scanning [61]. The key point to remember is that changes in activation pattern rarely point to the mechanism of the treatment itself, but rather reflect the behavioural improvement that has taken place, irrespective of which treatment was used. The field of functional imaging and language recovery after stroke is rapidly catching up with its counterpart in the motor domain in terms of numbers of publications. The details of numerous studies has been extensively and recently reviewed elsewhere [61–66].

Imaging cerebral consequences of spinal cord injury

Studies in animals with spinal cord injury (e.g. transection of the dorsal columns) demonstrate extensive reorganization of sensory inputs into the CNS [67–69]. In humans, functional brain imaging studies of those with spinal cord injury also provide evidence that distant neuronal damage has an impact on organization of the whole sensorimotor system. Studies that have examined brain activity during unaffected hand movements in paraplegic patients have shown a variety of changes [70]. Some, but not all, have demonstrated expansion or overrepresentation of one body part in the sensorimotor cortex at the expense of another. The magnitude and topography of cortical reorganization is variable and probably depends on a number of factors, in particular the characteristics of the anatomical damage. To examine these relationships explicitly, a recent study looked at the relationships between structural and functional changes following spinal cord injury [71] and found: (i) cortical thickness in sensorimotor areas was reduced in patients with spinal cord injury; (ii) task-related brain activation during hand grip was greater in M1 (leg) in spinal cord injury subjects with greater cord damage; and (iii) subjects with greater cord damage and greater reduction in tactile sensitivity showed greater brain activation of the face area of left S1 during right median nerve stimulation. Overall then, it is likely that variability of brain reorganization is driven by differences in anatomical damage. Failure to account for this in studies with small numbers of subjects is likely to lead to contradictory results. These caveats are of course true in stroke studies too, but more recently these problems have been addressed [8].

Assessing network connectivity

Many of the studies described use a 'voxel-wise' or region-of-interest approach. In other words, inferences are made about activity in certain parts of the brain independently of others. However, we know that the brain is organized in circuits and that brain regions influence one another. Assessing changes in connectivity within surviving networks is an interesting and biologically plausible way to go, but this approach is really only just starting. Two terms are often used—functional and effective connectivity.

The most important difference between these two analysis approaches is that effective connectivity analyses (e.g. dynamic causal modelling, structural equation modelling,) allows inference to be made about the influence that one brain area exerts over another, that is there is directionality in the data [72, 73]. Functional connectivity analyses (e.g. coherence or correlation analyses, graph theory) describes coupling between brain regions, but does not allow one to say that either area is influencing activity in the other (for example the coupling may be driven by another separate region) [74]. This is most commonly performed on fMRI data collected at rest, without the performance of a task.

Resting state data is most likely to reflect the consequences of changes in structural connectivity, since no actual task is performed. For example, stronger (functional) connectivity between ipsilesional M1 and other brain areas (i.e. more normal) in the early post-stroke phase is associated with better functional recovery 6 months later [75]. In particular, interhemispheric connectivity appears important, with reduced functional connectivity between ipsilesional M1 and contralesional M1 associated with greater motor impairment [76, 77].

Whichever approach is used, it is always important to find a link with behaviour, something that is intrinsically easier to do in pathological states than in healthy controls, because of the greater variability in performance. It is also useful to compare techniques (usually in the absence of a 'gold standard' metric). For example, Boudrias and colleagues [78] examined the influence of left M1 on right M1 during right hand squeeze, with both TMS and dynamic causal modelling (DCM) of fMRI data. The variability in this cohort came from the range of ages rather than pathology. The influence of left M1 on right M1 diminished with advancing age, and importantly, the assessment of interhemispheric inhibition with TMS correlated with that measured with DCM-fMRI, thus providing face validity for the DCM approach, at least in the cortical motor system.

Dynamic causal modelling of fMRI data has been used to show that effective connectivity between premotor areas and ipsilesional M1 was significantly reduced in the early post-stroke stages [36]. Another finding was of reduced coupling from ipsilesional SMA and PMd to ipsilesional M1 very early (less than 72 hours) after stroke. In patients who improved the most, these coupling parameters returned towards normal over the first few weeks [56].

The results from such studies have yet to converge in a way that provides convincing insights into network reorganization after CNS damage, but continued careful studies with larger numbers of subjects may lead to further insights.

Future applications for neuroimaging in neurorehabilitation

So far, we have considered studies that have examined brain organization at different stages of recovery after CNS injury. Although these findings are likely to reflect changes occurring as a consequence of neuroplasticity, it is not clear that they have led to different ways of thinking about how to treat patients with CNS injury. There are two ways that neuroimaging may contribute more directly to clinical care. First, by helping to predict likely outcomes and second, to indicate whether a particular treatment approach might benefit an individual patient.

Predicting outcomes with neuroimaging

The most obvious way to use neuroimaging to predict outcome after stroke is to assess CNS structure. DTI is able to assess integrity of white matter tracts and several studies have demonstrated that greater damage to the corticospinal tract (CST) is associated with more impairment [79], whilst the arcuate fasciculus is being examined in aphasia [80]. These measures may also be used to predict future outcome. CST integrity measured within three weeks of subcortical stroke correlate with both initial and 6 month upper limb impairment [81]. In a separate study, damage to the CST at the posterior limb of the internal capsule (PLIC) 12 hours post-stroke correlated well with motor impairment at 30 and 90 days [82]. These measures were superior to lesion volume and baseline clinical scores in their predictive power. TMS is also used to assess CST integrity and when combining it with DTI within 4 weeks of stroke, TMS had higher positive predictive value than DTI for upper limb function 6 months later, while DTI had higher negative predictive value [83]. Stinear and colleagues are currently developing an algorithm for sequentially combining simple clinical, TMS, and DTI measures to predict upper limb function [84]. The PREP (Predicting REcovery Potential) algorithm was tested in a sample of 40 subacute stroke patients and performed well in predicting motor function based on Action Research Arm Test scores at 12 weeks post-stroke. The performance of DTI in this setting should be improved by making the tracts specific to particular functions (e.g. upper limb [85]) (Figure 15.4), and developing ways for the assessment of tract integrity to be done in a standardized [86] and automatic [87] manner.

A more recent approach to predicting language outcome and recovery after stroke (PLORAS) uses the whole structural brain scan from which voxel-wise estimates of the likelihood of damaged tissue are derived. This 'lesion-map' for each patient is added to (i) time since stroke and (ii) a detailed assessment of various language capabilities. A new subject's lesion image is compared with those from all the other patients already in the database to find one with a similar lesion. The language scores for all the similar patients are plotted over time, enabling the time course of recovery for the new patient to be estimated (see Chapter 21) [88, 89]. The potential for such an approach extend to many domains including motor and cognitive outcomes. Using this type of neuroimaging complex biomarker discovery [90] we should be aiming to provide accurate prognostic models allowing accurate goal setting in neurorehabilitation and stratification in clinical trials [39].

Functional MRI data acquired in the first few days after stroke has been used to try to predict a subsequent change in motor performance [91]. A particular pattern of brain activation was highly predictive of clinical change over the subsequent 3 months, a finding that was independent of initial stroke severity and lesion volume. Although the multivariate analysis used did not allow anatomical inference to be made, it is clear that there is something about the way the function of the brain responds to injury, over and above the anatomy of the damage, that holds clues about future clinical progression. The pattern was distributed and certainly not confined to the motor system, even though clinical improvement was measured in the motor domain. This result suggests that motor improvement may not be solely related to the integrity of the corticospinal system but also with other characteristics of the post-stroke brain.

A similar approach was used to predict outcome in language using fMRI data acquired within 2 weeks of stroke in patients with aphasia [92]. A multivariate machine learning approach was used and demonstrated 76% accuracy in predicting good and bad outcome at 6 months. This accuracy was improved to 86% when age and baseline language impairment was added to the classification model.

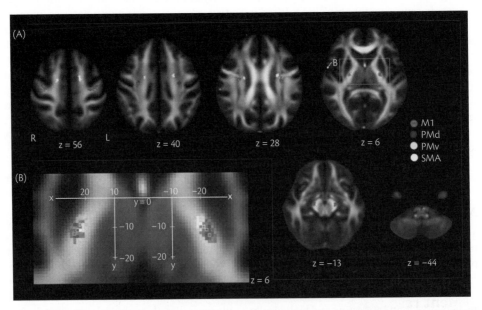

Fig. 15.4 (A) Corticospinal tract (CST) originating from primary motor cortex (M1), dorsolateral premotor cortex (PMd), ventrolateral premotor cortex (PMv), and supplementary motor area (SMA) connecting cortical areas known to be active during hand grip and a caudal pontine target zone. (B) The topographical distribution of CST fibres within posterior limb of the internal capsule (PLIC), with M1 located posteriorly and PMd, PMv, and SMA following in a posteroanterior direction.
Schulz R, Park C-H, Boudrias M-H, Assessing the integrity of corticospinal pathways from primary and secondary cortical motor areas after stroke, Stroke, 43, 2248–51 ©2012.

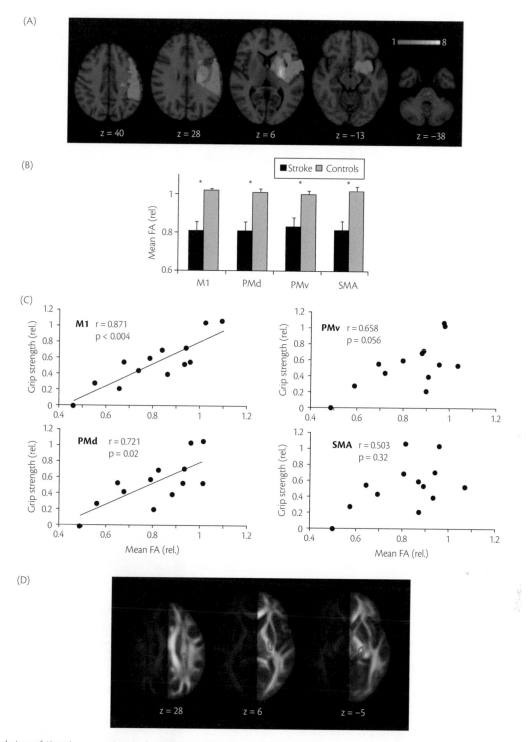

Fig. 15.5 (A) Stroke lesions of 13 patients superimposed, overlaid on a MNI-T1 template. Scale indicates number of patients overlapping. (B) One-way ANOVA revealed a significant reduction of proportional fractional anisotropy (FA) for corticospinal tract (CST) originating from M1, PMd, PMv, and SMA after stroke compared with controls. (C) Tract-specific proportional FA plotted against grip strength. (D) White-matter regions exhibiting significant positive correlation between proportional FA and grip strength (shown on axial sections).
Schulz R, Park C-H, Boudrias M-H, Assessing the integrity of corticospinal pathways from primary and secondary cortical motor areas after stroke, Stroke, 43, 2248–51 ©2012.

Predicting treatment response with neuroimaging

Predicting outcome will be useful for clinical and research stratification, but what a clinician would like to know is what are the chances of a patient responding to a specific intervention. Stinear and colleagues [93] set out to determine whether characterizing the state of the motor system would help in predicting an individual patient's capacity for further functional improvement at least 6 months post-stroke in a subsequent motor practice programme.

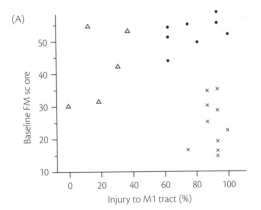

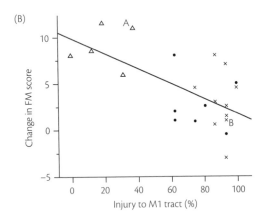

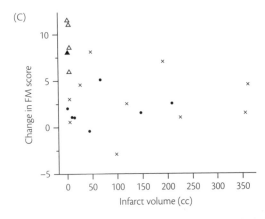

Fig. 15.6 Relationships between anatomical damage after stroke and motor improvement with training. (a) Injury to the tract descending from M1 in relation to baseline Fugl-Meyer (FM) score. A significant linear correlation was not present ($p > 0.25$). However, three subject clusters are apparent on inspection of the data: a subgroup of subjects with mild tract injury has mild–moderate motor deficits (marked as triangle); subjects with moderate-severe injury have either mild–moderate (marked as circles) or severe (marked as 'x') deficits. This injury/behaviour subgrouping was also apparent for the other three tracts. b) Injury to the tract descending from M1 correlates ($r = -0.65$, $p < 0.002$) with the treatment-induced change in FM score. Subjects with mild tract injury had greater gains from treatment. A and B indicate the two subjects whose images appear in Figure 15.7. (c) A global measure of stroke-induced injury, infarct volume, did not show a significant relationship with the treatment-induced change in FM score ($p > 0.2$).

Riley JD, Le V, Der-Yeghiaian L, See J, et al., Anatomy of stroke injury predicts gains from therapy, Stroke, 42, 421–6. ©2011.

In an approach similar to the subsequent PREP algorithm [84], TMS, structural MRI, and on this occasion, functional MRI were used. In patients with MEPs, meaningful gains with motor practice were still possible 3 years after stroke. The situation in patients without MEPs has always been more difficult to predict in the clinical setting but is often taken as a poor prognostic sign [94]. DTI assessment of CST integrity allowed further stratification into responders and non-responders. Interestingly, the patients also performed a simple motor task during fMRI, but the results as assessed by the degree of lateralization to one hemisphere or the other did not contribute to the predictive model. This kind of study illustrates how multimodal imaging and neurophysiological data could be used to assess the state of the motor system and predict the potential for therapy driven functional improvements.

Cramer and colleagues [95] assessed 13 baseline clinical/radiological measures and asked whether each was able to predict subsequent gains made during 6 weeks of robotic rehabilitation therapy. In the first analysis only two baseline measures were significant

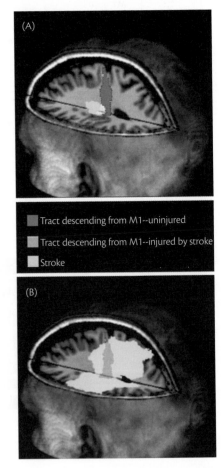

Fig. 15.7 Examples of stroke injury to the tract descending from M1. (A) This subject had 37.5% of the M1 tract injured by stroke and had a gain of 11 points on the FM scale across the period of therapy. (B) This subject had 93.4% of the M1 tract injured by stroke and had a gain of 1 point on the FM scale across the period of therapy.

Riley JD, Le V, Der-Yeghiaian L, See J, et al., Anatomy of stroke injury predicts gains from therapy, Stroke, 42, 421–6. ©2011.

and independent predictors of clinical improvement. The first was a lower level of impairment and the second was lower motor cortex activation, as measured with fMRI. The result tells us that there is something in the imaging data which is independent of baseline clinical impairment which can predict response to therapy.

In a second analysis, structural rather than functional imaging was used to try to explain differences in response to intensive rehabilitation [96]. The likely extent of damage to descending pathways from each of M1, PMd, PMv, and SMA was calculated from an overlap between the lesion map and the 'normal' map for each of the descending pathways (Figure 15.6). Less damage to M1 and PMd related pathways correlated well with treatment gains, but infarct volume and baseline behaviour did not. Linderberg and colleagues [97] also demonstrated that preserved tract integrity was associated with greater functional gains with bihemispheric cortical stimulation and physical therapy. This result is in keeping with the findings of Riley [96] that a more normal anatomy allows greater change. The anatomy of the damage is likely to set a limit on how well individual patents will respond.

At present, we are not able to tailor therapies to individual patients, but these studies illustrate the way forward. Clearly, there needs to be progression from proof-of-principle to incorporating predictive tools into larger trials and there is some evidence that it is possible to attempt this [98].

Conclusion

In summary, CNS damage leads to reconfiguration of brain networks with some brain regions adopting the characteristics of damaged or disconnected regions. This reorganization varies across patients, but does so in a way that appears to be at least partially predictable. Reorganization of regions and networks is often not successful in returning performance back to pre-injury levels—the extent of anatomical damage plays a significant limiting role—but it probably helps an individual to achieve some of their potential level of recovery. The potential for functionally relevant change to occur will depend on a number of other factors beyond the anatomy of the damage, not least the biologic age of the subject and the premorbid state of their based on levels of neurotransmitters and growth factors which are able to influence the ability of the brain to respond to afferent input might be determined by their genetic status [99]. Predicting treatment effects will be based on understanding the interactions between these factors [39]. It is clear that individual differences will have a major influence on how a patient might respond to restorative therapies, and it is in this context that modern neuroimaging (together with neurophysiological) techniques may be able to shed light on brain reorganization after CNS damage in individual subjects. Future work should aim to use these kinds of approaches to determine whether assessment of individual post-injury residual functional architecture can be a major predictor of outcome, opening the way for stratification of patients based on the likely response to an intervention

Acknowledgements

N.S.W. is supported by The Wellcome Trust, Medical Research Council and the European Commission (FP7).

References

1. Murphy TH, Corbett D. Plasticity during stroke recovery: from synapse to behaviour. Nat Rev Neurosci. 2009;**10**(12):861–872.
2. Cramer SC, Chopp M. Recovery recapitulates ontogeny. Trends Neurosci. 2000;**23**(6):265–271.
3. Dyrby TB, Søgaard LV, Parker GJ, et al. Validation of in vitro probabilistic tractography. NeuroImage. 2007 1;**37**(4):1267–1277.
4. Cramer SC, Nelles G, Benson RR, et al. A functional MRI study of subjects recovered from hemiparetic stroke. Stroke. 1997;**28**(12):2518–2527.
5. Chollet F, DiPiero V, Wise RJ, Brooks DJ, Dolan RJ, Frackowiak RS. The functional anatomy of motor recovery after stroke in humans: a study with positron emission tomography. Ann Neurol. 1991;**29**(1):63–71.
6. Seitz RJ, Höflich P, Binkofski F, Tellmann L, Herzog H, Freund HJ. Role of the premotor cortex in recovery from middle cerebral artery infarction. Arch Neurol. 1998;**55**(8):1081–1088.
7. Weiller C, Chollet F, Friston KJ, Wise RJ, Frackowiak RS. Functional reorganization of the brain in recovery from striatocapsular infarction in man. Ann Neurol. 1992;**31**(5):463–472.
8. Rehme AK, Eickhoff SB, Rottschy C, Fink GR, Grefkes C. Activation likelihood estimation meta-analysis of motor-related neural activity after stroke. NeuroImage. 2012;**59**(3):2771–2782.
9. Baron J-C, Cohen LG, Cramer SC, et al. Neuroimaging in stroke recovery: a position paper from the First International Workshop on Neuroimaging and Stroke Recovery. Cerebrovasc Dis. 2004;**18**(3):260–267.
10. Ward NS, Brown MM, Thompson AJ, Frackowiak RSJ. Neural correlates of outcome after stroke: a cross-sectional fMRI study. Brain. 2003;**126**(Pt 6):1430–1448.
11. Ward NS, Newton JM, Swayne OBC, et al. Motor system activation after subcortical stroke depends on corticospinal system integrity. Brain. 2006;**129**(Pt 3):809–819.
12. Ward NS, Brown MM, Thompson AJ, Frackowiak RSJ. The influence of time after stroke on brain activations during a motor task. Ann Neurol. 2004;**55**(6):829–834.
13. Staudt M, Grodd W, Gerloff C, Erb M, Stitz J, Krägeloh-Mann I. Two types of ipsilateral reorganization in congenital hemiparesis: a TMS and fMRI study. Brain. 2002;**125**(Pt 10):2222–2237.
14. Calautti C, Leroy F, Guincestre JY, Baron JC. Dynamics of motor network overactivation after striatocapsular stroke: a longitudinal PET study using a fixed-performance paradigm. Stroke. 2001;**32**(11):2534–2542.
15. Marshall RS, Perera GM, Lazar RM, Krakauer JW, Constantine RC, DeLaPaz RL. Evolution of cortical activation during recovery from corticospinal tract infarction. Stroke. 2000;**31**(3):656–661.
16. Ward NS, Brown MM, Thompson AJ, Frackowiak RSJ. Neural correlates of motor recovery after stroke: a longitudinal fMRI study. Brain. 2003;**126**(Pt 11):2476–2496.
17. Calautti C, Jones PS, Naccarato M, et al. The relationship between motor deficit and primary motor cortex hemispheric activation balance after stroke: longitudinal fMRI study. J Neurol Neurosurg Psychiatry. 2010;**81**(7):788–792.
18. Rehme AK, Eickhoff SB, Wang LE, Fink GR, Grefkes C. Dynamic causal modeling of cortical activity from the acute to the chronic stage after stroke. NeuroImage. 2011;**55**(3):1147–1158.
19. Tombari D, Loubinoux I, Pariente J, et al. A longitudinal fMRI study: in recovering and then in clinically stable sub-cortical stroke patients. NeuroImage. 2004;**23**(3):827–839.
20. Donahue MJ, Near J, Blicher JU, Jezzard P. Baseline GABA concentration and fMRI response. NeuroImage. 2010 1;**53**(2):392–398.
21. Hodics T, Cohen LG, Cramer SC. Functional imaging of intervention effects in stroke motor rehabilitation. Arch Phys Med Rehabil. 2006;**87**(12 Suppl 2):S36–42.

22. Whitall J, Waller SM, Sorkin JD, et al. Bilateral and unilateral arm training improve motor function through differing neuroplastic mechanisms: a single-blinded randomized controlled trial. Neurorehabil Neural Repair. 2011;**25**(2):118–129.

23. Rossiter HE, Eaves C, Davis E, et al. Changes in the location of cortico-muscular coherence following stroke. NeuroImage Clin. 2013;**2**(0):50–55.

24. Fridman EA, Hanakawa T, Chung M, Hummel F, Leiguarda RC, Cohen LG. Reorganization of the human ipsilesional premotor cortex after stroke. Brain. 2004;**127**(Pt 4):747–758.

25. Johansen-Berg H, Rushworth MFS, Bogdanovic MD, Kischka U, Wimalaratna S, Matthews PM. The role of ipsilateral premotor cortex in hand movement after stroke. Proc Natl Acad Sci U S A. 2002;**99**(22):14518–14523.

26. Lotze M, Markert J, Sauseng P, Hoppe J, Plewnia C, Gerloff C. The role of multiple contralesional motor areas for complex hand movements after internal capsular lesion. J Neurosci. 2006;**26**(22):6096–6102.

27. Riecker A, Gröschel K, Ackermann H, Schnaudigel S, Kassubek J, Kastrup A. The role of the unaffected hemisphere in motor recovery after stroke. Hum Brain Mapp. 2010;**31**(7):1017–1029.

28. Ward NS, Newton JM, Swayne OBC, et al. The relationship between brain activity and peak grip force is modulated by corticospinal system integrity after subcortical stroke. Eur J Neurosci. 2007;**25**(6):1865–1873.

29. Ward NS, Frackowiak RSJ. Age-related changes in the neural correlates of motor performance. Brain. 2003;**126**(Pt 4):873–888.

30. Ward NS, Swayne OBC, Newton JM. Age-dependent changes in the neural correlates of force modulation: an fMRI study. Neurobiol Aging. 2008;**29**(9):1434–1446.

31. Newton J, Sunderland A, Butterworth SE, Peters AM, Peck KK, Gowland PA. A pilot study of event-related functional magnetic resonance imaging of monitored wrist movements in patients with partial recovery. Stroke. 2002;**33**(12):2881–2887.

32. Verleger R, Adam S, Rose M, Vollmer C, Wauschkuhn B, Kömpf D. Control of hand movements after striatocapsular stroke: high-resolution temporal analysis of the function of ipsilateral activation. Clin Neurophysiol. 2003;**114**(8):1468–1476.

33. Serrien DJ, Strens LHA, Cassidy MJ, Thompson AJ, Brown P. Functional significance of the ipsilateral hemisphere during movement of the affected hand after stroke. Exp Neurol. 2004;**190**(2):425–432.

34. Bestmann S, Swayne O, Blankenburg F, Ruff CC, Teo J, Weiskopf N, et al. The role of contralesional dorsal premotor cortex after stroke as studied with concurrent TMS-fMRI. J Neurosci. 2010 8;**30**(36):11926–11937.

35. Murase N, Duque J, Mazzocchio R, Cohen LG. Influence of interhemispheric interactions on motor function in chronic stroke. Ann Neurol. 2004;**55**(3):400–409.

36. Grefkes C, Nowak DA, Eickhoff SB, al. Cortical connectivity after subcortical stroke assessed with functional magnetic resonance imaging. Ann Neurol. 2008;**63**(2):236–246.

37. Takeuchi N, Izumi S-I. Noninvasive brain stimulation for motor recovery after stroke: mechanisms and future views. Stroke Res Treat. 2012;**2012**:584727.

38. Talelli P, Wallace A, Dileone M, Hoad D, Cheeran B, Oliver R, et al. Theta burst stimulation in the rehabilitation of the upper limb: a semirandomized, placebo-controlled trial in chronic stroke patients. Neurorehabil Neural Repair. 2012;**26**(8):976–987.

39. Ward NS. Getting lost in translation. Curr Opin Neurol. 2008 ;**21**(6):625–627.

40. Heald A, Bates D, Cartlidge NE, French JM, Miller S. Longitudinal study of central motor conduction time following stroke. 2. Central motor conduction measured within 72 h after stroke as a predictor of functional outcome at 12 months. Brain. 1993;**116** (Pt 6):1371–1385.

41. Pennisi G, Rapisarda G, Bella R, et al. Absence of response to early transcranial magnetic stimulation in ischemic stroke patients: prognostic value for hand motor recovery. Stroke. 1999;**30**(12):2666–2670.

42. Soteropoulos DS, Edgley SA, Baker SN. Lack of evidence for direct corticospinal contributions to control of the ipsilateral forelimb in monkey. J Neurosci. 2011;**31**(31):11208–11219.

43. Boudrias M-H, Belhaj-Saïf A, Park MC, Cheney PD. Contrasting properties of motor output from the supplementary motor area and primary motor cortex in rhesus macaques. Cereb Cortex. 2006;**16**(5):632–638.

44. Maier MA, Armand J, Kirkwood PA, Yang H-W, Davis JN, Lemon RN. Differences in the corticospinal projection from primary motor cortex and supplementary motor area to macaque upper limb motoneurons: an anatomical and electrophysiological study. Cereb Cortex. 2002;**12**(3):281–296.

45. Boudrias M-H, McPherson RL, Frost SB, Cheney PD. Output properties and organization of the forelimb representation of motor areas on the lateral aspect of the hemisphere in rhesus macaques. Cereb Cortex. 2010;**20**(1):169–186.

46. Boudrias M-H, Lee S-P, Svojanovsky S, Cheney PD. Forelimb muscle representations and output properties of motor areas in the mesial wall of rhesus macaques. Cereb Cortex. 2010;**20**(3):704–719.

47. Baker SN. The primate reticulospinal tract, hand function and functional recovery. J Physiol. 2011;**589**(Pt 23):5603–5612.

48. Mazevet D, Meunier S, Pradat-Diehl P, Marchand-Pauvert V, Pierrot-Deseilligny E. Changes in propriospinally mediated excitation of upper limb motoneurons in stroke patients. Brain. 2003;**126**(Pt 4):988–1000.

49. Stinear JW, Byblow WD. Modulation of human cervical premotoneurons during bilateral voluntary contraction of upper-limb muscles. Muscle Nerve. 2004;**29**(4):506–514.

50. Mazevet D, Pierrot-Deseilligny E. Pattern of descending excitation of presumed propriospinal neurones at the onset of voluntary movement in humans. Acta Physiol Scand. 1994;**150**(1):27–38.

51. Pierrot-Deseilligny E. Transmission of the cortical command for human voluntary movement through cervical propriospinal premotoneurons. Prog Neurobiol. 1996;**48**(4–5):489–517.

52. Dum RP, Strick PL. The origin of corticospinal projections from the premotor areas in the frontal lobe. J Neurosci. 1991;**11**(3):667–689.

53. Rouiller EM, Moret V, Tanne J, Boussaoud D. Evidence for direct connections between the hand region of the supplementary motor area and cervical motoneurons in the macaque monkey. Eur J Neurosci. 1996;**8**(5):1055–1059.

54. Crinion JT, Leff AP. Recovery and treatment of aphasia after stroke: functional imaging studies. Curr Opin Neurol. 2007;**20**(6):667–673.

55. Saur D, Lange R, Baumgaertner A, et al. Dynamics of language reorganization after stroke. Brain. 2006;**129**(Pt 6):1371–1384.

56. Rehme AK, Fink GR, von Cramon DY, Grefkes C. The role of the contralesional motor cortex for motor recovery in the early days after stroke assessed with longitudinal FMRI. Cereb Cortex. 2011;**21**(4):756–768.

57. Winhuisen L, Thiel A, Schumacher B, et al. The right inferior frontal gyrus and poststroke aphasia: a follow-up investigation. Stroke. 2007;**38**(4):1286–1292.

58. Hillis AE, Kleinman JT, Newhart M, et al. Restoring cerebral blood flow reveals neural regions critical for naming. J Neurosci. 2006;**26**(31):8069–8073.

59. Hillis AE, Gold L, Kannan V, et al. Site of the ischemic penumbra as a predictor of potential for recovery of functions. Neurology. 2008;**71**(3):184–189.

60. Crinion JT, Warburton EA, Lambon-Ralph MA, Howard D, Wise RJS. Listening to narrative speech after aphasic stroke: the role of the left anterior temporal lobe. Cereb Cortex. 2006;**16**(8):1116–1125.

61. Rapp B, Caplan D, Edwards S, Visch-Brink E, Thompson CK. Neuroimaging in aphasia treatment research: issues of experimental design for relating cognitive to neural changes. NeuroImage. 2013;**73**:200–207.

62. Meinzer M, Beeson PM, Cappa S, et al. Neuroimaging in aphasia treatment research: consensus and practical guidelines for data analysis. NeuroImage. 2013;73:215–224.

63. Smits M, Visch-Brink EG, van de Sandt-Koenderman ME, van der Lugt A. Advanced magnetic resonance neuroimaging of language function recovery after aphasic stroke: a technical review. Arch Phys Med Rehabil. 2012;93(1 Suppl):S4–14.

64. Saur D, Hartwigsen G. Neurobiology of language recovery after stroke: lessons from neuroimaging studies. Arch Phys Med Rehabil. 2012;93(1 Suppl):S15–25.

65. Berthier ML, García-Casares N, Walsh SF, et al. Recovery from post-stroke aphasia: lessons from brain imaging and implications for rehabilitation and biological treatments. Discov Med. 2011;12(65):275–289.

66. Cappa SF. The neural basis of aphasia rehabilitation: evidence from neuroimaging and neurostimulation. Neuropsychol Rehabil. 2011;21(5):742–754.

67. Ghosh A, Haiss F, Sydekum E, Schneider R, Gullo M, Wyss MT, et al. Rewiring of hindlimb corticospinal neurons after spinal cord injury. Nat Neurosci. 2010;13(1):97–104.

68. Kaas JH, Qi H-X, Burish MJ, Gharbawie OA, Onifer SM, Massey JM. Cortical and subcortical plasticity in the brains of humans, primates, and rats after damage to sensory afferents in the dorsal columns of the spinal cord. Exp Neurol. 2008;209(2):407–416.

69. Tandon S, Kambi N, Lazar L, Mohammed H, Jain N. Large-scale expansion of the face representation in somatosensory areas of the lateral sulcus after spinal cord injuries in monkeys. J Neurosci. 2009;29(38):12009–12019.

70. Kokotilo KJ, Eng JJ, Curt A. Reorganization and preservation of motor control of the brain in spinal cord injury: a systematic review. J Neurotrauma. 2009;26(11):2113–2126.

71. Freund P, Weiskopf N, Ward NS, Hutton C, Gall A, Ciccarelli O, et al. Disability, atrophy and cortical reorganization following spinal cord injury. Brain. 2011;134(Pt 6):1610–1622.

72. Kahan J, Foltynie T. Understanding DCM: Ten simple rules for the clinician. NeuroImage. 2013;83C:542–549.

73. Seghier ML, Zeidman P, Neufeld NH, Leff AP, Price CJ. Identifying abnormal connectivity in patients using dynamic causal modeling of FMRI responses. Front Syst Neurosci. 2010;4:p. ii, 142.

74. Grefkes C, Fink GR. Reorganization of cerebral networks after stroke: new insights from neuroimaging with connectivity approaches. Brain. 2011;134(Pt 5):1264–1276.

75. Park C, Chang WH, Ohn SH, et al. Longitudinal changes of resting-state functional connectivity during motor recovery after stroke. Stroke. 2011;42(5):1357–1362.

76. Carter AR, Patel KR, Astafiev SV, et al. Upstream dysfunction of somatomotor functional connectivity after corticospinal damage in stroke. Neurorehabil Neural Repair. 2012;26(1):7–19.

77. Carter AR, Astafiev SV, Lang CE, et al. Resting interhemispheric functional magnetic resonance imaging connectivity predicts performance after stroke. Ann Neurol. 2010;67(3):365–375.

78. Boudrias M-H, Gonçalves CS, Penny WD, et al. Age-related changes in causal interactions between cortical motor regions during hand grip. NeuroImage. 2012;59(4):3398–3405.

79. Jang SH. Prediction of motor outcome for hemiparetic stroke patients using diffusion tensor imaging: A review. NeuroRehabilitation. 2010;27(4):367–372.

80. Kim SH, Lee DG, You H, et al. The clinical application of the arcuate fasciculus for stroke patients with aphasia: a diffusion tensor tractography study. NeuroRehabilitation. 2011;29(3):305–310.

81. Radlinska B, Ghinani S, Leppert IR, Minuk J, Pike GB, Thiel A. Diffusion tensor imaging, permanent pyramidal tract damage, and outcome in subcortical stroke. Neurology. 2010;75(12):1048–1054.

82. Puig J, Pedraza S, Blasco G, et al. Acute damage to the posterior limb of the internal capsule on diffusion tensor tractography as an early imaging predictor of motor outcome after stroke. Am J Neuroradiol. 2011;32(5):857–863.

83. Kwon YH, Son SM, Lee J, Bai DS, Jang SH. Combined study of transcranial magnetic stimulation and diffusion tensor tractography for prediction of motor outcome in patients with corona radiata infarct. J Rehabil Med. 2011;43(5):430–434.

84. Stinear CM, Barber PA, Petoe M, Anwar S, Byblow WD. The PREP algorithm predicts potential for upper limb recovery after stroke. Brain. 2012;135(Pt 8):2527–2535.

85. Schulz R, Park C-H, Boudrias M-H, Gerloff C, Hummel FC, Ward NS. Assessing the integrity of corticospinal pathways from primary and secondary cortical motor areas after stroke. Stroke. 2012;43(8):2248–2251.

86. Park C, Kou N, Boudrias M-H, Playford ED, Ward NS. Assessing a standardised approach to measuring corticospinal integrity after stroke with DTI. NeuroImage Clin. 2013;2:521–533.

87. Kou N, Park C-H, Seghier ML, Leff AP, Ward NS. Can fully automated detection of corticospinal tract damage be used in stroke patients? Neurology. 2013;80(24):2242–2245.

88. Price CJ, Seghier ML, Leff AP. Predicting language outcome and recovery after stroke: the PLORAS system. Nat Rev Neurol. 2010;6(4):202–210.

89. Hope TMH, Seghier ML, Leff AP, Price CJ. Predicting outcome and recovery after stroke with lesions extracted from MRI images. NeuroImage Clin. 2013;2(0):424–433.

90. Atluri G, Padmanabhan K, Fang G, et al. Complex biomarker discovery in neuroimaging data: Finding a needle in a haystack. NeuroImage Clin. 2013;3(0):123–131.

91. Zarahn E, Alon L, Ryan SL, et al. Prediction of motor recovery using initial impairment and fMRI 48 h poststroke. Cereb Cortex. 2011;21(12):2712–2721.

92. Saur D, Ronneberger O, Kümmerer D, Mader I, Weiller C, Klöppel S. Early functional magnetic resonance imaging activations predict language outcome after stroke. Brain. 2010;133(Pt 4):1252–1264.

93. Stinear CM, Barber PA, Smale PR, Coxon JP, Fleming MK, Byblow WD. Functional potential in chronic stroke patients depends on corticospinal tract integrity. Brain. 2007;130(Pt 1):170–180.

94. Heald A, Bates D, Cartlidge NE, French JM, Miller S. Longitudinal study of central motor conduction time following stroke. 2. Central motor conduction measured within 72 h after stroke as a predictor of functional outcome at 12 months. Brain. 1993;116 (Pt 6):1371–1385.

95. Cramer SC, Parrish TB, Levy RM, et al. Predicting functional gains in a stroke trial. Stroke. 2007;38(7):2108–2114.

96. Riley JD, Le V, Der-Yeghiaian L, et al. Anatomy of stroke injury predicts gains from therapy. Stroke. 2011;42(2):421–426.

97. Lindenberg R, Zhu LL, Rüber T, Schlaug G. Predicting functional motor potential in chronic stroke patients using diffusion tensor imaging. Hum Brain Mapp. 2012;33(5):1040–1051.

98. Pomeroy VM, Ward NS, Johansen-Berg H, et al. FAST INdiCATE Trial protocol. Clinical efficacy of functional strength training for upper limb motor recovery early after stroke: Neural correlates and prognostic indicators. Int J Stroke. 2014 9(2):240–245;

99. Kleim JA, Chan S, Pringle E, et al. BDNF val66met polymorphism is associated with modified experience-dependent plasticity in human motor cortex. Nat Neurosci. 2006;9(6):735–737.

CHAPTER 16

Enhancement of neuroplasticity by cortical stimulation

Orlando Swayne and John Rothwell

Introduction

Recent years have witnessed a dramatic increase in understanding of the pathophysiological mechanisms underlying neurorehabilitation, as detailed in the chapters of this volume. Some of these advances, though not all, relate to the role thought to be played by neuroplasticity, the process by which prior experience can alter the structure and function of the nervous system. This concept is an attractive one, as it raises the possibility that interventions which interact with neuroplasticity may be able to alter the outcome of neurorehabilitation. Non-invasive brain stimulation is one such intervention; its ready availability in the research setting, its relatively benign safety profile and a wealth of literature over the last two decades relating to its uses and mechanisms has prompted intense interest in its potential to augment the outcome of neurorehabilitation. The rationale behind this approach is that the application of cortical stimulation at or around the time of conventional therapy may enhance the associated neuroplasticity, with behavioural gains that would outlive the period of stimulation and therapy.

There is a growing literature describing the use of cortical stimulation in clinical settings. Its most established clinical application at present is in the treatment of depression, but although this has received the approval of the US Food and Drug Administration its role and efficacy remain controversial [1, 2]. In the context of neurorehabilitation most research has related to improving the motor deficit after stroke [3–5], but there is interest also in the use of cortical stimulation for non-motor stroke deficits and in other conditions including traumatic brain injury, Parkinson's disease, chronic pain, Tourette syndrome, and dystonia [6–10].

Despite extensive interest and much research, however, cortical stimulation is yet to find an established role in neurorehabilitation. There are a number of reasons for this, which we will review in the course of this chapter.

1. The most effective way to use cortical stimulation in a clinical context depends upon what we think it is doing, and at present this is far from clear. Much of what is known regarding the effects of cortical stimulation in humans comes from experiments measuring changes in excitability of motor cortex, itself often measured by brain stimulation. However it is not necessarily the case that excitability changes are accompanied by beneficial effects on a given behaviour, such as motor skill, and dissociations have frequently been observed [11].

2. Likewise when clear effects of stimulation on behaviour have been documented they are most commonly studied in the context of learning in the healthy brain [12]. The process of healthy learning is taken here as being analogous to neurorehabilitation: while there are sound arguments for this analogy it remains to some extent an assumption, and efficacy in the context of the normal brain will not necessarily translate into benefit for patients.

3. There are an increasing number of cortical stimulation protocols and each contains several variables (stimulation duration, frequency, intensity, site). Clinical studies of cortical stimulation in patient groups rarely employ an identical protocol to previous studies, making it hard to replicate or extend prior results. The result of this diversity of approach is that a consensus is currently lacking as to the most promising stimulation protocols, a necessary precursor to larger scale clinical trials.

4. Finally the clinical application of cortical stimulation is beset by the significant inter- and even intra-subject variability of effect commonly observed with most protocols.

In this chapter we review the currently available stimulation protocols and their likely mechanisms, the effects of stimulation on healthy learning and the current evidence in neurorehabilitation. We finally consider the combination of cortical stimulation with other interventions and future research directions.

Cortical stimulation techniques

Stimulation protocols

The two most widely studied forms of non-invasive cortical stimulation are transcranial magnetic stimulation (TMS) and transcranial direct current stimulation (tDCS)—see Figure 16.1. Transcranial electrical stimulation was a precursor to TMS and is rarely employed now in view of scalp pain induced by stimulation. Implanted stimulation devices have been studied in the context of stroke but will not be considered in this chapter. In TMS an extracranial magnetic coil is discharged while resting on the subject's scalp. A brief, rapidly changing electrical current within the coil induces a strong and localized magnetic field perpendicular to the brain's surface: this itself induces an electrical field parallel to the cortical surface. A suprathreshold stimulus may cause trans-synaptic depolarization of corticofugal neurons, in the case of the motor cortex giving rise to a corticospinal volley which

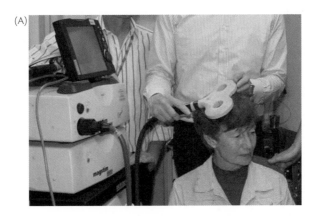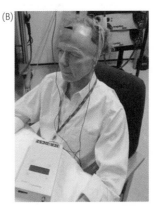

Fig. 16.1 (A) Transcranial magnetic stimulation is delivered here through a figure-of-eight coil resting on the subject's scalp. Resulting motor evoked potentials are monitored by electromyograph recording from the subject's hand. (B) Transcranial direct current stimulation electrodes arranged in a typical montage targeting the left hemisphere.

may be measured peripherally as a motor evoked potential (MEP) recorded by electromyography. As the preferential site of neuronal depolarization is the axon (rather than the cell body) the effect of TMS on cortical function is sensitive to coil orientation and position in relation to underlying gyri. In tDCS a low amplitude direct current, typically 1–2 mA, is applied via two surface conductive rubber electrodes typically of 25–35 cm^2 applied to the scalp. The constant electrical field modifies membrane potentials in the underlying cerebral cortex, altering firing thresholds without triggering depolarization. Both TMS and tDCS may induce 'offline' effects on brain excitability and function, which outlast the period of stimulation and which appear to depend on synaptic modulation. The effects of stimulation in humans have been most widely studied in relation to the motor cortex, as this region's excitability may be readily assessed by measuring the peripheral MEP amplitude.

Repetitive TMS (rTMS) at a frequency greater than around 0.1 Hz can induce transient changes in cortical excitability—these are summarized in Figure 16.2. Although a great number of protocols have been described, with a range of effects, it is generally the case that stimulation at low frequencies (around 1 Hz) induces a period of reduced excitability (i.e. smaller MEPs in response to a suprathreshold stimulus), whereas stimulation at higher frequencies (>5 Hz) induces a transient excitability increase. In a

typical inhibitory protocol, stimulation at 1 Hz for 5–15 minutes may reduce excitability for between 10 and 30 minutes [13–15]. Stimulation at 5 Hz for 5 minutes increases excitability in some studies for up to 30 minutes [16, 17], although other studies have found a shorter effect or none at all [18, 19]. The relatively poor reproducibility of the effects of 'conventional' rTMS led to the development of novel stimulation protocols, most notably theta burst stimulation (TBS) in which short high frequency bursts at low intensity are delivered every 200 milliseconds [20]. Continuous delivery of this pattern for 30 seconds (continuous TBS) in most subjects reduces excitability for up to 30 minutes, whereas intermittent delivery for 3 minutes (intermittent TBS) increases excitability for around 15 minutes [21].

The effects of tDCS on cortical excitability are summarized in Figure 16.3. The direction of effect depends on the polarity of stimulation: in many circumstances, anodal stimulation increases and cathodal stimulation decreases excitability of the underlying cortex. The amplitude of MEPs evoked by a suprathreshold stimulus is modulated during the period of stimulation and for a period of time afterwards which depends upon the duration of stimulation. For example, anodal stimulation at 1 mA for 13 minutes may increase excitability for 90 minutes 22. As an example of a more recent novel stimulation protocol, transcranial random noise stimulation (tRNS) involves the application of an electrical

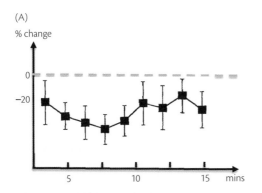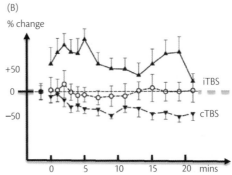

Fig. 16.2 Commonly used repetitive TMS protocols. (A) Data illustrating the effect of low frequency (0.9 Hz) repetitive TMS, delivered for 15 minutes, on post-stimulation motor cortex excitability as measured by motor evoked potential amplitude. Transient inhibition is seen lasting 15 minutes. A group mean is shown—individual results are variable. (B) Data adapted from Huang et al 2005 [21] illustrating the effects of intermittent (iTBS: upright black triangles) or continuous theta burst stimulation (cTBS: inverted black triangles) on motor cortex excitability.

(A) Adapted from Robert Chen, with permission. (B) Adapted with kind permission from Yingzu Huang.

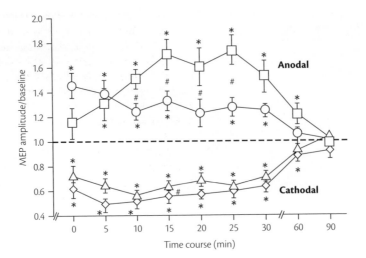

Fig. 16.3 Effects of transcranial direct current stimulation on motor cortex excitability. The after-effects of tDCS are shown, following anodal stimulation for 11 minutes (above x-axis) or cathodal stimulation for 9 minutes (below x-axis). Circles show effects of stimulation without additional medication, while square and triangles illustrate effects in presence of lorazepam.
Adapted with kind permission from Nitsche, Liebetanz et al. 2004 [217].

oscillation spectrum via standard electrodes sited over the cortex. The authors report an excitability increase in the stimulated motor cortex lasting 60 minutes following 10 minutes' stimulation [23], although follow-up studies are awaited to confirm the reproducibility of these effects.

Mechanism of stimulation effects

The excitability changes induced by rTMS appear to reflect the induction of a form of synaptic plasticity within the stimulated motor cortex [24]. Spinal recordings suggest that the element of the corticospinal volley reduced by low-frequency rTMS is primarily the late I-waves (indirect waves), which is evoked by trans-synaptic stimulation of the pyramidal cells [25]. Taken together with the lack of change in the stimulus threshold required to induce a response, a measure which is felt to reflect membrane excitability, this suggests that low frequency stimulation exerts its effect by changing the synaptic properties of interneurons within the cortex [26, 27]. The same observation applies to the effects of higher frequency 'conventional' rTMS at 5 Hz, which increases MEP amplitudes in several studies without affecting thresholds [28, 29]. Several studies have also demonstrated that 5 Hz rTMS reduces gamma-aminobutyric acid (GABA)-mediated inhibition within the motor cortex, lending further support to the notion that this form of stimulation produces its effects by modulating synaptic transmission within the cortex [17, 18]. Pharmacological studies of the 5 Hz effect suggest that the synaptic change is more likely to resemble post-tetanic potentiation (N-methyl-D-aspartate (NMDA) receptor-independent) than long-term potentiation (LTP) [30].

Spinal recordings following TBS suggest that the excitability increase induced by the intermittent form, and the decrease induced by the continuous form, reflect modulation of the late and early I-waves respectively. The synaptic changes believed to underlie the effects of TBS depend on the action of NMDA receptors and on modifiable calcium currents [31, 32], and resemble in some respects the early stages of LTP and long-term depression (LTD), by which lasting changes in synaptic efficacy may be induced experimentally by simultaneous stimulation of the

pre- and postsynaptic neurons [33]. As the effects of TBS on cortical excitability are relatively short lived, however, the modulation of synaptic strength may perhaps be described as LTP/LTD-like. It is suggested that the contrasting results of intermittent versus continuous TBS occurs because repetitive burst stimulation simultaneously induces a mixture of facilitatory and inhibitory effects, with differing time courses [34].

tDCS induces a polarity-dependent modulation of cortical excitability, which outlasts the period of stimulation. The change in excitability during stimulation does not depend on NMDA receptor function but is attenuated by sodium channel or calcium channel blockade, implicating the action of voltage-gated channels [35]. It is thus likely that the intrastimulation effects are mediated by the effect of direct current on axonal membrane potentials, rather than by synaptic modulation [36]. The lack of change in motor thresholds suggests that the current primarily affects the axons of interneurons rather than pyramidal cells [37]. The post-stimulation effects of tDCS, by contrast, are likely to depend on changes in synaptic efficacy. Pharmacological studies and changes in GABA-mediated inhibition within the cortex suggest that the excitability increase following anodal stimulation depends upon changes at glutamatergic synapses and reduced GABAergic inhibition [38, 39]. The excitability decrease following cathodal stimulation is likewise NMDA receptor-dependent but the role of changes in GABAergic synapses is less clear [35, 39]. Magnetic resonance spectroscopy has demonstrated changes in neurotransmitter availability following tDCS, with reduced GABA following anodal and reduced glutamate following cathodal stimulation [40]. It is interesting to note that direct current induces synaptic plasticity without itself causing the stimulated neurons to discharge. There is endogenous background synaptic activity even at rest, and it is presumed that the depolarization/hyperpolarization of tDCS causes this activity to induce changes in synaptic efficacy. This may be considered analogous to the altered efficacy of high frequency tetanic stimulation in experimental LTP induction preparation when given during the application of a depolarizing exogenous current [41].

Factors influencing the outcome of stimulation

One of the greatest impediments to the potential use of non-invasive brain stimulation techniques for neuroplasticity induction in a clinical context is the significant variability of response. This phenomenon is routinely encountered when the outcome being measured is a cortical excitability change in the healthy brain [42], and may be expected to be even more problematic when attempting to induce behavioural changes in patients undergoing neurorehabilitation. This point is effectively illustrated by a recent physiological study in which the authors applied continuous TBS to 56 healthy volunteers, using a standard protocol which typically reduces excitability at the group level [21]. The post-stimulation MEP amplitudes in individual subjects normalized to baseline are shown in Figure 16.4, and demonstrate that not only the size but also the direction of effect varies considerably between subjects [43]. A number of factors are thought to drive this variability of response, and understanding these is likely to be important when trying to use brain stimulation in a clinical setting.

There is now considerable evidence that both recent and current synaptic activity within the stimulation target have profound influences on the resulting neuroplasticity. This may be observed following 'priming' by another form of artificial plasticity induction and is often interpreted against the backdrop of the 'sliding threshold' model of synaptic modification proposed by Bienenstock et al. [44]. In this model the threshold for induction of LTP- or LTD-like synaptic plasticity varies according to the time-averaged post-synaptic activity: greater recent or current activity raises the threshold for further synaptic strengthening, while less activity has the opposite effect [45]. The self-limiting properties of such a system have given rise to the term 'homeostatic plasticity', and this phenomenon has been invoked to explain the outcome of cortical stimulation in a variety of circumstances. Thus when cathodal tDCS was used to 'prime' the motor cortex with an inhibitory stimulus the effect of subsequent 1 Hz TMS (usually inhibitory) was reversed to facilitation [46]. Using a similar priming approach, the response to 1 Hz TMS can be enhanced by preceding high frequency TMS [47], while the direction of change in response to 20 Hz stimulation can be defined by the polarity of preceding tDCS [19]. Priming effects

may also be observed following TBS, with the inhibitory effects of continuous TBS being enhanced by priming with (usually facilitatory) intermittent TBS [48]. It is also possible to induce priming effects by stimulation of brain regions distant from but connected to the subsequent target region [49]. Priming effects may also be responsible for the fact that prolonged administration of some protocols can reverse the outcome. For example, 13 min of anodal 1 mA TDCS increases corticospinal excitability in motor cortex, whereas 26 min stimulation reduces excitability [50].

Voluntary motor activity may be considered a form of behavioural priming and has important effects on the outcome of plasticity induction protocols. This phenomenon was demonstrated previously in rats, in whom training in a motor task altered the outcome of subsequent experimental LTP/LTD induction in horizontal connections of rat motor cortex [51]. The direction of an excitability change following TBS may be reversed if stimulation is preceded by either isometric contraction of the target hand muscle for 5 minutes [52] or a brief period of phasic finger movements [53]. If paired associative stimulation (PAS), a plasticity induction protocol that combines cortical and peripheral sensory stimulation, is applied soon after a period of motor training its effect on excitability reverses from facilitatory to inhibitory [54]. The outcome of a plasticity induction protocol is likewise sensitive to motor activity occurring during the period of stimulation. The effects of both common TBS protocols are attenuated by concurrent voluntary contraction [55], while performance of a motor task during tDCS reverses and enhances respectively the effects of anodal and cathodal stimulation [56].

A number of other factors, many of which are recognized to affect the capacity for learning, also influence the response to cortical stimulation in healthy subjects. Old age is associated with an attenuated response to PAS [57, 58], while the physiological response to cathodal tDCS is prolonged in female subjects when compared to males [59]. There has been recent interest in the genetic determinants of neuroplasticity, with variation in response to training [60] and artificial plasticity induction [61] linked to a common polymorphism of the BDNF (brain derived neurotrophic factor) gene. A more recent study demonstrated that an interaction between polymorphisms in the genes for BDNF and catechol-O-methyltransferase determines not only the response to PAS but also the level of skill in learning grammar, demonstrating a behavioural correlate of the physiological observation [62], although other studies suggest that there is unlikely to be a simple genetic determinant of plasticity induction [63, 64].

While age, sex, and genes may not be modifiable in the rehabilitation setting, factors found to favour neuroplasticity induction also include cardiovascular fitness [65], attentional focus on training [66], and training in the afternoon rather than the morning [67]. However, the influence on plasticity induction with perhaps the greatest potential significance in the rehabilitation setting, is that of pharmacological modulation. As previously detailed, the effects of several cortical stimulation protocols are attenuated in the presence of NMDA receptor blockade. Dopaminergic modulation exerts complex effects on several plasticity protocols, with a dopamine agonist extending the inhibitory effect of 1 Hz rTMS [68] but a single dose of L-Dopa reversing it [69]. Dopaminergic stimulation exerts a dose-dependent influence on the outcome of tDCS, with a high or low dose of a dopamine agonist suppressing the effects of anodal stimulation [70] while levodopa suppresses

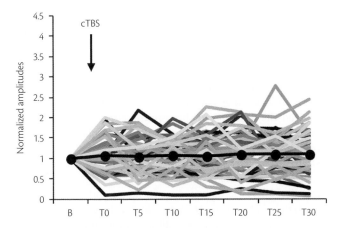

Fig. 16.4 Inter-subject variability: the effects of continuous theta burst stimulation. The after-effects of continuous TBS on motor cortex excitability are shown (200 bursts over 40 seconds) in 52 subjects. Thick black line and dots indicate mean, with no overall effect of stimulation in this group.

Adapted with kind permission from Hamada et al. 2013 [43].

both anodal and cathodal stimulation [71]. At a medium dose, by contrast, levodopa reverses the excitability change following anodal stimulation and prolongs the inhibitory cathodal effect [71, 72]. Promoting cholinergic transmission using the cholinesterase inhibitor rivastigmine attenuates both the anodal and cathodal tDCS effects but enhances the effects of PAS, in a study whose authors suggested that these divergent effects may reflect the difference in topographical focality between these two plasticity protocols [73]. The excitability increase following TBS is enhanced and prolonged in the presence of nicotine [74]. The catecholaminergic system also influences in the outcome of tDCS, with anodal facilitation prolonged by D-amphetamine and reduced by propranolol [75]. There is a growing literature regarding the pharmacological modulation of plasticity induction protocols (for reviews see [76] or [77]).

Influencing learning in the healthy brain

Cortical stimulation protocols such as those described have become widely used as means of inducing transient changes in cortical function. As well as being useful research tools they also provide a potential means of altering and perhaps enhancing specific aspects of brain function. In general the means by which non-invasive cortical stimulation may enhance a behaviour are either direct, by enhancing cortical function mediating the task in hand, or indirect, by reducing cortical activity that may compete or interfere with task performance. This approach has been applied not only in the field of motor control but also outside the motor cortex in cognitive neuroscience. It is important to remember however that the majority of information regarding the effects of cortical stimulation and their mechanisms comes from studies of the motor system, and that direct evidence that stimulation has equivalent effects in other cortical regions is at present lacking. We will focus here primarily on the effects of stimulation on motor learning and training, which are summarized in Figure 16.5.

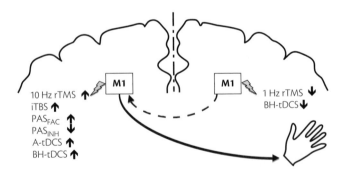

Fig. 16.5 Brain stimulation protocols that enhance motor training. Brain stimulation protocols are shown targeting the motor cortex either contralateral or ipsilateral to the training hand. Repetitive transcranial magnetic stimulation (rTMS) and paired associative stimulation (PAS) protocols are delivered before the start of training, 'priming' the cortical target region, whereas transcranial direct current stimulation (tDCS) is delivered during training. PAS protocols may be facilitatory (FAC) or inhibitory (INH), while the tDCS protocols here are either anodal (A-tDCS) or bihemispheric (BH-tDCS). The known effect of each protocol on cortical excitability is shown as an arrow. All protocols which successfully enhance training either facilitate the contralateral (active) motor cortex or inhibit the ipsilateral motor cortex, with one exception in which inhibitory PAS to the active motor cortex is also effective.

Stages and forms of learning

When subjects learn a new motor skill there is usually an improvement in performance during training itself (skill acquisition) which is associated with a rapid increase in motor cortex excitability [78, 79]. The motor memories acquired may then be strengthened further after training has finished, with increased resistance to interference by subsequent motor activity and even offline performance gains (consolidation) [80, 81]. This process may be blocked by interference in primary motor cortex function immediately after training but not 6 hours [82]: an implied role for this region may in fact not be specific as interference may also be induced by peripheral afferent input, suggesting that competing plasticity in overlapping circuits may disrupt early consolidation [83]. An already consolidated motor memory may become susceptible to further alteration while it is reactivated [84] (reconsolidation) and modulation of motor cortex activity also influences this process, suggesting that this region may transiently interact with the stored memory trace during movement execution [85]. These stages of learning have generally been defined in relation to the acquisition of a new motor skill, where incremental improvements in performance accrue over a relatively long period of training. Such tasks are sometimes termed 'non-rule-based' learning since participants do not know in advance how to improve their performance. They can be distinguished from a more rapid form of learning in which a previously learned movement is performed in the presence of a visuomotor or tactile perturbation—motor adaptation. In this case, participants are aware of the error and can use this information to update a previously learned skill. This type of learning relies upon contributions from both cortico-basal and cortico-cerebellar circuits for skill acquisition [86], but differentially upon corticocerebellar circuits for consolidation [87].

The motor cortex is important in both forms of learning, which suggests that artificially enhancing synaptic plasticity in this region by non-invasive stimulation may improve the outcome of a variety of types of motor training. Two approaches have been used to enhance excitability within the motor cortex: either directly by facilitatory stimulation of the target motor cortex, or indirectly by inhibitory stimulation of the contralateral motor cortex, preventing ongoing interference by reducing any ongoing transcallosal inhibition [88, 89].

Evidence from repetitive TMS

The practicalities of rTMS make it difficult to deliver during the course of training. In one study subjects made regular thumb movements to encode a directional motor memory trace, and the synchronous delivery of TMS pulses to the motor cortex prolonged the duration of the training effect [90]. The authors argued that in this case TMS provided a Hebbian input, which promoted synaptic plasticity. Most studies however have used rTMS to 'prime' the target cortical region for subsequent learning, such that training occurs during a period of increased excitability. Ten Hz rTMS delivered to the motor cortex for 2 seconds immediately before each training block enhanced training in a sequential motor learning task, although the effect duration was not tested [91]. Teo and colleagues tested the influence of intermittent TBS on subsequent training in a ballistic thumb movement task and found that iTBS enhanced the rate and extent of performance gains [92]. Interestingly, behavioural improvements were unrelated to changes in cortical excitability in that study and correlated instead with variability of performance, which increased after stimulation, suggesting a beneficial role for such variability in some forms of learning. Such a dissociation was also observed in another study testing the effects of 5 Hz rTMS, emphasizing that physiological and behavioural effects do not necessarily go hand in hand. No effect of iTBS on learning was observed when it was delivered half way through a training session [93].

PAS can either increase or decrease motor cortical excitability, depending on the interval between the peripheral stimulus and the TMS pulse. Interestingly, either facilitatory or inhibitory PAS enhanced performance in a motor learning task if the task was performed immediately after stimulation, suggesting that homeostatic rules do not always govern the interaction between stimulation and behaviour [94]. Stimulation of remote but connected regions may also influence training. Inhibitory 1 Hz rTMS applied to the motor cortex ipsilateral to the training hand (i.e. contralateral to the active motor cortex) enhanced subsequent training in a sequential key pressing task, presumably by suppressing transcallosal inhibition [95]. Delivering 1 Hz rTMS to the dorsal premotor cortex (ipsilateral to the active motor cortex) immediately after the completion of motor training over 4 consecutive days specifically improved overnight consolidation, with greater offline performance gains [96]. Less is known about the modulation of motor adaptation by rTMS: while continuous (inhibitory) TBS delivered to the primary motor cortex did not affect immediate adaptation to a visuomotor perturbation it appeared to impair re-adaptation after an interval [97]. The potential to enhance adaption using rTMS is not clear at present.

Evidence from transcranial direct current stimulation

There is now evidence that tDCS can influence the outcome of motor training. Although in the most commonly used montages the anode is placed over the primary motor cortex, the field of influence is considerably less focal than that resulting from rTMS and is likely to modulate excitability in several nodes of the network engaged in training. The observed effect depends crucially upon the timing of stimulation relative to training. When delivered immediately before training in a sequence learning task both anodal and cathodal stimulation reduced the rate of learning, whereas when delivered concurrently the effect on learning was polarity-dependent: faster with anodal, slower with cathodal [36]. A similar beneficial effect on sequence learning may be observed using bihemispheric stimulation, with the anode placed over the motor cortex contralateral to the training hand and the cathode over the homologous ipsilateral motor cortex, although there was no additional benefit over the more usual electrode montage [98]. Reis and colleagues studied the effect of applying anodal tDCS to the active motor cortex during training in an isometric pinch task over 5 days, and found that learning was enhanced over sham and that the benefit was sustained at 3 months [12]. Interestingly, tDCS in this study specifically enhanced offline gains between sessions, suggesting an effect on subsequent consolidation. Anodal stimulation delivered immediately after the completion of motor sequence learning also enhanced subsequent performance of the learned sequence [99]. Anodal tDCS applied to the cerebellum during a motor adaptation task was associated with faster error correction during training [100]. When applied to the primary motor cortex, on the other hand, anodal tDCS had no effect on

immediate adaptation but impaired de-adaptation on removal of the perturbation, implying stronger retention of the learned field [101]. Thus with regard to motor adaptation, stimulation of the cerebellum modulates learning whereas stimulation of motor cortex modulates retention.

Summary of effects on motor training

The potential of cortical stimulation to interact with motor training is suggested by common features of the believed mechanisms of these two processes. While it is clearly the case that they do indeed interact, the principles governing the effect of stimulation on training in a given individual are yet to be fully determined. A single subject's physiological response to one plasticity induction protocol does not reliably correlate with their response to another for example [102]. It is also unknown at present whether an individual's physiological response to brain stimulation predicts their capacity for training. While a subject's neurochemical response to tDCS (change in GABA levels as assessed by MR spectroscopy) has been correlated with their capacity to learn a finger sequence task [103], the effect of brain stimulation on cortical excitability does not appear to predict the effect on training [63, 92, 104]: as stimulation protocols are often chosen for application in rehabilitation according to their effect on excitability this dissociation may be important. The variables at play are increasingly becoming understood; however, including inter-individual factors, differences between stimulation protocols and the stages of motor learning being targeted. Fuller characterization of these factors is likely to be an essential prerequisite to successful clinical application.

Non-motor forms of learning

Non-invasive brain stimulation has proved a powerful tool in cognitive neuroscience where it is often employed to induce a 'virtual lesion' in a brain region subserving a specific cognitive function. There is also, however, a large and growing literature regarding the enhancement of cognitive function by this approach. While this is too extensive to be reviewed fully here, certain studies are of potential relevance to neurorehabilitation and these primarily employ tDCS. A polarity- and timing-specific beneficial effect of tDCS on acquisition of a visuomotor task may be induced not only by stimulation of the motor cortex, but alternatively the V5 region of extrastriate visual cortex, although the non-focal nature of tDCS should be kept in mind when interpreting the specific region said to be stimulated [105]. Stimulation of anterior temporal regions has been reported to improve visual memory [106] and name recall [107]. Stimulation of the left posterior perisylvian region enhances both performance in a language task and the learning of new words [108, 109]. Fregni and colleagues targeted the left dorsolateral prefrontal cortex and found that anodal but not cathodal stimulation improved performance of a task testing working memory [110], while stimulation of the same region has also been noted to improve planning in the Tower of London task in a manner dependent on the polarity of stimulation and the phase of training targeted [111]. When applied during slow wave sleep, stimulation of frontal regions also improved consolidation of learning in a declarative memory task [112]. A number of studies have targeted the parietal lobes, and investigators have reported beneficial effects on numerical processing [113], visuospatial attention [114], and spatial tactile acuity [115]. Novel stimulation techniques also show promise for cognitive enhancement, for example in the recent demonstration of improved learning of complex arithmetic tasks with the application of tRNS to the dorsolateral prefrontal cortices, with retention of behavioural gains at 6 months [116]. Interestingly, there appears in general to be less specificity of effect according to the polarity of stimulation in cognitive as compared to motor training [117].

Applying cortical stimulation to neurorehabilitation

Strategies for stimulation

As detailed in the previous sections, cortical stimulation may be used to alter synaptic properties within the cerebral cortex and may enhance the capacity for synaptic plasticity to occur in relation to training in a variety of tasks. Patients who are undergoing neurorehabilitation are commonly exposed to training over multiple sessions aimed primarily at their neurological deficit. There is evidence to support the idea that training during rehabilitation has a similar neurophysiological basis to that occurring in the healthy brain.

Rapid somatotopic reorganization is observed adjacent to an experimental infarct in the motor cortex of monkeys, similar to that which may be induced by motor training [118, 119]. This reorganization is underpinned by synaptic plasticity within the horizontal intracortical connections, which are thought to define motor map characteristics [120, 121]. This key role for synaptic plasticity has formed the rationale for a great many studies attempting to improve the recovery of neurological function by using non-invasive cortical stimulation to prime the patient's brain and enhance the response to therapy.

Most clinical studies of brain stimulation in the context of neurorehabilitation have focused on patients with stroke. This is likely to relate partly to the high prevalence of stroke, which as the leading cause of adult disability in the developed world has an enormous social and economic cost [122, 123]. Stroke is also attractive as a model for stimulation-enhanced neurorehabilitation as it presents a relatively focal lesion in what may be an otherwise intact system, at least macroscopically. Following an ischaemic stroke resulting in a motor deficit a number of abnormalities may be observed within the remaining cortical network. Functional imaging studies have revealed increased activation of non-primary motor cortical regions and of a number of regions in the contralesional hemisphere during movement of the paretic limb [124, 125]. Physiological studies using TMS have demonstrated that excitability of the corticospinal tract is commonly depressed in the stroke hemisphere but may be pathologically increased in the intact hemisphere [126, 127]. By contrast, disinhibition may be observed in the GABAergic intracortical circuits which regulate corticospinal output, both in the stroke hemisphere and the intact hemisphere [128–130]. These haemodynamic and physiological abnormalities are not static but evolve over the weeks and months following an acute stroke [131].

The idea of a pathological imbalance in excitability favouring the intact hemisphere was further advanced by an influential TMS study by Murase and colleagues [132], in which the interhemispheric influence of one primary motor cortex on its homologous counterpart was tested as subjects prepared to make a voluntary movement. In healthy subjects the interhemispheric interaction is inhibitory at rest but switches to causing facilitation immediately before movement onset; in patients with stroke, by contrast, inhibition is removed but not replaced by facilitation prior to movement onset. These and other observations [133] argue for a therapeutic approach, which seeks either to increase cortical excitability in the stroke hemisphere, or to reduce it in the intact hemisphere.

Motor stroke: effects of rTMS

There have been a number of promising studies in which motor performance or clinical status have been improved by the application of an rTMS intervention, seeking either to increase excitability in the primary motor cortex of the stroke hemisphere (Table 16.1) or to reduce it in the intact hemisphere (Table 16.2). Investigators have demonstrated immediate beneficial effects in stroke patients on reaction times [135], power [146, 147], movement kinematics [151], tone [146], and clinical scores [138]. In protocols which increase stroke hemisphere excitability, behavioural improvements have correlated with observed increases in MEP amplitude [134] and in movement-related activation of the ipsilesional motor cortex and corticobasal circuits [147]. In one study, however, this approach proved beneficial for patients with subcortical stroke but detrimental to those with cortical involvement [136]—interestingly stimulation was associated with a reduction in contralesional motor activation in the subcortical stroke group but an increase in the cortical group. In protocols which reduce intact hemisphere excitability, behavioural improvements have correlated with reduced transcallosal inhibition (of the stroke hemisphere by the intact hemisphere [153]) and with increased stroke hemisphere excitability [159]. Overall these results provide some support for the two principal strategies of stimulation and their proposed mechanism.

Trials of brain stimulation in both the stroke hemisphere and the intact hemisphere have produced several positive and a few negative results [144, 158], and it is not yet clear if either approach is more effective. The few direct comparisons that have been attempted have not been conclusive: Khedr and colleagues [139] found greater behavioural improvements with high frequency (stroke hemisphere) than low frequency (intact hemisphere) stimulation while Sasaki and colleagues [143] found the reverse, both studies testing patients in the subacute phase. A further study with chronic stroke patients found that stimulation of both hemispheres within a single session was more effective than either alone [164].

All repetitive TMS protocols have a relative short duration of physiological effect and, as discussed, their use in a clinical setting relies upon a presumed interaction of this effect with training in order to induce lasting behavioural improvements. A common approach more recently has been to deliver stimulation in combination with therapy or training over multiple sessions, aiming to derive a cumulative benefit. While some studies have demonstrated lasting gains in this way, persisting in one case at 1 year [141], others have shown no benefit using protocols with previously shown beneficial short-term effects [148]. Possible explanations for a lack of benefit may include clinical heterogeneity (and unrecognized variability of response to stimulation) and the fragility of the effects of stimulation to interference. Another possibility is that a small effect size of stimulation is lost when combined with

Table 16.1 Motor stroke: rTMS applied to increase excitability in the stroke hemisphere

	N	Time post-stroke	Active protocol	Sessions	Outcome measure	Clinical outcome
Single session						
Acute/subacute stroke						
No studies						
Chronic stroke						
Kim 2006 [134]	15	> 3m	10 Hz intermittent	1	Precision typing	Improvement vs sham
Talelli 2007 [135]	6	12–108 months	Intermittent TBS	1	Reaction time	Improvement vs sham
Ameli 2009 [136]	29	1–88 weeks	10 Hz intermittent	1	Hand/finger tapping	Improvement in subcortical but not cortical strokes
Ackerly 2010 [137]	10	7–86 months	Intermittent TBS	1	Grip lift task training	Improvement vs sham
Multiple sessions						
Acute/subacute stroke						
Khedr 2005 [138]	52	5–10 days	3 Hz intermittent	10	Barthel, SSS	Benefit at 10 days
					NIHSS	
Khedr 2009 [139]	24	<1 week	3 Hz intermittent	5	Keyboard task	Improvement at 3 months
Chang 2010 [140]	28	< 1m	10 Hz	10	FM, MI	Improved motor scores (but not function)
Khedr 2010 [141]	24	< 1 week	3 Hz/10 Hz	5	Motor Imp Scale, NIHSS	Improved hand strength & NIHSS with 3 Hz at 1 yr
Hsu 2013 [142]	12	16–28 days	Prolonged intermittent TBS	10	NIHSS, UE-Fugl-Meyer, ARAT	Improvement vs sham in NIHSS and UE-FM, not ARAT (combined with standard therapy)
Sasaki 2013 [143]	18	< 3 weeks	10 Hz intermittent	5	Grip strength, finger tapping	Greater improvement vs sham
Chronic stroke						
Malcolm 2007 [144]	19	> 1 yr	20 Hz intermittent	10	Wolf MFT, Motor Activity Log	No additional benefit over CIMT alone
Emara 2010 [145]	40	2–5 months	5 Hz continuous	10	Finger tapping, mRS	Improvement, sustained at 12 weeks
Koganemaru 2010 [146]	18	> 5m	5 Hz intermittent	12	Wrist spasticity, range & strength	All improved
Chang 2012 [147]	17	5–17 months	10 Hz intermittent	10	Sequential motor learning task	Improved accuracy with real rTMS, not sham
Talelli 2012 [148]	25	> 1 year	Intermittent theta burst stimulation	10	NHPT, JTT, Grip strength	No additional benefit over physio alone

All have a sham condition and target ipsilesional motor cortex.

a relatively powerful baseline intervention (e.g. physiotherapy). It is not yet clear which factors may predict a more successful response to a given stimulation strategy (cortical vs subcortical stroke, stage of recovery, age, stroke severity, etc.) although one meta-analysis suggests that most benefit is seen following subcortical stroke and targeting the intact hemisphere [165]. Further understanding of factors predicting the response to stimulation is likely to be important in taking this approach forward.

Motor stroke: effects of tDCS

There is now evidence from a number of studies demonstrating beneficial effects of tDCS on motor function in patients with stroke.

Investigators have aimed to increase excitability in the stroke hemisphere (Table 16.3) or to reduce it in the intact hemisphere (Table 16.4), with some studies testing both approaches. Clinical improvements following anodal stimulation of the stroke hemisphere have been shown to correlate with a stimulation-induced increase in motor cortex excitability [168], although only six patients were tested in this study, and with movement-related cortical activation [172] in the stimulated motor cortex. Nair et al. [181] examined clinical benefits following cathodal stimulation of the intact hemisphere, and demonstrated a correlation with reduced activation in the contralesional motor cortex during movement of the paretic hand, although both treatment and sham

Table 16.2 Motor stroke: rTMS applied to reduce excitability in the intact hemisphere

	N	Time post-stroke	Active protocol	Sessions	Outcome measure	Clinical outcome
Single session						
Acute/subacute stroke						
Liepert 2007 [149]	12	Mean 7 days	1 Hz continuous	1	Grip strength, NHPT	Improved NHPT
Dafotakis 2008 [150]	12	1–4 m	1 Hz continuous	1	Pincer grip task	Improved kinematics
Nowak 2008 [151]	15	1–4 m	1 Hz continuous	1	Pincer grip task	Improved kinematics (additional fMRI)
Chronic stroke						
Mansur 2005 [152]	10	< 1 year	1 Hz continuous	1	Reaction times, Pegboard test	Both improved
Takeuchi 2005 [153]	20	7–60 m	1 Hz continuous	1	Pinch task	Improved performance
Talelli 2007 [135]	6	12–108 months	Continuous TBS	1	Reaction Time	No effect
Takeuchi 2008 [154]	20	7–88 m	1 Hz continuous	1	Pinch task	Improved training in task
Grefkes 2010 [155]	11	1–3 m	1 Hz continuous	1	Fist closure frequency	Small improvement
Ackerly 2010 [137]	10	7–86 months	Continuous TBS	1	Grip lift task training	Improvement vs sham (but worse ARAT)
Meehan 2011 [156]	8	> 1 year	Continuous TBS	1	Motor targeting task	Faster movements after TBS vs sham
Multiple sessions						
Acute/subacute stroke						
Pomeroy 2007 [157]	27	Mean 27 days	1 Hz intermittent	8	ARAT	No effect
Khedr 2009 [139]	24	<1 week	1 Hz continuous	5	Keyboard task	Improvement at 3 months
Seniow 2012 [158]	33	12–129 days	1 Hz continuous	15	Wolf MFT, NIHSS, UE-Fugl-Meyer	No effect (combined with physio)
Sasaki 2013 [143]	20	< 3 weeks	1 Hz continuous	5	Grip strength, finger tapping	No effect
Chronic stroke						
Fregni 2006 [159]	15	> 1 year	1 Hz continuous	5	JTT, Reaction times	Improved
Emara 2010 [145]	40	2–13 months	1 Hz continuous	10	Finger tapping, mRS	Improvement, sustained at 12 weeks
Theilig 2011 [160]	24	2w–58m	1 Hz continuous	10	Motor function, Spasticity	No additional effect over FNMS
Avenanti 2012 [161]	30	6–88 months	1 Hz continuous	10	NHPT, JTT, box & block, grip strength	Improvement vs sham, sustained if rTMS before physio
Conforto 2012 [162]	30	5–45 days	1 Hz continuous	10	JTT, Fugl-Meyer Pinch force	JTT improved in active group
Talelli 2012 [148]	24	> 1 year	Continuous Theta Burst stimulation	10	NHPT, JTT, Grip strength	No additional benefit over physio alone
Wang 2012 [163]	24	> 6 months	1 Hz continuous	10	LE-Fugl-Meyer, gait spatial asymmetry	Improved vs sham (combined with gait training)

All have a sham condition and target contralesional motor cortex.

groups were included in the correlation. In studies of bihemisperic stimulation (simultaneous facilitation of stroke and inhibition of intact motor cortices) improvements after stimulation were related to normalization of the functional MRI 'laterality index', a measure of motor activation asymmetry between the two hemispheres [177], and to a reduction of interhemispheric inhibition targeting the stroke hemisphere as measured by TMS [178]. Interpretation of this result is difficult as the correlation was only present for movements of the elbow and not the wrist. In the majority of studies beneficial effects of stimulation were seen immediately, but when Kim and colleagues [174] combined tDCS with physical and occupational therapy there was no additional benefit over sham stimulation at 10 days but a marked difference at 6 months. These studies lend a degree of support for the proposed mechanism of action whereby the balance of excitability between the two homologous motor cortices is redressed by stimulation in favour of the stroke hemisphere. It is difficult to reach a firm conclusion on this front in view of the small sample sizes used for regression.

Despite many promising proof-of-principle studies and small clinical trials, however, there has been a notable failure to reproduce clinical benefit when testing larger patient numbers. Two separate trials of anodal stimulation in the acute post-stroke period, using a similar protocol but higher current to that applied successfully to the subacute period [166], showed no beneficial effect of stimulation vs sham on functional scores. In the study of Hesse and colleagues [175] a significant proportion of patients were severely affected at baseline (mean Fugl-Meyer score approximately 8/66, several patients with total anterior circulation infarction), which may potentially explain the lack of effect, but this did not apply to the patients studied by Rossi and colleagues [176] who had a wider range of baseline impairment. It seems likely that differing effects of stimulation may be observed depending on severity and stroke location, and this is supported by the results obtained by Bradnam and colleagues [180], in whose study cathodal stimulation of the intact hemisphere was beneficial to performance in an isometric biceps task in patients with milder impairment but detrimental in more impaired patients. This observation may perhaps reflect the collateral inclusion of contralesional non-primary motor areas such as the premotor cortex in the field of stimulation, which are recognized to support recovered motor function in the face of greater corticospinal tract disruption [182, 183].

A number of specific questions remain regarding the optimum tDCS strategy after stroke. Comparisons of anodal vs cathodal stimulation have found variably in favour of the former [172] or the latter [167]. The importance of stimulation intensity used remains unclear, with a range from 1 to 2 mA commonly employed, but no formal comparison available in stroke patients. The most effective duration of stimulation is not known, ranging in patient studies from 7 to 30 minutes [177, 179]. Worryingly, while most patient studies employ a longish period of stimulation such as 25 minutes, a recent study in healthy subjects demonstrated that the facilitatory effects of anodal tDCS may in fact be reversed when it is prolonged [50]. The lack of success with larger patient number emphasises the importance of resolving these questions before Phase III trials would be feasible or ethical.

Stimulation for non-motor impairments after stroke

A number of efforts have been made to apply an equivalent treatment strategy to patients with non-motor stroke deficits. As for the motor system the aim of stimulation in these studies is to alter the excitability balance between the stroke and intact hemispheres, and to combine stimulation with a form of training in the hope that these two processes may interact to induce lasting benefit. Investigators have shown benefit in patients with mild-to-moderate aphasia from anodal DC stimulation (excitatory) to the stroke hemisphere [184], targeting the perilesional cortex, whereas patients with a more severe deficit may respond to anodal stimulation of the intact

parietotemporal lobe [185]. However, one study demonstrated improvement following cathodal (inhibitory) stimulation of the stroke hemisphere, which runs counter to accepted treatment strategies [186] and perhaps emphasises how little is known regarding the mechanism of action. A recent Cochrane review made no attempt to allow for patient heterogeneity, but concluded that there is currently no convincing evidence for the efficacy of tDCS in post-stroke aphasia [187]. Repetitive TMS studies have likewise aimed to inhibit activity in the intact hemisphere in patients with chronic aphasia, with sustained improvement after multiple sessions of 1 Hz stimulation [188]. One study improved language task performance by applying 50 Hz (excitatory) stimulation to the stroke hemisphere [189]. There are no data for patients with acute aphasia.

Patients with visuospatial neglect have shown transient improvements in a range of psychological measures after receiving inhibitory rTMS to the contralesional hemisphere in the acute/subacute stage [190, 191] and in the chronic stage [192]. Kim and colleagues [193] produced beneficial effects by excitatory rTMS (10 Hz) of the stroke hemisphere. Only two studies have examined the efficacy of tDCS for neglect, but both demonstrated improved task performance, one following anodal stimulation of the stroke hemisphere [194] and the other with additional cathodal stimulation on the contralesional hemisphere [195].

Recent studies have attempted to use brain stimulation to treat post-stroke dysphagia. Excitatory rTMS delivered to the stroke hemisphere representation on five consecutive days induced an improvement in dysphagia in one study [196]. Anodal (excitatory) tDCS delivered to the stroke hemisphere, in combination with swallow training over 10 days, induced a delayed improvement at 3 months [197], while anodal stimulation to the intact hemisphere induced a measurable improvement after a single session [198]. The rationale for using non-invasive brain stimulation to treat post-stroke dysphagia differs from that for other deficits in that the motor component of swallowing is bilaterally represented, so the likely effect of altering an interhemispheric balance is less clear.

Summary of cortical stimulation after stroke: does it work?

For most forms of neurological deficit evident after stroke there are one or more studies demonstrating a beneficial effect of non-invasive brain stimulation. Earlier studies tend to have used stimulation to induce a transient behavioural enhancement, while more recently investigators have tended to combine stimulation with a form of training. Considering these studies together there is enormous heterogeneity of design with regard to chronicity of stroke, single vs multiple sessions, severity of baseline impairment, involvement of cortical structures, outcome measures used and stimulation protocol. It is thus difficult for review articles and formal meta-analyses to draw meaningful conclusions. With regard to motor function, reviews have variously concluded that 'it might be possible to harness effects (of stimulation) in a therapeutic setting' [199], or that stimulation 'may be beneficial in enhancing motor recovery' [3]. One recent meta-analysis of rTMS after stroke [165] found a significant positive effect of stimulation on motor function, with an effect size of 0.55, although both single- and multiple-session studies were included and a variety of outcome measures employed, while another by contrast concluded that that 'the routine use of rTMS for patients with stroke

Table 16.3 Motor stroke: tDCS applied to increase excitability in the stroke hemisphere

	N	Time post-stroke	Active protocol	Sessions	Outcome measure	Clinical outcome
Single session						
Acute/subacute stroke						
Kim 2009 [166]	10	3–12 weeks	20 min 1 mA anodal to stroke hemisphere	1	Box & Block Test, Finger acceleration	B&BT improved for 60 mins, Finger acceleration for 30 mins
Chronic stroke						
Fregni 2005 [167]	6	12–72 months	20 min 1 mA anodal to stroke hemisphere	1	JTT	Improvement vs sham (transient)
Hummel 2005 [168]	6	23–107 months	20 min 1 mA anodal to stroke hemisphere	1	JTT	Improvement vs sham (transient)
Celnik 2009 [169]	9	31–87 months	20 min 1 mA anodal to stroke hemisphere	1	Finger sequence training	Improved if with peripheral stim, but no effect of tDCS alone
Madhavan 2011 [170]	9	1–23 years	15 min 0.5 mA anodal (small electrode)	1	Ankle tracking task	Improved training in task vs sham
Mahmoudi 2011 [171]	10	1–16 months	20 min 1 mA anodal to stroke hemisphere	1	JTT	Immediate improvement JTT (not with sham)
Stagg 2012 [172]	13	18–70m	20 min 1 mA anodal to stroke hemisphere	1	Response times	Improved immediately after stimulation
Tanaka 2011 [173]	8	3–38 months	10 min 2 mA anodal	1	Knee extension power	Increased during anodal stimulation but not 30 mins later
Multiple sessions						
Acute/subacute stroke						
Kim 2010 [174]	13	34 days (mean)	20 min 2 mA anodal to stroke hemisphere	10	Fugl-Meyer	Non-significant improvement vs sham at 6 months
Hesse 2011 [175]	56	3 weeks (mean)	20 min 2 mA anodal to stroke hemisphere	30	Fugl-Meyer	No effect of stimulation (with robot assisted training)
Rossi 2012 [176]	50	Day 2	20 min 2 mA anodal to stroke hemisphere	5	NIHSS, Fugl-Meyer	No effect of tDCS (acute period: no adverse events)
Chronic stroke						
Lindenberg 2010 [177]	20	5–81 months	Bihemispheric 30 min anodal: stroke, cathodal: intact (1.5 mA)	5	Fugl-Meyer, Wolf MF test	Improved vs sham (combined with PT/OT)
Bolognini 2011 [178]	14	7–105 months	Bihemispheric 40 min 2 mA	10	JTT, Fugl-Meyer, Hand strength	Greater improvement vs sham (combined with CIMT)
Geroin 2011 [179]	20	16–34 months	7 mins 1.5 mA anodal leg area (stroke hemi)	10	Walking speed	No effect of tDCS (combined with robot-assisted gait training)

All have a sham condition and target the ipsilesional hemisphere.

is not recommended until its efficacy is verified in high-quality, large-scale RCTs' [5].

There is little doubt in our view that non-invasive stimulation is capable of inducing beneficial behavioural effects in some patients, but certain obstacles must be overcome before such an approach can enter routine clinical practice: (1) In view of the non-specific effects of stimulation on underlying structures it is important that studies are designed with the aim not to restore a particular function, but rather to interact with the normal processes of brain plasticity occurring after focal damage; (2) there needs to be increased understanding of the effects of brain stimulation, and crucially the development of protocols with less variability of effect than currently observed; (3) there is a need for greater understanding of the

pathophysiological mechanisms underpinning recovery: this may allow for the identification of patient subgroups who have greater or lesser capacity to respond to stimulation, and thus an improved effect size in treated patients; (4) finally, there is a need for the standardization of stimulation parameters under investigation and of outcome measures employed. Until these objectives are achieved it is unlikely to be possible to conduct a clinical trial that is sufficiently powerful to influence routine clinical practice after stroke.

Cortical stimulation for non-stroke neurological pathologies

While stroke neurorehabilitation is in many ways the paradigmatic clinical application for non-invasive brain stimulation, there

Table 16.4 Motor stroke: tDCS applied to decrease excitability in the intact hemisphere

	N	Time post- stroke	Active protocol	Sessions	Outcome measure	Clinical outcome
Single session						
Acute/subacute stroke						
No studies						
Chronic stroke						
Fregni 2005 [167]	6	12–72 months	20 min 1 mA cathodal to intact hemisphere	1	JTT	Improvement vs sham
Hesse 2011 [175]	56	3 weeks (mean)	20 min 2 mA cathodal to intact hemisphere	30	Fugl-Meyer	No effect of stimulation (with robot assisted training)
Mahmoudi 2011 [171]	10	1–16 months	20 min 1 mA cathodal to intact hemisphere	1	JTT	Immediate improvement JTT (not with sham)
Stagg 2012 [172]	13	18–70 months	20 min 1 mA cathodal to intact hemisphere	1	Response times	No improvement but better than sham
Bradnam 2012 [180]	12	2–34 months	20 min 1 mA cathodal to intact hemisphere	1	Selectivity of muscle control during UL task	Improved control with mild impairment, but worse with severe
Multiple sessions						
Acute/subacute stroke						
Kim 2010 [174]	12	19 days (mean)	20 min Cathodal 2 mA	10	Fugl-Meyer	Improved vs sham at 6 months (no immediate effect)
Chronic stroke						
Lindenberg 2010 [177]	20	5–81 months	Bihemispheric 30 min Anodal: stroke, Cathodal: intact (1.5 mA)	5	Fugl-Meyer, Wolf MF test	Improved vs sham (combined with PT/OT)
Bolognini 2011 [178]	14	7–105 months	Bihemispheric 40 mins 2 mA	10	JTT, Fugl-Meyer, Hand strength	Greater improvement vs sham (combined with CIMT)
Nair 2011 [181]	14	33 months (mean)	30 min cathodal 1 mA to intact hemisphere	5	UE-Fugl-Meyer, 3 joint range of movt	Improved scores vs sham (combined with OT)

All have a sham condition and target the ipsilesional hemisphere.

is evidence for beneficial effects across a range of neurological and psychiatric disorders. In Parkinson's disease cortical stimulation may be used to modulate activity within corticobasal loops and thereby influence the motor state. Some studies have delivered excitatory stimulation to the primary motor cortex [200, 201] with beneficial effects on bradykinesia. Others have delivered inhibitory stimulation to the primary motor cortex [202], the supplementary motor area [203] or the cerebellum [204], with transient improvements in levodopa-induced dyskinesia. In patients with writer's cramp inhibitory stimulation of the premotor cortex transiently improves symptoms [205]. Inhibitory stimulation applied to the motor cortex appeared in a preliminary study to slow clinical progression in patients with motor neurone disease [206], but a larger trial with 20 patients showed no effect [207]. Inhibitory rTMS delivered over multiple sessions shows promise as a strategy to reduce seizure frequency in patients with intractable epilepsy [208, 209]. Non-invasive stimulation has further been applied in efforts to treat a range of neuropsychiatric conditions, beyond the scope of this chapter, the most prominent of which is depression (for review see George et al. [210]).

The context in which patients with these largely chronic conditions undergo rehabilitation tends to differ from that in which recovering stroke patients are treated. However, the principle of using cortical stimulation to interact with therapy-induced plasticity is likely to apply as much here as in stroke. One recent study perhaps illustrates this approach, in which excitatory repetitive TMS was delivered to the leg area of the motor cortex in combination with treadmill training in a group of patients with Parkinson's disease with beneficial effects on walking performance [211]. Overall, the potential role for brain stimulation in neurological rehabilitation for these diverse neurological disorders is unclear at present.

Combining cortical stimulation with medication

As the effects of non-invasive stimulation depend at least in part on changes in synaptic strength it is perhaps not surprising that they are subject to modulation by the principal neuromodulatory systems of the brain. Such influences have been most extensively studied with regard to tDCS but some information is also available for repetitive TMS protocols: these are summarized in Table 16.5. It is interesting to note that in some cases the effect of a stimulation protocol on cortical excitability may be inverted by the presence of a medication, from facilitation to inhibition (e.g. levodopa on anodal tDCS) or vice versa

Table 16.5 Pharmacological modulation of the after-effects of transcranial direct current stimulation (tDCS) and theta burst stimulation (TBS) on corticospinal excitability

Neurotransmitter system	Drug	Principal action		Anodal tDCS (excitatory)	Cathodal tDCS (inhibitory)	iTBS (excitatory)	cTBS (inhibitory)	Reference
Glutamatergic	Dextromethorphan	NMDA antagonist		↓↓	↓↓	?	↓↓	212, 213
	Memantine	NMDA antagonist		?	?	↓↓	↓↓	214
	D-Cycloserine	NMDA partial agonist		Prolong	-	Invert	?	215, 216
GABA-ergic	Lorazepam	GABA$_A$ agonist		↑Prolong	?	?	?	217
Cholinergic	Nicotine	Nicotinic agonist		↓↓	↓↓	↑	?	218, 219
	Rivastigmine	Cholinesterase inhibitor		↓↓	↓ Prolong	?	?	220
Dopaminergic	Levodopa	Dopamine precursor	Low	↓↓	↓↓			221
			Med	Invert	Prolong	?	?	
			High	↓↓	↓↓			
	Ropinirole	D2 agonist	Low	↓↓	↓↓			222
			Med	-	Prolong	?	?	
			High	↓	↓↓			
	Sulpiride	D2 antagonist		↓↓	↓↓	↓↓	↓↓	223, 224
Noradrenergic	Propranolol	Beta-blocker		Shorten	Shorten	?	?	225
Serotonergic	Citalopram	Serotonic Specific Reuptake Inhibitor		↑ Prolong	Invert	?	?	226
Other	Amphetamine	Monoamine promoter		↑ Prolong	-	?	?	225
	Carbamazepine	Calcium blocker		↓↓	-	?	?	212
	Flunarazine	Calcium blocker		↓↓	-	?	?	227

All have a sham condition and target the intact hemisphere.

iTBS = intermittent TBS; cTBS = continuous TBS.

(e.g. citalopram on cathodal tDCS). Dopaminergic stimulation exerts a non-linear dose-dependent effect on effects of stimulation, with abolition of excitability change at low or high dosage but inversion or prolongation of the effect at medium dosage. This inverted U-shaped curve emphasizes that dosage is likely to be crucially important when trying to influence plasticity with medication. Of particular note perhaps are the significant prolongations of stimulation effect noted in the presence of citalopram and amphetamine, both of which groups of medication themselves have some evidence for benefit after stroke in humans or animal models. It is important to remember that effects of stimulation on corticospinal excitability do not necessarily translate into improvements in behavioural measures. Notwithstanding this cautionary note, the approach of combining brain stimulation with medication is certainly promising as an avenue of investigation but is currently in its infancy as a therapeutic strategy.

Conclusion

It is clear that non-invasive brain stimulation is capable of interacting with training-associated brain plasticity, and potentially of altering the outcome of neurological rehabilitation. It is less clear which protocols are most effective, how they should be delivered, in which patients and at what stage of rehabilitation. At present, the principal obstacles to translating this approach into clinical practice are the interindividual variability of response with current stimulation protocols, and the heterogeneity of protocols tested (and outcome measures used) across different centres. Resolving these key issues is essential before it will be feasible or ethical to conduct clinical trials of sufficient size to influence clinical practice. It is likely that the efficacy of brain stimulation in the clinical setting may be increased by using it in combination with neuromodulatory medication or other pharmacological promoters of endogenous plasticity, and this represents a promising future direction for research. The rewards of developing non-invasive stimulation as a clinical tool are potentially great. Together with other branches of restorative neuroscience this approach provides the opportunity to reduce neurological impairment, and hence disability, in patients undergoing rehabilitation. Applying such techniques correctly to appropriate patients has the potential to produce clinical benefits whose magnitude equals or exceeds that observed in other branches of clinical neuroscience. If this can be achieved then neurological rehabilitation as a discipline may shed its undeserved inferiority complex, and join the ranks of neurological specialties in which advances in neuroscience translate into benefit for patients.

References

1. Berlim MT, Van den Eynde F, Daskalakis ZJ. Efficacy and acceptability of high frequency repetitive transcranial magnetic stimulation (rTMS) versus electroconvulsive therapy (ECT) for major depression: a systematic review and meta-analysis of randomized trials. Depress Anxiety. 2013;30(7):614–623.

2. Hovington CL, McGirr A, Lepage M, Berlim MT.Repetitive transcranial magnetic stimulation (rTMS) for treating major depression and schizophrenia: a systematic review of recent meta-analyses.Ann Med. 2013;45(4):308–321.

3. Adeyemo BO, Simis M, Macea DD, Fregni F.Systematic review of parameters of stimulation, clinical trial design characteristics, and motor outcomes in non-invasive brain stimulation in stroke.Front Psychiatry. 2012;3:88.

4. Kandel M, Beis JM, Le Chapelain L, Guesdon H, Paysant J. Non-invasive cerebral stimulation for the upper limb rehabilitation after stroke: a review.Ann Phys Rehabil Med. 2012;55(9–10):657–680.

5. Hao Z, Wang D, Zeng Y, Liu M. Repetitive transcranial magnetic stimulation for improving function after stroke.Cochrane Database Syst Rev. 2013;5:CD008862.

6. Bonnì S, Mastropasqua C, Bozzali M, Caltagirone C, Koch G. Theta burst stimulation improves visuo-spatial attention in a patient with traumatic brain injury.Neurol Sci. 2013;34:2053–2056.

7. Koch G, Brusa L, Caltagirone C, et al. rTMS of supplementary motor area modulates therapy-induced dyski- nesias in Parkinson disease. Neurology. 2005;654:623–625.

8. Khedr EM, Kotb H, Kamel NF, Ahmed MA, Sadek R, Rothwell JC. Longlasting antalgic effects of daily sessions of repetitive transcranial magnetic stimulation in central and peripheral neuropathic pain.J Neurol Neurosurg Psychiatry. 2005;76:833–838.

9. Le K, Liu L, Sun M, Hu L, Xiao N. Transcranial magnetic stimulation at 1 Hertz improves clinical symptoms in children with Tourette syndrome for at least 6 months.J Clin Neurosci. 2013;20(2):257–262.

10. Murase N, Rothwell JC, Kaji R, et al. Subthreshold low-frequency repetitive transcranial magnetic stimulation over the premotor cortex modulates writer's cramp.Brain. 2005;128(Pt 1):104–115.

11. Teo JT, Swayne OB, Cheeran B, Greenwood RJ, Rothwell JC. Human θ burst stimulation enhances subsequent motor learning and increases performance variability. Cereb Cortex. 2011;21(7):1627–1638.

12. Reis J, Schambra HM, Cohen LG, et al. Noninvasive cortical stimulation enhances motor skill acquisition over multiple days through an effect on consolidation. Proc Natl Acad Sci U S A. 2009;106(5):1590–1595.

13. Fitzgerald PB, Brown TL, Daskalakis ZJ, Chen R, Kulkarni J. Intensity-dependent effects of 1 Hz rTMS on human corticospinal excitability. Clin Neurophysiol. 2002;113:1136–1141.

14. Romero JR, Anschel D, Sparing R, Gangitano M, Pascual-Leone A. Subthreshold low frequency repetitive transcranial magnetic stimulation selectively decreases facilitation in the motor cortex. Clin Neurophysiol. 2002;113:101–107.

15. Chen R, Classen J, Gerloff C, et al. Depression of motor cortex excitability by low-frequency transcranial magnetic stimulation.Neurology. 1997;48(5):1398–1403.

16. Peinemann A, Reimer B, Loer C, et al. Long-lasting increase in corticospinal excitability after 1800 pulses of subthreshold 5 Hz repetitive TMS to the primary motor cortex. Clin Neurophysiol. 2004;115:1519–1526.

17. Quartarone A, Bagnato S, Rizzo V, et al. Distinct changes in cortical and spinal excitability following high-frequency repetitive TMS to the human motor cortex. Exp Brain Res. 161: 114–124, 2005.

18. Di Lazzaro V, Oliviero A, Mazzone P, et al. Short-term reduction of intracortical inhibition in the human motor cortex induced by repetitive transcranial magnetic stimulation. Exp Brain Res. 2002;147:108–113.

19. Lang N, Siebner HR, Ernst D, et al. Preconditioning with transcranial direct current stimulation sensitizes the motor cortex to rapid-rate transcranial magnetic stimulation and controls the direction of after-effects. Biol Psychiatry. 2004;56:634–639.

20. Huang YZ, Rothwell JC. The effect of short-duration bursts of high-frequency, low-intensity transcranial magnetic stimulation on the human motor cortex. Clin Neurophysiol. 2004; 115(5):1069–1075.

21. Huang YZ, Edwards MJ, Rounis E, Bhatia KP, Rothwell JC. Theta burst stimulation of the human motor cortex. Neuron 2005; 45(2):201–206.

22. DC motor cortex stimulation in humans. Neurology. 2001;57(10):1899–1901.

23. Terney D, Chaieb L, Moliadze V, Antal A, Paulus W. Increasing human brain excitability by transcranial high-frequency random noise stimulation. J Neurosci. 2008;28(52):14147–14155.

24. Ziemann U, Paulus W, Nitsche MA, et al. Consensus: Motor cortex plasticity protocols. Brain Stimul. 2008;1:164–182.

25. Di Lazzaro V, Pilato F, Dileone M, et al. Low-frequency repetitive transcranial magnetic stimulation suppresses specific excitatory circuits in the human motor cortex.J Physiol. 2008;586(Pt 18):4481–4487.

26. Chen R. Studies of human motor physiology with transcranial magnetic stimulation. Muscle Nerve Suppl. 2000;9:S26–32.

27. Fitzgerald PB, Benitez J, Oxley T, Daskalakis JZ, de Castella AR, Kulkarni J. A study of the effects of lorazepam and dextromethorphan on the response to cortical 1Hz repetitive transcranial magnetic stimulation. Neuroreport. 2005;16:1525–1528.

28. Siebner HR, Mentschel C, Auer C, Lehner C, Conrad B. Repetitive transcranial magnetic stimulation causes a short-term increase in the duration of the cortical silent period in patients with Parkinson's disease. Neurosci Lett. 2000;284:147–150.

29. Peinemann A, Reimer B, Loer C, et al. Long-lasting increase in corticospinal excitability after 1800 pulses of subthreshold 5 Hz repetitive TMS to the primary motor cortex. Clin Neurophysiol. 2004;115:1519–1526.

30. Sommer M, Rummel M, Norden C, Rothkegel H, Lang N, Paulus W. Mechanisms of human motor cortex facilitation induced by subthreshold 5-Hz repetitive transcranial magnetic stimulation. J Neurophysiol. 2013;109(12):3060–3066.

31. Huang YZ, Chen RS, Rothwell JC, Wen HY.The after-effect of human theta burst stimulation is NMDA receptor dependent.Clin Neurophysiol. 2007;118(5):1028–1032.

32. Wankerl K, Weise D, Gentner R, Rumpf JJ, Classen J. L-type voltage-gated Ca2+ channels: a single molecular switch for long-term potentiation/long-term depression-like plasticity and activity-dependent metaplasticity in humans. J Neurosci. 2010;30(18):6197–6204.

33. Lømo T. Frequency potentiation of excitatory synaptic activity in the dentate area of the hippocampal formation. Acta Physiol Scand. 1966;68 (Suppl 277):128.

34. Huang YZ, Rothwell JC, Chen RS, Lu CS, Chuang WL. The theoretical model of theta burst form of repetitive transcranial magnetic stimulation. Clin Neurophysiol. 2011;122(5):1011–1018.

35. Nitsche MA, Fricke K, Henschke U, et al. Pharmacological modulation of cortical excitability shifts induced by transcranial direct current stimulation in humans. J Physiol. 2003;553(Pt 1):293–301.

36. Stagg CJ, Jayaram G, Pastor D, Kincses ZT, Matthews PM, Johansen-Berg H. Polarity and timing-dependent effects of transcranial direct current stimulation in explicit motor learning. Neuropsychologia. 2011;49(5):800–804.

37. Nitsche MA, Seeber A, Frommann K, et al. Modulating parameters of excitability during and after transcranial direct current stimulation of the human motor cortex.J Physiol. 2005;568 (Pt 1):291–303.

38. Liebetanz D, Nitsche MA, Tergau F, Paulus W. Pharmacological approach to the mechanisms of transcranial DC-stimulation-induced after-effects of human motor cortex excitability. Brain. 2002;125(Pt 10):2238–2247.

39. Nitsche MA, Jaussi W, Liebetanz D, Lang N, Tergau F, Paulus W. Consolidation of human motor cortical neuroplasticity by D-cycloserine. Neuropsychopharmacology. 2004;29(8):1573–1578.

40. Stagg CJ, Best JG, Stephenson MC, et al. Polarity-sensitive modulation of cortical neurotransmitters by transcranial stimulation. J Neurosci. 2009;29(16):5202–6.

41. Artola A, Bröcher S, Singer W. Different voltage-dependent thresholds for inducing long-term depression and long-term potentiation in slices of rat visual cortex.Nature. 1990;347(6288):69–72.

42. Ridding MC, Ziemann U. Determinants of the induction of cortical plasticity by non-invasive brain stimulation in healthy subjects. J Physiol. 2010;588(Pt 13):2291–2304.

43. Hamada M, Murase N, Hasan A, Balaratnam M, Rothwell JC. The role of interneuron networks in driving human motor cortical plasticity. Cereb Cortex 2013;23(7):1593–1605.

44. Bienenstock EL, Cooper LN, Munro PW. Theory for the development of neuron selectivity: orientation specificity and binocular interaction in visual cortex. J Neurosci. 1982;2(1):32–48.

45. Abraham WC. Metaplasticity: tuning synapses and networks for plasticity. Nat Rev Neurosci. 2008;9:387.

46. Siebner HR, Lang N, Rizzo V, et al. Preconditioning of low-frequency repetitive transcranial magnetic stimulation with transcranial direct current stimulation: evidence for homeostatic plasticity in the human motor cortex. J Neurosci. 2004;24(13):3379–3385.

47. Iyer MB, Schleper N, Wassermann EM. Priming stimulation enhances the depressant effect of low-frequency repetitive transcranial magnetic stimulation. J Neurosci. 2003;23:10867–10872.

48. Todd G, Flavel SC, Ridding MC. Priming theta-burst repetitive transcranial magnetic stimulation with low- and high-frequency stimulation. Exp Brain Res. 2009;195:307–315.

49. Ragert P, Camus M, Vandermeeren Y, Dimyan MA, Cohen LG. Modulation of effects of intermittent theta burst stimulation applied over primary motor cortex (M1) by conditioning stimulation of the opposite M1. J Neurophysiol. 2009;102:766–773.

50. Monte-Silva K, Kuo MF, et al. Induction of late LTP-like plasticity in the human motor cortex by repeated non-invasive brain stimulation.Brain Stimul. 2013;6(3):424–432.

51. Rioult-Pedotti MS, Friedman D, Donoghue JP. Learning-induced LTP in neocortex. Science. 2000; 290(5491):533–536.

52. Gentner R, Wankerl K, Reinsberger C, Zeller D, Classen J. Depression of human corticospinal excitability induced by magnetic theta-burst stimulation: evidence of rapid polarity-reversing metaplasticity. Cereb Cortex. 2008;18:2046–2053.

53. Iezzi E, Conte A, Suppa A, et al. Phasic voluntary movements reverse the after effects of subsequent theta-burst stimulation in humans. J Neurophysiol. 2008;100:2070–2076.

54. Rosenkranz K, Kacar A, Rothwell JC. Differential modulation of motor cortical plasticity and excitability in early and late phases of human motor learning. J Neurosci. 2007;27:12058–12066.

55. Huang YZ, Rothwell JC, Edwards MJ, Chen RS. Effect of physiological activity on an NMDA-dependent form of cortical plasticity in human. Cereb Cortex. 2008;18:563–570.

56. Antal A, Terney D, Poreisz C, Paulus W. Towards unravelling task-related modulations of neuroplastic changes induced in the human motor cortex. Eur J Neurosci. 2007;26:2687–2691.

57. Muller-Dahlhaus JF, Orekhov Y, Liu Y, Ziemann U. Interindividual variability and age-dependency of motor cortical plasticity induced by paired associative stimulation. Exp Brain Res. 2008;187:467–475.

58. Fathi D, Ueki Y, Mima T, et al. Effects of aging on the human motor cortical plasticity studied by paired associative stimulation. Clin Neurophysiol. 2010;121:90–93.

59. Kuo MF, Paulus W, Nitsche MA. Sex differences in cortical neuroplasticity in humans. Neuroreport. 2006;17:1703–1707.

60. Kleim JA, Chan S, Pringle E, et al. BDNF val66met polymorphism is associated with modified experience-dependent plasticity in human motor cortex. Nat Neurosci. 2006;9:735–737.

61. Cheeran B, Talelli P, Mori F, et al. A common polymorphism in the brain-derived neurotrophic factor gene (BDNF) modulates human cortical plasticity and the response to rTMS. J Physiol. 2008;586 (Pt 23):5717–5725.

62. Witte AV, Kürten J, Jansen S, et al. Interaction of BDNF and COMT polymorphisms on paired-associative stimulation-induced cortical plasticity. J Neurosci. 2012;32(13):4553–4561.

63. Li Voti P, Conte A, Suppa A, et al. Correlation between cortical plasticity, motor learning and BDNF genotype in healthy subjects. Exp Brain Res. 2011;212(1):91–99.

64. Nakamura K, Enomoto H, Hanajima R, et al. Quadri-pulse stimulation (QPS) induced LTP/LTD was not affected by Val66Met polymorphism in the brain-derived neurotrophic factor (BDNF) gene. Neurosci Lett. 2011;487(3):264–267.

65. Cirillo J, Lavender AP, Ridding MC, Semmler JG. Motor cortex plasticity induced by paired associative stimulation is enhanced in physically active individuals. J Physiol. 2009;587:5831–5842.

66. Antal A, Terney D, Poreisz C, Paulus W. Towards unravelling task-related modulations of neuroplastic changes induced in the human motor cortex. Eur J Neurosci. 2007;26:2687–2691.

67. Sale MV, Ridding MC, Nordstrom MA. Factors influencing the magnitude and reproducibility of corticomotor excitability changes induced by paired associative stimulation. Exp Brain Res. 2007;181:615–624.

68. Lang N, Speck S, Harms J, Rothkegel H, Paulus W, Sommer M. Dopaminergic potentiation of rTMS-induced motor cortex inhibition.Biol Psychiatry. 2008;63(2):231–233.

69. Koch G, Esposito Z, Codecà C, et al. Altered dopamine modulation of LTD-like plasticity in Alzheimer's disease patients. Clin Neurophysiol. 2011;122(4):703–707.

70. Monte-Silva K, Kuo MF, Thirugnanasambandam N, Liebetanz D, Paulus W, Nitsche MA. Dose-dependent inverted U-shaped effect of dopamine (D2-like) receptor activation on focal and nonfocal plasticity in humans. J Neurosci. 2009;29(19):6124–6131.

71. Monte-Silva K, Liebetanz D, Grundey J, Paulus W, Nitsche MA. Dosage-dependent non-linear effect of L-dopa on human motor cortex plasticity. J Physiol. 2010;588(Pt 18):3415–3424.

72. Kuo MF, Paulus W, Nitsche MA. Boosting focally-induced brain plasticity by dopamine.Cereb Cortex. 2008;18(3):648–651.

73. Kuo MF, Grosch J, Fregni F, Paulus W, Nitsche MA. Focusing effect of acetylcholine on neuroplasticity in the human motor cortex. J Neurosci. 2007;27(52):14442–14447.

74. Swayne OB, Teo JT, Greenwood RJ, Rothwell JC. The facilitatory effects of intermittent theta burst stimulation on corticospinal excitability are enhanced by nicotine. Clin Neurophysiol. 2009;120(8):1610–1615.

75. Nitsche MA, Grundey J, Liebetanz D, Lang N, Tergau F, Paulus W. Catecholaminergic consolidation of motor cortical neuroplasticity in humans. Cereb Cortex. 2004;14(11):1240–1245.

76. Ziemann U, Meintzschel F, Korchounov A, Ilić TV. Pharmacological modulation of plasticity in the human motor cortex. Neurorehabil Neural Repair. 2006;20(2):243–251.

77. Ridding MC, Ziemann U. Determinants of the induction of cortical plasticity by non-invasive brain stimulation in healthy subjects. J Physiol. 2010;588(Pt 13):2291–2304.

78. Nudo RJ, Milliken GW, Jenkins WM, Merzenich MM. Use-dependent alterations of movement representations in primary motor cortex of adult squirrel monkeys. J Neurosci. 1996;16(2):785–807

79. Muellbacher W, Ziemann U, Boroojerdi B, Cohen L, Hallett M. Role of the human motor cortex in rapid motor learning. Exp Brain Res. 2001;**136**(4):431–438

80. Brashers-Krug T, Shadmehr R, Bizzi E. Consolidation in human motor memory. Nature. 1996;**382**:252–255.

81. Walker MP, Brakefield T, Morgan A, Hobson JA, Stickgold R. Practice with sleep makes perfect: Sleep-dependent motor skill learning. Neuron. 2002;**35**:205–211.

82. Muellbacher W, Ziemann U, Wissel J, et al. Early consolidation in human primary motor cortex. Nature. 2002;**415**:640–644.

83. Lundbye-Jensen J, Petersen TH, Rothwell JC, Nielsen JB. Interference in ballistic motor learning: specificity and role of sensory error signals. PLoS One. 2011;**6**(3):e17451.

84. Nader K, Hardt O. A single standard for memory: the case for reconsolidation. Nat Rev Neurosci. 2009;**10**:224–234.

85. Censor N, Dimyan MA, Cohen LG. Primary cortical processing during memory reactivation enables modification of existing human motor memories. Curr Biol. 2010;**20**:1545–1549.

86. Doyon J, Penhune V, Ungerleider LG. Distinct contribution of the cortico-striatal and cortico-cerebellar systems to motor skill learning. Neuropsychologia. 2003;**41**(3):252–262.

87. Debas K, Carrier J, Orban P, et al. Brain plasticity related to the consolidation of motor sequence learning and motor adaptation. Proc Natl Acad Sci U S A. 2010;**107**(41):17839–17844.

88. Plewnia C, Lotze M, Gerloff C. Disinhibition of the contralateral motor cortex by low-frequency rTMS. Neuroreport.2003;**14**:609–612.

89. Schambra HM, Sawaki L, Cohen LG. Modulation of excitability of human motor cortex (M1) by 1 Hz transcranial magnetic stimulation of the contralateral M1. Clin Neurophysiol. 2003;**114**:130–133.

90. Bütefisch CM, Khurana V, Kopylev L, Cohen LG. Enhancing encoding of a motor memory in the primary motor cortex by cortical stimulation. J Neurophysiol. 2004;**91**(5):2110–2116.

91. Kim YH, Park JW, Ko MH, et al. Facilitative effect of high frequency subthreshold repetitive transcranial magnetic stimulation on complex sequential motor learning in humans. Neurosci Lett. 2004;**367**:181–185.

92. Teo JT, Swayne OB, Cheeran B, Greenwood RJ, Rothwell JC. Human theta burst stimulation enhances subsequent motor learning and increases performance variability. Cereb Cortex. 2011;**21**(7):1627–1638.

93. Agostino R, Iezzi E, Dinapoli L, et al. Effects of 5 Hz subthreshold magnetic stimulation of primary motor cortex on fast finger movements in normal subjects. Exp Brain Res. 2007;**180**(1):105–111.

94. Jung P, Ziemann U. Homeostatic and nonhomeostatic modulation of learning in human motor cortex. J Neurosci. 2009; **29**(17):5597–5604.

95. Kobayashi M. Effect of slow repetitive TMS of the motor cortex on ipsilateral sequential simple finger movements and motor skill learning. Restor Neurol Neurosci. 2010;**28**(4):437–448.

96. Meehan SK, Zabukovec JR, Dao E, Cheung KL, Linsdell MA, Boyd LA. One hertz repetitive transcranial magnetic stimulation over dorsal premotor cortex enhances offline motor memory consolidation for sequence-specific implicit learning. Eur J Neurosci. 2013;**38**:3071–3079;.

97. Riek S, Hinder MR, Carson RG. Primary motor cortex involvement in initial learning during visuomotor adaptation.Neuropsychologia. 2012;**50**(10):2515–2523.

98. Kang EK, Paik NJ. Effect of a tDCS electrode montage on implicit motor sequence learning in healthy subjects. Exp Transl Stroke Med. 2011;17;**3**(1):4.

99. Tecchio F, Zappasodi F, Assenza G, et al. Anodal transcranial direct current stimulation enhances procedural consolidation. J Neurophysiol. 2010;**104**(2):1134–1140.

100. Galea JM, Vazquez A, Pasricha N, de Xivry JJ, Celnik P. Dissociating the roles of the cerebellum and motor cortex during adaptive learning: the motor cortex retains what the cerebellum learns. Cereb Cortex. 2011;**21**(8):1761–1770.

101. Hunter T, Sacco P, Nitsche MA, Turner DL. Modulation of internal model formation during force field-induced motor learning by anodal transcranial direct current stimulation of primary motor cortex. J Physiol. 2009;**587**(Pt 12):2949–2961.

102. Vallence AM, Kurylowicz L, Ridding MC. A comparison of neuroplastic responses to non-invasive brain stimulation protocols and motor learning in healthy adults. Neurosci Lett. 2013;**549**:151–156.

103. Stagg CJ, Bachtiar V, Johansen-Berg H. The role of GABA in human motor learning. Curr Biol. 2011; **21**(6):480–484.

104. McAllister SM, Rothwell JC, Ridding MC. Cortical oscillatory activity and the induction of plasticity in the human motor cortex. Eur J Neurosci. 2011;**33**(10):1916–1924.

105. Antal A, Nitsche MA, Kruse W, Kincses TZ, Hoffmann K, Paulus W. Direct current stimulation over V5 enhances visuomotor coordination by improving motion perception in humans. J Cogn Neurosci. 2004;**4**(16):521–527.

106. Chi RP, Fregni F, Snyder AW. Visual memory improved by non-invasive brain stimulation. Brain Res. 2010;**1353**:168–175.

107. Ross L, McCoy D, Wolk DA, Coslett B, Olson IR. Improved proper name recall by electrical stimulation of the anterior temporal lobes. Neuropsychologia. 2010;**48**(12):3671–3674.

108. Sparing R, Dafotakis M, Meister IG, Thirugnanasambandam N, Fink GR. Enhancing language performance with non- invasive brain stimulation—a transcranial direct current stimulation study in healthy humans. Neuropsychologia. 2008;**46**:261–268.

109. Floel A, Rosser N, Michka O, Knecht S, Breitenstein C. Noninvasive brain stimulation improves language learning. J Cogn Neurosci. 2008;**20**(8):1415–1422.

110. Fregni F, Boggio PS, Nitsche MA, et al. Anodal transcranial direct current stimulation of prefrontal cortex enhances working memory. Exp Brain Res. 2005;**166**(1):23–30.

111. Dockery CA, Hueckel-Weng R, Birbaumer N, Plewnia C. Enhancement of planning ability by transcranial direct current stimulation. J. Neurosci. 2009;**29**:7271–7277.

112. Marshall L, Molle M, Hallschmid M, Born J. Transcranial direct current stimulation during sleep improves declarative memory. J Neurosci. 2004;**24**(44):9985–9992.

113. Cohen Kadosh R, Soskic S, Iuculano T, Kanai R, Walsh V. Modulating neuronal activity produces specific and long-lasting changes in numerical competence. Curr Biol. 2010;**20**:2016–2020.

114. Bolognini N, Fregni F, Casati C, Olgiati E, Vallar G. Brain polarization of parietal cortex augments training-induced improvement of visual exploratory and attentional skills. Brain Res. 2010;**1349**:76–89

115. Ragert P, Vandermeeren Y, Camus M, Cohen LG. Improvement of spatial tactile acuity by transcranial direct current stimulation. Clin Neurophysiol. 2008;**119**:805–811.

116. Snowball A, Tachtsidis I, Popescu T, et al. Long-term enhancement of brain function and cognition using cognitive training and brain stimulation. Curr Biol. 2013;**23**(11):987–992.

117. Jacobson L, Koslowsky M, Lavidor M. tDCS polarity effects in motor and cognitive domains: a meta-analytical review. Exp Brain Res. 2012;**216**(1):1–10.

118. Nudo RJ, Milliken GW. Reorganization of movement representations in primary motor cortex following focal ischemic infarcts in adult squirrel monkeys. J Neurophysiol. 1996;**75**:2144–2149.

119. Nudo RJ, Wise BM, SiFuentes F, Milliken GW. Neural substrates for the effects of rehabilitative training on motor recovery after ischemic infarct. Science. 1996;**272**(5269):1791–1794.

120. Ghosh S, Porter R. Morphology of pyramidal neurones in monkey motor cortex and the synaptic actions of their intracortical axon collaterals. J Physiol. 1988;**400**:593–615.

121. Cheney PD, Fetz EE, Palmer SS. Patterns of facilitation and suppression of antagonist forelimb muscles from motor cortex sites in the awake monkey. J Neurophysiol. 1985;**53**(3):805–820.

122. National Audit Office. Reducing brain damage: Faster access to better stroke care. NAO, London, 2005.

123. Saka O, McGuire A, Wolfe C. Cost of stroke in the United Kingdom. Age Ageing. 2009;**38**(1):27–32.

124. Chollet F, DiPiero V, Wise RJ, Brooks DJ, Dolan RJ, Frackowiak RS. The functional anatomy of motor recovery after stroke in humans: a study with positron emission tomography. Ann Neurol. 1991;**29**:63–71.

125. Ward NS, Brown MM, Thompson AJ, Frackowiak RSJ. Neural correlates of outcome after stroke: a cross-sectional fMRI study. Brain. 2003;**126**:1430–1448.

126. Catano A, Houa M, Caroyer JM, Ducarne H, Noel P. Magnetic transcranial stimulation in non-haemorrhagic sylvian strokes: interest of facilitation for early functional prognosis. Electroencephalogr Clin Neurophysiol. 1995;**97**(6):349–354.

127. Delvaux V, Alagona G, Gerard P, De Pasqua V, Pennisi G, de Noordhout AM. Post-stroke reorganization of hand motor area: a 1-year prospective follow-up with focal transcranial magnetic stimulation. Clin Neurophysiol. 2003;**114**:1217–1225.

128. Liepert J, Storch P, Fritsch A, Weiller C. Motor cortex disinhibition in acute stroke. Clin Neurophysiol. 2000;**111**:671–676.

129. Manganotti P, Patuzzo S, Cortese F, Palermo A, Smania N, Fiaschi A. Motor disinhibition in affected and unaffected hemisphere in the early period of recovery after stroke. Clin Neurophysiol. 2002;**113**:936–943.

130. Shimizu T, Hosaki A, Hino T, Sato M, Komori T, Hirai S, Rossini PM. Motor cortical disinhibition in the unaffected hemisphere after unilateral cortical stroke. Brain. 2002;**125**(Pt 8):1896–1907.

131. Swayne OB, Rothwell JC, Ward NS, Greenwood RJ. Stages of motor output reorganization after hemispheric stroke suggested by longitudinal studies of cortical physiology. Cereb Cortex. 2008;**18**:1909–1922.

132. Murase N, Duque J, Mazzocchio R, Cohen LG. Influence of interhemispheric interactions on motor function in chronic stroke. Ann Neurol. 2004;**55**:400–409.

133. Ward NS, Cohen LG. Mechanisms underlying recovery of motor function after stroke. Arch Neurol. 2004;**61**(12):1844–1848.

134. Kim YH, You SH, Ko MH, et al. Repetitive transcranial magnetic stimulation-induced corticomotor excitability and associated motor skill acquisition in chronic stroke. Stroke. 2006;**37**:1471–1476.

135. Talelli P, Greenwood RJ, Rothwell JC. Exploring theta burst stimulation as an intervention to improve motor recovery in chronic stroke. Clin Neurophysiol. 2007;**118**(2):333–342.

136. Ameli M, Grefkes C, Kemper F, et al. Differential effects of high-frequency repetitive transcranial magnetic stimulation over ipsilesional primary motor cortex in cortical and subcortical middle cerebral artery stroke. Ann Neurol. 2009;**66**(3):298–309

137. Ackerley SJ, Stinear CM, Barber PA, Byblow WD. Combining theta burst stimulation with training after subcortical stroke. Stroke. 2010;**41**:1568–1572

138. Khedr EM, Ahmed MA, Fathy N, Rothwell JC. Therapeutic trial of repetitive transcranial magnetic stimulation after acute ischemic stroke. Neurology. 2005;**65**:466–468.

139. Khedr EM, Abdel-Fadeil MR, Farghali A, Qaid M. Role of 1 and 3 Hz repetitive transcranial magnetic stimulation on motor function recovery after acute ischaemic stroke. Eur J Neurol. 2009;**16**(12): 1323–1330.

140. Chang WH, Kim YH, Bang OY, et al. Long-term effects of rTMS on motor recovery in patients after subacute stroke. J Rehabil Med. 2010;**42**:758–764.

141. Khedr EM, El Etraby A, Hemeda M, Nasef AM, Abd El Razek A. Long term effect of repetitive transcranial magnetic stimulation on motor function recovery after acute ischemic stroke. Acta Neurol Scand. 2010;**121**(1): 30–37.

142. Hsu Y-F, Huang Y-Z, Lin Y-Y, et al. Intermittent theta burst stimulation over ipsilesional primary motor cortex of subacute ischemic stroke patients: A pilot study. Brain Stim. 2013;**6**: 166–174.

143. Sasaki N, Mizutani S, Kakuda W, Abo M. Comparison of the effects of high- and low-frequency repetitive Transcranial magnetic stimulation on upper limb hemiparesis in the early phase of stroke. J Stroke Cerebrovasc Dis. 2013;**22**(4):413–418.

144. Malcolm MP, Triggs WJ, Light KE, et al. Repetitive transcranial magnetic stimulation as an adjunct to constraint- induced therapy: an exploratory randomized controlled trial. Am J Phys Med Rehabil. 2007;**86**:707–715.

145. Emara TH, Moustafa RR, Elnahas NM, et al. Repetitive transcranial magnetic stimulation at 1Hz and 5Hz produces sustained improvement in motor function and disability after ischaemic stroke. Eur J Neurol. 2010;**17**(9):1203–1209.

146. Koganemaru S, Mima T, Thabit MN, et al. Recovery of upper-limb function due to enhanced use-dependent plasticity in chronic stroke patients. Brain. 2010;**133**(11):3373–3384.

147. Chang WH, Kim YH, Yoo WK, et al. rTMS with motor training modulates cortico-basal ganglia-thalamocortical circuits in stroke patients. Restor Neurol Neurosci. 2012;**31**:1–11.

148. Talelli P, Wallace A, Dileone M, et al. Theta burst stimulation in the rehabilitation of the upper Limb: a semirandomized, placebo-controlled trial in chronic stroke patients. Neurorehabil Neural Repair. 2012;**26**:976–987.

149. Liepert J, Zittel S, Weiller C. Improvement of dexterity by single session low-frequency repetitive transcranial magnetic stimulation over the contralesional motor cortex in acute stroke: a double-blind placebo-controlled crossover trial. Restor Neurol Neurosci. 2007;**25**:461–465.

150. Dafotakis M, Grefkes C, Eickhoff SB, et al. Effects of rTMS on grip force control following subcortical stroke. Exp Neurol. 2008;**211**:407–412.

151. Nowak DA, Grefkes C, Dafotakis M, et al. Effects of low-frequency repetitive transcranial magnetic stimulation of the contralesional primary motor cortex on movement kine- matics and neural activity in subcortical stroke. Arch Neurol. 2008;**65**:741–747.

152. Mansur CG, Fregni F, Boggio PS, et al. A sham stimulation-controlled trial of rTMS of the unaffected hemisphere in stroke patients. Neurology. 2005;**64**:1802–1804.

153. Takeuchi N, Chuma T, Matsuo Y, Watanabe I, Ikoma K. Repetitive transcranial magnetic stimulation of contralesional primary motor cortex improves hand function after stroke. Stroke. 2005;**36**:2681–2686.

154. Takeuchi N, Tada T, Toshima M, Chuma T, Matsuo Y, Ikoma K. Inhibition of the unaffected motor cortex by 1 Hz repetitive transcranical magnetic stimulation enhances motor performance and training effect of the paretic hand in patients with chronic stroke. J Rehabil Med. 2008;**40**:298–303.

155. Grefkes C, Nowak DA, Wang LE, Dafotakis M, Eickhoff SB, Fink GR. Modulating cortical connectivity in stroke patients by rTMS assessed with fMRI and dynamic causal modeling. Neuroimage. 2010;**50**(1):233–242.

156. Meehan SK, Dao E, Linsdell MA, Boyd LA. Continuous theta burst stimulation over the contralesional sensory and motor cortex enhances motor learning post-stroke. Neurosci Lett. 2011;**500**:26–30.

157. Pomeroy V M, Cloud G, Tallis RC, Donaldson C, Nayak V, Miller S. Transcranial magnetic stimulation and muscle contraction to enhance stroke recovery: a ran- domized proof-of-principle and fea- sibility investigation. Neurorehabil. Neural Repair. 2007;**21**: 509–517.

158. Seniow J, Bilik M, Lesniak M. Transcranial magnetic stimulation combined with physiotherapy in rehabilitation of poststroke hemiparesis: a randomized, double-blind, placebo- controlled study. Neurorehabil Neural Repair. 2012;**26**:1072–1079.

159. Fregni F, Boggio PS, Valle AC, et al. A sham-controlled trial of a 5-day course of repetitive transcranial magnetic stimulation of the unaffected hemisphere in stroke patients. Stroke. 2006;**37**(8):2115–2122.

160. Theilig S, Podubecka J, Bösl K, et al. Functional neuromuscular stimulation to improve severe hand dysfunction after stroke: does inhibitory rTMS enhance therapeutic efficiency? Exp Neurol. 2011;**230**:149–155.

161. Avenanti A, Coccia M, Ladavas E, Provinciali L, Ceravolo MG. Low-frequency rTMS promotes use-dependent motor plasticity in chronic stroke: a randomized trial. Neurology. 2012;**78**, 256–264.

162. Conforto AB, Anjos SM, Saposnik G, et al. Transcranial magnetic stimulation in mild to severe hemiparesis early after stroke: a proof of principle and novel approach to improve motor function. J Neurol. 2012;**259**:1399–1405.

163. Wang R-Y, Tseng H-Y, Liao K-K, Wang C-J, Lai K-L, Yang Y-R. rTMS combined with task-oriented training to improve symmetry of interhemispheric corticomotor excitability and gait performance after stroke: a randomized trial. Neurorehabil Neural Repair. 2012;**26**:222–230.

164. Takeuchi N, Tada T, Toshima M, et al. Repetitive transcranial magnetic stimulation over bilateral hemispheres enhances motor function and training effect of paretic hand in patients after stroke. J Rehabil Med. 2009;**41**:1049–1054.

165. Hsu WY, Cheng CH, Liao KK, Lee IH, Lin YY. Effects of repetitive transcranial magnetic stimulation on motor functions in patients with stroke: a meta-analysis. Stroke. 2012;**43**(7):1849–1857.

166. Kim DY, Ohn SH, Yang EJ, et al. Enhancing motor performance by anodal transcranial direct current stimulation in subacute stroke patients. Am J Phys Med Rehabil. 2009;**88**:829–836.

167. Fregni F, Boggio PS, Mansur CG, et al. Transcranial direct current stimulation of the unaffected hemisphere in stroke patients. Neuroreport. 2005;**16**(14):1551–1555.

168. Hummel F, Celnik P, Giraux P, et al. Effects of non-invasive cortical stimulation on skilled motor function in chronic stroke. Brain. 2005;**128**:490–499.

169. Celnik P, Paik NJ, Vandermeeren Y, Dimyan M, Cohen LG. Effects of combined peripheral nerve stimulation and brain polarization on performance of a motor sequence task after chronic stroke. Stroke. 2009;**40**(5):1764–1771.

170. Madhavan S, Weber KA, Stinear JW. Non-invasive brain stimulation enhances fine motor control of the hemiparetic ankle: implications for rehabilitation. Exp Brain Res. 2011;**209**:9–17.

171. Mahmoudi H, Borhani Haghighi A, Petramfar P, et al. Transcranial direct current stimulation: electrode montage in stroke. Disabil Rehabil. 2011;**33**:1383–1388.

172. Stagg CJ, Bachtiar V, O'Shea J, et al. Cortical activation changes underlying stimulation-induced behavioural gains in chronic stroke. Brain. 2012;**135**:276–284.

173. Tanaka S, Takeda K, Otaka Y, et al. Single session of transcranial direct current stimulation transiently increases knee extensor force in patients with hemiparetic stroke. Neurorehabil Neural Repair. 2011;**25**:565–569.

174. Kim DY, Lim JY, Kang EK, et al. Effect of transcranial direct current stimulation on motor recovery in patients with subacute stroke. Am J Phys Med Rehabil. 2010;**89**:879–886.

175. Hesse S, Waldner A, Mehrholz J, et al. Combined transcranial direct current stimulation and robot-assisted arm training in subacute stroke patients: an exploratory, randomized multicenter trial. Neurorehabil Neural Repair. 2011;**25**:838–846.

176. Rossi C, Sallustio F, Di Legge S, et al. Transcranial direct current stimulation of the affected hemisphere does not accelerate recovery of acute stroke patients. Eur J Neurol. 2012; doi: 10.1111/j.1468–1331.2012.03703.x

177. Lindenberg R, Renga V, Zhu LL, et al. Bihemispheric brain stimulation facilitates motor recovery in chronic stroke patients. Neurology. 2010;**75**:2176–2184.

178. Bolognini N, Vallar G, Casati C, et al. Neurophysiological and behavioral effects of tDCS combined with constraint-induced movement therapy in poststroke patients. Neurorehabil Neural Repair. 2011;**25**:819–829.

179. Geroin C, Picelli A, Munari D, et al. Combined transcranial direct current stimulation and robot-assisted gait training in patients with chronic stroke: a preliminary comparison. Clin Rehabil. 2011;**25**:537–548.

180. Bradnam LV, Stinear CM, Barber PA, Byblow WD. Contralesional hemisphere control of the proximal paretic upper limb following stroke. Cereb Cortex. 2011; doi:10.1093/cercor/bhr344.

181. Nair DG, Renga V, Lindenberg R, et al. Optimizing recovery potential through simultaneous occupational therapy and non-invasive brain-stimulation using tDCS. Restor Neurol Neurosci. 2011;**29**:1–10.

182. Ward NS, Newton JM, Swayne OB, et al. The relationship between brain activity and peak grip force is modulated by corticospinal system integrity after subcortical stroke. Eur J Neurosci. 2007;**25**(6):1865–1873.

183. Bestmann S, Swayne O, Blankenburg F, et al The role of contralesional dorsal premotor cortex after stroke as studied with concurrent TMS-fMRI. J Neurosci. 2010;**30**(36):11926–11937.

184. Baker JM, Rorden C, Fridriksson J. Using transcranial direct-current stimulation to treat stroke patients with aphasia. Stroke. 2010;**41**:1229–1236.

185. Floel A, Meinzer M, Kirstein, R, Nijhof S, Deppe M, Knecht S, Breitenstein C Short-term anomia training and electrical brain stimulation. Stroke. 2011;**42**:2065–2067.

186. Monti A, Cogiamanian F, Marceglia S, et al. Improved naming after transcranial direct current stimulation in aphasia. J Neurol Neurosurg Psychiatry. 2008;**79**:451–453.

187. Elsner B, Kugler J, Pohl M, Mehrholz J. Transcranial direct current stimulation (tDCS) for improving aphasia in patients after stroke. Cochrane Database Syst Rev. 2013;**25**;6.

188. Naeser MA, Martin PI, Nicholas M, et al. Improved naming after TMS treatments in a chronic, global aphasia patient–case report. Neurocase. 2005;**11**(3):182–193.

189. Szaflarski JP, Vannest J, Wu SW, DiFrancesco MW, Banks C, Gilbert DL. Excitatory repetitive transcranial magnetic stimulation induces improvements in chronic post- stroke aphasia. Med Sci Monit. 2011;**17**(3):CR132–CR139.

190. Koch G, Bonnì S, Giacobbe V, et al. θ-burst stimulation of the left hemisphere accelerates recovery of hemispatial neglect. Neurology. 2012;**78**(1):24–30.

191. Kim BR, Chun MH, Kim DY, Lee SJ. Effect of high- and low-frequency repetitive transcranial magnetic stimulation on visuospatial neglect in patients with acute stroke: a double-blind, sham-controlled trial. Arch Phys Med Rehabil. 2013;**94**(5): 803–807.

192. Shindo K, Sugiyama K, Huabao L, Nishijima K, Kondo T, Izumi S. Long-term effect of low-frequency repetitive transcranial magnetic stimulation over the unaffected posterior parietal cortex in patients with unilateral spatial neglect. J Rehabil Med. 2006;**38**(1):65–67.

193. Kim BR, Chun MH, Kim DY, Lee SJ. Effect of high- and low-frequency repetitive Transcranial magnetic stimulation on visuospatial neglect in patients with acute stroke: a double-blind, sham-controlled trial. Arch Phys Med Rehabil. 2013;**94**(5): 803–807.

194. Ko MH, Han SH, Park SH, Seo JH, Kim YH. Improvement of visual scanning after DC brain polarization of parietal cortex in stroke patients with spatial neglect. Neurosci Lett. 2008;**448**(2):171–174.

195. Sparing R, Thimm M, Hesse MD, Küst J, Karbe H, Fink GR. Bidirectional alterations of interhemispheric parietal balance by non-invasive cortical stimulation. Brain. 2009;**132**(Pt 11):3011–3020.

196. Khedr EM, Abo-Elfetoh N, Rothwell JC. Treatment of post-stroke dysphagia with repetitive transcranial magnetic stimulation. Acta Neurol Scand. 2009;**119**(3):155–161.

197. Yang EJ, Baek SR, Shin J, et al. Effects of transcranial direct current stimulation (tDCS) on post-stroke dysphagia. Restor Neurol Neurosci. 2012;**30**:303–311.

198. Kumar S, Wagner CW, Frayne C, et al. Non- invasive brain stimulation may improve stroke-related dysphagia: a pilot study. Stroke. 2011;**42**:1035–1040.

199. Ridding MC, Rothwell JC. Is there a future for therapeutic use of transcranial magnetic stimulation? Nat Rev Neurosci. 2007;**8**(7):559–567.

200. Fregni F, Boggio PS, Santos MC, et al. Noninvasive cortical stimulation with transcranial direct current stimulation in Parkinson's disease. Movement Disorders. 2006; **21**(10): 1693–1702.

201. Khedr EM, Rothwell JC, Shawky OA, Ahmed MA, Hamdy A. Effect of daily repetitive transcranial magnetic stimulation on motor performance in Parkinson's disease. Movement Disorders 2006; **21**(12):2201–2205.

202. Filipovic SR, Rothwell JC, van de Warrenburg BP, Bhatia K. Repetitive transcranial magnetic stimulation for levodopa-induced dyskinesias in Par- kinson's disease. Movement Disorders 2009;**24**(2):246–253.

203. Koch G, Brusa L, Caltagirone C, et al. rTMS of supplementary motor area modulates therapy-induced dyskinesias in Parkinson disease. Neurology. 2005;**65**(4):623–625.

204. Koch G, Brusa L, Carrillo F, et al. Cerebellar magnetic stimulation decreases levodopa-induced dyskinesias in Parkinson disease. Neurology. 2009;**732**:113–119.

205. Murase N, Rothwell JC, Kaji R, et al. Subthreshold low-frequency repetitive transcranial magnetic stimulation over the premotor cortex modulates writer's cramp. Brain. 2005;**128**(Pt 1):104–115.

206. Di Lazzaro V, Dileone M, Pilato F, et al. Repetitive transcranial magnetic stimulation for ALS. A preliminary controlled study.Neurosci Lett. 2006;**408**(2):135–140.

207. Di Lazzaro V, Pilato F, Profice P, et al. Motor cortex stimulation for ALS: a double blind placebo-controlled study. Neurosci Lett. 2009;**464**(1):18–21.

208. Kinoshita M, Ikeda A, Begum T, Yamamoto J, Hitomi T, Shibasaki H. Low-frequency repetitive transcranial magnetic stimulation for seizure suppression in patients with extratemporal lobe epilepsy—a pilot study. Seizure. 2005; **14**(6):387–392.

209. Sun W, Mao W, Meng X, et al. Low-frequency repetitive transcranial magnetic stimulation for the treatment of refractory partial epilepsy: a controlled clinical study. Epilepsia. 2012;**53**(10):1782–1789.

210. George MS, Taylor JJ, Short EB.The expanding evidence base for rTMS treatment of depression.Curr Opin Psychiatry. 2013;**26**(1):13–18.

211. Yang YR, Tseng CY, Chiou SY, Liao KK, Cheng SJ, Lai KL, Wang RY. Combination of rTMS and treadmill training modulates corticomotor inhibition and improves walking in Parkinson disease: a randomized trial. Neurorehabil Neural Repair. 2013;**27**(1):79–86.

212. Liebetanz D, Nitsche MA, Tergau F, Paulus W. Pharmacological approach to the mechanisms of transcranial DC-stimulation-induced after-effects of human motor cortex excitability. Brain. 2002;**125**(Pt 10):2238–2247.

213. Wankerl K, Weise D, Gentner R, Rumpf JJ, Classen J. L-type voltage-gated Ca2+ channels: a single molecular switch for long-term potentiation/long-term depression-like plasticity and activity-dependent metaplasticity in humans. J Neurosci. 2010;**30**(18):6197–6204.

214. Huang YZ, Chen RS, Rothwell JC, Wen HY. The after-effect of human theta burst stimulation is NMDA receptor dependent. Clin Neurophysiol. 2007;**118**(5):1028–1032.

215. Chaieb L, Antal A, Terney D, Paulus W. Pharmacological modulation of the short-lasting effects of antagonistic direct current-stimulation over the human motor cortex. Front Psychiatry. 2012;**3**:67.

216. Teo JT, Swayne OB, Rothwell JC. Further evidence for NMDA-dependence of the after-effects of human theta burst stimulation. Clin Neurophysiol. 2007;**118**(7):1649–1651.

217. Nitsche MA, Liebetanz D, Schlitterlau A, et al. GABAergic modulation of DC stimulation-induced motor cortex excitability shifts in humans.,Eur J Neurosci. 2004;**19**(10):2720–2726.

218. Thirugnanasambandam N, Grundey J, Adam K, et al. Nicotinergic impact on focal and non-focal neuroplasticity induced by non-invasive brain stimulation in non-smoking humans. Neuropsychopharmacology. 2011;**36**(4):879–886.

219. Swayne OB, Teo JT, Greenwood RJ, Rothwell JC. The facilitatory effects of intermittent theta burst stimulation on corticospinal excitability are enhanced by nicotine. Clin Neurophysiol. 2009;**120**(8):1610–1615.

220. Kuo MF, Grosch J, Fregni F, Paulus W, Nitsche MA. Focusing effect of acetylcholine on neuroplasticity in the human motor cortex. J Neurosci. 2007;**27**(52):14442–14447.

221. Monte-Silva K, Liebetanz D, Grundey J, Paulus W, Nitsche MA. Dosage-dependent non-linear effect of L-dopa on human motor cortex plasticity. J Physiol. 2010;**588**(Pt 18):3415–3424.

222. Monte-Silva K, Kuo MF, Thirugnanasambandam N, Liebetanz D, Paulus W, Nitsche MA. Dose-dependent inverted U-shaped effect of dopamine (D2-like) receptor activation on focal and nonfocal plasticity in humans. J Neurosci. 2009;**29**(19):6124–6131.

223. Nitsche MA, Lampe C, Antal A, et al. Dopaminergic modulation of long-lasting direct current-induced cortical excitability changes in the human motor cortex.Eur J Neurosci. 2006 Mar;**23**(6):1651–1657.

224. Monte-Silva K, Ruge D, Teo JT, Paulus W, Rothwell JC, Nitsche MA. D2 receptor block abolishes θ burst stimulation-induced neuroplasticity in the human motor cortex. Neuropsychopharmacology. 2011;**36**(10):2097–2102.

225. Nitsche MA, Grundey J, Liebetanz D, Lang N, Tergau F, Paulus W. Catecholaminergic consolidation of motor cortical neuroplasticity in humans. Cereb Cortex. 2004;**14**(11):1240–1245.

226. Nitsche MA, Kuo MF, Karrasch R, Wächter B, Liebetanz D, Paulus W. Serotonin affects transcranial direct current-induced neuroplasticity in humans. Biol Psychiatry. 2009;**66**(5): 503–508.

227. Nitsche MA, Fricke K, Henschke U, et al. Pharmacological modulation of cortical excitability shifts induced by transcranial direct current stimulation in humans. J Physiol. 2003;**553** (Pt 1):293–301.

CHAPTER 17

Enhancement of neuroplasticity by drug therapy

Ulf Ziemann

Pharmacological modulation of stimulation-induced LTP in motor cortex: animal studies

In the rat motor cortex, long-term potentiation (LTP) usually requires activation of the *N*-methyl-D-aspartate (NMDA) receptor (NMDAR) [1–3]. Local disinhibition of rat motor cortex by iontophoretic application of bicuculline, an antagonist of the gamma-aminobutyric acid (GABA) type A receptor (GABAAR), results in unmasking of latent horizontal intracortical connections and rapid changes in representational organization [4]. This seminal paper, therefore, identified GABAA-ergic inhibitory cortical circuits as of crucial importance in regulating synaptic plasticity and map reorganization. Accordingly, LTP is facilitated if the rat motor cortex is locally disinhibited by bicuculline [2, 3, 5]. Similarly, LTP is facilitated in the disinhibited non-lesional surround tissue of experimentally induced focal infarction in rat sensorimotor cortex [6]. In contrast, diazepam, a benzodiazepine and positive allosteric modulator at the GABAAR, prevents the induction of LTP in rat motor cortex [7]. Neuromodulating transmitters such as dopamine (DA), norepinephrine (NE), acetylcholine (ACh), and serotonin (5-hydroxytryptamine, 5-HT) can exert significant effects on neocortical LTP (for review see [8]), but studies that have addressed pharmacological modulation of LTP in motor cortex are still limited. The dopamine D1 receptor antagonist SCH23390 and the dopamine D2 receptor antagonist raclopride reduce LTP induction in rat primary motor cortex, indicating an important supportive role of dopaminergic neurotransmission in synaptic plasticity [9]. Similarly, pharmacological blockade of muscarinic receptors by atropine prevented the induction of LTP and rather favoured the induction of long-term depression (LTD) by the same stimulation protocol [10].

Pharmacological modulation of stimulation-induced LTP in motor cortex: human studies

In human motor cortex, LTP-like plasticity can be induced by various non-invasive brain stimulation (NIBS) protocols (for reviews see [11–17]). LTP-like plasticity is typically expressed by long-term increase in the amplitude of the motor evoked potential (MEP), elicited by single-pulse transcranial magnetic stimulation (TMS) of the motor cortex, before and after the NIBS induction protocol,

and recorded by surface electromyography (EMG), typically from a hand muscle contralateral to the stimulated motor cortex [18, 19]. The term 'LTP-like' has been coined [20] because the increase in MEP amplitude exhibits close similarity compared to LTP as defined and studied at the cellular/molecular level, such as cooperativity, input-specificity, associativity, duration (>30 min), and dependence on NMDA receptor activation, but investigation is necessarily indirect at the systems level [14, 21].

LTP-like plasticity can be induced with several NIBS protocols and, although the detailed physiological mechanisms may be different between protocols, the effects of pharmacological modulation on LTP-like plasticity will be reviewed here from the perspective of classes of drugs with particular modes of action. All studies included in this review have been obtained in healthy subjects, and pharmacological modulation of LTP-like plasticity was typically assessed in placebo-controlled study designs by testing a single (oral) dose of study drug.

1. *GABAergic disinhibition*: no anti-GABAergic drugs are available for human use due to their adverse pro-convulsive effects. However, GABAergic disinhibition can be experimentally induced by transient limb ischaemic nerve block [22, 23]. This GABAergic disinhibition permits LTP-like plasticity induction to occur by low-frequency (0.1 Hz) repetitive TMS (rTMS) [24, 25] a protocol that does not produce overt MEP change when given alone [26].

2. *GABAergic inhibition*: Neurotransmission through the GABAAR is enhanced by benzodiazepines, allosteric positive modulators of the GABAAR. The permissive effect of GABAergic disinhibition on low-frequency rTMS induced LTP-like plasticity can be prevented by the benzodiazepine lorazepam [25]. Lorazepam reduces LTP-like plasticity induced by high-frequency (5 Hz) rTMS [27]. The benzodiazepine diazepam and the GABA-reuptake inhibitor tiagabine [28] and the GABAB receptor (GABABR) agonist baclofen [29] reduce LTP-like plasticity induced by paired associative transcranial magnetic stimulation (PAS). An additional subthreshold conditioning pulse 2 ms prior to the PAS test pulse, that would produce GABAA-ergic intracortical inhibition [30, 31], is also capable of blocking PAS-induce LTP-like plasticity [32]. Lorazepam attenuates LTP-like plasticity induced by anodal transcranial direct current stimulation (tDCS) in the first 10 min after stimulation [33], but MEP amplitude increases at later time points, an as of yet unexplained observation.

3. *NMDAR*: Dextromethorphan is a non-competitive partial antagonist at the NMDAR that results in blockade of PAS-induced [34], theta-burst stimulation (TBS)-induced [35] and anodal tDCS-induced [36] LTP-like plasticity. Similarly, the NMDAR antagonist memantine blocks LTP-like plasticity induced by TBS [37]. In contrast, D-cycloserine, a partial NMDAR agonist prolongs LTP-like plasticity induced by anodal tDCS [38].

4. *Blockers of voltage-gated sodium (Na+) and calcium (Ca2+) channels*: The voltage-gated Na+ and Ca2+ channel-blocking anticonvulsant lamotrigine prevents LTP-like plasticity induced by low-frequency rTMS in the context of transient limb ischaemic nerve block [25]. Similarly, lamotrigine or carbamazepine, another voltage-gated Na+ and Ca2+ channel blocking anticonvulsant, reduce PAS-induced [28, 39] and anodal tDCS-induced [36] LTP-like plasticity. Nimodipine, an L-type voltage-gated Ca2+ channel blocker abolishes TBS-induced LTP-like plasticity [35].

5. *Dopamine*: The effects of modulators of the dopaminergic system are complex. The DA precursor levodopa enhances PAS-induced LTP-like plasticity [40] but switches the LTP-like effect induced by anodal tDCS to an LTD-like effect [40, 41]. The enhancement of PAS-induced LTP-like plasticity by levodopa shows an inverted U-shaped dose dependency [42]. The DA D2 receptor agonist cabergoline has no effect on PAS-induced LTP-like plasticity while the D2 receptor antagonist haloperidol suppresses it [43]. Ropinirole, another D2 receptor agonist, demonstrates an inverted U-shaped dose dependent suppression of PAS- and anodal tDCS-induced LTP-like plasticity at low and high doses but no difference to placebo at intermediate doses [44]. The selective D2 receptor antagonist sulpiride blocks LTP-like plasticity induced by TBS [45] and anodal tDCS [46] but has no significant effect on LTP-like plasticity induced by PAS [47]. Addition of the D1/D2 receptor agonist pergolide does not prevent the suppression of anodal tDCS-induced LTP-like plasticity by sulpiride, underscoring the significance of D2 receptors in regulating LTP-like plasticity in human motor cortex [46]. In summary, agonists versus antagonists of the D2 receptor enhance or suppress, respectively, LTP-like plasticity in human motor cortex, but the results are not fully consistent and may depend non-linearly on dose, the balance of neurotransmission through D1 vs. D2 receptors, and the stimulation protocol to induce LTP-like plasticity.

6. *Norepinephrine*: Methylphenidate, an indirect NE agonist has no effect on PAS-induced LTP-like plasticity, whereas the NE antagonist and alpha-1-receptor antagonist prazosin suppresses it [43]. Amphetamine, a NE reuptake inhibitor enhances and prolongs anodal tDCS-induced plasticity, whereas the beta-adrenergic antagonist propranolol suppresses it [48].

7. *Acetylcholine*: The ACh esterase inhibitor tacrine has no effect on PAS-induced LTP-like plasticity, whereas the muscarinic (M1) receptor antagonist biperiden reduces it [43]. Rivastigmine, another ACh esterase inhibitor, increases PAS-induced LTP-like plasticity but, paradoxically, reduces anodal tDCS-induced LTP-like plasticity [49]. Similarly, nicotine results (in non-smokers) in enhancement of LTP-like effects induced by PAS [50] or TBS [51], but diminishes anodal tDCS-induced LTP-like plasticity [50, 52].

8. *Serotonin*: The selective 5-HT reuptake inhibitor citalopram enhances LTP-like plasticity induced by PAS [53] and anodal tDCS [54].

The overall picture of acute pharmacological effects on stimulation-induced LTP-like plasticity in human motor cortex is that anti-GABA-ergic manipulation and agonists of the neuromodulating neurotransmitter systems (DA, NE, Ach, and 5-HT) are usually enhancers (with few exceptions dependent on drug dose and stimulation protocol) while GABA-ergic drugs and antagonists of the neuromodulating neurotransmitter systems are suppressors. The currently available knowledge is summarized in Table 17.1.

Pharmacological modulation of practice-dependent plasticity in motor cortex: animal studies

In animal models, repeated practice or motor skill learning can be associated with substantial representational plasticity of the trained motor cortex [55–57]. There exists a wealth of animal studies on pharmacological alteration of (motor) learning behaviour in intact animals (for review see [58, 59]) and in animals after stroke lesion (for reviews see [59, 60]). It is beyond the scope of this chapter to provide a critical or even comprehensive review of this extensive research field. In addition, the problem with virtually all of these studies is that the observed behavioural effects were not submitted to investigation of the underlying mechanisms at the level of practice-dependent representational plasticity in the motor cortex. Therefore, these studies provide no link between neurophysiological mechanism and behavioural effect, and therefore, interpretation is rather limited. In the following, single studies will be reviewed that were influential in the field, serve as important examples for modulating effects of drugs with different modes of action, and as primers for the human studies in the following sub-chapter.

GABA-ergic inhibition

Infusion of muscimol, a GABAAR agonist, into the sensorimotor cortex of rats with surgical lesions in the ipsilateral anteromedial cortex significantly prolongs recovery from sensorimotor asymmetry when compared to animals with saline infusion [61]. Although the anteromedial cortex lesion creates a vulnerability to muscimol in the sensorimotor cortex, no detectable difference in the extent of cortical damage in this group accounts for the prolongation of behavioural asymmetry. These behavioural and anatomical data suggested for the first time that systemically delivered GABAA-ergic drugs might negatively interfere with restoration of function after cortical lesion.

Cortical GABA-ergic signalling through GABAARs is divided into phasic synaptic and tonic extrasynaptic components. Tonic extrasynaptic GABAA-ergic inhibition is mediated primarily by α5- or δ-subunit-containing GABAARs and sets an excitability threshold for neurons [62, 63]. Pharmacological and genetic knockdown of α5-GABAARs enhance LTP and improve performance on learning and memory tasks [64]. Tonic extrasynaptic GABAA-ergic inhibition is enhanced in the perilesional tissue in a photothrombotic mice stroke model (65). Reducing this excessive tonic inhibition by L655,708, a benzodiazepine inverse agonist of

Table 17.1 Acute pharmacological effects on LTP-*like* plasticity induced by non-invasive brain stimulation in human motor cortex

Drug (dose)	Mode of action	NIBS protocol	Effect	Reference
Ischaemic nerve block	Anti-GABAergic	0.1 Hz rTMS	↑	[24]
Lorazepam (2 mg)	Positive modulator of GABAAR	5 Hz rTMS	↓	[27]
Lorazepam (2 mg)		Anodal tDCS	↓↑	[33]
Diazepam (20 mg)	Positive modulator of GABAAR	PAS	↓	[28]
Tiagabine (15 mg)	GABA reuptake inhibitor	PAS	↓	[28]
Baclofen (50 mg)	GABABR agonist	PAS	↓	[29]
Dextromethorphan (150 mg)	NMDAR antagonist	PAS	↓	[34]
Dextromethorphan (150 mg)		Anodal tDCS	↓	[36]
Dextromethorphan (120 mg)		TBS	↓	[35]
Memantine (10 mg)	NMDAR antagonist	TBS	↓	[37]
D-Cycloserine (100 mg)	Partial NMDAR agonist	Anodal tDCS	↑	[38]
Lamotrigine (300 mg)	Voltage-gated Na+ channel blocker	PAS	↓	[28]
Lamotrigine (300 mg)		PAS	↓	[39]
Carbamazepine (600 mg)		Anodal tDCS	↓	[36]
Nimodipine (30 mg)	L-type Ca²⁺ channel blocker	TBS	↓	[35]
Levodopa (100 mg)	Precursor of dopamine	PAS	↑	[40]
Levodopa (25/100/200 mg)		PAS	↓/↑/↓	[42]
Levodopa (100 mg)		Anodal tDCS	↓	[40]
Levodopa (25/100/200 mg)		Anodal tDCS	●/↓/●	[41]
Cabergoline (2 mg)	D2 receptor agonist	PAS	●	[43]
Ropinirole (0.125/0.5/1.0 mg)	D2 receptor agonist	PAS	↓/●/↓	[44]
Ropinirole (0.125/0.5/1.0 mg)		Anodal tDCS	↓/●/↓	[44]
Pergolide (0.025 mg)	D1/D2 receptor agonist	Anodal tDCS	●	[46]
Haloperidol (2.5 mg)	D2 receptor antagonist	PAS	↓	[43]
Sulpiride (400 mg)	D2 receptor antagonist	TBS	↓	[45]
Sulpiride (400 mg)		PAS	●	[47]
Sulpiride (400 mg)		Anodal tDCS	↓	[46]
Methylphenidate (40 mg)	NE releaser	PAS	●	[43]
d-Amphetamine (20 mg)	NE reuptake inhibitor	Anodal tDCS	↑	[48]
Prazosin (1 mg)	a1-adrenergic receptor antagonist	PAS	↓	[43]
Propranolol (80 mg)	β-adrenergic receptor antagonist	Anodal tDCS	↓	[48]
Tacrine (40 mg)	ACh esterase inhibitor	PAS	●	[43]
Rivastigmine (3 mg)	ACh esterase inhibitor	PAS	↑	[49]
Rivastigmine (3 mg)		Anodal tDCS	↓	[49]
Nicotine (transdermal patch, 15 mg/16h release)	Nicotine receptor agonist	PAS	↑	[50]
Nicotine (lozenges, 4 mg)		TBS	↑	[51]
Nicotine (transdermal patch, 15 mg/16h release)		Anodal tDCS	↓	[50]
Nicotine (spray, 1 mg)		Anodal tDCS	↓	[52]
Biperiden (8 mg)	M1 muscarinic receptor antagonist	PAS	↓	[43]
Citalopram (20 mg)	Serotonin reuptake inhibitor	PAS	↑	[53]
Citalopram (20 mg)		Anodal tDCS	↑	[54]

Pharmacological effects on LTP-like plasticity are indicated as follows: ↑ Enhancement (increase and/or prolongation), ↓ Suppression, ● no effect, ↓↑ suppression followed by enhancement.

the α5-GABAAR, or by genetic reduction of the number of α5- or δ-subunit containing GABAARs has significant and sustained beneficial effects on motor recovery in this stroke model [65]. Specific antagonists of tonic extrasynaptic inhibition are not yet available for human use, but may constitute an interesting target for future drug development.

NMDAR

D-Cycloserine, a partial NMDAR agonist enhances sensorimotor and cognitive recovery in rats when given 24 hours after 90 min of temporary medial cerebral artery occlusion (MCAO), as measured by functional magnetic resonance imaging (fMRI) and behavioural assessments 30 days after lesion [66]. Despite these favourable effects, D-cycloserine, compared to saline injected control animals, does not affect final infarction size or secondary brain atrophy [66]. These data are of particular interest because it was long thought that excessive NMDAR activation in the acute stage after ischaemic stroke may contribute to delayed excitotoxic neuronal death [67]. However, all of the NMDAR antagonists studied so far have failed to show efficacy in large controlled clinical trials and, in some of these trials, NMDAR antagonists even worsened clinical outcome (for review see [68]). The findings from the D-cycloserine trial in the MCAO rat support a beneficial role for NMDAR stimulation during the recovery period after stroke, most likely caused by enhanced neuroplasticity rather than neuroprotection [66]. This may encourage testing of NMDAR agonists in clinical trials of human stroke rehabilitation.

Blockers of voltage-gated sodium (Na⁺) and calcium (Ca²⁺) channels

The antiepileptic drug lamotrigine acts by stabilizing voltage-sensitive Na⁺ channels in a usage-dependent manner, preventing glutamate release and reversibly blocking excitatory neurotransmission. Therefore, lamotrigine was tested in the rat MCAO model by application of different doses or saline at the time of reperfusion [69]. In disagreement with a neuroprotective effect, lamotrigine does not demonstrate any effect on the total infarction volume, and several behavioural tests even show a disadvantage of the lamotrigine treated rats in sensorimotor recovery 7 days after infarction [69]. This is an important negative study, which suggests that blockade of voltage-gated Na+ channels is not neuroprotective but potentially detrimental for plasticity processes that support behavioural recovery and relearning.

Dopamine

Elimination of dopaminergic terminals in rat primary motor cortex by intracortical injection of 6-hydroxydopamine in conjunction with desipramine to protect noradrenergic terminals results in impairment of motor skill learning (food pellet retrieval with the contralateral forepaw) [9]. This deficit is not observed when destruction of dopaminergic terminals is initiated at a time when the motor skill is already achieved through training. In addition, the learning deficit can be rescued by local infusion of levodopa [9]. A similar learning deficit can also be obtained by pharmacological treatment with specific antagonists at the dopamine D1 receptor (SCH02339) or D2 receptor (sulpiride, raclopride) when given early into the training period [9]. In the rat transient MCAO model, treatment with levodopa significantly and dose-dependently improves recovery of sensorimotor function as assessed by rotating pole test, a 28-point neuroscore, and a cylinder test 7 and 14 days after ischaemia without affecting the infarct volume [70]. These findings strongly corroborate the concept of recovery enhancing actions of levodopa treatment after ischaemic stroke.

Norepinephrine

A milestone publication in pharmacological enhancement of sensorimotor recovery was the investigation of the effects of the NE reuptake inhibitor d-amphetamine on sensorimotor recovery. Rats subjected to unilateral ablation of the motor cortex and placed on a narrow beam displays transient contralateral paresis. An immediate and enduring acceleration of recovery is produced by a single dose of d-amphetamine given 24 hours after injury. This effect is blocked by the dopamine D2 receptor antagonist haloperidol or by restraining the animals for 8 hours beginning immediately after amphetamine administration [71]. The dramatic effect of d-amphetamine vs. saline on walking beam performance in stroke rats can be appreciated in the Video 17.1 (http://www.unm.edu/~feeney/movicap.html).

Many subsequent studies in embolic and thrombotic stroke models in rats confirmed this original finding of a recovery promoting effect of d-amphetamine, in particular in conjunction with post-stroke motor skill training (e.g. [72–75]) and revealed that these effects on recovery are associated with increased structural plasticity in the contralesional [76, 77] and ipsilesional hemispheres [78].

Acetylcholine

ACh is important for practice-dependent motor cortical plasticity in rats because lesions of the basal forebrain cholinergic

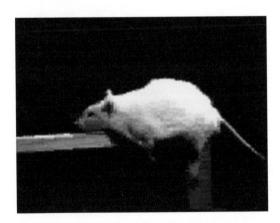

🎬 **Video 17.1** The first few seconds of the video is a close up illustrating hemiplegia in the rat 24 hours after suction ablation of the right sensorimotor cortex. When on the beam the affected limbs (especially hindlimb) are not placed on the surface as in normal rats. These symptoms are best observed by placing the rat on a narrow elevated beam as few deficits are apparent when the animal is on a flat surface. Recovery from hemiplegia can be quantified by utilization of a rating scale designed for this beam-walk task. In untreated rats, spontaneous recovery of locomotion occurs in about a week. Size and location of cortical lesions affect the symptoms and recovery rate. The remainder of the video illustrates the remarkable improvement in locomotion within 20 min after administering a drug increasing norepinephrine (NE) release. The treated rat was given a low dose of amphetamine compared to the control rat given saline.

system disrupt practice-dependent cortical map reorganization as assessed by intracortical microstimulation mapping, and at the same time, impair forepaw motor skill acquisition [79]. The potential of cholinergic drugs to enhance recovery in animal models of stroke has not been tested. Conversely, treatment with scopolamine, a muscarinic receptor antagonist, reinstates sensorimotor deficits in recovered rats after photothrombotic stroke [80].

Serotonin

Little evidence exists for the efficacy of serotonin-reuptake inhibitors to enhance practice-dependent recovery in animal models of stroke. Fluoxetine has no beneficial effect on sensorimotor recovery in rats with focal ischaemic lesions in motor cortex [81, 82]. Given this lack of preclinical evidence for a recovery-enhancing role of serotonin in animal models of stroke, it is interesting to note that the first successful prospective phase IIb randomized clinical trial (FLAME trial) investigated the effects of fluoxetine (20 mg/day) versus placebo on recovery of paretic arm/hand function in patients after ischaemic stroke [83] (for details, see the section 'Impact of pharmacological modulation on neurorehabilitation of stroke'). This adds to the well-known notion that animal models in stroke often face translational roadblocks that prevent prediction of successful interventions in clinical stroke trials [84].

Pharmacological modulation of practice-dependent plasticity in motor cortex: human studies

LTP is one important mechanism involved in motor learning. The strongest supporting evidence comes from interference experiments in rats: successful motor skill learning suppresses the subsequent induction of LTP in the training motor cortex when compared to LTP in an untrained motor cortex [85–88]. The same homeostatic interference between motor learning and subsequent induction of LTP-like plasticity is found in the intact human motor cortex [20, 89, 90]. From this tight interdependence of LTP and motor learning it is reasonable to assume that pharmacological modulation of LTP and motor learning are similar [91]. This paragraph will focus on the pharmacological modulation of learning of repetitive simple movements, a form of training that is particularly effective in motor rehabilitation after stroke [92, 93]. The following practice protocols will be reviewed systematically, as they have been studied most extensively with respect to pharmacological modulating effects:

PROTOCOL A: Practice of repetitive ballistic simple finger or arm movements results in an increase in corticospinal excitability of the trained movement representation as indexed by increase in MEP amplitude in the training muscle and an increase in the maximum peak acceleration of the trained movement [94, 95]. Virtual lesion experiments show that 1 Hz rTMS of the training motor cortex disrupts this form of practice-dependent learning, indicating that the primary motor cortex is essentially involved in this learning process [95].

PROTOCOL B (Figure 17.1A): Focal TMS of just suprathreshold intensity applied to the hand area of motor cortex results, in many subjects, in thumb movements consistently into one direction [96]. These subjects then train ballistic voluntary thumb movements into the opposite direction, typically for 30 min

at a rate of 1 Hz. During and after training, practice-induced plasticity is assessed by the shift of TMS induced thumb movements into the training direction [96]. This is an extremely elegant experimental protocol because the amount of learning is directly expressed by an electrophysiological measure of motor cortical plasticity.

PROTOCOL C: When subjects are requested to perform brisk movements of two different representations of one body side (either hand and leg [97], or hand and shoulder [98]) as synchronously as possible, motor learning occurs by improving synchronicity of the movement of the two trained motor representations, as can be assessed by the contraction onset delay of the two muscles in the electromyogram. The associated motor cortical plasticity is defined as the magnitude of the centre of gravity shifts of the two trained motor representations as assessed by MEP mapping towards each other [97, 98].

A critical comparison of the three protocols of practice-dependent plasticity leads to the conclusion that PROTOCOL B [96] bears several advantages over the other ones: it translates practice-dependent plasticity directly into an electrophysiological measure—that is the shift in direction of the TMS induced of thumb movement, that is closely related of the physiology of voluntary movement because the earliest signal emanating from motor cortex at voluntary movement onset encodes the direction of movement [99]. Furthermore, PROTOCOL B does not use MEP amplitude as an outcome measure for motor plasticity assessment. This is an advantage because MEP amplitude is rather indirectly linked to practice-dependent plasticity [100, 101]. Finally, all studies under PROTOCOL C report dissociation with effective pharmacological modulation of motor cortical representational plasticity, but lacking pharmacological effects on the improvement of motor performance. This suggests that motor cortical plasticity is not a sufficient prerequisite for motor learning. It may well be a prerequisite for motor memory formation and lasting improvement in motor performance, but this has not been tested in any of the PROTOCOL C studies. The following paragraph summarizes the pharmacological effects on practice-dependent motor learning, grouped according to pharmacological modes of action as already used in the section 'Pharmacological modulation of stimulation-induced LTP in motor cortex: human studies'.

1. *GABAergic disinhibition*: If subjects practise repeated ballistic elbow movements (PROTOCOL A) during transient forearm ischaemic nerve block—in the context of a disinhibited motor cortex [23]—then the increase in MEP amplitude and peak acceleration of the trained movement are enhanced compared to when the same training is performed in the absence of disinhibition [102]. In a recent study, GABA content in the training motor cortex was decreased by anodal tDCS and it was found that the amount of GABA decrease as measured with MRI spectroscopy directly correlates with the amount of improvement in reaction times in a visually instructed finger-sequence learning task [103], further corroborating the notion that GABA plays a fundamental role in regulating the extent of motor learning.

2. *GABAergic inhibition*: Application of lorazepam prior to practice abolishes motor learning in PROTOCOL A [102, 104], PROTOCOL B [105] and PROTOCOL C [98]. Similarly, diazepam and the GABABR agonist baclofen disrupt practice-dependent motor

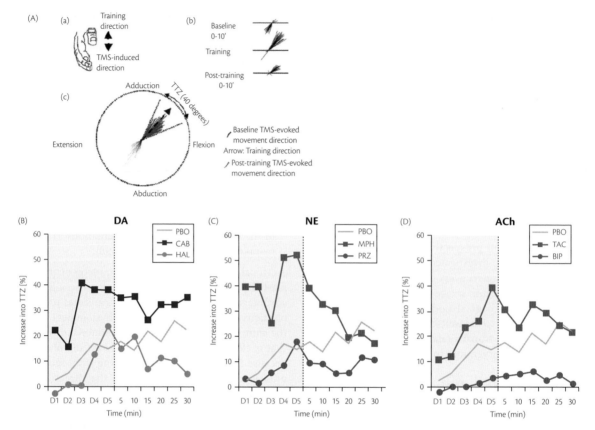

Fig. 17.1 Schematic diagram of the experimental design to measure practice-dependent motor plasticity (according to Protocol B, see text). (Aa) The direction of transcranial magnetic stimulation (TMS)-evoked or voluntary movement is derived from the first-peak acceleration in the two major axes (flexion–extension, abduction–adduction) of the movement measured by a two-dimensional accelerometer mounted on the proximal phalanx of the thumb. (Ab) Schematic diagram of the directional change of first-peak-acceleration vector of movements evoked by TMS after training. Before training (baseline), TMS evoked predominantly extension and abduction thumb movements. Training consisted of repetitive stereotyped brisk thumb movements in a flexion and adduction direction. Post-training, the direction of TMS-evoked thumb movements changed from the baseline direction to the trained direction. (Ac) Directional change of first peak acceleration vector of movements evoked by TMS before and after training. At baseline, TMS evoked predominantly extension and abduction thumb movements. Training movements (6 blocks × 300 movements, 1 Hz) are performed in a direction approximately opposite to baseline (dashed arrow, a combination of adduction and flexion). Post-training, the direction of TMS-evoked thumb movements changes from the baseline direction to the trained direction. The mean training direction (arrow) is at the centre of the training target zone (TTZ). TMS-induced thumb movement directions (red vectors, 60 trials, 0.1 Hz) after training largely fall within the TTZ, close to a 180-degree change from baseline direction. The increase of the proportion of TMS-evoked thumb movements into the TTZ post-training compared to baseline is an electrophysiological measure of practice-dependent motor plasticity (modified from [110], with permission). (B–D) Effects of single oral doses of neuromodulating drugs on practice-dependent motor plasticity tested in a randomized double-blind placebo-controlled crossover design in 6 healthy subjects. Plasticity is quantified by the percentage increase of TMS-induced thumb movements into the TTZ during (D1–D5) and over 30 min after practice compared to baseline. The dotted vertical lines indicate end of practice. The black curves in (B–D) show practice-dependent motor plasticity in the placebo (PBO) condition. (B) Effects of dopamine (DA) neuromodulators: D2 receptor agonist cabergoline (CAB, 2 mg) vs. D2 receptor antagonist haloperidol (HAL, 2.5 mg); (C) effects of norepinephrine (NE) neuromodulators: NE releaser methylphenidate (MPH, 40mg) vs. alpha-1-adrenergic blocker prazosin (PRZ, 1 mg); (D) effects of acetylcholine (ACh) neuromodulators: ACh esterase inhibitor tacrine (TAC, 40 mg) vs. muscarinic M1 receptor blocker biperiden (BIP, 8 mg). Note that agonists in the DA, NE, and ACh systems enhance practice-dependent motor plasticity while antagonists in these systems significantly reduce it (modified from [101], with permission).

learning and plasticity in a visuomotor skill acquisition task requiring to follow a force trajectory by adjusting voluntary ankle dorsiflexor torque [106], and lorazepam disrupts skill acquisition of arm movements in a force field [107]. On the other hand, zolpidem, a positive modulator selectively at the alpha-1 subunit bearing subtype of the GABAAR does not disrupt practice-dependent motor learning in Protocol, A suggesting that other GABAAR subtypes such as the alpha-2 subunit bearing subtype mediate the GABAAergic disruptive effect on motor learning [104].

3. *NMDAR antagonists:* Pretreatment with the NMDAR antagonist dextromethorphan suppresses practice-dependent plasticity in Protocol B [105] and skill acquisition of arm movements in a force field [107]. Similarly, the NMDAR antagonists amantadine [98] and memantine [108] reduced practice-dependent plasticity in Protocol C.

4. *Blockers of voltage-gated sodium (Na+) and calcium (Ca2+) channels:* Lamotrigine has no significant disruptive effect on motor learning in Protocol B [105] or learning arm movement trajectories in a force field [107].

5. *Dopamine:* Levodopa [100] and the D2 receptor agonist cabergoline [101] (Figure 17.1B) enhance motor learning in Protocol B, while the D2 receptor antagonist haloperidol decreases it [101] (Figure 17.1B). A recent study tested the impact of five genetic

polymorphisms with established effects on dopamine neuro-transmission on the effects of levodopa on practice-dependent motor learning and representational motor cortical plasticity in a marble navigation task, a skilled motor task that places intensive demands on the first dorsal interosseus muscle [109]. Levodopa results in enhancement in practice-dependent motor learning and motor cortex map enlargement of the trained motor representation in those individuals with polymorphisms associated with low dopamine neurotransmission, whereas levodopa is detrimental when compared to placebo in those individuals with polymorphisms associated with high dopa-mine neurotransmission [109]. These data are very important as they suggest that genetic variation in the dopamine system influences learning and its modulation by levodopa.

6. *Norepinephrine:* The indirect NE agonists d-amphetamine [110, 111] and methylphenidate [101] (Figure 17.1C) increase motor learning in PROTOCOL B, the selective NE reuptake inhibitor reboxetine enhances motor learning in PROTOCOL A [112], the selective NE reuptake inhibitor atomoxetine enhances motor learning in Protocol B [113], and d-amphetamine is an enhancer of motor learning in PROTOCOL C [114]. In contrast, the NE antagonist prazosin leads to suppression in PROTOCOL B [101, 115] (Figure 17.1C) and the beta-adrenergic blocker pro-pranolol shows a non-significant trend towards suppression [115]. Of note, the beneficial effects of increasing NE neuro-transmission on motor learning cannot be generalized to more complex practice tasks, such as finger-sequence learning, where reboxetine does not demonstrate a learning-enhancing effect [116].

7. *Acetylcholine:* The ACh esterase inhibitor tacrine enhances motor learning in PROTOCOL B [101] (Figure 17.1D), while the muscarinic receptor antagonists biperiden and scopolamine result in suppression of motor learning in PROTOCOL B [101, 117] (Figure 17.1D), but no effect of scopolamine in learning an arm movement trajectory in a force field [107].

8. *Serotonin:* Fluoxetine, a specific serotonin reuptake inhibitor enhances practice-dependent motor cortical representational plasticity but not motor learning in PROTOCOL C [118]. The spe-cific serotonin reuptake inhibitor paroxetine improved perfor-mance gain in the 9-hole peg test [119].

The acute pharmacological effects on practice-dependent plastic-ity in human motor cortex are summarized in Table 17.2. Of note, the pattern of effects is very similar to the acute pharmacological effects on LTP-like plasticity induced by NIBS supporting the view of overlapping mechanisms of LTP and learning in motor cortex.

Impact of pharmacological modulation on neurorehabilitation of stroke

The large body of preclinical studies in animal models of stroke on pharmacological modulation of recovery contrasts with the paucity of controlled studies in humans on pharmacotherapy for recovery after ischaemic stroke [120]. Almost all human stroke studies are based on either retrospective analyses, case reports, or controlled clinical trials with small numbers of patients (typi-cally less than 50 patients). Retrospective studies are the only way to obtain information in cases of suspected detrimental drugs

because prospective controlled clinical trials would be unethical. For instance, stroke patients were retrospectively divided into a 'detrimental group' and a 'neutral group' depending on whether or not they had received one or more drugs within the first 28 days after stroke that were identified to impair stroke recovery in ani-mal models, namely the antihypertensives clonidine and prazosin, neuroleptics, and other dopamine receptor antagonists, benzodi-azepines, and the anticonvulsants phenytoin and phenobarbital. Stepwise regression analyses incorporating other potential prog-nostic factors indicated that drug group independently influenced both the degree of upper-extremity motor impairment (as meas-ured by the Toronto Stroke Scale) and independence in activities of daily living (as measured by the Barthel Index) 84 days after stroke. These data are consistent with the detrimental effects of certain drugs on recovery in laboratory animals and suggest that similar effects may occur in humans [121].

It is another critical shortcoming of the available clinical stud-ies that only very rarely have mechanisms of pharmacological modulation of recovery been explored. In one study [122], treat-ment with a single oral dose of 100 mg of levodopa enhances practice-dependent motor cortical plasticity in chronic sub-cortical stroke patients, as assessed with the described (section 'Pharmacological modulation of practice-dependent plasticity in motor cortex: Human Studies') practice PROTOCOL B [96]. This enhancement is similar to the one observed when levodopa is administered to aged healthy subjects [100]. In another study [123], a single oral dose of 20 mg of the selective serotonin reuptake inhibitor fluoxetine enhances ipsilesional activation of the senso-rimotor cortex in lacunar stroke patients during movements of the paretic hand, as assessed with fMRI, and this enhancement corre-lates with the improvement in performance of finger tapping and dynamometer tests. These two studies are extremely important because, for the first time, they go beyond the purely clinical eval-uation of motor outcome and move pharmacological modulation of practice-dependent plasticity in healthy subjects (see section on 'Pharmacological modulation of practice-dependent plasticity in motor cortex: human studies') to the clinical stage. Exploration of pharmacological modulation of practice-dependent plastic-ity by electrophysiological and neuroimaging techniques may advance our knowledge on the mechanisms that enhance recovery of function after stroke lesion and, potentially, allow testing and predicting the responsiveness to a particular pharmacotherapy in individual patients.

The following detailed review on the effects of pharmacologi-cal modulation of practice-dependent recovery from stroke will focus on motor recovery, as practice-dependent plasticity in the motor domain has been the focus in the preceding sections, and motor impairment is the most prevalent disability after stroke [124]. Even after having completed standard motor rehabilita-tion in 50–60% of stroke patients at least some degree of motor impairment will persist [125–128]. Pharmacological modulation of recovery of other major disabilities after stroke, in particular aphasia, neglect and other cognitive deficits, has been surveyed in other recent authoritative reviews [129, 130].

GABAergic disinhibition

One trial tested the effects of GABAergic disinhibition as induced by selective upper brachial plexus anaesthesia of the paretic arm in seven chronic subcortical stroke patients

Table 17.2 Acute pharmacological effects on practice-dependent plasticity in human motor cortex

Drug (dose)	Mode of action	Learning protocol	Effect	Reference
Ischaemic nerve block	Anti-GABAergic	Protocol A	↑	[102]
Anodal tDCS	Decreases GABA concentration	SFM	↑	[103]
Lorazepam (2 mg)	Positive modulator of GABAAR	Protocol A	↓	[102]
Lorazepam (2.5 mg)		Protocol A	↓	[104]
Lorazepam (0.038 mg/kg)		Protocol B	↓	[105]
Lorazepam (2 mg)		Protocol C	↓	[98]
Lorazepam (0.038 mg/kg)		AFF	↓	[107]
Diazepam (10 mg)		FFT	↓	[106]
Zolpidem (10 mg)	α1-GABAAR agonist	Protocol A	●	[104]
Baclofen (20 mg)	GABABR agonist	FFT	↓	[106]
Dextromethorphan (2 mg/kg)	NMDAR antagonist	Protocol B	↓	[105]
Dextromethorphan (2 mg/kg)		AFF	↓	[107]
Amantadine (300 mg/day for 6 days)		Protocol C	↓	[98]
Memantine (10 mg)		Protocol C	↓	[108]
Lamotrigine (300 mg)	Voltage-gated Na⁺ channel blocker	Protocol B	●	[105]
Lamotrigine (300 mg)		AFF	●	[107]
Levodopa (100 mg)	Precursor of dopamine	Protocol B	↑	[100]
Levodopa (100 mg)		MNT	↑1)	[109]
Levodopa (100 mg)		MNT	↓2)	[109]
Cabergoline (2 mg)	D2 receptor agonist	Protocol B	↑	[101]
Haloperidol (2.5 mg)	D2 receptor antagonist	Protocol B	↓	[101]
Methylphenidate (40 mg)	NE releaser	Protocol B	↑	[101]
d-Amphetamine (10 mg)	NE reuptake inhibitor	Protocol B	↑	[110]
d-Amphetamine (10 mg)		Protocol B	↑	[111]
d-Amphetamine (20 mg)		Protocol C	↑	[114]
Reboxetine (8 mg)	Selective NE reuptake inhibitor	Protocol A	↑	[112]
Atomoxetine (40 mg)	Selective NE reuptake inhibitor	Protocol B	↑	[113]
Prazosin (1 mg)	α₁-adrenergic receptor antagonist	Protocol B	↓	[101]
Prazosin (5 mg)		Protocol B	↓	[115]
Propranolol (40 mg)	β-adrenergic receptor antagonist	Protocol B	↓3)	[115]
Tacrine (40 mg)	ACh esterase inhibitor	Protocol B	↑	[101]
Biperiden (8 mg)	Muscarinic receptor antagonist	Protocol B	↓	[101]
Scopolamine (transdermal patch, 1.5 mg)	Muscarinic receptor antagonist	Protocol B	↓	[117]
Scopolamine (transdermal patch, 1.5 mg)		AFF	●	[107]
Fluoxetine (20 mg)	Serotonin reuptake inhibitor	Protocol C	↑	[118]
Paroxetine (20/60 mg)	Serotonin reuptake inhibitor	9HPT	↑/↑	[119]

9HPT, 9-hole peg test; AFF, arm force field learning task; FFT, foot force trajectory learning task; MNT, marble navigation task; SFM, sequential-finger movement learning task. Pharmacological effects on LTP-like plasticity are indicated as follows: ↑ Enhancement (increase and/or prolongation), ↓ Suppression, ● no effect, ↑1) in a subgroup of subjects with polymorphisms associated with low dopamine neurotransmission, ↓2) in a subgroup of subjects with polymorphisms associated with high dopamine neurotransmission, ↓3) non-significant trend towards suppression.

on practice-dependent improvement of the kinematics of ballistic pincer-grip movements [131]. Out of a performance plateau that was reached through a 1-month long training, this intervention results in significant improvement of peak acceleration and strength of the trained movement including some activities of daily living. This improvement is associated with an increase in the MEP amplitude in practice hand muscles [131].

Dopamine

A single dose of 100mg/d of levodopa given over 3 weeks and combined with conventional physiotherapy improves motor recovery when compared to placebo in ischaemic stroke patients an effect that is maintained 3 weeks after the end of levodopa treatment [132]. This study was influential as it was one of the first prospective randomized double-blind placebo-controlled pharmacological trials in stroke rehabilitation, but also criticized because the levodopa vs. placebo groups were not balanced for age and stroke hemisphere, and other factors of importance for determining stroke outcome such as stroke location and stroke size were not even mentioned. Other more recent levodopa trials are listed in Table 17.3. The findings are inconsistent, so that the efficacy of levodopa in enhancing stroke rehabilitation is currently not clear.

Norepinephrine

Based on the early evidence on the recovery enhancing effects of d-amphetamine in the rat [71], the first controlled randomized clinical trial ever to enhance recovery in stroke patients tested the effects of d-amphetamine [133]. This prospective randomized double-blind placebo-controlled pilot study in acute stroke patients (less than 10 days after stroke) showed that a single dose of 10 mg of d-amphetamine coupled with physiotherapy enhances motor recovery as measured by the Fugl-Meyer Scale more than placebo. However, it is not clear to which extent spontaneous recovery differences in this small sample of acute stroke patients contributed to the results. Furthermore, this initial finding could not be replicated in several other trials (see Table 17.3) and d-amphetamine has potentially serious adverse effects (in particular blood pressure elevation, increased mortality) so that d-amphetamine is no longer considered as a primary choice in pharmacotherapy of stroke rehabilitation [134]. Novel selective NE reuptake inhibitors such as reboxetine may have a superior safety profile. One particularly interesting recent study showed that a single oral dose of 6 mg of reboxetine significantly increases maximum grip power and index finger-tapping speed of the paretic hand of subacute or chronic stroke patients [135]. This enhanced motor performance is associated with a reduction of cortical hyperactivity toward physiological levels, especially in the ipsilesional ventral premotor cortex and supplementary motor area. Connectivity analyses revealed that in stroke patients neural coupling of ipsilesional primary motor cortex with ventral premotor cortex and supplementary motor area is significantly reduced compared with healthy controls and that reboxetine treatment normalizes this deficient connectivity [135]. These findings underscore the capability of modern neuroimaging to further our understanding of the mechanisms that mediate pharmacological enhancement of function at the systems level of cortical networks.

Acetylcholine

No randomized clinical trials investigating the effects of ACh esterase inhibitors on stroke motor recovery have been published, as of August 2014.

Serotonin

The largest multicentre randomized clinical trial published to date to explore pharmacological enhancement of stroke rehabilitation is the Fluoxetine for Motor Recovery after Acute Ischaemic Stroke (FLAME) trial [83]. The trial showed that early (within the first 5–10 days after stroke) initiation of a daily dose of 20 mg of fluoxetine in combination with physiotherapy improves recovery, measured by the Fugl-Meyer Scale, 90 days after stroke compared to placebo. Although this is an impressive and clinically relevant result the mechanisms underlying this recovery enhancing effect remained unexplored. The fluoxetine group also shows a significantly lower occurrence of depression at 90 days compared to the placebo group, which may have contributed (non-specifically) to the enhanced motor recovery, even though the superiority of fluoxetine over placebo as measured by the Fugl-Meyer Scale was independent of the effect of fluoxetine on depression [83]. The finding that fluoxetine improves the rate of favourable outcomes measured by the modified Rankin Scale [83] has important public health implications as this rate improvement is similar to those achieved with thrombolytic therapy [136]. Unlike thrombolytic therapy, however, the usefulness of which is limited by having to give it within 4.5 h of stroke onset [137], an selective serotonin reuptake inhibitor (SSRI) could be given to a much larger cohort of stroke patients, as there is no (known) critical time window.

Limitations and outlook

Pharmacological enhancement of neuroplasticity and neurorehabilitation success is still an emergent field, despite its longstanding tradition in preclinical research. Evidence-based guidelines are not yet available and recent systematic reviews conclude that more evidence by adequately powered large-scale randomized controlled clinical trials is warranted before more definite recommendations can be given as the presently available evidence is promising but largely based on small-scale proof-of-principle studies [120, 155]. Also, the optimal interval after onset of brain injury to the start of pharmacological augmentation, the frequency and dose of medication, the optimal duration of medication and rehabilitation, and the intensity and components of concomitant skills practice, remain important features for the design of randomized clinical trials [156]. On the other hand, a recent Phase IIb randomized double-blind placebo-controlled parallel group clinical trial with 118 stroke patients demonstrated clinically relevant efficacy of early treatment with the selective serotonin reuptake inhibitor fluoxetine in enhancing stroke recovery [83]. The rate of improvement of disability as measured with the modified Rankin Scale 90 days post-stroke was comparable to the benefit obtained in thrombolysis trials for acute stroke treatment [136]. The effect size on the Fugl-Meyer Motor Score 90 days post-stroke in the fluoxetine trial, expressed by Cohen's d was 0.76, indicating a strong effect [83]. This opens up the realistic perspective that early pharmacotherapy for enhancing stroke recovery becomes a standard practice with clinically meaningful effects in the management of subacute stroke patients soon.

Table 17.3 Pharmacological modulation of motor recovery in stroke patients

Drug (dose)	Patients (number)	Design	Effect, Endpoint	Reference
Selective upper brachial plexus anaesthesia	Chronic stroke (7)	Non-controlled, open intervention	↑ Peak acceleration of trained movement	[131]
Levodopa (100 mg, single dose)	Chronic subcortical stroke (9)	Randomized, double-blind, placebo-controlled cross-over design	↑ Increase of TMS-induced thumb movements into TTZ	[122]
Levodopa (100 mg/d over 3 weeks) + PT	3 weeks to 6 months old stroke (26, placebo 27)	Randomized, double-blind, placebo-controlled parallel design	↑ Rivermead motor assessment	[132]
Levodopa (100 mg, single dose) + PT	Chronic stroke (10)	Randomized, double-blind, placebo-controlled cross-over design	• 9HPT, dynamometer strength, ARAT	[138]
Levodopa (100 mg/d over 5 weeks), no PT	Chronic cortical-subcortical or subcortical stroke (10)	Single-blind placebo-controlled crossover pilot study	↑ 9HPT • Rivermead motor assessment	[139]
Levodopa (100 mg/d) vs. d-amphetamine (10 mg/d) vs. combination over 2 weeks +PT	<10 days after stroke (total, 25)	Randomized, double-blind, placebo-controlled, parallel	• Fugl-Meyer Score, • Barthel index	[140]
Levodopa (125 mg/d) vs. Methylphenidate (20 mg/d) vs. combination over 3 weeks + PT	15–180 days after stroke (4 × 25)	Randomized, double-blind, placebo-controlled, parallel	↑ Barthel index and NIHSS at 6 months follow-up for all drug interventions compared to placebo	[141]
d-amphetamine (10 mg, single dose) + PT	<10 days after stroke (2 × 4)	Randomized, double-blind, placebo-controlled, parallel pilot study	↑ Fugl-Meyer Scale	[133]
d-amphetamine (10 mg for 10 sessions) + PT	16–30 days after stroke (2 × 5)	Randomized, double-blind, placebo-controlled, parallel pilot study	↑ Fugl-Meyer Scale	[142]
d-amphetamine (2.5, 5 or 10 mg for 5 days) + PT	<72 h after stroke (3 × 10, placebo 15)	Randomized, double-blind, placebo-controlled, parallel study	↑ LMAC motor function score during treatment • at 1 and 3 months follow-up	[143]
d-amphetamine (10 mg for 10 sessions) + PT	5–10 days after stroke (2 × 20)	Randomized, double-blind, placebo-controlled, parallel study	• Fugl-Meyer Scale	[144]
d-amphetamine (10 mg for 10 sessions) + PT	< 6 weeks after stroke (2 × 10)	Randomized, double-blind, placebo-controlled, parallel study	• Barthel index • Rivermead motor assessment	[145]
d-amphetamine (10 mg for 6 sessions) + PT	3 weeks–6 months after stroke (2 × 13)	Randomized, double-blind, placebo-controlled, parallel study	• Arm performance in TEMPA task	[146]
d-amphetamine (10 mg for 10 sessions) + PT	On average 8 days after stroke (31, placebo 36)	Randomized, double-blind, placebo-controlled, parallel study	• Fugl-Meyer Score	[147]
d-amphetamine (10 mg for 11 sessions) + PT	4–30 days after stroke (2 × 16)	Randomized, double-blind, placebo-controlled, parallel study	• Barthel index • Fugl-Meyer Score • mRS	[148]
d-amphetamine (10 mg for 10 sessions) + PT	14–60 days after stroke (2 × 8)	Randomized, double-blind, placebo-controlled, parallel study	↑ Arm function in Chedoke-McMaster Stroke Assessment	[149]
Methylphenidate (30 mg/d for 3 weeks) + PT	On average 18 days after stroke (10, placebo 11)	Randomized, double-blind, placebo-controlled, parallel study	↑ Fugl-Meyer Score ↑ FIM	[150]
Reboxetine (10 mg, single oral dose)	Chronic stroke (10)	Randomized, double-blind, placebo-controlled, crossover study	↑ Tapping speed and grip strength	[151]
Reboxetine (10 mg, single oral dose)	Sub-acute or chronic stroke (11)	Randomized, double-blind, placebo-controlled, crossover study	↑ Tapping speed and grip strength	[135]

(continued)

Table 17.3 (Continued)

Drug (dose)	Patients (number)	Design	Effect, Endpoint	Reference
Fluoxetine (20 mg, single oral dose)	Subcortical stroke (8)	Randomized, double-blind, placebo-controlled, crossover study	↑ Tapping speed ↑ Grip strength • 9HPT	[123]
Fluoxetine (20 mg/d for 3 months) + PT	1–6 months after stroke (2 × 16)	Randomized, double-blind, placebo-controlled, parallel study	↑ Barthel index	[152]
Citalopram (10 mg/d for 1 month)	< 10 days after cortical-subcortical or cortical stroke (2 × 10)	Randomized, double-blind, placebo-controlled, parallel study	↑ NIHSS • Barthel index	[153]
Citalopram (40 mg, single oral dose)	< 6 months after stroke (8)	Randomized, double-blind, placebo-controlled, crossover study	↑ 9HPT • Grip strength	[154]
Fluoxetine (20 mg/d for 3 months) + PT	5–10 days after stroke (2 × 59)	Randomized, double-blind, placebo-controlled, parallel study	↑ Fugl-Meyer Score ↑ mRS 0–2	[83]

FIM: Functional independence measure; mRS: modified Rankin scale; PT: physiotherapy; TTZ: training target zone; ↑ Enhancement (increase and/or prolongation), • no effect.

However, there are still important gaps of knowledge that need to be filled by further research. One important issue relates to the complexity of stroke pathobiology: 'therapy must acknowledge the "Janus-faced" nature of many stroke targets and must identify endogenous neuroprotective and repair mechanisms' [84]. That is, excitability decreasing pharmacotherapy (e.g. by anticonvulsants) in the acute phase of stroke may be neuroprotective but this positive effect may be overridden by detrimental effects on neuroplasticity and recovery [121, 157]. In addition, recovery-modulating drugs may have potentially serious adverse effects that limit their wide application, such as blood pressure elevation and increased mortality by d-amphetamine [134].

Furthermore, it is not clear to what extent effects of pharmacological modulation on ischaemic stroke recovery reviewed in this chapter can be generalized to other causes of acquired lesions of the central nervous system, such as traumatic brain injury or spinal cord injury. While it appears that there is large consistency for traumatic brain injury and ischaemic stroke (for reviews see [130, 158, 159]), there are also examples of divergence: For instance, patients with incomplete spinal cord injury do not benefit from adding levodopa to training of gait [160] while add-on treatment with levodopa improves motor recovery patients after ischaemic stroke [122, 132]. Clonidine, an α2-adrenergic receptor agonist, and therefore an inhibitor of presynaptic NE release, impairs recovery of function in an animal model of focal traumatic brain injury [161], and was identified as a 'detrimental drug' in motor recovery after ischaemic stroke in humans [121], while clonidine has demonstrated beneficial effects in combination with locomotor training in patients with severe but incomplete spinal cord injury (for review see [162]). The reasons for these discrepancies are only partly understood. Likely, they are related to the specific functions of neuromodulating neurotransmitters in neuronal circuits of cerebral cortex versus spinal cord. For instance, the presynaptic inhibition of NE release in spinal cord circuitry by clonidine can lead to relief from pain and spasticity, and induce concomitant changes towards normalization of the cyclic EMG locomotor activation pattern in incomplete spinal cord injury patients [162], while the same mechanism of presynaptic inhibition of NE release in cerebral cortex has detrimental effects on

motor recovery after ischaemic or traumatic brain lesions, most likely by its negative interference with cortical LTP [163].

Another issue relates to the neurobiological mechanisms underlying enhancement of neuroplasticity and recovery. This chapter demonstrates that animal models are generally very useful for identification of mechanisms that may be of translational value for clinical applications. However, this is not a straight avenue, and the chapter closes with the urgent recommendation that future clinical trials should include measurements of network reorganization, using fMRI, EEG, MEG, or TMS (for laudable examples, see [122, 123, 135]), in addition to clinical endpoints, in order to improve our understanding of the mechanisms underlying recovery enhancement and to open opportunities for applying more specific interventions to residual neuronal networks in individual stroke patients.

References

1. Aroniadou VA, Keller A. Mechanisms of LTP induction in rat motor cortex in vitro. Cereb Cortex. 1995;**5**(4):353–362.
2. Castro-Alamancos MA, Donoghue JP, Connors BW. Different forms of synaptic plasticity in somatosensory and motor areas of the neocortex. J Neurosci. 1995;**15**(7 Pt 2):5324–5333.
3. Hess G, Aizenman CD, Donoghue JP. Conditions for the induction of long-term potentiation in layer II/III horizontal connections of the rat motor cortex. J Neurophysiol. 1996;**75**(5):1765–1778.
4. Jacobs KM, Donoghue JP. Reshaping the cortical motor map by unmasking latent intracortical connections. Science. 1991;**251**(4996):944–947.
5. Hess G, Donoghue JP. Long-term potentiation of horizontal connections provides a mechanism to reorganize cortical motor maps. J Neurophysiol. 1994;**71**(6):2543–2547.
6. Hagemann G, Redecker C, Neumann-Haefelin T, Freund H-J, Witte O. Increased long-term potentiation in the surround of experimentally induced focal cortical infarction. Ann Neurol. 1998;**44**:255–258.
7. Trepel C, Racine RJ. GABAergic modulation of neocortical long-term potentiation in the freely moving rat. Synapse. 2000;**35**(2):120–128.
8. Gu Q. Neuromodulatory transmitter systems in the cortex and their role in cortical plasticity. Neuroscience. 2002;**111**(4):815–835.
9. Molina-Luna K, Pekanovic A, Rohrich S, et al. Dopamine in motor cortex is necessary for skill learning and synaptic plasticity. PloS One. 2009;**4**(9):e7082.

10. Hess G, Donoghue JP. Facilitation of long-term potentiation in layer II/III horizontal connections of rat motor cortex following layer I stimulation: route of effect and cholinergic contributions. Exp Brain Res Experimentelle Hirnforschung. 1999;**127**:279–290.

11. Ziemann U, Paulus W, Nitsche MA, et al. Consensus: Motor cortex plasticity protocols. Brain stimulation. 2008;**1**(3):164–182.

12. Müller-Dahlhaus F, Ziemann U, Classen J. Plasticity resembling spike-timing dependent synaptic plasticity: the evidence in human cortex. Front Syn Neurosci. 2010;**2**(34):1–11.

13. Thickbroom GW. Transcranial magnetic stimulation and synaptic plasticity: experimental framework and human models. Exp Brain Res Experimentelle Hirnforschung. 2007;**180**(4):583–593.

14. Cooke SF, Bliss TV. Plasticity in the human central nervous system. Brain. 2006;**129**(Pt 7):1659–1673.

15. Siebner HR, Rothwell J. Transcranial magnetic stimulation: new insights into representational cortical plasticity. Exp Brain Res Experimentelle Hirnforschung. 2003;**148**(1):1–16.

16. Hoogendam JM, Ramakers GM, Di Lazzaro V. Physiology of repetitive transcranial magnetic stimulation of the human brain. Brain Stim. 2010;**3**(2):95–118.

17. Stagg CJ, Nitsche MA. Physiological basis of transcranial direct current stimulation. The Neuroscientist. 2011;**17**(1):37–53. Epub 2011/02/24.

18. Hallett M. Transcranial magnetic stimulation and the human brain. Nature. 2000;**406**(6792):147–150.

19. Ziemann U, Hallett M. Basic neurophysiological studies with transcranial magnetic stimulation. In: George MS, Belmaker RH (eds)_Transcranial Magnetic Stimulation in Clinical Psychiatry. American Psychiatric Publishing, Inc., Washington, DC, 2007, pp. 59–84.

20. Ziemann U, Ilic TV, Pauli C, Meintzschel F, Ruge D. Learning modifies subsequent induction of LTP-like and LTD-like plasticity in human motor cortex. J Neurosci. 2004;**24**(7):1666–1672.

21. Classen J, Ziemann U. Stimulation-induced plasticity in the human motor cortex. In: Boniface SJ, Ziemann U (eds) Plasticity in the human nervous system Investigation with transcranial magnetic stimulation. Cambridge University Press, Cambridge, 2003, pp. 135–165.

22. Brasil-Neto JP, Cohen LG, Pascual-Leone A, Jabir FK, Wall RT, Hallett M. Rapid reversible modulation of human motor outputs after transient deafferentation of the forearm: a study with transcranial magnetic stimulation. Neurology. 1992;**42**(7):1302–1306.

23. Levy L, Ziemann U, Chen R, Cohen LG. Rapid modulation of GABA in sensorimotor cortex induced by acute deafferentation. Ann Neurol. 2002;**52**(6):755–761.

24. Ziemann U, Corwell B, Cohen LG. Modulation of plasticity in human motor cortex after forearm ischemic nerve block. J Neurosci. 1998;**18**(3):1115–1123.

25. Ziemann U, Hallett M, Cohen LG. Mechanisms of deafferentation-induced plasticity in human motor cortex. J Neurosci. 1998;**18**(17):7000–7007.

26. Chen R, Classen J, Gerloff C, et al. Depression of motor cortex excitability by low-frequency transcranial magnetic stimulation. Neurology. 1997;**48**:1398–1403.

27. Sommer M, Rummel M, Norden C, Rothkegel H, Lang N, Paulus W. Mechanisms of human motor cortex facilitation induced by subthreshold 5 Hz repetitive transcranial magnetic stimulation. J Neurophysiol. 2013. Epub 2013/03/29.

28. Heidegger T, Krakow K, Ziemann U. Effects of antiepileptic drugs on associative LTP-like plasticity in human motor cortex. Eur J Neurosci. 2010;**32**:1215–1222.

29. McDonnell MN, Orekhov Y, Ziemann U. Suppression of LTP-like plasticity in human motor cortex by the GABA(B) receptor agonist baclofen. Exp Brain Res Experimentelle Hirnforschung. 2007;**180**(1):181–186.

30. Kujirai T, Caramia MD, Rothwell JC, et al. Corticocortical inhibition in human motor cortex. J Physiol (Lond). 1993;**471**:501–519.

31. Ziemann U, Lönnecker S, Steinhoff BJ, Paulus W. The effect of lorazepam on the motor cortical excitability in man. Exp Brain Res Experimentelle Hirnforschung. 1996;**109**(1):127–135.

32. Elahi B, Gunraj C, Chen R. Short-interval intracortical inhibition blocks long-term potentiation induced by paired associative stimulation. J Neurophysiol. 2012;**107**(7):1935–1941. Epub 2012/01/13.

33. Nitsche MA, Liebetanz D, Schlitterlau A, et al. GABAergic modulation of DC stimulation-induced motor cortex excitability shifts in humans. Eur J Neurosci. 2004;**19**(10):2720–2726.

34. Stefan K, Kunesch E, Benecke R, Cohen LG, Classen J. Mechanisms of enhancement of human motor cortex excitability induced by interventional paired associative stimulation. J Physiol. 2002;**543**(Pt 2):699–708.

35. Wankerl K, Weise D, Gentner R, Rumpf JJ, Classen J. L-type voltage-gated Ca2+ channels: a single molecular switch for long-term potentiation/long-term depression-like plasticity and activity-dependent metaplasticity in humans. J Neurosci. 2010;**30**(18):6197–6204.

36. Nitsche MA, Fricke K, Henschke U, Schlitterlau A, Liebetanz D, Lang N, et al. Pharmacological modulation of cortical excitability shifts induced by transcranial direct current stimulation in humans. J Physiol. 2003;**553**(Pt 1):293–301.

37. Huang YZ, Chen RS, Rothwell JC, Wen HY. The after-effect of human theta burst stimulation is NMDA receptor dependent. Clin Neurophysiol. 2007;**118**(5):1028–1032.

38. Nitsche MA, Jaussi W, Liebetanz D, Lang N, Tergau F, Paulus W. Consolidation of human motor cortical neuroplasticity by D-cycloserine. Neuropsychopharmacology. 2004;**29**:1573–1578.

39. Delvendahl I, Lindemann H, Heidegger T, Normann C, Ziemann U, Mall V. Effects of lamotrigine on human motor cortex plasticity. Clin Neurophysiol. 2013;**124**(1):148–153. Epub 2012/07/04.

40. Kuo M-F, Paulus W, Nitsche MA. Boosting focally-induced brain plasticity by dopamine. Cereb Cortex. 2008;**18**(3):648–651.

41. Monte-Silva K, Liebetanz D, Grundey J, Paulus W, Nitsche MA. Dosage-dependent non-linear effect of L-dopa on human motor cortex plasticity. J Physiol. 2010;**588**(Pt 18):3415–3424.

42. Thirugnanasambandam N, Grundey J, Paulus W, Nitsche MA. Dose-dependent nonlinear effect of L-DOPA on paired associative stimulation-induced neuroplasticity in humans. J Neurosci. 2011;**31**(14):5294–5299.

43. Korchounov A, Ziemann U. Neuromodulatory neurotransmitters influence LTP-like plasticity in human cortex: a pharmaco-TMS study. Neuropsychopharmacology. 2011;**36**(9):1894–1902.

44. Monte-Silva K, Kuo M-F, Thirugnanasambandam N, Liebetanz D, Paulus W, Nitsche M. Dose-dependent inverted U-shaped effect of dopamine (D2-like) receptor activation on focal and nonfocal plasticity in humans. J Neurosci. 2009;**29**(19):6124–6131.

45. Monte-Silva K, Ruge D, Teo JT, Paulus W, Rothwell JC, Nitsche MA. D2 Receptor block abolishes theta burst stimulation-induced neuroplasticity in the human motor cortex. Neuropsychopharmacology. 2011.

46. Nitsche MA, Lampe C, Antal A, et al. Dopaminergic modulation of long-lasting direct current-induced cortical excitability changes in the human motor cortex. Eur J Neurosci. 2006;**23**(6):1651–1657.

47. Nitsche MA, Kuo MF, Grosch J, Bergner C, Monte-Silva K, Paulus W. D1-receptor impact on neuroplasticity in humans. J Neurosci. 2009;**29**(8):2648–2653.

48. Nitsche MA, Grundey J, Liebetanz D, Lang N, Tergau F, Paulus W. Catecholaminergic consolidation of motor cortical neuroplasticity in humans. Cereb Cortex. 2004;**14**(11):1240–1245.

49. Kuo M-F, Grosch J, Fregni F, Paulus W, Nitsche MA. Focusing effect of acetylcholine on neuroplasticity in the human motor cortex. J Neurosci. 2007;**27**(52):14442–14447.

50. Thirugnanasambandam N, Grundey J, Adam K, et al. Nicotinergic impact on focal and non-focal neuroplasticity induced by non-invasive brain stimulation in non-smoking humans. Neuropsychopharmacology. 2011;**36**(4):879–886.

51. Swayne OB, Teo JT, Greenwood RJ, Rothwell JC. The facilitatory effects of intermittent theta burst stimulation on corticospinal excitability are enhanced by nicotine. Clin Neurophysiol. 2009;**120**(8):1610–1615.

52. Grundey J, Thirugnanasambandam N, Kaminsky K, et al. Rapid effect of nicotine intake on neuroplasticity in non-smoking humans. Front Pharmacol. 2012;**3**:186. Epub 2012/11/08.

53. Batsikadze G, Paulus W, Kuo MF, Nitsche MA. Effect of serotonin on paired associative stimulation-induced plasticity in the human motor cortex. Neuropsychopharmacology. 2013;**38**:2260–2267.

54. Nitsche MA, Kuo MF, Karrasch R, Wachter B, Liebetanz D, Paulus W. Serotonin affects transcranial direct current-induced neuroplasticity in humans. Biol Psychiatry. 2009;**66**(5):503–508.

55. Nudo RJ, Milliken GW, Jenkins WM, Merzenich MM. Use-dependent alterations of movement representations in primary motor cortex of adult squirrel monkeys. J Neurosci. 1996;**16**(2):785–807.

56. Kleim JA, Barbay S, Nudo RJ. Functional reorganization of the rat motor cortex following motor skill learning. J Neurophysiol. 1998;**80**(6):3321–3325.

57. Remple MS, Bruneau RM, VandenBerg PM, Goertzen C, Kleim JA. Sensitivity of cortical movement representations to motor experience: evidence that skill learning but not strength training induces cortical reorganization. Behav Brain Res. 2001;**123**(2):133–141.

58. Cain DP. Testing the NMDA, long-term potentiation, and cholinergic hypotheses of spatial learning. Neurosci Biobehav Rev. 1998;**22**(2):181–193.

59. Feeney DM, Sutton RL. Pharmacotherapy for recovery of function after brain injury. Crit Rev Neurobiol. 1987;**3**(2):135–197.

60. Hosp JA, Luft AR. Cortical plasticity during motor learning and recovery after ischemic stroke. Neural Plasticity. 2011;**2011**:871296. Epub 2011/12/03.

61. Hernandez TD, Schallert T. Long-term impairment of behavioral recovery from cortical damage can be produced by short-term GABA-agonist infusion into adjacent cortex. Restorat Neurol Neurosci. 1990;**1**:323–330.

62. Glykys J, Mody I. Hippocampal network hyperactivity after selective reduction of tonic inhibition in GABA A receptor alpha5 subunit-deficient mice. J Neurophysiol. 2006;**95**(5):2796–2807. Epub 2006/02/03.

63. Farrant M, Nusser Z. Variations on an inhibitory theme: phasic and tonic activation of GABA(A) receptors. Nat Rev Neurosci. 2005;**6**(3):215–229. Epub 2005/03/02.

64. Collinson N, Kuenzi FM, Jarolimek W, et al. Enhanced learning and memory and altered GABAergic synaptic transmission in mice lacking the alpha 5 subunit of the GABAA receptor. J Neurosci. 2002;**22**(13):5572–5580. Epub 2002/07/05.

65. Clarkson AN, Huang BS, Macisaac SE, Mody I, Carmichael ST. Reducing excessive GABA-mediated tonic inhibition promotes functional recovery after stroke. Nature. 2010;**468**(7321):305–309. Epub 2010/11/05.

66. Dhawan J, Benveniste H, Luo Z, Nawrocky M, Smith SD, Biegon A. A new look at glutamate and ischemia: NMDA agonist improves long-term functional outcome in a rat model of stroke. Future Neurol. 2011;**6**(6):823–834. Epub 2011/12/06.

67. Choi DW, Rothman SM. The role of glutamate neurotoxicity in hypoxic-ischemic neuronal death. Annu Rev Neurosci. 1990;**13**:171–182. Epub 1990/01/01.

68. Hoyte L, Barber PA, Buchan AM, Hill MD. The rise and fall of NMDA antagonists for ischemic stroke. Curr Mol Med. 2004;**4**(2):131–136. Epub 2004/03/23.

69. Traystman RJ, Klaus JA, DeVries AC, Shaivitz AB, Hurn PD. Anticonvulsant lamotrigine administered on reperfusion fails to improve experimental stroke outcomes. Stroke. 2001;**32**(3):783–787. Epub 2001/03/10.

70. Ruscher K, Kuric E, Wieloch T. Levodopa treatment improves functional recovery after experimental stroke. Stroke. 2012;**43**(2):507–513. Epub 2011/11/19.

71. Feeney DM, Gonzalez A, Law WA. Amphetamine, haloperidol, and experience interact to affect rate of recovery after motor cortex injury. Science. 1982;**217**(4562):855–857.

72. Hurwitz BE, Dietrich WD, McCabe PM, et al. Amphetamine promotes recovery from sensory-motor integration deficit after thrombotic infarction of the primary somatosensory rat cortex. Stroke. 1991;**22**(5):648–654.

73. Stroemer RP, Kent TA, Hulsebosch CE. Enhanced neocortical neural sprouting, synaptogenesis, and behavioral recovery with D-amphetamine therapy after neocortical infarction in rats. Stroke. 1998;**29**(11):2381–2393; discussion 93–5. Epub 1998/11/06.

74. Adkins DL, Jones TA. D-amphetamine enhances skilled reaching after ischemic cortical lesions in rats. Neurosci Lett. 2005;**380**(3):214–218. Epub 2005/05/03.

75. Gilmour G, Iversen SD, O'Neill MF, O'Neill MJ, Ward MA, Bannerman DM. Amphetamine promotes task-dependent recovery following focal cortical ischaemic lesions in the rat. Behav Brain Res. 2005;**165**(1):98–109. Epub 2005/08/18.

76. Ramic M, Emerick AJ, Bollnow MR, O'Brien TE, Tsai SY, Kartje GL. Axonal plasticity is associated with motor recovery following amphetamine treatment combined with rehabilitation after brain injury in the adult rat. Brain Res. 2006;**1111**(1):176–186. Epub 2006/08/22.

77. Papadopoulos CM, Tsai SY, Guillen V, Ortega J, Kartje GL, Wolf WA. Motor recovery and axonal plasticity with short-term amphetamine after stroke. Stroke. 2009;**40**(1):294–302. Epub 2008/11/29.

78. Liu HS, Shen H, Harvey BK, et al. Post-treatment with amphetamine enhances reinnervation of the ipsilateral side cortex in stroke rats. NeuroImage. 2011;**56**(1):280–289. Epub 2011/02/26.

79. Conner JM, Culberson A, Packowski C, Chiba AA, Tuszynski MH. Lesions of the Basal forebrain cholinergic system impair task acquisition and abolish cortical plasticity associated with motor skill learning. Neuron. 2003;**38**(5):819–829.

80. De Ryck M, Duytschaever H, Pauwels PJ, Janssen PA. Ionic channels, cholinergic mechanisms, and recovery of sensorimotor function after neocortical infarcts in rats. Stroke. 1990;**21**(11 Suppl):III158–163.

81. Windle V, Corbett D. Fluoxetine and recovery of motor function after focal ischemia in rats. Brain Res. 2005;**1044**(1):25–32. Epub 2005/05/03.

82. Zhao CS, Puurunen K, Schallert T, Sivenius J, Jolkkonen J. Behavioral and histological effects of chronic antipsychotic and antidepressant drug treatment in aged rats with focal ischemic brain injury. Behav Brain Res. 2005;**158**(2):211–220. Epub 2005/02/09.

83. Chollet F, Tardy J, Albucher JF, et al. Fluoxetine for motor recovery after acute ischaemic stroke (FLAME): a randomised placebo-controlled trial. Lancet Neurol. 2011;**10**(2):123–130.

84. Endres M, Engelhardt B, Koistinaho J, et al. Improving outcome after stroke: overcoming the translational roadblock. Cerebrovasc Dis. 2008;**25**(3):268–278.

85. Rioult-Pedotti M-S, Friedman D, Hess G, Donoghue JP. Strengthening of horizontal cortical connections following skill learning. Nat Neurosci. 1998;**1**(3):230–234.

86. Rioult-Pedotti MS, Friedman D, Donoghue JP. Learning-induced LTP in neocortex. Science. 2000;**290**(5491):533–536.

87. Monfils MH, Teskey GC. Skilled-learning-induced potentiation in rat sensorimotor cortex: a transient form of behavioural long-term potentiation. Neuroscience. 2004;**125**(2):329–336.

88. Hodgson RA, Ji Z, Standish S, Boyd-Hodgson TE, Henderson AK, Racine RJ. Training-induced and electrically induced potentiation in the neocortex. Neurobiol Learn Mem. 2005;**83**(1):22–32.

89. Stefan K, Wycislo M, Gentner R, et al. Temporary occlusion of associative motor cortical plasticity by prior dynamic motor training. Cereb Cortex. 2006;**16**(3):376–385.

90. Rosenkranz K, Kacar A, Rothwell JC. Differential modulation of motor cortical plasticity and excitability in early and late phases of human motor learning. J Neurosci. 2007;27(44):12058–12066.

91. Nathan PJ, Cobb SR, Lu B, Bullmore ET, Davies CH. Studying synaptic plasticity in the human brain and opportunities for drug discovery. Curr Opin Pharmacol. 2011;11(5):540–548. Epub 2011/07/09.

92. Bütefisch C, Hummelsheim H, Denzler P, Mauritz K-H. Repetitive training of isolated movements improves the outcome of motor rehabilitation of the centrally paretic hand. J Neurol Sci. 1995;130(1):59–68.

93. Woldag H, Hummelsheim H. Evidence-based physiotherapeutic concepts for improving arm and hand function in stroke patients: a review. J Neurol. 2002;249(5):518–528.

94. Muellbacher W, Ziemann U, Boroojerdi B, Cohen LG, Hallett M. Role of the human motor cortex in rapid motor learning. Exp Brain Res Experimentelle Hirnforschung. 2001;136(4):431–438.

95. Muellbacher W, Ziemann U, Wissel J, et al. Early consolidation in human primary motor cortex. Nature. 2002;415:640–644.

96. Classen J, Liepert J, Wise SP, Hallett M, Cohen LG. Rapid plasticity of human cortical movement representation induced by practice. J Neurophysiol. 1998;79(2):1117–1123.

97. Liepert J, Terborg C, Weiller C. Motor plasticity induced by synchronized thumb and foot movements. Exp Brain Res Experimentelle Hirnforschung. 1999;125(4):435–439.

98. Tegenthoff M, Witscher K, Schwenkreis P, Liepert J. Pharmacological modulation of training-induced plastic changes in human motor cortex. Electroencephalogr Clin Neurophysiol Suppl. 1999;51:188–196.

99. Fu QG, Flament D, Coltz JD, Ebner TJ. Temporal encoding of movement kinematics in the discharge of primate primary motor and premotor neurons. Journal of neurophysiology. 1995;73(2):836–854.

100. Flöel A, Breitenstein C, Hummel F, et al. Dopaminergic influences on formation of a motor memory. Ann Neurol. 2005;58(1):121–130.

101. Meintzschel F, Ziemann U. Modification of practice-dependent plasticity in human motor cortex by neuromodulators. Cereb Cortex. 2006;16:1106–1115.

102. Ziemann U, Muellbacher W, Hallett M, Cohen LG. Modulation of practice-dependent plasticity in human motor cortex. Brain. 2001;124(6):1171–1181.

103. Stagg CJ, Bachtiar V, Johansen-Berg H. The role of GABA in human motor learning. Curr Biol. 2011;21(6):480–484. Epub 2011/03/08.

104. Teo JT, Terranova C, Swayne O, Greenwood RJ, Rothwell JC. Differing effects of intracortical circuits on plasticity. Exp Brain Res Experimentelle Hirnforschung. 2009;193(4):555–563.

105. Bütefisch CM, Davis BC, Wise SP, et al. Mechanisms of use-dependent plasticity in the human motor cortex. Proc Natl Acad Sci U S A. 2000;97(7):3661–3665.

106. Willerslev-Olsen M, Lundbye-Jensen J, Petersen TH, Nielsen JB. The effect of baclofen and diazepam on motor skill acquisition in healthy subjects. Exp Brain Res Experimentelle Hirnforschung. 2011;213(4):465–474.

107. Donchin O, Sawaki L, Madupu G, Cohen LG, Shadmehr R. Mechanisms influencing acquisition and recall of motor memories. J Neurophysiol. 2002;88(4):2114–2123.

108. Schwenkreis P, Witscher K, Pleger B, Malin JP, Tegenthoff M. The NMDA antagonist memantine affects training induced motor cortex plasticity—a study using transcranial magnetic stimulation. BMC Neurosci. 2005;6(1):35.

109. Pearson-Fuhrhop KM, Minton B, Acevedo D, Shahbaba B, Cramer SC. Genetic variation in the human brain dopamine system influences motor learning and its modulation by L-dopa. PloS One. 2013;8(4):e61197. Epub 2013/04/25.

110. Bütefisch CM, Davis BC, Sawaki L, et al. Modulation of use-dependent plasticity by d-amphetamine. Ann Neurol. 2002;51(1):59–68.

111. Sawaki L, Cohen LG, Classen J, Davis BC, Bütefisch CM. Enhancement of use-dependent plasticity by D-amphetamine. Neurology. 2002;59(8):1262–1264.

112. Plewnia C, Hoppe J, Cohen LG, Gerloff C. Improved motor skill acquisition after selective stimulation of central norepinephrine. Neurology. 2004;62(11):2124–2126.

113. Foster DJ, Good DC, Fowlkes A, Sawaki L. Atomoxetine enhances a short-term model of plasticity in humans. Arch Phys Med Rehabil. 2006;87(2):216–221.

114. Tegenthoff M, Cornelius B, Pleger B, Malin JP, Schwenkreis P. Amphetamine enhances training-induced motor cortex plasticity. Acta Neurol Scand. 2004;109(5):330–336.

115. Sawaki L, Werhahn KJ, Barco R, Kopylev L, Cohen LG. Effect of an alpha(1)-adrenergic blocker on plasticity elicited by motor training. Exp Brain Res Experimentelle Hirnforschung. 2003;148(4):504–508.

116. Plewnia C, Hoppe J, Gerloff C. No effects of enhanced central norepinephrine on finger-sequence learning and attention. Psychopharmacology. 2006;187(2):260–265.

117. Sawaki L, Boroojerdi B, Kaelin-Lang A, Burstein AH, Bütefisch CM, Kopylev L, et al. Cholinergic influences on use-dependent plasticity. J Neurophysiol. 2002;87(1):166–171.

118. Pleger B, Schwenkreis P, Grunberg C, Malin JP, Tegenthoff M. Fluoxetine facilitates use-dependent excitability of human primary motor cortex. Clin Neurophysiol. 2004;115(9):2157–2163.

119. Loubinoux I, Pariente J, Rascol O, Celsis P, Chollet F. Selective serotonin reuptake inhibitor paroxetine modulates motor behavior through practice. A double-blind, placebo-controlled, multi-dose study in healthy subjects. Neuropsychologia. 2002;40(11):1815–1821.

120. Berends HI, Nijlant JM, Movig KL, Van Putten MJ, Jannink MJ, Ijzerman MJ. The clinical use of drugs influencing neurotransmitters in the brain to promote motor recovery after stroke; a Cochrane systematic review. Eur J Phys Rehabil Med. 2009;45(4):621–630.

121. Goldstein LB. Common drugs may influence motor recovery after stroke. The Sygen In Acute Stroke Study Investigators. Neurology. 1995;45(5):865–871.

122. Flöel A, Hummel F, Breitenstein C, Knecht S, Cohen LG. Dopaminergic effects on encoding of a motor memory in chronic stroke. Neurology. 2005;65(3):472–474.

123. Pariente J, Loubinoux I, Carel C, Albucher JF, Leger A, Manelfe C, et al. Fluoxetine modulates motor performance and cerebral activation of patients recovering from stroke. Ann Neurol. 2001;50(6):718–729.

124. Dobkin BH. Clinical practice. Rehabilitation after stroke. N Engl J Med. 2005;352(16):1677–1684.

125. Hendricks HT, van Limbeek J, Geurts AC, Zwarts MJ. Motor recovery after stroke: a systematic review of the literature. Arch Phys Med Rehabil. 2002;83(11):1629–1637. Epub 2002/11/08.

126. Wade DT, Langton-Hewer R, Wood VA, Skilbeck CE, Ismail HM. The hemiplegic arm after stroke: measurement and recovery. J Neurol Neurosurg Psychiatry. 1983;46(6):521–524. Epub 1983/06/01.

127. Sunderland A, Tinson D, Bradley L, Hewer RL. Arm function after stroke. An evaluation of grip strength as a measure of recovery and a prognostic indicator. J Neurol Neurosurg Psychiatry. 1989;52(11):1267–1272. Epub 1989/11/01.

128. Kwakkel G, Kollen BJ, van der Grond J, Prevo AJ. Probability of regaining dexterity in the flaccid upper limb: impact of severity of paresis and time since onset in acute stroke. Stroke. 2003;34(9):2181–2186.

129. Berthier ML, Pulvermuller F, Davila G, Casares NG, Gutierrez A. Drug therapy of post-stroke aphasia: a review of current evidence. Neuropsychol Rev. 2011;21(3):302–317. Epub 2011/08/17.

130. Parton A, Coulthard E, Husain M. Neuropharmacological modulation of cognitive deficits after brain damage. Curr Opin Neurol. 2005;18(6):675–680. Epub 2005/11/11.

131. Muellbacher W, Richards C, Ziemann U, Wittenberg G, Weltz D, Boroojerdi B, et al. Improving hand function in chronic stroke. Arch Neurol. 2002;59(8):1278–1282.

132. Scheidtmann K, Fries W, Muller F, Koenig E. Effect of levodopa in combination with physiotherapy on functional motor recovery after stroke: a prospective, randomised, double-blind study. Lancet. 2001;358(9284):787–790.

133. Crisostomo EA, Duncan PW, Propst M, Dawson DV, Davis JN. Evidence that amphetamine with physical therapy promotes recovery of motor function in stroke patients. Ann Neurol. 1988;23(1):94–97.

134. Engelter ST. Safety in pharmacological enhancement of stroke rehabilitation. Eur J Phys Rehabil Med. 2013;49(2):261–267. Epub 2013/02/27.

135. Wang LE, Fink GR, Diekhoff S, Rehme AK, Eickhoff SB, Grefkes C. Noradrenergic enhancement improves motor network connectivity in stroke patients. Ann Neurol. 2011;69(2):375–388.

136. NINDS-rt-PA-Stroke-Study-Group. Tissue plasminogen activator for acute ischemic stroke. The National Institute of Neurological Disorders and Stroke rt-PA Stroke Study Group. N Engl J Med. 1995;333(24):1581–1587. Epub 1995/12/14.

137. Hacke W, Kaste M, Bluhmki E, et al. Thrombolysis with alteplase 3 to 4.5 hours after acute ischemic stroke. N Engl J Med. 2008;359(13):1317–1329. Epub 2008/09/26.

138. Restemeyer C, Weiller C, Liepert J. No effect of a levodopa single dose on motor performance and motor excitability in chronic stroke. A double-blind placebo-controlled cross-over pilot study. Restorat Neurol Neurosci. 2007;25(2):143–150.

139. Acler M, Fiaschi A, Manganotti P. Long-term levodopa administration in chronic stroke patients. A clinical and neurophysiologic single-blind placebo-controlled cross-over pilot study. Restorat Neurol Neurosci. 2009;27(4):277–283. Epub 2009/09/10.

140. Sonde L, Lokk J. Effects of amphetamine and/or L-dopa and physiotherapy after stroke—a blinded randomized study. Acta Neurol Scand. 2007;115(1):55–59. Epub 2006/12/13.

141. Lokk J, Salman Roghani R, Delbari A. Effect of methylphenidate and/or levodopa coupled with physiotherapy on functional and motor recovery after stroke—a randomized, double-blind, placebo-controlled trial. Acta Neurol Scand. 2011;123(4):266–273. Epub 2010/06/24.

142. Walker-Batson D, Smith P, Curtis S, Unwin H, Greenlee R. Amphetamine paired with physical therapy accelerates motor recovery after stroke. Further evidence. Stroke. 1995;26(12):2254–2259.

143. Martinsson L, Wahlgren NG. Safety of dexamphetamine in acute ischemic stroke: a randomized, double-blind, controlled dose-escalation trial. Stroke. 2003;34(2):475–481.

144. Sonde L, Nordstrom M, Nilsson CG, Lokk J, Viitanen M. A double-blind placebo-controlled study of the effects of amphetamine and physiotherapy after stroke. Cerebrovasc Dis. 2001;12(3):253–257.

145. Treig T, Werner C, Sachse M, Hesse S. No benefit from D-amphetamine when added to physiotherapy after stroke: a randomized, placebo-controlled study. Clin Rehabil. 2003;17(6):590–599.

146. Platz T, Kim IH, Engel U, Pinkowski C, Eickhof C, Kutzner M. Amphetamine fails to facilitate motor performance and to enhance motor recovery among stroke patients with mild arm paresis: interim analysis and termination of a double blind, randomised, placebo-controlled trial. Restorat Neurol Neurosci. 2005;23(5–6):271–280. Epub 2006/02/16.

147. Gladstone DJ, Danells CJ, Armesto A, et al. Physiotherapy coupled with dextroamphetamine for rehabilitation after hemiparetic stroke: a randomized, double-blind, placebo-controlled trial. Stroke. 2006;37(1):179–185. Epub 2005/12/03.

148. Sprigg N, Willmot MR, Gray LJ, et al. Amphetamine increases blood pressure and heart rate but has no effect on motor recovery or cerebral haemodynamics in ischaemic stroke: a randomized controlled trial (ISRCTN 36285333). J Hum Hypertens. 2007;21(8):616–624. Epub 2007/04/20.

149. Schuster C, Maunz G, Lutz K, Kischka U, Sturzenegger R, Ettlin T. Dexamphetamine improves upper extremity outcome during rehabilitation after stroke: a pilot randomized controlled trial. Neurorehabil Neural Repair. 2011;25(8):749–755. Epub 2011/06/30.

150. Grade C, Redford B, Chrostowski J, Toussaint L, Blackwell B. Methylphenidate in early poststroke recovery: a double-blind, placebo-controlled study. Arch Phys Med Rehabil. 1998;79:1047–1050.

151. Zittel S, Weiller C, Liepert J. Reboxetine improves motor function in chronic stroke: A pilot study. J Neurol. 2007;254(2):197–201.

152. Dam M, Tonin P, De Boni A, et al. Effects of fluoxetine and maprotiline on functional recovery in poststroke hemiplegic patients undergoing rehabilitation therapy. Stroke. 1996;27(7):1211–1214.

153. Acler M, Robol E, Fiaschi A, Manganotti P. A double blind placebo RCT to investigate the effects of serotonergic modulation on brain excitability and motor recovery in stroke patients. J Neurol. 2009;256(7):1152–1158.

154. Zittel S, Weiller C, Liepert J. Citalopram improves dexterity in chronic stroke patients. Neurorehabil Neural Repair. 2008;22(3):311–314. Epub 2008/01/26.

155. Mead GE, Hsieh CF, Lee R, Kutlubaev MA, Claxton A, Hankey GJ, et al. Selective serotonin reuptake inhibitors (SSRIs) for stroke recovery. Cochrane Database Syst Rev. 2012;11:CD009286. Epub 2012/11/16.

156. Dobkin BH. Rehabilitation and functional neuroimaging dose-response trajectories for clinical trials. Neurorehabi Neural Repair. 2005;19(4):276–282.

157. Carmichael ST. Brain excitability in stroke: the yin and yang of stroke progression. Arch Neurol. 2012;69(2):161–167. Epub 2011/10/12.

158. Goldstein LB. Neuropharmacology of TBI-induced plasticity. Brain Injury: [BI]. 2003;17(8):685–694. Epub 2003/07/10.

159. Liepert J. Pharmacotherapy in restorative neurology. Curr Opin Neurol. 2008;21(6):639–643. Epub 2008/11/08.

160. Maric O, Zörner B, Dietz V. Levodopa therapy in incomplete spinal cord injury. J Neurotrauma. 2008;25(11):1303–1307. Epub 2008/12/09.

161. Goldstein LB, Davis JN. Clonidine impairs recovery of beam-walking after a sensorimotor cortex lesion in the rat. Brain Res. 1990;508(2):305–309.

162. Barbeau H, Norman KE. The effect of noradrenergic drugs on the recovery of walking after spinal cord injury. Spinal Cord. 2003;41(3):137–143. Epub 2003/03/04.

163. Mondaca M, Hernandez A, Perez H, et al. Alpha2-adrenoceptor modulation of long-term potentiation elicited in vivo in rat occipital cortex. Brain Res. 2004;1021(2):292–296. Epub 2004/09/03.

SECTION 4

Clinical concepts

CHAPTER 18

Rehabilitation of gait and balance after CNS damage

Jacques Duysens, Geert Verheyden, Firas Massaad, Pieter Meyns, Bouwien Smits-Engelsman, and Ilse Jonkers

Introduction

For SCI (spinal cord injury) patients the rehabilitation of gait has focused on treadmill or locomotor training. This refers to intensive assisted locomotor training on a treadmill in combination with body weight support (BWS). The idea behind this therapy stems from animal studies, in which it has been shown that load feedback is essential for the regulation of gait and that training on a treadmill with assistance can restore gait even after complete transection of the spinal cord. The theoretical background of treadmill training has been described in several papers and therefore only a brief summary is given here in this chapter. The theory states that activation of sensory pathways, which have direct access to the central pattern generator (CPG), can re-establish basic locomotor rhythmicity.

Treadmill training has been used for stroke as well, but generally there have been much wider rehabilitation efforts. In fact, stroke is a condition for which there is no universally accepted rehabilitation approach, yet the integration of basic and clinical research provides new therapeutic concepts for the recovery of motor function after stroke. Studying brain function by means of non-invasive techniques such as transcranial magnetic stimulation has led to the development of new sensorimotor system rehabilitation approaches, but these should further be evaluated in large clinical trials to demonstrate statistical as well as clinical efficacy.

Bidirectional translational science—that is interactive science between basic and clinical research—is necessary to further develop strategies for sensorimotor system rehabilitation after CNS damage. Eventually, established proof-of-concepts and subsequently positive pilot studies should lead to adequately powered randomized controlled trials (RCTs) in order to establish clinical efficacy and provide the foundation for implementation studies.

Pathophysiology

SCI

Damage to the spinal cord can result either from a traumatic injury, for instance due to a motor vehicle accident, or from a non-traumatic cause, for instance due to a disease to the vertebral column like amyotrophic lateral sclerosis. The primary causes of traumatic SCI in the USA are traffic accidents, falls, and violence, where they result in an incidence rate of 39 per million inhabitants. Incidence rates of non-traumatic SCI are less clear because of the multitude of possible causes. The term SCI is commonly used for an injury to the spinal cord caused by trauma.

The pathophysiology of a SCI involves both a primary and secondary injury. The initial mechanical trauma results in damage of both central and peripheral neural pathways by the traction and compression of displaced bone fragments, disc material and ligaments. Micro-hemorrhages immediately occur which will expand in the spinal cord to fill up the entire diameter of the spinal canal at the level of the injury. This expansion, in turn, will lead to secondary ischemia (i.e. release of toxic chemicals from disrupted neural membranes), which will then trigger the secondary injury cascade. During the secondary injury, toxic chemicals released by previously damaged structures (e.g. axons, blood vessels) attack neighbouring cells (excitotoxicity).

Regardless of the type of SCI, damage to the spinal cord results in an impaired, or even a complete loss of, function. The symptoms (and their severity) vary among SCI patients and are dependent on the location of the lesion of the spinal cord and the severity of injury. SCI can affect the conduction of both sensory and motor signals, but also the autonomic nervous system. The International Standards for Neurological Classification of Spinal Cord Injury (ISNCSCI) is widely used to document the sensory and motor impairments in a SCI person [1]. The American Spinal Injury Association (ASIA) classes range from A (complete) to E (normal). This classification is based on an extensive neurological examination of the sensations in each dermatome (area of the skin mainly innervated by the sensory axons within one segmental nerve) and the strength of the muscles in several myotomes (collection of muscle fibres supplied by the motor axons within one segmental nerve). Such examination allows classifying SCI persons (with varying symptoms) into several categories. Based on the tests, one can then know the sensory level (the neurologically lowest, normally innervated dermatome) and motor level (the most caudal key muscle function with a grade of 3 or higher [on manual muscle testing], providing the key muscle functions more cranial are intact), the completeness of the lesion (a complete injury is defined as the absence of sacral sparing; that is no sensory or motor function in the lowest sacral segments), and whether there is a zone of partial preservation (dermatomes and myotomes caudal to the sensory and motor levels that remain partially innervated). Injuries at the cervical root level result in tetraplegia (loss of function and/or sensory problems in all four limbs and in the trunk), whereas paraplegia (function of the arms, neck, and breathing are usually unaffected) is caused by a deficit in motor and/or sensory function in thoracic, lumbar, or sacral spinal levels.

Stroke

Stroke is the leading cause of disability in human adults in the developed world. Roughly two thirds of survivors have residual neurological impairments, mainly hemiparesis affecting balance and gait. Some of the main gait impairments following stroke are characterized by a poor postural control, higher fall risk, slow walking speed, and higher energy consumption.

Research on a Canadian population showed that at three months after stroke, 85% of people were still impaired on gait speed (as measured by a 10-metre walk test), and 29% were still impaired on balance (as measured by the Berg balance scale) [2]. At 1 year post-stroke, the most noticeable area of difficulty appeared to be endurance, as measured by the 6-minute walk test. Only 50% of their sample was able to complete this test, and to walk, on average, about 250 metres, which is equivalent to 40% of their predicted ability. Geurts and colleagues reviewed recovery of standing balance after stroke and reported that recovery shows considerable inter-individual variability, depending on initial deficits [3]. Nevertheless, recovery is noted by improvement of stability in the anteroposterior and mediolateral plane, the ability to compensate for perturbations, and the ability to voluntary control posture. The review suggests that true restoration through recovery of paretic leg muscles in the first 3 months may improve standing balance but alternatively, mechanisms are suggested that improve standing balance without clear signs of improved support function or balance reaction in the paretic leg. Possible mechanisms suggested by the authors are improved core stabilisation, compensation through the non-paretic leg, and increased self-confidence [3].

Principles of therapy and management

Gait and balance training in SCI

After a transection of the spinal cord, the locomotor behaviour depends on automaticity from circuits in the lumbosacral spinal cord (i.e. CPGs; [4]). An additional important component of automaticity is the sensory input to the spinal cord from the periphery [5, 6]. This sensory input from cutaneous and proprioceptive sources is needed to assist the CPGs, to automatically switch from one phase to another. It has been argued that such mechanisms are important for humans as well and that this is the basis for the use of treadmill training as this provides the essential sensory stimulation to activate the spinal CPGs (see previous section; also [7–9]). Experimental evidence was obtained by the Harkema group for the contention that the isolated human spinal cord can interpret both loading [10] and velocity signals [11]. Most rehabilitation strategies employ repetitive and intensive practice of gait (for instance using [body weight supported] treadmill training). This training then provides task-specific sensory input associated with appropriate stepping movements.

Treadmill training proved to be more successful in incomplete versus complete spinal cord lesions (for review see [7, 12]). In the

group of incomplete SCI, clear positive effects can be obtained even for training long after the injury [13, 14]. Recovery also depends on the level of the lesion. For example, a relationship was reported between the level of the lesion in motor complete SCI patients and their orthotic gait performance [15]. Their results indicated that the slower gait speed and higher energy cost in patients with the SCI at a higher thoracic level was due to their limited hip motion and presumed increased upper limb load.

In daily life, the use of treadmill training can mean that patients can switch locomotor aids. Without training many patients with SCI need (powered) wheelchairs for locomotion. Therefore, promoting the recovery of (independent) gait has been one of the major topics of research [16]. Initially, it was suggested that repetitive gait retraining was more beneficial when applied sooner rather than later after the onset of injury in people with motor-incomplete lesions [16]. However, there is a limit and very early training can even be detrimental unless it is aimed at an enhancement of appropriate proprioceptive input [6]. Conversely, if no training is given in chronic SCI patients, the locomotor activity in the leg muscles exhausts rapidly during assisted locomotion. This is accompanied by a shift from early to dominant late spinal reflex components [17].

One important issue is the quantitative assessment of the progress made during gait rehabilitation. Functional tests are able to demonstrate the changes in behaviour, for example the maximum walking speed. In the first pioneering studies of this kind, these tests were the only ones available [18]. However, such measures are often crude and unreliable. Therefore there was a need to use more sophisticated assessment measures in order to better understand the underlying mechanisms of improvement. Thus, it was proposed to use objective measurements, such as measures of electromyography (EMG), to better document the progress made during the training. There are different ways to measure the changes in EMG activity during the training programme. First, one can measure the EMG as the performance level of the SCI person improves. This means that one measures EMGs at higher walking speeds and lower BWS when training progresses. The disadvantage of this method is that one cannot clearly distinguish between the influence of the training effect and the changing walking speed and BWS on the EMG muscle activity. The other strategy consists of performing measurements at a constant walking speed and constant BWS. The approach was successfully pioneered by Dietz et al [7, 12]. As training evolved there was a clear increase in the amplitude of the EMG in several leg muscles during walking on a treadmill at a constant speed.

One consistent finding observed in various laboratories, including ours, was that the EMG measured during walking far exceeded in amplitude the maximum activity in the same subjects during voluntary maximum contractions (as illustrated in Figure 18.1). Such observation strongly supports the notion that treadmill training can evoke spinal generated activity much better than cortical commands, and this is presumably through the activation of spinal CPGs.

Gait and balance training in stroke rehabilitation

Balance

Rehabilitation of postural control following stroke is very important in the context of independent mobility. Furthermore, falls

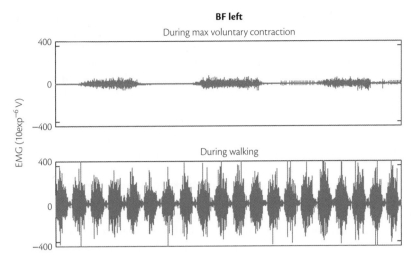

BF left

Fig. 18.1 Typical results of treadmill training in a SCI subject. When the subject was asked to produce a maximum voluntary contraction the resulting EMG was substantially lower than when the same subject later performed treadmill training. BF: Biceps Femoris
From: van de Crommert HWAA, Rijken H, Nienhuis B, van Kuppevelt D, Mulder T, Duysens J. Effects of locomotor training with body-weight support in spinal cord injured patients long after injury. In: Duysens J, Smits-Engelsman BCM, Kingma H, editors. Control of posture and gait. 2001. p. 773–6.

are very frequent in this population and a recent Cochrane review showed that up to date, there are no accepted and effective motor therapies for preventing falls in people after stroke [19], thereby increasing the need for effective training of postural control strategies, both early or in a later phase. The deficit in postural control is apparent in many everyday conditions. Stroke patients have difficulties when leaning their body as far as possible in a given direction, but mostly in the direction of their paretic leg [20]. Similarly, these patients have problems when shifting from a two-legged to a one-legged stance [21]. When postural perturbations are tested stroke patients show delayed responses [22].

The process of recovery of balance after a stroke has been reviewed by Geurts et al, while Pinter and Brainin provided a review on stroke rehabilitation, in particular in elderly [3, 23]. Here, a short overview and update is given. For a proper rehabilitation intervention it is crucial to have a good understanding of the scientific background, yet '. . . the neurophysiology underpinning stroke rehabilitation is often poorly established' [23]. Some reviews are available, summarizing the work on animal models [24] or on humans [3, 23]. In short, such studies emphasize that stable standing requires a combination of elements, including muscle strength, proper afferent input, and the ability to incorporate this input into one's own body scheme. Recovery of one of the elements is not sufficient and this may explain, for example, why physiological recovery of paretic leg muscle functions (particularly during the first 3 months post-stroke) does not necessarily predict improvement in support and balance functions [3]. Other mechanisms are likely to be just as important. In particular, the normal sensory integration appears to be critical for balance recovery. Hence, brain lesions involving the parietotemporal junction are especially devastating for poor postural control. Nevertheless, the majority of stroke patients show considerable improvement in standing balance after rehabilitation. Most of them have unilateral supratentorial brain infarction or haemorrhage and there may be some effect of lateralization as well since studies on stroke have indicated that the right hemisphere plays a more dominant role in postural control than the left hemisphere [25].

For rehabilitation of standing balance an important issue is to apply the appropriate training and assessment tools to measure improvement (for review see [26]). Several training programmes and assessment methods have been proposed, but we will focus here on just a few which we consider especially important. The ability to make voluntary weight shifts has long been known to be essential for gait initiation and the evaluation of this ability can be performed quite reliably [21]. Since one of the major deficits in standing balance in stroke is asymmetrical weight-bearing, it is evident that training and assessment has been targeted often at such weight-shifting tasks [27]. Typically, with this type of training, stroke patients increased both their walking speed and their precision of weight shifting. Even severe stroke patients (selected for inpatient rehabilitation) improved significantly. However, both old age and the presence of hemineglect affected progress. Nevertheless, most patients improved but some degree of weight-transfer time asymmetry persisted. Similar results were obtained in a more recent study on chronic stroke subjects, based on a 4-week training programme using both static and dynamic balance exercises with visual feedback [28]. Balance control was assessed with clinical measures (Berg Balance Scale) and with a pressure platform to register the centre of pressure (CoP) during quiet stance and during a forward reach task. The stroke patients improved their Berg Balance score and their performance on quiet standing, but again the weight distribution remained somewhat abnormal. Hence, this type of training programme improves balance control but not weight distribution.

Other approaches to restore balance

In contrast to weight-shifting, restoring balance control in stroke using whole-body vibration has not been very successful. Short-term beneficial effects on postural control can be obtained in unilateral chronic stroke patients [29] but long-term effects have been disappointing [30]. The addition of whole-body vibration to dynamic leg exercises was not more effective in improving neuromotor performance or reducing the incidence of falls compared to performing the leg exercises alone (without whole-body vibration) in chronic stroke patients with mild to moderate motor impairments [31].

Although only explored recently and awaiting further experimentation, it appears that a more promising approach is the use of game-based training [32]. In addition, an interesting new approach involves biofeedback with a force plate or a moving platform [33]. Typically, these approaches improve symmetry of standing but they do not necessarily have much effect on active functional activities, such as gait. The latter requires specific training as outlined in the following section.

Walking

The abnormalities of gait in stroke have been well-documented. Stroke patients walk with reduced speed and have difficulty to increase walking speed [34]. Impaired ankle power generation combined with saturation of hip power generation limits their potential to increase walking speed, especially in lower functioning hemiparetic subjects [34]. The abnormalities in the temporal patterning of lower extremity muscle activity have also been well-described in hemiparetic gait [35]. In the upper leg, durations of activity in hamstrings and rectus femoris were significantly prolonged. In the lower leg, longer total durations of gastrocnemius activity were found. Interestingly most of these disturbances are not limited to the paretic leg, but muscle activation patterns of the non-paretic leg also display some clear abnormalities. Such strong links between paretic and non-paretic side have also been noted in studies during obstacle avoidance in gait [36]. Over time, electromyographic abnormalities change only slightly. In particular, the durations of muscle (co-)activity and the level of swing phase asymmetry does not change much during rehabilitation [37]. In contrast, the level of ambulatory independence, body mobility, and maximum walking speed increases significantly, indicating that substantial improvements in gait ability occur. Apparently, physiological processes other than improved temporal muscular coordination must be important determinants of the restoration of ambulatory capacity after stroke.

Improvement of the function of walking is clearly one of the primary goals in stroke rehabilitation. Currently, most efforts include training on a treadmill with or without partial BWS but other physiotherapy approaches have been used as well, with limited success however (e.g. Glasgow Augmented Physiotherapy after Stroke (GAPS) Study Group; [38]). To evaluate the recovery, several measures have been used such as gait speed or stride length. The benefit of treadmill training has been well documented [39] and it was shown that there is a clear effect of the intensity of the training. Lamontagne and Fung (2004) demonstrated that fast walking on a treadmill induced marked speed-related improvements in body and limb kinematics and muscle activation patterns [40]. In contrast, BWS during overground walking increased gait speed to a lesser extent and only in low-functioning subjects. Nevertheless, it should be mentioned that one large study showed that locomotor training, including the use of BWS in stepping on a treadmill, was not superior to progressive exercises at home managed by a physical therapist [41].

In addition, several authors have attempted to further improve treadmill training by adding extra features. For example, Regnaux et al [2008] studied the effects of loading the unaffected limb during locomotor training and found that stroke participants significantly improved in walking speed, step length and cadence [42].

Weight-bearing on the paretic leg increased as well, along with kinematic improvements (greater hip and knee excursion). However, these adaptations were short-lived (20 min) and, therefore, the effects of longer-term locomotor retraining still need to be investigated. Similarly, in the future one may expect to see more combinations of treadmill training with dual tasks [43]. Indeed for stroke patients one has to take into account that asymmetric walking adds cognitive load by itself (as demonstrated by walking on a split-belt to simulate limping, see [44]).

Furthermore, walking is often associated with secondary tasks, such as obstacle avoidance. Post-stroke persons demonstrate markedly decreased obstacle avoidance success rates, in particular when time pressure is added [45]. They show normal avoidance strategies but have delayed and reduced muscle responses, smaller joint angle deviations from unperturbed walking, and smaller horizontal margins from the foot to the obstacle. In addition, it was shown that community-dwelling people with chronic stroke need disproportionate attention while walking and negotiating obstacles [46]. Proper selection of the best dual task will be required though since positive effects were not equally obtained with the various tasks tested so far.

Sitting balance and trunk control

Sitting balance and trunk control have been established as independent predictors of motor and functional outcome after stroke [47, 48]. The ability to regain sitting balance and trunk control is a core component of stroke rehabilitation, especially early after stroke. Trunk control is more than just sitting balance; it includes selective movements of shoulder and pelvic girdle as well and an important component is counter (i.e. the alternating) rotation between shoulder and pelvic girdle during normal and fast walking. Evidence of effective strategies to improve selective trunk control is scarce. Verheyden and colleagues showed that additional trunk rehabilitation exercises performed in supine and sitting have a beneficial effect on selective trunk movements in a sample of 33 people in the rehabilitation phase after stroke [49]. Saeys et al. provided a similar rehabilitation programme as the previously-mentioned study but for a longer period of time to 33 people in an earlier phase after stroke [50]. Their results showed again beneficial effects on trunk performance, but also on standing balance and mobility. Finally, Karthikbabu and colleagues showed stronger effects of trunk control exercises performed on a dynamic surface (i.e. physio ball) in comparison to the same exercises performed on a static surface (i.e. physio plinth) [51]. The effects were also not just seen in measures of trunk control but in assessments of functional balance as well. Possible reasons of increased effects of dynamic practice are an increased muscle activity with increased demands on (and thus learning of) postural control and voluntary trunk movements, and an increased response to postural perturbations when practising on a dynamic surface. This might positively influence the recruitment of high-threshold motor units of trunk muscles and have a positive effect on anticipatory postural adjustments [51].

Energy demands in stroke gait

Elevated energy demands are also of particular concern in stroke patients, especially in elderly individuals, because they promote activity intolerance with lower walking speed and a sedentary lifestyle that leads to physical deconditioning. This, in turn, compromises the patients' capacity to meet the energy-demanding gait, thus increasing the risk of cardiovascular disease and restraining social participation. Normal walking seems easy because it costs less than 50% of the maximal aerobic capacity and does not require anaerobic activity. A hemiparetic gait, however, draws on 75% of the maximal oxygen capacity, leaving little in reserve [52]. To this end, a physical conditioning programme can increase aerobic capacity, but decreasing the walking energy cost is quite challenging because it represents the ambulation task as such and is directly related to gait impairments. Effects on fitness have been assessed, using measures of cardiorespiratory physical fitness and gait endurance [53]. For example, using peak exercise capacity (VO$_2$ peak) and rate of oxygen consumption, studies of treadmill training with or without BWS convincingly showed that treadmill training improves physiological fitness in chronic stroke patients and decreased energy cost by 10% [54, 55].

Recent advances in gait rehabilitation using high doses of botulinum toxin injections, sophisticated orthoses of the lower or upper limbs and functional electrical stimulation combined with conventional rehabilitation programme have proven to be effective in enhancing impairments and locomotion ability in patients with stroke and have also been able to decrease the energy cost by 10% to 20% [56]. Many of these techniques also induced an improvement in gait speed; therefore gait assessments after training were often done at higher speed. However, mechanical energy levels and physiological energy cost were found to be higher in subjects with stroke who walked slower, as compared to those who walked faster [57]. When hemiparetic subjects following stroke are instructed to walk at faster speeds, the relative energy cost (per unit of distance travelled) actually decreased, suggesting that faster walking speeds may promote a more cost-effective gait pattern [58]. Indeed, in normal walking a minimum energy cost is reached at intermediate speeds (~4–5 km/h), which is the result of both mechanical factors (better exchange between potential and kinetic energy that reduces the mechanical muscle work) but also metabolic factors (greater efficiency of muscle contraction to provide mechanical work at intermediate speeds).Therefore, patients with pathological gait do not seem to necessarily choose the walking style that minimizes their metabolic energy costs. Furthermore, considering that the energy cost decreases with speed up to 4 km/h it is possible that the decrease seen in energy cost after many of the previous treatments was simply related to the change in gait speed. Hence it is important for future studies to consider assessing patients at similar speed before and after treatment.

Interventions to reduce energy costs

Despite considerable advances in treatments that have aimed at improving ambulation function in hemiparetic patients, the energy cost showed a limited decrease. Accordingly, effective and cost-efficient interventions that more specifically reduce energy costs are of the utmost need. Therefore, some recent techniques tried to address directly the main cause of the increased energy consumption in stroke in order to decrease the energy cost. The increased energy cost in hemiparetic gait seems to be primarily due to substantial muscle work provided by the non-paretic lower limb to excessively lift the body's centre of mass (CM) against gravity [57]. This excessive vertical CM is apart from the classical picture we usually have of people with gait deficits lumbering and limping, which is indirectly the expression of their CM

movement. This increase in the CM displacement is due to a compromised plantigrade movement of their ankle with a decreased knee flexion during the swing phase. Therefore, the CM vertical excursion is a compensatory strategy and may be increased up to three times more than normal to clear the limb during the swing phase and avoid stumbling. However, this strategy costs two to three times more energy [57]. Interestingly, energy consumption also doubled in able-bodied subjects when provided with a biofeedback of their CM displacement and asked to walk with excessive vertical displacement like stroke patients [59]. It has been postulated that humans would consume the least energy if they walk with their CM flat like a rolling wheel [60]. Hence the concept was adopted that fundamentally locomotion is the translation of the CM through space along a pathway requiring the least expenditure of energy. However, healthy Healthy subjects adopt an intermediate strategy of vertical CM displacement (3–4 cm at intermediate speeds) that is not as flat as a wheel but that minimizes energy consumption [59]. A pilot/feasibility study has thus been carried out in which six stroke patients were trained to decrease their vertical CM displacement with the help of a biofeedback to see if they could reduce their excessive CM displacement and so their energy cost ([61]; see Figure 18.2). The results indeed revealed that after only 6 weeks of training, stroke patients showed a marked decrease in their vertical CM displacement and their energy cost decreased by 30% (that is three times more decrease in three times less time than what has been reported for treadmill alone). The marked decrease in the energy cost was due to the parallel decrease in the total mechanical work provided by the muscles but also to the increase in the muscle efficiency to provide this work. As the patient gets closer to the intermediate optimal strategy that healthy individuals usually adopt, his energy consumption decreased. This suggests that the strategy the patient used before training was not necessarily the cheapest or most efficient one. This also contradicts the commonly held notion that a pathological gait may be viewed as an attempt to preserve the lowest level of energy consumption possible by exaggerations of the motions at unaffected levels [60]. It would thus be interesting to see the optimization constraints that may have led the patients to adopt this uneconomical strategy in the beginning. However, further RCTs are now underway by our group to validate this new promising treadmill training with the CM biofeedback which can also be combined with other aforementioned treatments to further improve walking and decrease energy consumption.

Treadmill training as task-specific training

An efficacious intervention that induces a motor skill acquisition would require active practice of close-to-normal movements, task-specificity, intensive practice (repetition), and focused attention [62, 63]. Modern concepts of gait rehabilitation favour a task-specific repetitive training—the patient who wants to relearn walking has to walk. Treadmill training enables the patient to perform repetitive and rhythmic stepping up to 1,000 steps in a 20-minute treadmill training session, compared to only 50 to 100 steps during a 20-minute session of conventional physiotherapy [64].

Biofeedback therapy

Biofeedback can be defined as the use of instrumentation to make covert physiological processes more overt. It provides patients with sensorimotor impairments with opportunities to regain

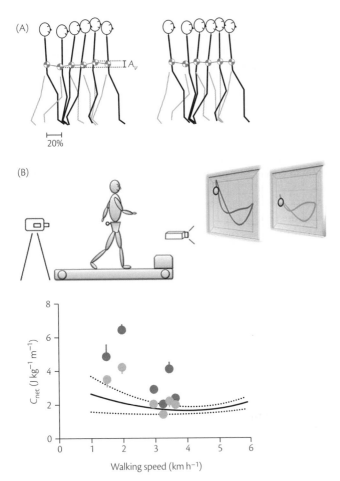

Fig. 18.2 Gait training with biofeedback of the body's centre of mass. (A) The stick figures show the segments' positions (right limb in thick lines) every 20% of a walking stride (i.e. beginning and ending with the paretic foot contact) for a patient with right hemiparesis walking naturally at self-selected speed (left figure) and trying to reduce his vertical CM displacement at the same speed (right figure). Av represents the vertical amplitude of the centre of mass. (B) The hourglass circle depicts the movement of the marker on the sacrum that represents the CM displacement and that is projected in front of the subject during the different conditions. This depicts the net energy cost as a function of walking speed in six stroke patients before (dark grey) versus after training (light grey). The results are compared with normal values of healthy adults walking at the same speed (solid line with dotted area (mean ± SD)).

Massaad F, Lejeune TM, Detrembleur C, Neurorehabil Neural Repai (24:4) pp. 338–47., copyright © 2010. Reprinted by Permission of SAGE Publications.

the ability to better assess different physiological responses and possibly to learn self-control of those responses. Many studies investigated the effects of biofeedback therapy on the treatment of motor deficits. The physiological sources to be fed back mainly included EMG to improve muscular control over a joint and angular or positional biofeedback to improve the patient's ability to self-regulate the movement of a specific joint. Parameters such as the CM or CoP were also often used as feedback sources during balance retraining programmes. Biofeedback provided during function-related task training is defined as task-oriented or 'dynamic biofeedback' (in comparison to static biofeedback). Effective biofeedback should re-educate the motor control system during dynamic movements that are functionally goal-oriented rather than relying primarily upon static control of a single

muscle or joint activity. During the training of functional tasks, it is important to choose the best information for feedback. The choice of a biofeedback vehicle should depend upon the training task and therapeutic goal. Often many variables should be considered, but using multiple indices provides another difficulty to patients whose cognition and perception may also be impaired. Designing a biofeedback system that overcomes the 'information overloading' obstacle is a challenge. An information/sensory fusion approach is one way to reduce information overload to patients during biofeedback therapy. Actually, an effective task-oriented biofeedback system requires: (i) orchestrated feedback of multiple variables that characterize the task performance without overwhelming a patient's perception and cognitive ability; (ii) attractive and motivating feedback to keep the subject attentive; and (iii) easy-to-understand cues to avoid the information overloading problem. The global approach using the whole body CM as a dynamic biofeedback appears to resolve this issue by simplifying the variables to be controlled by the patients [61].

One inherent limitation of biofeedback therapy is that patients with more severe motor or cognitive deficits cannot participate due to an inability to initiate any functional movement or understand the instructions, thus preventing utilization of biofeedback for improving performance. Rehabilitation robots or other devices could solve the problem in part by providing mechanical assistance for movement. However, as pointed out by Agrawal et al, moving the body through predetermined movement patterns rather than under the patient's own control would prevent relearning of typical patterns [65]. Possibly the most challenging question for all feedback approaches is whether the effect of feedback training is transferable to task performance in the real world. If this transition cannot be acquired, the biofeedback may not be applicable in motor rehabilitation.

In summary, future studies should probably be able to further improve walking in stroke by combining different treatment techniques (local or active training) and validating them into randomized controlled design. This would set the limits of any rehabilitation approach and validate its combination with the plethora of other treatments in stroke patients.

Can arm swing contribute to locomotor training?

Often arm swing is neglected in gait rehabilitation. Here the question I asked whether this is inappropriate and whether one should encourage arm swing instead. Some time ago, the point was made that bipedal and quadrupedal locomotion may share common spinal neuronal control mechanisms [66–68] (see Figure 18.3 for illustration).

During evolution, humans started to walk bipedally but the circuitry, previously used to drive the forelimbs during locomotion, remained functional to assist arm swing during gait (for review see [69]). Actually, Jackson and colleagues were the first to suggest that CPGs could be responsible for arm swing during locomotion [70], but evidence in support of this contention has only been obtained recently, mostly due to studies from the laboratories of Dietz and Zehr (reviewed in [69]).

Given this background it is natural that one has wondered whether one could not make use of interlimb facilitation for rehabilitation of locomotor activities. In fact, some studies on treadmill walking of SCI patients [71] or stroke [72] have claimed that arm movements could facilitate gait (for review see [69]). In one of

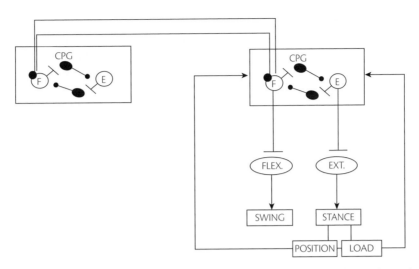

Fig. 18.3 Schematic representation of the current hypothesis about the spinal organization of locomotion and its reflex regulation. The central pattern generator (CPG) as originally described, contains F and E: flexor and extensor half-centre, controlling flexors (Flex.) and extensors (Ext.) respectively. Each limb is controlled by such a CPG (top: two arms, bottom two legs). Furthermore there are interconnections between these various CPGs. Some of these are schematically shown for the legs. Adapted from Swinnen S.P. & Duysens J. 2004 'Neuro-behavioral determinants of interlimb coordination – a multidisciplinary approach, with kind permission of Springer Science+Business Media.

these studies, the stroke patients walked while holding onto handles that could slide along handrails [72]. In such experiments it is difficult, however, to exclude that some of the effects are due to improved postural stability due to holding the rails. This complication can be avoided by using recumbent stepping, since subjects are sitting under these conditions, yet they can perform alternating arm and leg movements [73–75]. Muscle activity in passively moved legs was found to be increased by maximal arm exertion [73]. In contrast, arm movements did not facilitate muscle activity of maximally active legs either in control subjects [74] or in patients with SCI [75]. However, a ceiling effect (maximum muscle activation) could explain these negative findings and, therefore, there was a need to repeat these experiments with submaximally active legs [76]. In the latter study, it was found that in healthy controls the leg muscle activity was increased by active arm movements in most muscles investigated. In SCI patients such facilitation is much harder to prove because of the large variability. Nevertheless, in a recent study a group of nine SCI patients was tested and clear indications were found for a facilitation of some leg muscles by arm movements [76]. In particular, when the arm movements were decoupled from the stepper there was a significant facilitation in biceps femoris.

This raises the question whether arm movement need to be included in gait training. The use of gait assistance with robotic devices makes this question even more urgent as some of these devices do not allow arm movements to be performed while walking. In fact, subjects are often encouraged to hold the rails with their hands for additional support. However, this recent work on recumbent stepping suggests that for SCI it might be beneficial to combine rhythmic arm and leg movements while training on a treadmill.

Another approach taken to demonstrate the beneficial effect of combining arm and leg movements was the use of metabolic measurements. Meyns et al have studied whether the synchronous or asynchronous coordination between the arms would have a differential effect on measures of exercise intensity (i.e. oxygen

uptake, perceived exertion) either when cycling with the arms only or when combining arm cycling and leg cycling [77]. Their results indicate a clear metabolic benefit of combining arm and leg cycling rather than arm cycling only, especially when asynchronous arm cycling is used. Combining the results from previous studies in both spinal and healthy man, there appears to be growing evidence for the inclusion of arm movements in rehabilitation of gait, however, studies confirming these results in patients are currently scarce.

One such study, using a hybrid tricycle, clearly showed physical fitness and other benefits of combining rhythmic arm movements with functional electrical stimulation (FES)-induced leg cycling [78].

Practical treatment: some basic principles

Treatment is based on patient-centred goal setting, and the delivery of interventions aims to restore lost function or compensate for lost function when it cannot be restored, and importantly to support the individual to maintain optimal quality of life. It is widely accepted that motor training and exercises for gait and posture are absolutely essential ('use it or never get it (back)') for various types of neurology patients. Training rules are the same as for any type of training, but one has to be realistic in expectations (because of the presence of brain damage and decreased levels of fitness). For the same reason one should not underestimate the effort needed to relearn motor activity for these patients and adapt the frequency and duration of the training and recovery periods accordingly.

With respect to training, the focus here is on general principles of rehabilitation and motor learning of gait and posture. One of the important lessons from basic studies is that learning is context dependent (see also section. 'Neurorehabilitation and learning'). Therefore it is recommended to use 'task-oriented training', embedded in the environmental context of the individual (for example, compare task requirements for walking in a busy traffic environment or quiet hallway). In addition, the 'task' should be interpreted broadly enough. If the task is to relearn gait, the training should include not only leg movements but also the accompanying arm swing, walking at different speeds, various terrains, and with or without carrying objects.

Rehabilitation can never be seen to be independent of the natural environment of the patients and information about these constraints is thus mandatory for treatment planning. Clinical symptoms, such as spasticity, should not be the main focus of treatment. Rather, it is important to consider the implications of these clinical symptoms for training and the activities to be learned. In this respect it is important to consider the 'positive' value of some of these symptoms (spasticity as used for support for example, co-activation as a means to increase accuracy). Indeed sometimes patients can make use of their spasticity to support their motor actions. Failure to recognize this can lead to disappointing functional outcomes of medical treatments that focus mainly on clinical symptoms (surgery, botulinus toxin). Therefore it is recommended to make a complete movement analysis prior to such interventions. Careful assessments, based on advanced 3D recordings of posture and gait, can assist in making proper decisions about planned interventions, aimed at alleviating some clinical symptoms such as spasticity. In cases where spasticity is used to the advantage of the function of the patient, this should be taken into account before antispastic interventions are made.

Stroke

Despite convincing arguments that motor learning principles are relevant for stroke recovery and neurorehabilitation [79], information from large, multi-centre randomized controlled phase III trials is limited when it comes to balance and gait rehabilitation and results have not always been as expected. In fact, results from only one such trial were recently reported by Duncan and colleagues, who conducted the LEAPS trial, which tested the effect of locomotor training in 408 people more than 2 months after stroke with a moderate to severe walking deficit [41]. The LEAPS trial included three arms: a group initiating locomotor training by means of BWS and treadmill at 2 months post stroke, a group receiving a home exercise programme at 2 months post stroke, and a control group receiving usual care at 2 months and locomotor training at 6 months post stroke. Results showed no significant difference between any of the groups at 12 months post stroke. At 6 months post stroke, both the treadmill and home exercise group yielded significant better results than the control group. Despite non-significant differences between active conditions in the three trials discussed, these trials provide also convincing arguments that active therapy is better than 'usual' care. The challenge for neurorehabilitation after stroke remains to unravel the active and working component of therapy in relation to neurophysiological recovery and translate findings to areas and sample populations which have not profited from large multicentre trials yet. After all, differential effects for motor learning principles were suggested by the systematic review of Timmermans and colleagues [80]; the components 'distributed practice' and 'feedback' seem to be related to larger post-intervention effect sizes, and 'random practice' and 'use of clear functional goals' were more strongly related to follow-up effect sizes in 16 RCTs (528 people after stroke) evaluating the effect of task-oriented training, albeit for skilled arm-hand performance.

A recently updated Cochrane review by Mehrholz and colleagues investigated electromechanical and robot-assisted gait training devices for improving walking after stroke [81]. The authors included 17 trials with in total 837 participants and concluded that electromechanical-assisted gait training in combination with physiotherapy increased the chance of becoming an independent walker (odds ratio 2.21, 95% confidence interval 1.52 to 3.22). There was no significant effect on walking velocity or capacity. Heterogeneity of the studies included warrants caution when generalizing these findings. In summary, trials have been conducted where rehabilitation strategies incorporated principles of motor learning but overall, the level of evidence arising from these studies varies and limitations warrant caution when considering generalizability and implementation into clinical practice. Therefore, the different stages of research should be addressed in order to advance knowledge about motor learning in balance and gait rehabilitation after stroke (for a more in-depth discussion about aspects of the research pipeline, see [82]). Small-scale studies targeting individuals based on mechanistic principles might provide important first-step results. In a later stage, multicentre RCTs, which are sufficiently powered are needed to evaluate effectiveness in a more heterogeneous population.

Perspectives

To update rehabilitation tools it is essential to keep track of new technological developments. This includes new assessment tools as well. For example, from basic science studies on gait and balance it is increasingly clear that the motor system makes use of basic motor synergies that can be identified using advanced analytical tools. Identifying such synergies in patients allow to assess how well a given patient has returned to the use of 'normal' synergies. Furthermore, new insights in the neurophysiology of reflexes can assist the evaluation of progress of rehabilitation.

Modulation of reflexes as a marker of gait rehabilitation

From animal studies it is known that the motor control of locomotion involves not only the activation of motoneurones and muscles in an appropriate order, but also the control over the input to the motoneurons (Figure 18.4).

This requires a continuous regulation of the strength of reflexes during the gait cycle ('phase-dependent modulation' [83, 84]). Some of this modulation can be achieved already at the spinal level (through CPGs), while other aspects require supraspinal input [85]. Since these structures are essential for reflex modulation, it follows that one can assess damage and recovery of locomotor control through the study of the modulation of reflexes during gait.

Most work along this line has been performed using the study of H-reflexes during gait. In healthy people with no neurological impairments, the soleus H-reflex increases during the stance phase and depresses during the swing phase. However, in patients with central nervous system lesions the size of the soleus H-reflex is typically altered when compared to a healthy control group [86]. The modulation pattern can also be abnormal [86]. Hence, one can have a benefit from studying the reflex modulation in this type of patients since this can provide information on the recovery of supraspinal input.

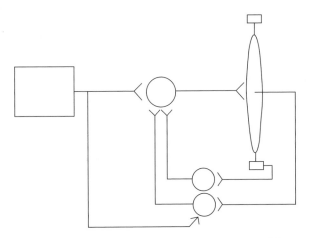

Fig. 18.4 Illustration of the control of reflex pathways. The output of the central nervous system is not only to motoneurones but also to pathways feeding into these motoneurons (and providing feedback from muscle receptors as well as from cutaneous or joint afferents).

Challenging locomotor tasks

Gait as trained on a treadmill has its limitations. In daily life the patients have to walk over uneven terrain, clear obstacles and listen to accompanying persons. Hence it can be argued that the use of more challenging locomotor tasks (obstacle avoidance, looking sideways, precision stepping, dual tasking, etc.) can enrich gait training by making it more realistic and related to daily life circumstances (Figure 18.5). Treadmill training can be adapted to include stepping over real obstacles [87, 88] (Figure 18.5).

Virtual obstacles on a treadmill were used by the group of Brown and compared to the use of real obstacles on a walkway [89]. They found that poststroke patients showed clinically meaningful changes in gait characteristics and in obstacle clearance capacity as a result of either training method but virtual obstacle training was superior (greater improvements in gait velocity compared with real training). These changes persisted for 2 weeks post-training. Virtual obstacle training can now be performed on a treadmill with commercial systems [90].

Subject-specific modelling

The use of integrated 3D motion capture has been advantageous in objectifying gait impairments in stroke subjects in terms of joint angles, joint moments, and powers. Based on these parameters and in combination with surface EMG measurements, classification studies aim to relate neural damage, control impairment and gross motor function [91, 92]. However, the use of these descriptive studies to understand gait impairments has some important limitations [93]. Measuring EMG activity gives information on the relative timing of muscle activations; however it is complicated to relate this directly to individual muscle force. Furthermore, due to dynamic coupling [94] muscles are able to act on joints that they do not span and on segments they are not attached to. It is therefore difficult to relate the contribution of an individual muscle to the resulting motion of the body (e.g. CM or individual joint angles). To determine causal relationships between muscle activity and the resulting motion, forward simulation studies are needed. Currently, dedicated algorithms (e.g. CMC; [95]) are available that

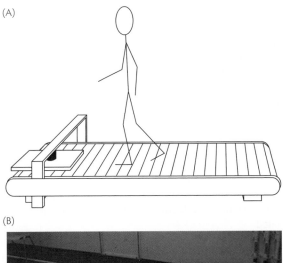

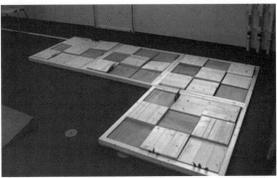

Fig. 18.5 Example of set-up to test and train obstacle avoidance on a treadmill (A) or to train stepping on uneven terrain (B), as was used by the authors in their laboratory in Nijmegen.

calculate muscle excitations based on numerical optimization. When applied on a complex dynamic model, these excitations are able to track experimentally measured kinematics with high accuracy and to reproduce the gait impairments observed in individual stroke subjects.

Studies by Petersen et al. and Higginson et al. used simulations to investigate how impaired muscle coordination after stroke influences support and progression of the COM during hemiplegic gait [96–98]. They found that during mid stance, both paretic and non-paretic leg plantarflexors contributed less to support than in the speed-matched control subject. This was compensated for by larger paretic leg knee extensors and gluteus maximus contributions to support [99]. Peterson et al. also found a decreased contribution of paretic leg plantarflexors and gluteus medius to propulsion during preswing [97]. Even though an increased contribution to propulsion was found of non-paretic knee extensors, this was counteracted by a simultaneous increased deceleration contribution of the non-paretic hamstrings. Jansen et al. furthered these insights by comparing the changes in muscle contributions observed in stroke subjects to muscle contributions during asymmetric gait in control subjects walking on a split-belt treadmill [100]. They conclude that the observed contributions in gluteus maximus, knee extensors, plantar-, and dorsiflexors may relate more to the limping-pattern itself, as they were also present during asymmetric gait in control subjects. However, modulations in gluteus medius and hamstrings found after stroke were different from modulations in split-belt walking, and these are therefore related to concomitant motor deficits.

The dynamic simulations presented so far, calculate muscle excitations and forces that underlie the experimental kinematics using specific tracking algorithms that are based on pure mechanical criteria. The human body is therefore considered as a pure mechanical system, while it is inherently a cybernetic system with information-based feedback by neural processes playing an important role. Therefore, incorporation of a neural control model is necessary to elucidate the relation between neural damage, control impairment and gross motor function during gait.

Some highly detailed models were defined in the past that included different types of neural feedback [101, 102] to generate a stable gait pattern rather than accurately reproducing the joint kinematics during normal gait. Furthermore, the performance of these models in reproducing specific gait impairments was not evaluated.

To investigate the complexity of the neural control strategy involved in controlling gait, a low-dimensional modular organization of muscle activation was incorporated in simulations of normal gait by using muscle activation modules that drive the muscle excitations [103]. Whereas five modules satisfy the sagittal plane biomechanical sub-tasks of 2D walking, a sixth module, which contributes primarily to mediolateral balance control and contralateral leg swing, is needed to account for the non-sagittal plane demands of 3D walking [104, 105]. These results provide evidence that a simple neural control strategy involving muscle activation modules may be used to control gait in healthy control subjects. Experimentally, it is confirmed that stroke subjects rely on fewer muscle activation modules that are composed from merging modules observed in healthy controls. However, so far, it could not be confirmed that imposing these reduced number of activation modules is likely to induce hemiparetic gait features. These simulations would confirm that the reduced independence of neural control signals contributes to the specific gait impairments observed in stroke subjects.

To investigate the contribution of increased length and velocity feedback, and altered reflex modulation pattern to hemiparetic gait impairments, Jansen et al. extended the classic musculoskeletal model with a neural model and a foot-ground contact model 106]. They used this neuromechanical model to examine the effect of increased muscle spindle feedback of soleus, gastrocnemius, rectus femoris, and vasti, along with altered modulation patterns on gait kinematics. They showed that increased length and velocity feedback induced gait deviations which are in accordance with previously reported hemiparetic gait impairments—that is, either an 'extended' pattern (in case of increased vastus, rectus femoris and soleus feedback)—or a 'flexed' pattern (increased gastrocnemius feedback [92]). Furthermore, altered modulation patterns of the reflex feedback loop were found to play an important role in controlling the expression of the increased length and velocity feedback, especially in the swing phase. They were unable to confirm phase dependency for the effect of increased length and velocity feedback on joint kinematics.

Conclusion

Simulation studies are only beginning to reach the level of neurophysiologic detail needed to understand the relation between neural damage, control deficit, and gait impairments. Nevertheless, the insights obtained are promising and encouraging that in the future they may provide a useful tool supporting clinical decision making by predicting treatment outcome in an individual stroke patient.

Final remarks

In view of the limited space there is no room here to discuss some other exciting new approaches. For example, currently high expectations are present with respect to new methods such as tDCS (transcranial direct current stimulation). This technique generates a wide scientific interest nowadays, probably because of the fact that the application of tDCS is relatively easy and simple, not overly expensive, has little to no adverse effects and shows potential to improve motor outcome after stroke. In fact, its application may go wider. For example, many patients who have stroke will have small vessel disease and leukoaraiosis, leading to gait apraxia. Recent evidence suggests that combined anodal tDCS and physical therapy improves gait and balance in this patient group, suggesting that tDCS could be an effective tool in patients with leukoaraiosis, for whom no treatment is currently available [107].

Acknowledgements

This project was supported by grant OT/08/034 & PDMK/12/180. JD was supported by grants from IDO (07/012) and F.W.O. (grant G.0901.11), FM by a Postdoctoral fellowship and a Navorser grant of FWO, an F+ fellowship from KU Leuven and a scientific prize (Van Goethem-Brichant).

References

1. Kirshblum SC, Burns SP, Biering-Sorensen F, et al. International standards for neurological classification of spinal cord injury revised 2011. J Spinal Cord Med. 2011;**34**(6):535–546.
2. Mayo NE, Wood-Dauphinee S, Ahmed S, et al. Disablement following stroke. Disabil Rehabil. 1999;**21**(5–6):258–268.
3. Geurts ACH, de Haart M, van Nes IJW, Duysens J. A review of standing balance recovery from stroke. Gait Posture. 2005;**22**(3):267–281.
4. Grillner S. Neurobiological bases of rhythmic motor acts in vertebrates. Science. 1985;**228**(4696):143–148.
5. Duysens J, Clarac F, Cruse H. Load-regulating mechanisms in gait and posture: Comparative aspects. Physiol Rev. 2000;**80**(1):83–133.
6. Dietz V. Neuronal plasticity after a human spinal cord injury: Positive and negative effects. Exp Neurol. 2012;**235**(1):110–115.
7. Dietz V, Colombo G, Jensen L. Locomotor activity in spinal man. Lancet. 199;**344**(8932):1260–1263.
8. Hubli M, Dietz V. The physiological basis of neurorehabilitation—locomotor training after spinal cord injury. J Neuroeng Rehabil. 2013 ;**10**:5. doi: 10.1186/1743-0003-10-5.
9. Dietz V. Body weight supported gait training: From laboratory to clinical setting. Brain Res Bull. 2008 Jul 30;**76**(5):459–463.
10. Harkema SJ, Hurley SL, Patel UK, Requejo PS, Dobkin BH, Edgerton VR. Human lumbosacral spinal cord interprets loading during stepping. J Neurophysiol. 1997;**77**(2):797–811.
11. Beres-Jones JA, Harkema SJ. The human spinal cord interprets velocity-dependent afferent input during stepping. Brain. 2004;**127**:2232–2246.
12. Dietz V, Colombo G, Jensen L, Baumgartner L. Locomotor capacity of spinal cord in paraplegic patients. Ann Neurol. 1995;**37**(5):574–582.
13. Protas EJ, Holmes SA, Qureshy H, Johnson A, Lee D, Sherwood AM. Supported treadmill ambulation training after spinal cord injury: a pilot study. Arch Phys Med Rehabil. 2001;**82**(6):825–831.

14. van de Crommert HWAA, Rijken H, Nienhuis B, van Kuppevelt D, Mulder T, Duysens J. Effects of locomotor training with body-weight support in spinal cord injured patients long after injury. In: Duysens J, Smits-Engelsman BCM, Kingma H (eds) Control of Posture and Gait, NPI, Maastricht, The Netherlands, 2001, pp. 773–776.

15. Kawashima N, Taguchi D, Nakazawa K, Akai M. Effect of lesion level on the orthotic gait performance in individuals with complete paraplegia. Spinal Cord. 2006;**44**(8):487–494.

16. Lam T, Eng JJ, Wolfe DL, Hsieh JT, Whittaker M. A systematic review of the efficacy of gait rehabilitation strategies for spinal cord injury. Top Spinal Cord Inj Rehabil. 2007;**13**(1):32–57.

17. Dietz V, Grillner S, Trepp A, Hubli M, Bolliger M. Changes in spinal reflex and locomotor activity after a complete spinal cord injury: a common mechanism. Brain. 2009;**132**:2196–2205.

18. Wernig A, Muller S. Laufband locomotion with body weight support improved walking in persons with severe spinal cord injuries. Paraplegia. 1992;**30**(4):229–238.

19. Verheyden GS, Weerdesteyn V, Pickering RM, Kunkel D, Lennon S, Geurts AC, Ashburn A. Interventions for preventing falls in people after stroke. Cochrane Database Syst Rev. 2013;**5**:CD008728.

20. Goldie PA, Matyas TA, Spencer KI, McGinley RB. Postural control in standing following stroke: test-retest reliability of some quantitative clinical tests. Phys Ther. 1990;**70**(4):234–243.

21. Eng JJ, Chu KS. Reliability and comparison of weight-bearing ability during standing tasks for individuals with chronic stroke. Arch Phys Med Rehabil. 2002;**83**(8):1138–1144.

22. Dietz V, Berger W. Interlimb coordination of posture in patients with spastic paresis—impaired function of spinal reflexes. Brain. 1984;**107**:965–978.

23. Pinter MM, Brainin M. Rehabilitation after stroke in older people. Maturitas. 2012;**71**(2):104–108.

24. Krakauer JW, Carmichael ST, Corbett D, Wittenberg GF. Getting neurorehabilitation right: what can be learned from animal models? Neurorehabil Neural Repair. 2012;**26**(8):923–931.

25. Ioffe ME, Chernikova LA, Umarova RM, Katsuba NA, Kulikov MA. Learning postural tasks in hemiparetic patients with lesions of left versus right hemisphere. Exp Brain Res. 2010 Apr;**201**(4):753–761.

26. Bronstein AM, Pavlou M. Balance. Handb Clin Neurol 2013;**110**:189–208.

27. de Haart M, Geurts AC, Dault MC, Nienhuis B, Duysens J. Restoration of weight-shifting capacity in patients with postacute stroke: A rehabilitation cohort study. Arch Phys Med Rehabil. 2005;**86**(4):755–762.

28. Tsaklis PV, Grooten WJA, Franzen E. Effects of weight-shift training on balance control and weight distribution in chronic stroke: a pilot study. Top Stroke Rehabil. 2012;**19**(1):23–31.

29. van Nes IJW, Geurts ACH, Hendricks HT, Duysens J. Short-term effects of whole-body vibration on postural control in unilateral chronic stroke patients: Preliminary evidence. Am J Phys Med Rehabil. 2004;**83**(11):867–873.

30. van Nes IJW, Latour H, Schils F, Meijer R, van Kuijk A, Geurts ACH. Long-term effects of 6-week whole-body vibration on balance recovery and activities of daily living in the postacute phase of stroke—A randomized, controlled trial. Stroke. 2006;**37**(9):2331–2335.

31. Lau RWK, Yip SP, Pang MYC. Whole-Body Vibration Has No Effect on Neuromotor Function and Falls in Chronic Stroke. Med Sci Sports Exerc. 2012;**44**(8):1409–1418.

32. Cho KH, Lee KJ, Song CH. Virtual-Reality Balance Training with a Video-Game System Improves Dynamic Balance in Chronic Stroke Patients. Tohoku J Exp Med. 2012;**228**(1):69–74.

33. Van Peppen RPS, Kortsmit M, Lindeman E, Kwakkel G. Effects of visual feedback therapy on postural control in bilateral standing after stroke: A systematic review. J Rehabil Med. 2006;**38**(1):3–9.

34. Jonkers I, Delp S, Patten C. Capacity to increase walking speed is limited by impaired hip and ankle power generation in lower functioning persons post-stroke. Gait Posture. 2009;**29**(1):129–137.

35. den Otter AR, Geurts ACH, Mulder T, Duysens J. Abnormalities in the temporal patterning of lower extremity muscle activity in hemiparetic gait. Gait Posture. 2007;**25**(3):342–352.

36. Kloter E, Wirz M, Dietz V. Locomotion in stroke subjects: interactions between unaffected and affected sides. Brain. 2011;**134**:721–731.

37. den Otter AR, Geurts ACH, Mulder T, Duysens J. Gait recovery is not associated with changes in the temporal patterning of muscle activity during treadmill walking in patients with post-stroke hemiparesis. Clin Neurophysiol. 2006;**117**(1):4–15.

38. van de Port IG, Wevers LE, Lindeman E, Kwakkel G. Effects of circuit training as alternative to usual physiotherapy after stroke: randomised controlled trial. Br Med J. 2012;**344**:e2672.

39. Kwakkel G, van Peppen R, Wagenaar RC, et al. Effects of augmented exercise therapy time after stroke—A meta-analysis. Stroke. 2004;**35**(11):2529–2536.

40. Lamontagne A, Fung J. Faster is better—Implications for speed-intensive gait training after stroke. Stroke. 2004;**35**(11):2543–2548.

41. Duncan PW, Sullivan KJ, Behrman AL, et al. Body-weight-supported treadmill rehabilitation after stroke. N Engl J Med. 2011;**364**(21):2026–2036.

42. Regnaux JP, Pradon D, Roche N, Robertson J, Bussel B, Dobkin B. Effects of loading the unaffected limb for one session of locomotor training on laboratory measures of gait in stroke. Clin Biomech Bristol, Avon. 2008;**23**(6):762–768.

43. Regnaux JP, David D, Daniel O, Ben Smail D, Combeaud M, Bussel B. Evidence for cognitive processes involved in the control of steady state of walking in healthy subjects and after cerebral damage. Neurorehabil Neural Repair 2005;**19**(2):125–132.

44. McFadyen BJ, Hegeman J, Duysens J. Dual task effects for asymmetric stepping on a split-belt treadmill. Gait Posture. 2009;**30**(3):340–344.

45. van Swigchem R, van Duijnhoven HJR, den Boer J, Geurts AC, Weerdesteyn V. Deficits in motor response to avoid sudden obstacles during gait in functional walkers poststroke. Neurorehabil Neural Repair. 2013;**27**(3):230–239.

46. Smulders K, van Swigchem R, de Swart BJM, Geurts ACH, Weerdesteyn V. Community-dwelling people with chronic stroke need disproportionate attention while walking and negotiating obstacles. Gait Posture. 2012;**36**(1):127–132.

47. Verheyden G, Nieuwboer A, De WL, et al. Trunk performance after stroke: an eye catching predictor of functional outcome. J Neurol Neurosurg Psychiatry. 2007;**78**(7):694–698.

48. Kwakkel G, Kollen BJ. Predicting activities after stroke: what is clinically relevant? Int J Stroke. 2013;**8**(1):25–32.

49. Verheyden G, Vereeck L, Truijen S, et al. Additional exercises improve trunk performance after stroke: a pilot randomized controlled trial. Neurorehabil Neural Repair. 2009;**23**(3):281–286.

50. Saeys W, Vereeck L, Truijen S, Lafosse C, Wuyts FP, Heyning PV. Randomized controlled trial of truncal exercises early after stroke to improve balance and mobility. Neurorehabil Neural Repair. 2012;**26**(3):231–238.

51. Karthikbabu S, Nayak A, Vijayakumar K, et al. Comparison of physio ball and plinth trunk exercises regimens on trunk control and functional balance in patients with acute stroke: a pilot randomized controlled trial. Clin Rehabil. 2011;**25**(8):709–719.

52. Waters RL, Mulroy S. The energy expenditure of normal and pathologic gait. Gait Posture. 1999;**9**(3):207–231.

53. Saunders DH, Greig CA, Mead GE, Young A. Physical fitness training for stroke patients. Cochrane Database Syst Rev. 2009;(4):CD003316.

54. Macko RF, Smith GV, Dobrovolny CL, Sorkin JD, Goldberg AP, Silver KH. Treadmill training improves fitness reserve in chronic stroke patients. Arch Phys Med Rehabil. 2001;**82**(7):879–884.

55. Mackay-Lyons M, McDonald A, Matheson J, Eskes G, Klus MA. Dual effects of body-weight supported treadmill training on

cardiovascular fitness and walking ability early after stroke: a randomized controlled trial. Neurorehabil Neural Repair. 2013;27(7):644–653.

56. Thijssen DH, Paulus R, van Uden CJ, Kooloos JG, Hopman MT. Decreased energy cost and improved gait pattern using a new orthosis in persons with long-term stroke. Arch Phys Med Rehabil. 2007;88(2):181–186.

57. Detrembleur C, Dierick F, Stoquart G, Chantraine F, Lejeune T. Energy cost, mechanical work, and efficiency of hemiparetic walking. Gait Posture. 2003;18(2):47–55.

58. Hesse S, Werner C, Paul T, Bardeleben A, Chaler J. Influence of walking speed on lower limb muscle activity and energy consumption during treadmill walking of hemiparetic patients. Arch Phys Med Rehabil. 2001;82(11):1547–1550.

59. Massaad F, Lejeune TM, Detrembleur C. The up and down bobbing of human walking: a compromise between muscle work and efficiency. J Physiol. 2007 Jul 15;582(Pt 2):789–799.

60. Saunders JB, Inman VT, Eberhart HD. The major determinants in normal and pathological gait. J Bone Joint Surg Am. 1953;35-A3:543–558.

61. Massaad F, Lejeune TM, Detrembleur C. Reducing the energy cost of hemiparetic gait using center of mass feedback: a pilot study. Neurorehabil Neural Repair. 2010;24(4):338–347.

62. Nudo RJ, Wise BM, SiFuentes F, Milliken GW. Neural substrates for the effects of rehabilitative training on motor recovery after ischemic infarct. Science. 1996;272(5269):1791–1794.

63. Dobkin BH. Strategies for stroke rehabilitation. Lancet Neurol. 2004;3(9):528–536.

64. Hesse S. Gait training after stroke: a critical reprisal. Ann Readapt Med Phys. 2006;49(8):621–624.

65. Agrawal SK, Banala SK, Fattah A, et al. Assessment of motion of a swing leg and gait rehabilitation with a gravity balancing exoskeleton. IEEE Trans Neural Syst Rehabil Eng. 2007;15(3):410–420.

66. Zehr EP, Duysens J. Regulation of arm and leg movement during human locomotion. Neuroscientist. 2004;10(4):347–361.

67. Dietz V. Do human bipeds use quadrupedal coordination? Trends Neurosci. 2002;25(9):462–467.

68. Dietz V. Quadrupedal coordination of bipedal gait: implications for movement disorders. J Neurol 2011 Aug;258(8):1406–1412.

69. Meyns P, Bruijn SM, Duysens J. The how and why of arm swing during human walking. Gait Posture 2013;38(4):555–562.

70. Jackson KM, Joseph J, Wyard SJ. A mathematical model of arm swing during human locomotion. J Biomech. 1978;11(6–7):277–289.

71. Behrman AL, Harkema SJ. Locomotor training after human spinal cord injury: a series of case studies. Phys Ther. 2000;80(7):688–700.

72. Stephenson JL, De Serres SJ, Lamontagne A. The effect of arm movements on the lower limb during gait after a stroke. Gait Posture. 2010;31(1):109–115.

73. Huang HJ, Ferris DP. Neural coupling between upper and lower limbs during recumbent stepping. J Appl Physiol. 2004;97(4):1299–1308.

74. Huang HJ, Ferris DP. Upper and lower limb muscle activation is bidirectionally and ipsilaterally coupled. Med Sci Sports Exerc. 2009;41(9):1778–1789.

75. Huang HJ, Ferris DP. Upper limb effort does not increase maximal voluntary muscle activation in individuals with incomplete spinal cord injury. Clin Neurophysiol. 2009;120(9):1741–1749.

76. de Kam D, Rijken H, Manintveld T, Nienhuis B, Dietz V, Duysens J. Arm movements can increase leg muscle activity during sub-maximal recumbent stepping in neurologically intact individuals. J Appl Physiol. 2013;115(1):34–42.

77. Meyns P, Van de Walle P, Hoogkamer W, Kiekens C, Desloovere K, Duysens J Coordinating arms and legs on a hybrid rehabilitation tricycle: the metabolic benefit of asymmetrical compared to symmetrical arm movements. Eur J Appl Physiol. 2014;114(4):743–750.

78. Heesterbeek PJC, Berkelmans HWA, Thijssen DHJ, van Kuppevelt HJM, Hopman MTE, Duysens J. Increased physical fitness after

79. Krakauer JW. Motor learning: its relevance to stroke recovery and neurorehabilitation. Curr Opin Neurol. 2006;19(1):84–90.

80. Timmermans AA, Spooren AI, Kingma H, Seelen HA. Influence of task-oriented training content on skilled arm-hand performance in stroke: a systematic review. Neurorehabil Neural Repair. 2010;24(9):858–870.

81. Mehrholz J, Werner C, Kugler J, Pohl M. Electromechanical-assisted training for walking after stroke. Cochrane Database Syst Rev. 2007;(4):CD006185.

82. Ward NS. Getting lost in translation. Curr Opin Neurol. 2008;21(6):625–627.

83. Forssberg H, Grillner S, Rossignol S. Phase dependent reflex reversal during walking in chronic spinal cats. Brain Res. 1975;85(1):103–107.

84. Duysens J, Pearson KG. The role of cutaneous afferents from the distal hindlimb in the regulation of the step cycle of thalamic cats. Exp Brain Res. 1976;24:245–255.

85. Duysens J, Baken BC, Burgers L, Plat FM, den Otter AR, Kremer HP. Cutaneous reflexes from the foot during gait in hereditary spastic paraparesis. Clin Neurophysiol. 2004;115(5):1057–1062.

86. Hodapp M, Klisch C, Mall V, Vry J, Berger W, Faist M. Modulation of soleus H-reflexes during gait in children with cerebral palsy. J Neurophysiol. 2007;98(6):3263–3268.

87. Lam T, Dietz V. Transfer of motor performance in an obstacle avoidance task to different walking conditions. J Neurophysiol. 2004;92(4):2010–2016.

88. van Hedel HJA, Biedermann A, Erni T, Dietz V. Obstacle avoidance during human walking: transfer of motor skill from one leg to the other. J Physiol. 2002;543(2):709–717.

89. Jaffe DL, Brown DA, Pierson-Carey CD, Buckley EL, Lew HL. Stepping over obstacles to improve walking in individuals with poststroke hemiplegia. J Rehabil Res Dev. 2004;41(3A):283–292.

90. van Ooijen MW, Roerdink M, Trekop M, Visschedijk J, Janssen TW, Beek PJ. Functional gait rehabilitation in elderly people following a fall-related hip fracture using a treadmill with visual context: design of a randomized controlled trial. BMC Geriatr. 2013;13:34.

91. Knutsson E, Richards C. Different types of disturbed motor control in gait of hemiparetic patients. Brain. 1979;102(2):405–430.

92. Mulroy S, Gronley J, Weiss W, Newsam C, Perry J. Use of cluster analysis for gait pattern classification of patients in the early and late recovery phases following stroke. Gait Posture. 2003;18(1):114–125.

93. Delp SL, Anderson FC, Arnold AS, et al. OpenSim: open-source software to create and analyze dynamic simulations of movement. IEEE Trans Biomed Eng. 2007;54(11):1940–1950.

94. Zajac FE, Gordon ME. Determining muscle's force and action in multi-articular movement. Exerc Sport Sci Rev. 1989;17:187–230.

95. Thelen DG, Anderson FC. Using computed muscle control to generate forward dynamic simulations of human walking from experimental data. J Biomech. 2006;39(6):1107–1115.

96. Peterson CL, Cheng J, Kautz SA, Neptune RR. Leg extension is an important predictor of paretic leg propulsion in hemiparetic walking. Gait Posture. 2010;32(4):451–456.

97. Peterson CL, Kautz SA, Neptune RR. Muscle work is increased in pre-swing during hemiparetic walking. Clin Biomech Bristol, Avon. 2011;26(8):859–866.

98. Higginson JS, Zajac FE, Neptune RR, Kautz SA, Burgar CG, Delp SL. Effect of equinus foot placement and intrinsic muscle response on knee extension during stance. Gait Posture. 2006;23(1):32–36.

99. Higginson JS, Zajac FE, Neptune RR, Kautz SA, Delp SL. Muscle contributions to support during gait in an individual with post-stroke hemiparesis. J Biomech. 2006;39(10):1769–1777.

100. Jansen K, De Groote F, Aerts W, De Schutter J, Duysens J, Jonkers I. Altering length and velocity feedback during a

4-week training on a new hybrid FES-cycle in persons with spinal cord injury. Technol Disabil. 2005;17(2):103–110.

neuro-musculoskeletal simulation of normal gait contributes to hemiparetic gait characteristics. J Neuroeng Rehabil. 2014;**11**:78.

101. Ogihara N, Yamazaki N. Generation of human bipedal locomotion by a bio-mimetic neuro-musculo-skeletal model. Biol Cybern. 2001;**84**(1):1–11.

102. Paul C, Bellotti M, Jezernik S, Curt A. Development of a human neuro-musculo-skeletal model for investigation of spinal cord injury. Biol Cybern. 2005;**93**(3):153–170.

103. Clark DJ, Ting LH, Zajac FE, Neptune RR, Kautz SA. Merging of healthy motor modules predicts reduced locomotor performance and muscle coordination complexity post-stroke. J Neurophysiol. 2010;**103**(2):844–857.

104. Allen JL, Neptune RR. Three-dimensional modular control of human walking. J Biomech. 2012;**45**(12):2157–2163.

105. Neptune RR, Clark DJ, Kautz SA. Modular control of human walking: a simulation study. J Biomech. 2009;**42**(9):1282–1287.

106. Jansen K, De Groote F, Duysens J, Jonkers I. Muscle contributions to center of mass acceleration adapt to asymmetric walking in healthy subjects. Gait Posture. 2013;**38**(4):739–744.

107. Kaski D, Dominguez RO, Allum JH, Bronstein AM. Improving gait and balance in patients with leukoaraiosis using transcranial direct current stimulation and physical training: an exploratory study. Neurorehabil Neural Repair. 2013;**27**(9):864–871.

CHAPTER 19

Neurorehabilitation approaches for disorders of the peripheral nervous system

William Huynh, Michael Lee, and Matthew Kiernan

Introduction

Disorders of the peripheral nervous system (PNS), either traumatic or non-traumatic in nature, may involve various levels from motor neurons in the spinal cord, emerging spinal nerve roots, brachial or lumbosacral plexus, to the peripheral nerves. Lesions can be focal, as in most cases of traumatic aetiology, or multifocal or generalized as commonly seen in non-traumatic causes. Current therapy aims at reversing the underlying cause of the nerve lesion, whilst at the same time, treat symptoms such as pain that may arise as a consequence of the lesion. In the case of traumatic lesions, surgery may be considered to remove the insult (such as nerve compression) or repair the nerve, to thereby facilitate the process of nerve regeneration. As such, the focus of this chapter relates to rehabilitation in patients diagnosed with lesions affecting the PNS. Depending on the nature of the underlying disorder, treatment goals are directed at the maintenance of strength and function, particularly in disorders that are reversible, or in the case of chronic disease, to prevent the progression of weakness and thereby resultant disability.

Traumatic lesions of the peripheral nervous system

Trauma disrupts the structural integrity of the axon and its surrounding myelin sheath. Traumatic nerve lesions may induce scattered damage, with distal axonal degeneration (Wallerian degeneration), a process known as *axonotmesis* [1]. In such an instance, regeneration of axons from the lesion site to the target is required before full clinical recovery may develop. However, a shorter period of recovery may be possible in the case of collateral sprouting and reinnervation for partial lesions [2]. *Neurotmesis* involves lesions of the entire nerve and its supportive sheath, that usually requires nerve grafting for effective treatment, although tends to have a poor prognosis with only partial recovery [1]. On the other hand, *neuropraxia* has a better prognosis as there is no loss of axonal continuity [2], although typically there is conduction block at the lesion site determined by electrophysiological studies (e.g. compressive lesions such as ulnar neuropathy at the elbow or peroneal neuropathy at the fibular neck). Neuropraxis may induce focal demyelination at the site of trauma with subsequent conduction slowing or block. Functional improvements are typically accompanied by resolution of conduction block within days or weeks following removal of the initial insult.

Non-traumatic lesions of the peripheral nervous system

PNS disorders of a non-traumatic nature are a heterogeneous group, in which one or more elements of the peripheral nervous system architecture become damaged, typically the myelin, the axon, or a mixture of the two. Demyelination produces dysfunction which may be rapidly reversed, while axonal damage with repair by regeneration or sprouting from intact elements may take many months, with recovery often incomplete [3]. In this chapter, the term *peripheral neuropathy* will be used to denote non-traumatic disorders of the PNS.

Peripheral neuropathies may be genetic or acquired in nature, some with insidious onset, whilst others tend to be more acute [3]. The natural history of neuropathy is dependent on the underlying aetiology, with acute neuropathies such as acute inflammatory demyelinating polyradiculoneuropathy (Guillain–Barré syndrome) reaching their maximal deficit acutely, followed by gradual recovery. Conversely, chronic inflammatory demyelinating polyradiculoneuropathy (CIDP) tends to relapse and remit, or gradually deteriorate over years (e.g. hereditary motor sensory neuropathy and alcohol-related neuropathy). The most common presentation for peripheral neuropathies is a symmetrical length-dependent polyneuropathy with variable sensory and motor components, depending on the aetiology. Most peripheral neuropathies begin by first affecting sensory nerve fibres, with gradual involvement of motor axons as the disease progresses. There are certain disorders, however, that only have motor involvement, such as multifocal motor neuropathy and some forms of inherited distal motor neuropathies.

Diabetes remains the most common cause of peripheral neuropathy and is present in more than 50% of patients with diabetes [4, 5]. Other common systemic causes include a range of metabolic disorders such as kidney disease, infectious agents such as human immunodeficiency virus (HIV), toxic processes such as chemotherapy and alcohol, immune-mediated and vasculitic disorders, and inherited polyneuropathies such as hereditary motor sensory neuropathy (also known as Charcot–Marie–Tooth disease, CMT). A substantial proportion of peripheral neuropathies (estimated around 30%) remain idiopathic [6].

Pathophysiology and clinical symptoms

Wallerian degeneration

Disruption of axonal integrity results in stereotypical nerve fibre degeneration distal to the focus of injury, with the earliest changes observed at the motor terminal of the neuromuscular junction [7]. Normal end-plate structures become altered within 3 to 5 hours after loss of spontaneous end-plate potentials. Axonal degeneration with collapse of the supportive microtubules and neurofilaments, accompanied by diminishing axoplasmic volume, rapidly ensues. Changes within the soma and proximal stump become evident within days, reaching a peak over weeks.

Weakness and muscle atrophy

Structural and chemical changes take place in denervated muscle, with progressive atrophy of contractile tissue and increased intermuscular fibrosis [8]. As a result, changes in muscle function and morphology parallel the gradual reduction in muscle fibre calibre [7]. Cross-sectional area of muscle fibres decrease over the initial 60–90 days and then plateau at about 70–90% atrophy [9, 10]. Gross muscle and fibre atrophy continues up to 7 months with dense collagen formation surrounding remaining muscle fibres [11]. By 18 months, a substantial reduction in sarcoplasmic reticulum may be observed, and at 2 years muscle fibre fragmentation and disintegration become evident. Adipose and fibrous connective tissue substitution occurs between 1 and 3 years after denervation, resulting in irreversible muscle fibre replacement (scar tissue) [11].

Slow-twitch muscle fibres are typically first involved following denervation, whilst fast-twitch fibres maintain myosin integrity up to five times longer [12]. A 5% decrement per day from initial strength levels has been observed as the functional consequence of muscle atrophy, which slowed to 25% at 7 days [13]. Over a 6-week period, the overall loss was estimated as 48% of baseline strength, averaging approximately 8% per week [14]. Non-denervated muscles, which may be part of the affected limb, may also reduce in size as a result of disuse, although the extent is usually not as pronounced as those in neurogenic atrophy. Studies have estimated that 60% of muscle atrophy after denervation is attributable to disuse [15].

Fatigue

Fatigue may be defined as the failure to maintain the required or expected force from a muscle following repeated muscle activity [16]. In the context of peripheral nerve disorders, the development of fatigue may be multifactorial: impaired muscular activation, generalized deconditioning, and diminished cardiopulmonary performance due to immobility [17, 18].

Pain and somatosensory deficits

Neuropathic pain is a common complaint of patients with disorders of the peripheral nervous system, and can hinder active participation in rehabilitation. According to the International Association for the Study of Pain (IASP), neuropathic pain is initiated or caused by a primary lesion of the nervous system [19]. The definition does not exclude pain that is due to secondary neuroplastic changes in the nociceptive system arising from inflammation, nor does it distinguish a musculoskeletal origin that may arise indirectly following a neurological disorder.

Neuropathic pain is associated with aberrant or increased afferent input and ectopic discharges from hypersensitive, damaged or regenerating sensory nerve fibres. The unpleasant sensation may be constant, intermittent, lancinating, burning, tingling, crawling or electrical in character [7]. The management of neuropathic pain is based on four physiological processes involved in the pain experience, namely transduction, transmission, modulation and perception [7]. It is also important to acknowledge when managing patients with neuropathy, that pain may encompass an emotional component, hence early and adequate emphasis on both physical and psychological aspects of pain remain important to achieve control of symptoms and thereby successful participation in the rehabilitation programme.

Balance and gait disturbance

In patients with disorders affecting the PNS, disturbance of balance and gait is a challenging, yet vital, aspect of the rehabilitation programme that requires intervention in order to maintain mobility and functional independence. Altered sensorimotor function, causing proprioceptive deficits in particular, may lead to impaired control of stance and increased postural sway [6], with resultant impairment of functional gait performance and risk of falling [20]. Diminished ankle strength and reduced rate of force production may lead to balance impairment, as normal recovery from perturbation involves rapid production of adequate muscle force to maintain the body's centre of mass over its base of support [5] (for further discussion see Chapter 18).

Joint and soft tissue changes

The equilibrium between intravascular and interstitial fluid volumes is maintained partly through contraction of skeletal muscles [7]. Following peripheral nerve lesions, immobility of the limb, and associated changes in local circulation, resultant oedema may develop [8]. Once chronic oedema develops, collagen formation and fibrosis may ensue, leading to joint stiffness and contractures [8, 21]. In addition, collagen biosynthesis increases following denervation, with tightening of the ordinarily loose meshwork that surrounds myofibres [7].

Spasticity may arise from a lesion that concurrently affects the spinal cord as well as the exiting nerve roots, such as a cervical disc protrusion, and will affect muscles arising from spinal levels below the lesion due to involvement of the dorsal reticulospinal tract that normally inhibits spinal reflex activity [22]. This may in turn lead to an imbalance of inhibition and excitation, with enhanced motor neuronal excitability developing through the loss of descending control. The resultant increase in limb tone will contribute to muscle shortening and the development of contractures, thereby worsening the functional impairment, often associated with pain.

Goals of rehabilitation for peripheral nervous system disorders

As a general principle, rehabilitation aims to maximize functional independence, locomotion, prevent physical deformity, facilitate integration into society, and overall, improve quality of life [4, 23].

Rehabilitation programmes can be divided into three phases [8]: (i) an initial phase aims to maintain nutrition, prevent muscle atrophy and deformities, and support the affected area with splints, to prevent overstretching of weak muscles as well as shortening of the normal antagonistic muscle (see section on Splints); (ii) second phase comprises functional re-education with a combination of progressive resistive and functional exercises; (iii) the final phase remains primarily functional, with the goal of preparing the patient for return to their normal home environment and employment life, and usually consists of a supervised, individually tailored home exercise programme that may adjust according to further improvement of the patient.

Delay in commencing rehabilitation may be associated with the development of complications, particularly contractures that may further hinder the success of rehabilitation [8]. The rehabilitation team must also formulate a realistic goal for the patient. The degree of impairment is not solely related to recovery of nerve function [24], with psychosocial factors such as the perception of impact of the deficit on activities of daily living and poor social adjustment, all contributing to the rate and extent of functional recovery [3].

Treatment is goal-oriented and impairment may be evaluated by measurements of strength, range of motion, and musculoskeletal deformity. Disability can be assessed by measures of mobility and limb function, physical adaptations, and psychosocial adjustment [4]. The best evidence for rehabilitation interventions for peripheral nerve disorders favours a multidisciplinary approach that is patient-centred, time-based, functionally oriented aiming to maximize activity, participation and social integration [25]. Ideally, such interventions includes coordinated delivery by two or more disciplines (physiotherapy, occupational therapy, social work, dietitian, speech pathologist, and psychologist) under medical supervision (e.g. neurologist, rehabilitation, or general physician).

Rehabilitative therapies

General considerations

An initial consideration relates to the timing of any required surgical intervention. In the vast majority of traumatic injuries, nerves remain in continuity, and so decisions regarding surgery may often be postponed for 8–12 weeks [7]. Whilst sharp lacerations are commonly explored early in view of surgical repair, only 15–20% are observed to be complete [26]. In those latter cases, surgical repair and nerve grafting procedures remain a consideration, particularly before any retraction of the nerve endings has developed.

Prevention of further injury is critical and patients must be educated about protecting anaesthetic skin regions to avoid injuries, such as burns, that may arise from trauma. It may be advisable for patients who have reduced skin sensibility to wear protective gloves and stockings. Appropriately fitted shoes will minimize the risk of secondary injury leading to ulcers, and adequate foot hygiene will help avoid infections. Patients should be encouraged to examine their splints, casts, footwear, and any device that is in contact with the skin, for signs of excessive pressure on the skin, such as erythema or blisters. Referral to a podiatrist may be worthwhile for regular assessment for such complications.

Physical therapy

General principles will focus on maintaining range of motion through the affected joints, in order to prevent the development of joint contractures and deformities, combined with muscle strengthening exercises to maintain adequate function. In the setting of traumatic nerve injuries, this process may only be required until recovery following the insult, either through appropriate surgery or conservative management. In contrast, physical therapy for non-traumatic nerve disorders such as chronic generalized peripheral neuropathy (e.g. immune-mediated or metabolic disorders), physical therapy may be longer term with the view to maintaining muscle function, or to reduce the rate of deterioration to prevent the progression to disability.

Traumatic peripheral nerve injuries

Range of motion exercises

The first step in the rehabilitation process is initiating a set of exercises to increase and maintain range of motion (ROM) and flexibility [27], with the simplest and most effective program incorporating slow, steady stretch that places the joint and muscle in the extreme range of available motion, maintained for 10–30 seconds, and repeated 10 times. These cycles may be performed either passively or actively, and the amount of force used to stretch the joint or muscle will depend on the length of time since injury or surgery, the severity of the injury, the surgical procedure, the joint, the length of immobilisation, as well as patient tolerance. Moist heat, such as the use of warm showers and heat packs, prior to range of motion exercises will facilitate the exercise programme.

Passive movements are best performed to the affected joint through the full range of motion at least once, but preferably several times a day [21]. Passive exercise before reinnervation develops may preserve structure of the motor end-plate and thereby enhance reinnervation [28]. In addition, passive muscle stretching early in the course of the injury may help muscle atrophy. It has been shown that stretch related mechanical loading of the muscle acts through up-regulation of signal pathways that result in transcription of certain genes, and subsequent production of actin and myosin filaments, with addition of new sarcomeres. In rat models, the cross-sectional area of denervated soleus muscle fibres after repetitive stretching, were significantly larger than controls [11].

Active movements are encouraged for the prevention of oedema, maintenance of full range of motion, and for preservation of muscle strength [21].

Proprioceptive neuromuscular facilitation (PNF): is a technique utilized to regain range of motion, flexibility and neuromuscular function, based on stimulation of Golgi tendon organs and nerve endings [27]. Three types of PNF stretching techniques may be directed at the 'target muscle' (TM), or the muscle group on the opposite side, referred to as the 'opposing muscle' (OM) as follows:

(i)   Contract–relax: The patient is asked to perform a submaximal (20–50% maximum voluntary contraction, MVC) contraction of the TM (for 3–10 seconds) at the end of range followed by relaxation. The therapist then moves the TM into further elongation and holds at end of range for 5–10 seconds, with stretch maintained until perceived sensation of the stretch diminishes (Figure 19.1, left).

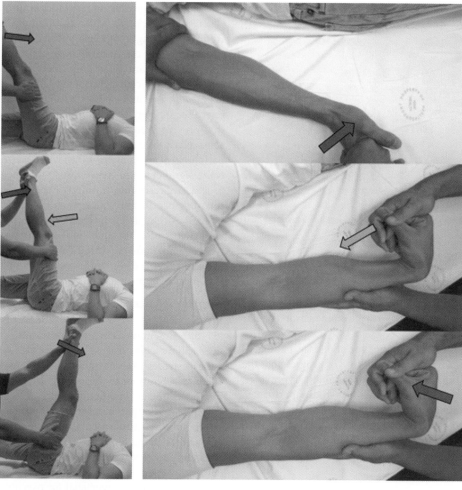

Fig. 19.1 Proprioceptive neuromuscular facilitation.
(Left column) Agonist–contract relax technique: top, therapist stretches target muscle (hamstrings) to end of range; middle, patient contracts target muscle at end of range; bottom, therapist further stretches the target muscle following release of agonist contraction. (Right column) Antagonist–contract technique: top. Therapist stretches target muscle (wrist extensors) to end of range; middle, patient contracts opposing muscles (wrist flexors) at end of range; bottom, therapist further stretches the target muscle following release of antagonist contraction. Red arrow, therapist direction of motion; yellow arrow, patient direction of motion.

(ii) Antagonist–contract: The therapist passively stretches the TM to end of range and then asks the patient to contract the OM (20% MVC) for 3–10 seconds. The patient then relaxes and the therapist stretches the TM further and holds at end of range for 5–10 seconds (Figure 19.1, right).

(iii) Contract–relax–antagonist–contract: Combination of techniques 1 and 2 consecutively.

Moving the TM into a position of stretch, should be undertaken at slow velocity to avoid muscle spindle excitation and viscous resistance. A minimum of one to five repetitions of PNF twice weekly is typically required to improve ROM.

Resistance exercises

Despite tremendous growth in the variety of equipment available for strengthening, the basic principles remain unchanged. In the early stages of peripheral nerve injury, maintenance of strength is vitally important to overcome disuse atrophy. Muscle strengthening can be divided as follows [27]:

Isometric exercise defined as muscle contraction without movement of the joint or limb upon which the muscle acts, is most effective in the early phases of rehabilitation when joint motion is restricted;

Isotonic exercise occurs when a joint moves through a range of motion against a constant resistance, such as with the use of dumbbells. Progressive resistance may be developed through the addition of weights as the muscle adapts. This usually requires a minimum of three sets of 6 to 10 repetitions of each exercise performed during each session of training (Figure 19.2);

Isokinetic exercise is similar to isotonic in that it is dynamic and involves movement of the joint. In addition, this form of exercise provides maximum resistance to the muscle throughout the entire range of motion for every repetition and is achieved by controlling the speed at which the exercise is performed.

Non-traumatic peripheral nerve disorders

Randomized controlled trials are lacking in this area and a recent Cochrane review failed to demonstrate significance in relation to functional outcome. However, there is evidence to suggest that patients may benefit from strengthening and aerobic fitness training programs, at least with respect to increasing muscle strength [3].

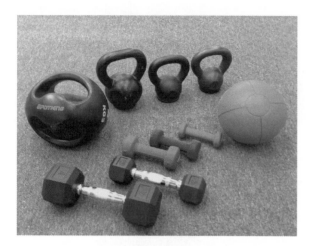

Fig. 19.2 Resistance training with weights. Different forms of hand-held weights of varying mass for use in progressive resistance training exercises.

Several studies have investigated the effects of exercise as a means to improve strength in peripheral neuropathy and neuromuscular disorders [29–37].

As disability depends on the specific type of disease, pathogenesis, extent of clinical involvement, and rate of progression, the ideal level of exercise training will also depend on the type, stage, and severity of disease. Results from aerobic studies performed on patients that are mildly affected demonstrated short-term cardiopulmonary improvements, whilst those with more severe disability may be unable to respond positively to either resistive or aerobic exercise [23].

Resistance exercise

Strength training or progressive resistance exercise increases lean body mass, muscle protein mass, contractile force, power, and improves physical function [23], in patients with peripheral neuropathy. Resistance training induces adaptations in both the muscular [38–42] and the nervous systems [43–46] and both contribute to the development of strength (Figure 19.2). Lifting weights during concentric or eccentric exercise places stress on muscles, inducing hypertrophy by increasing the DNA content of myofibrils and hence the number of muscle proteins, especially actin and myosin [23].

Improvements in functional measures and an increased type 1 fibre diameter were observed after the institution of a home-based progressive strength-training programme (3 days per week for 12 weeks) [47]. Choosing the right resistance and intensity is critical to ensure that the target muscles are loaded sufficiently to produce the appropriate training response (e.g. hypertrophy and hyperplasia) but not to provoke injury or aggravate pain. To guide such choices, a study that investigated patients with hereditary neuropathy, a 12-week moderate resistance programme (30% of maximal isometric force) resulted in strength gains up to 20% without deleterious effects [31], whilst a 12-week high resistance programme (maximal weight a subject could lift) showed no added benefit with evidence of overwork weakness in some participants [31]. Overwork weakness develops when the patient feels weaker rather than stronger within 30 minutes after exercise; or experiences excessive muscle soreness and cramping 24 to 48 hours after exercise [35].

Cross-education: during resistance training, a 'cross education' effect, may develop in which training of one limb may increase voluntary strength of the opposite, untrained limb [48, 49]. Cross education can occur in both upper and lower limb muscles [50–55], with training accomplished by voluntary effort, electrically stimulated contractions, or mental imagery training of unilateral contractions [55–57]. Cross education has potential clinical relevance in exercise rehabilitation for patients with conditions that prevent exercise of the affected or injured limb, including acute phase of painful neuropathy, forced immobilization after peripheral nerve injury or surgery, and neurological disorders that cause significant unilateral muscle weakness. In these instances, progressive resistance training of the opposite healthy limb may retard disuse atrophy and maintain strength of the injured limb [58–60]. Although it is reasonable to speculate the potential clinical benefits of cross education, it is premature to make formal recommendations regarding a role in exercise rehabilitation for peripheral nerve disorders because the underlying mechanisms of this effect remain largely unknown.

Aerobic exercises

Involvement of large muscle groups for sufficient intensity (50–85% VO_2 max) during aerobic training induces adaptations in the cardiovascular and skeletal muscular systems [23]. Treadmill running undertaken in reinnervating muscles may induce histochemical alterations in the muscle fibre, which include contractile properties and enzyme activity [61].

Gentle, low-impact aerobic exercises such as walking and swimming, improve cardiovascular performance and increases muscle efficiency, helping to reduce fatigue [17] (Figure 19.3). Subjective pain and functional abilities were also observed to improve after aerobic training in patients with neuropathy [62]. Aerobic exercises may also prove beneficial for psychological aspects such as depression, and improving pain tolerance, as well as reducing cardiovascular risk factors that may be associated with disability and consequent sedentary lifestyle, such as obesity, hypertension, glucose dysmetabolism, and dyslipidaemia. Hydrotherapy, particularly for those with musculoskeletal comorbidities such as arthritis, remains a good alternative, which also has the added benefit of muscle conditioning and strength-training achieved through water resistance.

Balance and gait training

Most patients with peripheral neuropathy will have some degree of balance and gait impairment, either directly from the underlying disorder affecting muscle strength or proprioceptive sensory processing, or indirectly from complications such as oedema or contractures. Balance and gait training exercises are important to maintain mobility and functional independence in these patients.

Subjective and objective improvements in balance were observed following participation in physiotherapist-supervised balance exercises or instrumental rehabilitation with an oscillating powered platform, with the suggestion of a synergistic effect when the two modalities were combined [63]. The proposed mechanisms for the improvements were thought to relate to an increased vestibulospinal responsiveness, to enable functional sensory substitution [64], following disruption to postural support.

Lower limb strengthening exercises, particularly those aimed at improving ankle strength, present the best clinical evidence for treating balance dysfunction in diabetic patients with neuropathy

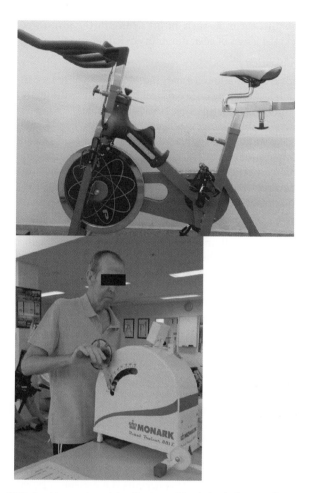

Fig. 19.3 Aerobic exercise training. Stationary bicycle (top) allows gentle low-impact aerobics exercising, whilst the arm ergometer (bottom) offers similar training in patients with lower limb difficulties, such as severe weakness or rheumatological conditions.

[5, 65]. Mind–body exercises such as Tai-Chi and yoga that emphasize movement control have demonstrated improvements in ankle-joint proprioception as well as sensibility in the feet and mobility [6, 66, 67]. Other interventions shown to have some limited benefit for balance and gait problems in patients with peripheral neuropathy include vibratory insoles 68 and monochromatic infrared energy therapy [5] (Figure 19.4), although definitive mechanisms of effect and positive results from large clinical trials remain lacking.

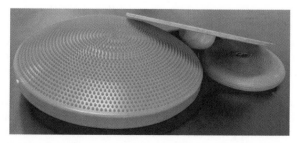

Fig. 19.4 Balance training. Top, different forms of balancing boards predominantly used for static balancing exercises. Bottom, novel machine with vibrating base for more advanced balance training using vibratory perturbations.

Combined exercise programmes

There is evidence to suggest that a supervised, community-based exercise programme that combines aerobic, resistance, and functional (balance and task-specific activity) components may prove beneficial for patients with peripheral neuropathy, leading to improvements in activity, function, balance, fatigue, and anxiety [65, 69, 70]. Strengthening exercises, involving functional movements such as sit to stand, lifting, and reaching, should be implemented as early as practically possible. The effects of a combined programme seem to outlast the strength gains achieved from the resistance component, suggesting that this approach to physical therapy is more likely of benefit than any of the individual components performed in isolation.

Prostheses, orthotics and equipment

Neuromuscular electrical stimulation

There are two types of neuromuscular electrical stimulation (NMES) systems in clinical use: transcutaneous and implantable systems. Implanted electrodes require open surgical procedures and are beyond the scope of this chapter. Transcutaneous systems are more commonly used in clinical rehabilitation, where electrodes are connected to an external portable stimulator. Current is then delivered directly through the skin over the motor point or peripheral nerve in either bipolar or monopolar arrangement. Conventional NMES techniques use low pulse frequencies (typically between 10–40 Hz) with narrow pulse duration (typically 50–200 µs), to produce fused tetanic contractions. Most commercially available transcutaneous units allow adjustment of stimulation parameters such as pulse width, frequency, intensity and duration. Therefore, stimulation paradigms can be customized for an individual patient.

A problem commonly encountered with electrical stimulation relates to accelerated fatigue during training. This is likely to be attributed to physiological differences in temporal and spatial recruitment of motor units between voluntary and electrically stimulated contractions. Transcutaneous electrical stimulation will recruit the same population of muscle fibres synchronously (i.e. those closest to the stimulating electrodes) [71], whereas voluntary contractions recruit motor units asynchronously [72, 73]. Specifically, electrically stimulated contractions require a non-physiological, extremely high firing rate to maintain smooth tetanus and therefore, a higher energy demand, making such interventions prone to rapid fatigue. Synaptic recruitment of motor units can be enhanced through modifying stimulation parameters including: stimulating over the peripheral nerve rather than muscle belly, using higher frequencies (e.g. 100 Hz), longer pulse duration (e.g. 1 ms), and low stimulation intensity to minimize antidromic block [74–77]. Synaptic recruitment of motoneurons resembles the recruitment pattern that underlies voluntary contraction, and may produce the most fatigue-resistant contractions [75, 76, 78]. However, the effectiveness of this type of stimulation paradigm remains to be validated through future longitudinal training studies and clinical trials.

The majority of NMES studies have focused on central nervous system disorders such as stroke and spinal cord injury. To date, there have been no large randomized control studies to valid... the benefits of NMES in peripheral nerve disorders. Despi... NMES is commonly used in the treatment and rehabi...

these conditions. Anecdotal evidence suggests that NMES therapy improves clinical and functional outcome in brachial plexus and peripheral nerve injuries [79–82], facial nerve palsy [83], painful nerve, and various muscle disorders [84–86]. Repetitive electrically stimulated contractions may help to maintain or improve range of motion [87], increase muscle strength [80, 84–86] and offset secondary complications such as muscle atrophy [88, 89]. As such, NMES may help to prevent the development of complications such as contractures as result of peripheral nerve disorders (see 'Joint and soft tissue changes').

NMES has also been shown to be a useful modality in the reversal of denervation [61, 90–92]. However, stimulation is only effective if an appropriate stimulation parameter is used [90, 93] and the therapy is commenced shortly after the onset of injury [93]. It must be emphasized that most of the evidence in support of stimulating denervated muscles were derived from animal experiments, and only a few studies have investigated the benefits of NMES in human subjects [88, 89, 94]. Because of the limited number of human studies and the heterogeneity in the stimulation protocols used, there is currently no consensus amongst clinicians with respect to the most appropriate stimulation protocol. For this reason, there is currently insufficient evidence to support or refute the use of NMES in the rehabilitation of peripheral nerve disorders. More research in this population group will be required to further elucidate the most appropriate stimulation parameters, as well as stimulation duration, onset and placement of electrodes. Only then, the most efficacious stimulation protocol can be developed and tested in subsequent human clinical trials.

Electrically stimulated contractions:

In peripheral nerve disorders, weakness may preclude voluntary contraction of the affected muscles and nearby joint. In such instances, electrical stimulation may be applied to either the muscle or nerve to generate contraction. An intensive daily regimen of electrical stimulation therapy may prevent atrophy and improve muscle architecture in denervated muscles [61, 89–92, 94], and chronic paraplegics [88]. With regard to peripheral nerve disorders, clinical intuition suggests that daily electrical stimulation may help to offset disuse atrophy if implemented shortly after injury [93], and should be continued until such point that the patient could engage in active exercise therapy [21].

Functional electrical stimulation (FES):

The delivery of electrical current to activate paretic muscles in a coordinated sequence and timely magnitude to produce a functionally purposeful movement may be accomplished via a neuroprosthetic device such as FES. For example, electrical stimulation of the tibialis anterior muscle or the peroneal nerve can be coordinated with a computer sensor during the swing phase of the gait cycle to improve walking in patients with foot drop [95, 96]. Several types of FES systems have been developed to specifically [improve perfo]rmance of tasks of daily living such as grasping, [standing, and wa]lking [97, 98]. Clinical studies have shown that [these walk]ing devices improve walking speed, endurance, [and mu]scle strength [99–102].

[A major drawback o]f the FES system is that the majority of these [devices are designe]d solely to improve performance of a single [task. Given th]e enormous costs involved, FES neuroprosthe[tics remain impractic]al and unaffordable to most consumers

who require them. As such, future neuroprosthetic research must address the issues of cost, durability, reliability and functionality.

Neuroplasticity

Electrical stimulation is emerging as a therapeutic tool to drive central plasticity, encouraged by a small but expanding body of evidence demonstrating that NMES is capable of inducing rapid and long-lasting changes in neural excitability [75, 78, 103–110]. Electrical stimulation induced neuroplasticity has important clinical implications, particularly for patients with peripheral nerve disorders where enhanced plasticity may lead to better functional outcomes derived from rehabilitation.

Slings

Slings are generally not recommended for patients with upper limb nerve injury who are ambulatory because they encourage arm dependency, which increases oedema. It also discourages use of the extremity, increasing the risk of muscle atrophy, and again oedema, and may result in joint contractures particularly around the elbow and shoulders because of the immobilisation [111].

Biofeedback

Biofeedback can be utilized in those patients with difficulty learning to use the reinnervated muscles [111], and in some patients it is difficult to selectively activate the weakened muscles without excessive activation of the agonists or antagonists. Small surface electrodes attached to the affected muscle produce an electromyographic signal that can be displayed to the patient either in audio or visual forms, while the patient executes the movement using the target muscle. This permits the patient to learn when a particular muscle is activated, and the threshold required for activation of the signal may be changed as the strength improves. Biofeedback can also be used to monitor activity of the antagonists during functional movement retraining.

Orthoses and ambulatory aids

A significant proportion of patients with disorders of the peripheral nervous system will require some form of assistive devices, due to various symptoms including muscle weakness, sensory and balance impairment, and fatigue. Options include shoe modifications, ankle–foot appliances or orthoses, canes, crutches, walkers, and power wheelchairs, and the selection will depend on the patient's strength, stability, coordination, cardiovascular capacity and cognitive status, all with the goal to optimizing residual motor function [25].

A systematic review that examined the relation between balance and ankle and foot appliances, demonstrated that facilitation of tactile sensation using tubing or vibrating insoles improved balance [112]. Vibrating insoles reduced sway via a proposed mechanism, which improved early detection of change in pressure distribution under the soles and hence earlier reaction and better control of balance. Flexible polyethylene tubing attached to the plantar surface boundaries of the feet improved stepping reactions after perturbations that result from sensory facilitation provided by the boundaries of the plantar surface. Standardized shoes with thick (16–27 mm) and soft insoles showed negative impact on static and dynamic balance, likely related to reduced

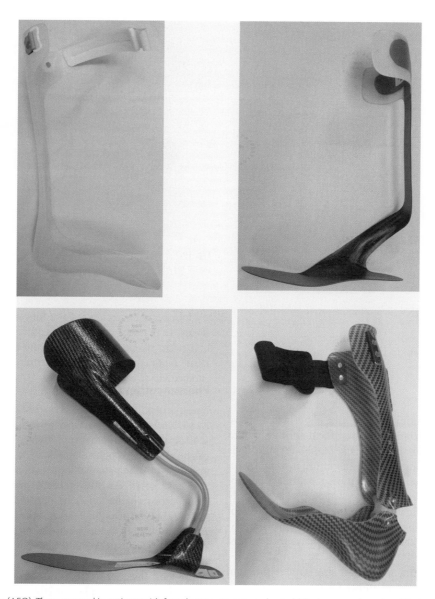

Fig. 19.5 Ankle–foot orthoses (AFO). These are used in patients with foot drop to prevent mechanical falls due to weakness in ankle dorsiflexion during walking. Different forms of AFOs are available, but plastic AFOs with articulated ankle joints (bottom two) are preferred as they offer improved shock absorption and smoothness of gait over non-articulated forms (top two).

foot proprioception [112]. However, such insoles may be beneficial for the effects on peak pressure, comfort and preventing ulcers.

Of interest, ankle immobilization has a negative impact on balance performance immediately after application, although improved thereafter following a period of training, likely as a result of an alternative motor control mechanism (hip strategy rather than ankle), as well as central adaptation [112]. This has implications for the type of physical therapy instituted early on in the rehabilitation process depending on the type of ankle-foot appliance used (Figure 19.5).

Oedema

Active movement of joints through their full range of motion may aid in reducing oedema. Elevation of the injured limb, with the use of a sling during the day and suspension in a roller towel at night are also useful strategies for the upper limbs [21]. Similarly, elevation of the leg whilst seated or in bed may help encourage venous return and reduce the extent of lower limb oedema.

Tight casts and constrictive splints or dressings that may be contributing to oedema should be loosened or changed to a more appropriate fitting. Gradient pressure elastic sleeves and stockings, or intermittent pneumatic compression at no more than the patient's diastolic blood pressure with the limb elevated, may also prove beneficial. Particular care should be applied when using compression devices on patients with peripheral vascular disease. Massage and compression in a retrograde manner to assist in mobilizing tissue fluid and proximal return to the intravascular circulation may also reduce oedema associated with trauma [7].

Contractures

The prevention and management of contractures usually requires a multimodal approach using a combination of splinting, stretching and medication depending upon the severity and response.

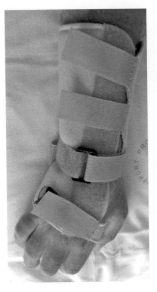
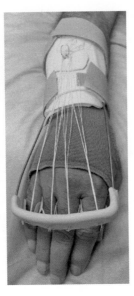

Fig. 19.6 Hand and wrist splints. The use of soft splints (left) permits the normal range of motion and prevents capsular contractures and joint stiffness, whilst the elastic splints (right) changes the hand and wrist from a position of non-function (flexion) into a position that facilitates functional use of the joint.

Splints

The three purposes for splinting in the setting of peripheral nerve injuries are to prevent deformity, to correct the deformity, and to improve and restore function [111]. The use of mobile splinting is preferred over rigid splinting to the joints in order to maintain their normal range of motion, and thus prevent capsular contractures that precede joint stiffness [8]. If contractures have already developed, dynamic splinting is useful to stretch out both the joint and musculotendinous stiffness. Such serial casting involves prolonged stretch in a cast and changed every 5 to 7 days with further stretch [113].

With proper design and fit, splints can also provide function lost by the muscle weakness and allows for improved function prior to muscle reinnervation and recovery. Splints with external power such as devices with springs or rubber bands can substitute for the weakened muscle until the function of that muscle returns. This may avoid muscle imbalance particularly those from the unaffected antagonist, which can lead to joint contractures and permanent deformity [111] (Figure 19.6).

Stretching

Stretching remains the essential principle of management of all patients with peripheral nerve lesions, and should form the basis from which further treatments are added. Stretching is helpful to reduce spasticity as well as other local changes such as stiffness, contractures and fibrosis, commonly associated with the immobilized joint.

Stretching should be steady, continuous and directional, with the physical therapist initially involved in the passive stretching but ultimately performed by the educated patient and caregiver ideally on a daily basis [113] (Figure 19.7. The use of elastic traction coupled with periods of active and passive exercises around the affected joint performed under heat may be helpful to manage more resilient contractures.

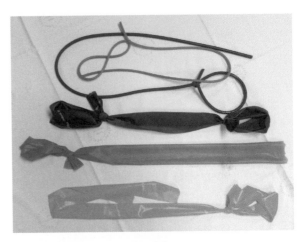

Fig. 19.7 Stretching. A variety of tubes, rubber tubes, and bands are commercially available for stretching exercises.

Tight scars can often restrict movement around the joint and the use of massage with oil or lanolin can achieve results in mobilizing scar tissue and free them from adhering to underlying soft tissue that may contribute to deformities [21].

Pharmacotherapy

Pharmacological agents are primarily used for muscle hyperactivity such as occurs in spasticity when the peripheral nerve disorder is associated with a spinal cord lesion. A variety of oral medication can be utilised to modulate spasticity but these effects need to be balanced against the potential for functional decline, reduced strength and adverse effects. The available medications are used either alone or in combination in an individualised regimen, and include γ-aminobutyric acid (GABA) agonists (baclofen, benzodiazepines), alpha-2 adrenergic agents acting on the central nervous system (tizanidine, clonidine), and peripheral inhibition at the neuromuscular or muscular level (dantrolene) [113].

The local injection with botulinum toxin type A as a means of chemodenervation, can be a useful adjunct together with occupational and physiotherapy, for the treatment of spasticity as well as contractures and dystonic posturing of the affected limb caused by an altered cocontraction from antagonist muscles [11]. It is also commonly used in combination with serial casting to reduce tone of the affected joint. Botulinum toxin acts by providing local muscle relaxation, but proposed additional effects on spasticity include modulation of abnormal central reorganization in the brain that may be maintaining the spasticity [114].

Pain and somatosensory disturbance
Physical therapy

Sensory desensitization

In those patients with certain degrees of hypersensitivity or dysaesthesia associated with the peripheral nerve disorder, 'desensitization' early in the rehabilitation programme is important to achieve compliance and active ongoing participation for successful physical therapy. Desensitisation involves the use of differing modalities to decrease sensitivity of the affected extremity to peripheral stimulation [111]. The patient can immerse the sensitive region into

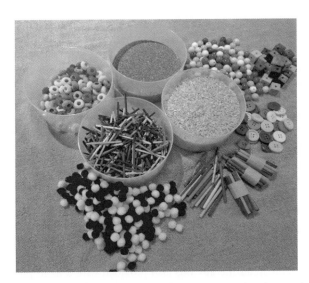

Fig. 19.8 Sensory desensitization and re-education. The use of mediums and objects of varying texture, consistency and shape for use in the process of sensory desensitization and re-education.

a medium such as styrofoam balls, rice, beans, or sand to begin with, and progress to manipulating the medium as the patient's tolerance increases during the therapy sessions. Thereafter, increasing force, duration and frequency as well the use of more irritating medium as desensitization takes effect. When the patient has achieved adequate tolerance to having the affected limb manipulated, sensory re-education can begin to take place (Figure 19.8).

Sensory re-education

The focus of sensory re-education is to retrain the patient to use what residual function remains [7], and in the setting of traumatic nerve injuries, whilst the nerve is undergoing regeneration. In normal subjects, sensory impulses from the limb reach the cortex and are associated with previous memories and experiences. Following peripheral nerve injury and repair, neural impulse profiles may be altered and not matched with previous experiences in the association cortex, hence the experience is not recognized [11]. Sensory re-education is based on cortical plasticity with remapping of the cortex by experience, and defined as the gradual and progressive process of reprogramming the brain through the use of cognitive learning techniques such as visualisation and verbalisation, the use of alternate senses such as vision or hearing and the use of graded tactile stimuli designed to restore sensory areas affected by nerve injury [115].

In patients with traumatic lesions, pain and temperature sensibilities return first, followed by vibration, then touch. Patients with profound sensory loss are at greatest risk of injuring the affected limb, and may be educated in increasing awareness of situations and stimuli that may place their limb in danger of further injury. The early phase of discriminative sensory re-education may focus on improving the ability to distinguish light touch from constant touch, as well as cortical hand representation maintenance using audio-tactile and visuotactile interactions, such as mirror therapy [7, 115]. In the late phase, the goal is to encourage recovery of texture discrimination and object recognition, as well as enhancing sensory re-education results from then earlier phase [7, 11]. Other

cortical functions such as memory and attention, are also involved during the learning process [11].

Sensory re-education may involve activities associated with day-to-day living such as self-care, kitchen activities (caution with heat), and cleaning, or recreational activities such as hold cards, golfing, wood carving and arts and craft, all with the intention of integrating the affected limb into daily use. Following this, late sensory re-education involves using the extremity in vision-occluding activities. This may include a home-kit containing items of different textures and shapes, and the patient required to identify them with and without vision.

Pharmacological therapy

Pharmacological treatment for neuropathic pain have largely been based on studies in patients with diabetic painful polyneuropathy, but symptomatology and treatment response are essentially the same amongst all patients regardless of aetiology, except for those with HIV-induced neuropathy [116]. The treatment regimen usually encompasses the use of antidepressants, antiepileptics, opioids and others, either alone or in combination.

The 2nd European Federation of Neurological Societies Task Force (EFNS) [116] guidelines on the pharmacological treatment of neuropathic pain, have recommended tricyclic antidepressants (TCAs; e.g. amitriptyline and nortriptyline), gabapentin, pregabalin, and serotonin-noradrenaline reuptake inhibitors (SNRIs; e.g. duloxetine, venlafaxine), as first line treatment (level A). Tramadol (level A) is recommended as second line except for exacerbations of pain, and third line agents include stronger opioids such as oxycodone. Other options to consider include nitrate derivatives and nicotinic agonists, and topical agents such as lidocaine and capsaicin [116]. More recently, researches have studied the use intradermal injection of botulinum toxin type A for the treatment diabetic neuropathic pain. Results have shown that injection into multiple sites of the feet produced a good response in terms of pain reduction [117]. The mechanism of action may be through the inhibition of glutamate release by nociceptive afferents. If proven effective in phase III trials, the toxin can be a useful adjunct in the management for patients with focal neuropathic pain.

Electrical stimulation

Transcutaneous electrical nerve stimulation (TENS) is commonly used in the management of many acute and chronic pain conditions such rheumatoid arthritis [118], chronic low back pain [119, 120], and pain during labour [121]. TENS treatment is rarely associated with adverse side effects and has been shown to be effective in patients with neuropathic pain [122–124]. It is thought that repetitive stimulation activates descending pain inhibitory system and the spinal gating mechanism to produce an analgesic effect. Two main stimulation parameters are used clinically: high-frequency (100 Hz) at intensity just below motor threshold or low-frequency (<20 Hz) set at an intensity above motor threshold [125, 126]. Low-frequency TENS has been shown to be a promising treatment option for symptomatic diabetic neuropathy [127], trigeminal neuralgia [128], and neuropathic pain after spinal cord injury [124, 129]. TENS is an inexpensive and non-invasive treatment that can be self-administered and may be included as an adjunct to pharmacotherapy in the management of neuropathic pain [130].

Illustrative case

A 67-year-old man presented with numbness and persistent weakness of the right upper limb after a total shoulder replacement 2 weeks previously. On initial examination, the patient had complete paralysis of the right biceps, deltoids, and triceps, whilst moderate weakness was present in the wrist extensors and flexors, and as well as the intrinsic hand muscles. Deep tendon reflexes of the right biceps and brachioradialis were absent. Sensory examination revealed numbness involving the upper arm and forearm, and the patient complained of persistent pins and needles in the right hand.

A magnetic resonance image of the right brachial plexus and cervical spine demonstrated perineural oedema around all three trunks of the brachial plexus, consistent with neuropraxia likely caused by a traction injury.

Main problems

Profound weakness and paralysis of multiple right upper limb and shoulder girdle muscles secondary to the brachial plexopathy may result in progressive inferior subluxation of the shoulder prosthesis in the absence of active muscle support. Furthermore, inability to participate in active exercise rehabilitation may contribute to the development of joint stiffness and pain later. Whilst the neuropraxia itself may take up to several months to recover, rehabilitation of the shoulder must begin immediately in order to maximise functionality and prevent complications such as muscle wasting and contractures, particularly in the context of the recent shoulder replacement.

Goals of rehabilitation

1. Improve muscle strength and stability of the shoulder and prevent disuse atrophy

2. Improve passive and active ROM of the shoulder

3. Maintain full ROM in elbow, wrist, and intrinsic hand muscles

4. Sensory desensitization and re-education

5. Prevent joint contractures

6. Prevent inferior subluxation of the shoulder joint

7. Maintain cardiovascular fitness and improve strength

Rehabilitation strategy and rationale

1. Improve muscle strength and prevent atrophy
   In this case, the use of NMES is ideal to activate the weak muscles such as the biceps, triceps, deltoids and the wrist extensors. Electrical stimulation can be delivered directly over the motor points of the muscles or over the peripheral nerves that innervate these muscles. Peripheral nerve stimulation (especially at high frequencies) may also promote neuroplasticity and is less prone to training fatigue. During NMES training, the patient was encouraged to 'try' and contract the same muscles being stimulated or at the very least, 'imagine' contracting the same muscles. Active strengthening exercises for the unaffected left arm takes place concurrently to maximise the 'cross education' effect.

2. Improve ROM of the shoulder
   Passive stretching and ROM exercises are an important part of the rehabilitation programme and must be performed by a trained therapist. The main goals are to gradually improve range of motion of passive and active shoulder flexion and abduction, as well as internal and external rotation of the glenohumeral joint. Passive stretches involving sustained static holds are most effective when performed by a therapist. The patient must also perform active shoulder flexion, abduction and rotation ROM exercises at home daily. These can be performed with the assistance of the unaffected arm or using props such as a broomstick or stretch bands (Figure 19.7). In addition, ROM of the elbow, wrist, and fingers were monitored regularly.

3. Sensory desensitization and re-education
   This process is important prior to manipulating the limb and engaging in active physical therapy in this patient with significant sensory impairment and dysaesthesia. The hand and fingers were immersed initially into a gentle medium such as soft foam, and progressive changed to more irritating mediums such as grain or sand as the hand desensitizes. Following this, specific hand therapy was also provided with a hand physical therapist once per fortnight, to improve dexterity and hand function in the form of sensory re-education that incorporates the functional manipulation of the hands and fingers using items with different shapes, sizes and texture to provide varying sensory stimulation (Figure 19.8).

4. Prevent contractures and subluxation
   The patient was encouraged to wear an arm sling during activities where he is required to stand or walk for long periods of time. The sling will help support the new prosthesis in the absence of active muscle control. In this case, the wrist extensors are much weaker than the wrist flexors. He was also fitted with a non-rigid wrist splint to maintain the wrist joint in neutral position to prevent the development of flexion contracture as well as to allow functional movement around the joint (Figure 19.6).

5. Maintain cardiovascular fitness and improve strength
   To maintain cardiovascular fitness, the patient was encouraged to brisk walk daily between 45–60 minutes. In addition, 2-3 sessions of moderate intensity cycling on a stationary bike was also recommended (Figure 19.3). The patient also attended hydrotherapy supervised by a trained physical therapist twice per week. The buoyancy of the water is a useful medium for both ROM and strengthening exercises. In addition, progressive resistance training with hand held weights Figure 19.2) was incorporated into the rehabilitation programme as the patient's muscle strength improved.

Outcome

The patient's upper limb muscle strength slowly improved over the next 3 months and by the 4th month was sufficiently strong to engage in active resistance exercises. He made a full recovery 6 months later and has resumed weekly golf and ocean swimming. The patient still complained of intermittent pins and needles and numbness over the lateral forearm and dorsum of his hand, but without significant impact on his activities of daily living.

Conclusion

Successful neurorehabilitative management of peripheral nerve disorders, whether traumatic or non-traumatic in aetiology, requires a multidisciplinary approach to the coordinated delivery of interventions that is integrated early on in the rehabilitation process. Unnecessary delays to initiation of treatment should be avoided to prevent the development of complications such as contractures and joint deformities that may hinder the physical therapy process. The best outcome occurs in patients who receive a goal-oriented and individualized programme that is formulated by both the administering health care professional as well as the well-informed patient in order to facilitate participation and adherence, and not only addresses the physical aspects of the disability or impairment but also the psychosocial ramifications of the disorder on the patient.

References

1. Seddon HJ. A classification of nerve injuries. Br Med J. 1942;**2**(4260):237–239.
2. Beric A. Peripheral nerve disorders. Adv Neurol. 2002;**90**:227–240.
3. White CM, Pritchard J, Turner-Stokes L. Exercise for people with peripheral neuropathy. Cochrane Database Syst Rev. 2004(4):CD003904.
4. Carter GT. Rehabilitation management of peripheral neuropathy. Semin Neurol. 2005;**25**(2):229–237.
5. Ites KI, Anderson EJ, Cahill ML, Kearney JA, Post EC, Gilchrist LS. Balance interventions for diabetic peripheral neuropathy: a systematic review. J Geriatr Phys Ther. 2011;**34**(3):109–116.
6. Li L, Hondzinski JM. Select exercise modalities may reverse movement dysfunction because of peripheral neuropathy. Exerc Sport Sci Rev. 2012;**40**(3):133–137.
7. Robinson MD, Shannon S. Rehabilitation of peripheral nerve injuries. Phys Med Rehabil Clin N Am. 2002;**13**(1):109–135.
8. Aldes JH, Bockstahler AC, Lieberman LI. Rehabilitation of peripheral nerve injuries. Ann W Med Surg. 1952;**6**(7):418–422.
9. Bowden RE. Muscle changes in denervation and re-innervation. Br Med J. 1945;**2**(4423):487–488.
10. Gutmann E, Young JZ. The re-innervation of muscle after various periods of atrophy. J Anat. 1944;**78**(Pt 1–2):15–43.
11. Smania N, Berto G, La Marchina E, et al. Rehabilitation of brachial plexus injuries in adults and children. Eur J Phys Med Rehabil. 2012;**48**(3):483–506.
12. Jakubiec-Puka A. Changes in myosin and actin filaments in fast skeletal muscle after denervation and self-reinnervation. Comp Biochem Physiol. Comp Physiol. 1992;**102**(1):93–98.
13. Muller EA. Influence of training and of inactivity on muscle strength. Arch Phys Med Rehabil. 1970;**51**(8):449–462.
14. MacDougall JD, Elder GC, Sale DG, Moroz JR, Sutton JR. Effects of strength training and immobilization on human muscle fibres. Eur J Appl Physiol Occup Physiol. 1980;**43**(1):25–34.
15. Davis HL, Kiernan JA. Neurotrophic effects of sciatic nerve extract on denervated extensor digitorum longus muscle in the rat. Exp Neurol. 1980;**69**(1):124–134.
16. Edwards RH. Human muscle function and fatigue. Ciba Foundation Symp. 1981;**82**:1–18.
17. Carter GT, Kikuchi N, Abresch RT, Walsh SA, Horasek SJ, Fowler WM, Jr. Effects of exhaustive concentric and eccentric exercise on murine skeletal muscle. Arch Phys Med Rehabil. 1994;**75**(5):555–559.
18. Videler AJ, Beelen A, Aufdemkampe G, de Groot IJ, Van Leemputte M. Hand strength and fatigue in patients with hereditary motor and sensory neuropathy (types I and II). Arch Phys Med Rehabil. 2002;**83**(9):1274–1278.
19. Treede RD, Jensen TS, Campbell JN, et al. Neuropathic pain: redefinition and a grading system for clinical and research purposes. Neurology. 2008;**70**(18):1630–1635.
20. Akbari M, Jafari H, Moshashaee A, Forugh B. Do diabetic neuropathy patients benefit from balance training? J Rehabil Res Dev. 2012;**49**(2):333–338.
21. Dyer L. Rehabilitation following peripheral nerve injuries. Physiotherapy. 1964;**50**:61–63.
22. Sheean G. The pathophysiology of spasticity. Eur J Neurol. 2002;**9** Suppl 1:3–9; dicussion 53-61.
23. Abresch RT, Han JJ, Carter GT. Rehabilitation management of neuromuscular disease: the role of exercise training. J Clin Neuromusc Dis. 2009;**11**(1):7–21.
24. Molenaar DS, Vermeulen M, de Visser M, de Haan R. Impact of neurologic signs and symptoms on functional status in peripheral neuropathies. Neurology. 1999;**52**(1):151–156.
25. Khan F, Amatya B. Rehabilitation interventions in patients with acute demyelinating inflammatory polyneuropathy: a systematic review. Eur J Phys Rehabil Med. 2012;**48**(3):507–522.
26. Aldea PA, Shaw WW. Management of acute lower extremity nerve injuries. Foot Ankle. 1986;**7**(2):82–94.
27. Vegso JJ, Torg E, Torg JS. Rehabilitation of cervical spine, brachial plexus, and peripheral nerve injuries. Clin Sports Med. 1987;**6**(1):135–158.
28. Pachter BR, Eberstein A. Passive exercise and reinnervation of the rat denervated extensor digitorum longus muscle after nerve crush. Am J Phys Med Rehabil. 1989;**68**(4):179–182.
29. Lindeman E, Leffers P, Reulen J, Spaans F, Drukker J. Quadriceps strength and timed motor performances in myotonic dystrophy, Charcot–Marie–Tooth disease, and healthy subjects. Clin Rehabil. 1998;**12**(2):127–135.
30. Kilmer DD, Aitkens SG, Wright NC, McCrory MA. Simulated work performance tasks in persons with neuropathic and myopathic weakness. Arch Phys Med Rehabil. 2000;**81**(7):938–943.
31. Aitkens SG, McCrory MA, Kilmer DD, Bernauer EM. Moderate resistance exercise program: its effect in slowly progressive neuromuscular disease. Arch Phys Med Rehabil. 1993;**74**(7):711–715.
32. Kilmer DD, McCrory MA, Wright NC, Aitkens SG, Bernauer EM. The effect of a high resistance exercise program in slowly progressive neuromuscular disease. Arch Phys Med Rehabil. 1994;**75**(5):560–563.
33. Kilmer DD. Response to aerobic exercise training in humans with neuromuscular disease. Am J Phys Med Rehabil. 2002;**81**(11 Suppl):S148–150.
34. Kilmer DD. Response to resistive strengthening exercise training in humans with neuromuscular disease. Am J Phys Med Rehabil. 2002;**81**(11 Suppl):S121–126.
35. Kilmer DD. The role of exercise in neuromuscular disease. Phys Med Rehabil Clin N Am. 1998;**9**(1):115–125, vi.
36. Lindeman E, Leffers P, Spaans F, et al. Strength training in patients with myotonic dystrophy and hereditary motor and sensory neuropathy: a randomized clinical trial. Arch Phys Med Rehabil. 1995;**76**(7):612–620.
37. Cheah BC, Boland RA, Brodaty NE, et al. INSPIRATIonAL—INSPIRAtory muscle training in amyotrophic lateral sclerosis. Amyotrophic Lateral Sclerosis. 2009;**10**(5–6):384–392.
38. Abernethy PJ, Jurimae J, Logan P. Acute and chronic response of skeletal muscle to resistance exercise. Sports Med. 1994;**17**(1):22–38.
39. Baldwin KM, Haddad F. Effects of different activity and inactivity paradigms on myosin heavy chain gene expression in striated muscle. J App Physiol. 2001;**90**:345–357.
40. Del Balso C, Cafarelli E. Adaptations in the activation of human skeletal muscle induced by short-term isometric resistance training. J Appl Physiol. 2007;**103**(1):402–411.
41. Moore DR, Phillips SM, Babraj JA, Smith K, Rennie MJ. Myofibrillar and collagen protein synthesis in human skeletal muscle in young men after maximal shortening and lengthening contractions. Am J Physiol Endocrinol Metab. 2005;**288**(6):E1153–1159.
42. Willoughby DS, Taylor L. Effects of sequential bouts of resistance exercise on androgen receptor expression. Med Sci Sports Exerc. 2004;**36**(9):1499–1506.
43. Carroll TJ, Riek S, Carson RG. The sites of neural adaptation induced by resistance training in humans. J Physiol. 2002;**544**(Pt 2):641–652.

44. Carroll TJ, Selvanayagam VS, Riek S, Semmler JG. Neural adaptations to strength training: moving beyond transcranial magnetic stimulation and reflex studies. Acta Physiol. 2011;**202**(2):119–140.

45. Enoka RM. Neural adaptations with chronic physical activity. J Biomech. 1997;**30**(5):447–455.

46. Sale DG. Neural adaptation to resistance training. Med Sci Sports Exerc. 1988;**20**(5):S135–S145.

47. Chetlin RD, Gutmann L, Tarnopolsky M, Ullrich IH, Yeater RA. Resistance training effectiveness in patients with Charcot–Marie–Tooth disease: recommendations for exercise prescription. Arch Phys Med Rehabil. 2004;**85**(8):1217–1223.

48. Carroll TJ, Herbert RD, Munn J, Lee M, Gandevia SC. Contralateral effects of unilateral strength training: evidence and possible mechanisms. J Appl Physiol. 2006;**101**(5):1514–1522.

49. Lee M, Carroll TJ. Cross education: possible mechanisms for the contralateral effects of unilateral resistance training. Sports Med. 2007;**37**(1):1–14.

50. Carolan B, Cafarelli E. Adaptations in coactivation after isometric resistance training. J Appl Physiol. 1992;**73**(3):911–917.

51. Davies CTM, Dooley P, McDonagh MJN, White MJ. Adaptation of mechanical properties of human to high force training. J Physiol. 1985;**365**:277–284.

52. Evetovich TK, Housh TJ, Housh DJ, Johnson GO, Smith DB, Ebersole KT. The effect of concentric isokinetic strength training of the quadriceps femoris on electromyography and muscle strength in the trained and untrained limb. J Strength Cond Res. 2001;**15**(4):439–445.

53. Ploutz P, Tesch PA, Biro RL, Dudley GA. Effect of resistance training on muscle use. J Appl Physiol. 1994;**76**(4):1675–1681.

54. Shima N, Ishida K, Katayama K, Morotome Y, Sato Y, Miyamura M. Cross education of muscular strength during unilateral resistance training and detraining. Eur J Appl Physiol. 2002;**86**(4):287–294.

55. Yue G, Cole KJ. Strength increases from the motor program: comparison of training with maximal voluntary and imagined muscle contractions. J Neurophysiol, 1992;**67**(5):1114–1123.

56. Ranganathan VK, Siemionow V, Liu JZ, Sahgal V, Yue GH. From mental power to muscle power- gaining strength by using the mind. Neuropsychologia. 2004;**42**:944–956.

57. Hortobagyi T, Scott K, Lambert NJ, Hamilton G, Tracy J. Cross-education of muscle strength is greater with stimulated than voluntary contractions. Motor Control. 1999;**3**:205–219.

58. Farthing JP, Krentz JR, Magnus CR. Strength training the free limb attenuates strength loss during unilateral immobilization. J Appl Physiol. 2009;**106**(3):830–836.

59. Hendy AM, Spittle M, Kidgell DJ. Cross education and immobilisation: mechanisms and implications for injury rehabilitation. J Sci Med Sport. 2012;**15**(2):94–101.

60. Magnus CR, Barss TS, Lanovaz JL, Farthing JP. Effects of cross-education on the muscle after a period of unilateral limb immobilization using a shoulder sling and swathe. J Appl Physiol. 2010;**109**(6):1887–1894.

61. Marqueste T, Alliez J-R, Alluin O, Jammes Y, Decherchi P. Neuromuscular rehabilitation by treadmill running or electrical stimulation after peripheral nerve injury and repair. J Appl Physiol. 2004;**96**(5):1988–1995.

62. El Mhandi L, Millet GY, Calmels P, et al. Benefits of interval-training on fatigue and functional capacities in Charcot–Marie–Tooth disease. Muscle Nerve. 2008;**37**(5):601–610.

63. Nardone A, Godi M, Artuso A, Schieppati M. Balance rehabilitation by moving platform and exercises in patients with neuropathy or vestibular deficit. Arch Phys Med Rehabil. 2010;**91**(12):1869–1877.

64. Horak FB, Hlavacka F. Somatosensory loss increases vestibulospinal sensitivity. J Neurophysiol. 2001;**86**(2):575–585.

65. Richardson JK, Sandman D, Vela S. A focused exercise regimen improves clinical measures of balance in patients with peripheral neuropathy. Arch Phys Med Rehabil. 2001;**82**(2):205–209.

66. Malhotra V, Singh S, Singh KP, Gupta P, Sharma SB, Madhu SV, Tandon OP. Study of yoga asanas in assessment of pulmonary function in NIDDM patients. Ind J Physiol Pharmacol. 2002;**46**(3):313–320.

67. Li L, Manor B. Long term Tai Chi exercise improves physical performance among people with peripheral neuropathy. Am J Chinese Med. 2010;**38**(3):449–459.

68. Priplata AA, Niemi JB, Harry JD, Lipsitz LA, Collins JJ. Vibrating insoles and balance control in elderly people. Lancet. 2003;**362**(9390):1123–1124.

69. Graham RC, Hughes RA, White CM. A prospective study of physiotherapist prescribed community based exercise in inflammatory peripheral neuropathy. J Neurol. 2007;**254**(2):228–235.

70. Kruse RL, Lemaster JW, Madsen RW. Fall and balance outcomes after an intervention to promote leg strength, balance, and walking in people with diabetic peripheral neuropathy: 'feet first' randomized controlled trial. Phys Ther. 2010;**90**(11):1568–1579.

71. Enoka RM. Activation order of motor axons in electrically evoked contractions. Muscle Nerve. 2002;**25**(6):763–764.

72. Henneman E. Relation between size of neurons and their susceptibility to discharge. Science. 1957;**126**(3287):1345–1347.

73. Henneman E. The size-principle: a deterministic output emerges from a set of probabilistic connections. J Exp Biol. 1985;**115**:105–112.

74. Bergquist AJ, Clair JM, Collins DF. Motor unit recruitment when neuromuscular electrical stimulation is applied over a nerve trunk compared with a muscle belly: triceps surae. J Appl Physiol. 2011;**110**(3):627–637.

75. Collins DF. Central contributions to contractions evoked by tetanic neuromuscular electrical stimulation. Exerc Sport Sci Rev. 2007;**35**(3):102–109.

76. Collins DF, Burke D, Gandevia SC. Large involuntary forces consistent with plateau-like behavior of human motoneurons. J Neurosci. 2001;**21**(11):4059–4065.

77. Lagerquist O, Collins DF. Influence of stimulus pulse width on M-waves, H-reflexes, and torque during tetanic low-intensity neuromuscular stimulation. Muscle Nerve. 2010;**42**(6):886–893.

78. Dean JC, Yates LM, Collins DF. Turning on the central contribution to contractions evoked by neuromuscular electrical stimulation. J Appl Physiol. 2007;**103**(1):170–176.

79. Ramos LE, Zell JP. Rehabilitation program for children with brachial plexus and peripheral nerve injury. Semin Pediatr Neurol. 2000;**7**(1):52–57.

80. Boonstra AM, van Weerden TW, Eisma WH, Pahlplatz VB, Oosterhuis HJ. The effect of low-frequency electrical stimulation on denervation atrophy in man. Scand j rehabil. Med. 1987;**19**(3):127–134.

81. Williams HB. A clinical pilot study to assess functional return following continuous muscle stimulation after nerve injury and repair in the upper extremity using a completely implantable electrical system. Microsurgery. 1996;**17**(11):597–605.

82. Williams HB. The value of continuous electrical muscle stimulation using a completely implantable system in the preservation of muscle function following motor nerve injury and repair: an experimental study. Microsurgery. 1996;**17**(11):589–596.

83. Targan RS, Alon G, Kay SL. Effect of long-term electrical stimulation on motor recovery and improvement of clinical residuals in patients with unresolved facial nerve palsy. Otolaryngol Head Neck Surg. 2000;**122**(2):246–252.

84. Colson SS, Benchortane M, Tanant V, et al. Neuromuscular electrical stimulation training: a safe and effective treatment for facioscapulohumeral muscular dystrophy patients. Arch Phys Med Rehabil. 2010;**91**(5):697–702.

85. Zupan A. Long-term electrical stimulation of muscles in children with Duchenne and Becker muscular dystrophy. Muscle Nerve. 1992;**15**(3):362–367.

86. Scott OM, Hyde SA, Vrbova G, Dubowitz V. Therapeutic possibilities of chronic low frequency electrical stimulation in children with Duchenne muscular dystrophy. J Neurol Sci. 1990;**95**(2):171–182.

87. Ramos LE, Zell JP. Rehabilitation program for children with brachial plexus and peripheral nerve injury. Semin Pediatr Neurol. 2000;**7**(1):52–57.

88. Gargiulo P, Vatnsdal B, Ingvarsson P, et al. Restoration of muscle volume and shape induced by electrical stimulation of denervated degenerated muscles: qualitative and quantitative measurement of changes in rectus femoris using computer tomography and image segmentation. Artif Organs. 2008;32(8):609–613.

89. Osborne SL. The retardation of atrophy in man by electrical stimulation of muscles. Arch Phys Med Rehabil. 1951;32(8):523–528.

90. Ashley Z, Sutherland H, Russold MF, et al. Therapeutic stimulation of denervated muscles: the influence of pattern. Muscle Nerve. 2008;38(1):875–886.

91. Ashley Z, Salmons S, Boncompagni S, et al. Effects of chronic electrical stimulation on long-term denervated muscles of the rabbit hind limb. J Muscle Res Cell Motil. 2007;28(4–5):203–217.

92. Asensio-Pinilla E, Udina E, Jaramillo J, Navarro X. Electrical stimulation combined with exercise increase axonal regeneration after peripheral nerve injury. Exp Neurol. 2009;219(1):258–265.

93. Eberstein A, Eberstein S. Electrical stimulation of denervated muscle: is it worthwhile? Med Sci Sports Exerc. 1996;28(12):1463–1469.

94. Valencic V, Vodovnik L, Stefancic M, Jelnikar T. Improved motor response due to chronic electrical stimulation of denervated tibialis anterior muscle in humans. Muscle Nerve. 1986;9(7):612–617.

95. Liberson WT, Holmquest HJ, Scot D, Dow M. Functional electrotherapy: stimulation of the peroneal nerve synchronized with the swing phase of the gait of hemiplegic patients. Arch Phys Med Rehabil. 1961;42:101–105.

96. Moe JH, Post HW. Functional electrical stimulation for ambulation in hemiplegia. Lancet. 1962;82:285–288.

97. Doucet BM, Lam A, Griffin L. Neuromuscular electrical stimulation for skeletal muscle function. Yale J Biol Med. 2012;85(2):201–215.

98. Sheffler LR, Chae J. Neuromuscular electrical stimulation in neurorehabilitation. Muscle Nerve. 2007;35(5):562–590.

99. Hesse S, Malezic M, Schaffrin A, Mauritz KH. Restoration of gait by combined treadmill training and multichannel electrical stimulation in non-ambulatory hemiparetic patients. Scand J Rehabil Med. 1995;27(4):199–204.

100. Kesar TM, Perumal R, Jancosko A, et al. Novel patterns of functional electrical stimulation have an immediate effect on dorsiflexor muscle function during gait for people poststroke. Phys Ther. 2010;90(1):55–66.

101. Thrasher TA, Flett HM, Popovic MR. Gait training regimen for incomplete spinal cord injury using functional electrical stimulation. Spinal Cord. 2006;44(6):357–361.

102. Thrasher TA, Popovic MR. Functional electrical stimulation of walking: function, exercise and rehabilitation. Annales de readaptation et de medecine physique. 2008;51(6):452–460.

103. Van Boxtel A. Differential effects of low-frequency depression, vibration-induced inhibition, and posttetanic potentiation on H-reflexes and tendon jerks in the human soleus muscle. J Neurophysiol. 1986;55(3):551–568.

104. Ridding MC, Brouwer B, Miles TS, Pitcher JB, Thompson PD. Changes in muscle responses to stimulation of the motor cortex induced by peripheral nerve stimulation in human subjects. Exp Brain Res. 2000;131:135–143.

105. Ridding MC, McKay DR, Thompson PD, Miles TS. Changes in corticomotor representations induced by prolonged peripheral nerve stimulation in humans. Clinical Neurophysiol. 2001;112(8):1461–1469.

106. Khaslavskaia S, Ladouceur M, Sinkjaer T. Increase in tibialis anterior motor cortex excitability following repetitive electrical stimulation of the common peroneal nerve. Exp Brain Res. 2002;145(3):309–315.

107. Knash ME, Kido A, Gorassini M, Chan KM, Stein RB. Electrical stimulation of the human common peroneal nerve elicits lasting facilitation of cortical motor-evoked potentials. Exp Brain Res. 2003;153(3):366–377.

108. Mima T, Oga T, Rothwell J, et al. Short-term high-frequency transcutaneous electrical nerve stimulation decreases human motor cortex excitability. Neurosc Lett. 2004;355(1–2):85–88.

109. Murakami T, Sakuma K, Nomura T, Nakashima K. Short-interval intracortical inhibition is modulated by high-frequency peripheral mixed nerve stimulation. Neurosci Lett. 2007;420(1):72–75.

110. Schabrun SM, Ridding MC, Galea MP, Hodges PW, Chipchase LS. Primary sensory and motor cortex excitability are co-modulated in response to peripheral electrical nerve stimulation. PloS One. 2012;7(12):e51298.

111. Frykman GK, Waylett J. Rehabilitation of peripheral nerve injuries. Orthoped Clin N Am. 1981;12(2):361–379.

112. Hijmans JM, Geertzen JHB, Dijkstra PU, Postema K. A systematic review of the effects of shoes and other ankle or foot appliances on balance in older people and people with peripheral nervous system disorders. Gait Posture. 2007;25(2):316–323.

113. Strommen JA. Management of spasticity from spinal cord dysfunction. Neurolo Clin. 2013;31(1):269–286.

114. Huynh W, Krishnan AV, Lin CSY, et al. Botulinum toxin modulates cortical maladaptation in post-stroke spasticity. Muscle Nerve. 2013;48(1):93–99.

115. Jerosch-Herold C. Sensory relearning in peripheral nerve disorders of the hand: a web-based survey and delphi consensus method. J Hand Ther. 2011;24(4):292–298; quiz 299.

116. Attal N, Cruccu G, Baron R, Haanpaa M, Hansson P, Jensen TS, Nurmikko T. EFNS guidelines on the pharmacological treatment of neuropathic pain: 2010 revision. Eur J Neurol. 2010;17(9):1113-e1188.

117. Yuan RY, Sheu JJ, Yu JM, et al. Botulinum toxin for diabetic neuropathic pain: a randomized double-blind crossover trial. Neurology. 2009;72(17):1473–1478.

118. Brosseau L, Judd MG, Marchand S et al. Transcutaneous electrical nerve stimulation (TENS) for the treatment of rheumatoid arthritis in the hand. Cochrane Database Syst Rev. 2003(3):CD004377.

119. Khadilkar A, Odebiyi DO, Brosseau L, Wells GA. Transcutaneous electrical nerve stimulation (TENS) versus placebo for chronic low-back pain. Cochrane Database Syst Rev. 2008(4):CD003008.

120. Nnoaham KE, Kumbang J. Transcutaneous electrical nerve stimulation (TENS) for chronic pain. Cochrane Database Syst Rev. 2008(3):CD003222.

121. Dowswell T, Bedwell C, Lavender T, Neilson JP. Transcutaneous electrical nerve stimulation (TENS) for pain relief in labour. Cochrane Database Syst Rev. 2009(2):CD007214.

122. Johnson MI, Bjordal JM. Transcutaneous electrical nerve stimulation for the management of painful conditions: focus on neuropathic pain. Exp Rev Neurother. 2011;11(5):735–753.

123. Raphael JH, Raheem TA, Southall JL, Bennett A, Ashford RL, Williams S. Randomized double-blind sham-controlled crossover study of short-term effect of percutaneous electrical nerve stimulation in neuropathic pain. Pain Med. 2011;12(10):1515–1522.

124. Norrbrink C. Transcutaneous electrical nerve stimulation for treatment of spinal cord injury neuropathic pain. J Rehabil Res Dev. 2009;46(1):85–93.

125. Barr JO. Transcutaneous electrical nerve stimulation for pain management. In: Nelson RM, Hayes KW, Currier DP (eds). Clinical Electrotherapy, 3rd edn. Appleton and Lange, Stamford, 1999, pp. 291–354.

126. Robertson V, Ward A, Low J, Reed A. Electrotherapy Explained: Principles and Practice. Elsevier, Edinburgh, 2006.

127. Forst T, Nguyen M, Forst S, Disselhoff B, Pohlmann T, Pfutzner A. Impact of low frequency transcutaneous electrical nerve stimulation on symptomatic diabetic neuropathy using the new Salutaris device. Diabetes Nutr Metab. 2004;17(3):163–168.

128. Singla S, Prabhakar V, Singla RK. Role of transcutaneous electric nerve stimulation in the management of trigeminal neuralgia. J Neurosci Rural Pract. 2011;2(2):150–152.

129. Celik EC, Erhan B, Gunduz B, Lakse E. The effect of low-frequency TENS in the treatment of neuropathic pain in patients with spinal cord injury. Spinal Cord. 2013.

130. Siddall PJ. Management of neuropathic pain following spinal cord injury: now and in the future. Spinal Cord. 2009;47(5):352–359.

CHAPTER 20

Treatment of arm and hand dysfunction after CNS damage

Nick Ward

Introduction

Residual upper limb dysfunction after injury to the central nervous system (CNS) is a major clinical, socioeconomic, and societal problem. The inability to incorporate an upper limb in activities of daily living has an enormous impact on an individual's ability to live independently. Neurorehabilitation has traditionally adopted a holistic approach in order to help a person acquire the knowledge and skills needed for optimum physical, psychological, and social function. However, there is growing interest in combining traditional and novel treatments to focus on specific clinical problems such as upper limb dysfunction.

It is estimated that 77% of stroke survivors will have upper limb symptoms after acute stroke [1]. Only 5% to 20% achieve full recovery of the paretic upper limb in terms of activities at 6 months [2–5]. Initial severity of upper limb impairment and function are the most significant predictors of upper limb recovery [6]. Between 33% to 66% of stroke patients with an initially paretic upper limb do not show any recovery in upper limb function 6 months after stroke [4, 5]. Patients showing some (synergistic) movement in the upper limb within 4 weeks post stroke had a greater than 90% chance of improving, whereas this probability remained below 10% in those who failed to show any return of motor control [2]. These data have been used to argue that after stroke there is a critical period for aggressive neurorehabilitation particularly when it comes to upper limb function [7].

After cervical spinal cord injury (C-SCI) arm and hand impairments play a major role in rehabilitation [8] and contribute significantly to the level of functioning [9]. Those with a motor incomplete lesion tend to achieve better outcomes than those with motor complete lesions [10], but overall, upper limb performance and activity can be improved by specific rehabilitation even if not commenced until 6 months after injury [10]. Furthermore, performance levels do not tend to decline after rehabilitation. Exercise therapy appears to be effective in C-SCI [11, 12] and there is increasing interest in the use of technology, including neuromuscular electrical stimulation and robotic devices [13], although the evidence base remains small.

In multiple sclerosis (MS) upper limb dysfunction is reported in at least two-thirds of patients [14]. As in other conditions, the level of arm and hand functioning plays a major role in determining the level of independence in daily activities like eating, dressing, grooming [15]. Despite this, there is relatively limited clinical experience in upper limb rehabilitation in MS. Patients with MS

may have both spinal cord and brain lesions and so have clinical characteristics of stroke and/or C-SCI. In contrast to patients with stroke and C-SCI, patients with MS may show temporal fluctuations in impairment or may exhibit a progressive course, and their upper limb symptoms may be either unilateral or bilateral. For these reasons, direct translation of findings from upper limb neurorehabilitation studies in stroke or C-SCI patients is not straightforward. A recent systematic review of motor training programmes of arm and hand in MS patients found that overall, most studies demonstrated improvements in upper limb in medical stable MS patients with different degrees of severity [16]. However, a consensus on the optimal content of upper limb training programmes for patients with MS is lacking.

This chapter reviews current approaches to promoting upper limb recovery after CNS damage, particularly stroke. In many instances it will be seen that treatment studies are performed in the chronic rather than 'critical' phase (likely to be the first few months) and on relatively unselected patients. The crucial questions of when is best to deliver a treatment and who is most likely to benefit are largely unanswered [17]. In future, clinical trials of rehabilitation strategies might cross disease boundaries to develop and test the most optimal methods for training patients based on impairments and disabilities rather than diseases [18]. At present, however, there is a stronger evidence base for upper limb rehabilitation strategies in stroke than for other conditions.

General approaches to upper limb therapy

There is an appreciation that neurorehabilitation strategies that aim to restore as much arm and hand function as possible do not provide adequate dose or intensity of treatment [7]. A recent study determined that during inpatient rehabilitation patients were engaged in activities with the potential to prevent complications and improve recovery of mobility only 13% of the time, and were alone over 60% of the time [19]. Furthermore, practice of task-specific, functional upper-extremity movements occurred in only 51% of the rehabilitation sessions that were meant to address upper-limb rehabilitation [20]. There is conflicting evidence about whether providing additional upper limb therapy improves outcomes, but the design of many studies investigating this question varies quite significantly, and so inconsistent results are not surprising. For example, it is likely that the amount of extra therapy is important but ranges from 2 hours per week to 3 hours a day. Furthermore, extra treatment was sometimes initiated early after stroke, but sometimes in the chronic phase. One influential study initiated an extra 30 min of rehabilitation with an emphasis on either arm or leg training within 14 days after stroke [21]. Although it is suggested that the study provided evidence for a task-specific effect, there was no difference in dexterity, walking ability or activities of daily living at 26 weeks. Other studies using a similar dose of extra therapy failed to find benefits in upper limb function [22–24]. A recent study that looked for a dose effect, found that an additional 2–3 hours of arm training a day for 6 weeks improved both Fugl-Meyer and Action Research Arm Test scores when started 1–2 months after stroke [25]. It seems likely that when it comes to upper limb therapy, more is better.

Dose of therapy can also mean number of repetitions. Data from the animal literature suggest that changes in synaptic density in the primary motor cortex occur after 400 but not 60 reaches [26, 27]. In most rodent models of stroke, animals strokewill typically reach several hundred times in a training session. It is possible that there is threshold for activity below which motor recovery is unlikely to occur [28]. In human stroke patients, the typical number or repetitions in a therapy session is much lower, approximately 30 [20]. The ability to perform repeated movements during rehabilitation is likely to be related to the functional level and it appears that there may be a functional threshold above which upper limb use improves, but below which it decreases [29].

One way of increasing dose is to implement a treatment programme that patients can administer themselves. The self-administered graded repetitive arm supplementary programme (GRASP) has the advantage of being flexible enough to use in patients with a range of impairments [30]. When started early after stroke in an in-patient setting, 4 weeks of GRASP led to improvements in upper limb function (as assessed by the Chedoke Arm and Hand Activity Inventory, CAHAI) compared patients undergoing an education program. These gains were maintained at 5 months post-stroke. The GRASP is easy to administer, cost-effective and feasible to implement in a number of health care settings on a large scale [31].

Additional therapy may be task-specific, and it is often suggested that task-specificity is required for motor learning to occur. However, to learn complex everyday tasks almost certainly requires that instruction and knowledge combine with adaptation, reinforcement, and acuity mechanisms. To be useful, task-specific training must be both retained and generalizable [32]. A number of underlying training components have been identified in task oriented training after stroke (Table 20.1). The elements 'distributed practice' and 'feedback' were associated with the largest post-intervention effect sizes, wheras 'random practice' and 'use of clear functional goals' were associated with the largest follow-up effect sizes [33]. In other words, applying some of the principles of motor learning (particularly in promoting skill retention and generalizability) are important aspects of designing the optimum therapeutic approach [32]. However, study variability led a Cochrane review of repetitive task-specific training to conclude that there was no evidence to support any beneficial effects upper limb function [34]. Several studies have been performed since 2007, including one large randomized controlled trial (RCT) comparing 4 weeks of task specific training with a Bobath approach in 103 stroke patients recruited 4 to 24 weeks after [35]. Patients in the task-specific group achieved significantly greater gains compared to the control group on a range of tests including Fugl-Meyer and

Table 20.1 Task-oriented training components used in upper limb rehabilitation

1. *Functional movements:* A movement involving task execution that is not directed towards a clear activities of daily living goal (e.g. moving blocks from one location to another, stacking rings over a cone).

2. *Clear functional goal:* A goal that is set during everyday life activities (e.g. washing dishes, grooming activity, dressing oneself, playing golf).

3. *Client-centred patient goal:* Therapy goals that are set through the involvement of the patient himself/herself in the therapy goal decision process. The goals respect patients' values, preferences, and expressed needs and recognize the clients' experience and knowledge.

4. *Overload:* Training that exceeds the patient's metabolic muscle capacity. Overload is determined by the total time spent on therapeutic activity, the number of repetitions, the difficulty of the activity in terms of coordination, muscle activity type and resistance load, and the intensity (i.e. number of repetitions per time unit).

5. *Real-life object manipulation:* Manipulation that makes use of objects that are handled in normal everyday-life activities (eg, cutlery, hairbrush, etc.).

6. *Context-specific environment:* A training environment (supporting surface, objects, people, room, etc.) that equals or mimics the natural environment for a specific task execution, in order to include task characteristic sensory/perceptual information, task-specific context characteristics, and cognitive processes involved.

7. *Exercise progression:* Exercises on offer have an increasing difficulty level that is in line with the increasing abilities of the patient, in order to keep the demands of the exercises and challenges optimal for motor learning.

8. *Exercise variety:* A variety of exercises offered to support motor skill learning of a certain task because of the person experiencing different movement and context characteristics (within task variety) and problem-solving strategies.

9. *Feedback:* Specific information on the patient's motor performance that enhances motor learning and positively influences patient motivation.

10. *Multiple movement planes:* Movement that uses more than 1 degree of freedom of a joint, therefore occurring around multiple joint axes.

11. *Total skill practice:* The skill is practiced in total, with or without preceding skill component training (eg, via chaining).

12. *Patient-customized training load:* A training load that suits the individualized treatment targets e.g, endurance, coordination, or strength training as well as the patient's capabilities (e.g. 65% of 1 repetition maximum or 85% of 1 repetition maximum for the specific patient).

13. *Random practice:* In each practice session, the exercises are randomly ordered.

14. *Distributed practice:* A practice schedule with relatively long rest periods.

15. *Bimanual practice:* Tasks where both arms and hands are involved.

Timmermans AAA, Spooren AIF, Kingma H, Seelen HAM, Neurorehabil Neural Repair (24:9), pp. 858–70, copyright © 2010. Reprinted by Permission of SAGE Publications.

Action Research Arm Test that were maintained at an 8-week follow up. Overall, it seems that task-specific training might improve upper limb function in some patients, but important questions remain concerning how to maximize retention of new skills and whether improvement in taught tasks generalizes to other tasks. It is still not clear whether there is a real mechanistic difference between different approaches, or whether the key variable is simply time on task(s).

When considering the established neurodevelopmental approaches (e.g. Bobath, Brunnstrom's Movement Therapy, and Proprioceptive Neuromucular Facilitation (PNF)), there is no evidence to suggest that on average, one is superior to the other [36, 37] or that neurodevelopmental techniques are superior to other therapeutic approaches [38, 39].

Robotic training

A specific example of task-specific upper limb training is the recent use of robotic technology. It is hoped that the use of robots in guiding highly specific training regimes will allow a sufficient number of repetitions to be delivered [40, 41]. Robotic devices also offer the prospect of very detailed assessment of changes in motor control [42]. Most clinical trials have been small and have involved chronic stroke patients. Overall, there is evidence of improvement in the Fugl-Meyer score of 2–4 points when compared to usual care [43], which falls below the level of a clinically meaningful change [44]. In one of the largest studies to date, chronic stroke patients with a Fugl-Meyer score of between 7 and 38 (range 0–66) were included. The robotic treatment did achieve a large number of repetitions (over 1,000 per session), but the Fugl-Meyer score only improved by just over 2 points compare to usual (less intense) therapy, and was no different to therapy matched for dose [45]. Others have argued that this intensity of therapy needs to be delivered much earlier than 6 months post stroke [7, 46], and it may also be that certain subgroups of patients would be more likely to benefit [47, 48], but this is currently not clear. There are a number of devices available and these are discussed in detail elsewhere in this book (Chapter 31). The relationship between robotic technology and motor learning is also addressed in detail elsewhere in this book (Chapter 7).

Strength training

Loss of muscle strength has significant negative impact on functional recovery of the upper limb after stroke [49, 50]. Two meta-analyses of strength training of the upper limb after stroke concluded that there was evidence to support a positive effect on grip strength, but also on upper limb function and activity, without adverse effects on spasticity or pain [51, 52].

It has been argued that increases in muscle strength may not translate into improvements in functional activity unless strengthening activity is provided as part of training of everyday functional activities [53]. Muscle strength training can be combined with functional training. The resulting functional strength training (FST) emphasizes improving the power of shoulder and elbow muscles to enable appropriate placing of the hand and improving the production of appropriate force in different muscles to achieve a specific grasp. Preliminary data from a phase II trial suggest that FST may be more effective than standard therapy of equal intensity [54] and a larger trial is underway [55].

Trunk restraint

Many stroke patients use compensatory trunk or shoulder girdle movements to extend the reach of the affected arm [56]. These compensatory trunk movements may improve reaching in the short term but are likely to be detrimental to long-term recovery. A number of studies have investigated whether restraining the trunk in combination with task-specific training can promote more 'normal' patterns of reaching. Additional trunk-restraint appears to improve upper limb impairment assessed with the Fugl-Meyer score, but had a less certain effect on function [57].

Somatosensory training

After stroke, somatosensory deficits are common, with proprioceptive impairment and asterognosis in particular occurring in as many as one to two thirds of patients [58]. Sensory impairment is associated with slower recovery after stroke because it is important for motor function. Although many of the approaches described incorporate sensory stimulation with motor training, there have been specific attempts to examine whether additional sensory training can influence motor recovery. Systematic reviews have generally included a wide variety of techniques including transcutaneous electrical nerve stimulation (TENS), acupuncture, thermal stimulation, repetitive passive movement therapy, intermittent pneumatic compression, and learning based sensorimotor training [59]. Each may have a different mechanism of action and so evaluating the effect of these therapies together may not be appropriate. Currently, there is insufficient evidence to support or refute effectiveness of these sensory interventions in improving sensory impairment, upper limb function, or participants' functional status and participation after stroke [59].

Constraint-induced movement therapy

Constraint-induced movement therapy (CIMT) is an approach to upper limb rehabilitation that comprises two key features. First, patients are required to wear a sling or mitten restricting use of the unaffected hand/arm (Figure 20.1). Second, increased use of the affected hand/arm in functional tasks, a form of training that has been termed 'shaping'. This approach was first introduced in 1994 after Taub and colleagues [60] noted that monkeys with a peripherally deafferented upper limb did not use the affected limb even after neurological injury had resolved. They proposed that 'excess' motor disability could be caused through negative reinforcement and learned nonuse and that changing the contingencies of reinforcement could lead to improvement in limb function. The biological mechanisms underpinning CIMT in those with damage to the central nervous system (compared to peripheral deafferentation) are unclear. Indeed, whether learned nonuse is a major contributor to 'excess motor disability' after stroke is unproven, partly because learned nonuse cannot be measured. Furthermore, the relative contributions of increasing the amount of affected limb practice and constraining the unaffected side, are not known. Nevertheless, CIMT has been widely studied.

The largest and most rigorous of all the CIMT trials was Extremity Constraint Induced Therapy Evaluation (EXCITE) [61], which recruited patients 3 to 9 months after stroke. Active treatment was provided to 106 patients consisting of wearing a restraining mitt on the unaffected hand while engaging in repetitive task practice and behavioural shaping with the hemiplegic hand for 6 hours a day for 10 days. They were compared to 116 patients receiving usual care (ranging from no treatment after concluding formal rehabilitation to pharmacologic or physiotherapeutic interventions). Those receiving CIMT had superior scores on the Wolf Motor Function test and the Motor Activity Log (a self-report of performance in activities of daily living), and these gains were maintained 2 years after treatment [62]. On the other hand CIMT does not appear to reduce impairment or lead to recovery of lost motor control [63, 64].

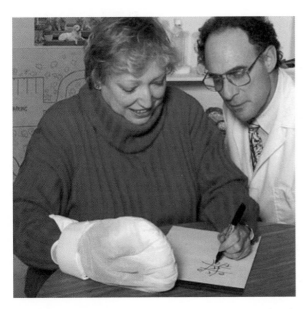

Fig. 20.1 A mitten is worn on the right hand as part of constraint induced movement therapy (CIMT)

There have been 13 RCTs of CIMT in the subacute or chronic phase of stroke, but EXCITE remains the largest by far. The results are generally supportive of a benefit of CIMT over usual care on motor function in those with some preserved wrist (20 degrees of extension) and hand (10 degrees of metacarpophalangeal and interphalangeal) movement. CIMT might also be more effective in those with neglect or sensory loss, impairments that might contribute to diminished use of a functional limb.

Since EXCITE, there have been a number of CIMT protocols in use. The commonest variation is modified CIMT (mCIMT), introduced because some patients found it difficult to wear the mitten for 90% of waking hours in the standard protocol. Modified CIMT is generally less intense, with periods of restriction for 5 hours a day combined with structured ½ hour therapy sessions for 3 days a week [65]. Other variations are in use, for example increasing the duration of treatment from 2 to 10 weeks [64]. In general, these mCIMT studies in the chronic stroke phase have been small with quite different protocols. It is therefore difficult to draw firm conclusions about mCIMT in chronic stroke.

A smaller number of studies have tested whether CIMT can be introduced earlier. The Very Early Constraint-Induced Movement during Stroke Rehabilitation (VECTORS) study randomized 52 patients at about 10 days post-stroke to 2 weeks of therapy consisting of two levels of intensity of CIMT (2 hours shaping/mitt for 6 hours per day versus 3 hours of shaping/mitt for 90% of waking hours per day) or standard therapy (1 hour of training on activities of daily living plus 1 hour of bilateral arm training) [66]. Upper limb function measured with the Action Research Arm Test (ARAT) improved in all groups, but the improvement was less for the intense CIMT group compared to the other two groups, which were comparable in their gains. In other words, the intense CIMT group was worse off at 90 days, although there was no difference compared to the control group at 30 days. It is unclear why intense CIMT might have had a late effect on upper limb function.

The only comparable study enrolled 23 patients within one week of stroke onset. Here, the intensity of the control group therapy was matched (3 hours a day for 6 days a week over 2 weeks). At 3 months, the Fugl-Meyer score and reported quality of hand function were improved in the CIMT group, but other measures were not significant. This study is likely to have been underpowered. Modified CIMT has also been examined in the early post-stroke phase, with one study including 28 patients with any level of arm paresis [67]. Both mCIMT and control groups received an hour of therapy per day for 2 weeks, but the mCIMT group improved more on novel measures of upper limb function. Overall, there is conflicting evidence on the effect of CIMT in the very early phase after stroke.

In summary, CIMT might be suitable for patients with residual wrist and hand function. It is worth bearing in mind that only 6.3% of the patients screened for EXCITE were eligible [61], and so CIMT is only likely to be an adjunct to other approaches. Although there is little evidence that CIMT leads to either significant reductions in impairment or a return to closer to normal levels of motor control [63], it appears to be able to improve some aspects of motor function over and above standard care. Function may improve through learning to compensate for deficits better by practicing particular tasks using intact residual capacities. Many studies do not provide a matched dose or intensity of a control therapy and so it remains unclear what the 'active ingredient' of CIMT might be, or whether this is just a useful way to increase therapy time in motivated patients.

Bilateral arm training

Bilateral arm training (BAT) techniques involve the practice of the same movement with both upper limbs simultaneously. Bilateral arm function is important because much of what we do every day involves the use of both arms. Recovery of bilateral arm function is best facilitated through training of both arms together rather than separately, since different mechanisms are involved in unilateral and bilateral arm movement [68, 69]. However, it is also suggested that practising bilateral activities may have a positive effect on unilateral (affected) arm function, although the justification is usually in terms of neurophysiological changes perceived as being beneficial (i.e. reduced intracortical inhibition and/or increased intracortical facilitation affected hemisphere motor cortex [70]).

There are a number of factors to consider in evaluating studies of BAT. Most clinical studies have examined the effects of BAT on unilateral affected arm function, with little emphasis on recovery of bilateral movements. Furthermore, the type of bilateral movement varies between studies. Bilateral tasks may be symmetrical or complementary. Most clinical studies use symmetrical movements, which can be in-phase or anti-phase, although there are only limited examples of functional tasks using each (folding a towel for in-phase, climbing a ladder for anti-phase). The most common bilateral tasks used day to day require non-identical but complementary movements (e.g. using a knife and fork), in which the dominant hand manipulates, whilst the non-dominant hand stabilizes, but this type of task is rarely used in BAT studies.

Repetitive reaching with fixed hand approaches include bilateral arm training with rhythmic auditory cueing (BATRAC) (Figure 20.2) and mirror image movement enabling (MIME). In both, movements are symmetrical but can be in phase or anti-phase.

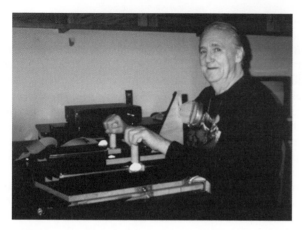

Fig. 20.2 Bilateral arm trainer used in BACTRAC.
Whitall J, McCombe Waller S, Silver KH, Macko RF, Repetitive bilateral arm training with rhythmic auditory cueing improves motor function in chronic hemiparetic stroke. Stroke, 31 (10), 2390–5. © 2000.

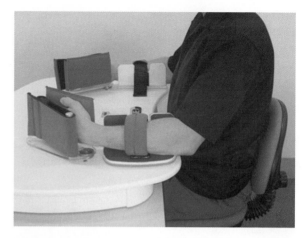

Fig. 20.3 Device used for active–passive bilateral arm training.
Stinear CM, Petoe MA, Anwar S, Barber PA, Byblow WD, Bilateral priming accelerates recovery of upper limb function after stroke: a randomized controlled trial, Stroke, 45 (1), 205–10. © 2014.

BATRAC involves two unyoked handles, which are moved forwards and backwards [71]. One relatively large study found similar effects with BATRAC and dose-matched therapeutic exercise in chronic stroke patients treated for 6 weeks. The improvements were small (1–2 points on the upper limb Fugl-Meyer scale), and so probably not clinically meaningful [72]. MIME involves strapping both arms into splints connected to a robotic manipulator. Movement of the unaffected arm is translated by the robot into mirrored movements of the affected arm. It appeared to improve proximal function compared to a neurodevelopmental approach in mild to moderately impaired chronic stroke patients [73], but when started 7–21 days after stroke, MIME (15 or 30 hours) provided no additional benefit assessed with the Fugl-Meyer scale [74].

Another approach is to train a specific muscle group or joint movement bilaterally. For example, active–passive bilateral training (APBT) (Figure 20.3), in which active movement of unaffected wrist moves the affected wrist via a manipulandum), or wrist and finger extension combined with electrical stimulation. Overall, some benefits in impairment have been seen in those with moderate to severe paresis, but improvements in function were less convincing [75, 76]. APBT may also be used as a way of priming the motor system—that is, it disinhibits motor cortex contralateral to the paretic limb [76]. APBT prior to standard upper limb therapy can accelerate recovery but may not improve long term outcomes [77]. Nevertheless, accelerated recovery on its own would be beneficial in terms of reduced hospital stays, earlier return to activities including work and possibly avoidance of complications.

The last category of study includes those that train grasp, reach, and release during BAT [78–81]. This type of approach is perhaps closest to what might happen in a standard therapy session. Overall, these studies are relatively small and show most benefits in those with mild paresis.

On the basis of the studies performed to date, there is little consistent evidence that BAT is superior to unilateral arm training [82] or dose-matched conventional treatment [83]. However, many of the studies that have been compared have quite different approaches. The success of the intervention is likely to depend on the severity of upper limb paresis and time of intervention post stroke.

Interventions for improving coordination of reach to grasp

There is an argument that the conventional approaches described have not taken into account the fact that the hand and arm are coordinated as one unit during skilled everyday use. Patients with more severe stroke may suffer a breakdown in spatial and temporal inter-segmental coordination between reaching and grasping [84], resulting in a smaller number of stereotypical movement patterns, which themselves may be abnormal [85, 86]. Patients may develop unwanted elbow flexion or abduction and forward flexion of the shoulder during attempted reach. There may be abnormalities of anticipatory hand shaping, premature hand closure, inadequate opening, dysmetria, as well as segmented and slowed movements, all of which can all contribute to clumsy upper limb function or disuse [87].

A recent systematic review examined rehabilitation strategies in which a key aim was to improve coordination of the arm during reach and grasp [88]. Three main categories of intervention were identified: (i) functional training, (ii) robot therapy or computerized training, (iii) biofeedback or electrical stimulation. Although there were examples of studies targeting improvements reach and grasp together, overall, the results were disappointing with no clear evidence that interventions led to specific benefit in reach and grasp. The reasons were most likely to be the variability in the intensity or dose of the training, in the specificity of the training, the provision of feedback to promote learning and heterogeneity of the subjects enrolled.

Mental imagery, mirror training, action observation

The use of mental imagery to enhance motor recovery (performance) has been adopted from the field of sports psychology. A recent Cochrane review looked at six RCTs and concluded that the addition of mental practice regimes to standard therapy did not convincingly improve upper limb outcomes [89]. One of the problems here is the diversity of approaches used. Anecdotal evidence also suggests that the degree to which patients find it helpful varies greatly, with up to 40% being unable to perform motor imagery [90]. Without having a way to stratify patients in clinical trials, then any positive treatment effect will be diluted by these non-responders.

The use of action observation as an adjunct to upper limb therapy has also gained some interest. Here, unlike mental imagery, action observation is seen as a way of priming the motor system (i.e. it disinhibits motor cortex contralateral to the paretic limb), so that subsequent therapy is more likely to lead to motor memory encoding [91]. A large RCT involving 102 patients examined the effect of asking patients view particular upper limb actions with a view to imitating these actions with a therapist afterwards [92]. In comparison to the control group, the treatment group performed better at the box and blocks test after 2 weeks.

Mirror box therapy (Figure 20.4) is often confused with the previous two approaches. Here, subjects place both arms outstretched on a table, with the affected hand behind a mirror. When looking at the affected hand, subjects will see the unaffected hand. Subjects are asked to move both hands simultaneously, and the mirror creates an illusion that the affected hand is moving normally. A Cochrane review examined 14 RCTs of mirror therapy after stroke and concluded that there was a modest benefit in terms of motor function, although the nature of the studies was quite diverse. One of the benefits of mirror therapy is that it is simple to set up and so could easily be performed by patients in their own home. However, as with mental imagery, it is likely that there are some people for whom it just does not work. Anecdotal evidence suggests that the formation of a strong illusion that the unaffected hand is moving normally, is important for a therapeutic effect.

Little is known about which patients are likely to benefit most from any of these three interventions. Each has some theoretical underpinnings which relate to particular brain regions and so it ought to be possible to determine whether there are responders and non-responders. As with many of these approaches, stratification based on mechanistic principles in future will be important [17].

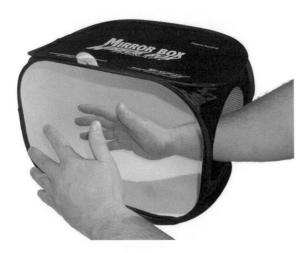

Fig. 20.4 Device used in Mirror Box Training.
From http://www.ireflex.co.uk/mirrorboxtherapy.com/howitworks/

Neuromuscular electrical stimulation

Neuromuscular electrical stimulation (NMES) refers to the electrical stimulation of lower motor neurons to cause muscle contraction. When combined with attempts to perform functional movements, it is referred to as functional electrical stimulation (FES).

There are a range of approaches that come under the banner of NMES:

(i) Cyclical NMES uses a set cyclical schedule of electrical stimulation but does not require attempted movement from the participant.

(ii) EMG-triggered NMES couples intent to move (generating an EMG response) and NMES-induced muscle contraction.

(iii) NMES controlled neuroprostheses that aid the completion of functionally relevant tasks.

A number of RCTs have examined whether the addition of cyclical NMES to standard physiotherapy is superior to standard physiotherapy. When delivered within the first weeks of months after stroke there is clear evidence of improvement in motor function, activities of daily living and dexterity [93–95] and that this early improvement is sustained at 6 months [94].

A systematic review of studies examining the effects of electromyographic (EMG)-triggered NMES found evidence of improvements in a range of upper limb impairments and activities, but reported that the effects were non-significant [96]. However, many of these studies were performed in chronic stroke, but when applied early after stroke it appears that the effects are more likely to be significant [97]. Direct comparison of cyclic and EMG-triggered NMES has not found any significant differences in the benefits of each approach [98, 99].

NMES delivered with a variety of neuroprosthetic devices also show benefit [100–102]. More sophisticated devices are under development including implantable microstimulators allowing sequential activation of affected muscles to facilitate functional reach and grasp [103, 104] and contralaterally controlled FES (i.e. with the 'unaffected' upper limb) [105]. Understanding interactions between voluntary effort and FES assistance should also lead to improved devices. For example, recent work suggests that FES-produced hand opening is often overpowered by finger flexor coactivation in response to patient attempts to reach and open the hand. Devices that can stimulate both reach and hand opening allow reduced levels of voluntary effort in these muscles and consequently facilitate useful amounts of simultaneous reach and hand opening [106].

Overall, surface NMES appears to be effective in reducing motor impairment, although the evidence of an effect on upper limb-related activities remains less strong. The effect appears to be more significant for those with milder impairments and is also likely to be more robust and enduring in the weeks and months after stroke rather than in the chronic phase.

Avoiding complications—treatment for spasticity or contracture

Most activity-based therapies assume that patients have avoided the complications of CNS damage, specifically marked spasticity with reduction of joint range or even fixed contractures. Spasticity is defined as a velocity dependent increase in muscle tone or tonic stretch reflexes. Roughly a quarter to a third of first-ever stroke patients have evidence of spasticity 1 year after the acute event [107] with lower scores on the Barthel Index at 7 days predicting more severe spasticity [108]. In the first few days, spasticity is most likely to appear in the arm, but after 3 months is equally likely to be present in both arm and leg [109]. Spasticity in the leg alone appears to be uncommon after stroke. Overall, severe disability was found in a similar proportion of patients with and without spasticity [109].

Physical approaches

A number of approaches to reducing spasticity are available from physical therapies (such as stretching, splinting and occasionally surgery), oral antispasticity agents, intramuscular botulinum toxin, or intrathecal drug therapies. The effects of centrally acting antispasticity medication tend to be limited by side effects such as muscle weakness and sedation and so physical therapies together with botulinum toxin are the most commonly used treatments.

The use of splinting to counteract or prevent spasticity in the upper limb is common, but a recent systematic review examined four trials including 126 stroke patients and found no evidence that upper limb orthoses improve upper limb function, range of movement at the wrist, fingers, or thumb, nor pain [110]. Another commonly used approach is to use stretching regimes, and one study has shown some benefit in terms of increasing joint angles, reducing pain and improving activities of daily living in chronic stroke patients [111] but there is less evidence in the early post-stroke phase [112]. One of the problems with trials in both splinting and stretching is that the optimum dose is not clear and one solution to this that is routinely employed is to encourage patients or carers to perform stretching themselves.

Botulinum toxin

Botulinum toxin selectively blocks the release of acetylcholine at the neuromuscular junction, leading to muscle weakness and reduction in spasticity. It is used to selectively target overactive muscles often with the help of electromyographic guidance. The effects are dose dependent and typically last between 2 and 4 months [113]. It appears to be safer, better tolerated and more effective than tizanidine in treating upper limb spasticity [114]. Two early systematic reviews supported the finding that botulinum toxin is effective at reducing spasticity and improving passive range of movement, but not upper limb function [115, 116]. Another systematic review, however, reported a relationship between the maximum change in spasticity and the maximum change in arm function suggesting that reduction in spasticity is associated with improved arm function [117]. This supported by a systematic review of 16 trials, which found that the use of botulinum toxin was associated with moderate improvement in upper-extremity performance after stroke [118].

Muscle weakness, rather than spasticity, appears to be the main contributor to reduced upper limb function after stroke. Reducing spasticity might therefore allow strength training in appropriate muscles thereby improving function. Several studies have therefore combined botulinum toxin with upper limb training. The BoTULS trial enrolled 333 stroke patients with stroke with upper limb spasticity and reduced arm function and examined the effect of botulinum toxin plus a 4-week therapy programme compared to therapy alone [119]. Improvements were seen in muscle tone, pain, upper limb strength, and basic functional tasks, but not in the primary outcome of the ARAT. The majority of the subjects in this study had little if any distal hand function to begin with which might account for the lack of effect on the ARAT, which has prominent pinch and grasp components. A recent systematic review of studies combining botulinum toxin and multidisciplinary care looked at three trials involving 91 patients and found low-level evidence to support this combination in improving upper limb function and /or impairment. Clearly, patient selection, choice of adjunctive therapy, and appropriate outcomes are important in assessing the impact of these studies. The most obvious cohort would appear to be those patients who have evidence of muscle activity that is 'unmasked' by botulinum toxin. It would also seem important that the subsequent physical therapy includes some form of (functional) strength training.

Intrathecal baclofen

Baclofen is a derivative of gamma-aminobutyric acid (GABA). It is an agonist of the $GABA_B$ receptor and can exert some of its beneficial effects on spasticity by restoring the balance of excitatory and inhibitory input in the spinal cord and so reducing muscle hypertonus. Baclofen is relatively poorly tolerated as an oral

Table 20.2 Stages of motor recovery of the Chedoke–McMaster Stroke Impairment Inventory

Stage	Characteristics
1	Flaccid paralysis is present. Phasic stretch reflexes are absent or hypoactive. Active movement cannot be elicited reflexively with a facilitory stimulus or volitionally.
2	Spasticity is present and is felt as a resistance to passive movement. No voluntary movement is present but a facilitatory stimulus will elicit the limb synergies reflexively. These limb synergies consist of stereotypical flexor and extensor movements.
3	Spasticity is marked. The synergistic movements can be elicited voluntarily but are not obligatory.
4	Spasticity decreases. Synergy patterns can be reversed if movement takes place in the weaker synergy first. Movement combining antagonistic synergies can be performed when the prime movers are the strong components of the synergy.
5	Spasticity wanes, but is evident with rapid movement and at the extremes of range. Synergy patterns can be revised even if the movement takes place in the strongest synergy first. Movements that utilize the weak components of both synergies acting as prime movers can be performed.
6	Coordination and patterns of movement can be near normal. Spasticity as demonstrated as resistance to passive movement is no longer present. Abnormal patterns of movement with faulty timing emerge when rapid or complex actions are requested.
7	Normal. A 'normal' variety of rapid, age appropriate complex movement patterns are possible with normal timing, coordination, strength and endurance.There is no evidence of functional impairment compared to the normal side. There is a 'normal' sensory-perceptual motor system.

Gowland C, Stratford P, Ward M, et al, Measuring physical impairment and disability with the Chedoke-McMaster Stroke Assessment, Stroke, 24 (1), 58–63 © 1993.

Table 20.3 Consensus on treatment of upper limb impairment after stroke

A. Recommendations for patients with severe impairment

For stroke patients with severe motor, sensory and functional deficits in the involved limb after stroke (Chedoke–McMaster Stroke Impairment Inventory score less than stage 4):

1. Maintain a comfortable, pain-free, mobile arm and hand

   ◆ Emphasize proper positioning, support while at rest and careful handling of the upper limb during functional activities.

   ◆ Engage in classes overseen by professional rehabilitation clinicians in an institutional or community setting that teach the patient and caregiver to perform self-range of motion exercises.

   ◆ Avoid use of overhead pullies that appear to contribute to shoulder tissue injury

   ◆ Use some means of external support for the upper limb in stages 1 or 2 (of Chedoke–McMaster Stroke Impairment Inventory) during transfers and mobility

   ◆ Place upper limb in a variety of positions that include placing arm and hand within the patient's visual field.

   ◆ Use some means of external support to protect the upper limb during wheelchair use.

2. To maximize functional independence, stroke patients with persistent motor and sensory deficits and their caregivers should be taught compensatory techniques and environmental adaptations that enable performance of important tasks and activities with the less affected arm and hand.

B. Recommendations for patients with moderate impairment

For patients with moderate impairments (Chedoke–McMaster Stroke Impairment Inventory score of stage 4 or better):

1. Engage in repetitive and intense use of novel tasks that challenge the patient to acquire necessary motor skills to use the involved upper limb during functional tasks and activities.

2. Engage in motor-learning training including the use of imagery.

Data from Barreca S, et al. [136].

agent but it can be delivered via the intrathecal route. Intrathecal baclofen (ITB) is increasingly used to treat intractable spasticity, particularly in spinal cord injury, cerebral palsy and multiple sclerosis. Despite evidence of its efficacy, it is not commonly used in stroke [120]. There is evidence that intrathecal baclofen used in post-stroke spastic hemiparesis reduces muscle tone, facilitates muscle strength, and is associated with improvements in functional independence and quality of life [121, 122].

Overall, the goals of treatment aimed at reducing spasticity will depend on the individual patient. Whilst in some in may be that unmasking of weak muscles followed by strength training will lead to improvements in upper limb function, it is certainly the case that in others, the goal may not be to restore function (at least of the hand), but to prevent further complications, reduce pain, and facilitate use of the arm in activities of daily living. Specialist multidisciplinary goal-centred management is essential to beneficial outcomes [123].

Enhancing plasticity

Training works through mechanisms of experience-dependent plasticity [124], but what do we understand about manipulating plasticity therapeutically ('plasticity-enhancement') to increase the efficacy of motor-skills training after stroke? A key determinant of the potential for plasticity in adults is the balance between cortical inhibition and excitation [125]. Reduced GABAergic-inhibition and/or enhanced glutamatergic-excitation increase spike-timing dependent plasticity [126], long-term potentiation (LTP), and enhance a number of downstream effects, including induction of brain-derived neurotrophic factor (BDNF) and cortical structural remodelling [127]. This balance is, consequently, an exciting therapeutic target in restorative neurology. After cortical infarcts in animals, there is conflicting evidence of both early perilesional hyper-[128] and hypoexcitability (129). The timing and extent of similar changes after human stroke is unclear. Knowing the profile of these longitudinal

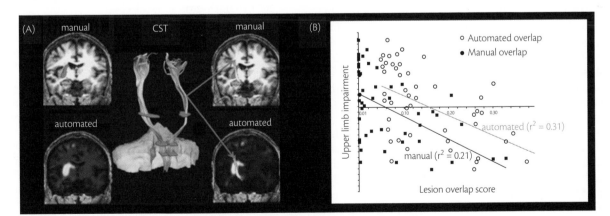

Fig. 20.5 Automated assessment of corticospinal tract integrity after stroke. (A) Infarcts were defined manually (top left in red) or automatically (bottom left in light grey). Normal template corticospinal tracts were reconstructed through the regions of interest (posterior limb of internal capsule, and upper and lower pons), and with an exclusion mask (CST). Template corticospinal tracts were then overlapped with the manually (top right) and automatically (top left) defined infarcts. (B) Overlap of corticospinal tract from the primary motor cortex (M1) and infarct determined from manual (black squares) and automated (open circles) methods plotted against motor impairment. Similar correlations with motor impairment between the two overlap methods are supported by a Fisher r–z transformation (M1: $p = 0.509$).
From Kou et al. [138].

changes is crucial because it will impact on plasticity-mediated recovery, influence when training is best delivered and when plasticity-enhancement might be attempted [7].

Several approaches to plasticity-enhancement to promote the effects of training are of interest in stroke, including neuropharmacological [130, 131] (see Chapter 17) and non-invasive brain stimulation [132, 133] (see Chapter 16). We have come across other examples of this approach with action observation and active-passive bilateral training. Currently, there is no clear rationale for patient selection or optimal timing [134]. Future studies require a mechanistic framework for understanding how to use putative plasticity-enhancing treatments more effectively in stroke neurorehabilitation.

Overall approach

On the basis of a synthesis of the available evidence, clinicians need to determine consistent approaches to managing patients with upper limb paresis. One key factor that appears in most of the studies is that the baseline degree of severity of impairment is important in determining whether a particular approach works. For example, the Chedoke–McMaster Stroke Impairment Inventory (Table 20.2) [135] has been used as a way of dividing stroke patients into those who are more likely to benefit from intensive therapy (Table 20.3) [136].

In future, other metrics, including brain imaging or neurophysiology, might be helpful [137,138] (Figure 20.5).

Conclusion

The appropriate approach to upper limb treatment after CNS injury is most likely to be determined by the level of severity of impairment and the chronicity of the stroke. Patients with severe impairment beyond several months have less chance for restoration of normal motor function, although improvement of function through compensatory strategies is certainly possible. Those with less severe impairment, for example preservation of activity in the elbow, wrist and/or finger extensors, are more likely to have the necessary neural infrastructure to support further recovery. There is increasing evidence that the first few months are a critical period, with greater potential for recovery, possibly through enhanced neuroplastic processes. Resources should be maximally directed at patients in these first few months. Unfortunately, this is the time in most health care systems around the world that patients do not get upper limb rehabilitation, increasing the chances of the complications of CNS injury setting in.

There are many approaches being investigated, but all too often the studies are too small, or they have not employed reasonable patient stratification based on an understanding of the mechanisms involved. It is clear that at present there is no clear idea, who each of these approaches is best suited to. Currently, treatment approaches such as CIMT or motor imagery are used on an ad hoc basis. Future strategies require studies at all stages of the translational pipeline [134] in order to understand how interventions work, who they wo11.339 ptk best in, what the clinical effects of these interventions are, and whether they can be delivered on a large scale in diverse healthcare systems.

References

1. Lawrence ES, Coshall C, Dundas R, et al. Estimates of the prevalence of acute stroke impairments and disability in a multiethnic population. Stroke. 2001;**32**(6):1279–1284.
2. Kwakkel G, Kollen BJ, van der Grond J, Prevo AJH. Probability of regaining dexterity in the flaccid upper limb: impact of severity of paresis and time since onset in acute stroke. Stroke. 2003;**34**(9):2181–2186.
3. Nakayama H, Jørgensen HS, Raaschou HO, Olsen TS. Recovery of upper extremity function in stroke patients: the Copenhagen Stroke Study. Arch Phys Med Rehabil. 1994;**75**(4):394–398.
4. Sunderland A, Fletcher D, Bradley L, Tinson D, Hewer RL, Wade DT. Enhanced physical therapy for arm function after stroke: a one year follow up study. J Neurol Neurosurg Psychiatry. 1994;**57**(7):856–858.
5. Wade DT, Langton-Hewer R, Wood VA, Skilbeck CE, Ismail HM. The hemiplegic arm after stroke: measurement and recovery. J Neurol Neurosurg Psychiatry. 1983;**46**(6):521–524.
6. Coupar F, Pollock A, Rowe P, Weir C, Langhorne P. Predictors of upper limb recovery after stroke: a systematic review and meta-analysis. Clin Rehabil. 2012;**26**(4):291–313.
7. Krakauer JW, Carmichael ST, Corbett D, Wittenberg GF. Getting neurorehabilitation right: what can be learned from animal models? Neurorehabil Neural Repair. 2012;**26**(8):923–931.
8. Snoek GJ, IJzerman MJ, Hermens HJ, Maxwell D, Biering-Sorensen F. Survey of the needs of patients with spinal cord injury: impact and priority for improvement in hand function in tetraplegics. Spinal Cord. 2004;**42**(9):526–532.
9. Yarkony GM, Roth EJ, Heinemann AW, Lovell L, Wu YC. Functional skills after spinal cord injury rehabilitation: three-year longitudinal follow-up. Arch Phys Med Rehabil. 1988;**69**(2):111–114.
10. Spooren AIF, Janssen-Potten YJM, Snoek GJ, Ijzerman MJ, Kerckhofs E, Seelen HAM. Rehabilitation outcome of upper extremity skilled performance in persons with cervical spinal cord injuries. J Rehabil Med. 2008;**40**(8):637–644.
11. Valent L, Dallmeijer A, Houdijk H, Talsma E, van der Woude L. The effects of upper body exercise on the physical capacity of people with a spinal cord injury: a systematic review. Clin Rehabil. 2007;**21**(4):315–3130.
12. Kloosterman MGM, Snoek GJ, Jannink MJA. Systematic review of the effects of exercise therapy on the upper extremity of patients with spinal-cord injury. Spinal Cord. 2009;**47**(3):196–203.
13. Kowalczewski J, Prochazka A. Technology improves upper extremity rehabilitation. Prog Brain Res. 2011;**192**:147–159.
14. Johansson S, Ytterberg C, Claesson IM, et al. High concurrent presence of disability in multiple sclerosis. Associations with perceived health. J Neurol. 2007;**254**(6):767–773.
15. Yozbatiran N, Baskurt F, Baskurt Z, Ozakbas S, Idiman E. Motor assessment of upper extremity function and its relation with fatigue, cognitive function and quality of life in multiple sclerosis patients. J Neurol Sci. 2006;**246**(1–2):117–122.
16. Spooren AIF, Timmermans AAA, Seelen HAM. Motor training programs of arm and hand in patients with MS according to different levels of the ICF: a systematic review. BMC Neurol. 2012;**12**:49.
17. Ward NS. Getting lost in translation. Curr Opin Neurol. 2008;**21**(6):625–627.
18. Dobkin BH. Motor rehabilitation after stroke, traumatic brain, and spinal cord injury: common denominators within recent clinical trials. Curr Opin Neurol. 2009;**22**(6):563–569.
19. Bernhardt J, Dewey H, Thrift A, Donnan G. Inactive and alone: physical activity within the first 14 days of acute stroke unit care. Stroke. 2004;**35**(4):1005–1009.

20. Lang CE, Macdonald JR, Reisman DS, et al. Observation of amounts of movement practice provided during stroke rehabilitation. Arch Phys Med Rehabil. 2009;**90**(10):1692–1698.

21. Kwakkel G, Wagenaar RC, Twisk JW, Lankhorst GJ, Koetsier JC. Intensity of leg and arm training after primary middle-cerebral-artery stroke: a randomised trial. Lancet. 1999;**354**(9174):191–196.

22. Lincoln NB, Parry RH, Vass CD. Randomized, controlled trial to evaluate increased intensity of physiotherapy treatment of arm function after stroke. Stroke. 1999;**30**(3):573–579.

23. Rodgers H, Mackintosh J, Price C, et al. Does an early increased-intensity interdisciplinary upper limb therapy programme following acute stroke improve outcome? Clin Rehabil. 2003;**17**(6):579–589.

24. Duncan P, Studenski S, Richards L, et al. Randomized clinical trial of therapeutic exercise in subacute stroke. Stroke. 2003;**34**(9):2173–2180.

25. Han C, Wang Q, Meng P, Qi M. Effects of intensity of arm training on hemiplegic upper extremity motor recovery in stroke patients: a randomized controlled trial. Clin Rehabil. 2013;**27**(1):75–81.

26. Luke LM, Allred RP, Jones TA. Unilateral ischemic sensorimotor cortical damage induces contralesional synaptogenesis and enhances skilled reaching with the ipsilateral forelimb in adult male rats. Synap N Y N. 2004;**54**(4):187–199.

27. Remple MS, Bruneau RM, VandenBerg PM, Goertzen C, Kleim JA. Sensitivity of cortical movement representations to motor experience: evidence that skill learning but not strength training induces cortical reorganization. Behav Brain Res. 2001;**123**(2):133–141.

28. MacLellan CL, Keough MB, Granter-Button S, Chernenko GA, Butt S, Corbett D. A critical threshold of rehabilitation involving brain-derived neurotrophic factor is required for poststroke recovery. Neurorehabil Neural Repair. 2011;**25**(8):740–748.

29. Schweighofer N, Han CE, Wolf SL, Arbib MA, Winstein CJ. A functional threshold for long-term use of hand and arm function can be determined: predictions from a computational model and supporting data from the Extremity Constraint-Induced Therapy Evaluation (EXCITE) Trial. Phys Ther. 2009;**89**(12):1327–1336.

30. Harris JE, Eng JJ, Miller WC, Dawson AS. A self-administered Graded Repetitive Arm Supplementary Program (GRASP) improves arm function during inpatient stroke rehabilitation: a multi-site randomized controlled trial. Stroke. 2009;**40**(6):2123–2128.

31. Connell LA, McMahon NE, Watkins CL, Eng JJ. Therapists' use of the Graded Repetitive Arm Supplementary Program (GRASP) intervention: a practice implementation survey study. Phys Ther. 2014;**94**(5):632–643

32. Krakauer JW. Motor learning: its relevance to stroke recovery and neurorehabilitation. Curr Opin Neurol. 2006;**19**(1):84–90.

33. Timmermans AAA, Spooren AIF, Kingma H, Seelen HAM. Influence of task-oriented training content on skilled arm-hand performance in stroke: a systematic review. Neurorehabil Neural Repair. 2010;**24**(9):858–870.

34. French B, Thomas L, Leathley M, et al. Does repetitive task training improve functional activity after stroke? A Cochrane systematic review and meta-analysis. J Rehabil Med. 2010;**42**(1):9–14.

35. Arya KN, Verma R, Garg RK, Sharma VP, Agarwal M, Aggarwal GG. Meaningful task-specific training (MTST) for stroke rehabilitation: a randomized controlled trial. Top Stroke Rehabil. 2012;**19**(3):193–211.

36. Barreca S, Wolf SL, Fasoli S, Bohannon R. Treatment interventions for the paretic upper limb of stroke survivors: a critical review. Neurorehabil Neural Repair. 2003;**17**(4):220–226.

37. Van Peppen RPS, Kwakkel G, Wood-Dauphinee S, Hendriks HJM, Van der Wees PJ, Dekker J. The impact of physical therapy on functional outcomes after stroke: what's the evidence? Clin Rehabil. 2004;**18**(8):833–862.

38. Luke C, Dodd KJ, Brock K. Outcomes of the Bobath concept on upper limb recovery following stroke. Clin Rehabil. 2004;**18**(8):888–898.

39. Paci M. Physiotherapy based on the Bobath concept for adults with post-stroke hemiplegia: a review of effectiveness studies. J Rehabil Med. 2003;**35**(1):2–7.

40. Schweighofer N, Choi Y, Winstein C, Gordon J. Task-oriented rehabilitation robotics. Am J Phys Med Rehabil. 2012;**91**(11 Suppl 3): S270–279.

41. Krebs HI, Volpe BT. Rehabilitation robotics. Handb Clin Neurol. 2013;**110**:283–294.

42. Balasubramanian S, Colombo R, Sterpi I, Sanguineti V, Burdet E. Robotic assessment of upper limb motor function after stroke. Am J Phys Med Rehabil. 2012;**91**(11 Suppl 3):S255–269.

43. Kwakkel G, Kollen BJ, Krebs HI. Effects of robot-assisted therapy on upper limb recovery after stroke: a systematic review. Neurorehabil Neural Repair. 2008;**22**(2):111–121.

44. Gladstone DJ, Danells CJ, Black SE. The fugl-meyer assessment of motor recovery after stroke: a critical review of its measurement properties. Neurorehabil Neural Repair. 2002;**16**(3):232–240.

45. Lo AC, Guarino PD, Richards LG, Haselkorn JK, Wittenberg GF, Federman DG, et al. Robot-assisted therapy for long-term upper-limb impairment after stroke. N Engl J Med. 2010;**362**(19):1772–1783.

46. Zeiler SR, Krakauer JW. The interaction between training and plasticity in the poststroke brain. Curr Opin Neurol. 2013;**26**(6):609–616.

47. Riley JD, Le V, Der-Yeghiaian L, et al. Anatomy of stroke injury predicts gains from therapy. Stroke. 2011;**42**(2):421–426.

48. Cramer SC, Parrish TB, Levy RM, et al. Predicting functional gains in a stroke trial. Stroke. 2007;**38**(7):2108–2114.

49. Harris JE, Eng JJ. Individuals with the dominant hand affected following stroke demonstrate less impairment than those with the nondominant hand affected. Neurorehabil Neural Repair. 2006;**20**(3):380–389.

50. Kamper DG, Fischer HC, Cruz EG, Rymer WZ. Weakness is the primary contributor to finger impairment in chronic stroke. Arch Phys Med Rehabil. 2006;**87**(9):1262–1269.

51. Ada L, Dorsch S, Canning CG. Strengthening interventions increase strength and improve activity after stroke: a systematic review. Aust J Physiother. 2006;**52**(4):241–248.

52. Harris JE, Eng JJ. Strength training improves upper-limb function in individuals with stroke: a meta-analysis. Stroke. 2010;**41**(1):136–140.

53. Bohannon RW. Muscle strength and muscle training after stroke. J Rehabil Med. 2007;**39**(1):14–20.

54. Donaldson C, Tallis R, Miller S, Sunderland A, Lemon R, Pomeroy V. Effects of conventional physical therapy and functional strength training on upper limb motor recovery after stroke: a randomized phase II study. Neurorehabil Neural Repair. 2009;**23**(4):389–397.

55. Pomeroy VM, Ward NS, Johansen-Berg H, van Vliet P, Burridge J, Hunter SM, et al. FAST INdiCATE Trial protocol. Clinical efficacy of functional strength training for upper limb motor recovery early after stroke: Neural correlates and prognostic indicators. Int J Stroke. 2014; **9**(2):240–245 ;

56. Cirstea MC, Levin MF. Compensatory strategies for reaching in stroke. Brain. 2000;**123** (Pt 5):940–953.

57. Wee SK, Hughes A-M, Warner M, Burridge JH. Trunk restraint to promote upper extremity recovery in stroke patients: a systematic review and meta-analysis. Neurorehabil Neural Repair. 2014; **28**(7):660–677 ;

58. Connell LA, Lincoln NB, Radford KA. Somatosensory impairment after stroke: frequency of different deficits and their recovery. Clin Rehabil. 2008;**22**(8):758–767.

59. Doyle S, Bennett S, Fasoli SE, McKenna KT. Interventions for sensory impairment in the upper limb after stroke. Cochrane Database Syst Rev. 2010;(6):CD006331.

60. Taub E, Crago JE, Burgio LD, et al. An operant approach to rehabilitation medicine: overcoming learned nonuse by shaping. J Exp Anal Behav. 1994;**61**(2):281–293.

61. Wolf SL, Winstein CJ, Miller JP, Taub E, Uswatte G, Morris D, et al. Effect of constraint-induced movement therapy on upper extremity function 3 to 9 months after stroke: the EXCITE randomized clinical trial. JAMA 2006;**296**(17):2095–2104.

62. Wolf SL, Winstein CJ, Miller JP, et al. Retention of upper limb function in stroke survivors who have received constraint-induced movement therapy: the EXCITE randomised trial. Lancet Neurol. 2008;**7**(1):33–40.

63. Kitago T, Liang J, Huang VS, et al. Improvement after constraint-induced movement therapy: recovery of normal motor control or task-specific compensation? Neurorehabil Neural Repair. 2013;**27**(2):99–109.

64. Page SJ, Levine P, Leonard A, Szaflarski JP, Kissela BM. Modified constraint-induced therapy in chronic stroke: results of a single-blinded randomized controlled trial. Phys Ther. 2008;**88**(3):333–340.

65. Page SJ, Sisto SA, Levine P, Johnston MV, Hughes M. Modified constraint induced therapy: a randomized feasibility and efficacy study. J Rehabil Res Dev. 2001;**38**(5):583–590.

66. Dromerick AW, Lang CE, Birkenmeier RL, et al. Very Early Constraint-Induced Movement during Stroke Rehabilitation (VECTORS): A single-center RCT. Neurology. 2009;**73**(3):195–201.

67. Treger I, Aidinof L, Lehrer H, Kalichman L. Modified constraint-induced movement therapy improved upper limb function in subacute poststroke patients: a small-scale clinical trial. Top Stroke Rehabil. 2012;**19**(4):287–293.

68. Cardoso de Oliveira S. The neuronal basis of bimanual coordination: recent neurophysiological evidence and functional models. Acta Psychol (Amst). 2002;**110**(2–3):139–159.

69. Weiss PH, Jeannerod M, Paulignan Y, Freund HJ. Is the organisation of goal-directed action modality specific? A common temporal structure. Neuropsychologia. 2000;**38**(8):1136–1147.

70. McCombe Waller S, Forrester L, Villagra F, Whitall J. Intracortical inhibition and facilitation with unilateral dominant, unilateral non-dominant and bilateral movement tasks in left- and right-handed adults. J Neurol Sci. 2008;**269**(1–2):96–104.

71. Whitall J, McCombe Waller S, Silver KH, Macko RF. Repetitive bilateral arm training with rhythmic auditory cueing improves motor function in chronic hemiparetic stroke. Stroke. 2000;**31**(10):2390–2395.

72. Whitall J, Waller SM, Sorkin JD, et al. Bilateral and unilateral arm training improve motor function through differing neuroplastic mechanisms: a single-blinded randomized controlled trial. Neurorehabil Neural Repair. 2011;**25**(2):118–129.

73. Lum PS, Burgar CG, Shor PC, Majmundar M, Van der Loos M. Robot-assisted movement training compared with conventional therapy techniques for the rehabilitation of upper-limb motor function after stroke. Arch Phys Med Rehabil. 2002;**83**(7):952–959.

74. Burgar CG, Lum PS, Scremin AME, et al. Robot-assisted upper-limb therapy in acute rehabilitation setting following stroke: Department of Veterans Affairs multisite clinical trial. J Rehabil Res Dev. 2011;**48**(4):445–458.

75. Hesse S, Werner C, Pohl M, Rueckriem S, Mehrholz J, Lingnau ML. Computerized arm training improves the motor control of the severely affected arm after stroke: a single-blinded randomized trial in two centers. Stroke. 2005;**36**(9):1960–1966.

76. Stinear JW, Byblow WD. Rhythmic bilateral movement training modulates corticomotor excitability and enhances upper limb motricity poststroke: a pilot study. J Clin Neurophysiol. 2004;**21**(2):124–131.

77. Stinear CM, Petoe MA, Anwar S, Barber PA, Byblow WD. Bilateral priming accelerates recovery of upper limb function after stroke: a randomized controlled trial. Stroke. 2014;**45**(1):205–210.

78. Desrosiers J, Bourbonnais D, Corriveau H, Gosselin S, Bravo G. Effectiveness of unilateral and symmetrical bilateral task training for arm during the subacute phase after stroke: a randomized controlled trial. Clin Rehabil. 2005;**19**(6):581–593.

79. Mudie MH, Matyas TA. Can simultaneous bilateral movement involve the undamaged hemisphere in reconstruction of neural networks damaged by stroke? Disabil Rehabil. 2000;**22**(1–2):23–37.

80. Platz T, Bock S, Prass K. Reduced skilfulness of arm motor behaviour among motor stroke patients with good clinical recovery: does it indicate reduced automaticity? Can it be improved by unilateral or bilateral training? A kinematic motion analysis study. Neuropsychologia. 2001;**39**(7):687–698.

81. Summers JJ, Kagerer FA, Garry MI, Hiraga CY, Loftus A, Cauraugh JH. Bilateral and unilateral movement training on upper limb function in chronic stroke patients: A TMS study. J Neurol Sci. 2007;**252**(1):76–82.

82. Van Delden AEQ, Peper CE, Beek PJ, Kwakkel G. Unilateral versus bilateral upper limb exercise therapy after stroke: a systematic review. J Rehabil Med. 2012;**44**(2):106–117.

83. Van Delden ALEQ, Peper CLE, Nienhuys KN, Zijp NI, Beek PJ, Kwakkel G. Unilateral versus bilateral upper limb training after stroke: the Upper Limb Training After Stroke clinical trial. Stroke. 2013;**44**(9):2613–2616.

84. Van Vliet PM, Sheridan MR. Coordination between reaching and grasping in patients with hemiparesis and healthy subjects. Arch Phys Med Rehabil. 2007;**88**(10):1325–1331.

85. Ellis MD, Holubar BG, Acosta AM, Beer RF, Dewald JPA. Modifiability of abnormal isometric elbow and shoulder joint torque coupling after stroke. Muscle Nerve. 2005;**32**(2):170–178.

86. Zackowski KM, Dromerick AW, Sahrmann SA, Thach WT, Bastian AJ. How do strength, sensation, spasticity and joint individuation relate to the reaching deficits of people with chronic hemiparesis? Brain. 2004;**127**(Pt 5):1035–1046.

87. Lang CE, Wagner JM, Bastian AJ, Hu Q, Edwards DF, Sahrmann SA, et al. Deficits in grasp versus reach during acute hemiparesis. Exp Brain Res. 2005;**166**(1):126–136.

88. Pelton T, van Vliet P, Hollands K. Interventions for improving coordination of reach to grasp following stroke: a systematic review. Int J Evid Based Healthc. 2012;**10**(2):89–102.

89. Barclay-Goddard RE, Stevenson TJ, Poluha W, Thalman L. Mental practice for treating upper extremity deficits in individuals with hemiparesis after stroke. Cochrane Database Syst Rev. 2011;(5):CD005950.

90. Simmons L, Sharma N, Baron J-C, Pomeroy VM. Motor imagery to enhance recovery after subcortical stroke: who might benefit, daily dose, and potential effects. Neurorehabil Neural Repair. 2008;**22**(5):458–467.

91. Celnik P, Webster B, Glasser DM, Cohen LG. Effects of action observation on physical training after stroke. Stroke. 2008;**39**(6):1814–1820.

92. Franceschini M, Ceravolo MG, Agosti M, et al. Clinical relevance of action observation in upper-limb stroke rehabilitation: a possible role in recovery of functional dexterity. A randomized clinical trial. Neurorehabil Neural Repair. 2012;**26**(5):456–462.

93. Chae J, Bethoux F, Bohine T, Dobos L, Davis T, Friedl A. Neuromuscular stimulation for upper extremity motor and functional recovery in acute hemiplegia. Stroke. 1998;**29**(5):975–979.

94. Lin Z, Yan T. Long-term effectiveness of neuromuscular electrical stimulation for promoting motor recovery of the upper extremity after stroke. J Rehabil Med. 2011;**43**(6):506–510.

95. Powell J, Pandyan AD, Granat M, Cameron M, Stott DJ. Electrical stimulation of wrist extensors in poststroke hemiplegia. Stroke. 1999;**30**(7):1384–1389.

96. Meilink A, Hemmen B, Seelen HAM, Kwakkel G. Impact of EMG-triggered neuromuscular stimulation of the wrist and finger extensors of the paretic hand after stroke: a systematic review of the literature. Clin Rehabil. 2008;**22**(4):291–305.

97. Bello AI, Rockson BEA, Olaogun MOB. The effects of electromyographic-triggered neuromuscular electrical muscle stimulation on the functional hand recovery among stroke survivors. Afr J Med Med Sci. 2009;38(2):185–191.

98. Boyaci A, Topuz O, Alkan H, et al. Comparison of the effectiveness of active and passive neuromuscular electrical stimulation of hemiplegic upper extremities: a randomized, controlled trial. Int J Rehabil Res 2013;36(4):315–322.

99. De Kroon JR, IJzerman MJ. Electrical stimulation of the upper extremity in stroke: cyclic versus EMG-triggered stimulation. Clin Rehabil. 2008;22(8):690–697.

100. Alon G, Ring H. Gait and hand function enhancement following training with a multi-segment hybrid-orthosis stimulation system in stroke patients. J Stroke Cerebrovasc Dis. 2003;12(5):209–216.

101. Alon G, Levitt AF, McCarthy PA. Functional electrical stimulation enhancement of upper extremity functional recovery during stroke rehabilitation: a pilot study. Neurorehabil Neural Repair. 2007;21(3):207–215.

102. Popovic DB, Popovic MB, Sinkjaer T, Stefanovic A, Schwirtlich L. Therapy of paretic arm in hemiplegic subjects augmented with a neural prosthesis: a cross-over study. Can J Physiol Pharmacol. 2004;82(8–9):749–756.

103. Merrill DR, Davis R, Turk R, Burridge JH. A personalized sensor-controlled microstimulator system for arm rehabilitation poststroke. Part 1: System architecture. Neuromodulation 2011;14(1):72–79; discussion 79.

104. Turk R, Burridge JH, Davis R, Cosendai G, Sparrow O, Roberts HC, et al. Therapeutic effectiveness of electric stimulation of the upper-limb poststroke using implanted microstimulators. Arch Phys Med Rehabil. 2008 Oct;89(10):1913–1922.

105. Knutson JS, Harley MY, Hisel TZ, Hogan SD, Maloney MM, Chae J. Contralaterally controlled functional electrical stimulation for upper extremity hemiplegia: an early-phase randomized clinical trial in subacute stroke patients. Neurorehabil Neural Repair. 2012;26(3):239–246.

106. Makowski NS, Knutson JS, Chae J, Crago PE. Functional electrical stimulation to augment poststroke reach and hand opening in the presence of voluntary effort: a pilot study. Neurorehabil Neural Repair. 2014;28(3):241–249.

107. Watkins CL, Leathley MJ, Gregson JM, Moore AP, Smith TL, Sharma AK. Prevalence of spasticity post stroke. Clin Rehabil. 2002;16(5):515–522.

108. Leathley MJ, Gregson JM, Moore AP, Smith TL, Sharma AK, Watkins CL. Predicting spasticity after stroke in those surviving to 12 months. Clin Rehabil. 2004;18(4):438–443.

109. Sommerfeld DK, Eek EU-B, Svensson A-K, Holmqvist LW, von Arbin MH. Spasticity after stroke: its occurrence and association with motor impairments and activity limitations. Stroke. 2004;35(1):134–139.

110. Tyson SF, Kent RM. The effect of upper limb orthotics after stroke: a systematic review. NeuroRehabilitation. 2011;28(1):29–36.

111. Tseng C-N, Chen CC-H, Wu S-C, Lin L-C. Effects of a range-of-motion exercise programme. J Adv Nurs. 2007;57(2):181–191.

112. Turton AJ, Britton E. A pilot randomized controlled trial of a daily muscle stretch regime to prevent contractures in the arm after stroke. Clin Rehabil. 2005;19(6):600–612.

113. Bell KR, Williams F. Use of botulinum toxin type A and type B for spasticity in upper and lower limbs. Phys Med Rehabil Clin N Am. 2003;14(4):821–835.

114. Simpson DM, Gracies JM, Yablon SA, Barbano R, Brashear A, BoNT/TZD Study Team. Botulinum neurotoxin versus tizanidine in upper limb spasticity: a placebo-controlled study. J Neurol Neurosurg Psychiatry. 2009;80(4):380–385.

115. Cardoso E, Rodrigues B, Lucena R, Oliveira IR de, Pedreira G, Melo A. Botulinum toxin type A for the treatment of the upper limb spasticity after stroke: a meta-analysis. Arq Neuropsiquiatr. 2005;63(1):30–33.

116. Van Kuijk AA, Geurts ACH, Bevaart BJW, van Limbeek J. Treatment of upper extremity spasticity in stroke patients by focal neuronal or neuromuscular blockade: a systematic review of the literature. J Rehabil Med. 2002;34(2):51–61.

117. Francis HP, Wade DT, Turner-Stokes L, Kingswell RS, Dott CS, Coxon EA. Does reducing spasticity translate into functional benefit? An exploratory meta-analysis. J Neurol Neurosurg Psychiatry. 2004;75(11):1547–1551.

118. Foley N, Pereira S, Salter K, et al. Treatment with botulinum toxin improves upper-extremity function post stroke: a systematic review and meta-analysis. Arch Phys Med Rehabil. 2013;94(5):977–989.

119. Shaw LC, Price CIM, van Wijck FMJ, et al. Botulinum Toxin for the Upper Limb after Stroke (BoTULS) Trial: effect on impairment, activity limitation, and pain. Stroke. 2011;42(5):1371–1379.

120. Dvorak EM, Ketchum NC, McGuire JR. The underutilization of intrathecal baclofen in poststroke spasticity. Top Stroke Rehabil. 2011;18(3):195–202.

121. Ivanhoe CB, Francisco GE, McGuire JR, Subramanian T, Grissom SP. Intrathecal baclofen management of poststroke spastic hypertonia: implications for function and quality of life. Arch Phys Med Rehabil. 2006;87(11):1509–1515.

122. Schiess MC, Oh IJ, Stimming EF, et al. Prospective 12-month study of intrathecal baclofen therapy for poststroke spastic upper and lower extremity motor control and functional improvement. Neuromodulation. 2011;14(1):38–45; discussion 45.

123. Graham LA. Management of spasticity revisited. Age Ageing. 2013;42(4):435–441.

124. Murphy TH, Corbett D. Plasticity during stroke recovery: from synapse to behaviour. Nat Rev Neurosci. 2009;10(12):861–872.

125. Bavelier D, Levi DM, Li RW, Dan Y, Hensch TK. Removing brakes on adult brain plasticity: from molecular to behavioral interventions. J Neurosci. 2010 ;30(45):14964–14971.

126. Paille V, Fino E, Du K, et al. GABAergic circuits control spike-timing-dependent plasticity. J Neurosci. 2013;33(22):9353–9363.

127. Chen JL, Lin WC, Cha JW, So PT, Kubota Y, Nedivi E. Structural basis for the role of inhibition in facilitating adult brain plasticity. Nat Neurosci. 2011;14(5):587–594.

128. Witte OW, Stoll G. Delayed and remote effects of focal cortical infarctions: secondary damage and reactive plasticity. Adv Neurol. 1997;73:207–227.

129. Clarkson AN, Huang BS, Macisaac SE, Mody I, Carmichael ST. Reducing excessive GABA-mediated tonic inhibition promotes functional recovery after stroke. Nature. 2010;468(7321):305–309.

130. Chollet F, Tardy J, Albucher J-F, et al. Fluoxetine for motor recovery after acute ischaemic stroke (FLAME): a randomised placebo-controlled trial. Lancet Neurol. 2011;10(2):123–130.

131. Engelter ST, Frank M, Lyrer PA, Conzelmann M. Safety of pharmacological augmentation of stroke rehabilitation. Eur Neurol. 2010;64(6):325–330.

132. Hsu W-Y, Cheng C-H, Liao K-K, Lee I-H, Lin Y-Y. Effects of repetitive transcranial magnetic stimulation on motor functions in patients with stroke: a meta-analysis. Stroke. 2012;43(7):1849–1857.

133. Butler AJ, Shuster M, O'Hara E, Hurley K, Middlebrooks D, Guilkey K. A meta-analysis of the efficacy of anodal transcranial direct current stimulation for upper limb motor recovery in stroke survivors. J Hand Ther 2013;26(2):162–170; quiz 171.

134. Cumberland Consensus Working Group, Cheeran B, Cohen L, Dobkin B, et al. The future of restorative neurosciences in stroke: driving the translational research pipeline from basic science to rehabilitation of people after stroke. Neurorehabil Neural Repair. 2009;23(2):97–107.

135. Gowland C, Stratford P, Ward M, et al. Measuring physical impairment and disability with the Chedoke-McMaster Stroke Assessment. Stroke. 1993;**24**(1):58–63.

136. Barreca S, Bohannon R, Charness A, et al. Management of the post-stroke hemiplegic arm and hand: treatment recommendations of the 2001 consensus panel. Heart and Stroke Foundation of Ontario, Canada, 2001.

137. Stinear CM, Ward NS. How useful is imaging in predicting outcomes in stroke rehabilitation? Int J Stroke. 2013;**8**(1):33–37.

138. Kou N, Park C, Seghier ML, Leff AP, Ward NS. Can fully automated detection of corticospinal tract damage be used in stroke patients? Neurology. 2013;**80**(24):2242–2245.

CHAPTER 21

Acquired disorders of language and their treatment

Alex Leff and Jenny Crinion

Introduction

Aphasia is more common than multiple sclerosis or Parkinson's disease, with around 80,000 new aphasic patients per annum from stroke alone in the United States, and about 20,000 in the UK [1]. Together with functional activities of daily living (ADL) performance, age and gender, aphasia leads to reduced long-term social participation [2]. Yet in spite of its high incidence aphasia is still a hidden disability, isolating patients and relatives. A third of aphasic stroke patients have associated depression 12 months after their stroke [3–5]. As such aphasia is one of the most feared consequences of stroke according to surveys of those who are most at risk [6] and persisting aphasia correlates with poor health outcomes [7]. Therefore, effective aphasia treatment approaches are urgently needed. The major acquired disease categories in terms of aetiological cause are: (1) acquired focal brain injury, we will use stroke as the archetypical example but tumours, and to some extent, head injury, can also present in a similar manner; (2) degenerative diseases, primary progressive aphasia is often cited as the archetypical example, but Alzheimer's disease is much more common and is often associated with aphasic symptoms, such as word finding problems (anomia).

Aphasia therapy that is properly selected, carefully targeted to specific aphasic symptoms and administered with sufficient dosage does work in cases of acquired brain injury ([8–11]. Therapy for dementia syndromes has somewhat lagged behind focal syndromes, but using similar approaches evidence is growing that therapy can be effective at maintaining aspects of language performance in the face of a more general decline in cognitive function [12–14]. Most language interventions are administered by speech and language therapists (SALTs) that evaluate patients' individual needs, and then use a combination of face–to–face and computer delivered techniques tailored to the individual patient's impairment profile.

This is an exciting time for SALT. The evidence-base for its effectiveness is growing and promising adjuvant treatments (non-invasive brain stimulation and drug therapy) are emerging. In this chapter we will first briefly cover the classification and testing of patients with acquired aphasia before moving on to the main sections where we attempt to answer key questions about SALT, for example: Does it work? What dose is required? What intensity? Is it ever too late? We then turn to adjuvant treatments (brain stimulation and drugs) before ending with sections on e-rehabilitation, alternative and augmentative communication and what the future might hold.

Classification of aphasia

The traditional classification of aphasia tends to be a two-step process: (1) description of the aphasic patient's language impairment and then (2) labelling the patient as belonging to one of the current main clinical syndrome subgroups: Broca's, Wernicke's, global, transcortical, conduction, and anomic. We agree with the first step but question the utility of the second on both conceptual and practical grounds. Conceptually the case for the 'double-dissociation' between Broca's (primarily an output disorder, with impaired grammar) and Wernicke's aphasia (primarily a disorder of speech comprehension at the lexico/semantic level, often associated with a jargon output) is weak, and the similarities, in terms of error frequency and type, are often as striking as the differences [15]. On the practical side, diagnostic tests designed to categorize patients to help guide therapy, such as the Boston Diagnostic Aphasia Examination [16] or Western Aphasia Battery [17], have poor agreement with clustering algorithms [18]. Recent attempts to revamp these aphasia syndrome classifications have perhaps created more heat than light [19].

Clinically it is important to quantify patients' language impairment as this can be helpful for patients, their carers and others to understand their condition; and importantly, it can help guide therapy. We advocate always testing the two main language output routes (speaking and writing); the two main inputs (speech comprehension and reading); as well as basic tests of semantic association to gain a global picture of the patient's language functioning. There are several test batteries clinicians can use to do this. In the UK the Comprehensive Aphasia Battery is preferred as it has aphasic norms, from a UK population, and is a useful tool for assessing change over time [20]. Other more detailed tests are needed if one wants greater definition in terms of a psycholinguistic model [21] or if there are concomitant, lower-level motor components such as speech apraxia [22], which complicates a fair proportion of cases of post-stroke aphasia [23], particularly those with lesions in the anterior portion of the middle cerebral artery (MCA) territory.

It is important that characterization of the language profile detailing which language functions and related cognitive functions are impaired or intact is carried out both pre and post treatment to evaluate its effectiveness. This diagnostic work can be done with different degrees of specificity. For example, in the domain of speech production, a naming deficit may be described broadly as anomia, or more precisely e.g., as a disruption involved in the linking of semantic information with its corresponding phonological word form. Diagnostic testing can be based on the theoretical view that the spoken word production system consists of multiple stages of processing that allow word semantics, lexical retrieval, phonemic encoding and motor production to be distinguished from one another e.g., for a review see [24]. Given this, the diagnostic work for characterizing speech deficits would involve testing hearing, auditory language comprehension, object naming, word fluency, and repetition. Spoken naming can be further evaluated to determine error profiles. For example, are naming errors phonemic (e.g. the patient says /mat/ when asked to name a picture of a cat); or semantic (e.g. /dog/ for cat)? Are subjects helped by phonological cueing (e.g. after failing to name the picture of the cat, when given the first sound /ca/ do they name it correctly)? The reasoning is as follows: intact auditory comprehension rules out a semantic deficit, good repetition rules out motor speech problems and only mild (if any) apraxia of speech, whereas difficulties with picture naming, decreased fluency, production of semantic errors, and sensitivity to phonemic cueing point to a disruption in the link between word meaning and word form. In addition, a more comprehensive evaluation of related language and cognitive abilities will include tests of written language, short-term memory (verbal and visual), attention and executive functions. To capture speech production beyond the single word level composite picture description (e.g. a picture from the Comprehensive Aphasia Test (CAT) of a sitting room scene that a patient is asked to describe (see Video 21.1) would allow the patient some latitude of expression, which confrontation naming of an individual item does not, while keeping them focused on a specific task that has been quantified. For example, in the CAT the patient's spoken picture description over a one minute period is transcribed and then analysed using measures such as the number of appropriate and inappropriate information carrying words (both nouns and verbs), as well more global variables such as syntactic variety and grammatical well-formedness [20]. Almost all aphasic patients have an anomic component, and a classification of their naming errors (phonological, semantic, jargon, absent response) and the type of cueing they best respond to (phonological or semantic), can help characterize what level within a model of language processing the patient's speech deficit is and then guide therapy and monitor the patient's progress and response to SALT.

Patient videos

To illustrate some aphasic speech production errors, the reader is referred to two videos of a patient with post-stroke aphasia (Videos 21.1 and 21.2 online). She is trilingual (German, English and Spanish), and had been living and working in the UK for several years prior to her left-hemisphere stroke. The videos (in English only) were recorded 21 months after her stroke. She has kindly given her written permission for the videos to be viewed.

Spoken picture description

This is taken from the CAT. Her speech is generally fluent and she clearly knows what she wants to say (i.e. what is going on in the

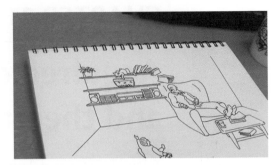

Video 21.1. Spoken picture description from a patient with aphasia caused by a thromboembolic stroke of the posterior portion of the left MCA.

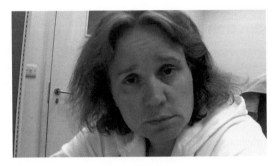

Video 21.2. Repetition of single words from a patient with aphasia caused by a thromboembolic stroke of the posterior portion of the left MCA.

picture), but she has problems finding the right words. Listen out for the following errors:

1. 00.15: 'The dogs, the bok, the book are falling dow..' This appears to be a mixture of a semantic error (dog instead of cat) interfering with the target word -book. She attempts to self correct and makes a vowel-based phonemic error to produce 'bok' and then misses out the final phoneme of (down).

2. 00.22 'The man is sleeping, over the paper, and he used to have a cup of tea, or . . . sleeping, em there are . . . sleeping, the man is still sleeping.' Here she makes an agrammatic error missing the noun (feet) and makes a preposition selection error (over instead of on), and then a tense error (used to have instead of has). The rest of the sentence looks like perseveration, but we think she is temporizing while trying to construct the next sentence, which finally arrives.

3. 1.10: 'Everybody is going to call down everything is going coreflawe on the floor.' Here she makes some phonemic errors with blends of fall/floor/cat.

Repetition

Again this is taken from the CAT. She is considerably worse than one might expect given her performance on the spoken picture description task. Interestingly, she makes occasional semantic errors on repetition. These are rarely seen and have been termed deep-dysphasic errors [25].

1. [Radio] 'Say again.' [Radio] 'Oh, the radio.'

2. [Crucifix] 'Fff- Cross cross the fff-fros fr-crooks frooks . . . forix frooks.'

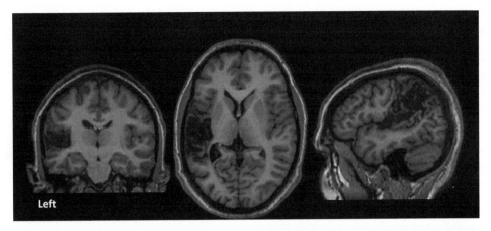

Fig. 21.1 High-resolution, volumetric, T1 MRI brain image for the patient shown in the videos. She had a thromboembolic stroke affecting the posterior portion of the left MCA artery and centered on the temporoparietal junction (Wernicke's area). Temporal cortex including Heschl's gyrus (primary auditory cortex) and cortex lateral and anterior to this is affected (superior temporal gyrus and superior temporal sulcus). Supramarginal gyrus, angular gyrus, and inferior parietal lobule are affected, as is post-central sulcus but motor strip and frontal regions are spared. The posterior half of the insula is also affected.

3. [Trade] 'Train.'

4. [Etiquette] 'People who walk properly.'

5. [Plant] 'Flower.'

6. [Tomato] 'Tomato.'

There are other examples. She makes semantic errors and phonemic errors. She finds longer words (polysyllabic) more difficult but there is also a frequency and imageability effect as well, so she is able to repeat high frequency, concrete nouns that are polysyllabic (such as tomato). She has a digit span of two and thus cannot 'hold on' to phonemic representations for long. Her MRI brain scan is shown in Figure 21.1.

Speech and language therapy: assessing the evidence

There are two important general study design issues that we would like to highlight in this section. While neither are specific to SALT research, they do affect most SALT studies and how the evidence for SALT interventions are viewed by non-specialists. (i) What is the correct control condition for assessing the efficacy of SALT input? (ii) What are the most appropriate SALT outcome measures?

What is the correct control?

SALT is a complex intervention. The Medical Research Council have defined this as follows:

> Complex interventions are built up from a number of components, which may act both independently and inter-dependently. The components usually include behaviours, parameters of behaviours (e.g. frequency, timing), and methods of organising and delivering those behaviours (e.g. type(s) of practitioner, setting and location). It is not easy to precisely define the 'active ingredients' of a complex intervention. For example, although research suggests that stroke units work, what exactly, is a stroke unit? What are the active ingredients that make it work? The physical set-up? The mix of care providers? The skills of the providers? The technologies available? The organisational arrangements? [26]

This causes a problem when it comes to designing studies testing SALT, namely, what is the correct control to compare therapy

with? The answer to this depends on the hypothesis one is testing. If the hypothesis is mechanistic, that is, what is the key element of the complex intervention that makes a difference? Then the control therapy should contain all but this element, e.g.: semantic versus phonological treatment [27–29]. However, if the hypothesis relates to the efficacy of a given, perhaps novel therapy (which may rest on multiple elements), then the appropriate control is likely to be standard clinical practice. 'Comparing the new intervention with standard treatment, if there is one, is more informative than comparing it to placebo [p. 29]' [30]. This approach may have been a better approach in studies that were not mechanistic in nature and compared SALT to a bespoke, non-standard 'control' therapy [31, 32].

There should be no hard and fast rules about study design, but between-subject variability is a pervasive issue and one that needs to be considered by producers and consumers of aphasia research. It has been demonstrated that, as far as stroke studies are concerned, the between-subject variability is usually greater than the within-subject variability. Or, as Bath and colleagues put it, 'In stroke trials, the impact of covariates such as severity on outcome is typically much larger than the treatment effect that is being measured' [33]. This argues for either repeated measures designs (multiple baseline measures prior to the intervention which everyone gets, or a cross-over design); or, if only one group is to receive the therapy, that great care be taken to ensure that the groups do not become unbalanced on key baseline variables, such as severity. Minimization is one technique that can be applied to randomization algorithms to address this [34].

What outcomes should be measured?

Clinical studies of the prevention of a second stroke often have very simple outcomes that most people agree are clinically relevant: for example, occurrence of a second vascular event, or death. Aphasia research can never be like this because aphasia is not a unitary entity and there is a major distinction, in terms of therapy targets, between the two main types of SALT treatment. Those that target specific aspects of language functions/difficulties, with effect specificity being the rule rather than the exception, and those that target communication skills more broadly [35]. The former type of approach assumes that improvement in language impairment will lead to improvements in communication ability and quality of life, while the latter assumes that the communication system and, therefore, the overall language network should be the target of treatment see [36], for in-depth discussion of these approaches and their integration. To date, most meta-studies of aphasia treatment have been undertaken within the 'language functions' framework, however even within a language domain (e.g. naming ability) there are a variety of standardized tests for assessing response to therapy, but no gold standard. This causes a problem for meta-analysis studies, when attempting to assess questions like 'Does speech and language therapy work?'

Assessments of functional outcome or of social participation address efficacy from a different perspective; that is, does the therapy have a 'real-world' effect on language function? This is obviously an important aspect of any translatable therapy but again, it is not clear exactly how best this should be measured. Is a questionnaire model the best? If so, should the patient be rating their own performance (e.g. SAQOL-39 [37]); or should we be asking a relative or someone who knows them best for their view (e.g. ASHA FACS [38]). Some tests have been adapted for both (e.g. COAST [39]). Generally, these tests are ordinal rather scalar and thus potentially limit the type of statistical tests that can be carried out on them. Ordinal data should not usually be subjected to parametric tests, at least not without tests of normality being performed first. A reasonable compromise for focused therapy is to have both: a test of impairment tailored to the specific intervention and a more global measure of functional communication to assess 'real-world' impact.

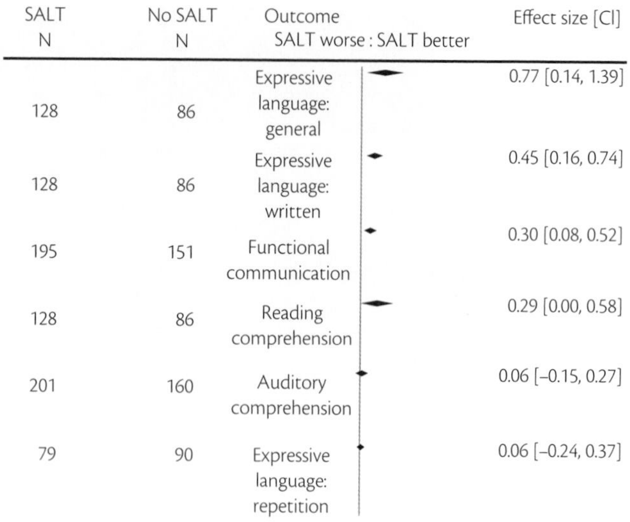

Speech therapy for aphasia: does it work?

The answer is **yes**.

Despite potential pitfalls, as mentioned earlier, meta-analyses are probably the best way to assess overall or average effect sizes for SALT interventions. The challenge is, which ones to trust. Cochrane reviews are generally more rigorous than others [40], but because of the very stringent requirements for study inclusion, they can end up with biased results based on a very small proportion of the actual research studies carried out in the field. Thankfully, the current Cochrane review on speech therapy for aphasic stroke is helpful in assessing the evidence here [41].

This review is up-to-date (three revisions since the original one in 2000) and positive. They reviewed the evidence from all RCTs (randomized controlled trials) from 1966 to 2009. Thirty-nine out of over 100 trials passed their inclusion criteria providing data from 2518 randomised participants; certainly the largest review currently available. The main result is that SALT vs. no SALT significantly improves patients' performance on most of the main outcome measures (Figure 21.2). This may seem trivial, but while this comparison obviously includes no behavioural control therapy, it does control for the effects of time alone, and thus the effects of any spontaneous 'natural' recovery, itself a complex and poorly understood process [42]. The authors were concerned that the meta-analysis may have been biased by a few Chinese studies where the effect sizes were relatively high and they were unable to contact the original study authors to confirm individual subject data. Notwithstanding this, the results show a significant average effect of SALT on: general expressive spoken language,

SALT N	No SALT N	Outcome SALT worse : SALT better	Effect size [CI]
128	86	Expressive language: general	0.77 [0.14, 1.39]
128	86	Expressive language: written	0.45 [0.16, 0.74]
195	151	Functional communication	0.30 [0.08, 0.52]
128	86	Reading comprehension	0.29 [0.00, 0.58]
201	160	Auditory comprehension	0.06 [−0.15, 0.27]
79	90	Expressive language: repetition	0.06 [−0.24, 0.37]

Fig. 21.2 Summary of the Cochrane review forest plots of SALT vs. no SALT [41]. Rows are ordered by effect size for each language function (third column). The first two columns show the number of subjects (N) in the SALT and No SALT groups garnered from the studies included. The forth column shows the 'diamond' or summary statistic for each of the six language functions. The vertical line represents the line of no effect, 'The lateral points of [the diamond] . . . indicate confidence intervals for this estimate. If the points of the diamond overlap the line of no effect the overall meta-analysed result cannot be said to differ from no effect at the given level of confidence.'
Brady MC, Kelly H, Godwin J, Enderby P, Speech and language therapy for aphasia following stroke, Cochrane Database of Systematic Reviews by permission of John Wiley Sons.

writing, overall functional communication and reading, with non-significant effects on auditory perception and repetition.

The rest of the Cochrane review meticulously documents studies where SALT was compared against some other 'active' control (e.g.: SALT (A) vs. SALT (B)). These analyses (102!) are all non-conclusive and provide no good evidence for one approach over another. This may seem surprising, but is probably due to two main factors: the differential effect size between one SALT therapy and another is smaller than the effect size of SALT versus no SALT; most studies are under-dosed in terms of amount of therapy given. We shall explore this issue in the next section.

What is the correct dose of therapy?

We have touched on how a behavioural therapy like SALT cannot be simply likened to a drug, at least not in terms of controlling for its effects in standard trial designs; however, it is an intervention that unfolds over time and presumably has a dose effect (the more therapy you receive the greater your chances of recovery) and yet we find it extraordinary that no systematic dose-ranging studies have been published. Recommendations from august bodies such as the Royal College of Physicians Intercollegiate Stroke Working Party make for depressing reading. The 2008 guidelines mention intensity but nothing about total dose, 'Any patient with aphasia persisting for more than two weeks should be considered for early intensive (2–8 hours/week) speech and language' [43: p. 141]. The question any reasonable patient or carer would have at this point would be, 'OK, but for how many weeks?'. The 2012 guidelines have reneged on even this, making no recommendations about

Table 21.1 Conflation of intensity and dose in Bhogal et al. 2003 [45]

	Therapy measures mean (SD)			Outcome measures mean (SD)	
	Length (weeks)	Hours (per week)	Total (hours)	PICA	Token test
Positive studies n = 259	11.2 (1.7)	8.8 (2.0)	98.4 (28.2)	15.1 (3.1)	13.74 (6.67)
Negative studies n = 574	22.9 (2.3)	2.0	43.6 (8.3)	1.37 (1.37)	0.59 (0.79)
t statistic	12.80	8.72	5.61	8.79	2.561
P value	0.001	0.001	0.001	0.001	0.05

Both intensity (hours per week, second column) and total dose (third column) were associated with better outcomes on the PICA and Token test (last two columns)
Bhogal SK, Teasell R, Speechley M. (2003). Intensity of aphasia therapy, impact on recovery. Stroke, 34(4), 987–993.

either intensity or dose, instead offering the decidedly unhelpful, '[aphasic] patients . . . should be given the opportunity to practice their language and communication skills as tolerated by the patient' [44: p. 174].

Actually, there is good evidence available about therapy dose. In 2003 Bhogal et al. produced a meta-analysis comparing speech therapy trials that had shown a positive effect against those that were negative in order to look for any systematic differences. They found 10 suitable studies, half of which were positive and half negative. There were more subjects in the negative studies (574 vs. 259). Their findings were very clear: the positive studies provided 98.4 hours of therapy in total compared with the negative studies that provided 43.6 hours [45]. Intensity and dose were confounded (the high dose studies got to the higher dose targets by providing four times as much therapy per week as the low dose studies) and could not be separated by this analysis (columns two and three of Table 21.1). As such it is surprising the authors chose to focus on intensity in their title when the main message appears to be total dose. Interestingly, as an aside, the measures that were sensitive to change across these studies were impairment based ones: the Token Test [46] and the Porch Index of Communicative Ability [47]; whereas more general functional measures did not come out as significant, suggesting that change in this domain may be harder to capture.

Bhogal's review makes it much easier to understand the results from high profile negative studies, such as those comparing SALT therapy with that provided by carers: it is under-dosing until proven otherwise. In the study by David et al., both groups (SALT vs. relatives) received low-intensity therapy (2 hours per week) to a total of 30 hours [32]. In the recent ACTNoW study, where SALT in the acute post-stroke phase was compared with carers providing 'everyday communication', the SALT group only received an average total dose of 18 hours of SALT input. Furthermore only half of that could be described as impairment-based therapy, the rest being assessment and advice [31, 48].

Given what we know about human learning and deliberate practice for skill learning, is it reasonable to expect a patient with aphasia to improve their significant language impairment with only a handful of therapy sessions? We think not. Indeed the discipline of neurological rehabilitation in general, and speech and language therapy in particular, can learn a lot from the lessons contained in the human expert performance literature. It is perhaps not fair to compare aphasia therapy (language re-learning) in a damaged brain with language acquisition, e.g., an adult learning a second language. Nevertheless, no-one is surprised that the

later takes many years with many hours of exposure, repetition and feedback to achieve a high level of proficiency. The evidence from the American Foreign Service Institute, summarized in Omaggio's book [49], suggests that even to get to the most basic level of proficiency (level 1 of 4), in the easiest of second languages takes 240 hours of practice. This is multiplied by a factor of two for a 'hard' language, with each level of proficiency costing a further doubling of time-on-task. There are many other examples in the literature which has been somewhat simplistically summarized as the '10,000 hours rule' popularized by Malcolm Gladwell in his book *Outliers* [50]. Gladwell leans heavily on the large body of work produced by Ericsson, whose summary from a recent review effectively sums up what most rehabilitation therapists will recognize:

> In sum, our empirical investigations and extensive reviews show that the development of expert performance will be primarily constrained by individuals' engagement in deliberate practice and the quality of the available training resources [51].

Perhaps the august UK bodies are reticent about dose because they know how much the average patient actually receives in the National Health Service (NHS). There is clearly a lot of variability dependent on local service provision, and aphasic patients can often re-access therapy in the chronic phase if they or an advocate pushes for it, but it is difficult to get away from the fact that the average available dose in the UK on the NHS is less than 10 hours in total [52]. Barring a huge change in UK funding, the amount of face-to-face time that a SALT can provide an individual patient is unlikely to change much; but that doesn't mean that we bury our heads in the sand. The challenge for clinicians is to find ways of delivering the appropriate treatment dose patients need using other means. These approaches will be covered in later sections (brain stimulation, drugs and electronic therapies).

What is the correct intensity of therapy?

Given that more appears to be better, one would assume that high-intensity is better than low-intensity. Cherney et al. produced a review on aphasia treatment intensity and found that it is not so simple [53]. Reviewing evidence from 10 studies that met their inclusion criteria, they found beneficial intensity effects (where dose had been controlled for) in the majority of chronic studies [53], but this effect disappeared for the more acute studies. Although modest evidence exists for the efficacy of more intensive treatment and constraint induced language therapy (CILT) in

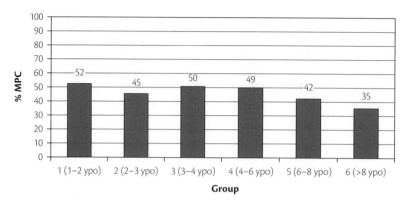

Fig. 21.3 Percentage of maximum possible change (%MPC), *y*-axis, vs. time since stroke, *x*-axis, for patients more than a year post-onset (ypo).

individuals with chronic stroke-induced aphasia [54–58], extensive language therapy whether delivered intensively or not, is difficult to administer with limited clinical resources not least because significantly more people withdraw from intensive SALT than conventional SALT [11]. Some of the recent Cochrane sub-analyses also hint that an intense treatment schedule may be beneficial but the main finding was that patients allocated to high-intensity SALT arms were less likely to comply with the protocol and were more likely to drop out of the study. The reasons for this are not clear but it is a concern particularly in the acute phase post stroke [41]. Interestingly, previous studies reported half of their elderly aphasic patients were unwilling to participate in intensive behavioural training, particularly if they received therapy before, and still others initiated rehabilitation but abandoned before the minimum period required for improvement [59]. Our view is that different patients at different points in their recovery trajectory will be amenable to intensive therapy. It is probably the easiest way to ensure that patients get the right dose of therapy, but it should not preclude others who cannot tolerate this approach from accruing their practice slowly but surely.

Is it ever too late for SALT?

Despite a seemingly popular belief that the patient's age matters, with younger patients having a better outcome after aphasic stoke, there is actually very little evidence to support this [60]. Old people learn (the oldest recorded recipient of a master's degree at age is Nola Ochs who received her MSc in liberal studies from Fort Hays State University in August 2007 aged 98 years: http://tinyurl.com/a8t7cbu). While working memory and processing speed tend to decrease with advancing age, some forms of memory remain static or even increase (e.g. vocabulary), which relies in part on semantic memory [61]. Indeed, a rehabilitation study of 38 stroke patients, split into older (70–84 years) and younger (20–34 years) age groups receiving eye movement based therapies for visual search and text reading found both groups improved a similar amount [62]. The interventions were software-based 'e-rehabilitation' and also go some way to dispelling another myth that older people cannot manage with electronic media.

To investigate whether time post stroke matters for SALT Moss and Nicholas [63] reviewed a whole series of case studies (*n* = 57) all in the chronic phase >1 year post onset. Partly because outcomes differed across studies and partly to try and control for

ceiling effects, they calculated a measure called percent of maximum possible change. For a subject who improved from a baseline of 40 to 60 on a score with a ceiling of 100, one could argue that they have improved by an absolute 20% [60–40], or that they had improved by a relative percentage of 50% [(60 – 40/40) × 100]. Moss and Nicholas's measure divided the amount of change by the amount of change possible, which penalizes more severely affected patients somewhat. For example their measure would be [(60 – 40/40 – 100) × 100] = 33%. They split their subjects into 2-year time buckets and asked whether response to therapy changed with years post stroke: it didn't (Figure 21.3).

> There is no correlation between time post onset and amount of change seen with treatment in people with aphasia who are >1 year post onset. Therefore, expectations of how well individuals will respond to aphasia treatment, which are based solely on time post onset, are not warranted [63].

So contrary to what many anecdotally believe, it is **never too late** for SALT input. Improvement of language function should be expected if the right treatment and correct dose is delivered irrespective of the patient's age and time post stroke.

Brain stimulation

Extensive SALT can be costly and difficult to achieve with limited resources. In addition recovery is frequently incomplete, and frustratingly slow for patients and their families. Improved rehabilitation methods are therefore needed to achieve higher levels of recovery within a shorter time frame. This has lead researchers to consider complementary brain stimulating strategies to treat aphasia such as noninvasive (transcranial electrical or magnetic) brain stimulation techniques (NIBS). The aim with these techniques is to change brain function and thereby promote neuroplasticity to enhance recovery and supplement the effects of aphasia rehabilitation.

Chief among these used in stroke rehabilitation include repetitive transcranial magnetic stimulation (rTMS) and anodal or cathodal transcranial direct current stimulation (tDCS), delivered to the ipsilesional, or contralesional hemisphere. The goals being to either increase ipsilesional excitability (increase local neuronal excitation) or decrease contralesional excitability (reduce distant neuronal inhibition). The functional improvement from noninvasive brain stimulation methods alone in stroke patients is reported to be small, in the region of 10% to 30%, and the effects short-lasting [64–66]. However, animal studies in the motor domain have shown that the combination of peripheral and central stimulation enhances synaptic plasticity more than central stimulation alone [67]. This suggests that in the search for more effective and longer-lasting interventions, NIBS, not as a complete therapy in itself but in combination with rehabilitation, seems a reasonable approach to magnify therapeutic outcomes.

It is early days in this field but the small number of aphasia studies that have applied tDCS or TMS to investigate its therapeutic effects—primarily on speech production– have obtained mixed but mostly positive results. The TMS findings from placebo-controlled trials ($n = 4$ to date) [68–71] have collectively found inhibitory rTMS to the right Broca's area homologue effective in the treatment of non-fluent aphasia. Whereas tDCS as an adjunct to SALT treatment for aphasia has been applied to the perilesional left hemisphere [72–76] or non-dominant right hemisphere [77–79] as a treatment of speech production and comprehension impairments. Each of these two techniques brings with them a set of relative advantages and disadvantages that may affect their potential wider clinical use. We direct the interested readers to a recent special issue of *Aphasiology* for details about both and their application to aphasia [80]. Particular focus in clinical trials is now on tDCS as it is portable, non-expensive, regarded as safe (lower risk of seizures than TMS) and involves a relatively simple set-up. These features together with the fact it can easily be delivered concurrently with SALT without adversely affecting the patient make tDCS a putative candidate for home treatment as an add-on to behavioural training or substitutive therapy for pharmacological treatments. Applying stimulation during SALT has the potential to influence both the immediate language performance and the consolidation phases of relearning. Using these NIBS methods in clinical practice could bring enormous gains for the treatment of aphasia in the future.

Drug therapy

Unfortunately the Cochrane review of drug therapy for aphasia is not helpful in assessing the evidence here [81]. Published in 2001 and yet to be updated, they searched for studies from 1966 to 1998, finding over 300 abstracts from which they extracted 55 studies. 45 of these were rejected on methodological grounds, and of the 10 remaining in the review, 'only one trial reported sufficient detail for analysis (abstract)'. A quantitative meta-analysis based on only one trial is clearly not useful. A recent dedicated special issue of *Aphasiology*, Volume 28, issue 2 (Special Issue: Pharmacology and Aphasia) (2014), provides a more rounded update on the surprising amount of studies published on this topic over many decades. We recommend this to interested parties as a full review is beyond the scope of this chapter. Overall, many different classes of drug have been tried with roughly half of the studies pairing a drug with behavioural therapy in an attempt to boost language relearning. The rationale behind those studies that did not pair drugs with SALT is that the drug will provide a simple main effect of general improvement in speech and language function that presumably will be lost if the drug were to be stopped (a tonic effect). Over half of the literature reports single-case studies or small case series (hence they don't meet the criteria for Cochrane), such studies are not necessarily unhelpful but care needs to be taken with study design as they can be plagued by bias. The better ones include a form of control (placebo if possible) which means the patient(s)

can be blinded. Those that do not (drug blocks alternated with no drug blocks) should certainly blind the assessors. Alternating drug blocks with placebo/no drug blocks is important; if nothing else, a baseline must be clearly established with preferably more than one assessment prior to the intervention as this will help estimate any test-retest or practice effects on the outcome measures, as well as give a handle on any background or 'natural' recovery rates (patients don't have to be stable over time, rates of change across blocks can be used instead of raw scores). Lastly, it is often useful to have a drug holiday or final block where the drug is withdrawn. If the theory is that the drug is having a tonic effect on language behaviour, then performance should drop off when the drug is stopped (thus providing evidence that, if effective, patients need to remain on it indefinitely). If the drug works by enhancing learning in a phasic manner, then there should be some behavioural carry over into the drug-free block. The implication here is that the drug may only be required during learning/therapy phases.

Dopaminergic drugs have probably been tried the most. Unfortunately, the commonest form has been bromocriptine (an ergot derived dopamine agonist) that is not used much by movement disorder specialists as it can cause long-term problems with lung and cardiac fibrosis. The other drug to be trialed in this class is L-dopa. The overall evidence is mixed, with about half of all published studies showing a beneficial effect of dopaminergic therapy. Dopamine, as might be expected, has an effect on the motor system *per se* so with some of the studies it is difficult to disentangle purely motoric effects from linguistic ones [82]. The study that provides the best evidence that L-dopa improves language learning was actually carried out in healthy controls. Knecht et al. used a randomized double-blind and parallel-group design in 40 subjects. L-dopa was used in a phasic way, paired with a computer-delivered task that required subjects to learn a novel vocabulary (nouns) associated with pictures of familiar objects. One group got L-dopa and the other placebo, 90 minutes prior to high-frequency, repetitive training. L-dopa significantly enhanced the speed, overall success, and long-term retention of novel word learning in a dose-dependent manner [83]. The most recent positive study in aphasic patients used a very similar approach to Knecht's pairing L-dopa or placebo with 15 daily computer-based therapy sessions. The main effect was of practice, with the placebo group improving on confrontation naming by 25% and the L-dopa group by 35% (a statistically non-significant difference). There were significant differences on repetition and verbal fluency, suggesting a main motoric effect on speech production but also hinting at a smaller language learning effect as well.

Cholinergic therapy has also been shown to improve speech output [84, 85] with a more recent study demonstrating a positive effect using Mementine (an *N*-methyl-D-aspartate receptor antagonist, licensed for use in treating patients with dementia). In this latter study, both groups ($n = 14$ in both the placebo and drug groups, all in the chronic phase) received intensive therapy (30 hours over 2 weeks). Both groups improved significantly with the drug having an additive effect on therapy [86]. The main outcome was the total score on the Western Aphasia Battery's Aphasia Quotient (WAB-AQ) [17]. Effect sizes were reported using Cohen's *d* where the difference between the groups is divided by the pooled standard deviation. In this study the variance was surprisingly small (severely affected patients were excluded) so the Cohen's *d* values are impressively large, but the actual average change in the WAB-AQ was modest: an improvement from a baseline in the mid-sixties by four in the placebo group and eight in the Mementine group. There was a washout period (the drug group dipped but remained significantly better than controls), and a partial crossover after washout where both groups moved to Mementine, improving again (although there was no SALT or blinding in this block). We highlight this study as a good example of how these complex studies can be well designed. One could argue that an extra cell (group) could have been added, drug alone, so that the interaction between drug and therapy could have been more formally assessed.

E-rehabilitation

Given what we know about total dose required and the lack of SALT time, computer-based or web-based therapies are perhaps one of the most promising ways of delivering enough dose of appropriate SALT to aphasic patients. There are many e-therapy devices or programmes available, over 50 software programs and over 40 apps: http://www.aphasiasoftwarefinder.org/. Unfortunately, almost none have been subject to a clinical trial. One that has is 'Step-by-Step', and moderate gains were demonstrated [87]. This was a two-group study ($n = 17$ in each, all chronic aphasic patients) comparing 'Step-by-Step' with standard clinical care. The 'Step-by-Step' group amassed 25 hours of practice over a three-month period (low intensity), but this came at a 'cost' of ~5 hours of SALT time and 4 hours of volunteer time ('Step-by-Step' is not adaptive and the appropriate exercises need to be chosen and loaded by a SALT). The main clinical outcome was the increased ability of patients to name practiced pictures. The 'Step-by-Step' group was more impaired at baseline (39% correct compared with the control group at 52%) and improved 20% more than the controls (who didn't improve at all).

For this burgeoning field to move forward, there needs to be much a more rigorous testing of the effectiveness of these e-programmes, particularly as some are relatively expensive to buy. The ideal product (not yet available) should allow patients to use it independently with no or minimal help from others, would adapt to their behaviour (i.e. get harder as they get better), and provide feedback so the patients can see how they are doing and learnt from their mistakes. All should have prominent user involvement in the alpha and beta testing (development) phases. Claims over general 'brain training' effects of e-therapy packages should be taken with a large pinch of salt. E-practice, just like most standard practice, results in task-specific and not generalized 'cognitive' improvements [88]. If you practice Sudoku puzzles a lot, you'll probably just get better at Sudoku. Clearly not helpful if you are aphasic and want to improve your speech production!

Augmentative and alternative communication (AAC)

Therapy, by definition, aims to improve behaviour in a way that persists outside the intervention period. Whatever the exact mechanism of therapy (restoration of function or strategic changes in behaviour), any successful change in behaviour will be mediated by neuroplastic processes. While recovery of language is the goal sometimes this cannot be achieved, or may take significant time and this is where AAC plays a role. AAC can include any strategy used to express thoughts, needs, wants, and ideas. Examples of common AAC strategies might include gesture, picture communication boards and voice output communication devices. Many AAC strategies use pictures, symbols, letters, words, and phrases to represent the messages, objects, people and places needed to talk about. Individuals with aphasia can benefit from the use of AAC tools to overcome functional communication challenges, develop language and literacy skills, make choices, speak their minds, lead productive lives and participate more fully in society. Depending on the severity of the stroke, the AAC solution may range from low-tech (paper and pen) to high-tech (computer devices), as part of or as a complete communication strategy.

For example, communicating during social situations may be particularly challenging for people with aphasia. An individual with expressive aphasia may have difficulties creating a complete sentence when ordering what they want at a restaurant. Another person, one with receptive aphasia, may not understand what the waiter is telling them about the menu. In the case of an aphasic with speech problems an AAC device can be used to supplement their existing speech or replace non-functional speech by providing vocabulary words, phrases and sentences on topics (e.g. food) when they have trouble finding the words that they want to say. When the person with speech comprehension problems uses AAC devices displaying written words and pictures under topic pages for adult social settings it can aid the aphasic's understanding and at the same time allow them to show their understanding and comprehension of what is being communicated, keeping them in the conversation. Other ways AAC devices can support aphasic's recovery are by: (1) providing a voice so they can listen to words being spoken and practice their own speech, just like in the e-rehabilitation section earlier; (2) giving them a tool to practice writing, spelling and building phrases and sentences; (3) providing a means to control their home environment, send email/ texts (e.g. using text to speech apps), and re-connect to the world.

Future directions

Predicting the likely recovery trajectory of individual patients is an important goal that may be achievable in the next decade or so. Stroke has a variable effect across patients and recovery is clearly dependent on several key factors that are either intrinsic (site of lesion, cognition) or extrinsic (time, therapy) to the individual; these factors necessarily interact, but what are the important ones? As mentioned, age itself is not one but initial severity is clearly important. As Anna Basso remarked in an early review of the topic which focused on demographic variables and found no role for age, sex or handedness: 'The factors that really do influence outcome are initial severity of aphasia (which is inextricably associated with the extent and the location of the lesion) and rehabilitation' [89]. Almost all surviving stroke patients improve over time and as well as tracing these 'natural' recovery curves, we also wish to be able to predict the effect of therapy on these curves; that is, to identify why some patients respond better to a given therapy dose than others [90]. Some work has already been done on this and cognitive factors such as working memory [91], and a combination of attention, semantic memory, and phonological skills [92] have been found to be important. The main challenge, which is now becoming tractable, is to investigate how demographic, cognitive, and neural factors interact to determine response to therapy.

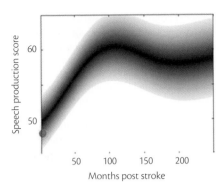

Fig. 21.4 An example of predicted prognoses was made after removing the 'test patient' from the data, and then training with the rest; the prognoses are then constructed by making 240 individual predictions for the test patient, by replacing their 'time post-stroke' value first. In the plot, the actual data measured at assessment is plotted in light gray, on the y-axis (at 1 year post stroke. The prediction is expressed as a probability distributions through time, with the mean prediction in black, and borders at 2 standard deviations from that mean prediction (i.e. 95% confidence).

Current research is working towards identifying neural factors that may be useful in predicting the recovery of aphasic stroke patients or may influence their treatment. Both the structural and functional anatomy of the aphasic stroke patient's brain will be important. For example, knowing where the lesion is and what perilesional tissue is anatomically intact is critical for identifying which part of the brain to stimulate when using NIBS to augment SALT. Knowing the residual functional connectivity may help explain why patients with seemingly similar lesions vary in both their baseline severity, and in their recovery over time [93]. Lesion location is clearly an important factor in this. Structural brain imaging contains a wealth of complex information, but when this is reduced to a single number, such as the volume of tissue damaged by the stroke, the prognostic value becomes useless [94]. Advances in computer processing power have meant that much more detailed multivariate analyses of imaging and behavioural data are now possible [95]. This means that the location, shape and number of regions included in the lesion can be factored into prediction algorithms along with behavioural measures. Many of the studies addressing prediction to date have opted for a binarized outcome ('good' versus 'poor'); however, we question the utility of this for both patients and therapists. It is likely to be much more informative to predict recovery trajectories on a continuous measure of outcome. Although more technically challenging, this is possible [96] (see Figure 21.4).

In terms of planning for the future, what would the perfect interventional study look like? The patients would be carefully characterized in terms of their behavioural measures, along with structural and possibly functional brain imaging. The intervention would be targeted at either their impairment or aimed to improve social participation, preferably both; and would be delivered at a high enough dose. The patients would have been involved in the development of the intervention, and perhaps even its funding. Perhaps a cognitive enhancer (NIBS or drug therapy) would be added into the design. If the study proves successful, then a translational plan will be in place so that current and future patients may benefit from any positive findings. If that sounds futuristic, think again, as William Gibson says, 'The future is already here— it's just not very evenly distributed' [97].

References

1. Albert ML. Aphasia therapy works! Stroke. 2003;**34**(4):987–993.
2. Dalemans RJP, De Witte LP, Beurskens AJHM Van den Heuvel WJA, Wade DT. An investigation into the social participation of stroke survivors with aphasia. Disabil Rehabil. 2010;**32**(20):1678–1685.
3. Cruice M, Worrall L, Hickson L, Murison R. Finding a focus for quality of life with aphasia: Social and emotional health, and psychological well-being. Aphasiology. 2003;**17**(4):333–353.
4. Hilari K. The impact of stroke: are people with aphasia different to those without? Disabil Rehabil. 2011;**33**(3):211–218.
5. Kauhanen, M. L., Korpelainen, J. T., Hiltunen, P., Maatta, R., Mononen, H., Brusin, E., et al. Aphasia, depression, and non-verbal cognitive impairment in ischaemic stroke. Cerebrovasc Dis. 2000;**10**(6):455–461.
6. Samsa GP, Matchar DB, Goldstein L, et al. Utilities for major stroke: results from a survey of preferences among persons at increased risk for stroke. Am Heart J. 1998;**136**(4 Pt 1):703–713.
7. Wade DT, Hewer RL, David RM, Enderby PM. Aphasia after stroke: natural history and associated deficits. J Neurol Neurosurg Psychiatry. 1986;**49**(1):11–16.
8. Bhogal SK, Teasell RW, Foley NC, Speechley MR. Rehabilitation of aphasia: more is better. Top Stroke Rehabil. 2003;**10**(2):66–76.
9. Cicerone KD, Langenbahn DM, Braden C, et al. Evidence-based cognitive rehabilitation: updated review of the literature from 2003 through 2008. Arch Phys Med Rehabil. 2011;**92**(4):519–530.
10. Code C. (2012;Apportioning time for aphasia rehabilitation. Aphasiology. **26**(5):729–735.
11. Kelly H, Brady MC, Enderby P. Speech and language therapy for aphasia following stroke. [Meta-Analysis Review]. Cochrane Database Syst Rev. 2010; (5):CD000425.
12. Jokel R, Rochon E, Anderson ND. Errorless learning of computer-generated words in a patient with semantic dementia. Neuropsychol Rehabil. 2010;**20**(1):16–41.
13. Noonan KA, Pryer LR, Jones RW, Burns AS, Ralph MAL. A direct comparison of errorless and errorful therapy for object name relearning in Alzheimer's disease. Neuropsychol Rehabil. 2012;**22**(2):215–234.
14. Ousset PJ, Viallard G, Puel M, Celsis P, Demonet JF, Cardebat D. Lexical therapy and episodic word learning in dementia of the Alzheimer type. Brain Language. 2002;**80**(1):14–20.
15. Bastiaanse R, Edwards S. Word order and finiteness in Dutch and English Broca's and Wernicke's aphasia. Brain Language. 2004;**89**(1):91–107.
16. Goodglass H, Kaplan E. Boston diagnostic aphasia examination booklet. Lea & Febiger, Philadelphia, 1983.
17. Kertesz A. The Western Aphasia Battery. Grune and Stratton, New York, 1982.
18. Crary MA, Wertz RT, Deal JL. Classifying aphasias— cluster-analysis of Western Aphasia Battery and Boston diagnostic aphasia examination results. Aphasiology. 1992;**6**(1):29–36.
19. Ardila A. A proposed reinterpretation and reclassification of aphasic syndromes. Aphasiology. 2010;**24**(3):363–394.
20. Swinburn K, Porter G, Howard D. Comprehensive Aphasia Test. Psychology Press, Hove and New York, 2004.
21. Kay J, Lesser R, Coltheart M. Psycholinguistic assessments of language processing in aphasia (PALPA): reading and spelling. Lawrence Erlbaum Associates, Hove, 1992.
22. Duffy J. Motor speech disorders: substrates. differential diagnosis and management. Elsevier, St Louis, 2005.
23. Square-Storer PA, Roy EA, Hogg SC. The dissociation of aphasia from apraxia of speech, ideomotor limb, and buccofacial apraxia. In Hammond GR (ed.) Cerebral Control of Speech and Limb Movements. North-Holland, Amsterdam, 1990, pp. 451–474.
24. Rapp B, Goldrick M. Speaking words: Contributions of cognitive neuropsychological research. Cogn Neuropsychol. 2006;**23**(1):39–73.

25. Katz RB, Goodglass H. Deep dysphasia: analysis of a rare form of repetition disorder. Brain Lang. 1990;**39**(1):153–185.

26. Campbell M, Fitzpatrick R, Haines A, et al. Framework for design and evaluation of complex interventions to improve health. Br Med J. 2000;**321**(7262):694–696.

27. Doesborgh SJ, van de Sandt-Koenderman MW, Dippel DW, van Harskamp F, Koudstaal PJ, Visch-Brink EG. Effects of semantic treatment on verbal communication and linguistic processing in aphasia after stroke: a randomized controlled trial. Stroke. 2004;**35**(1):141–146.

28. Howard D, Patterson K, Franklin S, Orchard-Lisle V, Morton J. Treatment of word retrieval deficits in aphasia. A comparison of two therapy methods. Brain. 1985;**108** (Pt 4):817–829.

29. Wambaugh JL, Doyle PJ, Martinez AL, Kalinyak-Fliszar M. Effects of two lexical retrieval cueing treatments on action naming in aphasia. J Rehabil Res Dev. 2002;**39**(4):455–466.

30. MRC. Developing and evaluating complex interventions:new guidance. Medical Research Council, London, 2008.

31. Bowen A, Hesketh A, Patchick E, et al. Effectiveness of enhanced communication therapy in the first four months after stroke for aphasia and dysarthria: a randomised controlled trial. Br Med J. 2012;**345**, e4407.

32. David R, Enderby P, Bainton D. Treatment of acquired aphasia: speech therapists and volunteers compared. J Neurol Neurosurg Psychiatry. 1982;**45**(11):957–961.

33. Bath PM, Lees KR, Schellinger PD, et al. Statistical analysis of the primary outcome in acute stroke trials. Stroke. 2012;**43**(4):1171–1178.

34. Altman DG, Bland JM. Treatment allocation by minimisation. Br Med J. 2005;**330**(7495):843.

35. Byng S, Duchan JF. Social model philosophies and principles: Their applications to therapies for aphasia. Aphasiology. 2005;**19**(10–11):906–922.

36. Martin N, Thompson CK, Worrall L. Aphasia Rehabilitation: the Impairment and Its Consequences. Plural Publishing Company, San Diego, CA, 2008.

37. Hilari K, Byng S, Lamping DL, Smith SC. Stroke and Aphasia Quality of Life Scale-39 (SAQOL-39): evaluation of acceptability, reliability, and validity. Stroke. 2003;**34**(8):1944–1950.

38. Frattali CM, Thompson CK, Holland AL, Wohl CB, Ferketic MM. American speech-language hearing association functional assessment of communication skills for adults. ASHA Fulfilment Operations, Rockville, MD, 1995.

39. Long A, Hesketh A, Bowen A. Communication outcome after stroke: a new measure of the carer's perspective. Clin Rehabil. 2009;**23**(9):846–856.

40. Moher D, Tetzlaff J, Tricco AC, Sampson M, Altman DG. Epidemiology and reporting characteristics of systematic reviews. PLoS Med. 2007;**4**(3):e78.

41. Brady MC, Kelly H, Godwin J, Enderby P. Speech and language therapy for aphasia following stroke. Cochrane Database Syst Rev. 2012; (5).

42. Cramer SC. Repairing the human brain after stroke: I. Mechanisms of spontaneous recovery. Ann Neurol. 2008;**63**(3):272–287.

43. Intercollegiate Stroke Working Party. National clinical guideline for stroke. 2008; available from https://www.rcplondon.ac.uk/resources/stroke-guidelines (accessed 29 September 2014).

44. Intercollegiate Stroke Working Party. National clinical guideline for stroke. 2012; available from https://www.rcplondon.ac.uk/resources/stroke-guidelines (accessed 29 September 2014).

45. Bhogal SK, Teasell R, Speechley M. Intensity of aphasia therapy, impact on recovery. Stroke. 2003;**34**(4):987–993.

46. De Renzi, E., Vignolo, L. A. (1962;The token test: A sensitive test to detect receptive disturbances in aphasics. Brain. **85**, 665–678.

47. Porch B. Porch Index of Communicative Ability (PICA). Consulting Psychologists Press, Palo Alto, 1981.

48. Leff AP, Howard D. Stroke: Has speech and language therapy been shown not to work? Nat Rev Neurol. 2012;**8**(11):600–601.

49. Omaggio AC. Teaching language in context: proficiency-oriented instruction. Heinle, University of California, 1986;

50. Gladwell M. Outliers: the story of sucess. Penguin, London, 2008;

51. Ericsson KA, Nandagopal K, Roring RW. Toward a science of exceptional achievement: attaining superior performance through deliberate practice. Ann N Y Acad Sci. 2009;**1172**, 199–217.

52. Code C, Heron C. Services for aphasia, other acquired adult neurogenic communication and swallowing disorders in the United Kingdom, 2000. Disabil Rehabil. 2003;**25**(21):1231–1237.

53. Cherney LR, Patterson JP, Raymer A, Frymark T, Schooling T. Evidence-based systematic review: effects of intensity of treatment and constraint-induced language therapy for individuals with stroke-induced aphasia. J Speech Lang Hear Res. 2008a;**51**(5):1282–1299.

54. Barthel G, Meinzer M, Djundja D, Rockstroh B. Intensive language therapy in chronic aphasia: Which aspects contribute most? Aphasiology. 2008;**22**(4):408–421.

55. Cherney LR, Patterson JP, Raymer A, Frymark T, Schooling T. Evidence-based systematic review: effects of intensity of treatment and constraint-induced language therapy for individuals with stroke-induced aphasia. J Speech. Lang Hear Res. 2008b;**51**(5):1282–1299.

56. Meinzer M, Djundja D, Barthel G, Elbert T, Rockstroh B. Long-term stability of improved language functions in chronic aphasia after constraint-induced aphasia therapy. Stroke. 2005;**36**(7):1462–1466.

57. Meinzer M, Elbert T, Wienbruch C, Djundja D, Barthel G, Rockstroh B. Intensive language training enhances brain plasticity in chronic aphasia. BMC Biol. 2004;**2**, 20.

58. Pulvermuller F, Neininger B, Elbert T, et al. Constraint-induced therapy of chronic aphasia after stroke. Stroke. 2001;**32**(7):1621–1626.

59. Basso A, Macis M. Therapy efficacy in chronic aphasia. Behavioural Neurol. 2011; **24**(4):317–325.

60. Plowman E, Hentz B, Ellis C. Post-stroke aphasia prognosis: a review of patient-related and stroke-related factors. J Eval Clin Pract. 2012;**18**(3):689–694.

61. Park DC, Lautenschlager G, Hedden T, Davidson NS, Smith AD, Smith PK. Models of visuospatial and verbal memory across the adult life span. Psychol Aging. 2002;**17**(2):299–320.

62. Schuett S, Zihl J. Does age matter? Age and rehabilitation of visual field disorders after brain injury. Cortex. 2013;**49**(4):1001–1012.

63. Moss A, Nicholas M. Language rehabilitation in chronic aphasia and time postonset: a review of single-subject data. Stroke. 2006;**37**(12):3043–3051.

64. Hummel FC, Cohen LG. Non-invasive brain stimulation: a new strategy to improve neurorehabilitation after stroke? Lancet Neurol. 2006;**5**(8):708–712.

65. Talelli P, Rothwell J. Does brain stimulation after stroke have a future? Curr Opin Neurol. 2006;**19**(6):543–550.

66. Webster BR, Celnik PA, Cohen LG. Noninvasive brain stimulation in stroke rehabilitation. NeuroRx. 2006;**3**(4):474–481.

67. Fritsch B, Reis J, Martinowich K, et al. Direct current stimulation promotes BDNF-dependent synaptic plasticity: potential implications for motor learning. Neuron. 2010;**66**(2):198–204.

68. Barwood CHS, Murdoch BE, Whelan BM, et al. The effects of low frequency repetitive transcranial magnetic stimulation (rTMS) and sham condition rTMS on behavioural language in chronic non-fluent aphasia: Short term outcomes. Neurorehabilitation. 2011;**28**(2):113–128.

69. Barwood CHS, Murdoch BE, Whelan BM, et al. Longitudinal modulation of N400 in chronic non-fluent aphasia using low-frequency rTMS: A randomised placebo controlled trial. Aphasiology. 2012;**26**(1):103–124.

70. Kindler J, Schumacher R, Cazzoli D, et al. Theta burst stimulation over the right broca's homologue induces improvement of naming in aphasic patients. Stroke. 2012;**43**(8):2175-U2270.

71. Weiduschat N, Thiel A, Rubi-Fessen I, et al. Effects of repetitive transcranial magnetic stimulation in aphasic stroke a randomized controlled pilot study. Stroke. 2011;**42**(2):409–415.

72. Baker JM, Rorden C, Fridriksson J. Using transcranial direct-current stimulation to treat stroke patients with aphasia. Stroke. 2010;**41**(6):1229–1236.

73. Cattaneo Z, Pisoni A, Papagno C. Transcranial direct current stimulation over Broca's region improves phonemic and semantic fluency in healthy individuals. Neuroscience. 2011;**183**, 64–70.

74. Fiori V, Coccia M, Marinelli CV, et al. Transcranial direct current stimulation improves word retrieval in healthy and nonfluent aphasic subjects. J Cogn Neurosci. 2011;**23**(9):2309–2323.

75. Fridriksson J, Richardson JD, Baker JM, Rorden C. Transcranial direct current stimulation improves naming reaction time in fluent aphasia a double-blind, sham-controlled study. Stroke. 2011;**42**(3):819–821.

76. Monti A, Cogiamanian F, Marceglia S, et al. Improved naming after transcranial direct current stimulation in aphasia. J Neurol Neurosurg Psychiatry. 2008;**79**(4):451–453.

77. Floel A, Meinzer M, Kirstein R, et al. Short-term anomia training and electrical brain stimulation. Stroke. 2011;**42**(7):2065–2067.

78. Kang EK, Kim YK, Sohn HM, Cohen LG, Paik NJ. Improved picture naming in aphasia patients treated with cathodal tDCS to inhibit the right Broca's homologue area. Restorat Neurol Neurosci. 2011;**29**(3):141–152.

79. Vines BW, Norton AC, Schlaug G. Non-invasive brain stimulation enhances the effects of melodic intonation therapy. Front Psychol. 2011;**2**, 230.

80. Crinion J. Shocking speech. Aphasiology. 2012;**26**(9):1077–1081.

81. Greener J, Enderby P, Whurr R. Pharmacological treatment for aphasia following stroke (Cochrane review). The Cochrane Library. 2003;2.

82. Goberman AM, Coelho C. Acoustic analysis of parkinsonian speech I: speech characteristics and L-Dopa therapy. NeuroRehabilitation. 2002;**17**(3):237–246.

83. Knecht S, Breitenstein C, Bushuven S, et al. Levodopa: faster and better word learning in normal humans. Ann Neurol. 2004;**56**(1):20–26.

84. Berthier ML, Hinojosa J, Martin Mdel C, Fernandez I. Open-label study of donepezil in chronic poststroke aphasia. Neurology. 2003;**60**(7):1218–1219.

85. Berthier ML, Green C, Higueras C, Fernandez I, Hinojosa J, Martin MC. A randomized, placebo-controlled study of donepezil in post-stroke aphasia. Neurology. 2006;**67**(9):1687–1689.

86. Berthier ML, Green C, Lara J P, et al. Memantine and constraint-induced aphasia therapy in chronic poststroke aphasia. Ann Neurol. 2009;**65**(5):577–585.

87. Palmer R, Enderby P, Cooper C, et al. Computer therapy compared with usual care for people with long-standing aphasia poststroke: a pilot randomized controlled trial. Stroke. 2012;**43**(7):1904–1911.

88. Owen AM, Hampshire A, Grahn JA, et al. Putting brain training to the test. Nature. 2010;**465**(7299):775-U776.

89. Basso A. Prognostic factors in aphasia. Aphasiology. 1992;**6**(4):337–348.

90. Lazar RM, Antoniello D. Variability in recovery from aphasia. Curr Neurol Neurosci Rep. 2008;**8**(6):497–502.

91. Caspari I, Parkinson SR, LaPointe LL, Katz RC. Working memory and aphasia. Brain Cogn. 1998;**37**(2):205–223.

92. Ralph MAL, Snell C, Fillingham JK, Conroy P, Sage K. Predicting the outcome of anomia therapy for people with aphasia post CVA: Both language and cognitive status are key predictors. Neuropsychol Rehabil. 2010;**20**(2):289–305.

93. Schofield TM, Penny WD, Stephan KE, et al. Changes in auditory feedback connections determine the severity of speech processing deficits after stroke. J Neurosci. 2012;**32**(12):4260–4270.

94. Coupar F, Pollock A, Rowe P, Weir C, Langhorne P. Predictors of upper limb recovery after stroke: a systematic review and meta-analysis. Clin Rehabil. 2012;**26**(4):291–313.

95. Price, C. J., Seghier, M. L., Leff, A. P. (2010;Predicting language outcome and recovery after stroke: the PLORAS system. Nat Rev Neurol. **6**(4):202–210.

96. Hope TMH, Seghier ML, Leff AP, Price CJ. Predicting outcome and recovery after stroke with lesions extracted from MRI images. NeuroImage: Clinical. 2013;**1**(2):424–433.

97. Gibson W. The Science in Science Fiction: National Public Radio (USA), 1999.

CHAPTER 22

Neuropsychological rehabilitation of higher cortical functions after brain damage

Radek Ptak and Armin Schnider

Introduction

Motor rehabilitation after central lesions follows certain principles. The main one is that focused training, shaped according to the patient's current capacities, improves motor function and is associated with reorganization of the cerebral representation of motor control [1, 2]. Medication and electrical or magnetic stimulation of the brain may modulate the underlying processes [3, 4]. When retraining is insufficient or impossible, external aids are introduced—for example, a wheelchair—to allow mobility despite lost motricity.

Cognitive rehabilitation follows the same principles, although a main difference is the higher degree of freedom in cognitive functions. Independent of the function that has to be trained, intensive training is critical. It has been used successfully to improve language functions and has invoked methods such as constraint-induced therapy in aphasia [5] or computer training for anomia [6]. Spatial attention in hemispatial neglect or spatial alexia may benefit from repetitive exploration through intensive training [7, 8]. In some situations, the exploitation of physiological principles improves cognitive functions. For example, neck-muscle vibration or prism-adaptation improve spatial exploration in hemispatial neglect. However, lasting effects generally require the coupling of such manipulations with active, intensive training [9].

Similar to motor function, recovery of cognitive functions may be modulated by medication [3], although the effects may vary individually. Accordingly, dopaminergic medication has been beneficial [10] or deleterious [11] for hemispatial neglect, possibly because treatment response may depend on the preserved brain tissue available to respond to medication. Similarly, the effects of electrical or magnetic stimulation have varied. Promising results of potential clinical relevance have been obtained with inhibition of the contralesional hemisphere by theta-burst stimulation (TBS) in hemispatial neglect [12].

Retraining is not always possible and compensation of lost functions may be necessary. This concerns basic functions such as the automatic encoding of information in memory. While patients with moderately severe amnesia may profit from mnemonic strategies [13], many instances of severe amnesia need external aids such as notes or electronic agendas to effectively replace the lost function [14].

Thus, in many aspects cognitive rehabilitation is fundamentally similar to motor rehabilitation. In the following paragraphs, we will present specific treatment strategies for the main groups of cognitive deficits (memory impairment, spatial neglect, attentional deficits, and dysexecutive problems), with an emphasis on neuropsychological interventions. The rehabilitation of language functions is treated in Chapter 21.

Memory rehabilitation

Memory problems are frequent consequences of brain damage, though they may go undetected due to the absence of specific complaints. Memory is a complex function that involves distinct cognitive processes related to how information is registered (encoding), how it is rendered stable (consolidation), how memory traces are accessed (retrieval), and how traces related to distinct events are distinguished (source memory). In addition, the term 'memory' relates to several, largely independent systems that may be distinguished based on whether content is accessed consciously (explicit versus implicit memory), whether learning is abrupt or incremental (declarative versus procedural memory), or whether memory contents are linked to a spatiotemporal context (episodic versus semantic memory). Patients with severe memory problems may have largely intact performance in procedural learning, classical conditioning or priming, and some of these capacities are relevant for memory rehabilitation [15–17].

Diverse functions of memory depend on various brain regions, such as the medial temporal lobe, the diencephalon, the dorsolateral prefrontal cortex, and the orbitofrontal cortex. The degree and quality of memory impairment varies as a function of the affected brain area. For example, stroke in the territory of the posterior cerebral artery typically affects the storage of information because of the importance of the hippocampus in memory consolidation. Conversely, prefrontal cortex damage may particularly affect acquisition and recall of information due to the importance of this region for encoding and strategic organisation of retrieval. Orbitofrontal damage may induce an inability to sense whether evoked memories relate to present reality, as evidenced in confabulation and disorientation [18, 19].

Two distinct classes of memory problems deserve special attention in neurorehabilitation as they interfere particularly strongly with patients' independence. The first relates to acquisition of new, domain-specific information, such as learning names or a new vocabulary. Anterograde amnesia discribes this failure. Given the reduced capacity of patients with memory problems to acquire new information the aim of memory rehabilitation is to find ways to enhance learning and to reduce errors during recall. The second problem has to do with failures of prospective memory, which is the reduced ability of memory-impaired patients to maintain in memory behavioural goals over prolonged time periods.

Acqusition of new memory contents

The traditional method to improve acquisition and retention of new information, that is, to compensate for anterograde amnesia, in patients with memory problems are mnemonics, such as building an acronym or creating rhymes [20]. However, most of these techniques are inflexible and can only be used for very specific material. In addition, mnemonics rely on a systematic effort and are therefore only of use for patients with relatively slight memory impairment [21] while patients with severe impairment do better only when new information is presented in a special format (e.g. a word combined with a picture [22]). Some mnemonic strategies use visual imagery, and one of the rare randomized studies in the domain of memory rehabilitation compared systematic training of visual imagery during encoding with a 'pragmatic' therapy including face-name associations and the use of memory notebooks [23]. Each group consisted of 12 patients who were trained for 30 sessions. Imagery training started with simple exercises (imaging of single objects), went gradually through more difficult tasks (imaging of actions) and ended with transfer to the use of imagery in everyday situations. Imagery training resulted in improved retention of stories and appointments and better ratings of everyday memory by the relatives (Figure 22.1). Thus, this study shows that systematic training of an 'internal' mnemonic technique can have beneficial effects on everyday memory function. Such techniques have therefore been recommended for patients with mild to moderate memory problems [24, 25].

Regarding severely amnesic patients mnemonics are generally not applicable and new information must be presented in a

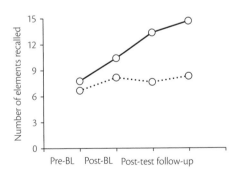

Fig. 22.1 Outcome of systematic training of mental imagery on delayed story recall. The black line shows data of the experimental group before (pre-BL) and after base-line (post-BL), after 30 sessions of imagery training (post-test) and 3 months later (follow-up). The stippled line shows data of control patients who received 'pragmatic' memory rehabilitation (e.g. they were taught how to use memory notebooks).

Imagery mnemonics for the rehabilitation of memory: A randomised group controlled trial, Kaschel R, Della Sala S, Cantagallo A et al., Neuropsychol Rehab, 2002, reprinted by permission of Taylor & Francis Ltd.

special format in order to enhance retention. Glisky et al. [26] presented computer-related terms (a simplified programming language allowing patients to process forms by interacting with a computer) while gradually diminishing the number of letters consituting each word. This 'vanishing cues' technique lead to slow, incremental learning and eventually resulted in correct retention across several weeks or months. However, learning was laborious (memory-impaired patients required many more trials than healthy subjects), and the success at retrieval strongly depended on whether recall was tested in conditions similar to acquisition or not [27]. This latter finding suggests that new knowledge acquired using the vanishing cues technique is hyperspecific, mainly associative, largely inflexible and possibly depends on implicit memory systems [28]. An additional problem with the technique is that it promotes the production of errors, which is particularly deleterious in patients with impaired memory. The reason is that actively produced errors during learning may remain activated in implicit memory and therefore re-emerge whenever the patient attempts to access a specific memory content. Baddeley and Wilson [29] therefore suggested that memory rehabilitation should use techniques that, whenever possible, eliminate errors ('errorless learning'). Several studies have demonstrated an advantage of errorless learning as compared to conditions that did not prevent wrong answers. This applies to the acquisition of verbal associations [30, 31] or the learning of more complex procedural knowledge [32]. Overall the effect size of interventions using errorless learning is higher compared to the vanishing cues technique [33]. Recent studies have emphasized the advantages of both techniques (that is, active and effortful learning with the vanishing cues technique and error prevention in errorless learning) and attempted to combine them [34, 35]. A conclusion from these studies is that acquisition of new information in patients with memory problems should be active rather than passive, and should prevent errors as much as possible. The latter is particularly important for patients with severe amnesia who are likely to repeatedly produce wrong answers.

Rehabilitation of prospective memory

The primary objective of memory rehabilitation is to render patients independent in everyday life. In activities of daily living memory expresses itself often in the ability to remember to do things at a particular moment in time (prospective memory) [36]. It seems straightforward that prospective memory is best supported by external memory aids and agendas; however, systematic use of a notebook may prove extremely difficult for patients with severe memory problems who never used external memory aids before injury [37, 38]. A systematic training programme is therefore necessary that divides training into an acquisition phase (learning to know the function of the agenda), an application phase (exercises how to note fake or real appointments), and a transfer phase (use of the agenda in everyday life) [37, 39, 40].

Given the wide accessibility of electronic devices some newer studies have examined whether such devices can be helpful in memory rehabilitation. In a large group study Wilson et al. [41, 42] tested an electronic pager system that received short text messages reminding patients of appointments or specific tasks. This simple system lead to an increase of completed target tasks from 37% before therapy to 85% after introduction of the pager. In addition, in at least some of the treated patients the proportion of completed tasks did not decrease after withdrawal of the pager, suggesting that the regular reminders lead to increased attention to prospective tasks and appointments. Recent single-case studies showed similar findings when a commercial smartphone was used [43, 44]. Finally, some studies have explored the use of a wearable camera (SenseCam) that automatically takes pictures (approximately every 30 s), which can later be viewed at accelerated speed. A patient with severe memory problems due to encephalitis showed improved retention of everyday memories when wearing the camera and reviewing the film as compared to written notes in a diary [45].

In conclusion, the use of internal mnemonics (in particular, imagery training) can be recommended for patients with mild to moderate memory problems [46], while acquisition of new material in severe amnesia can be enhanced when coupling the vanishing cues technique with errorless learning [24, 47]. Finally, the future of ecological memory rehabilitation belongs to smartphones and other electronic memory aids, since these can easily be programmed to signal upcoming appointments and prospective tasks [48].

Spatial neglect

Spatial neglect is a significant predictor of prolonged hospital stay, worse recovery of motor and sensory function, and greater dependence in activities of daily living [49, 50]. The rehabilitation of spatial neglect has therefore received special attention. Initial studies have focused on the deficits of contralesional awareness and involved systematic training of visual scanning, reading and reorienting of attention [51, 52]. These studies revealed positive effects of training on classic neglect measures (cancellation, line bisection, reading, etc.), but lacked adequate control and follow-up measures. These findings have also been criticized for the lack of effect on neglect expressed in activities of daily living [53]. More recent studies have examined the impact of diverse physiological modulations, and some of these have reported significant and lasting effects on standard neglect measures as well as independence in everyday life. Dramatic attenuation of neglect may be observed under caloric stimulation with cold water, but the effect is short-lived (approximately 15 min) and not well tolerated [54]. Schindler et al. [9] examined the effect of neck muscle vibration on neglect recovery in a cross-over design. Vibratory stimulation of the neck muscles at 80–100 Hz mimics a head-turn contralateral to vibration and thus biases perceived head-on-trunk signals. During 2 weeks (15 sessions) one group of 10 neglect patients received visual exploration training combined with neck muscle vibration, followed by 2 weeks of exploration training alone. The other group received the same treatment in reversed order. Both groups showed improved performance in cancellation, tactile exploration, reading, and the judgement of where the subjective straight ahead is following neck muscle vibration, while no significant changes were observed following exploration training. In addition, there was also an effect on activities of daily living that remained stable 2 months after the end of the therapy. These findings suggest that neck muscle vibration ameliorates neglect by recalibrating a biased egocentric reference system.

Another technique that is thought to have effects by recalibrating the biased egocentric reference frame in neglect is prismatic adaptation. This technique requires patients to point to visual targets while wearing prismatic goggles that deviate the field of view by 10–15 degrees to the right. This deviation introduces an error signal between the perceived position and the actual position of the target that must be compensated by pointing further to the left. This compensatory effect is evidenced following adaptation, where pointing is biased to the left after removal of the prisms. Rossetti et al. [55] showed that a single session of prismatic adaptation (50–60 pointing movements) had positive effects on spatial neglect immediately following adaptation and even better effects two hours later. A more systematic study [56] revealed beneficial effects on neglect symptoms up to 5 weeks following the therapy. More recently Serino et al. [57] tested the effects of prismatic adaptation in a randomized controlled trial involving 20 neglect patients. Ten patients were adapted during 10 sessions while the other 10 patients exercised pointing with non-prismatic goggles. Results showed a specific effect of prismatic adaptation on diverse measures of neglect, but no effect of pointing without prisms.

Although these results are encouraging, some findings preclude unconditional recommendation of prismatic adaptation therapy. First, Rousseaux et al. [58] failed to replicate the initial resuls of Rossetti et al. [55], suggesting that a single session of adaptation may not be sufficient to improve neglect. Turton et al. [59] used a very similar design as the study of Serino et al. [57] and observed comparable improvement of neglect after prismatic adaptation and neutral pointing. The main difference between these two studies was that Turton et al. [59] tested patients at earlier stages of the disease while Serino et al. [57] included patients with chronic neglect. It is therefore possible that prismatic adaptation acts differently in post-acute and chronic neglect. A recent meta-analysis [60] has shown that prismatic adaptation has significant positive effects immediately after the end of the therapy (mean effect size: 0.89), but not at follow-up (effect size: 0.15). Finally, the finding of positive adaptation effects appears to depend on the presence of intentional motor deficits in neglect [61], suggesting that the therapy may only be useful for patients with a special variant of neglect.

A number of studies have explored the possibility of using transcranial magnetic stimulation (TMS) to ameliorate neglect. The rationale is that neglect is partially due to an imbalance of interhemispheric inhibition [62], which can be corrected by applying inhibitory stimulation over the intact (left) hemisphere. Of particular interest is a stimulation consisting of continuous trains of rapid bursts of pulses (TBS), which has been shown to decrease brain excitation for a prolonged period [63]. Nyffeler et al. [64] reported a decrease of neglect symptoms for 8 hours following two trains (each 44 s) of TBS applied over the left posterior parietal cortex. The duration of effects could be extended up to 32 h post-stimulation when four trains of TBS were applied. This finding supports the view that a decrease of cortical excitability directly affects the degree of inhibition of the damaged right by the intact left hemisphere. The principle was extended in two recent single-blind studies. Koch et al. [65] treated nine neglect patients during 2 weeks with continuous TBS over the posterior parietal cortex while a control group received sham stimulation. Results showed that the TBS group increased their scores in various neglect tests following therapy and at follow-up (2 weeks later) while the sham group showed no significant changes. In addition, the authors showed that TBS leads to a decrease of cortical excitability as evidenced by decreased potentiation of motor evoked potentials by a conditioning TMS pulse applied over the parietal

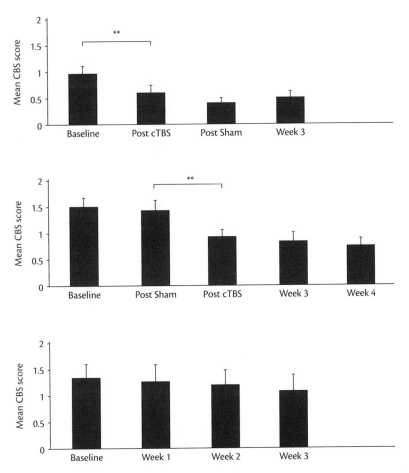

Fig. 22.2 Effect of theta-burst stimulation (TBS) on spatial neglect as assessed with the Catherine Bergego Scale (CBS), a rating scale of neglect signs in everyday behaviour. Eight neglect patients received eight TBS trains over the left parietal cortex, followed 1 week later by sham stimulation (upper row). Eight neglect patients received sham stimulation first, followed by TBS (middle row) and eight patients received no stimulation. Neglect signs assessed with the CBS diminished after TBS, but not after sham stimulation or no stimulation (bottom row).

Figure adapted from Cazzoli et al. [12], with permission from Oxford University Press.

cortex. This finding strongly supports the hypothesis that beneficial effects of TMS on neglect are directly linked to decreased excitability of the left cerebral hemisphere.

In the second study eight trains of TBS were applied over 2 days in one neglect group while a second group received sham stimulation and a third group no stimulation [12]. Following the first stimulation period the TBS group received sham stimulation and the sham group received TBS. The findings showed that TBS not only leads to a significant improvement in cancellation, reading and picture comparison, but also to improved neglect symptoms, as assessed through behavioural observation by hospital staff (Figure 22.2). Together, the findings from these recent studies show that TBS is an effective method for the rehabilitation of spatial neglect with effects that may last for 2–4 weeks.

Neglect is a relatively frequent disorder and efficient interventions are needed that can be applied without special training and precautions. In a pilot study Kerkhoff et al. [66] observed that repetitive optokinetic stimulation with random dots moving at varying speed from right to left may significantly improve neglect symptoms. In a recent large randomized-controlled trial these authors compared the effects of five sessions of optokinetic

stimulation (each 50 min) to visual exploration training [67]. They found strong effects of optokinetic stimulation on cancellation, reading, line bisection, but also on auditory midline judgment, while no changes were observed after exploration training (Figure 22.3). Kerkhoff et al. [68] further extended their findings by demonstrating that optokinetic stimulation is feasible at bedside and that its effects extend to measures of functional independence. These results support the view that oculomotor deficits in neglect are central [69] and that stimulation of the oculomotor system may improve spatial attention and recalibrate the egocentric reference frame. The finding that optokinetic stimulation improves a measure of auditory neglect is particularly interesting, as it suggests that a purely visual stimulation may have multimodal effects, and thus supports the view that neglect reflects impairment of modality-independent spatial representations [70, 71].

In conclusion, several techniques are available that have proven efficient for the rehabilitation of spatial neglect. While some contradictory findings have been reported for prismatic adaptation the technique is easy to use and may be particularly recommended for chronic patients with motor-intentional deficits. Continuous

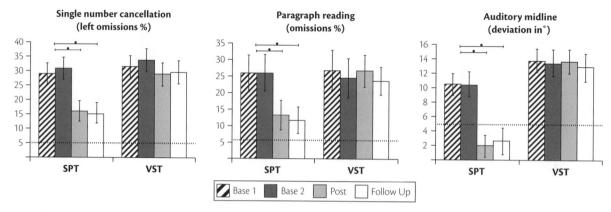

Fig. 22.3 Effect of optokinetic (or smooth-pursuit) stimulation on spatial neglect. One neglect group received five sessions smooth-pursuit training (SPT) while the second group trained visual scanning (VST). Only the SPT group improved significantly in the post-test and at follow-up in visual (cancellation, reading) and auditory neglect measures (auditory midline judgment).
Figure adapted from Kerkhoff et al. [67], with permission from Sage Publications.

TBS has positive effects on neglect symptoms as assessed with paper-and-pencil tests as well as neglect behaviour in everyday life. There is evidence from one controlled study that neck muscle vibration may have lasting effects on neglect symptoms. Finally, optokinetic stimulation is a simple method for the improvement of neglect that can be applied at bedside and has effects on neglect symptoms as well as on functional independence.

Attention

The term attention does not refer to a single, isolated function, but to a collection of skills and processes. Most models of attention distinguish between the ability to focus attention (selective attention), to divide attention (divided attention), and to maintain attention over time (sustained attention).

Attention deficits are present in 30–50% of brain-injured patients [72] and are a significant predictor of decreased quality of life and greater functional impairment [73]. Niemann et al. [74] compared the efficacy of a specialized attention training program to a control training centred on memory problems. Thirteen randomly allocated chronic head-injured patients practised computerized attention tasks in 18 sessions, which probed focused attention (identifying coloured targets) or set-shifting (moving attention away from one stimulus feature to another), both in the visual and the auditory modality. The authors found that patients participating in the attention training had significantly improved scores in several neuropsychological tests evaluating speed of processing, selective attention and sustained attention, while no generalization to tests evaluating memory was found. Indeed, attention training may have specific effects on the trained attentional dimension but may not generalize to other dimensions. Sturm et al. [75] selected specific training programs according to the most impaired domains of attention in a group of stroke patients. Training of attention tasks (e.g. alertness or vigilance) lead to relatively specific improvements in the trained function. Vigilance training improved measures of vigilance, but also reaction time in a task evaluating selective attention. The authors concluded that specific attention problems need very specific training.

Sohlberg and Mateer [39] developed a comprehensive rehabilitation programme termed Attention Process Training that targets different components of attention and uses hierarchically structured tasks that are gradually introduced and practiced with increasing degrees of complexity. The proposed exercises include a wide range of tasks with components of sustained attention (detecting visual or auditory targets, mental mathematics, sequencing), alternating attention (switching targets, generating alternating responses), selective attention (performing a foreground task while ignoring background noise), and divided attention (reading text and simultaneously scanning for target words). However, when testing this programme in head-injured patients, Park et al. [76] found improved performance on two attention tests after 40 hours of training, but the improvement was not better than in an untreated control group. A more recent controlled trial examined the effects of Attention Process Training in 38 post-acute stroke patients who received 30 h of training over four weeks [73]. Compared to non-treated controls the trained patients showed significantly better scores on tests of auditory and visual attention 5 weeks after the end of the training. However, no difference between groups was observed for secondary measures, suggesting that the best effects were obtained in tasks that were similar to the trained tasks. Similar results were observed in a study in which head-injured patients were trained to divide attention in tasks whose difficulty progressively increased [77]. After 24 h of training significant increases of performance were observed in a divided attention task, but only slight training-related effects in executive measures, and none in simple reaction time tasks.

An important question raised by these studies is whether training attention transfers to everyday life. Unfortunately, there are virtually no data available that could answer this question; when transfer to everyday life was tested it was done with observational rating scales [77]. The best answer so far comes from a study which reported that specific training targeting an enlargement of the 'attentional field of view' had no specific effect on measures of attention than visuoperceptual training [78]. Nevertheless, in patients with right-hemisphere damage this type of attention training increased the rate of success in an on-road driving evaluation.

In sum, studies with brain-injured patients suggest that attention training has specific practice effects that are greatest for tasks closely resembling the practised task, but do not notably generalize to other attentional domains, and even less so to other functions such as memory [79]. However, the evidence is based on a small number of controlled studies. It is also largely unknown whether there are long-term benefits of attention training and whether training gains transfer to attention functions in everyday life [80].

Executive functions

The term executive functions refers to a variety of cognitive capacities required in novel, non-habitual and non-routine situations that have a large degree of freedom for the implementation of decisional processes [81, 82]. These capacities include the initiation of new actions, inhibition of inappropriate behaviour, maintenance of specific behaviour, planning and organization, and generative thinking [39, 83]. Patients with dysexecutive symptoms may exhibit impairment in one or several functions, often in domains that appear contradictory. For example, a patient may have difficulty initiating an activity, but once started may fail to interrupt the activity when an alternative reaction is required. Another characteristic of these patients is that they may not verbally report their cognitive failures, which may become evident only when the patients attempt to execute an action. For example, a patient may adequately describe what is required from him in a given task, yet fail to follow his own action plan, a behaviour that has been termed 'goal neglect' [84]. Rehabilitation programmes mainly target disorganized behaviour through acquisition of new routines, training of problem-solving and metacognitive strategies. In addition, recent work has focused on the failures of some patients with executive dysfunctions to regulate emotion and to anticipate the outcomes of their behaviour, in particular in social situations.

Acquisition of new routines

Many daily actions become habits when performed repetitively. The acquisition of new habits (such as operating a new TV set) may require decomposition of a complex task into discrete components that can be followed step by step. Patients with perseverative behaviour or impulsivity may fail to implement and follow a simple action-plan. The aim of the intervention is therefore to brake down the task into logically structured steps, to develop a simple checklist allowing the patient to follow these steps, and to practise the routine repeatedly [39]. Unfortunately, this approach has not been evaluated in clinical studies. It is therefore unknown whether it leads to improved retention of new routines. However, there is good evidence that a much simpler method may improve temporal routines: Patients with executive dysfunctions often show difficulty respecting time schedules, even if these are repetitive [85]. These failures have been successfully treated with a pager system that permitted to send brief messages shortly before the appointment or the task that had been scheduled. The study included a group of patients who failed in prospective memory tasks due to memory problems or executive failures [41]. The fact that patients continued to complete scheduled tasks even after withdrawal of the pager suggests that simple prompting is a powerful way to acquire new routines.

Training problem-solving skills

A few controlled studies evaluated the efficacy of interventions to improve problem-solving. Von Cramon et al. [86] trained a group of brain-injured patients to decompose complex problems into smaller and better manageable portions. After 25 therapy sessions the experimental group scored better than a control group receiving memory training on measures of action-planning and received better ratings of everyday problem-solving capacities. In a more recent study [87] chronic head-injury patients received problem-solving training in small groups that focused on the systematic recognition, anticipation, and analysis of real-life problems, often within an interpersonal context. The intervention also emphasized self-observation of emotional and behavioural reactions of participants during problem solving in order to anticipate emotional overreactions. The intervention group improved their scores in neuropsychological tests evaluating problem-solving skills, but also in measures of verbal and visual memory. In addition, problem-solving training improved scores on several self-observational scales evaluating emotional regulation and 'clear thinking'. These improvements were maintained at follow-up 6 months after the end of the intervention.

Robertson [88] developed a step-by-step training for disorganized behaviour termed goal-management training (GMT). The programme has five steps: direct attention to the relevant task (Step 1), select and define an action goal (Step 2), partition the goal into sub-goals (Step 3), encode and retain sub-goals (Step 4), and compare the action outcome with the target goal (Step 5). Levine et al. [89] examined in traumatic brain-injury patients the effects of a single session of GMT as compared to a session of motor-skill learning and found significantly improved performance after GMT for three ecological tasks that might be part of daily routines of a secretary (e.g. proofreading). However, such effects of a very short intervention are unlikely to be maintained in the long run. Thus, this study provides a proof-of-principle result but is no proof of clinical effectiveness [82]. A more recent study examined the effects of 14 hours of GMT immediately after the end of the therapy and at follow-up 4 months later [90]. The study involved patients who had suffered from traumatic brain injury at least 6 months before the study, all of whom had shown good recovery, were independent in everyday activities, but reported executive problems. The GMT group showed a decreased number of attentional lapses and better problem-solving performance after the therapy and at follow-up compared to a group receiving a control intervention (Figure 22.4). Thus, the GMT programme may be beneficial, in particular for patients who are already relatively independent and have good insight into their executive problems. A similar treatment program to the GMT, but with a greater focus on attentional errors during problem solving was tested by Miotto et al. [91]. Patients were selected on the basis of the presence of damage in the left or right frontal lobes. The intervention improved action planning in a multiple errands task. However, neither side nor site of damage predicted whether a patient benefited from the intervention or not. Finally, Fish et al. [92] showed that teaching some of the GMT steps improved prospective memory in a group of patients who failed to recall tasks and appointments.

In conclusion, several studies have provided evidence that training problem-solving skills through a structured programme such as GMT has enduring effects on problem-solving in real-life situations. The different approaches examined in clinical studies share some components, such as the teaching of steps to decompose a problem, self-monitoring during task execution, and verification of action outcomes [93]. These abilities support a whole variety of

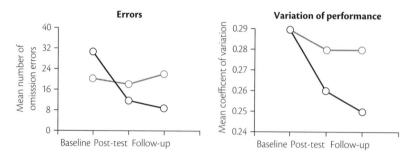

Fig. 22.4 Effect of goal-management training (GMT) on a computerized measure of sustained attention. The test requires the maintenance of attention over time on task goals, a capacity that is specifically trained in GMT. Patients receiving GMT (black line) showed improved performance after the therapy and 4 months later (follow-up) while no significant changes were observed for patients receiving psychoeducation (grey line).
Figure modified from Levine et al. [90].

tasks; generalization can thus be expected for the rehabilitation of problem-solving deficits. Accordingly, some studies observed improved performance in executive tasks that had not been specifically trained. On the other hand, programmes such as GMT are relatively complex and require a high degree of awareness of one's own deficits as well as a good capacity to monitor one's own actions. Such programmes may therefore be only applicable to patients with relatively slight impairments.

Neurobehavioural symptoms and impaired emotional regulation

Along with cognitive impairment, deficits of emotional regulation are crucial predictors of social functioning and integration [94]. Neurobehavioural deficits include apathy and lack of drive, carelessness, and social isolation, as well as disinhibition, irritability, aggressiveness, or sexually inappropriate behaviour. Although some of these deficits are linked to specific cognitive impairments or to a difficulty in comprehending actions, intentions, and emotions of others ('theory of mind') [95], they may occur in isolation or become evident during recovery following brain damage. These symptoms are generally perceived by the family and by the patient (if she/he has sufficient insight) as extremely disturbing and are important sources of caregiver stress. Interventions used to treat severe neurobehavioural symptoms apply principles of operant learning, such as reinforcement, interruption, and the analysis and modulation of contextual variables favouring dysfunctional behaviour. The effects of an intervention based on behavioural and contextual analysis were examined in a randomized trial including caregivers of patients with behavioural problems following traumatic brain injury [96]. Patients and their caregivers received special education concerning the behavioural sequelae of traumatic brain injury as well as assistance with the definition and treatment of problematic behaviour. For example, an intervention strategy for the control of outbursts of anger included identification of anger-eliciting cues, relaxation training, and reinforcement of verbal expression versus acting out strong emotions. The results showed a reduction of disruptive and aggressive behaviour 3 months after termination of the intervention.

A detailed analysis of behaviour and context is fundamental to cognitive-behavioural interventions. The goal of cognitive-behavioural therapy (CBT) is to increase awareness of problematic emotions/behaviour, adapt dysfunctional thoughts, and teach coping strategies. These interventions have been successful in reducing anger in patients with traumatic brain injury [97, 98], but showed mixed effects on depressive symptoms in post-acute stroke patients [99]. Future studies should evaluate whether etiology, chronicity and type of behavioural symptom (e.g. depression versus anger and irritability) are significant predictors of positive effects of CBT or other interventions. Due to mixed findings, these approaches are considered practice options as there is currently no formal confirmation of their efficacy.

Conclusion and perspectives

Neurorehabilitation of higher cognitive functions is confronted with several problems that may complicate conclusions regarding the efficacy of specific interventions. One problem is the lack of evidence that training—even if it generates better performance in a specific task—transfers to daily activities. This is mainly due to the difficulty to evaluate trained functions in standardized ecological situations. Evidence for a transfer mainly comes from observational scales, which are sources of bias and do not necessarily measure all significant changes. Another problem is that most studies included small groups or single patients, making randomization difficult or impossible. Finally, behavioural interventions are often incompatible with blinding of the patient and the therapist since the objectives of the intervention are clear from the outset. For these reasons, the common quality criteria for therapeutic trials (e.g. placebo control, blinding of patients and therapists) are often not applicable to cognitive intervention studies.

Despite these drawbacks, data accumulated in the last 15 years show that neuropsychological rehabilitation may lead to significant improvement of the trained functions. The evidence is particularly strong for spatial neglect, where physiological stimulation techniques (such as optokinetic stimulation) and transcranial stimulation lead to long-lasting improvements. The training of attention generally shows specific improvements in the trained task, but little or no generalization to other tasks. In the domain of memory and executive function compensatory strategies and goal management can be recommended. Whatever the domain, intensive training is necessary to obtain significant and lasting effects on performance and independence.

References

1. Woldag H, Stupka K, Hummelsheim H. Repetitive training of complex hand and arm movements with shaping is beneficial for motor improvement in patients after stroke. J Rehabil Med. 2010;**42**(6):582–587.

2. Wolf SL, Thompson PA, Winstein CJ, et al. The EXCITE stroke trial: comparing early and delayed constraint-induced movement therapy. Stroke. 2010;41(10):2309–2315.

3. Liepert J. Pharmacotherapy in restorative neurology. Curr Opin Neurol. 2008;21(6):639–643.

4. Sandrini M, Cohen LG. Noninvasive brain stimulation in neurorehabilitation. Handb Clin Neurol. 2013;116:499–524.

5. Pulvermuller F, Neininger B, Elbert T, et al. Constraint-induced therapy of chronic aphasia after stroke. Stroke; a journal of cerebral circulation. 2001;32(7):1621–1626.

6. Laganaro M, Di Pietro M, Schnider A. Computerised treatment of anomia in acute aphasia: treatment intensity and training size. Neuropsychol Rehabil. 2006;16(6):630–640.

7. Kerkhoff G, Schenk T. Rehabilitation of neglect: an update. Neuropsychologia. 2012;50(6):1072–1079.

8. Schuett S. The rehabilitation of hemianopic dyslexia. Nat Rev Neurol. 2009;5(8):427–437.

9. Schindler I, Kerkhoff G, Karnath H-O, Keller I, Goldenberg G. Neck muscle vibration induces lasting recovery in spatial neglect. J Neurol Neurosurg Psychiatry. 2002;73:412–419.

10. Geminiani G, Bottini G, Sterzi R. Dopaminergic stimulation in unilateral neglect. J Neurol Neurosurg Psychiatry. 1998;65:344–347.

11. Grujic Z, Mapstone M, Gitelman DR, et al. Dopamine agonists reorient visual exploration away from the neglected hemispace. Neurology. 1998;51(5):1395–1398.

12. Cazzoli D, Muri RM, Schumacher R, et al. Theta burst stimulation reduces disability during the activities of daily living in spatial neglect. Brain. 2012;135(Pt 11):3426–3439.

13. Wilson B. Recovery and compensatory strategies in head injured memory impaired people several years after insult. J Neurol Neurosurg Psychiatry. 1992;55(3):177–180.

14. Fish J, Manly T, Emslie H, Evans JJ, Wilson BA. Compensatory strategies for acquired disorders of memory and planning: differential effects of a paging system for patients with brain injury of traumatic versus cerebrovascular aetiology. J Neurol Neurosurg Psychiatry. 2008;79(8):930–935.

15. Tate RL. Beyond one-bun, two-shoe: recent advances in the psychological rehabilitation of memory disorders after acquired brain injury. Brain Injury. 1997;11(12):907–918.

16. Wilson B. Memory Rehabilitation. Integrating Theory and Practice. Guilford Press, New York, 2009.

17. Ptak R, Van der Linden M, Schnider A. Cognitive rehabilitation of episodic memory disorders: From theory to practice. Front Human Neurosci. 2010;4.

18. Nahum L, Bouzerda-Wahlen A, Guggisberg A, Ptak R, Schnider A. Forms of confabulation: dissociations and associations. Neuropsychologia. 2012;50(10):2524–2534.

19. Schnider A. The Confabulating Mind. How the Brain Creates Reality. Oxford University Press, Oxford, 2008.

20. Harris JE. Ways to help memory. In: Wilson BA, Moffat N, eds. Clinical Management of Memory Problems. Chapman & Hall, London, 1992, pp. 59–85.

21. Doornheim K, De Haan EHF. Cognitive training for memory deficits in stroke patients. Neuropsychol Rehabil. 1998;8(4):393–400.

22. Ptak R, Gutbrod K, Schnider A. Association learning in the acute confusional state. J Neurol Neurosurg Psychiatry. 1998;65(3):390–392.

23. Kaschel R, Della Sala S, Cantagallo A, Fahlböck A, Laaksonen R, Kazen M. Imagery mnemonics for the rehabilitation of memory: A randomised group controlled trial. Neuropsychol Rehabil. 2002;12(2):127–153.

24. Cicerone KD, Dahlberg C, Malec JF, et al. Evidence-based cognitive rehabilitation: Updated review of the literature from 1998 through 2002. Arch Phys Med Rehabil. 2005;86:1681–1692.

25. Cicerone KD, Dahlberg C, Kalmar K, et al. Evidence-based cognitive rehabilitation: Recommendations for clinical practice. Arch Phys Med Rehabil. 2000;81:1596–1615.

26. Glisky EL, Schacter DL, Tulving E. Computer learning by memory impaired patients: acquisition and retention of complex knowledge. Neuropsychologia. 1986;24:313–328.

27. Glisky EL. Acquisition and transfer of declarative and procedural knowledge by memory-impaired patients: A computer data-entry task. Neuropsychologia. 1992;30(10):899–910.

28. Riley GA, Sotiriou D, Jaspal S. Which is more effective in promoting implicit and explicit memory: The method of vanishing cues or errorless learning without fading? Neuropsychol Rehabil. 2004;14(3):257–283.

29. Baddeley A, Wilson BA. When implicit learning fails: amnesia and the problem of error elimination. Neuropsychologia. 1994;32(1):53–68.

30. Hamann SB, Squire LR. On the acquisition of new declarative knowledge in amnesia. Behav Neurosci. 1995;109(6):1027–1044.

31. Hunkin NM, Squires EJ, Aldrich FK, Parkin AJ. Errorless learning and the acqisition of word processing skills. Neuropsychol Rehabil. 1998;8(4):433–449.

32. Andrewes D, Gielewski E. The work rehabilitation of a herpes simplex encephalitis patient with anterograde amnesia. Neuropsychol Rehabil. 1999;9(1):77–99.

33. Kessels RPC, de Haan EHF. Implicit learning in memory rehabilitation: A meta-analysis on errorless learning and vanishing cues methods. J Clin Exp Neropsychol. 2003;25(6):805–814.

34. Evans JJ, Wilson BA, Schuri U, et al. A comparison of 'errorless' and 'trial-and-error' learning methods for teaching individuals with acquired memory deficits. Neuropsychol Rehabil. 2000;10(1):67–101.

35. Tailby R, Haslam C. An investigation of errorless learning in memory-impaired patients: improving the technique and clarifying theory. Neuropsychologia. 2003;41:1230–1240.

36. Fish J, Mandly T, Wilson BA. Rehabilitation for prospective memory problems resulting from acquired brain injury. In: Oddy M, Worthington A, eds. The Rehabilitation of Executive Disorders A guide to theory and practice. Oxford University Press, Oxford, 2009. p. 75–95.

37. Schmitter-Edgecombe M, Fahy JF, Whelan JP, Long CJ. Memory remediation after severe closed head injury: notebook training versus supportive therapy. J Consult Clin Psychol. 1995;63(3):484–489.

38. Squires EJ, Hunkin NM, Parkin AJ. Memory notebook training in a case of severe amnesia: Generalising from paired associate learning to real life. Neuropsychol Rehabil. 1996;6(1):55–65.

39. Sohlberg MM, Mateer CA. Cognitive Rehabilitation. An Integrative Neuropsychological Approach. Guilford Press, New York, 2001.

40. Burke JM, Danick JA, Bemis B, Durgin CJ. A process approach to memory book training for neurological patients. Brain Injury. 1994;8(1):71–81.

41. Wilson BA, Emslie HC, Quirk K, Evans JJ. Reducing everyday memory and planning problems by means of a paging system: a randomised control crossover study. J Neurol Neurosurg Psychiatry. 2001;70:477–482.

42. Wilson BA, Evans JJ, Emslie H, Malinek V. Evaluation of NeuroPage: a new memory aid. J Neurol Neurosurg Psychiatry. 1997;63:113–115.

43. Svoboda E, Richards B. Compensating for anterograde amnesia: A new training method that capitalizes on emerging smartphone technologies. J Int Neuropsychol Soc. 2009;15:629–638.

44. Svoboda E, Richards B, Polsinelli A, Guger S. A theory-driven training programme in the use of emerging commercial technology: Application to an adolescent with severe memory impairment. Neuropsychol Rehabil. 2010:1–25.

45. Berry E, Kapur N, Williams L, et al. The use of a wearable camera, SenseCam, as a pictorial diary to improve autobiographical memory in a patient with encephalitis: A preliminary report. Neuropsychol Rehabil. 2007;17:582–601.

46. Gade A. Imagery as a mnemonic aid in amnesia patients: effects of amnesia subtype and severity. In: Riddoch MJ, Humphreys GW, eds. Cognitive Neuropsychology and Cognitive Rehabilitation. Lawrence Erlbaum Associates, Hove, 1994, pp. 571–589.

47. das Nair R, Lincoln N. Cognitive rehabilitation for memory deficits following stroke. Cochrane Database of Systematic Reviews. 2007;**3**, No. CD002293.

48. LoPresti EF, Mihailidis A, Kirsch N. Assistive technology for cognitive rehabilitation: state of the art. Neuropsychol Rehabil. 2004;**14**(1/2):5–39.

49. Kalra L, Perez I, Gupta S, Wittink M. The influence of visual neglect on stroke rehabilitation. Stroke. 1997;**28**:1386–1391.

50. Denes G, Semenza C, Stoppa E, Lis A. Unilateral spatial neglect and recovery from hemiplegia. Brain. 1982;**105**:543–552.

51. Weinberg J, Diller L, Gordon WA, et al. Visual scanning training effect on reading-related tasks in acquired right brain damage. Arch Phys Med Rehabil. 1977;**58**:479–486.

52. Làdavas E, Menghini G, Umiltà C. A rehabilitation study of hemispatial neglect. Cogn Neuropsychol. 1994;**11**(1):75–95.

53. Bowen A, Lincoln NB. Rehabilitation for spatial neglect improves test performance but not disability. Stroke. 2007;**38**(10):2869–2870.

54. Rubens AB. Caloric stimulation and unilateral visual neglect. Neurology. 1985;**35**:1019–1024.

55. Rossetti Y, Rode G, Pisella L, Farné A, Li L, Boisson D, et al. Prism adaptation to a rightward optical deviation rehabilitates left hemispatial neglect. Nature. 1998;**395**:166–169.

56. Frassinetti F, Angeli V, Meneghello F, Avanzi S, Làdavas E. Long-lasting amelioration of visuospatial neglect by prism adaptation. Brain. 2002;**125**:608–623.

57. Serino A, Barbiani M, Rinaldesi ML, Ladavas E. Effectiveness of prism adaptation in neglect rehabilitation: a controlled trial study. Stroke. 2009;**40**(4):1392–1398.

58. Rousseaux M, Bernati T, Saj A, Kozlowski O. Ineffectiveness of prism adaptation on spatial neglect signs. Stroke. 2006;**37**:542–543.

59. Turton AJ, O'Leary K, Gabb J, Woodward R, Gilchrist ID. A single blinded randomised controlled pilot trial of prism adaptation for improving self-care in stroke patients with neglect. Neuropsychol Rehabil. 2010;**20**(2):180–196.

60. Yang NY, Zhou D, Chung RC, Li-Tsang CW, Fong KN. Rehabilitation interventions for unilateral neglect after stroke: a systematic review from 1997 through 2012. Front Hum Neurosci. 2013;**7**:187.

61. Goedert KM, Chen P, Boston RC, Foundas AL, Barrett AM. Presence of motor-intentional aiming deficit predicts functional improvement of spatial neglect with prism adaptation. Neurorehabil Neural Repair. 2014.

62. Corbetta M, Kincade MJ, Lewis C, Snyder AZ, Sapir A. Neural basis and recovery of spatial attention deficits in spatial neglect. Nat Neurosci. 2005;**8**(11):1603–1610.

63. Hallett M. Transcranial magnetic stimulation: a primer. Neuron. 2007;**55**(2):187–199.

64. Nyffeler T, Cazzoli D, Hess CW, Müri RM. One session of repeated parietal theta burst stimulation trains induces long-lasting improvement of visual neglect. Stroke. 2009;**40**:2791–2796.

65. Koch G, Bonni S, Giacobbe V, et al. Theta-burst stimulation of the left hemisphere accelerates recovery of hemispatial neglect. Neurology. 2012;**78**(1):24–30.

66. Kerkhoff G, Keller I, Ritter V, Marquardt C. Repetitive optokinetic stimulation induces lasting recovery from visual neglect. Restorat Neurol Neurosci. 2006;**24**:357–369.

67. Kerkhoff G, Reinhart S, Ziegler W, Artinger F, Marquardt C, Keller I. Smooth pursuit eye movement training promotes recovery from auditory and visual neglect: a randomized controlled study. Neurorehabil Neural Repair. 2013;**27**(9):789–798.

68. Kerkhoff G, Bucher L, Brasse M, et al. Smooth pursuit 'bedside' training reduces disability and unawareness during the activities of daily living in neglect: a randomized controlled trial. Neurorehabil Neural Repair. 2014;**28**(6):554–563.

69. Ptak R, Müri RM. The parietal cortex and saccade planning: lessons from human lesion studies. Front Human Neurosci. 2013;**7**:254.

70. Ptak R, Fellrath J. Spatial neglect and the neural coding of attentional priority. Neurosci Biobehav Rev. 2013;**37**(4):705–722.

71. Golay L, Hauert CA, Greber C, Schnider A, Ptak R. Dynamic modulation of visual detection by auditory cues in spatial neglect. Neuropsychologia. 2005;**43**(9):1258–1265.

72. Hyndman D, Pickering RM, Ashburn A. The influence of attention deficits on functional recovery post stroke during the first 12 months after discharge from hospital. J Neurol Neurosurg Psychiatry. 2008;**79**:656–663.

73. Barker-Collo SL, Feigin VL, Lawes CM, Parag V, Senior H, Rodgers A. Reducing attention deficits after stroke using attention process training: a randomized controlled trial. Stroke. 2009;**40**(10):3293–3298.

74. Niemann H, Ruff RM, Baser CA. Computer-assisted attention retraining head-injured individuals: a controlled efficacy study of an outpatient program. J Consult Clin Psychol. 1990;**58**(6):811–817.

75. Sturm W, Willmes K, Orgass B, Hartje W. Do specific attention deficits need specific training? Neuropsychol Rehabil. 1997;**7**(2):81–103.

76. Park NW, Proulx G-B, Towers WM. Evaluation of the attention process training programme. Neuropsychol Rehabil. 1999;**9**(2):135–154.

77. Couillet J, Soury S, Lebornec G, et al. Rehabilitation of divided attention after severe traumatic brain injury: a randomised trial. Neuropsychol Rehabil. 2010;**20**(3):321–339.

78. Mazer BL, Sofer S, Korner-Bitensky N, Gelinas I, Hanley J, Wood-Dauphinee S. Effectiveness of a visual attention retraining program on the driving performance of clients with stroke. Arch Phys Med Rehabil. 2003;**84**(4):541–550.

79. Park NW, Ingles JL. Effectiveness of attention rehabilitation after an acquired brain injury: A meta-analysis. Neuropsychology. 2001;**15**(2):199–210.

80. Lincoln N, Majid M, Weyman N. Cognitive rehabilitation for attention deficits following stroke. Cochrane Database Syst Rev. 2000;**4**: No. CD002842.

81. Lezak MD. Neuropsychological Assessment, 3rd edn. Oxford University Press, New York, 1995.

82. Cicerone K, Levin H, Malec J, Stuss D, Whyte J. Cognitive rehabilitation interventions for executive function: moving from bench to bedside in patients with traumatic brain injury. J Cogn Neurosci. 2006;**18**(7):1212–1222.

83. Norman DA, Shallice T. Attention to Action. Willed and automatic control of behavior. In: Davidson RJ, Schwartz GE, Shapiro D, eds. Consciousness and Self-Regulation. 4. Plenum Press, New York, 1986, pp. 1–18.

84. Duncan J, Emslie H, Williams P, Johnson R, Freer C. Intelligence and the frontal lobe: the organization of goal-directed behavior. Cogn Psychol. 1996;**30**:257–303.

85. Ptak R, Schnider A. Disorganised memory after right dorsolateral prefrontal damage. Neurocase. 2004;**10**(1):52–59.

86. von Cramon DY, Matthes-von-Cramon G, Mai N. Problem solving deficits in brain injured patients. A therapeutic approach. Neuropsychol Rehab. 1991;**1**:45–64.

87. Rath JF, Simon D, Langenbahn DM, Sherr RL, Diller L. Group treatment of problem-solving deficits in outpatients with traumatic brain injury: A randomised outcome study. Neuropsychol Rehab. 2003;**13**(4):461–488.

88. Robertson I. Goal Management Training: A clinical manual. PsyConsult, Cambridge, UK, 1996.

89. Levine B, Robertson IH, Clare L, et al. Rehabilitation of executive functioning: an experimental-clinical validation of goal management training. J Int Neuropsychol Soc. 2000;**6**(3):299–312.

90. Levine B, Schweizer TA, O'Connor C, et al. Rehabilitation of executive functioning in patients with frontal lobe brain damage with goal management training. Front Hum Neurosci. 2011;**5**:9.

91. Miotto EC, Evans JJ, de Lucia MC, Scaff M. Rehabilitation of executive dysfunction: a controlled trial of an attention and problem solving treatment group. Neuropsychol Rehabil. 2009;**19**(4):517–540.

92. Fish J, Evans JJ, Nimmo M, et al. Rehabilitation of executive dysfunction following brain injury: 'content-free' cueing improves everyday prospective memory performance. Neuropsychologia. 2007;**45**(6):1318–1330.

93. Kennedy MR, Coelho C, Turkstra L, et al. Intervention for executive functions after traumatic brain injury: a systematic review, meta-analysis and clinical recommendations. Neuropsychol Rehabil. 2008;**18**(3):257–299.

94. Cattelani R, Zettin M, Zoccolotti P. Rehabilitation treatments for adults with behavioral and psychosocial disorders following acquired brain injury: a systematic review. Neuropsychol Rev. 2010;**20**(1):52–85.

95. Aboulafia-Brakha T, Christe B, Martory MD, Annoni JM. Theory of mind tasks and executive functions: a systematic review of group studies in neurology. J Neuropsychol. 2011;**5**(Pt 1):39–55.

96. Carnevale GJ, Anselmi V, Johnston MV, Busichio K, Walsh V. A natural setting behavior management program for persons with acquired brain injury: a randomized controlled trial. Arch Phys Med Rehabil. 2006;**87**(10):1289–1297.

97. Aboulafia-Brakha T, Greber Buschbeck C, Rochat L, Annoni JM. Feasibility and initial efficacy of a cognitive-behavioural group programme for managing anger and aggressiveness after traumatic brain injury. Neuropsychol Rehabil. 2013;**23**(2):216–233.

98. Medd J, Tate RL. Evaluation of an anger management therapy program following acquired brain injury: A preliminary study. Neuropsychol Rehab. 2000;**10**(2):185–201.

99. Lincoln NB, Flannaghan T, Sutcliffe L, Rother L. Evaluation of cognitive behavioral treatment for depression after stroke: A pilot study. Clin Rehabil. 1997;**11**(2):114–122.

CHAPTER 23

The clinical neurology of problems with oral feeding

Tom Hughes

Introduction

Hydration and nutrition are basic human requirements but their provision to people with acute and chronic neurological conditions is a very real challenge. A person who is unable to maintain good sitting posture and has ineffective upper limb function is unlikely to be able to participate normally in festive social occasions, but with the right sort of care they may be able to feed by mouth. If vigilance, conscious level, coughing, respiratory function, or swallowing is impaired, alone or in combination, they may require feeding and hydration using artificial enteral, or parenteral, methods.

One of the provider compliance assessment tools (Outcome 5 (Regulation 14): Meeting nutritional needs) developed by the Care Quality Commision [1] focuses on basic hydration and nutrition. A separate section on nutrition and hydration in the Francis report [2] highlights its relevance to clinical practice and that failure of provision is a valid and very obvious sign of ineffective or negligent clinical practice. The National Patient Safety Agency and The Royal College of Nursing [3] have confirmed that hydration is a fundamental aspect of care and everyone in a healthcare environment has a role to play in ensuring patients do not become dehydrated. In the fourth Nutrition Screening Week survey (spring 2011) malnutrition (medium and high risk according to MUST (Malnutrition Universal Screening Tool)) was found to affect one in four adults on admission to hospital, more than one in three adults admitted to care homes in the previous 6 months, and up to one in five adults on admission to Mental Health Units in the United Kingdom [4]. Unfortunately, it is clear that admission to hospital may further compromise nutritional problems that have developed in the community, with obvious detrimental effects on the presenting medical or surgical problem. At a time of rapid scientific and technological development in all medical specialties, it seems improbable that we should not be succeeding in meeting such well-described and basic needs.

In some patients dehydration and malnutrition can be anticipated—and possible remedies discussed—in advance, for example in a progressive neurological disorder involving the bulbar and respiratory musculature. In some it may relate to one easily identifiable problem, such as oesophageal obstruction or a blocked gastrostomy, for which there is an obvious solution. Often it is multifactorial in origin, a common situation in patients with conditions affecting posture, vigilance, swallowing, and breathing. Sometimes

it is a product of the environment in which they are being cared for; a strict 'Nil By Mouth' policy applied unthinkingly on a Friday afternoon adds to patients' vulnerability. Occasionally problems with eating and drinking, and an underlying neurological condition (e.g. Arnold–Chiari malformation), are recognized for the first time only after a presentation with aspiration pneumonia [5].

If a problem with oral feeding is recognized there are usually four important issues that require careful consideration: the underlying diagnosis of the disease process, the mechanism of the problem, the most appropriate interventions, and the prognosis. The latter is usually closely linked to the prognosis of the underlying disease. It is common for diagnostic and management issues to require attention concurrently, often involving a range of healthcare professionals; a nasogastric tube may be required whilst investigations get underway to establish a diagnosis of both the underlying condition and the exact mechanism of the feeding problem. The consequences of even short periods without adequate hydration and nutrition justify considering the different diagnostic and management issues in parallel rather than in series.

Although problems with oral feeding are often discussed in relation to the disease (e.g. stroke, motor neuron disease, dementia, etc.) from a mechanistic perspective, and in common with some other forms of neurological disability, the anatomical location of the disease is a more important determinant of the mechanism of the disability than is the disease process itself. Stroke illustrates this. The residual oral feeding problem in patients who have made some progress after lateral medullary syndrome has more in common with a recurrent laryngeal nerve palsy than it has with other stroke syndromes, because airway closure during swallowing is a prerequisite for sustainable oral feeding. Similarly, a pure corticobulbar palsy causing profound slowing of tongue movements and impaired oral control of a bolus has comparable effects on oral feeding whether it is due to motor neurone disease, multiple sclerosis, or cerebrovascular disease. The mechanism of the swallowing problem, rather than the underlying disease process is also the most important determinant of the techniques used to enhance oral feeding.

With these thoughts in mind the chapter will start with a detailed description of the mechanism of successful oral feeding in adults, with an emphasis on the innervation of the involved structures and how their function is integrated. If the importance of the individual components and their integration is appreciated, the nature of oral feeding problems can be understood and sometimes predicted. An appreciation of the neuroanatomy of the process also informs the approach to management, including techniques to enhance swallowing and the effect of different consistencies of the presented bolus. Although the emphasis will be on a generic approach, a number of conditions will be used to illustrate important points.

The subject matter requires of clinicians a challenging mix of perspectives and skills, but also a healthy dollop of common sense. Anybody involved with a patient should be able to say whether they are being adequately nourished and hydrated: relatives can. If a patient has not had 2 litres of fluid and 1,500 calories in the preceding 24 hours, something needs to be done, regardless of how many specialists are involved, and regardless of what investigations may be outstanding. A nasogastric tube is relatively easy to insert and highly effective in delivering food and water and it is questionable whether remedial action, by resident nursing and medical staff, about such basic requirements can be postponed because of protocols requiring referral to more specialist services, especially when those services are not immediately available. However, as problems of a very practical nature are being addressed, there are often difficult decisions to be made which require a working and detailed knowledge of the neuroanatomy of oral feeding as well as the more traditional insights required to diagnose the underlying disease process. Once in the midst of a complex case, the responsible team needs microscopic, telescopic, and periscopic perspectives, as well as an array of very practical skills, to ensure that patients get both adequate sustenance and an accurate diagnosis.

The neurology of oral feeding in health

Oral feeding is a composite function comprising a number of other composite functions. To help structure the clinical approach it can be useful to break it down in to four territories or domains of clinical practice: swallowing, breathing, general medical issues, and the situation in which the patient is being cared for. A detailed description of the process in health will inform a discussion of the changes that occur in disease, many of which can be anticipated based on a sound appreciation of the mechanisms involved.

Swallowing

The cutting up of food, and the accurate and timely placement of food in the mouth with fork or spoon is a considerable challenge for the neurologically impaired. Retention of the bolus in the mouth requires lip closure (seventh (VII) cranial nerve). Chewing depends on jaw closure and jaw opening (respectively temporalis and masseter, and the pterygoids, both supplied by the fifth cranial nerve (V)). Common intraoral sensation is also dependent on the Vth nerve, including common sensation to the tongue. The mobility and range of movement of the tongue (twelfth (XII) nerve) combined with its rich sensory innervation make it a powerful tool for exploration of the bolus and for its manipulation and control.

With the bolus suitably prepared, it has to be moved to the oesophagus, without entering the larynx and because the pharynx is a conduit for both air and food (it is an aerodigestive tract) defects in this part of the process can lead to food and drink entering the upper airway and beyond.

The safe passage of bolus involves the opening of the upper oesophagus (the 'foodway') and the closing of the larynx (the airway). These two quintessential functions involve, respectively, the suprahyoid muscles, sometimes referred to as the external muscles of the larynx (innervated by segments 1–3 of the cervical cord and the Vth and VIIth cranial nerves) and the internal muscles of the larynx (all innervated by the tenth cranial nerve).

So many neurological conditions manifest for the first time as a consequence of involvement of the internal and external muscles of the larynx that further explanation is justified [6].

During swallowing the larynx must shut; this ensures that oropharyngeal content does not enter the airway. The closure of the larynx is referred to as its sphincteric action. The larynx closes at four levels as a result of apposition of the true vocal cords, the false vocal cords, the arytenoids, and the apposition of the epiglottis with the superior surface of the larynx. All of the involved muscles are innervated by the tenth cranial nerve (Xth), the majority by its recurrent laryngeal branch. There are upper airway reflexes which leave the larynx in a state of readiness as a result of stimulation of neighbouring structures, for example the glottopharyngeal reflex which, in response to stimulation of the pharynx produces partial adduction of the cords without producing laryngeal closure. This may be exaggerated in diseases involving the corticobulbar tracts and contribute to choking episodes not obviously related to eating or drinking (e.g. in corticobulbar involvement in motor neuron disease).

However, the external muscles of the larynx are also very important in swallowing, because they are responsible for the opening of the upper oesophageal sphincter. During swallowing the larynx, connected above and below by appropriately named ligaments to the hyoid and cricoid, moves upwards and forwards. A swallow with two fingers resting on the larynx (the Adam's apple) allows the reader to demonstrate this to themselves. The muscles that suspend the larynx from the skull base attach mainly to the hyoid, and they are sometimes referred to as the suprahyoid muscles. Anteriorly they include the anterior belly of digastric, mylohyoid and geniohyoid (Vth cranial nerve), and posteriorly the posterior belly of digastric and stylohyoid (VIIth).

The cricopharyngeus, the main muscle of the upper oesophageal sphincter, is attached to the posterior cricoid; its name is the giveaway. Movement of the cricoid will therefore result in a change in the conformation of the upper oesophageal sphincter. Anterior movement of the cricoid results in traction on the anterior cricopharyngeus and its opening. In patients with inactive suprahyoid muscles (e.g. in acute bilateral styloid fractures), elevation of the hyolaryngeal complex is very reduced, and patients can be aphagic.

The associated drop in pressure in the sphincter, as it opens, creates suction (the 'hypopharyngeal suction pump'), which pulls the bolus in to the pharynx and upper oesophagus.

Apposition of the tongue base with the posterior pharyngeal wall follows and this initiates a stripping wave of peristalsis which, by acting on the tail of the bolus, ensures that its remnants in the pharynx are encouraged to move on down in to the oesophagus. As the suprahyoid muscles relax the larynx returns to its starting position, aided by contraction of the infrahyoid (strap) muscles, innervated by cervical roots C1–3.

So this is mere swallowing: following suitable preparation of the bolus the larynx closes and moves upwards and forwards, and as it opens the associated drop in pressure in the upper oesophageal sphincter propels the bolus into the oesophagus by

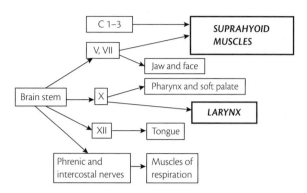

Fig. 23.1 Cranial nerve involvement in swallowing, with the laryngeal contribution (internal and external muscles) in bold to emphasize their importance.

hypopharyngeal suction. A clearing wave of peristalsis starts with the tongue base against the contracting superior pharyngeal constrictor (Passavant's cushion). When this is complete, and with the bolus is safely in the oesophagus, the involved structures stand down, passively or with assistance. Figure 23.1 shows a schematic diagram of the important cranial nerve contribution to the swallowing process.

In a way analogous to timed measurement of walking, swallowing function can be measured; a known volume of water is swallowed as the time taken and number of swallows used is recorded. This produces indices of swallowing including average volume per swallow (mls) and swallowing capacity (ml/second). Normative data exists for adults which shows that 55% of the variance of swallowing capacity is accounted for by age, sex, and height, which is very similar to the determinants of forced vital capacity in adults. In a study of patients with motor neuron disease, those who answered 'Yes' to the question 'Do you have to be careful when you are swallowing?' had significantly slower swallowing, and the majority had a swallowing capacity of less than 10 ml per second [7].

Voluntary and reflex swallowing

The elegant experiments of Miller and Sherrington [8] established that this closure and elevation of the larynx, with (respectively) the resulting cessation of breathing and opening of the cricopharyngeus, can be elicited by stimulation with various phagetic agents (whisky was the most effective) applied to the territory of the superior laryngeal nerve (a sensory nerve apart from its innervation of cricothyroid). The experiments were done in decerebrate cats.

The relevance of these findings to clinical practice in humans is not clear, particularly in health. If laryngeal elevation and closure is elicited by a bolus appearing uninvited in the pharynx it is a very effective way of diverting the bolus away from the airway and into the oesophagus. This crude Sherringtonian swallow, which is not tailored to the size or consistency of the bolus, but simply a sequence of muscle contractions in response to a sensory stimulus, complements an array of other upper airway protective mechanisms including coughing, gagging, retching, and vomiting, all of which promote the egress of bolus away from the larynx and pharynx.

However, it is questionable whether alert adults rely on the bolus to elicit swallowing in the same way. Timing data from videofluoroscopy [9] suggests that before the bolus has left the mouth the

hyolaryngeal complex is starting to move upwards and forwards to create the necessary drop in pressure to draw the bolus in to the upper oesophagus. This suggests that, in keeping with the day-to-day experience of eating and drinking, we decide when and how to swallow, without having to rely on the bolus eliciting reflex laryngeal movement and closure, and that swallowing when eating and drinking is a behavioural or voluntary act rather than a reflex. It is true that once initiated the sequence of events is immutable, with the involved muscles activated in the same sequence every time, but it is a process, the initiation of which—like a deliberate hop or jump—remains largely under voluntary control.

Making a distinction between reflex protective (Sherringtonian) swallowing and bespoke voluntary swallowing may be less clear cut than portrayed here, but this way of thinking informs thinking about how patients maintain oral feeding in different conditions, and enriches thinking about the place and relevance of the different strategies used to promote continued oral feeding.

Breathing and coughing

Sherrington's work also established the elegant integration of breathing and swallowing, findings subsequently replicated by many others [10]. The swallowing described is, in healthy adults, preceded and followed by expiration (E).

This promotes clearing of the laryngeal inlet after swallowing. Inspiration (I) after a swallow could lead to the inhalation of bolus remnants, despite effective swallowing. So-called EE swallows are the norm (>90% of swallows); EI and IE the exceptions.

So a patient who is unable to coordinate their respiration around deglutition may suffer significant respiratory complications despite normal swallowing. Successful coughing is similarly important to preserve the airway. The volume of air inspired, the effectiveness of vocal cord apposition and the necessary control of head, neck, and trunk posture determine how well the cough clears the airways, and the viability of continued eating and drinking.

Voluntary and reflex coughing

A dissociation of reflex and voluntary coughing is common in diseases involving the central nervous system. Patients with isolated corticobulbar and corticospinal involvement lose voluntary control of their breathing, notably during attempts to estimate their forced vital capacity. However, in response to mucus or bolus in the larynx or airway, dramatic coughing can be elicited, often with associated eye watering and involuntary limb movement. Such projectile coughing is highly effective and helps maintain the patency of the airway; what is lost in voluntary control is partly compensated for by the dramatic preservation of elicitable reflex function.

So both swallowing and coughing can be thought of as highly effective upper airway reflexes, which very effectively remove any threats to the airway, and as functions to be deployed voluntarily to maintain successful oral feeding.

The general medical and surgical context

Impaired vigilance, drowsiness, pain, anxiety, vertigo, dry mouth, toothache, paranoia, mouth ulcers, oesophageal candidiasis, oesophageal reflux, visual neglect, and head tremor are just some of the long list of medical problems that can unhinge oral feeding in patients who have relatively well-preserved swallowing and breathing. Destructive lesions of the tongue, jaw, and larynx are just some of the surgical problems. Such problems can sometimes make oral feeding difficult in otherwise healthy adults, but their effect can be even greater in those with already compromised swallowing or breathing, sometimes leading to a significant decompensation and a requirement for adjunctive feeding techniques.

The caring environment

Successful oral feeding can be maintained in unlikely situations if the consistency of the food is changed accordingly. The consistency of food presented to the patients determines the nature of the challenge their swallowing and breathing has to overcome; steak and chips is a completely different kettle of fish to a pureed pudding with custard-thickened liquids. Thin liquids require careful control in the mouth and they easily breach laryngeal defences if there is untimely escape from the mouth. Food requiring chewing and significant tongue movement to prepare it to an appropriate consistency will be inedible for patients with weakness or slowing of bulbar structures. If liquids are thickened and food pureed, patients with considerable disability can continue to feed by mouth. The importance of food consistency is often revealed when a change of carers with deficient skills in food preparation uncover problems with eating and drinking for which other caring environments had compensated.

Oral feeding in neurological disease

Armed with a detailed understanding of the components of oral feeding it is possible to have insightful discussions about the mechanism of the problem and the interventions that are most likely to have a beneficial effect. For illustrative purposes a table of recognized stroke syndromes is included (Table 23.1) to emphasize how one disease process (infarction) can cause oral feeding problems through a variety of mechanisms, determined mainly by the anatomical location of the lesion. Stroke is perhaps the condition in which some of the most elegant work has been done to identify regions of cortex involved in swallowing, during health and the recovery from stroke.

Disorders of swallowing

It is self-evident that difficulty with movements of the tongue, defective chewing as a result of impaired sensory or motor function and poor function of the lips and cheek muscles will compromise oral control and preparation of the bolus. The more challenging the bolus is to prepare (e.g. tough steak), or to control (e.g. water), the more likely it is that a given impairment will manifest. The relevance of food consistency to the success or failure of oral feeding is obvious. A slow tongue, with reduced amplitude of movement, will not be able to move and retrieve bolus around the mouth, or complement mastication in the preparation of the bolus, but that same patient may be able to feed easily by mouth if presented with a puree diet.

If laryngeal elevation is compromised, as a result of tethering of the larynx (e.g. by a large thyroid (particularly with retrosternal extension), tracheostomy, scar tissue around a tracheostomy site, or a reduction in the excursion of movement as a result of hypokinesia or weakness) the opening of the upper oesophageal sphincter will be reduced with an associated reduction in the pressure drop and consequently less 'hypopharyngeal suction'. This

leads to impaired transit of the bolus through the pharynx and an increased risk of there being bolus residue in the pharynx after the swallow, with an obvious risk of aspiration when the larynx reopens and breathing (in, particularly) restarts.

Of even greater importance is laryngeal closure. The larynx is the sphincter of the airway. If it closes effectively the patient may 'get away' with terrible oral control, particularly if in addition to timely laryngeal closure there is a good cough. However, if laryngeal closure is defective the consequences are predictable. Acute occlusion of the larynx or chronic aspiration into the airways will produce a range of respiratory complications including asphyxiation, aspiration pneumonia, lobar collapse secondary to distal airway collapse, and a chemical pneumonitis if acidic gastric contents are involved. A unilateral vocal cord palsy, unaccompanied by any other symptoms such as vertigo or nausea, highlights the importance of the sphincteric action of the larynx. The four levels of laryngeal closure—true cords, false cords, arytenoids, and epiglottis—are all defective, and the bolus is free to enter the elevated larynx (laryngeal elevation should be normal in a Xth nerve palsy). To compound the problem, and in effect to make it an insurmountable problem in some patients, coughing is also unhinged because of the vocal cord palsy, and no amount of bovine coughing can effectively clear the airway of aspirated secretions, uninvited bolus, and oesophageal refluxate.

Therefore the larynx deserves to be considered centre stage when it comes to bulbar function. Not only is it responsible for the voicing of speech but its importance as the airway sphincter and as the device to create effective coughing means that it is difficult or impossible for other involved functions to compensate for loss of laryngeal function.

Disorders of breathing

Effective coughing depends on adequate pulmonary function, good posture control, preserved laryngeal function, and a preserved sensory system to trigger the necessary reflex or voluntary response; all of these functions are vulnerable to neurological disease. The integration of breathing and swallowing is also vulnerable and although abnormalities may be difficult to appreciate at the bedside, techniques which record the inspiration and expiration around the deglutition apnoea have established that disease can disrupt the control of breathing around deglutition [10]. Breathing in, rather than out, after swallowing increases the risk of bolus residue in the pharynx being aspirated, by inhalation effectively, into the airway. Persistent abnormalities of the respiratory cycle around deglutition may contribute to recurrent chest infections in some patients in whom mere swallowing—as described—is relatively preserved.

Medical and surgical problems

The long list of problems described, in patients with a given degree of impairment of swallowing and breathing, can compromise or completely unhinge oral feeding. Vertigo, nausea, and vomiting comprise a triad, which is common in neurological disease and immediately compromises oral feeding even in those with normal swallowing and breathing.

Situational factors

The quality of the caring environment, the consistency of the food presented, seating and utensils are just some of the very important factors determining whether people can maintain oral intake.

Table 23.1 Oral feeding problems after stroke

Neurological problem	Involved structures	Contribution to oral feeding problem
Lateral medullary syndrome	Cerebellar hemisphere and central connections	Vertigo, nausea, and vomiting
	Trigeminal sensory nucleus	Intraoral sensory loss
	Nucleus Ambiguus	Failure of laryngeal closure, impaired palatal elevation, and defective pharyngeal persistalsis
Medial medullary syndrome	Fascicle of twelfth nerve	Unilateral weakness of the tongue
	Medial lemniscus	Contralateral joint position sense loss
	Pyramidal tract	Contralateral limb and truncal weakness
Middle cerebral artery territory	Corticobulbar motorneurons	Slowing and imprecision of movement of tongue, lips and jaw
	Corticospinal neurones	Impaired posture and limb function
	Hemisphere swelling	Decreased vigilance and impaired conscious level
	Parietal lobe and its connections (left)	Apraxia of the tongue, lips and jaw
	Broca's and Wernicke's area	Impaired communication
	Parietal lobe (right)	Neglect of left side
		Anosagnosia (failure to acknowledge or recognise disability)
Extrcranial carotid artery dissection (within the carotid sheath)	Sympathetic plexus	No obvious effect on feeding (deglutition is not an autonomic function)
	Neuropraxia or ischaemia of the tenth nerve	Failure of laryngeal closure
	Neuropraxia or ischaemia of the twelfth cranial nerve	Impaired movement of the tongue in the mouth
	Subsequent embolization to middle cerebral arteries	Impaired peristalsis (the base of the tongue forms the anterior wall of the pharynx)
		Problems as previously described
Bilateral frontal opercular infarction (branch MCA occlusions)	Corticobulbar neurones, producing a bilateral corticobulbar palsy (Foix Chavany Marie syndrome)	Loss of voluntary movement of the face, tongue, jaw, and palate makes bolus control and preparation impossible
		Relative preservation of reflex functions including coughing, gagging, and retching

These issues are susceptible to intervention and for many patients it is attention to detail regarding the caring environment that determines the viability of oral feeding. The consistency of the diet is perhaps the most important, as discussed in the section on therapy interventions.

The mechanism of the problem is different depending on the area of infarction (see Table 23.1), raising important questions about the relevance of a uniform approach to dysphagia after stroke. In carotid dissection in the region of the carotid sheath, with associated Xth and XIIth cranial nerve palsies there can be severe dysphagia even if there is not associated secondary embolic cerebral infarction, highlighting again the need to make diagnoses of the disease process and the mechanism of the associated feeding problem.

Approach to the patient

A number of questions may arise when a patient presents with a problem eating and drinking, which often have to be managed in parallel rather than in series, to ensure that issues relating to nutrition and hydration are not neglected. There may also be more than one disease process to be diagnosed, and when the diagnosis is secure, a number of possible mechanisms to explain the oral feeding problem.

Management of immediate metabolic deficits

In most patients the priority is to ensure adequate hydration and nutrition using a nasogastric (NG) tube, to buy time to pursue investigations, which will allow a more informed approach to management. Is some cases in whom only intravenous access is available it may be possible only to hydrate and correct fluid imbalance, but this at least can defuse a situation for 24 hours whilst more information is acquired.

Management of major underlying diseases

The diagnosis of the underlying condition is obviously central to ensuring that the correct treatment is administered. Any underlying vascular, inflammatory, or infective condition, if treated, may lead to a complete resolution of the problem with oral feeding, as conscious level, or awareness, or nausea and vomiting improve. The discipline of the traditional diagnostic process—history, examination and investigation—has to be seen through to a final conclusion, a task made doubly difficult by the immediacy of feeding and hydration issues.

The process of diagnosis is beyond the scope of this chapter and the approach required is well described elsewhere. However, it is important to appreciate when approaching patients whose symptoms are confined to the bulbar region that the range of symptoms and signs may be limited and structural disease can easily mimic neurological disease, particularly malignancies infiltrating the floor of the mouth, the base of the tongue, the hypopharynx, the cricopharynx, and the retropharyngeal space. Therefore if there are no symptoms and signs in the limbs a high index of suspicion regarding structural disease is required. Sometimes, structural disease of the mouth, pharynx or oesophagus can be complicated by neurological disease, producing a diagnostic trap for the unwary. A carcinoma of the oesophagus complicated by polymyositis can produce a swallowing problem through both obstruction and weakness; a mediastinal mass in an older male can produce paraneoplastic myasthenia gravis as well as a recurrent laryngeal nerve palsy or compression of the oesophagus; hyperthyroidism can produce a myopathy and enlargement of the thyroid gland, both of which may affect laryngeal elevation during swallowing.

The concept of diagnosis has to be extended, however, to ensure that any marginal gains are aggregated in the pursuit of preserving oral feeding. Patients with a given neurological condition are vulnerable to routine problems such as concurrent infection, drug side effects and changes in mood and motivation, all of which can unhinge oral feeding without signs of the underlying disease having progressed. Patients with neurodegenerative disease may become unusually susceptible to the side effects of medication (e.g. Lewy Body disease and major tranquillisers). In very vulnerable patients, particularly those with advanced degenerative diseases, a banal problem can completely disrupt the oral feeding routine. New onset atrial fibrillation in patients with Freidrich's ataxia, oesophageal reflux in percutaneous endoscopic gastrostomy (PEG)-fed patients with multiple sclerosis, and constipation in patients with severe head injury, are just a few examples of situations in which precarious but established oral feeding may fail.

Mechanism of oral feeding failure

If these more traditional diagnostic questions have been successfully answered, there is also great merit in trying to diagnose the mechanism of the oral feeding problem. In some conditions this is very straightforward. Using the description of normal feeding and the examples of how it may be disrupted by different diseases, it should be possible, if the disease process has been identified, to anticipate the mechanism of the oral feeding problem, by methodically working through the four domains of clinical problems that may affect oral feeding: swallowing (including the preoral stage and chewing), respiratory function (including cough and control of respiration around deglutition), the additional neurological, general medical and surgical problems, and the situation in which the patient is being cared for. Muscle disease causes weakness, therefore the main impairments of laryngeal elevation, lip control, and head and neck posture, and of breathing, are likely to be a result of weakness. Common complications of the disease should also be anticipated, such as secondary musculoskeletal changes. However, even when the disease has been diagnosed with confidence, the mechanism of the feeding problem may not be evident. In patients with motor neuron disease upper motor neuron involvement may affect oral control and bolus preparation, but laryngeal function, particularly reflex closure of the larynx, may be relatively unaffected. In this situation reflex coughing may be effectively preserved and, as a result, oral feeding continues.

Magnitude of eating and drinking problem

Perhaps the most taxing question is whether it is possible to make quick decisions about the appropriateness of eating and drinking for a particular individual.

In long-term conditions, reliable witness accounts of feeding behaviour are invaluable, and have the advantage of being a reflection of a representative time period. Some patients with seemingly insurmountable disability involving the bulbar region are fed orally by devoted carers who become expert in catering for their idiosyncratic needs. Patients with basilar tip occlusions are an example, some of whom manage a pureed diet if it is placed carefully into their mouths; reflex swallowing and coughing is preserved and with the help of gravity and any residual control of head and neck posture, individuals are able to maintain an adequate intake.

In more acute situations a number of studies highlight the poor correlation between bedside tests of swallowing—using trials of swallowing and detailed clinical examination—and the results of investigations that allow one or more of the components of swallowing to be observed e.g. videofluoroscopy and fibreoptic endoscopic evaluation of swallowing [11]. This raises questions about the different approaches to assessment of oral feeding and the relative merits of tests that look only at swallowing. If oral feeding is considered rather than just swallowing, it immediately becomes apparent that, for example, the effectiveness of coughing and posture control may be as important as swallowing function in determining the success or safety of oral feeding. If the clinical assessment is confined to swallowing, the subsequent discussions are impoverished and are unlikely to lead to a comprehensive assessment of their feeding ability. The same applies to the use of ancillary investigations; the immediacy of videofluoroscopy images is arresting, but the presence or absence of aspiration in a few sequences in optimal conditions is unlikely to be representative of eating and drinking over a longer time period, and of course pulmonary function, cough, and control of respiration around deglutition are not part of a videofluoroscopy assessment. In this regard, the results of investigations that involve imaging or direct visualization of the structures involved in swallowing, or images tracking the course of the bolus, have to be interpreted with caution, particularly if there are observations garnered during a representative time period that suggest that oral feeding is, or is not, proceeding successfully. If someone is well nourished and has enjoyed or endured cautious oral feeding over a representative time period this information has obvious face validity and clinical relevance which is lacking in paraclinical assessments, many of which provide information about only one component of the oral feeding process. Similarly, if someone is losing weight and suffering recurrent chest infections, an intervention of some sort is required regardless of the presence or absence of abnormal tests of swallowing.

Therapy options

In keeping with the approach to any sort of therapy for people with neurological disability the basics of seating, sitting posture, pain control, minimization of distractions, and prompt attention to general medical problems are a platform on which therapist and patient thrive.

Directed at the mechanics of swallowing

In addition to the treatment of the underlying condition there are certain techniques and methods which may enhance swallowing function. These include deliberate repeat swallows, and techniques to improve the effectiveness of individual swallows (so called supraglottic swallows and super-supraglotic swallows), which involve the patient accentuating the apnoea during, and expiration following, the swallow [12].

Techniques designed to stimulate oral, palatal, and pharyngeal receptors involved in reflex swallowing, based on the original experiments of Sherrington, have involved trials with different stimuli in the hope of promoting a return of swallowing function [13–15].

Although techniques to drive cortical plasticity in the adult motor cortex have been associated with improved motor function after brain injury, the effects of pharmacological agents have been disappointing [16].

Directed at posture

These range from attempts to prevent bolus moving down the paralysed side of the pharynx in a Xth nerve palsy (head turning to the side of the lesion), to chin tuck (which is said to reduce the risk of aspiration and position the tongue base and pharynx more favourably), to side lying (which may help avoid aspiration by reducing the effect of gravity). The importance of good sitting posture, appropriate seating, and access to upper limb support at the right level is self-evident.

Directed at food texture

Perhaps the single most important issue in oral feeding problems is the consistency of the food. In his original work Sherrington, in decerebrate cats, described whisky as the most effective phagetic agent, as it seemed to elicit reflex swallowing (laryngeal elevation and closure) more reliably than water or liquids of an oily consistency [8]. Although the consistency of the food and liquid may be of relevance to the elicitation of reflex swallowing, the consistency of the bolus determines the challenge faced by the simple mechanics of ensuring the preparation and propulsion of the bolus in to the oesophagus without any of it reaching or breaching the sphincter of the airway, the larynx. Fluids with the consistency and viscosity of water are a stringent test of laryngeal closure and oral control; simply by thickening liquids they can become manageable in the mouth and less of a threat to the airway. Even the most tender meat can be impossible to chew for patients with impaired jaw function or intraoral sensation, but if it is pureed it can be consumed without the need for other interventions.

In Dysphagia Diet Food Texture Descriptors (March 2012) [17], the different types and textures of foods are described allowing all health professionals and food providers to communicate effectively; knowing the difference between a thin puree and a fork-mashable dysphagia diet should be essential for all members of the team.

Directed at carers and caring environment

The importance of carers who are attuned to the needs of the patient cannot be overstated. Some patients require help with cutting up of food; others require a formidable routine of food preparation and labour-intensive spoon feeding. Many patients are able to avoid gastrostomy feeding owing to the dedication of their carers, therefore any changes in management suggested by the therapists involved in care must be fully discussed with and channelled through the carers.

Artificial enteral and parenteral feeding

Regardless of the mechanism of failure, oral feeding can be replaced by tube feeding. NG, nasojejunal, PEG, radiologically inserted gastrostomy, percutaneous endoscopic jejunostomy, and surgically placed jejunostomy are the typical options, with NG and PEG the most frequently used devices. Over half of those patients established on home enteral feeding have conditions involving the nervous system, with stroke the most common diagnosis. The use of fine-bore tubes has improved the tolerance of NG tubes and some patients in the community continue to use them. Their placement is not without complication, typically as a result of trauma and abrasions to the lining of the nose and nasopharynx, and improbable outcomes of placement (e.g. intracranial placement through the cribriform plate), have been recorded. PEG placement is associated with more risks, including those of sedation (usually with midazolam), endoscopy and penetration of the peritoneal cavity and the wall of the stomach. The morbidity and mortality associated with PEG insertion suggests that it should be undertaken only in selected patients, ideally following a multidisciplinary discussion. Both NG and PEG tubes are associated with long-term complications after placement, notably blockage and displacement, and vigilant monitoring is required. Parenteral nutrition is an option for those patients who not eligible for tube feeding.

Many patients have a combination of tube feeding and limited oral intake, allowing them to enjoy the pleasure of oral feeding but not placing upon them the burden of having to swallow safely all of the calories they require.

Ethical and legal issues

The issues regarding the appropriateness of intervention are generic from an ethical and legal perspective; however, feeding issues in patients with complex neurological disability create some of the most difficult intellectual challenges for the neurorehabilitation team. An informed discussion about the best interests and the best medical interests of an individual are central to a reasoned and informed discussion between healthcare professionals and the family.

The approach to the patient has to be based on a sound appreciation of ethical principles and the legal framework within which health care professionals operate. The 2005 Mental Capacity Act [18] provides clear guidance about the issue-specific nature of capacity and the approach to the patient who has capacity—and therefore the absolute right to decline even life-preserving treatment—is obviously different to those patients who do not have capacity. The important clinical, ethical and legal issues are elegantly summarized in the report by the Royal College of Physicians entitled 'Oral feeding difficulties and dilemmas' [19] which includes invaluable advice ranging from succinct summaries of why NG and PEG feeding and hydration represents medical (not basic) care to examples of case law which inform current clinical practice (e.g. the Bolam test). It is a useful starting point for those who may be faced with the more complex discussions and need a sound understanding of the concepts of beneficence and non-maleficence, autonomy and justice, religious and secular beliefs regarding the sanctity of life and how it differs to vitalism, and the important difference between ordinary and extraordinary means. It is important to be sufficiently familiar with the doctrine of double effect to be able to articulate a version to a partner or family which helps explain why with the intention of relieving suffering a discussion is required about withdrawing feeding even though it can be foreseen that it will lead to their relative's death, and to be able to refer promptly to the guidance of the General Medical Council (GMC) on such matters. The importance of clinicians understanding the legal and ethical framework is no less important when dealing with patients who have written advanced directives; it can still be very difficult to judge the relevance of past instructions when patients emerge from an illness a very changed person.

However, with a sound appreciation of the common ethical issues such as capacity and the Mental Capacity Act, consent, confidentiality, and how to deal with conflict (between family members and within the healthcare team), and a detailed understanding of the prognosis of the condition and the mechanism of the feeding problem, the passage of time provides invaluable information, which usually inevitably informs decision making. Central to the decision making is the importance of a clear process, which ensures all parties have opportunities to express their opinion and that conclusions are reached following a period of serious reflection and thought.

The MEALTIME approach

Confronted with a complex patient it can be difficult to organize thinking in order to ensure that important issues are addressed in parallel. The following may provide some structure.

Metabolic requirements; mechanism of oral feeding problem; management of underlying disease process

Immediate metabolic requirements such as hydration and electrolyte and glycaemic abnormalities can usually be corrected fairly quickly with intravenous fluids, including insulin if necessary.

Using the framework already set out the mechanism of the failure of oral feeding should be established. It may not be possible to work out the mechanism until the underlying disease process has been diagnosed. It is not uncommon for these three Ms to be confronted and managed in parallel.

Ethical

The first question to ask of oneself is whether there are any ethical questions to address and what questions are likely to arise in the future, as the condition of the patient changes.

Achievable goals

The relative importance and urgency of the issues arising is dictated to some extent by the conclusions of the attending clinicians about the achievable goals. It is often in the attempt to set realistic goals that uncertainties about the case are revealed, and temporary goals may have to be set without knowing the details of the diagnosis or the prognosis.

Legal

If the ethical issues are discussed at length it is usually the case that the legal issues about what help and advice is required are discovered. If there are any doubts it is advisable to seek help immediately.

Therapy from team

In routine practice it is rare for a professional to face these problems alone, and it is important that a team approach is adopted to ensure a multidisciplinary approach. To maximize oral feeding ability therapy options should be considered at an appropriate time. In practice, patients may not be able to participate in exercises to maximize their swallowing and coughing ability until their condition has stabilized. A dietician will provide information about nutritional requirements and nurse specialists may be required to place NG tubes and devices to secure them in position.

Information; acquisition and dissemination

As much information as is possible must be acquired about the individual and the family to inform thinking about the achievable goals. This information must also be disseminated to other team members to ensure that the same goals are pursued by everyone and that there is not duplication of effort.

Monitoring

When goals have been set the patient needs to be monitored closely, so that goals can be revised as the clinical picture changes

End of involvement and end of life issues

Whatever the involvement of the team it is imperative that the lines of responsibility and accountability are clearly defined, particularly when one team is asked to take on management responsibilities.

It is not unusual for oral feeding failure, or a marked loss of interest in food and drink, to be a sign that the end of life is approaching and the goals may have to be changed from adequate feeding and hydration to ensuring a peaceful death, with the minimum of suffering.

Conclusion

The approach to patients with oral feeding problems requires of the clinician an approach that synthesizes information from a number of different sources to ensure that the diagnosis and prognosis of the underlying condition informs the setting of achievable goals. Decisions about intervention must include an informed discussion with the family about the ethics and legality of the proposals and all discussions are best carried out within a multidisciplinary team.

References

1. Care Quality Commission. Outcome 5 (Regulation 14); meeting nutritional needs. Care Quality Commission, London, 2010.
2. Mid Staffordshire NHS Foundation Trust Public Inquiry. Robert Francis, February 2013. The Stationery Office, London. ISBN 9780102981476

3. Water for health. Hydration best practice toolkit for hospitals and healthcare. Royal College of Nursing and National Patient Safety Agency, London, 2007.

4. Nutrition screening survey in the UK and Republic of Ireland. British Association for Parenteral and Enteral Nutrition (BAPEN), London, 2011.

5. Nathadwarawala KM, Richards CA, Lawrie B, Thomas GO, Wiles CM. Recurrent aspiration due to Arnold--Chiari type I malformation. Br Med J. 1992;**304**(6826):565–566.

6. Miller AJ. Deglutition. Physiol Rev. 1982;**62**:129–184.

7. Hughes TAT, Wiles CM. Clinical measurement of swallowing in health and in neurogenic dysphagia. Q J Med. 1996;**89**:109–116.

8. Miller FR, Sherrington CS. Some observations on the bucco-pharyngeal stage of reflex deglutition in the cat. Q J Exp Physiol. 1916;**9**:147–186.

9. Curtis DJ, Cruess DF, Dachman AH, Maso E. Timing in the normal pharyngeal swallow. Prospective selection and evaluation of 16 normal asymptomatic patients. Invest Radiol. 1984;**19**(6):523–529.

10. Selley WG, Flack FC, Ellis RE, Brooks WA. The Exeter Dysphagia Assessment Technique. Dysphagia. 1990;**4**(4):227–235.

11. Splaingard ML, Hutchins B, Sulton LD, et al Aspiration in rehabilitation patients: videofluoroscopy vs bedside clinical assessment. Arch Phys Med Rehabil. 1988;**69**(8):637–640.

12. Bülow M, Olsson R, Ekberg O. Videomanometric analysis of supra-glottic swallow, effortful swallow, and chin tuck in patients with pharyngeal dysfunction. Dysphagia. 2001. Summer;**16**(3):190–195.

13. Lazarra G, Lazarus C, Logemann J A. Impact of thermal stimulation on the triggering of the swallow reflex. Dysphagia. 1986;**1**(2):73–77.

14. Fraser C, Power M, Hamdy S, et al. Driving plasticity in human adult motor cortex is associated with improved motor function after brain injury. Neuron. 2002;**34**(5):831–840.

15. Hamdy S, Aziz Q, Rothwell JC, et al. Explaining oropharyngeal dysphagia after unilateral hemispheric stroke. Lancet. 1997;**350**(9079):686–692.

16. Perez I, Smithard DG, Davies H, et al. Pharmacological treatment of dysphagia in stroke. Dysphagia. 1998 Winter:**13**(1):12–16.

17. Dysphagia Diet Food Texture Descriptors. April 2011. National Patient Safety Agency, Royal College of Speech and Language Therapists, British Dietetic Association, National Nurses Nutrition Group, Hospital Caterers Association.

18. Mental Capacity Act 2005. Available from http://www.legislation.gov.uk/ukpga/2005/9/contents (accessed 1 October 2014).

19. Royal College of Physicians and British Society of Gastroenterology. Oral feeding difficulties and dilemmas: A guide to practical care, particularly towards the end of life. Royal College of Physicians, London, 2010.

CHAPTER 24

Management of bladder, bowel, and sexual dysfunction

Ulrich Mehnert

Introduction

Bladder, bowel, and sexual dysfunctions are frequent sequelae of neurotrauma and neurodegenerative diseases. Such dysfunctions have a significant impact on the patient's quality of life and—depending on the severity of the bladder and bowel dysfunction and the level of neurological disability—adequate management is often defined as primary rehabilitation goal by the patients [1].

If not adequately treated or managed, bladder and bowel dysfunctions can not only essentially interfere with other rehabilitation measures but might even become hazardous to health.

This chapter reviews the underlying pathophysiology of bladder, bowel, and sexual dysfunction in neurotrauma and neurodegenerative diseases and provides a comprehensive overview on the principles of their therapy and management with special emphasis to the practical management. The chapter will conclude with an outlook on current scientific findings and future directions of therapy.

The aim of the chapter is to sensitize physicians on this essential part/aspect of neurorehabilitation and to provide practical information for the management of patients with bladder, bowel, and sexual dysfunction.

Pathophysiology

Pathophysiology of bladder dysfunction in neurological disorders

The urinary bladder (including the detrusor muscle), the bladder neck, the urethra and the external urethral sphincter, which are in summary named the lower urinary tract (LUT), in differentiation to the upper urinary tract consisting of the ureters and kidneys, relies on a complex neuronal network for adequate functioning. Such functions are:

1. low pressure continent storage of urine and

2. periodically, self determined and more or less complete release of the stored urine.

The neuronal LUT control network involves different neurons, nerves, and fibre types from different levels of the spinal cord (Figure 24.1) forming reflex circuitries that are under supraspinal control [2]. The latter is essential to voluntarily control LUT function, that is to decide where and when to empty the bladder. Neurophysiological studies in animals and recent neuroimaging

studies in humans could reveal several supraspinal areas that are involved in LUT control including the pons, periaqueductal grey, thalamus, hypothalamus, insula, cingulated gyrus, cerebellum, frontal, and prefrontal cortical areas (Figure 24.2) [2].

Due to this complex neuronal innervation and control it is not surprising that next to traumatic (e.g. spinal cord injury with 91–99% prevalence of LUT dysfunction [3]) and congenital (e.g. meningomyelocele with 98% prevalence of LUT dysfunction [4]) neurogenic lesions, also various neurological diseases frequently compromise LUT function (Table 24.1). Such functional impairments usually affect LUT sensibility, detrusor contractility, and/ or urinary sphincter function. Each of these functional properties can be either over-, normo-, or underactive resulting in various different clinical findings and symptoms which can be functionally classified as storage or voiding symptoms (Table 24.2).

Based on observations and findings in spinal cord injury (SCI) patients, certain LUT dysfunctions and symptoms can be attributed to specific lesion sites (Figure 24.3, Table 24.2, and Table 24.3).

In general, but often related to the extent of the neuronal defects, lesions of peripheral nerves (i.e. pelvic or pudendal nerves), can result in hypo- or acontractile bladder and sphincter function, due to loss of connection to the sacral micturition centre (S2–S3), which contains important neurons for LUT control (i.e. parasympathetic neurons for bladder contraction or motor neurons in Onuf's nucleus for sphincter contraction (Figure 24.1)). The same applies for lesions at the subsacral spinal cord level.

Suprasacral lesions in contrast can result in detrusor overactivity (DO) due to an intact bladder reflex circuit on sacral level but interruption of LUT control from brainstem and suprapontine centres. Thus, DO is a kind of smooth muscle spasticity that was previously also termed detrusor hyperreflexia [5]. Again, the severity of DO depends on the extent of lesions. A patient with a complete spinal cord injury at thoracic level 10 will almost always develop a DO following spinal shock phase. In contrast, a small incomplete lesion at the frontal horn might not at all cause DO. Another severe dysfunction that can occur with suprasacral lesions is detrusor-sphincter-dyssynergia (DSD). In healthy conditions, detrusor contractions during voluntary micturition are usually accompanied by a synergistic sphincter relaxation to let the urine pass. This synergistic function of detrusor and external urethral sphincter is mainly coordinated by neurons in the dorsolateral pons [6]. In DSD, pontine input to the LUT is disrupted,

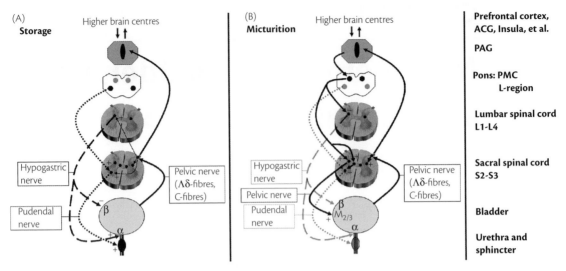

Fig. 24.1 Schematic illustration of spinal cord and brain stem regions involved in lower urinary tract (LUT) control and their most relevant neuronal connection to the LUT. The illustration summarizes the findings of neurophysiological animal studies from De Groat et al. [1] and early functional neuroimaging studies in humans from Blok et al. [2]. During the storage phase (a), which normally accounts for most of the daily time (98%), the detrusor is relaxed and the bladder neck closed due to a certain sympathetic tone on bladder body and bladder neck. Sympathetic fibres travel along the hypogastric nerve from the sympathetic nuclei in the intermediolateral column of the lumbar spinal cord to the LUT and provide adrenergic input to beta-receptors on intramural ganglia of the bladder body (→ relaxation) and alpha-receptors at the bladder neck (→ contraction/closure). Bladder afferents traverse through the pelvic nerve and enter the dorsal horn of the sacral spinal cord. At low filling volumes, there might be only little afferent activity and weak afferent signals might reach the PAG and diencephalic structures (e.g. thalamus), but bladder sensations do usually not reach consciousness during this state. With increasing bladder volumes, afferent activity might increase probably due to changes in intravesical pressure and at some degree of filling, bladder sensations will reach consciousness in form of a first desire to void. From the sacral dorsal horn, excitatory collaterals reach to the sympathetic nuclei in the lumbar intermediolateral column and to the sacral frontal horn, where the motor neurons of the external urethral sphincter (EUS) are located (Onuf's nucleus), to facilitate sympathetic input to the bladder and bladder neck, and somatic input to the EUS respectively. This supports continence during increasing bladder volumes, when voiding has to be postponed. Another region supposed to be responsible for continence is the pontine L-region (named L-region as it is lateral to the other relevant pontine structure named pontine micturition centre or M-region or Barrington's nucleus), which has excitatory input to the EUS motor neurons in Onuf's nucleus and thus facilitates the elevation of the EUS tone. If the decision to empty the bladder is made (in the higher brain centres), the periaqueductal grey (PAG) activates the pontine micturition centre (PMC) (b). The switch between L-region and PMC activation is sometimes model-likely simplified as moving a lever from one programme to the other. Only one region can be activated at a time. From the PMC strong inhibitory inputs reach the sympathetic nuclei in the intermediolateral lumbar cord to suppress the sympathetic input to bladder body and bladder neck to enable a synergic micturition. Simultaneously, the PMC has strong excitatory projections to the parasympathetic nuclei in the sacral spinal cord that in turn activate the detrusor muscle via muscarinic receptors. The parasympathetic fibres travel along the pelvic nerve. In addition to the parasympathetic activation, the PMC has excitatory collaterals to inhibitory interneurons in the sacral cord that reduce the activity of EUS motor neurons, and thus facilitate EUS relaxation and synergic micturition.

1. de Groat WC. Integrative control of the lower urinary tract: preclinical perspective. Br J Pharmacol. 2006;**147**(Suppl 2):S25–40.

2. Blok BF, Holstege G. The central control of micturition and continence: implications for urology. BJU Int. 1999;**83**(Suppl 2):1–6.

Figure and legend reprinted by permission from Springer-Verlag London Limited: Mehnert U (2009) Technologies for the rehabilitation of neurogenic lower urinary tractdysfunction. In: Dietz V, Nef T, Rymer Z (eds) Neurorehabilitation technology. Springer, Berlin Heidelberg New York, pp. 413–439

causing dyssynergic sphincter spasticity. The health related trouble with DSD are the extraordinary high intravesical pressures that occur during DO, as the spastic detrusor is now pressing against the outlet resistance of the spastic sphincter. Such elevated pressures will, in the long term, jeopardize lower and upper urinary tract function and morphology [7].

An especially hazardous complication that typically occurs with SCI above the splanchnic sympathetic outflow (T5–T6) is autonomic dysreflexia (AD) [8]. AD, most frequently elicited by bladder and/or bowel distension, is a severe and potentially life-threatening condition, characterized by an excessive rise in systolic blood pressure accompanied by a decrease in heart rate. The pathomechanism of AD relies on the decoupling of descending central (brain stem) inhibitory pathways to the sympathetic chain. This becomes especially eminent with SCI lesions above T6 due to the lack of central modulation on the splanchnic nerves that usually emanate below T5 but innervate the critical mass of blood vessels required to cause elevation of the blood pressure [8]. Thus, a noxious stimuli, such as bladder distension, causes uninhibited

sympathetic outflow to the splanchnic nerves that consequently results in peripheral and splanchnic vasoconstriction, followed by development of hypertension [8].

In return, baroreceptors above the lesion might counteract the excessive rise in blood pressure with an increased parasympathetic output resulting in slowing of heart rate, headache, flushing and sweating in the head and neck region [8].

Supraspinal lesions (i.e. stroke, Parkinson's disease (PD)), frequently cause DO but rarely DSD due to intact pontine control to the LUT (Table 24.1). However, it appears that certain cerebellar and/or basal ganglia lesions are associated with DSD as such regions seem to exert relevant functional control on the periaqueductal grey (PAG) and/or pons [9, 10].

Impairments of LUT sensation can occur with lesions along the whole neuronal axis. Peripheral and subsacral lesions rather result in decreased sensibility whereas suprasacral or supraspinal can cause decreased (i.e. complete SCI), or often increased sensibility such as urinary urgency (i.e. multiple sclerosis (MS), PD).

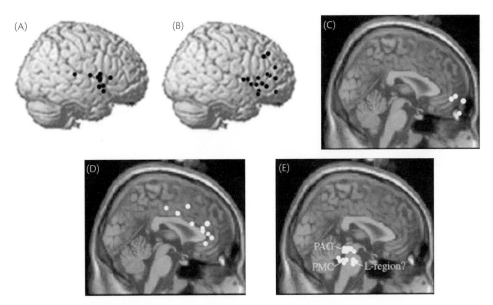

Fig. 24.2 For normal subjects, reported locations of peak activation (deactivation in a few cases) projected on a lateral surface or medial section of the brain, depending on which is closer to actual location; for simplicity, left and right activations are both projected on the same (right) side of the brain. Results are based on PET, fMRI, and one SPECT study, of which the latter may be less reliable. (A) Insula and adjacent lateral frontal areas activated during withholding of urine or full bladder (outlier on left is SPECT study). (B) Lateral (pre)frontal areas reported as activated during withholding of urine or full bladder (note there is some overlap with panel A). (C) Medial prefrontal areas activated during withholding of urine or full bladder (the two most anterior locations are from the SPECT study). (D) (Anterior) cingulate areas activated during withholding of urine or full bladder (the most posterior location is from the SPECT study and is close to the posterior cingulate activation described by DasGupta et al. [3]). (E) Brainstem areas activated during withholding of urine or full bladder, or during voiding (all but one of the PMC activations are from voiding studies; the PAG and putative L-region activations are from storage studies; the midbrain area located slightly anterior to the PAG by DasGupta et al. (2005) has not been included.

Dasgupta R, Critchley HD, Dolan RJ and Fowler CJ. Changes in brain activity following sacral neuromodulation for urinary retention. J Urol. 2005;**174**:2268–2272. Figure and legend reprinted by permission from John Wiley and Sons: Griffiths, D. and Tadic, S. D. (2008), Bladder control, urgency, and urge incontinence: Evidence from functional brain imaging. Neurourol. Urodyn. **27**: 466–474.

It is important to consider that LUT dysfunctions and symptoms may change over time, especially in progressive neurological diseases and thus, such patients require regular neuro-urological follow-up.

Pathophysiology of bowel dysfunction in neurological disorders

The gastrointestinal (GI) tract has three main functions:

1. Break up of food into smaller absorbable compounds/molecules (small intestine) and degradation of short fatty acids (colon).

2. Absorbtion of nutrients and vitamins (ileum) and of water and salts (colon).

3. Transit of faeces in distal direction and storage of faeces until defecation is appropriate.

Neurogenic control of the GI tract comprises an intrinsic (enteric) and extrinsic nervous system. The intrinsic nervous system is unique to the GI tract and can be divided into a myenteric and submucosal plexus, which are densely connected by interneurons. The myenteric plexus mainly controls the circular and longitudinal muscle layers while the submucosal plexus has secretomotor (small intestine) and sensory function and innervates the muscularis mucosa and submucosal vessles. Both plexus enable autonomic GI peristalsis and might in total contain up to 100 million neurons, which is similar to the amount of neurons in the human spinal cord [11].

The extrinsic nervous system corresponds to the autonomic nervous system with sympathetic input from T5–L3 and parasympathetic input via the vagus nerve (10th cranial nerve) and S2–4 (Figure 24.4). The sympathetic input is mainly responsible for slowing GI motility and increasing colonic wall compliance and internal anal sphincter tone while parasympathetic input causes mainly increase in GI motility and relaxation of the internal anal sphincter.

Both extrinsic and intrinsic nervous systems do not allow voluntary control. The only structure that can be voluntarily controlled is the striated external anal sphincter, that similar to the external urethral sphincter has its motor neurons in the ventral horn of the sacral spinal cord (Onuf's nucleus) that also travel via the pudendal nerve.

Defecation most probably depends on several factors and processes that are not all fully understood. Such factors and processes include sensation of rectal filling, amount of stool in the rectum, adequate colonic and rectal motility (i.e. high-amplitude propagated contractions), and adequate relaxation of sphincters and pelvic floor. Although most of such processes are not voluntarily controllable, it is, under healthy conditions, possible to voluntarily decide where and when to defecate. Thus, anorectal activity seems to be at least partly under supraspinal control similar to the LUT. Indeed, recent neuroimaging studies of anorectal control revealed involvement of very similar supraspinal areas as described for LUT control [12].

Traditionally, neurogenic bowel dysfunctions (NBD) are distinguished into supra- and subconal lesions, according to their functional impairment [13]. With supraconal lesions, sympathetic inhibitory influence might be impaired, resulting in reduced

Table 24.1 Prevalence of different neurogenic lower urinary tract dysfunctions (NLUTD) and symptoms in multiple sclerosis (MS), Parkinson's disease (PD), multiple system atrophy (MSA), and stroke. Table adapted from: Mehnert, U. and Nehiba, M. (2012), Neurourologische Funktionsstörungen des unteren Harntraktes bei Erkrankungen des ZNS. Der Urologe A. 51 (2): 189–197

	MS	PD	MSA	Stroke
Prevalence of NLUTD	34–99% [1]	27–71% [2,3]	78–96% [4]	38–94% [5,6]
Average time interval between diagnosis of neurological disease and onset of urological symptoms [years]	5.9 (4.6–7.8) [1]	5 [7]	2 [7]	
Urinary urgency	63.4% (32–86%) [1]	33–68% [2,3]	63% [8]	70% [5]
Urinary frequency	54.4% (25–99%) [1]	16–71% [2,3]	45% [8]	59% [5]
Nocturia		60–86% [2,3]	74% [8]	76% [5]
Urinary urgency incontinence	56.3% (19–80%) [1]	27% [3]	63% [8]	29% [5]
Dysuria	34.8% (6–79.5%) [1]	30% [7]	69% [7]	6% [5]
Retention/incomplete bladder emptying (PVRV > 100ml)	35.6% (8.3–73.8%) [1]		52% [8]	48% [5]
DO	65% (43–99%) [1]	45–93% [3]	35–56% [7,8]	36–82% [5]
DSD	35% (5–83%) [1]		47–98% (incl. bladder neck dyssynergia) [7,8]	
Reduced compliance	2–10% [1]		31% [8]	
Detrusor hypocontractility	25% (0–40%) [1]	53% [3]	52–67% [4,7]	33–40% [5]
Open bladder neck during filling cystometry		31% [4]	87% [4]	
Pathologic EUS–EMG		5% [4]	93% [4]	

Such specifications reflect only gross guide values due to sparse and/or heterogeneous data form investigations using different assessment methods.

PVRV post void residual volume, DO detrusor overactivity, DSD detrusor-sphincter-dyssynergia, EUS-EMG external urethral sphincter electromyogram.

[1] de Seze M, Ruffion A, Denys P, Joseph PA and Perrouin-Verbe B. The neurogenic bladder in multiple sclerosis: review of the literature and proposal of management guidelines. Multiple sclerosis 2007; **13**: 915–28.

[2] Winge K, Skau AM, Stimpel H, Nielsen KK and Werdelin L. Prevalence of bladder dysfunction in Parkinsons disease. Neurourol Urodyn 2006; **25**: 116–22.

[3] Sakakibara R, Uchiyama T, Yamanishi T, Shirai K and Hattori T. Bladder and bowel dysfunction in Parkinson's disease. Journal of neural transmission 2008; **115**: 443–60.

[4] Sakakibara R, Hattori T, Uchiyama T and Yamanishi T. Videourodynamic and sphincter motor unit potential analyses in Parkinson's disease and multiple system atrophy. Journal of neurology, neurosurgery, and psychiatry 2001; **71**: 600–6.

[5] Tibaek S, Gard G, Klarskov P, Iversen HK, Dehlendorff C and Jensen R. Prevalence of lower urinary tract symptoms (LUTS) in stroke patients: a cross-sectional, clinical survey. Neurourol Urodyn 2008; **27**: 763–71.

[6] Gupta A, Taly AB, Srivastava A and Thyloth M. Urodynamics post stroke in patients with urinary incontinence: Is there correlation between bladder type and site of lesion? Annals of Indian Academy of Neurology 2009; **12**: 104–7.

[7] Bloch F, Pichon B, Bonnet AM, Pichon J, Vidailhet M, Roze E et al. Urodynamic analysis in multiple system atrophy: characterisation of detrusor-sphincter dyssynergia. Journal of neurology 2010; **257**: 1986–91.

[8] Sakakibara R, Hattori T, Uchiyama T, Kita K, Asahina M, Suzuki A et al. Urinary dysfunction and orthostatic hypotension in multiple system atrophy: which is the more common and earlier manifestation? Journal of neurology, neurosurgery, and psychiatry 2000; **68**: 65–9.

Table 24.2 Summary of common storage and voiding symptoms that might occur due to LUT dysfunction in neurological diseases or lesions in association with their typically related urodynamical and clinical findings. Definitions of Symptoms are reproduced from the International Continence Society standardisation of terminology in lower urinary tract function [5].

	Symptom	Most typical urodynamical and clinical findings (listed are single findings that can also occur in combination)	Typical neurological lesion site
Storage symptoms	Urinary urgency *Complaint of a sudden compelling desire to pass urine, which is difficult to defer.*	- Detrusor overactivity[1, 2] - Low bladder compliance[1, 2]	1 suprasacral 2 supraspinal
	Urinary frequency (increased daytime frequency, pollakisuria) *Complaint by the patient who considers that he/she voids too often by day.*	- Detrusor overactivity[1, 2] - Low bladder compliance[1, 2] - Incomplete bladder emptying/elevated post void residual volume due to hypocontractile detrusor[3, 4] or bladder outlet obstruction (anatomical: prostate enlargement, urethral stricture; functional: detrusor-sphincter-dyssynergia[1, 2])	1 suprasacral 2 supraspinal 3 subsacral/lumbosacral 4 peripheral

(continued)

Table 24.2 Continued

	Symptom	Most typical urodynamical and clinical findings (listed are single findings that can also occur in combination)	Typical neurological lesion site
	Nocturia *Complaint that the individual has to wake at night one or more times to void.*	- Detrusor overactivity[1,2] - Low bladder compliance[1,2] - Incomplete bladder emptying/elevated post void residual volume due to hypocontractile detrusor[3,4] or bladder outlet obstruction (anatomical: prostate enlargement, urethral stricture; functional: detrusor-sphincter-dyssynergia[1,2])	1 suprasacral 2 supraspinal 3 subsacral/lumbosacral 4 peripheral
	Urgency urinary incontinence *Complaint of involuntary leakage accompanied by or immediately preceded by urgency.*	- Detrusor overactivity[1,2] - Low bladder compliance[1,2]	1 suprasacral 2 supraspinal
	Stress urinary incontinence *Complaint of involuntary leakage on effort or exertion, or on sneezing or coughing.*	- Urethral sphincter insufficiency[3,4] - Bladder neck incompetence[3,4]	3 subsacral/lumbosacral 4 peripheral
	Mixed urinary incontinence *Complaint of involuntary leakage associated with urgency and also with exertion, effort, sneezing or coughing.*	- Detrusor overactivity[1,2] - Low bladder compliance[1,2] **AND** - Urethral sphincter insufficiency[3,4] - Bladder neck incompetence[3,4]	1 suprasacral 2 supraspinal 3 subsacral/lumbosacral 4 peripheral
	Continuous urinary incontinence *Complaint of continuous urinary leakage.*	- Open bladder neck and flaccid urethral sphincter[3,4] **OR** - Overflow incontinence due to bladder outlet obstruction (anatomical: prostate enlargement, urethral stricture; functional: detrusor-sphincter-dyssynergia[1,2]) and/or acontractile[3,4], hyposensitive bladder[3,4]	1 suprasacral 2 supraspinal 3 subsacral/lumbosacral 4 peripheral
	Reduced or absent bladder sensation *The individual is aware of bladder filling but does not feel a definite desire to void or reports no sensation of bladder filling or desire to void.*	- Bladder distension during filling cystometry is not perceived or only at high volumes[1–4]	1 suprasacral 2 supraspinal 3 subsacral/lumbosacral 4 peripheral
	Increased bladder sensation *The individual feels an early and persistent desire to void.*	- Bladder distension during filling cystometry is perceived early, at low volumes[1,2]	1 suprasacral 2 supraspinal
Voiding symptoms	Urinary retention *Inability to pass urine to empty the bladder. This might occur acute or chronically, complete or incomplete.*	- Hypo- or acontractile detrusor muscle[3,4] - Bladder outlet obstruction (anatomical: prostate enlargement; functional: detrusor-sphincter-dyssynergia[1,2])	1 suprasacral 2 supraspinal 3 subsacral/lumbosacral 4 peripheral
	Urinary hesitancy *An individual describes difficulty in initiating micturition resulting in a delay in the onset of voiding after the individual is ready to pass urine.*	- Bladder outlet obstruction (anatomical: prostate enlargement, urethral stricture; functional: detrusor-sphincter-dyssynergia[1,2]) - Hypocontractile detrusor[3,4]	1 suprasacral 2 supraspinal 3 subsacral/lumbosacral 4 peripheral
	Urinary intermittency *An individual describes urine flow which stops and starts, on one or more occasions, during micturition.*	- Detrusor-sphincter-dyssynergia[1,2] - Hypocontractile detrusor[3,4]	1 suprasacral 2 supraspinal 3 subsacral/lumbosacral 4 peripheral
	Slow urinary stream *Perception of reduced urine flow, usually compared to previous performance or in comparison to others.*	- Bladder outlet obstruction (anatomical: prostate enlargement, urethral stricture; functional: detrusor-sphincter-dyssynergia[1,2]) - Hypocontractile detrusor[3,4]	1 suprasacral 2 supraspinal 3 subsacral/lumbosacral 4 peripheral

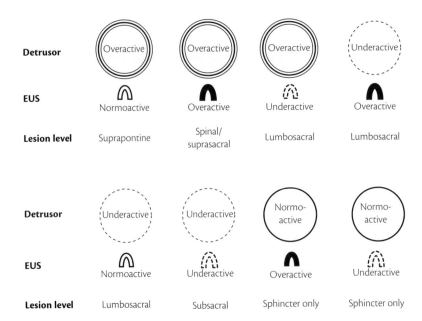

Fig. 24.3 Classification system according to Madersbacher H. The various types of neurogenic bladder dysfunction: an update of current therapeutic concepts. Paraplegia. 1990;28:217–29, showing different lesion levels of spinal cord injury and the according lower urinary tract dysfunction that can result from the spinal cord lesion.

Figure adapted from: Madersbacher H. The various types of neurogenic bladder dysfunction: an update of current therapeutic concepts. Paraplegia. 1990;28:217–29.

Table 24.3 Summary of a meta-analysis by Jeong et al. [3] on the associations between injury levels and urodynamic findings in patients with SCI

Level of spinal cord injury	Cervical	Thoracic	Lumbar	Sacral	Statistical difference (Pearson chi-sqare test)
No. of Patients	259	215	137	46	
DO [%]	65	78	49	22	p < 0.001
DSD [%]	63	72	33	13	p < 0.001
DA [%]	9	9	39	70	p < 0.001
Normal [%]	1	2	2	9	p = 0.002

Thoracic lesions are indicated to spinal cord level T9 or above, and injuries at the T10 through T12 levels are included in lumbar lesions. The combined suprasacral and sacral lesions have been excluded from this analysis.

DO detrusor overactivity. DSD detrusor-sphincter-dyssynergia, DA detrusor acontractility.

rectal compliance and hypertonia. Preserved reflex coordination and stool propulsion in conjunction with unaltered or elevated sphincter tone predisposes to constipation and faecal retention [14], but might also result in reflex defecation and incontinence. In contrast, subconal lesions (i.e. cauda equina lesions), typically result in rectal hypotonia and increased compliance, leading to slow stool propulsion. Subconal lesions are commonly associated with constipation and a significant risk of incontinence due to the atonic external anal sphincter and lack of control over the levator ani muscle [14]. However, this classical view does not always match with clinical findings, which might be due to the fact that the exact level and extent of autonomic nervous system lesions is difficult to assess and that the exact post-injury interaction of the intrinsic and extrinsic nervous system is unknown. Newer investigations demonstrated increased sigmoid and rectal compliance

in supraconal SCI, suggesting that supraconal lesions might also cause increased sympathetic input, potentially due to loss of supraspinal control [15].

Increased colonic transit time occurs with supraconal and subconal lesions, which is partly related to an interrupted or reduced gastrocolic reflex [16]. Supraconal lesions may affect whole colonic transit, whereas subconal lesions predominantly cause transit delay in the left colon and rectosigmoid [17]. The latter is also frequently associated with other neurological diseases such as PD and MS, causing constipation and defecation difficulties [18, 19]. In PD, however, pathophysiological processes in NBD seem to be very different to SCI or MS, as PD seems to directly affect also the intrinsic nervous system of the GI tract. This is supported by the reduced number of dopaminergic cells found in the colonic wall of PD patients [20] and Lewy body formation in the enteric ganglia [21].

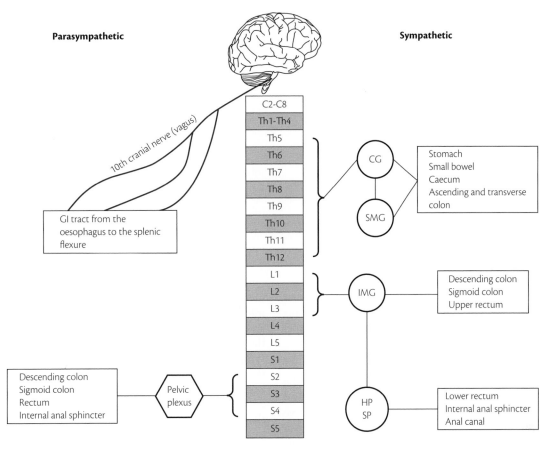

Fig. 24.4 Schematic display of autonomic nervous system innervation of the GI tract. CG celiac ganglion, HP hypogastric plexus, IMG inferior mesenteric ganglion, SMG superior mesenteric ganglion, SP sacral plexus.

Loss of anorectal sensation and external anal sphincter control rather depend on the extent of lesion than its level and are next to faecal retention key aspects that facilitate faecal incontinence.

Pathophysiology of sexual dysfunction in neurological disorders

Physiology of human sexual function

Sexual function plays an important role for the quality of life, body perception and self-esteem. Next to reproductive purposes of sexual function, it is an endogenous desire of humans to become involved in sexual activities and to sustain sexual relationships.

Human sexual function can be described to occur in different phases. Masters and Johnson identified four different phases: (1) sexual arousal/excitement, (2) plateau, (3) orgasm, and (4) satisfaction/resolution [22]. Later, Kaplan proposed three phases: (1) sexual drive, (2) sexual excitement, and (3) orgasm, with each of these phases requiring specific neurophysiological processes [23]. Generally, these phases are not strictly successive but rather they can strongly overlap and even vary in sequence.

Supraspinal neuronal processes are involved in each phase of sexual response and are a mandatory prerequisite to experience sexual arousal, sexual excitement, and orgasm. Supraspinal processes even allow humans to experience sexual arousal and excitement from spontaneous memory. In consequence, the brain can be regarded as the primary human sex organ [24]. Although

recent neuroimaging studies have provided valuable additional insight into supraspinal activity during different phases of human sexual response [25], the exact processes and neurophysiological mechanism are not yet fully known or understood. Findings from studies in animals and humans (predominantly lesion studies) propose a network of supraspinal key areas that are involved in sexual arousal and behaviour (Table 24.4) [26, 27]. This network influences spinal sexual reflexes and is itself modulated by sensory feedback (e.g. visual, tactile, olfactory, auditory), and by neuroendocrine effects of sex hormones. Dopamine, oxytocin, gonadotropin-releasing hormone, melanocyte-stimulating hormone, and norepinephrine (noradrenaline) act as excitatory neurotransmitters, whereas opioids, endocannabinoids, and serotonin act as inhibitory neurotransmitters within this network [28]. Lesion of one or more key areas can result in significant aberrant sexual function and behaviour [26].

The neuronal structures mediating the spinal sexual reflexes encompass sympathetic fibres originating from T12–L2, parasympathetic fibres from S2–S4, and somatosensory fibres from S2–S4 [27]. The sympathetic fibres travel via the sympathetic chain to the superior hypogastric plexus, from where they join the pelvic plexus via the hypogastric nerve. Parasympathetic fibres directly project to the pelvic plexus, from where both sympathetic and parasympathetic fibres travel within the cavernous nerve to the external genitalia [27]. Somatosensory fibres travel via the pudendal nerve that provides branches with motoric fibres that innervate pelvic

Table 24.4 Overview on key brain areas in sexual function and their probable role in human sexual function

Key brain regions	Sexual function
Subcortical regions	
Septal region (paraventricular nucleus)	Pleasurable response, orgasm
Hypothalamus (medial preoptic area)	Neuroendocrine and autonomic aspects of sexual drive, sexual orientation
Ansa lenticularis and pallidum	Sexual drive
Cortical regions	
Frontal lobes	Motor components of sexual behaviour, control of sexual response (disinhibition)
Parietal lobes (paracentral lobule)	Genital sensation
Temporal lobes (amygdala)	Sexual orientation, sexual drive, and arousal

Reproduced from Journal of neurology, neurosurgery, and psychiatry, Baird AD, Wilson SJ, Bladin PF et al., 78,1042–9, © 2007 with permission from BMJ Publishing Group Ltd.

floor musculature including bulbospongiosus and ischiocavernosus muscle and branches with sensory fibres that mediate afferent sensory information from the external genitalia to the dorsal roots of S2–S4, and from there to supraspinal centres such as the medial preoptic area via anterolateral spinothalamic pathways [27].

Male sexual function

In males, the cavernous nerves travel beneath the prostate to the corpora cavernosa to innervate vascular smooth muscles and endothelium. The dorsal nerve of the penis and the perineal nerve are both terminal branches of the pudendal nerve that provide sensory information from the glans and dorsal part of the penis (dorsal nerve of the penis) and from the ventral part of the penis, posterior scrotum and perineum (perineal nerve) [27]. In addition, the ilioinguinal nerve, which is a branch of the first lumbar nerve, provides sensory information form the skin of the anterior and upper part of the scrotum and penile root.

Although the exact relationship between sexual desire and arousal can be complex and is often influenced by different psychological and cognitive aspects, male sexual arousal is usually represented by penile erection. Since an erect penis is the main prerequisite to perform 'conventional' sexual intercourse, erectile function is often used as pars pro toto for male sexual function. In general, two types of erection can be distinguished: psychogenic and reflexogenic erection. Both forms of erections interact synergistically, improving the response of each other to achieve an erection that is adequate for penetration and sexual intercourse [29, 30].

Psychogenic erection is initiated by erotic stimuli (i.e. visual, tactile, olfactory, auditory, and/or imaginative). Such erotic stimuli can trigger responses in the brain that cause the release of neurotransmitters such as dopamine and oxytocin, which facilitate hypothalamic emission of pro-erectile signals to the sacral erectile centre (S2–S4). Parasympathetic outflow from the sacral erectile centre via the cavernous nerve to the arterial sinuses of the corpora cavernosa causes smooth muscle relaxation mainly by release of nitric oxide of the parasympathetic nerve terminals [29]. This causes arterial dilatation and increased arterial inflow with consequent expansion of the corpora cavernosa. Simultaneously, the expanding corpora cavernosa compress the intracavernosal and subtunical venous plexus, prohibiting outward flow of blood and thus allowing penile expansion to full erection [29].

The male sexual cycle usually climaxes with ejaculation and the perception of orgasm. Ejaculation requires emission of semen into the posterior urethra, which is sympathetically controlled and induced by peristaltic contractions of the smooth muscles of the vas deferens, seminal vesicles, and prostate [29]. In addition, sympathetic output provides closure of the bladder neck, which is required to prevent retrograde ejaculation. Intermittent relaxation of the external urethral sphincter allows semen to enter the bulbous urethra from where it is propelled outside through the urethral lumen (= ejaculation) by rhythmic contractions of the ischiocavernous and bulbocavernosus muscle, which are induced by a sacral reflex mediated by the pudendal nerve [29]. However, full erection is not always necessary for ejaculation and orgasm, and ejaculation is not necessarily accompanied by orgasm.

Next to the decrease in proerectile signals from the brain after achieving orgasm, penile detumescence is caused by the sympathetic output required for emission, resulting in contraction of the smooth muscles of the arterial sinuses in the corpora cavernosa by release of norepinephrine (noradrenaline) [29].

Reflexogenic erections are induced by genital stimulation and mediated by the dorsal nerve of the penis to the sacral erectile centre (afferent pathway) and from there via parasympathetic fibres in the cavernous nerve to the corpora cavernosa (efferent pathway) [30]. Reflexogenic erections alone are of short duration, and thus usually inadequate for sexual intercourse.

Female sexual function

In females, the cavernous nerves presumably travel along the lateral surface of the vaginal wall and innervate the vagina and the clitoral crus, which is part of the clitoral erectile tissue [31]. Sensory information is conveyed via the terminal branches of the pudendal nerve from the glans of the clitoris and vaginal introitus (dorsal clitoral nerve) and the posterior part of labia majora and perineum (perineal nerve). Sensory information from the anterior part of the labia majora and mons pubis is conveyed via the ilioinguinal nerve.

Female sexual function is generally less well understood and investigated compared to males. Nevertheless, there seems to be some similarity between males and females in regard to basic neural organization of sexual function and the subsequent genital responses [31]. The correlate of erection as response to sexual arousal and excitement in males is vaginal lubrification and clitoral erection in females, which are caused by increased blood flow to the vagina and clitoral cavernosal arteries. Engorgement of blood in the vaginal wall raises the pressure inside the capillaries and creates an increase in transudation of plasma through the vaginal epithelium [31]. In addition, the vagina lengthens and dilates during sexual arousal as a result of vaginal wall smooth muscle relaxation. Such processes are probably mediated via parasympathetic output of nitric oxide and vasoactive peptide. However, the exact mechanism remains to be elucidated and involvement of other neurotransmitter is matter of current investigations [31].

Towards orgasm, vaginal luminal pressure progressively increase and finally climax in a series of clonic contractions of striated and smooth muscles [31].

Despite some basic similarities, a major difference between male and female sexual function seems to be related to sexual drive and subjective perception of sexual arousal. In women, the feeling of sexual arousal might result more from cognitive processing of stimulus meaning and content [31]. Basson et al. observed that a women's motivation to engage in sexual activity is often responsive rather than spontaneous [32]. Especially in ongoing relationships, a woman's sexual motivation seems to be mainly driven by her wish for emotional intimacy with her partner and to enhance it. Once having perceived sexual stimuli, women started to become sexually excited and then developed the desire to continue the sexual experience [32].

Impact of different neurological disorders on sexual function

Stroke

Post stroke sexual activity significantly declines in both genders and seems to be mainly related to reduced or lost libido [33]. Strokes in certain brain areas can affect sexual desire; strokes affecting frontolimbic connections, and areas such as frontal lobe or thalamus, can result in disinhibited sexual behaviour, whereas strokes of basal ganglia and parietal areas seems to diminish sexual drive [33]. Ejaculatory dysfunction has also been reported [33].

However, stroke rarely cause sexual disorders alone and is mostly a consequence of factors associated with stroke such as psychological disorders, such as depression, and concomitant medication (i.e. antihypertensive medications such as beta-blockers) [34, 35]. In addition, most stroke patients have concomitant risk factors for sexual dysfunction such as diabetes and vascular disease. Other factors contributing to a decreased sexuality post stroke are sensorymotor and cognitive impairments with potentially 'unattractive' behaviours such as urinary incontinence and drooling, and psychological factors such as fear of relapse and anxiety by the patient and partner [34, 36].

Epilepsy

Epilepsy can provoke involuntary sexual gestures (i.e. self-fondling, grabbing, or scratching of the genitals), as part of a frontolimbic or temporolimbic complex partial seizure [34]. Temporal seizures may also generate sexual or erotic auras that can even result in ictal orgasms. During interictal intervals most patients are rather hyposexual [34]. Certain antiepileptic drugs, especially those that induce the hepatic enzyme P450 such as phenytoin, phenobarbitone, and carbamazepine, can cause sexual dysfunction due to changes in free testosterone by increasing the levels of sex-hormone-binding-globuline. Valproic acid, in contrast, has a P450-inhibiting function and can also elevate androgen levels as well as oestradiol [34]. If such effect is beneficial for the sexual function in epileptic patients remains controversial. Whether antiepileptic drugs without P450 enzyme activity, such as gabapentin, lamotrigine, and pregabalin, have less impact on sexual function remain to be clarified [34].

Sixty-four percent of epilepsy patients receiving temporal lobe resection, compared to 25% receiving extratemporal resection as treatment of epilepsy, reported changes in sexual function with a similar proportion of increase and decrease in sexual function [37].

Multiple sclerosis

MS frequently cause sexual dysfunctions, with about 50–75% erectile dysfunction, 50% ejaculatory and/or orgasmic dysfunction, 39% sexual interest dysfunction, and 37% anorgasmia in men [38]. For women with MS about 61% were reported with sensory genital dysfunction, 24–60% having difficulty achieving orgasm, 40% with reduced libido, and 36% having decreased vaginal lubrication [38]. Initially, symptoms may vary in severity due to incompleteness of lesion. However, especially in MS sexual dysfunction is not only caused by the direct neurogenic lesion but also due to secondary (i.e. fatigue, weakness, spams, cognitive impairments, pain, etc.), and tertiary (i.e. psychological, emotional, social and cultural aspects of having a debilitating chronic disease), factors of MS [38].

Demyelating lesions in the pons seems to be related to orgasmic dysfunctions, but otherwise clear correlations between MS lesion sites and specific sexual dysfunction could not yet been demonstrated [38]. The exact effect of the level of MS-related disability on sexual dysfunction remains also unclear [39].

Parkinson's disease

Sexual dysfunction is common in PD, with 54–79% erectile dysfunction and a high rate of men with difficulties to ejaculate and/or reach orgasm [40]. Women with PD frequently demonstrate vaginal tightness, loss of lubrication, involuntary urination, anxiety, and inhibition [40]. Although PD affects supraspinal areas relevant for sexual function and PD patients demonstrated a higher prevalence of sexual dysfunction compared to healthy controls, the same difference in prevalence could not be demonstrated compared to patients with a chronic non-neurological disease, thus questioning a decisive impact of the known brain 'lesions' related to PD on the prevalence of sexual dysfunction in PD [40].

Similar to MS there are secondary and tertiary concomitant factors of PD that additionally impair sexual function.

Dopaminergic treatment may increase sexual desire in PD patients, which may be related to inhibition of prolactin [34, 41] or excessive D3-receptor stimulation [42]. Following deep brain stimulation of the subthalamic nucleus, male PD patients, especially when under 60, appeared more satisfied with their sexual well-being over a short term follow up period [43].

Multiple system atrophy

Erectile dysfunction can be an early symptom of MSA before further neurological symptoms occur [34]. Especially, the ability for reflex erections can be lost due to the frequently MSA-affected intermediolateral cell columns of the sacral cord that convey efferent parasympathetic fibres of the erectile reflex arc [44].

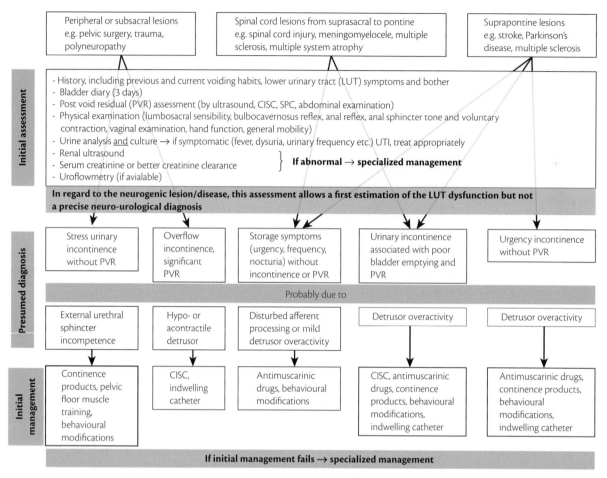

Fig. 24.5 Schematic overview on initial assessments and management options of different NLUTD according to the lesion site. Adapted from [62].

It is currently unclear if ejaculatory dysfunctions are equally common or if women demonstrate comparable symptoms [34].

Spinal cord injury

Sexual dysfunction is highly prevalent in SCI and patients might indicate their loss of sexual function as most devastating aspect of their neurological disorder [1]. The pattern and severity of sexual dysfunction largely depends on the level and extension of the lesion resulting in individual clinical manifestations.

Immediately post injury, during spinal shock, reflexive sexual responses are extinct. Thereafter, reflexogenic erections in men and reflexogenic lubrification in women can occur when the sacral erectile centre (S2–4) and the peripheral nerves are preserved. However, reflexogenic erections and lubrification is usually short lived and might not be sufficient for comfortable penetration or intercourse. The ability of psychogenic arousal seems to be usually preserved if the level of lesion is below T12 but not in lesions above T9 [45].

In men, ejaculatory dysfunction is more frequently observed than erectile dysfunction, of which the latter can be regained to some degree within 2 years after SCI [45]. With a complete lesion only 4–18% of patients had preserved ability to ejaculate during sexual activity [46]. Newer, but smaller, reports indicate that about 25% of men with complete lower motor neuron lesions of the sacral spinal segment may have psychogenic erections and may be

able to ejaculate despite lost reflexogenic erectile function [47] and that 38% of patients with complete tetraplegia were able to experience orgasm and ejaculation [48].

Orgasms can be perceived/experienced by SCI men and women, though more commonly in women than men [45]. In general, men with incomplete SCI are more likely to achieve simultaneous orgasm and ejaculation than those with complete SCI [49]. However, the quality of orgasm might vary substantially and is not necessarily associated with ejaculation. The ability to perceive orgasm cannot be determined by completeness of SCI [45].

Similarly, women with complete SCI can experience genital sensation and orgasm [49]. Reaching orgasm might require more time and might also require stimulation of other erogenous body areas above lesion level [45]. However, the quality of orgasm in SCI women seems to be comparable to non-injured controls [50]. Interestingly, women with complete spinal cord injury above T10 have been reported to experience sensations in response to vaginal-cervical mechanical self-stimulation [51]. The neuronal structure responsible for this phenomenon appears to be the vagus nerve that seems to permit sensory perception from the cervix and vagina bypassing the spinal cord.

Secondary and tertiary factors such as mobility impairments and psychological issues are highly relevant and need to be considered in sexual dysfunction due to SCI.

Fertility

Impairment of fertility due to neurogenic disease or lesion usually affects men with SCI due to ejaculatory dysfunction and/or reduced sperm quality and quantity. The decline of sperm quality occurs quite rapidly during the first few weeks following injury and remains stable on a low level in chronic SCI (>1 year) [52, 53]. SCI patients that were able to ejaculate by masturbation showed significantly better sperm motility than patients not able to ejaculate by masturbation [54]. Potential factors contributing to the decline in sperm quality following SCI include elevated scrotal temperature due to autonomic dysfunction, infrequency of ejaculation, and methods of bladder management [53].

Female fertility seems to be mainly unaffected by neurogenic disease or lesions, but sufficient data are lacking. During the spinal shock phase, amenorrhoea is observed in 50% to 60% of premenopausal women. Within 6 months and 1 year after SCI, 50% and 90% of women resume their normal menstrual cycle, respectively [49].

Principles of therapy and management

Therapeutical principles in the management of bladder dysfunction

The principal purpose of treatment of neurogenic lower urinary tract dysfunction (NLUTD) is threefold:

1. Protection and maintenance of upper urinary tract function and prevention of long-term complications
   Based on clinical observations and clinical long-term outcomes it is generally assumed that frequently or constantly elevated pressures in the lower urinary tract, will sooner or later compromise LUT and upper urinary tract function which is often accompanied by severe long-term sequelae and complications [55–58]. Such sequelae and complications include detrusor hypertrophy, recurrent symptomatic urinary tract infections, autonomic dysreflexia, vesicoureteral reflux, formation of urinary calculi, urosepsis, and renal failure, and were reported to be the primary cause of death in individuals with SCI until the mid 1970s [59].
   To protect upper urinary tract function and prevent long-term complications, it is necessary to maintain or restore the LUT as a low-pressure urinary reservoir and to provide unrestricted, low-pressure urinary drainage from the kidneys to this urinary reservoir and from the reservoir outwards.
   Therapeutic advances in the dynamic field of neuro-urology aiming at this important treatment goal have essentially contributed to a higher life expectancy of SCI patients and the fact that urinary tract complications are no longer the primary cause of death in SCI, at least in developed countries.
   However, there still remain many questions unanswered and the understanding of the exact pathomechanisms and interrelations between different NLUTD and their long-term complications is often poor. For example, it is still controversially discussed which level of intravesical pressure over which time is hazardous for upper urinary tract function or not. There is only one study suggesting an intravesical pressure of >40 cmH$_2$O to be a risk factor for upper urinary tract damage, i.e. vesicoureteral reflux and ureteral dilatation [56]. However, even in subjects without NLUTD intravesical pressures during micturition can easily exceed 40 cmH$_2$O without being characterized

abnormal or hazardous [60, 61]. Thus, not only the pressure level itself but also duration and frequency of upper urinary tract exposure to pressure exceeds seem to be relevant but reliable reference values are currently unknown.

2. Independency in the daily management of LUT function
   Independency in LUT management is important for the patient's self-esteem, a simpler integration into a work activity, and the relief of involved caregivers. To provide independency in the management of LUT function, it is important to use treatments that are adapted to the patient's individual situation. Thus it is often reasonable and necessary to involve rehabilitation specialists (e.g. ergo- and physiotherapists), into the discussion of individual neuro-urological therapy options. Urological treatments that advance the independent management of LUT (dys-) function include amongst others, clean intermittent self-catheterization (CISC), continent catheterizable abdominal stoma, sacral anterior root stimulator (SARS), and ileum conduit.

3. Improvement of the quality of life
   Improvement of quality of life in regard to NLUTD is a highly individual process but usually involves at least one of the following aspects: (a) achievement of continence, (b) low time consumption and high practicability of applied therapies, (c) recovery of spontaneous self-controlled micturition, (d) prevention of recurrent complications of LUT dysfunction such as urinary tract infrctions (UTIs), and (e) the reduction and/or abolishment of irritating and/or painful LUT sensations.

Therapeutic principles in the management of bowel dysfunction

The principal purpose of treatment of NBD is twofold:

1. Regular and timely bowel evacuation
   Depending on the severity and type of NBD, this therapeutic principle is important to prevent severe constipation, ileus, autonomic dysreflexia, feacal incontinence, haemorrhoids, and anal fissures. In consideration of mobility restrictions, especially hand function, management of NBD should be designed to be performed as independently as possible.

2. Prevention of faecal incontinence
   Faecal incontinence severely reduces quality of life and often impedes successful integration into social activities.

Therapeutical principles in the management of sexual dysfunction

The principal purpose treating sexual dysfunction is twofold:

1. Improving or maintaining sexual function that enables the patient to sustain a satisfactory sexual relationship
   Sexual dysfunctions can have a detrimental effect on the quality of life of each patient resulting in or further increasing frustration, anger, reduced self-esteem, anxiety, and depression concomitant to the neurological disease. Thus, treatment of sexual dysfunction is important to improve quality of life and to prevent further psychological sequelae.
   However, the ingredients for a 'satisfactory sexual relationship' are defined and selected on a highly individual basis and are not necessarily confined only to good penile erection and

vaginal lubrification. It is thus important to know and respect each patient's sexual attitude, orientation, and sociocultural background.

2. Providing fertility support

Fertility might be impaired, especially in male spinal cord injury patients, preventing them from having their own child. However, having a child can represent hope for the future and some normalcy for people with SCI and their partner [53]. Here, counselling is important, and when necessary or required, specialized support for fertility measures should be provided or initiated at according centres.

Practical treatment

Practical treatment and management of bladder dysfunction

In general, all patients with known neurological lesions should be assessed in regard to LUT dysfunction, as LUT dysfunctions are highly prevalent in this group of patients but do not always cause symptoms. In addition, symptoms might not correlate with severity of dysfunction.

Non-neurological causes of LUT dysfunction such as bladder outlet obstruction due to benign prostate enlargement, pelvic organ prolapse, and fistulas need to be considered and ruled out or treated accordingly.

In patients without known or obvious neurological disease or lesion who present symptoms of LUT dysfunction, a latent neurological cause should be considered and excluded or confirmed if possible.

To adequately treat NLUTD it is essential to understand the mechanism leading to the NLUTD which largely depends on the site and extent of the neurogenic lesion/disease. Figures 24.5 and 24.6 provide a simple but practical overview on initial and specialized assessments and management options of different NLUTD according to the lesion site.

It is often advisable to manage bladder and bowel dysfunctions at the same time as treatment outcomes are usually more successful due to frequent interactions between bladder and bowel function.

All treatments for NLUTD require regular and meticulous follow-up to evaluate treatment success and to be able to readjust treatment in case of failure, insufficient success, adverse events or altered prerequisites, i.e. progression of neurological disease.

In order to comply with the aforementioned principles of NLUTD treatment, the following therapeutic strategies are most relevant (for more detailed information and specific evidence based recommendations see also [62, 63]):

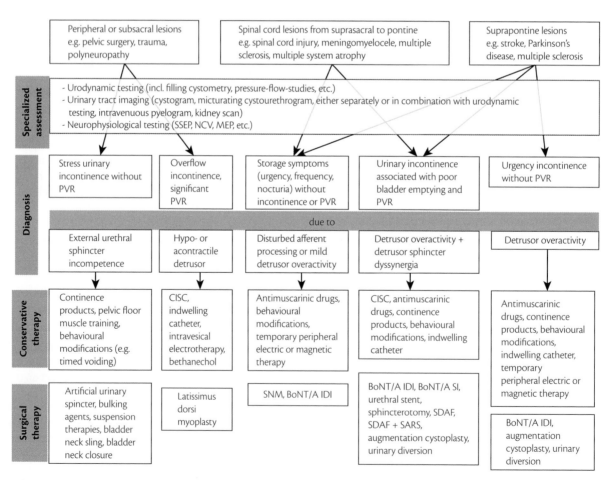

Fig. 24.6 Schematic overview on specialized assessments and management options of different NLUTD according to the lesion site. Adapted from [62].

Inhibition or reduction of detrusor overactivity

Inhibition or reduction of detrusor overactivity is relevant to decrease storage symptoms, urinary incontinence, intravesical pressures, and functional deterioration of lower and upper urinary tract. Inhibition or reduction of detrusor overactivity is mainly achieved by the following conservative or surgical measures:

Conservative treatment
Antimuscarinics

The first-line conservative measure to reduce NDO are antimuscarinic drugs [63] that can be applied either orally (oxybutynin, trospium chloride, tolterodine, solifenacin, darifenacin, propiverine, fesoterodine), transdermally (oxybutynin), or intravesically (oxybutynin, propiverine). Detrusor contractions are mainly elicited by parasympathetic input to the detrusor via acethylcholine release from parasympathetic nerve terminals, i.e. pelvic nerve, and subsequent activation of muscarinic M2 and M3 receptors on the detrusor [64]. Antimuscarinics cause a competitive blockage of the M2 and M3 receptors resulting in a reduction of parasympathetic influence on the detrusor and consequently a reduction in detrusor contractility [65].

With the exception of transdermal application via patch, antimuscarinics usually need to be applied on a daily basis. Extended-release formulations are usually better tolerable and enable a once daily treatment. Although antimuscarinics are generally regarded as safe, the most frequent side effects that are associated with antimuscarinic treatment include dry mouth, constipation, blurred vision, somnolence, dizziness, urinary retention, and cognitive impairment. Untreated, close-angle glaucoma is a contraindication for antimuscarinics. Using the intravesical or transdermal application, side effects of antimuscarinic drugs are supposed to be fewer than with oral application

but antimuscarinic patches might cause local skin reactions [66]. Although some large clinical trials could demonstrate statistically significant efficacy differences between certain antimuscarinics, such differences remain rather marginal form a clinical point of view [66]. Differences in the safety and tolerability profiles, depending on the selectivity for specific muscarinic receptor subtypes on other organs than the bladder, seems to be more relevant and should be considered when choosing an antimuscarinic drug for a specific patient. In example, darifenacin, trospium chloride, and fesoterodine cause none or only very few impairments of cognition and memory due to low central nervous system penetration, which is especially relevant when treating elderly or already cognitively impaired patients [66].

Patients with severe DO due to neurogenic lesions, i.e. complete SCI, might need higher antimuscarinic doses to adequately reduce DO than officially approved for overactive bladder symptoms (OABS) [67, 68]. However, with higher doses, adverse events might be more pronounced, decreasing the benefit/risk ratio and patient compliance with this therapy [69, 70]. In general, long-term results of antimuscarinic treatment are sparse.

Temporary, peripheral/external neuromodulation

Neuromodulative therapies do not stimulate a certain efferent nerve to cause a muscle contraction rather they cause modulation of afferent and efferent signals traveling in the nerve next to the source of stimulation. Thus, neuromodulation has effects on the periphery and the central nervous system [71–73]. However, the exact mechanism of action of neuromodulation for LUT dysfunction remains unknown. It is hypothesized that in the dorsal horn of the sacral spinal cord, bladder afferent activity may be inhibited through interneurones activated by somatic sensory pathways originating in the external genitalia, perineum, lower limb and muscles of the pelvic floor via the

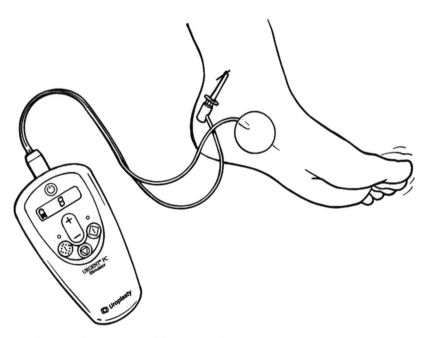

Fig. 24.7 Schematic display of electrode position for percutaneous tibial nerve stimulation.
Reprinted from The Journal of Urology, Volume 183, Issue 4, Kenneth M. Petersa, Donna J. Carricoa, Ramon A. Perez-Marreroc, Ansar U. Khand, Leslie S. Wooldridgeb, Gregory L. Davise, Scott A. MacDiarmidf, Randomized Trial of Percutaneous Tibial Nerve Stimulation Versus Sham Efficacy in the Treatment of Overactive Bladder Syndrome: Results From the SUmiT Trial, Pages 1438–1443, Copyright (2010), with permission from Elsevier.

pudendal and/or tibial nerve [74, 75]. This inhibitory interaction between larger somatic sensory fibres and small bladder afferents (A-delta or unmyelinated C fibres) could operate in a similar way to the 'gate control' theory of pain [76]. Animal studies suggest that pudendal nerve stimulation can elicit two effects [77]: (1) suppression of pelvic nerve activity to the detrusor by inhibition of the sacral micturition reflex at either the afferent input or the parasympathetic pre-ganglionic motoneurones and (2) activation of sympathetic neurones which run in the hypogastric nerves and cause inhibition of the parasympathetic efferent motoneurones at the level of the pelvic ganglia.

Dorsal genital nerve and percutaneous tibial nerve stimulation are currently the most frequently investigated temporary external neuromodulative methods. For dorsal genital nerve stimulation (DGNS), several techniques have been described, including usage of transcutaneous needle electrodes. Usually bipolar stimulation is applied using two self-attaching surface electrodes on the dorsal side of the penis or using two ring electrodes. In females, surface electrodes are usually attached to the labia majora and to the contralateral pubic skin. For percutaneous tibial nerve stimulation (PTNS), a 34-gauge needle electrode is inserted approximately 5 cm cephalad to the medial malleolus and posterior to the tibia (Figure 24.7) with a surface electrode on the arch of the foot [75]. Both methods provided promising initial results in the treatment of NDO and also demonstrate improvements of other urodynamic parameters [78–82]. However, there are few long-term results and larger randomized controlled trials, which might be, in addition to the handling and necessity for regular appliance of an external device, a reason that this kind of therapy is still not very commonly used, despite that commercially devices are available and adverse events are almost nonexistent.

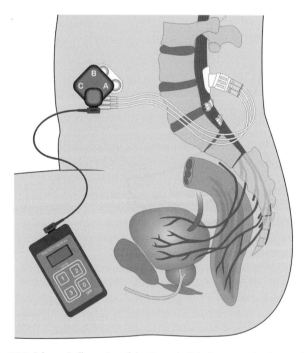

Fig. 24.8 Schematic illustration of the Finetech–Brindley neurostimulator and its position in the human body after implantation.
Reprinted by permission from Neurocontrol Inc.

Other conservative treatments

Other conservative treatments for NDO include pelvic floor muscle training with or without biofeedback [83], and intravesical electrostimulation [84, 85]. However, to be effective, such treatments often require at least some preserved motor and sensory control of the pelvic organs and muscles. In general, the current evidence for such treatments in NDO is rather poor and randomized controlled trials specifically investigating the efficacy of those therapies in NDO are needed to better evaluate their future potential in the treatment of NDO.

Minimally invasive treatment

There are two treatment options for NDO that require special attention, as they have drawn increasing attention during the last two decades: Botulinum toxin A (BoNT/A) intradetrusor injections and sacral neuromodulation (SNM). Although both require minor surgical intervention, such interventions are rather minimally invasive, reversible, and aim to preserve LUT structures and anatomy. Both therapies have significantly contributed to reduce the treatment gap between drug treatment and open surgery in the treatment of NDO.

BoNT/A intradetrusor injections

BoNT/A intradetrusor injections are performed using either a rigid or flexible cystoscope under local, spinal or general anesthesia. Spinal or general anesthesia is usually chosen if the patient has intact bladder sensibility or if the patient is prone to develop autonomic dysreflexia. Although there are still controversies in regard to the injection technique [86], the currently approved technique for treatment of NDO is the use of 200 units, as 1 ml (~6.7 units) injections across 30 sites into the detrusor, sparing the trigone [87].

BoNT/A is a 150 kDa molecule, consisting of a heavy and a light chain, of which the light chain destroys the docking molecules (SNAP-25) that are responsible for the release of the acetylcholine vesicles from the parasympathetic nerve terminals of the pelvic nerve into the neuromuscular junction [88, 89]. Thereby, BoNT/A causes a chemodenervation of the detrusor which is presumably not 100% but sufficient enough to cause a significant reduction in detrusor tone and pressure. However, this therapy is not self-applicable and patients have to return for reinjection, as the average duration of efficacy is 8 months [90] due to resprouting of the axon terminals [88, 89]. Despite their limited duration, BoNT/A intradetrusor injections are highly effective with only few and usually self-limited adverse events, including urinary retention, hematuria, injection site pain, procedure related urinary tract infection, and generalized muscle weakness [90]. Urinary retention has to be always considered and explained to the patient. Usually it is necessary that the patient learns how to perform CISC before the injections [91]. In SCI patients urinary retention might not be relevant in most cases, as patients are often already on CISC. Hematuria (2–21%) is usually very mild and self-limited, however, clotting parameters and concomitant medication (e.g. plavix, coumarin) should be checked to avoid a hemorrhagic vasical tamponade. Injection site pain is usually mild and can be avoided with adequate local, spinal or general anesthesia. Procedure related UTI (2–32%) can be treated with adequate antibiotic drugs following urine culture. Systematic antibiotic prophylaxis is not necessary and advisable, but might be considered in risk patients with recurrent pyelonephritis and vesico-ureteral reflux.

BoNT/A intradetrusor injections can be repeated without further adverse events, damage to bladder tissue or significant loss of efficacy [92, 93]. When using botulinum toxin A for NDO treatment, it should be considered that of the different botulinum toxin A formulations on the market only Onabotulinumtoxin A (Botox®) has been approved for the treatment of NDO by European and US governmental drug administrations.

Sacral neuromodulation (SNM)

SNM is a minimally invasive procedure that includes in a first step the placement of electrodes (tined lead, Medtronic, Minneapolis, Minnesota, USA) next to the sacral nerve roots, usually S3, by needle puncture of the S3 foramen under fluoroscopic control. During the procedure, repetitive test stimulations can be performed to find the optimal position for definitive electrode placement. Following the placement of the electrode, the electrode lead is passed subcutaneously and connected to an external temporary stimulator. Electrodes might be placed uni- or bilateral. The procedure can be performed in local or, if necessary, in general anaesthesia. Local anaesthesia has the advantage that the surgeon can obtain sensory feedback from the patient while placing the electrode. Using the external temporary stimulator, efficacy of SNM on LUT symptoms is evaluated using bladder diaries or even urodynamics on an outpatient basis. If SNM attributes to at least 50% improvement, a permanent neuromodulator (Interstim® or InterStim-II®, Medtronic, Minneapolis, Minnesota, USA) is implanted in a second step. The permanent stimulator is usually placed subcutaneously in the buttock. If the SNM test phase does not demonstrate successful symptom reduction, electrodes can be easily removed. During the test phase, adverse events appear to be extremely rare, whereas during the permanent SNM phase after neuromodulator implantation, adverse events such as lead migration (7%), pain at neuromodulator implantation site (5%), infection at neuromodulator implantation site (5%), hypersensitivity to stimulation (4%), infection at lead site (2%), pain at lead site (1%), lead fracture (1%), migration of neuromodulator (1%), malfunction of neuromodulator (1%), and other (4%) have been reported [94]. Surgical interventions that were required due to adverse events included explantation of the whole device (leads + neuromodulator) (11%), explantation of leads only (4%), drainage/evacuation of seroma/haematoma/abscess (1%), and other (4%) [94].

SNM does, similar to other neuromodulative procedures, not rely on stimulation of nerves to produce a contraction but rather on the influence of activity in one neural pathway that affects the pre-existing activity in another neural pathway by synaptic interaction. The stimulation applied by SNM reaches the S3 nerves and interferes with their neural activity, which seems to normalize LUT afferent and/or efferent signals, as OAB symptoms and DO can improve under SNM. The exact therapeutic mechanism of SNM in LUT dysfunction has not yet been completely understood but from the available evidence it is assumed that both, spinal reflexes and supraspinal networks are modulated [94, 95].

The current evidence for the use of SNM in NLUTD does not allow any definitive conclusion or recommendation, as only small prospective cohort studies or retrospective case series are available [94]. Nevertheless, recent studies could demonstrate promising results of SNM of treatment of NDO that should encourage to further pursue this technique and to perform a randomized controlled trial [94, 96].

Surgical treatment

Surgical measures to treat NDO include: sacral deafferentation, augmentation cystoplasty, and complete cystectomy with the creation of a new continent or incontinent urinary diversion.

Sacral deafferentation (with/without sacral anterior root stimulator)

The efficacy of the sacral deafferentation, also known as posterior rhizotomy, results from the direct interruption of the afferent part of the sacral reflex arc and consequently parasympathetic input to the detrusor muscle [97]. When properly done and complete transection of the sacral roots S2–S5 can be achieved, this operation leads to an acontractile or flaccid bladder, which can be emptied via CISC. In addition, sacral deafferentation can effectively abolish autonomic dysreflexia [97]. Disadvantage of this operation is that potentially preserved sensation of the pelvis and lower limbs and sexual function (e.g. reflex erections) will be lost [98]. In addition, the defecation reflex will be lost and secondary myoatrophy of buttock and lower limb musculature can occur, which in turn increases the risk of pressure ulcers.

However, in combination with a sacral anterior root stimulator (Finetech–Brindley bladder stimulation system, Fig. 24.8) patients can regain control of micturition and even improve erectile and defecation function [97]. Nevertheless, due to the sacral deafferentation, this procedure is mainly preserved for SCI patients [97, 98].

Augmentation cystoplasty

With an augmentation cystoplasty, overactive detrusor will be removed (sparing the trigone) or cleaved at the dome, and subsequently replaced or augmented by a pouch created from tissue of the gastrointestinal tract (usually ileum). This surgery is usually performed as open surgery and can be combined with a continent cutaneous urinary diversion to facilitate CISC via an abdominal site, when CISC via the urethra is not possible. An augmentation cystoplasty increases the bladder capacity and restricts detrusor contractility [99]. However, it requires a long hospitalization (2–4 weeks), some time to regenerate and readapt after discharge, and comes with the risks of an open abdominal surgery including bowl dysfunction (e.g. diarrhoea, obstruction), infection, and fistula formation [100]. Long-term complications can include changes in acid–base balance, urinary stone formation, and perforation of the augmentation [100]. Urinary incontinence via the urethra might still be possible in some cases and subsequent surgery might be necessary. Augmentation cystoplasty with or without continent cutaneous diversion should be only performed in patients who are able and willing to perform CISC. Otherwise the patient will gain nothing from this kind of surgery.

Cystectomy + urinary diversion

The complete bladder is removed and replaced by a newly created urinary reservoir. Operative and postoperative risks and complications are similar to those of the augmentation cystoplasty. However, complete cystectomy and creation of a new urinary reservoir might be more complex and time consuming and require the reimplantation of the ureters, which implies the risk of ureteral stenosis. The new urinary diversion can be constructed to be continent or incontinent. There are several different forms of continent urinary diversions available using different forms of pouches and neobladders [101, 102].

The construction of an incontinent urinary diversion is less complex and requires 'only' the connection of the ureters to the abdominal skin via a short ileum segment [103]. As the urine is now directly draining outwards, a urinary bag has to be placed on the stoma site to collect the draining urine. This latter operation, also known as ileum conduit, might appear radical, but is an excellent option for some patients with neurogenic LUT disorders. It requires usually less hospitalization than the augmentation cystoplasty or a continent urinary diversion, no CISC, no pads or diapers, no recurrent or daily drug treatment, and a urinary incontinence via the urethra is completely excluded. However, changes in kidney function and morphology, stenosis of the ureteroileal and ileocutaneous junction, and bowl dysfunctions are known postoperative complications [104, 105].

Reduction of bladder outlet resistance

The reduction of outlet resistance aims to improve bladder emptying, reduce post void residual, and to reduce intravesical pressures. It is mainly achieved by the following conservative or surgical measures:

Conservative treatment
Alpha-adrenoceptor antagonists
Alpha-adrenoceptor antagonists are traditionally used in bladder outlet obstruction due to benign prostate enlargement and are supposed to exert their effect by relaxation of smooth muscle in the prostate through a sympathetic response. However, recent studies have suggested that α receptors in the bladder, $α_{1D}$ receptors in the spinal cord, and dysfunction of the bladder neck or urethra could potentially be influenced by pharmacological manipulation of α receptors [106]. This might explain why selective and non-selective alpha-adrenoceptor antagonists have been demonstrated to be at least partially effective for decreasing bladder outlet resistance, residual urine and autonomic dysreflexia in NLUTD [63].

Indwelling catheter
An indwelling urethral catheter might appear as simple and handy solution, as it is easy to apply by trained/specialized personnel, nearly ubiquitarily available, immediately reduces bladder outlet resistance, and does not require surgery. However, to effectively reduce intravesical storage pressures in case of DO and/or DSD, the catheter needs to be on permanent drainage. In consequence, bladder capacity might decrease over time which often limits the later use of conservative therapies. Other frequent complications of indwelling urethral catheters are urethral trauma, scaring and bleeding, urethritis, bladder stones, recurrent or chronic urinary tract infections, epididymo-orchitis, bladder neck incompetence, urethral erosion, fistulas, discomfort and pain [62]. Long-term treatment using indwelling catheters seems to be associated with a higher incidence of bladder cancer [107, 108].

The use of a suprapubic catheter can overcome at least the uretheral complications and has the advantage that it can be much better used for diagnostic and training purposes if applicable, i.e. to assess post void residual volume if voluntary micturition can be initiated. Suprapubic catheters, however, require a minor surgical procedure in local or general anaesthesia with generally low but potential risk of injury to other pelvic organs and structures.

Indwelling catheters require regular changing every 4 to 6 weeks or earlier if the catheter is clogged or in case of recurrent symptomatic UTIs.

In conclusion, indwelling catheters, preferably suprapubic catheters, are an option especially for short-term use (i.e. during the evaluation phase of LUT dysfunction after SCI before CISC is established), and for some patients also as long-term treatment if other treatment concepts are not applicable or failed.

Surgical treatment
Surgical therapies for the reduction of the outflow resistance in case of NDO require the wearing of a condom catheter thereafter, as the patients are usually completely incontinent which needs to be explained to and comprehended by the patient. Before considering this therapy, the ability of using a condom catheter needs to be evaluated. Consequently, these treatment options are mainly preserved for men, as there is no adequate alternative for a condom catheter in women.

Endoscopic resection/transection
Under cystoscopic view, the functionally or anatomically obstructive structure (e.g. bladder neck, urethral sphincter, prostate) is either resected using an electrical resection sling or transected using a cold knife or an electrical knife. Very often a re-operation becomes necessary at some time during follow-up to achieve a continuous good functional result [109].

Urethral stents
Urethral stents are a very simple and potentially reversible technique to achieve a free urinary outflow and to keep the intravesical pressures low. Placed endoscopically into the urethra, they distend the functionally or anatomically obstructive structure in the urethra (e.g. bladder neck, urethral sphincter, prostate) and keep it open [110–112]. Urethral stents appear to be similar effective compared to surgical sphincterotomy with the advantage of reversibility [113, 114]. However, if the stent does not epithelialize well, dislocation and formation of urinary calculi frequently occur, rendering removal difficult. Temporary stents provide the possibility to assess the effect of reduced outlet resistance on bladder function and the necessity for further, more invasive therapy.

BoNT/A sphincter injections
Although off-label treatment, it might be a minimally invasive option in selected cases to decrease DSD by chemodenervation of the external urethral sphincter. However, the current evidence is still low and efficacy appears highly variable [115–117] which might be related to patient selection and injection technique, i.e. transurethral injection vs transperineal injections with or without EMG control [116, 118, 119]. Hence, this treatment requires further evaluation.

Promoting self-controlled bladder emptying or voluntary micturition
Clean intermittent self-catheterisztion (CISC)
Introduced in 1972 by Lapides [120], it is today's gold standard to regularly, efficiently, and autonomously empty the bladder in case of voiding dysfunction. During CISC, the patient introduces a catheter transurethrally into the bladder and drains the urine through the catheter into a urine bag or directly into the toilet. Catheter models and characteristics significantly improved during the last decades and today there is a wide selection of high-tech

catheters available, covering the needs of nearly every patient. Intelligent integrated insertion aids reduce additional material (e.g. disinfection material, sterile compresses, gloves) to a minimum and enable even patients with mild to moderate impaired hand function to perform CISC. This technique is atraumatic and allows an efficient and timely evacuation of urine, although preparation might be a little time-consuming in some cases (e.g. women who are wheelchair bound).

Intravesical electric stimulation

Already described in 1878 by the Danish surgeon Mathias Hieronymus Saxtorph [121] and later revisited by Francis Katona [122], intravesical electric stimulation is still the only conservative treatment that potentially can improve detrusor contractility and sensibility providing that the patient has unimpaired detrusor tissue and only incomplete neurogenic lesion with at least some preserved pathways between bladder and supraspinal centres [123]. Although more recent studies showed promising results [84, 124], the initial outstanding results of Katona et al. [125] in children with meningomyelocele could not be reproduced. Due to the overall heterogeneous data with partly conflicting results and the lack of randomized controlled trials, intravesical electric therapy is not considered a first line treatment but might be an option prior to more invasive treatments. However, intravesical electric therapy is extremely time-consuming and requires frequent urodynamic follow-up to control treatment success and potentially adjust stimulation parameters.

Continent catheterizable abdominal stoma

If CISC via the native urethra is not possible but would be possible if the bladder could be catheterized via the abdominal skin, a continent catheterizable abdominal stoma is a reasonable option. A continent catheterizable abdominal stoma is a construction of a catheterizable tube usually from the appendix (Mitrofanoff technique; [126, 127]) or a small segment of ileum (Monti technique; [128]). This tube is then implanted into the bladder or cystoplasty where required and connected to the abdominal skin (usually at the umbilicus). To prevent urinary leakage through the catherizable tube, the implantation into the bladder or cystoplasty can be performed through a sub-mucous tunnel (= antirefluxive) to create a valve-like continence mechanism.

Sacral anterior root stimulator (SARS)

In 1986, Brindley reported on the first implantation of a SARS for the treatment of LUT dysfunction in SCI patients [129]. Improvements and refinements of this technique became known as Finetech–Brindley bladder stimulation system. Today this technique is an FDA-approved therapy that has been applied in several thousand SCI patients for neurogenic LUT dysfunction in specialized centres throughout the world [130].

The electrodes are implanted intra- or extradurally on the anterior sacral nerve roots S2–S4 bilaterally [130, 131]. The electrodes are connected to a receiver that is implanted subcutaneously in the lower left- or right-sided abdomen (Figure 24.8). For stimulation, the patient places a transmitter pad, which is connected to a programmable stimulation generator, directly above the implanted receiver. The stimulation signal is then transmitted transcutaneously to the receiver and subsequently to the electrodes. Different stimulation programs can be set up to allow the patient to use

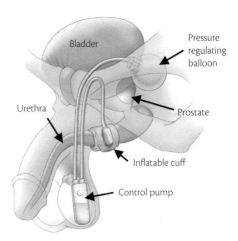

Fig. 24.9 Schematic illustration of the AMS 800® and its position in a male body after implantation. The AMS 800 consists of three components: the inflatable cuff, the balloon, and the pump. The cuff is placed around the bulbar urethra (in men) or bladder neck (in women and men after prostatectomy or in some neurogenic indications). The balloon is placed extraperitoneally into the lower abdomen. The pump is usually placed in the scrotum (in men) or labium majus (in women) for manual control of the sphincter.
Courtesy of American Medical Systems (American Medical Systems, Minnetonka, Minnesota, USA; www.AmericanMedicalSystems.com).

different stimulation parameters for different nerve roots. The stimulation of the anterior sacral nerve roots S3–S4 does not cause a single complete contraction of the bladder as during voiding in a healthy person. Rather a stimulation and hence contraction, of both detrusor and urethral sphincter results. However, due to the different characteristics of the muscle fibres in the detrusor and urethral sphincter (smooth vs striated muscle), intermittent stimulation bursts result in fast sphincter contraction with subsequent fatigue and relaxation while the detrusor shows a slower but more sustained contraction, allowing the urine to be evacuated until sphincter tonus increases again and detrusor contraction ceases [130]. This results in intermitted micturitions, usually requiring the application of intermittent stimulation bursts for several minutes.

This therapy is usually reserved to SCI patients, as implantation of a SARS is in most cases combined with a sacral posterior rhizotomy to abolish DO. Posterior rhizotomy causes irreversible loss of pelvic and lower limb sensibility.

Triggered voiding

Despite the aforementioned negative consequences of NDO, it can be used in certain circumstances to empty the bladder in association with voluntary maneuvers such as suprapubic tapping to provoke bladder contractions. However, this treatment approach is only reasonable in regard to lower and upper urinary tract safety if the bladder outlet resistance is adequately reduced to let urine pass during DO without significant intravesical pressure elevations and if the upper urinary tract is not already deteriorated.

Such therapy might be an interesting option especially for tetraplegic patients who cannot perform CISC but want to remain as independent as possible regarding management of LUT function. At given intervals (to be determined on an individual basis) the patient starts to repeatedly tap on his bladder until DO and subsequent urine leakage can be provoked. Usually, tapping for several minutes also beyond the first urine leakage is necessary to empty the bladder as far as possible. In consequence, a reliable possibility to collect the urine is required, which makes it a useful option only for male patients who can use a condom catheter.

Latissimus dorsi myoplasty

Although it is currently not a standardized or established therapy option for NLUTD, initial and medium-term results of latissimus dorsi myoplasty appear promising with complete spontaneous voiding in 71% of patients [132, 133], but further evidence and evaluation is needed.

Achievement of continence

Continence can be improved or achieved using the therapies mentioned for treatment of NDO, behavioural therapy, but also by applying therapies that improve sphincter function in cases of sphincter and bladder neck insufficiency. Insufficiency of the closing mechanisms at bladder neck or sphincter due to the lack or impairment of neurogenic innervation of these structures results in neurogenic stress urinary incontinence (nSUI).

Surgical therapy of nSUI aim to support or increase the closing function of sphincter or bladder neck. Three different types of surgical interventions can be distinguished: (1) injectables (e.g. bulking agents), (2) suspensions (e.g. Burch, suburethral tapes and slings), and (3) implants (e.g. artificial sphincter). To apply these therapies, it is absolutely mandatory that the patient has a normo- or hypotone detrusor and no or sufficiently treated NDO. Otherwise these therapies would be counterproductive to therapeutic principle (1).

Behavioural therapy

Behavioural therapy aims to adapt drinking and voiding behaviour. Such therapy does not actually treat the underlying cause of urinary incontinence but rather contribute to avoid urinary incontinence and helps to regain control of urinary continence. Timed voiding (= fixed time interval between micturitions that might be even indicated by alarm) might be useful in patients with impaired bladder sensation to prevent overflow incontinence or potentially in patients with mild terminal DO to prevent DO incontinence. In general, such behavioural regimens have to be adapted to the individual abilities and needs of the patient and suit best for patients in whom urinary incontinence is mainly due to cognitive or motor deficits. However, in such cases, caregivers need to provide additional support.

Adaption of drinking behaviour can positively influence LUT symptoms—that is shifting fluid intake from the evening to the morning and early afternoon in case of bothersome nocturia. Omittance of caffeinated or alcoholic drinks might improve frequency and/or DO. Restriction of excessive fluid intake might also be reasonable and useful but should not fall below a certain level, as that can result in other complications such as recurrent UTIs, urinary stones, and constipation.

Injectables

Injectables can consist of different materials (e.g. autologous fat, collagen, silicon, carbon, Teflon®, poly-acrylamide hydrogel) and they are injected transurethally below the bladder neck to create a sub-mucous cushion/bulking of the urethra that cause obstruction to withhold the urine. Despite some recent promising findings [134, 135], the current literature does not provide sufficient evidence for this kind of therapy [136].

Suspensions

Suspension therapies aim to restore or to improve urethral and/or bladder neck position and support, thereby enhancing the bladder neck or sphincteric closing mechanism. These are established treatment methods for female SUI [137, 138] and have been just recently introduced also for male SUI [139, 140]. Next to traditional techniques like a Burch colposuspension there are several different forms and materials of slings and tapes available. However, there are currently not many studies reporting results of suspension therapies in neurogenic patients. Most studies in neurological patients describe the use of autologous rectus abdominis fascia slings in children or adolescents usually in combination with an augmentation cystoplasty, demonstrating excellent results and low complication rates [141–147]. Only one study reports on the use of a polypropylene tape in 14–20-year-old boys with good initial results regarding continence but high complication rates [148].

Implants

Implants for SUI treatment are implantable devices that cause adjustable mechanical obstruction or closure of the urethra and/or bladder neck. There are currently two devices available, the artificial sphincter (AMS 800) and the inflatable paraurethral balloons (ACT/ProACT).

The currently most widely used artificial sphincter model (AMS 800®, American Medical Systems, Minnetonka, Minnesota, USA) consists of 3 major components, the inflatable cuff, the pump, and the pressure-regulating balloon (Figure 24.9). All three components are implanted and connected via special flexible but non-colliding tubes, allowing hydraulic functioning of the sphincter. The inflatable cuff is placed around the bulbar urethra (in men) or bladder neck (in men after prostatectomy and women or in some neurogenic indications) and connected to a control pump that is placed in the scrotum (in men) or labium majus (in women). The balloon is placed in the subperitoneal space lateral of the bladder. Activating the pump deflates the cuff by pumping the water from the cuff into the balloon, from where it flows back into the cuff due to the hydraulic gradient between balloon and cuff. The re-closing of the cuff takes 2–4 minutes during which the patients can empty the bladder via spontaneous voiding or CISC. The artificial sphincter is suitable for both men and women. Due to its high efficacy, the artificial sphincter is today's gold standard in the therapy of SUI [140]. Also patients with neurogenic SUI, in whom the natural sphincter is insufficiently working due to damage of its neuronal control, have greatly benefited from this therapy [149]. The success rate (proportion of continent patients) in patients with neurogenic SUI lies between 23% and 91% (mean 73%) [150–156]. However, Fulford et al. and Venn et al. investigated a mixed population (neurogenic and non-neurogenic SUI) [150, 156].

Frequent complications are erosion, infection, and mechanical/device-related failure that cause a re-operation rate for revisions and/or explantations of 16% to 80% [150, 151, 153–156].

Murphy et al. compared the treatment outcomes between patients with neurogenic SUI and patients with non-neurogneic SUI [152]. According to this study, patients with neurogenic SUI tend to have more frequently complications that were not related to mechanical or device-related failure [152].

A recently published study by Bersch et al. reported the very promising long-term results of a modified AMS800 system in patients with neurogenic SUI [157]. This modified system has the advantage that it works without the pump and is thus less

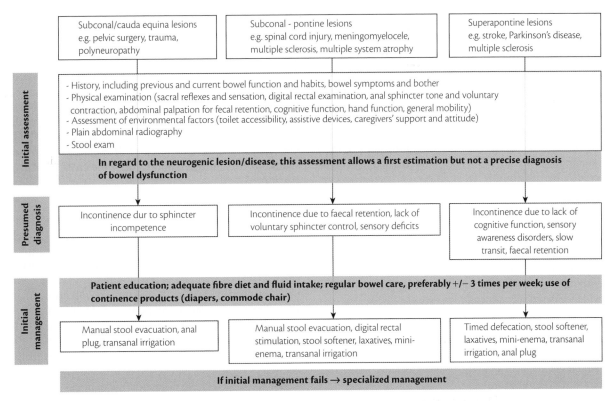

Fig. 24.10 Schematic overview on initial assessments and management options of neurogenic bowel dysfunction.
Adapted from [62].

susceptible to device-related defects and less costly [157]. Instead of the pump, a subcutaneous port is implanted that enables postoperative adjustments of the cuff-pressure. This system also seems to have some advantage in regard to the risk of pump-erosion in wheelchair bound female patients [157]. In addition, cuff pressure can be adjusted at any later time point via the subcutaneous port.

The inflatable paraurethral balloons are a rather new technique [158, 159] and only one study reports results in NLUTD [160]. The balloons are placed bilaterally of the urethra at the bladder neck (in women) or at the membranous urethra (in men) and can be inflated until the desired effect is achieved or the maximum capacity of the balloons is reached. Each balloon has a port that is placed into the ipsilateral scrotum or labium majus. The inflation is performed during follow-up visits with saline via the port of each balloon. Depending on the volume, the balloons cause a functional obstruction that should keep the urine within the bladder during situations of increased abdominal pressure.

Prevention of recurrent complications

Recurrent complications that cause health impairments and recurrent medical consultations reduce QoL. One of the most common recurrent complications occurring with NLUTD are symptomatic UTIs. Symptoms of UTIs include fever, general weakness, pain, dysuria, increased lower limb spasticity, urinary urgency, frequency, and incontinence. If the recurrent symptomatic UTIs are treatment related, i.e. frequently following BoNT/A intradetrusor injections, prophylactic antibiotic treatment prior to injection should be considered.

In case of recurrent UTIs it is important to re-evaluate and if necessary change the treatment concept of NLUTD in this patient, as recurrent UTIs might be a sign of inadequately treated NLUTD including inappropriate CISC technique. Identification of the responsible germ is necessary to evaluate if vaccination is an option and to adapt antibiotic therapy. Urine acidification and cranberry products are widely used prophylactic measures to prevent UTIs albeit poor evidence in the current literature [161]. In some refractory cases antibiotic long term treatment might be necessary [162].

Non-symptomatic UTIs that are detected by random urine analysis should not be arbitrarily treated if no urinary tract intervention is planned.

Another recurrent complication that might occur with NLUTD are urinary tract calculi which are in turn frequently associated with recurrent UTIs. Especially, SCI patients are at increased risk for recurrent urinary tract stones due to hypercalciuria resulting from immobilization, hypocitrituria, reduced fluid intake to reduce frequency of CISC, elevated urine pH, and a higher rate of indwelling catheters [163]. Prevention measures include adequate fluid intake (preferably pH neutral beverages resulting in a diuresis of 2.0–2.5 L/day and a specific urine weight of < 1010), dietary considerations (balanced diet rich in vegetable and fibre, normal calcium content of 1–1.2 g/day, limited NaCl content of 4–5 g/day, limited animal protein content of 0.8–1.0 g/kg/day, avoiding excessive consumption of vitamin supplements), and lifestyle considerations (BMI 18–25 kg/m^2) [164].

Practical treatment and management of bowel dysfunction

As NBD and resulting symptoms are mainly related to functional impairements of the descending colon, rectosigmoid and anus, therapeutic strategies ususally target these parts of the GI tract.

In general, conservative treatment is the mainstay of NBD management. However, most conservative measures are only successful if a regular routine of bowel management is established.

It should be always considered to include continence products (diapers, commode chair) into the therapeutic regime as patients might instantly benefit from it. In addition, perineal skin care should not be neglected as it can be essential to prevent skin ulcers that can easily lead to further complications.

Figures 24.10 and 24.11 provide a simple but practical overview on initial and specialized assessments and management options of NBD.

In order to comply with the aforementioned therapeutic principle, the following conservative and surgical therapeutic strategies are currently most relevant (for more detailed information and specific evidence based recommendations see also [62]):

Conservative treatment

Conservative treatments of NBD require adequate patient education and training and often more time and readjustments until success becomes evident. In severely disabled patients, caregivers need to help where required.

In case of decreased or even absent anorectal sensitivity, it is important to learn and perform digital rectal examination to improve awareness of rectal filling, as it is pointless trying to perform measures of stool evacuation with an empty rectum.

Optimizing stool consistency

This can be achieved by dietary measures (adequate fluid and fibre intake) or chemical stimulants such as laxatives (e.g. lactulose, bisacodyl, dioctyl, macrogol). Antidiarrheal drugs (e.g. loperamide, codeine phosphate) can be helpful to make faeces better manageable in cases of fluffy or watery stools [165] that are not related to infectious diseases. However, antidiarrheal drugs should be used only temporary until preferred stool consistency is achieved.

Facilitating stool evacuation

Manual stool extraction might be used as solitary measure for stool evacuation if appropriate or in addition to the following techniques for complete evacuation of stool if necessary: Suppositories (e.g. glycerin, sodium bicarbonate) [166] and mini-enemas (e.g. docusate enema) [167] can be used to trigger reflex evacuation and to facilitate controlled evacuation in conjunction with manual evacuation. Digital rectal stimulation can be also used to provoke a reflex contraction especially in supraconal lesions by inserting a finger into the rectum and performing circular motions for about 30 seconds [168]. Similarly, anal stimulation using pulsed water irrigation can be used to elicit reflex peristalsis for defecation with the additional advantage of facilitating disintegration of faecal deposits by irrigation [14]. Transanal colonic irrigation is also a safe and well tolerated method to effectively facilitate stool evacuation [169].

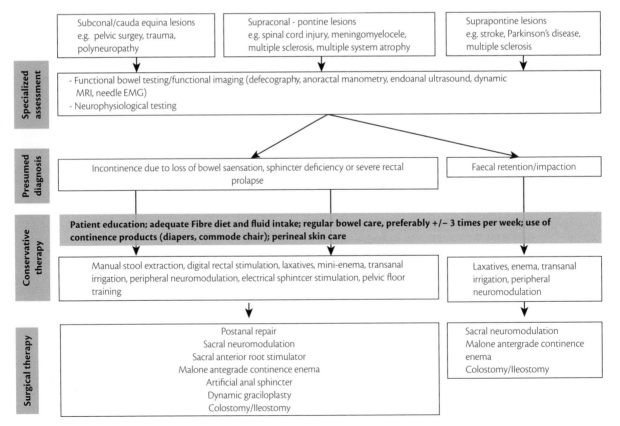

Fig. 24.11 Schematic overview on specialized assessments and management options of neurogenic bowel dysfunction. Adapted from [62].

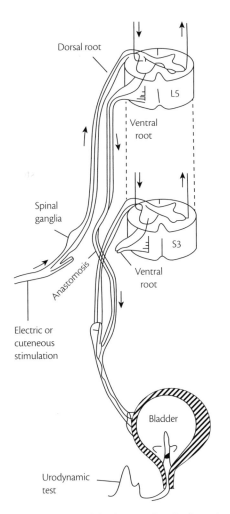

Fig. 24.12 Schematic illustration of the skin–spinal cord reflex pathway after re-rerouting the ventral roots of L5 with S3.
Reprinted from The Journal of Urology, Volume 170, Issue 4, Part 1, Chuan-Guo Xiao, Mao-Xin Du, An Artificial Somatic-Central Nervous System-Autonomic Reflex Pathway for Controllable Micturition After Spinal Cord Injury: Preliminary Results in 15 Patients, Pages 1237–1241, Copyright (2003), with permission from Elsevier.

Such measures should be done on a regular basis, i.e. daily or on alternate days, depending on pre-lesion defecation and dietary habits. However, caution should be paid in patients who tend to develop autonomic dysreflexia.

Temporary, peripheral/external neuromodulation
There are very few studies on temporary, peripheral/external neuromodulation for treatment of NBD. Two studies investigated the effect of neuromodulation in children with meningomyelocele using either transrectal [170] or transcutaneous interferential electrical stimulation [171] resulting in significant reduction of faecal incontinence [170] or significant improvements of constipation and defecation frequency [171]. Two other studies investigated the short-term effect of magnetic stimulation on NBD in PD and SCI patients, demonstrating a significant reduction in transit time and constipation [172, 173].

Other conservative measures
Pelvic floor mucle training with or without biofeedback might be beneficial for NBD, especially for sphincteric incompetence or insufficient relaxantion of pelvic floor and/or sphincter muscles during defecation. However, there is currently no study available that has investigated pelvic floor muscle training in NBD and such therapy requires at least partial voluntary control on pelvic floor muscles and sphincter. Continence products such as diapers, pads or anal plugs [174] should always accompany therapy regimes if applicable.

Surgical treatment
Perianal injectable bulking agents
So far, one large randomised controlled trial has shown that perianal injection of dextranomer in stabilised hyaluronic acid (NASHA Dx) improves continence for a little over half of patients in the short term [175]. Thus, it might be an option for selected patients. However, there are currently not data for the use of bulking agents in neurogenic faecal incontinence. Furthermore, this technique might worsen faecal evacuation, which potentially is the reason why this technique is rarely used in neurogenic faecal incontinence.

Postanal repair
A V-shaped incision is made posterior to the anal orifice. The tissues are dissected to the internal and external sphincters, which are separated. The puborectalis muscle is separated from the rectum providing direct access to the superior aspect of the pelvic floor muscles. A series of sutures are placed in the two limbs of the pelvic floor including the puborectalis, forming a lattice across the pelvis [176]. The original technique was described by Parks in 1975 [177] and aimed at restoration of an acute anorectal angle, improving continence by creating a flap valve effect of the puborectalis sling. However, other considerations suggest that the procedure attains its effect rather by increasing the functional length of the anal canal than by changing the anorectal angle [178]. Prospective evaluation of the technique in patients with neurogenic faecal incontinence demonstrated excellent short-term efficacy with favourable safety [179].

One recent study investigated the treatment outcome of this technique in 57 patients with neurogenic faecal incontinence > 9 years after surgery. Patients were selected for surgery after neurophysiological confirmation of neurogenic sphincter incompetence and failure of conservative therapy. Although efficacy declined over time with only 26% of patients reporting none to minimal incontinence after 9 years, patient satisfaction with treatment outcome remained high with 79% [178]. Similar results were also reported by earlier studies [180]. Despite the actually poor scientific evidence, this method might be an option for patients with significant comorbidities due to its low morbidity and high patient satisfaction.

Sacral neuromodulation
SNM is a minimally invasive therapy with few usually temporary complications (see also SNM for NLUTD) that appears to be an interesting option in the treatment of NBD at least in incomplete neurogenic lesions. Currently, there are only few studies reporting on outcomes in NBD but results were quite favourable with significant improvements of continence [181–183] and quality of life [181]. Nevertheless, larger randomized controlled trials are necessary to further evaluate and potentially establish this treatment for NBD.

Sacral anterior root stimulator (SARS)
As aforementioned for the treatment of NLUTD, SARS is almost always preceded by sacral deafferentation with irreversible loss

of pelvic and lower limb sensibility and colorectal reflex activity. Thus, this therapy is usually reserved for selected complete SCI patients.

Prolongation of intervals between the stimulation bursts on S2 has been demonstrated to facilitate colorectal motility and thereby reducing constipation and improving defecation [130, 184]; 55–70% of patients use their SARS to assist in defecation [185].

Malone antegrade continence enema (MACE)
The MACE procedure was first described by Malone et al. in 1990 [186] and aims to provide a permanent possibility for repeated antegrade colonic irrigation for faecal washout by creating a catheterisable non-refluxing channel (formed from the appendix or a small piece of ileum) between the colon and a cutaneous stoma usually at the lower abdomen. The almost complete colonic and rectal washout prevents faecal incontinence. This surgical intervention has been successfully used mainly in children with severe NBD/intractable faecal incontinence [187, 188], but also adult patients significantly benefited from this therapy [189, 190]. Despite long-term continence rates of up to 84% [191], this technique remains a major surgical intervention with stoma stenosis requiring revision as most common complication.

Artificial anal sphincter
The artificial anal sphincter (Acticon® Neosphincter, American Medical Systems, Minnetonka, Minnesota, USA) is a slightly modified version of the artificial sphincter used for SUI consisting of the same three components: the inflatable cuff, the pump, and the pressure regulating balloon. The placement of the components is nearly identical to the placement used with the AMS 800® for SUI with exemption of the cuff which is of course placed around the upper anal canal. Although most studies included few neurogenic patients, only few subgroup results were reported [192–194]. The overall success rate ranges from 47% to 90% [192–198] but seems to be lower in neurogenic patients [192, 193, 195]. Randomized controlled trials are lacking and the complication rate appears to be quite high [196]. Using the artificial anal sphincter it need to be considered that rectal evacuation can worsen. Thus, prior evaluation of transit and evacuation capability is recommended.

Dynamic gracioplasty
During this procedure, the gracilis muscle is transposed around the anal canal. In addition, a pacemaker is implanted for low-frequency intramuscular stimulation of the gracilis muscle to induce adaptive changes in means of transformation of fast-twitching type II muscle fibres into slow-twitching type I fibres that enable sustained contraction for anal closure [199–201]. Although there are several even larger studies evaluating this technique [202–204], there is only one study indicating inclusion of neurogenic patients with according subgroup results [205]. Overall there is a lack of randomized controlled trials and complication rate is high (>50%), including major infection, minor infection, thromboembolic events, pain, noninfectious gracilis problems, noninfectious wound-healing problems, treatment failure requiring revision [204, 206].

Colostomy/ileostomy
Colostomy or ileostomy might be the last option in severe intractable faecal incontinence. It is a surgical procedure that divert the colon or the ileum through an incision in the anterior abdominal wall. Hence, faeces are excreted via this new GI-outlet and collected in a stoma bag attached to it.

Although ostomy creation is an abdominal surgical intervention with all the associated risks and long term complications such as diversion colitis [207], it is a generally common surgical procedure that can significantly increase the patient's QoL especially due to improved faecal control and less time requirements for bowel management [208]. Creation of an ostomy in selected patients provides equivocal or superior QoL outcomes when compared to conservative bowel management strategies [208]. There are no clear advantages when functional, clinical, or QoL outcomes associated with colostomy are compared to those seen in SCI patients undergoing ileostomy [208].

Practical treatment and management of sexual dysfunction
Sexual dysfunctions can be classified according to four categories on the basis of the previously mentioned sexual response phases [209]:

(a) Sexual interest/desire disorder (reduced libido) with persistent or recurrent deficiency or absence of sexual fantasies/thoughts, and/or receptivity to sexual activity which causes personal distress.

(b) Sexual arousal disorder with persistent or recurrent inability to attain, or maintain sufficient sexual excitement causing personal distress.

(c) Orgasmic or ejaculatory disorders with persistent or recurrent difficulty in, delay in, or lack of attaining orgasm following sufficient sexual stimulation and arousal, which causes personal distress.

(d) Sexual pain disorders with dyspareunia (persistent or recurrent genital pain associated with sexual intercourse), vaginismus (recurrent or persistent involuntary spasms of the musculature of the outer third of the vagina that interferes with vaginal penetration and causes personal distress), and other sexual pain disorders (recurrent or persistent genital pain induced by non-coital sexual stimulation)

Although this classification has not been established specifically for patients with neurogenic disorders or lesions it provides a useful basis for patient evaluation and providing therapeutic concepts also in neurogenic cases.

Due to the fact that sexual dysfunction is already highly prevalent in the general population [210] as cause of other prevalent diseases and risk factors such as cardiovascular disease, diabetes, obesity, endocrine disorders, age, radiation therapy, polypharmacy, etc. it can be often challenging to differentiate if the sexual dysfunction is actually part of the neurological condition or not. In neurogenic disease, sexual dysfunctions might be multifactorial and can be described as (1) primary (i.e. resulting directly from the neurological lesion/disease), (2) secondary (i.e. resulting from non-sexual sequelae of the neurological lesion/disease that affect sexual function), or (3) tertiary (i.e. resulting from psychological, emotional or cultural impact of living with a neurological disease and sexual dysfunction) [38]. Counselling and treatment need to consider these secondary and tertiary factors.

Sexual dysfunction is a highly intimate and individually differently experienced aspect of human health that is strongly influenced by gender, age, and sociocultural background and requires an atmosphere of open-mindedness, confidence, and acceptance to be adequately discussed and evaluated. Thus, sensible counselling is of major importance and can alone already reduce the level of anxiety and frustration concerning sexual dysfunction. Patients with neurogenic lesions or diseases should know that sexual dysfunction can occur as a symptom of their neurological condition and that there are therapeutic options available that can help to alleviate or even abolish sexual dysfunction. However, approaching patients in the early phase of their neurogenic lesion or disease can be delicate and even appear inappropriate as patients might struggle with other, 'more important' matters of their neurological disease and disability. Nevertheless, counselling on sexual dysfunction should not be deferred to the very end of a rehabilitation or treatment course but rather be stepwise integrated for example into the counselling on other pelvic organ dysfunction such as bladder and bowel, giving the patient the time to become comfortable discussing also sex related health issues. Timely counselling on sexual dysfunction can help to prevent the development of misapprehension, prejudice, anxiety, and frustration in patients dealing with sexual dysfunction. Also, the patient's partner and/or caregiver should not be ignored and integrated into consultation if appropriate.

Certainly, patients should not be forced into counselling for sexual dysfunction and such counselling needs to be individually tailored with respect to the patient's sexual attitude and orientation. Useful models for approaching and managing patients regarding sexual dysfunction are BETTER and PLISSIT, which describe different levels of assessment and intervention [211]. The BETTER model serves for the health care professional who is not specialized in assessment and treatment of sexual dysfunction, whereas the PLISSIT model requires knowledge of assessment and treatment of sexual dysfunction.

BETTER (basic/general approach model):

B—Bring up the topic.

E—Explain that you are concerned with quality-of-life issues, including sexuality. Although you may not be able to answer all questions, you will want to convey that patients can talk about their concerns.

T—Tell patients that you will find appropriate resources to address their concerns.

T—Timing might not seem appropriate, but acknowledge that patients can ask for information at any time.

E—Educate patients about the side effects of their treatments.

R—Record your assessment and interventions in patient medical records.

PLISSIT (advanced/specialized approach model):

P (permission)—bringing the topic of sexual (dys)function to the patient's mind, e.g. by generally mentioning changes in sexual function as a frequent symptom of neurological disease, and thus legitimizing the topic and demonstrating the willingness to discuss sex related issues which in turn 'permits' the patient to think about sexuality in his/her situation and to potentially accept the offer for counselling.

LI (limited information)—providing first, 'limited information' to the patient, helping him/her to address more specific aspects of his/her neurological condition affecting sexual function.

SS (specific suggestions)—'specific suggestion' can be offered, e.g. using a vaginal lubricant for vaginal dryness.

IT (intensive therapy)—'intensive therapy' might be need to improve sexual dysfunction and involves specialized psychosexual management.

Assessment of sexual dysfunction is a mandatory prerequisite prior to initiation of adequate treatment. Such assessment includes in its basic form (1) a complete medical history including concomitant medication, of which the latter can often significantly alter sexual function, psychosocial evaluation, and sexual function evaluation. Psychosocial and sexual functions are best assessed using validated questionnaires such as the International Index for erectile Function (IIEF) [212] or the Female Sexual Function Index (FSFI) [213]. (2) A physical examination assessing general appearance and secondary sexual characteristics of the patient, cardiovascular function, appearance, size, and shape of the genitalia, digital rectal examination, and orienting neurological exam (e.g. perineal and genital sensibility, anal tone, bulbocavernosal reflex). (3) Laboratory tests (e.g. testosterone, other sex hormones and laboratory parameters as required from patient history and complaints).

Optional tests such as pharmacologic testing (intracavenosal vasoactive drug injection, i.e. PGE1) and color Doppler imaging can be used to distinguish between vasculogenic and non-vasculogenic erectile dysfunction or to evaluate genital perfusion, respectively.

The following therapy options are listed according to the category of sexual dysfunction they are supposed to treat:

Treatment of sexual interest/desire disorder (reduced libido)

Treatment of sexual interest disorders, which is mainly treatment of low libido, can be difficult, as there is no drug treatment available selectively activating the brain's sexual desire network or restoring its function when affected by neurological disorders. Hormone treatment has been demonstrated to have a positive effect on libido but not specifically in patients with neurogenic disease [214]. Long-term data on treatment effects and side effects are missing [215].

However, before adding new drugs to the patient's treatment it should be first considered to minimize endo- and exogenic factors with negative impact on libido but high prevalence among patients with neurogenic diseases, such as mood disorders or other psychological factors, concomitant medication, and physical disabilities.

Mood disorders, such as depression, can occur as a consequence of being diagnosed with a chronic neurological disease or as pathophysiological process of the neurological disease. In such cases, psychological support and antidepressant drug treatment should be considered. However, some antidepressant drugs itself, such as serotonin reuptake inhibitors, have negative effects on sexual desire, arousal, and orgasm. Bupropion (norepinephrine and dopamine reuptake inhibitor) and mirtazapine (presynaptic alpha-2-adrenergic receptor) might be valuable alternatives with fewer side effects on sexual function.

Other psychological disorder should be considered if indicated and treated accordingly. Again, many substances used for psychological treatments can impair sexual function.

If possible, drugs with negative impact on libido (e.g. tricyclic antidepressants, selective serotonin reuptake inhibitors, anticonvulsants, opioids) should be avoided or replaced by alternatives without or lesser effects on sexual function.

An altered body self-perception and/or reduced self-esteem due to physical disabilities and impairments, i.e. immobility, spasticity, sensory deficits, pain, and altered body functions, such as of bladder and bowel with fear of incontinence during sexual activity, can significantly reduce libido. Here, adequate treatment of bladder and bowel dysfunction (see earlier sections) and antispasticity treatment is necessary. It is important to provide counselling and reassurance to the affected patient and partner, if applicable. This can and should include advice on managing practical issues of sexual activity, such as optimized positioning for intercourse. Open communication and experimentation between patient and partner should be supported [45]. Additional psychological support can be helpful and should be offered.

Similar to the general population, reduced libido in patients with neurogenic disease might also be related to relationship and partner issues. Psychosexual and couple therapy is an option but the outcome mainly depends on patient and partner motivation.

Hypersexuality with increased libido can be an issue in PD patients under treatment with L-dopa or dopamine antagonists. In such cases, dose adjustment or change of medication usually resolves the symptoms [216].

Treatment of sexual arousal disorder

Treatment of sexual arousal disorder includes the treatment of erectile dysfunction (ED) in men which is the most prominent and best investigated part of sexual dysfunction therapy [217, 218].

Lifestyle modifications are a very useful measure and should at least accompany other forms of treatment. Smoking, obesity, limited physical activity, and alcohol consumption are factors commonly associated with erectile dysfunction and should be considered in the treatment regimen of sexual dysfunction [218]. Certainly, the level of physical activity needs to be adapted to the level of mobility impairment in patients with neurogenic disorders.

Phosphodiesterase type 5 (PDE-5) inhibitors such as sildenafil (Viagra®), vardenafil (Levitra®), and tadalafil (Cialis®) are the first-line treatment of ED. All PDE-5 inhibitors promote smooth muscle relaxation within the arterial sinuses of the corpora cavernosa and consequently penile erection by prolonging the effect of cyclic guanosine monophosphate (cGMP) in the smooth muscles. cGMP is the active component that causes smooth muscle relaxation and is converted from guanosine triphosphate by the enzyme guanylat cyclase under the influence of nitric oxide released from the parasympathetic nerve terminals of the cavernous nerve [217]. cGMP is usually hydrolyzed and inactivated to GMP by the PDE-5. All PDE-5 inhibitors have similar efficacy and tolerability but differ regarding onset and duration of action. Sildenafil and vardenafil are effective after 30–60 minutes and last for 4 hours, whereas tadalafil is effective after 30 minutes and lasts for up to 36 hours [218]. Treatment should be started with 50 mg/day using sildenafil or 10 mg/day using vardenafil or tadalafil. Dosing can be increased up to 100 mg/day using sildenafil and up to 20 mg/day

using vardenafil or tadalafil depending on tolerability and demand. Typical side effects are dyspepsia, headache, facial flushing, nasal congestion, abnormal vision, myalgia, and back pain [217]. Side effects are usually mild to moderate.

All PDE-5 inhibitors have been investigated in SCI patients and sildenafil also in MS and PD patients demonstrating good efficacy and safety [219–221]. Sildenafil seems to be more effective than using a vacuum constriction device in SCI patients and was preferred over vacuum constriction device or injection therapy [222].

None of the PDF-5 inhibitors has been approved for female sexual dysfunction but sildenafil demonstrated some beneficial effect on sexual arousal in women with SCI [223]. In female patients with MS such beneficial effect of sildenafil on sexual function could not be demonstrated [224].

It should be considered that PDE-5 inhibitors do not cause an erection per se. It still requires sexual stimulation.

Caution has to be paid in patients taking nitrates, as PDE-5 inhibitors are strictly contraindicated in combination with organic nitrates and nitric oxide donors due to an additive effect (relaxation) on the smooth muscles of blood vessels which can result in severe hypotension. Due to their hypotensive effects, PDE-5 inhibitors should be cautiously used in conditions of pre-existing hypotension, i.e. postural hypotension in MSA.

Apomorphine acts on the D2 dopaminergic receptors in the hypothalamus, thus requires intact spinal pathways to exert its effect on mild ED. The efficacy in ED treatment of Apomorphine has been demonstrated to be inferior to sildenafil but it might be a treatment option for patients who cannot take sildenafil [225]. Dosage starts with 2 mg and onset of action is about 20 minutes. Side effects are mild to moderate and include nausea, dizziness yawning and rare bradycardia. However it should be used cautiously in patients with postural hypotension.

Yohimbine is predominantly an alpha-2-adrenergic blocker that is supposed to act centrally and peripherally to improve erectile function [226]. The level of evidence for the use in ED is generally low and since the introduction of the PDE-5 inhibitors it has hardly any relevance in ED treatment. Side effects include palpitations, headache, nausea, indigestion, urinary frequency, and transient hypertension.

Intracorporeal or intraurethral drug applications can be alternatives in men if oral drug treatment is not effective or tolerated. Drugs for intracorporeal injections comprise substances such as prostaglandin E1 (PGE1), papaverine, and phentolamine [217]. However, only PGE1 is used as a single therapeutic agent (alprostadil, Caverject®), whereas papaverine and phentolamine are used in combination with (Trimix) or without (Bimix) additional PGE1. Only alprostadil is currently licensed and approved for therapy of erectile dysfunction. Bimix and trimix are not brand names and the preparations need to be individually mixed by a pharmacy.

PGE1 acts, similar to PDE-5 inhibitors, on the smooth muscles of the corpora cavernosa were it causes relaxation by increasing the level of cyclic adenosine monophosphate (cAMP) and subsequently decrease in intracellular calcium. Papaverine seems to act mainly as a non-selective PDE inhibitor that inhibits hydrolysis of cGMP and cAMP, causing decrease of intracellular calcium levels and thus smooth muscle relaxation but probably has also other mechanism of action [217]. Phentolamine has synergistic effects when combined with PGE1 and/or papaverine by inhibiting both, alpha-1 and alpha-2 adrenoceptors blocking sympathetic activity that would induce smooth muscle contraction, and consequently, detumescence [217].

The technique of injection is simple, safe, and painless if appropriately explained and taught to the patient. For patients with limited hand and arm function, the partner and/or primary care giver might be instructed instead. Following injection into the corpora cavernosa from either side, distribution of the substance should be facilitated by massaging the penile shaft. Erection usually occurs within 10–15 minutes. In contrast to PDE-5 inhibitors, erections occur without any additional sexual stimulation. Efficacy is high (70–80%) and duration of response ranges between 50 and 180 minutes [227]. Reasons for treatment failure despite maximum dosage might be severe vasculogenic erectile dysfunction. Adverse events include penile or inguinal pain, fibrosis of cavernous body, and priapism. Pain is more frequent with PGE1 (up to 50%) than with Bimix or Trimix [228]. However, bimix and trimix cause more fibrosis (6–12%) and priapism (7%) [227]. Priapism is defined as continuous erection for more than 4 hours and patients should immediately seek specialist medical help to prevent thrombosis, muscle necrosis, and fibrosis of the corpora cavernosa.

Intraurethral therapy include PGE1 application either using MUSE (medicated urethral system for erection) or intrameatal application (not very common). The MUSE applicator is inserted into the distal urethra and by pressing the release button a small pellet is placed into the urethral lumen [228]. From there PGE1 is absorbed and reaches the corpora cavernosa via venous channels between the corpus spongiosum and corpora cavernosa. Erection occurs within 30 minutes. Efficacy seems to be somewhat less than with intracevernosal injection or PDE-5 inhibitors [218, 228]. Side effects are similar as for PGE1 injections plus urethral irritation and burning [228]. Due to the urethral placement of the substance there might be PGE1 in the semen, which can be dangerous for pregnant women and requires the use of a condom.

Vacuum tumescence devices are a non-pharmacological treatment option of ED and consists of a vacuum pump and a penile constriction ring. The pump cylinder is placed over the penis and pressed against the pubis to prevent air entrance into the cylinder while applying a vacuum to the cylinder. The negative pressure leads to engorgement of the penis. To maintain this erected state after removing the pump, a constriction ring made of elastic rubber is placed around the base of the penis, preventing premature outflow of blood from the penis. It is important to select the correct size of the constriction ring as the whole procedure might be inefficient if the ring is too large or, if the ring is too tight, damage to the penis might occur. It is generally recommended that the constriction ring should not be used for more than 30 minutes. The vacuum pump plus constriction ring is effective in about 60–70% but requires some dexterity by the patient or partner [222]. It should not be used in bleeding conditions. Potential disadvantages are a rather cold penis, bruising of the penis, and block of ejaculate by the constriction ring. Some rings have a notch to facilitate ejaculation.

A vacuum device is also available for women. The EROS-CTD system has been demonstrated to improve orgasm and sexual satisfaction by increasing vaginal lubrification and genital sensation [229]. However, there are no data available in women with neurological disease.

'Sex toys', i.e. vibrators, can also be useful to improve sexual arousal.

Sacral neuromodulation seems be an option that can improve bladder dysfunctions as well as sexual dysfunctions in male and female patients with neurogenic disorders [230, 231]. However, current data are limited.

Implantation of a penile prosthesis can be considered as last resort when all other therapeutic approaches have failed or are contraindicated. Despite the high satisfaction rates for patients and partners (70–90%), it is an invasive procedure with irreversible damage to the corpora spongiosa as those are replaced by the prosthetic rods [218]. In general, two types of prosthesis can be differentiated, malleable, and inflatable. Malleable prostheses usually consist of a pair of flexible silicon rods that have sufficient rigidity for penetration. With this form of prosthesis, the penis is always in the 'erected mode' and intercourse could be immediately started just by bending the rods into the appropriate position. Inflatable prosthesis require three components: inflatable cylinder that provides erection sufficient for penetration when inflated, a reservoir, and a pump. The reservoir might exist as a separate part or might be integrated into the cylinder. Complications include pain, device infection (2–4%), mechanical device failure, and device perforation/arrosion [218].

Local vaginal oestrogen supply and/or vaginal lubricants are useful to prevent or reduce dyspareunia in women with vaginal atrophy and/or dryness [232, 233]. Vaginal lubricants should be water based for better tolerability and less interference with condoms and silicone-based sex toys [45].

Treatment of orgasmic or ejaculatory disorders

Some of the treatments mentioned for reduced libido and sexual arousal disorder can be also beneficial to improve orgasmic function (e.g. yohimbine, vacuum devices, vibrator). The ability to perceive orgasm is at least partly maintained in many neurological disorders but it might require more time and additional stimulation also of other 'ergogenous' body areas to reach orgasm. Again, counselling is important and it is often necessary for the patient to newly explore his/her abilities of body functions such as sexual function that might be altered by the neurological disease or lesion, rather than concentrating only on the disabilities.

Certainly, reaching orgasm is, with other factors (see earlier), dependent on sexual sensory inputs that, once completely lost due to neurological disease or lesion, are difficult to retrieve. However, it should be also considered that depending on the quality and level of relationship between the patient and his/her partner, reaching orgasm might not necessarily be the primary factor for achieving a satisfactory sex life.

Nerve re-routing surgery seems to be a promising option to restore or improve next to bladder and bowel function as well as sexual sensations, and has been successfully performed in SCI and spina bifida patients [234, 235]. If and how far this treatment helps to regain genital sensibility, improve the ability to reach orgasm, or improve the quality of orgasm, remains to be elucidated.

Premature ejaculation can be treated with behavioural therapy (stop/start and squeeze technique, sensate focus), relationship counselling, pharmacotherapy, and combination therapy. In general there are very limited data on patients with neurological disease, but it might be an issue in PD patients [236]. Behavioural therapy can be difficult for some patients with neurological diseases and requires a high level of motivation and compliance. Pharmacotherapy includes off-label use of selective serotonin reuptake inhibitors such as paroxetine, sertraline, or fluoxitine for 6–8 weeks and/or topical anesthetics [237]. However, all demonstrated only limited efficacy. Other drugs such as tramadol and PDE-5 inhibitors have also been evaluated [238, 239]. The currently only approved and licensed drug treatment for premature ejaculation is dapoxetine (Priligy®) which demonstrates favourable results [240].

An- or retrograde ejaculation can be an issue regarding fertility. In particular, men with SCI frequently have ejaculatory dysfunction. As mentioned earlier, semen quality can rapidly decrease in SCI and in combination with an- or retrograde ejaculation, specific techniques are required to retrieve semen for further reproductive measures (i.e. insemination, in vitro fertilization). In men with an intact ejaculatory reflex (i.e. lesions above Th12), vibratory stimulation to the dorsal side of the glans of the penis can provoke sufficient reflex ejaculation. Oral application of the alpha-agonist midodrine (Gutron®, Amatine®) using about 18.7 mg 30–120 minutes prior to vibratory stimulation has been shown to improve ejaculation and orgasm rates in SCI men, especially with complete lesions above Th10 [241]. Care should be taken in patients with hypertension and a tendency to develop autonomic dysreflexia.

If vibratory stimulation is not successful or applicable due to lesions affecting the ejaculatory reflex, electroejaculation is an option with high success rate (98%) related to direct stimulation of preganglionic efferent fibres using a rectal probe [242]. However, the procedure can be painful and requires general anaesthesia, or at least sedation.

Treatment of sexual pain disorders

Painful sexual intercourse or ejaculation might be related to infection (i.e. urethritis, cystitis, prostatitis), which should be ruled out or treated accordingly.

Local vaginal oestrogen supply and/or vaginal lubricants are useful to prevent or reduce dyspareunia in women with vaginal atrophy and/or dryness [232, 233]. Sometimes anesthetic gels can be useful.

More complex or chronic pain disorders, including neuropathic pain, require a multilevel specialized treatment comprising but not limited to physical therapy (e.g. pelvic floor training, peripheral electric neurostimulation, and neuromodulation), pharmacological therapy (e.g. analgesic drugs, antidepressant drugs), and psychotherapy (e.g. cognitive behavioural treatment). However, the detailed elaboration on treatment of pain disorders would be beyond the scope of this chapter and cannot be covered here.

Perspectives

Future improvements and therapeutic advances for NLUTD and NBD are to be expected in the following areas:

Neuromodulation

This area provides great potential but also an enormous diversity of therapeutic options and parameters. There are currently several ongoing trials investigating different forms of neuromodulation such as SNM and PTNS for lower urinary tract and bowel dysfunction. However, neurogenic patients are rarely considered. Only one randomized controlled trial is currently ongoing, investigating SNM in chronic NLUTD.

Just recently, Sievert et al. published the results of a very interesting approach using bilateral sacral neuromodulation in 10 patients with complete SCI and urodynamically proven DO [243]. The time after injury was on average 3 months and in regard to this, the technique was named early sacral neuromodulation. The underlying hypothesis was that sacral neuromodulation might be able to positively influence the neural plasticity of LUT relevant nerves below the lesion and thus can contribute in the reduction of DO [243]. The results were extraordinary, as all patients were continent, the DO abolished, and UTIs significantly reduced during a mean follow-up of 26 months [243]. In addition, bilateral SNM facilitated bowel and erectile function in some patients. Lead displacement and/or rupture in 5 of 10 patients caused recurrence of DO, which could be treated with replacement of the electrode [243]. Although these results are very preliminary in a small group, they might be a milestone in the treatment of LUT dysfunction in SCI and deserves further investigations.

Other recent studies used the InterStim® device to perform chronic pudendal nerve stimulation in patients with non-neurogenic and neurogenic DO, via placement of the tined lead electrodes directly to the pudendal nerve. This approach seems feasible, with first promising short-term results [244, 245]. Unfortunately, a randomized controlled trial had to be terminated due to recruitment difficulties [151]. A current investigation evaluated a new method to improve electrode placement [246].

A different approach has been described by Possover et al., with laparoscopic bilateral implantation of octapolar electrodes directly across the pudendal and sciatic nerves in complete SCI patients with DO [247]. Pudendal stimulation with 15–20 Hz caused an inhibition of DO up to 550 ml during filling cystometry [247]. Subsequently, the pudendal stimulation was switched off to unleash a detrusor reflex contraction. In patients with no or insignificant DSD this resulted in efficient bladder emptying [247]. However, DSD could get in the way of that outcome. Thus, Possover et al. tried not to switch off pudendal stimulation completely, but rather switch to high frequency pudendal stimulation with 1200 Hz, resulting in a reduction of DSD and nearly complete bladder emptying [247]. However, it has to be admitted that Possover et al. still used Fintech–Brindley electrodes in addition to the octapolar pudendal electrode to promote sufficient bladder emptying [247].

In addition to the promising effects on bladder control, this therapy seems to be also beneficial for erectile function, reduction of lower limb spasticity and even to enable short-term assisted standing by a sustained contraction of the quadriceps muscles via sciatic nerve stimulation [247].

However, this approach is still experimental and the results presented are very preliminary (only three patients with 3 months maximum follow-up). Nevertheless, this is the first therapy addressing multiple pelvic dysfunctions at the same time without destroying or remodeling any nerves or organs. Further refinements of the system and technique without additional implantation of a Finetech–Brindley electrode in a larger series of patients has been planned but not yet performed.

Other recent investigations strived for the development of an automated system that can identify a beginning DO and immediately trigger pudendal stimulation to suppress DO [248, 249]. Such a device in an implantable format would be a highly interesting treatment option for patients with NDO.

Pharmacotherapy

Just recently a new drug has been released for the treatment of overactive bladder. Mirabegron is a selective β3-adrenoceptor agonist that causes detrusor relaxation and increased stability during bladder storage through direct activation of β-adrenoceptors [250]. If mirabegron is a relevant alternative for the therapy of NDO compared or in addition to the current first line antimuscarinic treatment is matter of future investigations.

Other relevant targets for future pharmacological therapy of NDO that have been recently described are cannabinoid-2-receptors and fatty acid amide hydrolases in the LUT and spinal cord [251, 252].

Also properties of already available drugs are currently revisited that might lead to new applications in the treatment of NLUTD [253].

Nerve re-routing

Re-routing of LUT nerves after SCI has been investigated in animals and recently also in a quite large population of complete SCI patients. This technique is based on a microsurgical anastomosis between the L5 and S2/3 ventral root, leaving the dorsal roots intact (Figure 24.12) [254, 255]. The idea is that impulses delivered from the efferent neurons of a somatic reflex arc can be transferred to initiate responses of an autonomic effector [254, 255]. To elicit a bladder contraction, patients have to scratch or squeeze on the L5 dermatome [254, 255].

Xiao et al. reported a success rate of 67–88% in SCI and 85% in spina bifida patients after unilateral re-routing of the ventral nerve roots L5 with S3 [254, 255]. However, the therapy success was poorly defined. Post void residual significantly decreased from 332 ml to 31 ml and maximum urinary flow increased from 2.4 to 14.3 ml/s, but maximum detrusor pressure decreased, although significantly, only from 82 cmH_2O to 62 cmH_2O and bladder capacity remained nearly unchanged (364 ml preoperatively vs. 387 ml postoperatively) [254, 255]. Moreover, patients had to wait for approximately 1 year until improvements occur [254, 255]. Although this approach seems to be an interesting alternative with only few reported adverse events, it appears inferior in efficacy to previously described techniques like botulinum toxin intradetrusor injections, augmentation cystoplasty and SARS + posterior rhizotomy. Other groups currently do not confirm the initial results of Xiao et al. [256].

Although the main focus of those recent studies was on LUT function, the joint innervation of bladder and the distal colorectum from the sacral segments S2–S4 could form the basis for additional effect on bowel function [257]. The multiple stimuli on a daily basis might facilitate colorectal motility and emptying.

Tissue engineering

Tissue engineering is the umbrella term for a rapidly advancing and highly complex medical research field that aims to improve tissue and organ reconstruction using autologous cells and stem cells. Especially augmentation cystoplasty could be largely improved by using grown autologous bladder tissue instead of bowel segments.

However, the major difficulty in tissue engineering is to find the most suitable scaffold to develop a biodegradable three-dimensional construct that can accommodate adequate amounts of cells for functional tissue formation [258, 259].

Another challenge is to provide sufficient blood supply to the engineered tissue once it is implanted [258, 259].

First successful results have been reported in a small group of young patients with menigomyelocele requiring cystoplasty for the treatment of their LUT dysfunction [258].

To be able to advance further, to enhance product development, and make tissue engineering products widely available, current and upcoming research in this field need to be focused on the clinical applicability and capable to fulfil the ethical and legal regulations and to master the boundaries of licensing [259].

References

1. Anderson KD. Targeting recovery: priorities of the spinal cord-injured population. J Neurotrauma. 2004; **21**: 1371–1383.
2. Fowler CJ, Griffiths D, de Groat WC. The neural control of micturition. Nat Rev Neurosci. 2008;**9**:453–466.
3. Jeong SJ, Cho SY, Oh SJ. Spinal cord/brain injury and the neurogenic bladder. Urol Clin N Am. 2010; **37**: 537–546.
4. Torre M, Buffa P, Jasonni V, Cama A. Long-term urologic outcome in patients with caudal regression syndrome, compared with meningomyelocele and spinal cord lipoma. J Pediatr Surg. 2008; **43**: 530–533.
5. Abrams P, Cardozo L, Fall M, et al. The standardisation of terminology in lower urinary tract function: report from the standardisation sub-committee of the International Continence Society. Urology. 2003; **61**: 37–49.
6. Blok BF. Central pathways controlling micturition and urinary continence. Urology. 2002;**59**:13–17.
7. Karsenty G, Reitz A, Wefer B, Boy S, Schurch B. Understanding detrusor sphincter dyssynergia—significance of chronology. Urology. 2005;**66**:763–768.
8. Blackmer J. Rehabilitation medicine: 1. Autonomic dysreflexia. CMAJ. 2003; **169**: 931–935.
9. Sakakibara R, Tateno F, Kishi M, Tsuyuzaki Y, Uchiyama T, Yamamoto T. Pathophysiology of bladder dysfunction in Parkinson's disease. Neurobiol Dis. 2012; **46**: 565–571.
10. Dietrichs E, Haines DE. Possible pathways for cerebellar modulation of autonomic responses: micturition. Scand J Urol Nephrol. Supplementum 2002;16–20.
11. Gershon MD. The enteric nervous system: a second brain. Hospital Pract. 1999;**34**:31–32, 35–38, 41–42 passim.
12. Mayer EA, Naliboff BD, Craig AD. Neuroimaging of the brain-gut axis: from basic understanding to treatment of functional GI disorders. Gastroenterology. 2006;**131**:1925–1942.
13. Brading AF, Ramalingam T. Mechanisms controlling normal defecation and the potential effects of spinal cord injury. Progr Brain Res. 2006;**152**:345–358.
14. Krassioukov A, Eng JJ, Claxton G, Sakakibara BM, Shum S. Neurogenic bowel management after spinal cord injury: a systematic review of the evidence. Spinal Cord. 2010;**48**:718–733.
15. Trivedi PM, Bajwa A, Boulos PB, Craggs MD, Emmanuel AV. Increased sigmoid compliance may explain symptoms and response to treatment in supraconal spinal cord injury [abstract]. Gut. 2009; **58**: A34.
16. Aaronson MJ, Freed MM, Burakoff R. Colonic myoelectric activity in persons with spinal cord injury. Dig Dis Sci. 1985;**30**:295–300.
17. Krogh K, Mosdal C, Laurberg S. Gastrointestinal and segmental colonic transit times in patients with acute and chronic spinal cord lesions. Spinal Cord. 2000;**38**:615–621.
18. Weber J, Grise P, Roquebert M, et al. Radiopaque markers transit and anorectal manometry in 16 patients with multiple sclerosis and urinary bladder dysfunction. Dis Colon Rectum. 1987;**30**:95–100.
19. Sakakibara R, Odaka T, Uchiyama T, et al.Colonic transit time and rectoanal videomanometry in Parkinson's disease. J Neurol Neurosurg Psychiatry 2003;**74**:268–272.

20. Edwards LL, Quigley EM, Harned RK, Hofman R, Pfeiffer RF. Characterization of swallowing and defecation in Parkinson's disease. Am J Gastroenterol. 1994;**89**:15–25.

21. Kupsky WJ, Grimes MM, Sweeting J, Bertsch R, Cote LJ. Parkinson's disease and megacolon: concentric hyaline inclusions (Lewy bodies) in enteric ganglion cells. Neurology. 1987;**37**:1253–1255.

22. Masters WH, Johnson VE. Human sexual inadequacy. Little Brown, New York, 1970.

23. Kaplan HS. Sexual medicine. A progress report. Arch Intern Med. 1980;**140**:1575–1576.

24. McKenna K. The brain is the master organ in sexual function: central nervous system control of male and female sexual function. Int J Impotence Res. 1999;**11**(Suppl 1):S48–55.

25. Stoleru S, Fonteille V, Cornelis C, Joyal C, Moulier V. Functional neuroimaging studies of sexual arousal and orgasm in healthy men and women: a review and meta-analysis. Neurosci Biobehav Rev. 2012;**36**:1481–1509.

26. Baird AD, Wilson SJ, Bladin PF, Saling MM, Reutens DC. Neurological control of human sexual behaviour: insights from lesion studies. J Neurol Neurosurg Psychiatry. 2007;**78**:1042–1049.

27. Tajkarimi K, Burnett AL. The role of genital nerve afferents in the physiology of the sexual response and pelvic floor function. Journal Sex Med. 2011;**8**:1299–1312.

28. Pfaus JG, Kippin TE, Coria-Avila GA, et al. Who, what, where, when (and maybe even why)? How the experience of sexual reward connects sexual desire, preference, and performance. Arch Sex Behav. 2012;**41**:31–62.

29. Giuliano F. Neurophysiology of erection and ejaculation. J Sex Med. 2011;**8**(Suppl 4):310–315.

30. Sachs BD. Placing erection in context: the reflexogenic-psychogenic dichotomy reconsidered. Neurosci Biobehav Rev. 1995;**19**:211–224.

31. Giuliano F, Rampin O, Allard J. Neurophysiology and pharmacology of female genital sexual response. JSex Marital Ther. 2002;**28**(Suppl 1):101–121.

32. Basson R. Female sexual response: the role of drugs in the management of sexual dysfunction. Obstet Gynecol. 2001;**98**:350–353.

33. Jung JH, Kam SC, Choi SM, Jae SU, Lee SH, Hyun JS. Sexual dysfunction in male stroke patients: correlation between brain lesions and sexual function. Urology. 2008;**71**:99–103.

34. Rees PM, Fowler CJ, and Maas CP. Sexual function in men and women with neurological disorders. Lancet. 2007;**369**:512–525.

35. Kimura M, Murata Y, Shimoda K, Robinson RG. Sexual dysfunction following stroke. Comprehens Psychiatry. 2001;**42**:217–222.

36. Giaquinto S, Buzzelli S, Di Francesco L, Nolfe G. Evaluation of sexual changes after stroke. J Clin Psychiatry. 2003;**64**:302–307.

37. Baird AD, Wilson SJ, Bladin PF, Saling MM, Reutens DC. Sexual outcome after epilepsy surgery. Epilepsy Behav E&B. 2003;**4**:268–278.

38. Fletcher SG, Castro-Borrero W, Remington G, Treadaway K, Lemack GE, Frohman EM. Sexual dysfunction in patients with multiple sclerosis: a multidisciplinary approach to evaluation and management. Nature clinical practice. Urology. 2009;**6**:96–107.

39. McCabe MP. Exacerbation of symptoms among people with multiple sclerosis: impact on sexuality and relationships over time. Arch Sex Behav. 2004;**33**:593–601.

40. Bronner G, Vodusek DB. Management of sexual dysfunction in Parkinson's disease. Therapeut Adv Neurol Disord. 2011;**4**:375–383.

41. Uitti RJ, Tanner CM, Rajput AH, Goetz CG, Klawans HL, Thiessen B. Hypersexuality with antiparkinsonian therapy. Clinical Neuropharmacol. 1989;**12**:375–383.

42. Fenu S, Wardas J, Morelli M. Impulse control disorders and dopamine dysregulation syndrome associated with dopamine agonist therapy in Parkinson's disease. Behav Pharmacol. 2009;**20**: 363–379.

43. Castelli L, Perozzo P, Genesia ML, et al. Sexual well being in parkinsonian patients after deep brain stimulation of the subthalamic nucleus. J Neurol Neurosurg Psychiatry. 2004;**75**:1260–1264.

44. Sakakibara R, Kishi M, Ogawa E, et al. Bladder, bowel, and sexual dysfunction in Parkinson's disease. Parkinson's Dis. 2011; **2011**:924605.

45. Hess MJ, Hough S. Impact of spinal cord injury on sexuality: broad-based clinical practice intervention and practical application. J spinal Cord Med. 2012;**35**:211–218.

46. Bors E, Comarr A. Neurological disturbances of sexual function with special references to 529 patients with spinal cord injury. Urol Survey. 1960;**10**:191–222.

47. Linsenmeyer TA. Sexual function and infertility following spinal cord injury. Phys Med Rehabil Clin N Am. 2000;**11**:141–156, ix.

48. Alexander CJ, Sipski ML, Findley TW. Sexual activities, desire, and satisfaction in males pre- and post-spinal cord injury. Arch Sex Behav. 1993;**22**:217–228.

49. Ricciardi R, Szabo CM, Poullos AY. Sexuality and spinal cord injury. Nursing Clin N Am. 2007;**42**:675–684; viii–ix.

50. Sipski ML, Alexander CJ, Rosen R. Sexual arousal and orgasm in women: effects of spinal cord injury. Ann Neurol. 2001;**49**:35–44.

51. Komisaruk BR, Whipple B. Functional MRI of the brain during orgasm in women. Annu Rev Sex Res. 2005;**16**:62–86.

52. Iremashvili V, Brackett NL, Ibrahim E, Aballa TC, Lynne CM. Semen quality remains stable during the chronic phase of spinal cord injury: a longitudinal study. J Urol. 2010;**184**:2073–2077.

53. DeForge D, Blackmer J, Garritty C, Yazdi F, Cronin V, Barrowman N et al. Fertility following spinal cord injury: a systematic review. Spinal Cord. 2005;**43**:693–703.

54. Kathiresan AS, Ibrahim E, Modh R, Aballa TC, Lynne CM, Brackett NL. Semen quality in ejaculates produced by masturbation in men with spinal cord injury. Spinal Cord. 2012;**50**:891–894.

55. Steinhardt GF, Goodgold HM, Samuels LD. The effect of intravesical pressure on glomerular filtration rate in patients with myelomeningocele. J Urol. 1988;**140**:1293–1295.

56. McGuire EJ, Woodside JR, Borden TA, Weiss RM. Prognostic value of urodynamic testing in myelodysplastic patients. J Urol. 1981;**126**:205–209.

57. Shingleton WB, Bodner DR. The development of urologic complications in relationship to bladder pressure in spinal cord injured patients. J Am Paraplegia Soc. 1993;**16**:14–17.

58. Muller T, Arbeiter K, Aufricht C. Renal function in meningomyelocele: risk factors, chronic renal failure, renal replacement therapy and transplantation. Curr Opin Urol. 2002;**12**:479–484.

59. van den Berg ME, Castellote JM, de Pedro-Cuesta J, Mahillo-Fernandez I. Survival after spinal cord injury: a systematic review. J Neurotrauma. 2010;**27**:1517–1528.

60. Schmidt F, Shin P, Jorgensen TM, Djurhuus JC, Constantinou CE. Urodynamic patterns of normal male micturition: influence of water consumption on urine production and detrusor function. J Urol. 2002;**168**:1458–1463.

61. Cucchi A, Quaglini S, Rovereto B. Proposal for a urodynamic redefinition of detrusor underactivity. J Urol. 2009;**181**:225–229.

62. Drake MJ, Apostolidis A, Emmanuel A, et al. Committee 10: Neurologic Urinary and Faecal Incontinence. In: Abrams P, Cardozo L, Khoury S, Wein A (eds) Incontinence. EAU, Arnhem, The Netherlands, 2013, pp. 827–1000.

63. Pannek J, Blok BF, Castro-Diaz D, et al.Guidelines on neurogenic lower urinary tract dysfunction. In: European Association of Urology (EAU), Arnhem, The Netherlands, 2011. Available from //www.guideline.gov/content.aspx?id=34062 (accessed 3 October 2014).

64. Andersson KE, Appell R, Cardozo LD, et al. The pharmacological treatment of urinary incontinence. BJU Int. 1999;**84**:923–947.

65. Sellers DJ, Chess-Williams R. Muscarinic agonists and antagonists: effects on the urinary bladder. In: Rosenthal W (ed.) Handbook of Experimental Pharmacology. Springer, Berlin, 2012, pp. 375–400.

66. Athanasopoulos A, ad Giannitsas K. An overview of the clinical use of antimuscarinics in the treatment of overactive bladder. Adv Urol. 2011;**2011**:820816.

67. Amend B, Hennenlotter J, Schafer T, Horstmann M, Stenzl A, Sievert KD. Effective treatment of neurogenic detrusor dysfunction by combined high-dosed antimuscarinics without increased side-effects. Eur Urol. 2008;**53**:1021–1028.

68. Horstmann M, Schaefer T, Aguilar Y, Stenzl A, Sievert KD. Neurogenic bladder treatment by doubling the recommended antimuscarinic dosage. Neurourol Urodyn. 2006;**25**:441–445.

69. Menarini M, Del Popolo G, Di Benedetto P, et al. Trospium chloride in patients with neurogenic detrusor overactivity: is dose titration of benefit to the patients? Int J Clin Pharmacol Therapeut. 2006;**44**:623–632.

70. Schwantes U, Topfmeier P. Importance of pharmacological and physicochemical properties for tolerance of antimuscarinic drugs in the treatment of detrusor instability and detrusor hyperreflexia—chances for improvement of therapy. Int J Clin Pharmacol Therapeut.1999;**37**:209–218.

71. Blok BF, Groen J, Bosch JL, Veltman DJ, Lammertsma AA. Different brain effects during chronic and acute sacral neuromodulation in urge incontinent patients with implanted neurostimulators. BJU Int. 2006;**98**:1238–1243.

72. Kavia R, Dasgupta R, Critchley H, Fowler C, Griffiths D. A functional magnetic resonance imaging study of the effect of sacral neuromodulation on brain responses in women with Fowler's syndrome. BJU Int.2010;**105**:366–372.

73. Mehnert U, Boy S, Svensson J, et al. Brain activation in response to bladder filling and simultaneous stimulation of the dorsal clitoral nerve—an fMRI study in healthy women. Neuroimage. 2008;**41**:682–689.

74. Craggs M, McFarlane J. Neuromodulation of the lower urinary tract. Exp Physiol. 1999;**84**:149–160.

75. Staskin DR, Peters KM, MacDiarmid S, Shore N, de Groat WC. Percutaneous tibial nerve stimulation: a clinically and cost effective addition to the overactive bladder algorithm of care. Curr Urol Rep. 2012;**13**:327–334.

76. Melzack R, Wall PD. Pain mechanisms: a new theory. Science. 1965;**150**:971–979.

77. Lindstrom S, Fall M, Carlsson CA, Erlandson BE. The neurophysiological basis of bladder inhibition in response to intravaginal electrical stimulation. J Urol. 1983;**129**:405–410.

78. Dalmose AL, Rijkhoff NJ, Kirkeby HJ, Nohr M, Sinkjaer T, Djurhuus JC. Conditional stimulation of the dorsal penile/clitoral nerve may increase cystometric capacity in patients with spinal cord injury. Neurourol Urodyn. 2003;**22**:130–137.

79. Horvath EE, Yoo PB, Amundsen CL, Webster GD, Grill WM. Conditional and continuous electrical stimulation increase cystometric capacity in persons with spinal cord injury. Neurourol Urodyn. 2010;**29**:401–407.

80. Andrews BJ, Reynard JM. Transcutaneous posterior tibial nerve stimulation for treatment of detrusor hyperreflexia in spinal cord injury. J Urol. 2003;**170**:926.

81. Kabay SC, Kabay S, Yucel M, Ozden H. Acute urodynamic effects of percutaneous posterior tibial nerve stimulation on neurogenic detrusor overactivity in patients with Parkinson's disease. Neurourol Urodyn. 2009;**28**:62–67.

82. de Seze M, Raibaut P, Gallien P, et al.Transcutaneous posterior tibial nerve stimulation for treatment of the overactive bladder syndrome in multiple sclerosis: results of a multicenter prospective study. Neurourol Urodyn. 2011;**30**:306–311.

83. De Ridder D, Vermeulen C, Ketelaer P, Van Poppel H, Baert L. Pelvic floor rehabilitation in multiple sclerosis. Acta Neurol Belg. 1999;**99**:61–64.

84. Hagerty JA, Richards I, Kaplan WE. Intravesical electrotherapy for neurogenic bladder dysfunction: a 22-year experience. J Urol. 2007;**178**:1680–1683; discussion 1683.

85. Decter RM, Snyder P and Rosvanis TK. Transurethral electrical bladder stimulation: initial results. J Urol. 1992;**148**:651–643; discussion 654.

86. Apostolidis A, Dasgupta P, Denys P, et al. Recommendations on the use of botulinum toxin in the treatment of lower urinary tract disorders and pelvic floor dysfunctions: a European consensus report. Eur Urol. 2009;**55**:100–119.

87. Cruz F, Herschorn S, Aliotta P, et al. Efficacy and safety of onabotulinumtoxinA in patients with urinary incontinence due to neurogenic detrusor overactivity: a randomised, double-blind, placebo-controlled trial. Eur Urol. 2011;**60**:742–750.

88. Lam SM. The basic science of botulinum toxin. Facial Plast Surg Clin North Am. 2003;**11**:431–438.

89. Montal M. Botulinum neurotoxin: a marvel of protein design. Annu Rev Biochem. 2010;**79**:591–617.

90. Karsenty G, Denys P, Amarenco G, et al. Botulinum toxin A (Botox) intradetrusor injections in adults with neurogenic detrusor overactivity/neurogenic overactive bladder: a systematic literature review. Eur Urol. 2008;**53**:275–287.

91. Kessler TM, Khan S, Panicker J, Roosen A, Elneil S, Fowler CJ. Clean intermittent self-catheterization after botulinum neurotoxin type A injections: short-term effect on quality of life. Obstet Gynecol. 2009;**113**:1046–1051.

92. Dowson C, Khan MS, Dasgupta P and Sahai A. Repeat botulinum toxin-A injections for treatment of adult detrusor overactivity. Nat Rev Urol. 2010;**7**:661–667.

93. Yokoyama T, Chancellor MB, Oguma K, et al.Botulinum toxin type A for the treatment of lower urinary tract disorders. In J Urol. 2012;**19**:202–215.

94. Kessler TM, La Framboise D, Trelle S, et al.Sacral neuromodulation for neurogenic lower urinary tract dysfunction: systematic review and meta-analysis. Eur Urol. 2010;**58**:865–874.

95. Apostolidis A. Neuromodulation for intractable OAB. Neurourol Urodyn. 2011;**30**:766–770.

96. Sievert KD, Amend B, Gakis G, et al. Early sacral neuromodulation prevents urinary incontinence after complete spinal cord injury. Ann Neurol. 2010;**67**:74–84.

97. Kutzenberger J. Surgical therapy of neurogenic detrusor overactivity (hyperreflexia) in paraplegic patients by sacral deafferentation and implant driven micturition by sacral anterior root stimulation: methods, indications, results, complications, and future prospects. Acta Neurochir Suppl. 2007;**97**:333–339.

98. Madersbacher H, Fischer J. Sacral anterior root stimulation: prerequisites and indications. Neurourol Urodyn, 1993;**12**:489–494.

99. Reyblat P, Ginsberg DA. Augmentation cystoplasty: what are the indications? Curr Urol Rep. 2008;**9**:452–458.

100. Greenwell TJ, Venn SN, Mundy AR. Augmentation cystoplasty. BJU Int. 2001;**88**:511–525.

101. Fisch M, Thuroff JW. Continent cutaneous diversion. BJU Int. 2008;**102**:1314–1319.

102. Hautmann RE. Urinary diversion: ileal conduit to neobladder. J Urol. 2003;**169**:834–842.

103. Bricker EM. Bladder substitution after pelvic evisceration. Surg Clin North Am. 1950;**30**:1511–1521.

104. Madersbacher S, Schmidt J, Eberle JM, et al. Long-term outcome of ileal conduit diversion. J Urol. 2003;**169**:985–990.

105. Pagano S, Ruggeri P, Rovellini P, Bottanelli A. The anterior ileal conduit: results of 100 consecutive cases. J Urol. 2005;**174**:959–962; discussion 962.

106. Nitti VW. Is there a role for alpha-blockers for the treatment of voiding dysfunction unrelated to benign prostatic hyperplasia? Rev Urol. 2005;7(Suppl 4):S49–55.

107. Groah SL, Weitzenkamp DA, Lammertse DP, Whiteneck GG, Lezotte DC, Hamman RF. Excess risk of bladder cancer in spinal cord injury: evidence for an association between indwelling catheter use and bladder cancer. Arch Phys Med Rehabil. 2002;**83**:346–351.

108. Pannek J. Transitional cell carcinoma in patients with spinal cord injury: a high risk malignancy? Urology. 2002;**59**:240–244.

109. Juma S, Mostafavi M, Joseph A. Sphincterotomy: long-term complications and warning signs. Neurourol Urodyn. 1995;**14**:33–41.

110. Boone TB. External urethral sphincter stent for dyssynergia. J Urol. 2009;**181**:1538–1539.

111. Denys P, Thiry-Escudie I, Ayoub N, Even-Schneider A, Benyahya S, Chartier-Kastler E. Urethral stent for the treatment of detrusor-sphincter dyssynergia: evaluation of the clinical, urodynamic, endoscopic and radiological efficacy after more than 1 year. J Urol. 2004;**172**:605–607.

112. Game X, Chartier-Kastler E, Ayoub N, Even-Schneider A, Richard F, Denys P. Outcome after treatment of detrusor-sphincter dyssynergia by temporary stent. Spinal Cord. 2008;**46**:74–77.

113. Chancellor MB, Bennett C, Simoneau AR, et al. Sphincteric stent versus external sphincterotomy in spinal cord injured men: prospective randomized multicenter trial. J Urol. 1999;**161**:1893–1898.

114. Chancellor MB, Gajewski J, Ackman CF, et al. Long-term followup of the North American multicenter UroLume trial for the treatment of external detrusor-sphincter dyssynergia. J Urol. 1999;**161**:1545–1550.

115. Gallien P, Reymann JM, Amarenco G, Nicolas B, de Seze M, Bellissant E. Placebo controlled, randomised, double blind study of the effects of botulinum A toxin on detrusor sphincter dyssynergia in multiple sclerosis patients. J Neurol Neurosurg Psychiatry. 2005;**76**:1670–1676.

116. de Seze M, Petit H, Gallien P, et al. Botulinum a toxin and detrusor sphincter dyssynergia: a double-blind lidocaine-controlled study in 13 patients with spinal cord disease. Eur Urol. 2002;**42**:56–62.

117. Dykstra DD, Sidi AA, Scott AB, Pagel JM, Goldish GD. Effects of botulinum A toxin on detrusor-sphincter dyssynergia in spinal cord injury patients. J Urol. 1988;**139**:919–922.

118. Chen SL, Bih LI, Chen GD, Huang YH, You YH. Comparing a transrectal ultrasound-guided with a cystoscopy-guided botulinum toxin a injection in treating detrusor external sphincter dyssynergia in spinal cord injury. Am J Phys Med Rehabil. 2011;**90**:723–730.

119. Schulte-Baukloh H, Schobert J, Stolze T, Sturzebecher B, Weiss C, Knispel HH. Efficacy of botulinum-A toxin bladder injections for the treatment of neurogenic detrusor overactivity in multiple sclerosis patients: an objective and subjective analysis. Neurourol Urodyn. 2006;**25**:110–115.

120. Lapides J, Diokno AC, Silber SJ, Lowe BS. Clean, intermittent self-catheterization in the treatment of urinary tract disease. J Urol. 1972;**107**:458–461.

121. Saxtorph MH. Strictura urethrae, Fistula perinei, Retentio urinae. In: Chirurgiske Forelæsninger: Supplement til 'Clinisk Chirurgi' Copenhagen: Gyldendalske Baghandels Forlag, 1878, p. 265–280.

122. Katona F. Electric stimulation in the diagnosis and therapy of bladder paralysis.. Orvosi Hetilap. 1958;**99**:277–278.

123. Madersbacher H. Intravesical electrical stimulation for the rehabilitation of the neuropathic bladder. Paraplegia. 1990;**28**:349–352.

124. Primus G, Kramer G, Pummer K. Restoration of micturition in patients with acontractile and hypocontractile detrusor by transurethral electrical bladder stimulation. Neurourol Urodyn. 1996;**15**:489–497.

125. Katona F, Berenyi M. Intravesical transurethral electrotherapy in meningomyelocele patients. Acta Paediatr Acad Scientiarum Hungaricae. 1975;**16**:363–374.

126. Cendron M, Gearhart JP. The Mitrofanoff principle. Technique and application in continent urinary diversion. Urol Clin North Am. 1991;**18**:615–621.

127. Bihrle R, Adams MC, Foster RS. Adaptations of the Mitrofanoff principle in adult continent urinary reservoirs. Tech Urol. 1995;**1**:94–101.

128. Castellan MA, Gosalbez R, Jr., Labbie A, Monti PR. Clinical applications of the Monti procedure as a continent catheterizable stoma. Urology. 1999;**54**:152–156.

129. Brindley GS, Polkey CE, Rushton DN, Cardozo L. Sacral anterior root stimulators for bladder control in paraplegia: the first 50 cases. J Neurol Neurosurg Psychiatry. 1986;**49**:1104–1114.

130. Ragnarsson KT. Functional electrical stimulation after spinal cord injury: current use, therapeutic effects and future directions. Spinal Cord. 2008;**46**:255–274.

131. Kutzenberger J, Domurath B, Sauerwein D. Spastic bladder and spinal cord injury: seventeen years of experience with sacral deafferentation and implantation of an anterior root stimulator. Artif Organs. 2005;**29**:239–241.

132. Ninkovic M, Stenzl A, Schwabegger A, Bartsch G, Prosser R. Free neurovascular transfer of latisstmus dorsi muscle for the treatment of bladder acontractility: II. Clinical results. J Urol. 2003;**169**:1379–1383.

133. Gakis G, Ninkovic M, van Koeveringe GA, et al. Functional detrusor myoplasty for bladder acontractility: long-term results. J Urol. 2011;**185**:593–599.

134. Ghoniem G, Corcos J, Comiter C, Bernhard P, Westney OL, Herschorn S. Cross-linked polydimethylsiloxane injection for female stress urinary incontinence: results of a multicenter, randomized, controlled, single-blind study. J Urol. 2009;**181**:204–210.

135. Ghoniem G, Corcos J, Comiter C, Westney OL, Herschorn S. Durability of urethral bulking agent injection for female stress urinary incontinence: 2-year multicenter study results. J Urol. 2010;**183**:1444–1449.

136. Keegan PE, Atiemo K, Cody J, McClinton S, Pickard R. Periurethral injection therapy for urinary incontinence in women. Cochrane Database Syst Rev. 2007; CD003881.

137. Latthe PM. Review of transobturator and retropubic tape procedures for stress urinary incontinence. Curr Opin Obstet Gynecol. 2008;**20**:331–336.

138. Nilsson CG, Palva K, Rezapour M, Falconer C. Eleven years prospective follow-up of the tension-free vaginal tape procedure for treatment of stress urinary incontinence. Int Urogynecol J Pelvic Floor Dysfunct. 2008;**19**:1043–1047.

139. Romano SV, Metrebian SE, Vaz F, et al. An adjustable male sling for treating urinary incontinence after prostatectomy: a phase III multicentre trial. BJU Int. 2006;**97**:533–539.

140. Sandhu JS. Treatment options for male stress urinary incontinence. Nat Rev Urol. 2010;**7**:222–228.

141. Austin PF, Westney OL, Leng WW, McGuire EJ, Ritchey ML. Advantages of rectus fascial slings for urinary incontinence in children with neuropathic bladders. J Urol. 2001;**165**:2369–2371; discussion 2371–2.

142. Castellan M, Gosalbez R, Labbie A, Ibrahim E, Disandro M. Bladder neck sling for treatment of neurogenic incontinence in children with augmentation cystoplasty: long-term followup. J Urol. 2005;**173**:2128–2131; discussion 2131.

143. Chrzan R, Dik P, Klijn AJ, de Jong TP. Sling suspension of the bladder neck for pediatric urinary incontinence. J Pediatr Urol. 2009;**5**:82–86.

144. Dik P, Klijn AJ, van Gool JD, de Jong TP. Transvaginal sling suspension of bladder neck in female patients with neurogenic sphincter incontinence. J Urol. 2003;**170**:580–581; discussion 581–2.

145. Nguyen HT, Bauer SB, Diamond DA, Retik AB. Rectus fascial sling for the treatment of neurogenic sphincteric incontinence in boys: is it safe and effective? J Urol. 2001;**166**:658–661.

146. Snodgrass W, Keefover-Hicks A, Prieto J, Bush N, Adams R. Comparing outcomes of slings with versus without enterocystoplasty for neurogenic urinary incontinence. J Urol. 2009;**181**: 2709–2714; discussion 2714–6.

147. Snodgrass WT, Elmore J, Adams R. Bladder neck sling and appendicovesicostomy without augmentation for neurogenic incontinence in children. J Urol. 2007;**177**:1510–1514; discussion 1515.

148. Dean GE, Kunkle DA. Outpatient perineal sling in adolescent boys with neurogenic incontinence. J Urol. 2009;**182**:1792–1796.

149. Hussain M, Greenwell TJ, Venn SN, Mundy AR. The current role of the artificial urinary sphincter for the treatment of urinary incontinence. J Urol. 2005;174:418–424.

150. Fulford SC, Sutton C, Bales G, Hickling M, Stephenson TP. The fate of the 'modern' artificial urinary sphincter with a follow-up of more than 10 years. Br J Urol. 1997;79:713–716.

151. Lopez Pereira P, Somoza Ariba I, Martinez Urrutia MJ, Lobato Romero R, Jaureguizar Monroe E. Artificial urinary sphincter: 11-year experience in adolescents with congenital neuropathic bladder. Eur Urol. 2006;50:1096–1101; discussion 1101.

152. Murphy S, Rea D, O'Mahony J, et al. A comparison of the functional durability of the AMS 800 artificial urinary sphincter between cases with and without an underlying neurogenic aetiology. Ir J Med Sci. 2003;172:136–138.

153. Patki P, Hamid R, Shah PJ, Craggs M. Long-term efficacy of AMS 800 artificial urinary sphincter in male patients with urodynamic stress incontinence due to spinal cord lesion. Spinal Cord. 2006;44:297–300.

154. Simeoni J, Guys JM, Mollard P, et al. Artificial urinary sphincter implantation for neurogenic bladder: a multi-institutional study in 107 children. Br J Urol. 1996;78:287–293.

155. Singh G, Thomas DG. Artificial urinary sphincter in patients with neurogenic bladder dysfunction. Br J Urol. 1996;77:252–255.

156. Venn SN, Greenwell TJ, Mundy AR. The long-term outcome of artificial urinary sphincters. J Urol. 2000;164:702–706; discussion 706–7.

157. Bersch U, Gocking K, Pannek J. The artificial urinary sphincter in patients with spinal cord lesion: description of a modified technique and clinical results. Eur Urol. 2009;55:687–693.

158. Gilling PJ, Bell DF, Wilson LC, Westenberg AM, Reuther R, Fraundorfer MR. An adjustable continence therapy device for treating incontinence after prostatectomy: a minimum 2-year follow-up. BJU Int. 2008;102:1426–1430; discussion 1430–1.

159. Hubner WA, Schlarp OM. Adjustable continence therapy (ProACT): evolution of the surgical technique and comparison of the original 50 patients with the most recent 50 patients at a single centre. Eur Urol. 2007;52:680–686.

160. Mehnert U, Bastien L, Denys P, et al. Treatment of neurogenic stress urinary incontinence using an adjustable continence device: 4-year followup. J Urol. 2012;188:2274–2280.

161. Pannek J. [Prophylaxis of urinary tract infections in subjects with spinal cord injury and bladder function disorders—current clinical practice]. Aktuelle Urologie. 2012; 43: 55–58.

162. Salomon J, Denys P, Merle C, et al. Prevention of urinary tract infection in spinal cord-injured patients: safety and efficacy of a weekly oral cyclic antibiotic (WOCA) programme with a 2 year follow-up—an observational prospective study. J Antimicrob Chemother. 2006;57:784–788.

163. Welk B, Fuller A, Razvi H, Denstedt J. Renal stone disease in spinal-cord-injured patients. J Endourol. 2012;26: 954–959.

164. Türk C, Knoll T, Petrik A, et al. Guidelines on urolithiasis. European Association of Urology (EAU), Arnhem, The Netherlands, 2008 (updated 2013). Available from http://www.guideline.gov/content.aspx?id=45324&search=urolithiasis (accessed 3 October 2014).

165. Ehrenpreis ED, Chang D, Eichenwald E. Pharmacotherapy for fecal incontinence: a review. Dis Colon Rectum. 2007;50:641–649.

166. Correa GI, Rotter KP. Clinical evaluation and management of neurogenic bowel after spinal cord injury. Spinal Cord. 2000;38:301–308.

167. Dunn KL, Galka ML. A comparison of the effectiveness of Therevac SB and bisacodyl suppositories in SCI patients' bowel programs. Rehabil Nursing. 1994;19:334–338.

168. Emmanuel A. Managing neurogenic bowel dysfunction. Clin Rehabil. 2010;24:483–488.

169. Christensen P, Krogh K, Buntzen S, Payandeh F, Laurberg S. Long-term outcome and safety of transanal irrigation for constipation and fecal incontinence. Dis Colon Rectum. 2009;52:286–292.

170. Palmer LS, Richards I, Kaplan WE. Transrectal electrostimulation therapy for neuropathic bowel dysfunction in children with myelomeningocele. J Urol. 1997;157:1449–1452.

171. Kajbafzadeh AM, Sharifi-Rad L, Nejat F, Kajbafzadeh M, Talaei HR. Transcutaneous interferential electrical stimulation for management of neurogenic bowel dysfunction in children with myelomeningocele. Int J Colorectal Dis. 2012;27:453–458.

172. Chiu CM, Wang CP, Sung WH, Huang SF, Chiang SC, Tsai PY. Functional magnetic stimulation in constipation associated with Parkinson's disease. J Rehabil Med. 2009;41:1085–1089.

173. Tsai PY, Wang CP, Chiu FY, Tsai YA, Chang YC, Chuang TY. Efficacy of functional magnetic stimulation in neurogenic bowel dysfunction after spinal cord injury. J Rehabil Med. 2009;41:41–47.

174. Bond C, Youngson G, MacPherson I, et al. Anal plugs for the management of fecal incontinence in children and adults: a randomized control trial. J Clin Gastroenterol. 2007;41:45–53.

175. Maeda Y, Laurberg S, Norton C. Perianal injectable bulking agents as treatment for faecal incontinence in adults. Cochrane Database Syst Rev. 2013;2:CD007959.

176. Brown SR, Wadhawan H, Nelson RL. Surgery for faecal incontinence in adults. Cochrane Database Syst Rev. 2013;7:CD001757.

177. Parks AG. Royal Society of Medicine, Section of Proctology; Meeting 27 November 1974. President's Address. Anorectal incontinence. Proc Roy Soc Med. 1975; 68: 681–690.

178. Mackey P, Mackey L, Kennedy ML, et al. Postanal repair—do the long-term results justify the procedure? Colorectal Dis. 2010;12:367–372.

179. Womack NR, Morrison JF, Williams NS. Prospective study of the effects of postanal repair in neurogenic faecal incontinence. Br J Surg. 1988;75:48–52.

180. Setti Carraro P, Kamm MA, Nicholls RJ. Long-term results of postanal repair for neurogenic faecal incontinence. Br J Surg. 1994;81:140–144.

181. Holzer B, Rosen HR, Novi G, Ausch C, Holbling N, Schiessel R. Sacral nerve stimulation for neurogenic faecal incontinence. Br J Surg. 2007;94:749–753.

182. Lombardi G, Del Popolo G, Cecconi F, Surrenti E, Macchiarella A. Clinical outcome of sacral neuromodulation in incomplete spinal cord-injured patients suffering from neurogenic bowel dysfunctions. Spinal Cord. 2010;48:154–159.

183. Rosen HR, Urbarz C, Holzer B, Novi G, Schiessel R. Sacral nerve stimulation as a treatment for fecal incontinence. Gastroenterology. 2001;121:536–541.

185. Vastenholt JM, Snoek GJ, Buschman HP, van der Aa HE, Alleman ER, Ijzerman MJ. A 7-year follow-up of sacral anterior root stimulation for bladder control in patients with a spinal cord injury: quality of life and users' experiences. Spinal Cord. 2003;41:397–402.

186. Malone PS, Ransley PG, Kiely EM. Preliminary report: the antegrade continence enema. Lancet. 1990;336:1217–1218.

187. Herndon CD, Rink RC, Cain MP, et al. In situ Malone antegrade continence enema in 127 patients: a 6-year experience. J Urol. 2004;172:1689–1691.

188. Bar-Yosef Y, Castellan M, Joshi D, Labbie A, Gosalbez R. Total continence reconstruction using the artificial urinary sphincter and the Malone antegrade continence enema. J Urol. 2011;185:1444–1447.

189. Teichman JM, Zabihi N, Kraus SR, Harris JM, Barber DB. Long-term results for Malone antegrade continence enema for adults with neurogenic bowel disease. Urology. 2003;61:502–506.

190. Bruce RG, el-Galley RE, Wells J, Galloway NT. Antegrade continence enema for the treatment of fecal incontinence in adults: use of gastric tube for catheterizable access to the descending colon. J Urol. 1999;161:1813–1816.

191. Dey R, Ferguson C, Kenny SE, et al. After the honeymoon—medium-term outcome of antegrade continence enema procedure. J Pediatr Surg. 2003;38:65–68; discussion 65–8.

192. Lehur PA, Michot F, Denis P, et al. Results of artificial sphincter in severe anal incontinence. Report of 14 consecutive implantations. Dis Colon Rectum. 1996;**39**:1352–1355.

193. Parker SC, Spencer MP, Madoff RD, Jensen LL, Wong WD, Rothenberger DA. Artificial bowel sphincter: long-term experience at a single institution. Dis Colon Rectum. 2003;**46**:722–729.

194. Wong WD, Jensen LL, Bartolo DC, Rothenberger DA. Artificial anal sphincter. Dis Colon Rectum. 1996;**39**:1345–1351.

195. Christiansen J, Rasmussen OO, Lindorff-Larsen K. Long-term results of artificial anal sphincter implantation for severe anal incontinence. Ann Surg. 1999;**230**:45–48.

196. Wong WD, Congliosi SM, Spencer MP, et al. The safety and efficacy of the artificial bowel sphincter for fecal incontinence: results from a multicenter cohort study. Dis Colon Rectum. 2002;**45**:1139–1153.

197. Devesa JM, Rey A, Hervas PL, et al. Artificial anal sphincter: complications and functional results of a large personal series. Dis Colon Rectum. 2002;**45**:1154–1163.

198. Michot F, Costaglioli B, Leroi AM, Denis P. Artificial anal sphincter in severe fecal incontinence: outcome of prospective experience with 37 patients in one institution. Ann Surg. 2003;**237**:52–56.

199. Baeten C, Spaans F, Fluks A. An implanted neuromuscular stimulator for fecal continence following previously implanted gracilis muscle. Report of a case. Dis Colon Rectum. 1988;**31**:134–137.

200. Salmons S, Vrbova G. The influence of activity on some contractile characteristics of mammalian fast and slow muscles. J Physiol. 1969;**201**:535–549.

201. Salmons S, Henriksson J. The adaptive response of skeletal muscle to increased use. Muscle Nerve. 1981;**4**:94–105.

202. Rongen MJ, Uludag O, El Naggar K, Geerdes BP, Konsten J, Baeten CG. Long-term follow-up of dynamic graciloplasty for fecal incontinence. Dis Colon Rectum. 2003;**46**:716–721.

203. Wexner SD, Baeten C, Bailey R, et al. Long-term efficacy of dynamic graciloplasty for fecal incontinence. Dis Colon Rectum. 2002;**45**:809–818.

204. Madoff RD, Rosen HR, Baeten CG, et al. Safety and efficacy of dynamic muscle plasty for anal incontinence: lessons from a prospective, multicenter trial. Gastroenterology. 1999;**116**:549–556.

205. Ortiz H, Armendariz P, DeMiguel M, Solana A, Alos R, ad Roig JV. Prospective study of artificial anal sphincter and dynamic graciloplasty for severe anal incontinence. Int J Colorectal Dis. 2003;**18**:349–354.

206. Matzel KE, Madoff RD, LaFontaine LJ, et al. Complications of dynamic graciloplasty: incidence, management, and impact on outcome. DisColon Rectum. 2001;**44**:1427–1435.

207. Lai JM, Chuang TY, Francisco GE, Strayer JR. Diversion colitis: a cause of abdominal discomfort in spinal cord injury patients with colostomy. Arch Phys Med Rehabil. 1997;**78**:670–671.

208. Hocevar B, Gray M. Intestinal diversion (colostomy or ileostomy) in patients with severe bowel dysfunction following spinal cord injury. J Wound OstomyContinence Nursing. 2008;**35**:159–166.

209. Hatzimouratidis K, Hatzichristou D. Sexual dysfunctions: classifications and definitions. J Sex Med. 2007;**4**:241–250.

210. Lewis RW, Fugl-Meyer KS, Corona G, et al. Definitions/epidemiology/risk factors for sexual dysfunction. J Sex Med. 2010;**7**:1598–1607.

211. Southard NZ, Keller J. The importance of assessing sexuality: a patient perspective. Clin J Oncol Nursing. 2009;**13**:213–217.

212. Rosen RC, Riley A, Wagner G, Osterloh IH, Kirkpatrick J, Mishra A. The international index of erectile function (IIEF): a multidimensional scale for assessment of erectile dysfunction. Urology. 1997;**49**:822–830.

213. Rosen R, Brown C, Heiman J, et al. The Female Sexual Function Index (FSFI): a multidimensional self-report instrument for the assessment of female sexual function. J Sex Marital Therapy. 2000;**26**:191–208.

214. Davis SR, Moreau M, Kroll R, et al. Testosterone for low libido in postmenopausal women not taking estrogen. N Engl J Med. 2008;**359**:2005–2017.

215. Bolour S, Braunstein G. Testosterone therapy in women: a review. Int J Impotence Res. 2005;**17**:399–408.

216. Klos KJ, Bower JH, Josephs KA, Matsumoto JY, Ahlskog JE. Pathological hypersexuality predominantly linked to adjuvant dopamine agonist therapy in Parkinson's disease and multiple system atrophy. Parkinsonism Related Disorders. 2005;**11**:381–386.

217. Andersson KE. Mechanisms of penile erection and basis for pharmacological treatment of erectile dysfunction. Pharmacol Rev. 2011;**63**:811–859.

218. Shamloul R, Ghanem H. Erectile dysfunction. Lancet. 2013;**381**:153–165.

219. Lombardi G, Macchiarella A, Cecconi F, Del Popolo G. Ten years of phosphodiesterase type 5 inhibitors in spinal cord injured patients. J Sex Med. 2009;**6**:1248–1258.

220. Fowler CJ, Miller JR, Sharief MK, Hussain IF, Stecher VJ, Sweeney M. A double blind, randomised study of sildenafil citrate for erectile dysfunction in men with multiple sclerosis. J Neurol Neurosurg Psychiatry. 2005;**76**:700–705.

221. Hussain IF, Brady CM, Swinn MJ, Mathias CJ, Fowler CJ. Treatment of erectile dysfunction with sildenafil citrate (Viagra) in parkinsonism due to Parkinson's disease or multiple system atrophy with observations on orthostatic hypotension. J Neurol Neurosurg Psychiatry. 2001;**71**:371–374.

222. Moemen MN, Fahmy I, AbdelAal M, Kamel I, Mansour M, Arafa MM. Erectile dysfunction in spinal cord-injured men: different treatment options. IntJ Impotence Res. 2008;**20**:181–187.

223. Sipski ML, Rosen RC, Alexander CJ, Hamer RM. Sildenafil effects on sexual and cardiovascular responses in women with spinal cord injury. Urology. 2000;**55**:812–815.

224. Dasgupta R, Wiseman OJ, Kanabar G, Fowler CJ, Mikol D. Efficacy of sildenafil in the treatment of female sexual dysfunction due to multiple sclerosis. J Urol. 2004;**171**:1189–1193; discussion 1193.

245. Spinelli M, Malaguti S, Giardiello G, Lazzeri M, Tarantola J, Van Den Hombergh U. A new minimally invasive procedure for pudendal nerve stimulation to treat neurogenic bladder: description of the method and preliminary data. Neurourol Urodyn. 2005;**24**:305–309.

246. Heinze K, Hörmann R, Fritsch H and van Ophoven A: Kadaver-Studie zur Modifizierung der Elektrodenplatzierung bei pudendaler Neuromodulation [abstract]: 22.Jahrestagung des Forum Urodynamicum e.V.,2011.

247. Possover M, Schurch B, Henle K. New strategies of pelvic nerves stimulation for recovery of pelvic visceral functions and locomotion in paraplegics. Neurourol Urodyn. 2010;**29**(8):1433–1438.

248. Fjorback MV, Rijkhoff N, Petersen T, Nohr M, Sinkjaer T. Event driven electrical stimulation of the dorsal penile/clitoral nerve for management of neurogenic detrusor overactivity in multiple sclerosis. Neurourol Urodyn. 2006;**25**:349–355.

249. Opisso E, Borau A, Rodriguez A, Hansen J, Rijkhoff NJ. Patient controlled versus automatic stimulation of pudendal nerve afferents to treat neurogenic detrusor overactivity. J Urol. 2008;**180**:1403–1408.

250. Caremel R, Loutochin O and Corcos J. What do we know and not know about mirabegron, a novel beta3 agonist, in the treatment of overactive bladder? International Urogynecol J. 2014;**25**(2):165–170.

251. Gratzke C, Streng T, Stief CG, et al. Effects of cannabinor, a novel selective cannabinoid 2 receptor agonist, on bladder function in normal rats. Eur Urol. 2010;**57**:1093–1100.

252. Fullhase C, Russo A, Castiglione F, et al. Spinal cord FAAH in normal micturition control and bladder overactivity in awake rats. J Urol. 2013;**189**:2364–2370.

253. Fullhase C, Hennenberg M, Giese A, et al. Presence of phosphodiesterase type 5 in the spinal cord and its involvement in bladder outflow obstruction related bladder overactivity. J Urol. 2013;**190**(4):1430–1435.

254. Xiao CG. Reinnervation for neurogenic bladder: historic review and introduction of a somatic-autonomic reflex pathway procedure for patients with spinal cord injury or spina bifida. Eur Urol. 2006;**49**:22–28; discussion 28–9.

255. Xiao CG, Du MX, Dai C, Li B, Nitti VW, de Groat WC. An artificial somatic-central nervous system-autonomic reflex pathway for controllable micturition after spinal cord injury: preliminary results in 15 patients. J Urol. 2003;**170**:1237–1241.

256. Sievert KD, Amend B, Roser F, Tatagiba M, Stenzl A. Outcome of intraspinal nerve re-routing to re-establish bladder function in spinal cord injured patients: a single center experience. J Urol. 2010;**183**:392.

257. Worsoe J, Rasmussen M, Christensen P, Krogh K. Neurostimulation for neurogenic bowel dysfunction. Gastroenterol Res Pract. 2013;**2013**:563294.

258. Atala A, Bauer SB, Soker S, Yoo JJ, Retik AB. Tissue-engineered autologous bladders for patients needing cystoplasty. Lancet. 2006;**367**:1241–1246.

259. Sievert KD, Amend B, Stenzl A. Tissue engineering for the lower urinary tract: a review of a state of the art approach. Eur Urol. 2007;**52**:1580–1589.

CHAPTER 25

The assessment and treatment of pain syndromes in neurorehabilitation

Eva Widerström-Noga

Introduction

A person may experience several types of pain after a trauma involving the central nervous system (CNS) [1–5]. Persistent pains of various origins are common and serious consequences of spinal cord injury (SCI) and stroke [3, 6] with large numbers of patients reporting pain despite the availability of a variety of pharmacological and non-pharmacological treatments [7–12]. A few medications have shown to significantly reduce neuropathic pain severity in SCI clinical pain trials [13–18]; however, no treatments are currently available that completely relieve neuropathic pain [19–21]. Persistent pain is associated with lower well-being, higher levels of depression catastrophizing, affective distress [2, 22–27], significant psychosocial impact [28–31], and lower quality of life [22, 32–34].

Most persistent pains can be categorized into two principal types: nociceptive and neuropathic. Nociceptive pain is caused by the activation of nociceptors or pain receptors, and may be associated with inflammatory mechanisms [3]. This pain type is defined by the International Association for the Study of Pain (IASP) as: 'Pain that arises from actual or threatened damage to non-neural tissue and is due to the activation of nociceptors' (IASP Task Force on Taxonomy [35]). The IASP also added the critical statement that nociceptive pain is used to describe pain occurring within a normally functioning somatosensory nervous system. After SCI, it is generally accepted that pain above the neurological level injury (NLI) is nociceptive as it occurs in an area that has normal somatosensory function as measured with the American Spinal Injury Impairment scale [36]. However, nociceptive pain that is present in an area with significant sensory dysfunction (e.g. pain located either around or below the NLI), is more difficult to determine based on these criteria. Therefore, the determination of nociceptive pain below the NLI should include additional criteria such as changes in pain depending on movement or change in position, muscular tenderness, evidence of skeletal pathology that is consistent with the pain distribution, dull or aching pain qualities, or reduction in pain due to anti-inflammatory medication [4]. A common example of nociceptive pain in persons with SCI is musculoskeletal neck and shoulder pain due to overuse.

The other major category, neuropathic pain, is defined by the IASP as: 'Pain caused by a lesion or disease of the somatosensory nervous system'. The IASP definition states that neuropathic pain is a clinical description that requires evidence of a lesion or trauma, or neurological findings that indicate the presence of neurological trauma or disease. When determination of neuropathic after neurotrauma is difficult and/or inconclusive, a tentative diagnosis based on clinical judgment is recommended.

Neuropathic pain caused by an injury to the brain can present anywhere in the body such as in a hemiplegic shoulder after a stroke [37]. In contrast, neuropathic pain after SCI is primarily present at or below the level of injury. However, the recent SCI pain classification also includes other types of pain not directly caused by SCI to facilitate clinical utility ([4], see Figure 25.1). At-level neuropathic pain is either central in nature (e.g. central neuropathic pain; CNP) or peripheral and caused by injury to the spinal nerve roots. As a contrast, below-level neuropathic pain is a CNP type and a direct consequence of the SCI. CNP can also be a significant part of the complex clinical picture associated with different types of trauma and diseases involving the CNS, such as stroke, multiple sclerosis, epilepsy, tumours, syringomyelia, brain or spinal cord injury, or Parkinson's disease [38, 39]. CNP is often associated both with evoked non-painful and painful sensations such as hyperalgesia (exaggerated pain in response to a mild painful stimulus) and mechanical or thermal allodynia (pain in response to a non-painful stimulus such as light touch, pressure, cool or warm stimuli) [39, 40]. These sensory abnormalities should be routinely assessed as part of the pain evaluation. Although CNP is prevalent after SCI [3], the frequency of CNP in the general population is relatively low [38], and therefore standardized diagnostic and outcome measures are of critical importance since these can facilitate both multicentre trials and the interpretation and application of research results to improve clinical treatment.

Pathophysiology

Underlying pathophysiological mechanisms of chronic pain are dependent on the pain type. However, many underlying mechanisms such as central sensitization are commonly involved in a variety of pain conditions and are not specific to pain type [41]. Nociceptive pain types have similar mechanisms in neurotrauma populations as in the general population; these may include peripheral sensitization, decreased inhibition, increased facilitation, etc. [42].

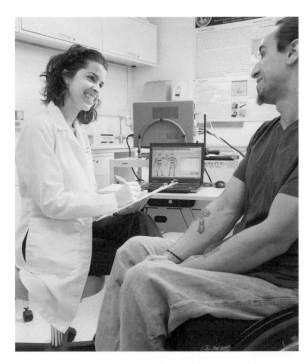

Fig. 25.1 The pain history is a valuable part of the pain evaluation and should be conducted in a relaxed setting.

Some nociceptive pain types may also develop secondary to the physical impairments associated with an injury. A common example of this is musculoskeletal pain in the upper body caused by the overuse and repetitive movements that are necessary for transfer and propulsion of wheelchairs [34, 43].

Injury to the CNS causes widespread changes in both sensory neurons and in various central pain pathways and brain structures and these changes have the potential to result in persistent neuropathic pain [44–48]. One hypothesis that has been proposed is that clinical pain phenotypes (specific combinations of pain symptoms and sensory signs) may reflect underlying mechanisms [48, 49]. Unfortunately, mechanisms of neuropathic pain after neurotrauma are complex with multiple combinations of contributing mechanisms, including loss of inhibition and increased hyperexcitability [50–56], making these translations more difficult. Preclinical research suggests that the development and maintenance of neuropathic pain after SCI is associated with multiple molecular and plastic changes in the central nervous system. These changes include: up-regulation of chemokines and chemokine receptors in the spinal cord [57]; changes in neurotrophic factors and in TrkB tyrosine kinase signalling pathways in the spinal cord [58]; brain plasticity caused by cannabinoid and vanilloid receptors, and chemokine interaction [59]; changes in calcium ion channel expression [60] and membrane transporter proteins [61]; loss of inhibitory interneurons in the spinal dorsal horn [62]; inflammatory mediators [63]; and activation of glial cells in the spinal cord and brain [64].

Assessment of pain and related psychosocial factors

Pain is a subjective phenomenon and self-reported pain symptoms, positive or negative sensory signs, and psychosocial factors are all critical components of the pain experience that should be routinely assessed as part of a comprehensive pain evaluation. There are also important interrelationships between these assessment domains. For example, pain symptoms and signs that are common in neuropathic pain conditions such as intense pain, presence of hyperalgesia or allodynia, electric pain quality, and constant pain, have been associated with greater psychosocial impact [24, 65, 66], perceived as particularly disturbing [67] and predictive of using prescription medication after SCI [68].

In order to accurately assess a specific type of pain in a person who may experience concomitant nociceptive and neuropathic pain types, he or she must be able to differentiate between these. Approximately 75% of people with SCI and chronic pain can differentiate between different types of pain [67, 69]. Therefore, a comprehensive pain evaluation should carefully evaluate each pain separately as part of the general pain assessment (Figure 25.1). For example, the International Spinal Cord Injury Basic Pain Dataset (ISCIBPD) [70] is designed to evaluate the worst, second worst, and third worst pain when a person experiences one or more pains. The ISCIBPD includes a pain classification made by a healthcare professional, and self-reported information regarding number of pain problems, pain location, intensity, and temporal pattern of pain (i.e. onset, presence, and number of days with pain over the last 7 days, duration, and variation in intensity) for each specific pain problem. In addition, the impact of pain on physical, social and emotional function, and sleep is evaluated. The ISCIBPD was reviewed and officially endorsed by major SCI and pain organizations (e.g. the International Spinal Cord Injury Society, the American Spinal Injury Association, the American Pain Society, and the International Association for the Study of Pain, and is now part of the National Institutes of Health (NIH) Common Data Elements http://www.commondataelements. ninds.nih.gov/SCI.aspx#tab=Data_Standards. A self-report version of the ISCIBPD was found to be valid with respect to questions about pain interference, pain intensity, pain location, frequency and duration of pain, and time of day of worst pain [69]. Because the classification of chronic pain after SCI was recently standardized—the International Spinal Cord Injury Pain Classification (ISCIP; [4]; Figure 25.2)—by a consensus group consisting of SCI and pain experts, the ISCIBPDS has been updated to reflect this change [71]. The ISCIP [4] provide a practical framework for classifying pain after SCI and its inter-rater reliability was established [72]. Similar pain taxonomies have also been proposed for other CNS conditions, such as Parkinson's disease [73].

Several self-report measures are available for assessment of general pain intensity or pain severity. The most commonly used is the numerical rating scale (NRS), which has been used widely to assess pain and has excellent reliability and validity [74]. An NRS usually consists of an 11-point scale for pain intensity, with the anchors labeled as 0 = no pain and 10 = most pain imaginable. Another example is the Pain Severity Subscale of the Multidimensional Pain Inventory (MPI) [75] which consist of three items concerning pain severity 'at the moment', during 'the past week', and suffering due to pain. Each item is rated on a scale from 0 to 6 and these are averaged to create a score. Other instruments are specifically designed to evaluate the severity of neuropathic pain symptoms. One example is the Neuropathic Pain Symptom Inventory (NPSI) [76]. The NPSI is sensitive to change and evaluates five common features of neuropathic pain: (1) *evoked pain* includes three questions related to pain evoked by brushing, pressure, or

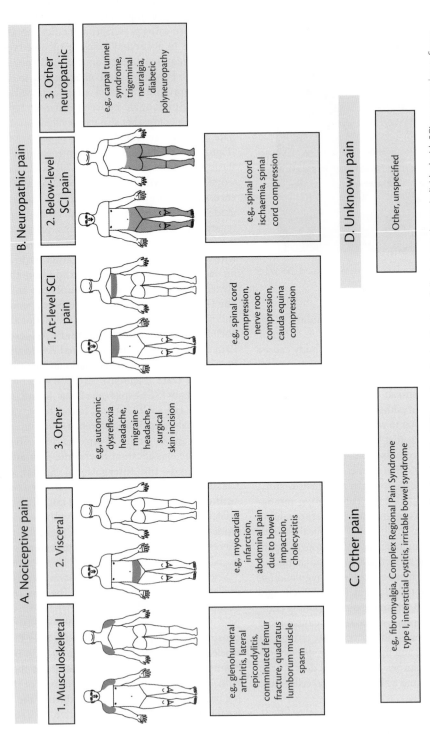

Fig. 25.2 The International Spinal Cord Injury Pain Classification. The ISCIP consists of a classification of all pain types that an individual with SCI may experience. Seven broad types of pain are specified in the ISCIP (possible locations are illustrated in the pain drawings). (A) Nociceptive: 1. Musculoskeletal; 2. Visceral, and 3. Other (pains that are less prevalent or not directly related to SCI and not categorized as musculoskeletal or visceral). (B) Neuropathic: 1. At-level SCI (includes level of neurological injury and three dermatomes below); 2. Below-level; and 3. Other (pains that are not associated with a lesion or disease affecting the spinal cord or nerve roots yet are nevertheless neuropathic). (C) Other category is used for defined pain syndromes of unknown aetiology. (D) Unknown category used when it is not possible to classify the pain into one of the categories listed above and the etiology is unknown.

Reprinted by permission from Macmillan Publishers Ltd: Spinal Cord (50: 404–12), copyright (2012).

cold; (2) *pressing (deep) pain* includes pressure or squeezing qualities; (3) *paroxysmal pain* includes electric shocks and stabbing; (4)
paraesthesia/dysaesthesia includes tingling and pins and needles;
and (5) *burning (superficial)* includes burning pain. The psychometric properties of the NPSI, including its sensitivity to change,
suggest that it may be useful in the evaluation of treatment outcome in clinical practice and in clinical trials [77]. Morover, the
NPSI overall shows many similarities among different patient
groups with peripheral or central lesions, which supports its utility as a method for pain evaluation in diverse neurotrauma populations [78]. However, the psychometric properties for NPSI have
not yet been evaluated for the SCI and other neurotrauma populations. The Neuropathic Pain Scale (NPS) [79] is another psychometric test that may be particularly useful for differentiating
between neuropathic and non-neuropathic pain [80]. It includes
ratings of pain intensity and unpleasantness, pain quality ('sharp,'
'dull,' 'sensitive,' 'hot,' 'cold,' and 'itchy pain'), and spatial qualities ('deep' and 'surface' pain). For recent NIH pain assessment
recommendations for SCI, please visit the NIH-NINDS common
data element website http://www.commondataelements.ninds.
nih.gov/SCI.aspx#tab=Data_Standards.

Quantitative sensory testing (QST)

QST is a common method to quantify positive and negative sensory signs in a standardized way. QST can be used to evaluate sensory function by applying a variety of mechanical and thermal
stimuli that can activate both large (Aβ) and small (Aδ and C)
nerve fibres and their central pathways. QST can assess detection
and pain thresholds and therefore quantify both decreased (negative sensory signs) and increased (positive sensory signs) sensory
function.

Semmes–Weinstein monofilaments can be used to evaluate tactile sensation mediated via the dorsal column medial lemniscus

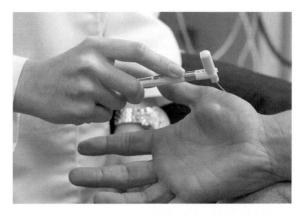

Fig. 25.3 The filament is calibrated to provide a specific amount of force when it bends.

pathway (DCML). This method is simple and one of the most
common non-invasive techniques used in animals and humans
(Figure 25.3). A set usually contains 20 filaments that are individually calibrated within a 5% standard deviation to deliver a target
force ranging from 0.008 to 300 g. A filament no. 5.17 with a bending force of 10 g in combination with a numerical rating scale can
be used to quantify static mechanical allodynia, which is a sensory
abnormality that may be associated with neuropathic pain.

Computer-controlled devices capable of generating and documenting responses to thermal and vibratory stimuli are commercially available. One of these is the TSA Neurosensory Analyzer
(Figure 25.4). This device can be used to quantify the function of
both small-calibre (Aδ and C) and large-calibre (Aβ) nerve fibres
and their central pathways.

Vibratory sense is mediated via the DCML and it can be evaluated
using the handheld probe of the computerized system (Figure 25.5).

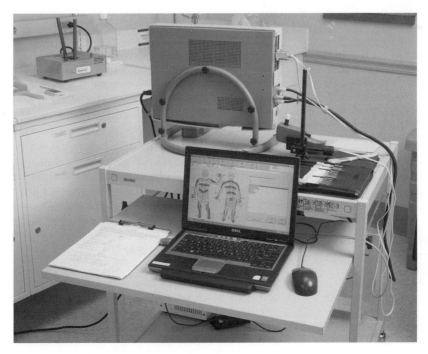

Fig. 25.4 The computer controlled Thermal Sensory Analyzer (TSA) NeuroSensory Analyzer (Medoc).

The vibratory amplitude typically starts at 0 µm at a rate of 0.5 µm/s at a 100 Hz stimulus frequency and is increased until the patient reports a sensation or until the maximum amplitude of 130 µm is reached. Using the same device but with a Peltier thermode, which produces either a cold or warm stimulus, the temperature sense mediated via Aδ and C and the spinothalamic tract (STT), can be evaluated. The examiner holds the thermode against the skin with light pressure during testing and each trial begins with the thermode temperature set at 32°C (Figure 25.6). Once the trial begins, the temperature decreases (for cold sensation) or increase (for warm sensation) at a rate of 1°C/s until the subject perceived the stimulus as either cool, warm or painful, or until the stimulus reaches the cutoff value (0°C or 50°C).

The German Network on Neuropathic Pain (DFNS) examined the test–retest reliability and the inter-observer reliability of QST modalities in a group of 60 individuals who experienced pain and

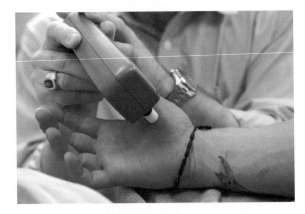

Fig. 25.5 The vibratory probe is held firmly in place during testing.

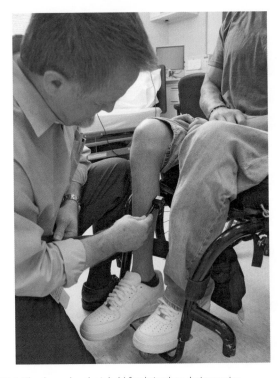

Fig. 25.6 The thermal probe is held firmly in place during testing.

sensory abnormalities due to lesions or diseases of nervous system [81]. Test–retest reliability and inter-observer reliability for test sites in the most painful area were excellent with coefficients ranging between 0.80 and 0.93 for thermal detection and pain thresholds, vibration detection threshold, mechanical detection threshold, mechanical pain threshold for pinprick, and dynamic mechanical allodynia, and pressure pain threshold. The study provides evidence to support that QST is a reliable method that is useful for assessing sensory disturbances in persons with lesions or diseases of the somatosensory nervous system.

Evidence for the reliability of QST over a 2 to 4 week period has also been provided for the SCI neuropathic pain population [82]. In this study, QST was applied in areas with and without neuropathic pain above, at, and below the neurological level of injury. The results from this study demonstrated excellent test–retest reliability for the light touch, vibration, cool, and warm modalities, with intraclass correlation coefficients (ICC) ranging from 0.84 to 0.95. The QST modalities cold pain and hot pain thresholds, however, exhibited lower reliability (ICC = 0.50). Thus, the test–retest reliability of QST in persons with SCI and chronic neuropathic pain appears to be adequate although the psychometric properties should be re-examined in a larger sample to confirm and expand on these results.

One potentially important and exciting application for QST is its ability to define specific clinical pain phenotypes that are generalizable with different chronic pain populations, since the hope is that these may lead to the uncovering of specific underlying pain mechanisms [83, 84]. The DFNS [85] used a standardized protocol for the assessment and analysis of QST data from 1236 patients with the clinical diagnosis of neuropathic pain. Common clinical phenotypes based on QST were found in several neurological syndromes; however, there were important differences with respect to how frequently they were observed. The most common clinical pain phenotype in 27.5% of persons with central neuropathic pain included mixed thermal/mechanical sensory loss without hyperalgesia. This was also the most common sensory profile identified in persons with polyneuropathy (26.2%), but less common in postherpetic neuralgia (13.9%), in peripheral nerve injuries (11.7%), in complex regional pain syndromes (3.5%), and in trigeminal neuralgia (7.6%). While most studies have concluded that injury of the STT is necessary for the development and maintenance of neuropathic pain it is less clear if damage to the DCML pathway is also required [86–94].The data from the DFNS suggests that a combination of STT damage and injury to the DCML pathways is an important mechanism represented by a specific clinical pain phenotype with mixed thermal/mechanical sensory loss. This particular phenotype has also recently been observed after SCI [93].

An important factor related to the usefulness of QST, is its validity, or to what extent QST findings are related to the presence and/or severity of neuropathic pain. This was examined in 17 persons with SCI and neuropathic pain in a multiple regression analysis [82]. The analysis showed that increased severity of neuropathic pain symptoms was significantly associated with increased thermal pain z-scores (i.e. greater sensitivity to thermal pain). The relationship between neuropathic pain severity and spinothalamic function was later confirmed in a significantly larger study group [93]. Consistent with these findings Wasner and colleagues [92] evoked heat pain in areas with experimentally induced peripheral sensitization below the level of injury in persons with clinically complete SCI and neuropathic pain. These authors suggested that neuropathic pain after SCI was associated with spontaneous activity in residual thermosensitive STT neurons triggered by inflammatory processes within the injured STT.

Another important question is to what extent QST can be used to predict the development of neuropathic pain. One study [95] indicated that increased sensitivity to pinprick within the first year of SCI predicted the development of neuropathic pain. Another study [96] assessed 30 persons with SCI and 27 normative controls for a period of 6 months after injury, or until central neuropathic pain developed. These results indicate that the best predictor of neuropathic pain development is dynamic mechanical allodynia below the level of injury and that neuronal hyperexcitability may precede the development of neuropathic pain. These findings are consistent with a recent prospective study in persons with SCI where early sensory hypersensitivity (assessed with SCI) predicted the development of below-level central neuropathic pain [97]. These results are also in agreement with basic research studies suggesting neuropathic pain may be caused by hyperactivity in residual STT neurons, partly due to complex molecular processes including up-regulation of intracellular signalling proteins that influence the phosphorylation of kinases, transcription factors, and/or changes in membrane excitability of receptors [98, 99].

In summary, QST is a very interesting method that may be useful for increasing the understanding of the mechanisms that contribute to the development of neuropathic pain, and facilitate the translation of basic research findings to clinical treatments tailored to specific underlying pain mechanisms.

Small fibre evoked potentials

Another interesting and promising method for determining sensory functionality includes the recording of scalp potentials in response to stimulation of small sensory fibres. Several methods are available for evoking cerebral responses that can be recorded (for a critical review regarding the advantages and limitations of the different methods, see [100]). The recorded responses—evoked potentials—are captured by electroencephalograph (EEG) electrodes placed in several locations on the scalp. Once recorded, the signals can be analysed with respect to specific characteristics (e.g. amplitude and latency), and interpretations regarding the functionality of a specific sensory modality can be made. Decrease in amplitude of specific EEG components, prolonged latencies, or absence of responses can occur in neuropathic pain conditions [101, 102].

One method of stimulation that is frequently used in this context includes the recording of potentials evoked by thermal stimuli (contact heat evoked potentials; CHEPs). CHEPs evoke cerebral responses to thermal stimuli by activating pain mediating Aδ or C-fibres. Recent research has investigated psychometric properties of this method. For example, test-retest reliability was examined in healthy normals, and the ICCs for both CHEPs' latencies and amplitudes were found to be adequate for cervical dermatomes [103]. Consistent with this, spinothalamic CHEPs were found to be a reliable and a sensitive component of the clinical determination of neurological injury after SCI [104]. The ability of CHEPs to evoke potentials in body areas initially not responsive to thermal

stimulation after SCI appears to be enhanced by increasing the baseline temperature [105].

An important question with regards to utility is whether CHEPs can provide information contributing to an increased mechanistic understanding of pain after SCI, and be sensitive to change and be appropriate for outcome measurement. Wydenkeller and colleagues [102] found that although CHEPs did not differ between persons with and without below level neuropathic pain, they were decreased in 94% of those with neuropathic pain. There was a slowing of EEG peak frequency in the 6–12-Hz range, in those with neuropathic pain, consistent with deafferentation. Interestingly, a discriminant analysis correctly classified 84% of subjects as having neuropathic pain versus not having neuropathic pain, based on their EEG peak frequency. In a recent study, Kumru and colleges [106], investigated the pain relieving effect of transcranial direct current stimulation (tDCS) combined with visual illusion (VI) in 18 persons with SCI (14 able-bodied people served as controls). Compared to baseline, two weeks of tDCS + VI, resulted in 13 persons reporting a mean decrease of 50% in neuropathic pain intensity. Similarly, evoked pain intensity, and CHEPs amplitudes (evoked by stimuli applied at C4 dermatome) were significantly reduced, whereas QST heat pain thresholds increased after treatment (i.e. less sensitivity to heat). These studies suggest that CHEPs could potentially be useful both for diagnosis and support the potential utility of these methods as biomarkers of treatment outcome for people with SCI and neuropathic pain.

Psychosocial factors

The biopsychosocial perspective on pain involves dynamic relationships among biological, psychological, social and cultural factors [107]. Biological mechanisms may initiate, maintain, and modulate pain, psychological factors may influence the perception of pain, and social factors may modulate each person's behaviour in response to pain (Figure 25.7).

Due to the difficulty in treating pain associated with CNS injuries and diseases [3, 10–12, 108, 109], a large proportion of people live with persistent pain, ranging from mild to severe, in addition to their physical impairment and other medical consequences. Therefore, personal adaptation and coping skills are crucial for optimal quality of life in these populations [110]. The Initiative on Methods, Measurement, and Pain Assessment in Clinical Trials group (IMMPACT; www.immpact.org) suggested that in addition to assessing the severity of pain, other important health related quality of life domains (e.g. physical and emotional functioning) should be included in a comprehensive evaluation of pain reflecting its multidimensionality. CNS injuries and diseases often cause

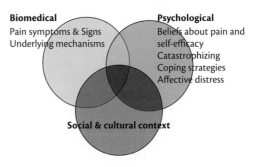

Fig. 25.7 The biopsychosocial perspective on pain.

physical impairments and other general health issues; therefore in these populations, the effect of pain on physical and emotional functioning may be confounded. In order to specifically determine the impact of persistent pain on physical activity in these populations, pain interference measures can be used. These instruments assess the effect of persistent pain on various aspects of life more accurately [66]. Common pain interference measures include the Brief Pain Inventory [111] and the Life Interference subscale of Multidimensional Pain Inventory [75]. Both these measures have demonstrated adequate psychometric properties in samples of persons with SCI and have been recommended as useful measures of pain interference [112]. A subset of these measures is included in the ISCIPBDS [71].

Chronic pain is a multifactorial problem influenced by a variety of interrelated psychological and cognitive factors. For example, affective distress, including depressed mood, anxiety and anger, is closely related to the experience of chronic pain in a variety of patient populations [113]. After SCI, greater psychological distress and excessive fatigue has been reported by individuals who experience persistent pain [114]. Anxiety and depression levels have been found to be higher in persons with greater pain severity and pain interference [26]. Similar to physical functioning, it is not always simple to determine to what extent persistent pain per se causes emotional distress in persons with significant diability after a neurological injury or disease. Since affective distress is a critical to the pain experience and may profoundly affect quality of life, it is important to assess this domain despite these limitations.

Multiaxial psychometric instruments, assessing multiple aspects of the pain experience and associated psychosocial factors, are versatile since their subscales can be either used separately or together to subgroup or classify persons with chronic pain [75, 115]. A cluster analysis of the SCI-version of the Multidimensional Pain Inventory (MPI-SCI) [116], identified three different psychosocial subgroups associated with SCI-related chronic pain [65]. The Dysfunctional subgroup (including persons with higher levels of pain severity, life interference, affective distress and lower levels of life control and activities) and the Adaptive Coper subgroup (including persons with lower levels of pain severity, life interference, and affective distress and greater levels of life control and activities) have been identified in several different chronic pain populations [115] After SCI, however, a new subgroup, the Interpersonally Supported, with high levels of perceived positive support from significant others and lower degree of pain interference and affective distress, despite moderately high pain severity was reported [65]. People belonging to this latter subgroup appeared to have the impact of their pain moderated by social support. Greater perceived social support often facilitate healthy behaviours such as adherence to treatment and adaptive coping. However, solicitous spouse behaviours and responses have also been associated with both increased pain severity and disability in heterogeneous chronic pain populations, [117] and with depression and pain interference after SCI [118]. Moreover, when responses from significant others are perceived to be negative, greater pain severity and disability is a common finding [119]. These psychosocial subgroups have also been found to be related to pain type after SCI. For example, the Dysfunctional subgroup included persons with more neuropathic pain types, suggested by higher frequencies of neuropathic pain symptoms and evoked pain [120], frequent exacerbation of pain [68], electric pain quality, and continuous pain, compared to the other subgroups

[24]. These findings suggest that in chronic pain populations who may experience neuropathic and nociceptive pain concomitantly, persistent neuropathic pain types are likely to have a more negative psychosocial impact than nociceptive pain types.

The relationship between cognitive factors, including catastrophizing thoughts, negative pain beliefs, and impact of pain after SCI has been investigated in several studies. For example, catastrophizing thoughts and negative pain beliefs were related to both greater pain interference and poorer mental health [121]. Consistent with these results, another study found that lower pain intensity was associated with greater levels of internal health locus of control and adaptive coping, and lower levels of catastrophizing thoughts [33]. Greater internal health locus of control orientation is important for greater productivity, satisfaction with performance of daily activities and community integration after CNS injuries [122]. Importantly, the sense of having control in one's life can be enhanced by incorporating education regarding pain as part of multidisciplinary pain management programs [123]. Jensen and colleagues [124], suggested that catastrophizing cognitions, task persistence, guarding and resting coping responses, and perceived social support, were important predictors of pain and dysfunction in physically impaired populations including SCI.

Research and clinical experience show that that psychosocial factors influence the severity of pain and the treatment response. For example, individuals who experience persistent pain, report more psychological distress and excessive fatigue than those who do not experience pain. For clinical pain management, therefore, it is important to determine the role of cognitive factors and beliefs for each individual's pain and psychosocial impact, and address these factors in order to reduce the pain and pain-related disability, and enhance the sense of control and adaptive coping [124].

Treatments

Principles
Psychological and social factors are major contributors to the pain experience. Therefore, a comprehensive treatment strategy targeting persistent pain should also consider pain-related psychosocial factors as important contributors to pain and pain-related disability. Increased knowledge regarding the relationships between underlying pathophysiology and clinical pain symptoms and signs and relevant psychosocial factors is needed to improve pain management for those who live with persistent pain after CNS injuries.

Pharmacological treatments
While nociceptive pain types may be pharmacologically treated with medications such as acetaminophen, non-steroidal anti-inflammatory drugs (NSAIDs) and weak opiods, the treatment of neuropathic pain types usually includes other medications. Unfortunately, treatments that have proven to be efficacious in reducing peripheral neuropathic pain may not relieve CNP conditions [108]. Indeed, treatments often fail to produce substantial relief of CNP; however, recent reviews [19, 52, 90, 125] suggest some beneficial effects of anticonvulsants (including gabapentin and pregabalin), intravenous analgesics (including lidocaine and ketamine), non-pharmacological interventions (such as neuro-stimulation), and cognitive approaches. Many studies include small sample sizes and are therefore unable to yield conclusive results, which highlights the need for large scale multicentre trials involving these populations. There is some evidence that different

clinical pain phenotypes based on symptom and signs may reflect specific underlying mechanisms as evidenced by clinical treatment response to pharmacological intervention [126, 127]. For example, in the latter study, which included 27 individuals with multiple sclerosis, the investigators conducted a responder analysis and found that patients with lancinating pain and those without mechanical allodynia obtained pain relief greater than placebo with the anticonvulsant levitiracetam. Despite these promising results, current evidence supporting that specific clinical phenotypes correspond to specific underlying mechanisms and positive treatment responses is still very limited and requires additional research.

The first line of treatment based on available clinical trial data for CNP recommended by the European Federation of Neurological Societies (EFNS; [128]) includes gabapentin, pregabalin, and tricyclic antidepressants (TCA). As a second line of treatments, cannabinoids (for MS), lamotrigine, opioids, and tramadol (for SCI) were recommended.

The analgesic effects of anticonvulsants are likely due to their ability to suppress neuronal hyperactivity [129]. Anticonvulsants have been shown to be effective in reducing the severity of of several different types of neuropathic pain conditions [130, 131], such as carbamazepine in individuals with multiple sclerosis [127], and gabapentin in diabetic peripheral neuropathy [132] and post-herpetic neuralgia [133].

There have also been several larger scale studies examining the pain relieving effect of anticonvulsants in CNP populations. For example, a multicentre 12-week study tested varying doses (150–600 mg/day) of pregabalin in 137 people with SCI and demonstrated significant effects compared to placebo in reducing pain intensity and anxiety, enhancing sleep and global improvement ratings [14]. These results were recently confirmed in another multicentre study, which also examined the effects of a daily dose of 150–600 mg of pregabalin or placebo over a 16-week period in 220 persons with SCI and below-level neuropathic pain [18]. This study showed significant improvements compared to placebo for duration-adjusted average change in pain and for secondary outcome measures including daily pain ratings and sleep interference. These results suggest that pregabalin is effective in reducing neuropathic pain in some persons with SCI. In contrast, another study examined the effects of pregabalin in 219 persons with post stroke CNP [134]. Although the results from this study showed significant improvements in pain scores compared to baseline, this difference was not significantly different compared to placebo. There were, however significant improvements compared to placebo with respect to sleep, anxiety, and general impression of change. Due to the positive effects on sleep and mood, the authors suggested that the effects on pain after stroke should be examined in more detail in other studies. Other anticonvulsants that have been tested in CNP populations include levetiracetam, which was not found to be effective in reducing either SCI-related [135] or poststroke neuropathic pain [136].

Combinations of anticonvulsants and other medications may increase the pain relieving effect of anticonvulsants by addressing several putative mechanisms simultaneously. For example, the combination of 300 mg gabapentin three times daily with adjuvant low-dose ketamine (N-methyl-D-aspartate (NMDA) receptor antagonist) infusion was compared with gabapentin in 40 persons with SCI and neuropathic pain [137]. While the early pain relieving effect was significantly greater in the group that received the combination with ketamine compared to those who received only gabapentin, there was no significant difference between the groups 2 weeks after infusion. Another study examined the effects of intravenous ketamine, an NMDA receptor antagonist, and found a significant reduction of SCI-related neuropathic pain after administration [138]. This result suggests that central sensitization via activation of NMDA receptors might have been a primary underlying mechanism in those subjects that experienced relief of pain in response to this treatment.

Another commonly used pharmacological treatment for neuropathic pain is antidepressant medication [139]. The pain-relieving effects of TCAs are thought to be mediated by enhancing endogenous pain inhibitory systems that include neurotransmitters such as serotonin and norepinephrine [140]. Clinical trials demonstrate that approximately 60% to 70% of people with heterogeneous neuropathic pain report at least moderate reductions in pain with TCAs [139]. A problem with older TCAs, such as imipramine and amitriptyline, is the presence of significant side effects that may hinder effective dosing [141]. However, the newer types of antidepressants with a balanced serotonin-norepinephrine reuptake inhibition are designed to cause fewer side effects than the older TCAs.

Several clinical trials have demonstrated relief of peripheral neuropathic pain (e.g. post-herpetic neuralgia, diabetic neuropathy) using antidepressant medication [128]. Unfortunately, clinical research does not support the effectiveness of tricyclic antidepressants in relieving CNP after stroke; however, Rintala and colleagues [15] found that amitriptyline was effective in reducing neuropathic pain intensity in participants who also had significant depressive symptomatology. In contrast, another study showed no significant pain relieving effects of amitriptyline in persons with SCI [142]. A recent study including 48 persons with either stroke or SCI [143] showed no significant reduction in pain intensity by duloxetine compared to placebo ($p = 0.056$). However, duloxetine reduced both mechanical ($p = 0.035$) and cold allodynia ($p < 0.001$) suggesting a biological effect, possibly via activation of endogenous pain inhibitory systems.

The analgesic effects of sodium channel blockers such as lidocaine, have been examined in persons with CNP. One study [144] showed a significant reduction in SCI-related pain after lidocaine administration into the subarachnoid space. Lidocaine has also been administered intravenously with beneficial effects on both spontaneous and evoked pain in stroke- or SCI-related neuropathic pain [145]. Specifically, intravenous lidocaine significantly reduced pain intensity, mechanical allodynia and hyperalgesia, but not thermal allodynia and hyperalgesia. The differential effects on sensory dysfunctions suggest that these may represent different underlying mechanisms and hence support a mechanisms-based approache to pain management. However, mexilitine, an oral drug structurally similar to lidocaine, does not appear to reduce SCI-related neuropathic pain [21].

Another class of medications commonly used to relieve severe CNP is opioid receptor agonists. These bind to opioid receptors in the brain, spinal cord, and primary sensory neurons involved in endogenous pain modulation. Therefore, systemic administration of opiods can thus produce pain relief on different levels along the neuroaxis. A study by Attal and colleagues [146] examined the effects of intravenous morphine in persons with neuropathic pain after either stroke or SCI. These investigators found a reduction in the intensity of brush-evoked allodynia but no significant reduction in perceived pain in response to the treatment. In a recent multicentre observational study the effects of oxycodone in combination with anticonvulsants were examined [147]. The study included 54 people with SCI and neuropathic pain, and the authors reported decreases in pain, improvement of health related quality of life, and decreased impact on physical activity and sleep after treatment. A randomized controlled study in 15 patients with SCI-related neuropathic pain examined the effects of intrathecal administration of morphine or clonidine (α-adrenergic agonist), either individually or in combination [148]. The study demonstrated that the combination of morphine and clonidine ($α_2$-adrenergic agonist) significantly reduced pain 4 h after administration compared to placebo or individual administration. In this study, 7 out of 15 patients received 50% or greater reduction in pain. The authors suggested that clonidine and opioid acted synergistically by influencing different mechanisms involving descending inhibitory systems. Similarly, a study involving nine individuals with SCI and neuropathic pain [138] found significant decreases in both spontaneous and evoked pain after intravenous alfentanil, a mu-opioid receptor agonist. In summary, these studies indicate that opioids can effectively reduce CNP when administered intravenously or intrathecally.

Marijuana is often mentioned by respondents with chronic pain as an effective pain treatment. A survey study [9] showed that 32% out of a group of 117 spinal cord injured individuals had used marijuana to reduce pain during some period after their SCI and 23% reported current use. Although several studies support the pain-relieving effects of cannabinoids in multiple sclerosis patients [149–151], a recent small clinical trial in SCI showed no pain-relieving effect on neuropathic pain below the level of injury of the oral cannabinoid, dronabinol, compared to active placebo [152]. The positive effects of cannabinoids on neuropathic pain associated with MS, and the positive patient reports, suggest that the effects of these treatments should be explored in larger studies and in different patient populations with CNP.

Non-pharmacological treatments

Many non-pharmacological treatments are available for the treatment of persistent pain whether it is nociceptive or neuropathic. These range from invasive (e.g. surgery, spinal cord and deep brain stimulation) to non-invasive treatments (e.g. various physical therapies, non-invasive electrical stimulation, and exercise).

When pain is caused or exacerbated by mechanical factors (e.g. peripheral nerve compression, tethering of nerve roots or of the spinal cord, and syringomyelia) surgical methods (e.g. stabilization of the spine, decompression, and un-tethering) may be effective. Other surgical methods include elimination of hyperactivity in the dorsal horn by dorsal root entry zone lesioning, which has produced pain relief in some patients with SCI and neuropathic pain [153]. Spinal cord and deep brain stimulation (DBS) has produced some pain relief both after SCI and stroke [154–156]. Two studies involving persons with post-stroke central neuropathic pain, one involving 15 [151] and the other 31 patients [156], applied DBS in the thalamus and/or the periaqueductal grey. DBS resulted in 48.8% improvement in pain scores but there was a wide variability in responses with about 70% responders for both studies.

Non-invasive therapies, such as transcranial motor cortex stimulation have shown positive results with regards to relief of SCI-related neuropathic pain [157–159]. For example, the latter randomized, sham controlled, double-blind, parallel group design study tested transcranial direct current stimulation and visual illusion in 39 patients with CNP. The best long-term effect (12 weeks after treatment) on pain intensity was obtained when the two interventions were combined. These studies suggest that both invasive and non-invasive treatments stimulating the brain and or spinal cord can be effective in reducing pain after CNS injuries and diseases.

The activation of somatic afferents via different modes (e.g. electrical, mechanical, or physiological) may be promising avenues as part of multidisciplinary treatment programs for both nociceptive and neuropathic pain. Massage and other physiotherapeutic interventions (e.g. application of heat, cold, transcutaneous electrical nerve stimulation (TENS)), are among the most common non-pharmacological methods used to relieve pain. In two survey studies physiotherapeutic interventions were perceived as providing 'considerable to complete' pain relief in 50% of an SCI sample [8], with pain relief often lasting hours to days [9]. Several studies suggest that acupuncture, TENS and massage, or combinations of these interventions may also be beneficial for neuropathic pain after CNS injuries [160–164]. Findings of a 10-week exercise study suggested beneficial effects on both musculoskeletal and neuropathic pain types associated with SCI [166]. Importantly, reductions in pain regardless of aetiology may have a profound effect on quality of life. For example, reduction in shoulder pain, after a 12-week, home exercise programme aimed to strengthen shoulder muscles and modify movements related to upper extremity weight bearing, resulted in significant increases in social participation and improvements in quality of life [34]. Similarly, another study including 80 individuals with paraplegia and musculoskeletal pain showed improvements in both pain and quality of life in response to a shoulder exercise programme [167].

An important part of a comprehensive approach to therapy-resistant pain is to increase individual coping skills with the goal of optimizing quality of life. Therefore, treatment strategies that include cognitive-behavioural interventions directed toward enhancing a person's coping ability and adaptation to pain are important components of a multidisciplinary pain management programme [123, 124, 168]. A recent multicentre trial [169] included 61 individuals with neuropathic pain and SCI. The participants were randomized to cognitive-behavioural therapy (CBT) or to wait-list control and the primary outcomes were pain intensity and pain-related disability and secondary outcomes were mood, participation in activities and life satisfaction. While CBT significantly reduced anxiety and participation in activities compared to control, there were no significant differences in pain intensity and pain-related disability. Another study in 22 people with MS examined the effects of self-hypnosis training and progressive relaxation [170]. Most of the participants reported that they found that both of these interventions caused pain relief. A more recent study also involving people with MS [69] suggested that a combination of self-hypnosis and cognitive restructuring may be more effective in reducing pain than either of the approaches alone. The results of these studies suggest that self-hypnosis and cognitive restructuring would be beneficial components of chronic pain management in a population with CNS injuries.

Conclusion

Severe, chronic pain of various origins is a serious consequence that affects many people after CNS injury or disease and one that can significantly interfere with daily activities and reduce quality of life. People who have sustained a spinal cord or brain injury or have a disease involving the CNS may also develop CNP. Unfortunately, currently available treatments for CNP are usually not effective, although anticonvulsants and antidepressants are often recommended as the first line of medication. The complex clinical presentation of pain in these populations with multiple simultaneous persistent pains of different origins and variable psychosocial impact suggest a critical need for individually tailored mechanism-based treatment approaches that also include psychosocial interventions. Although treating the underlying and contributing mechanisms of pain in each individual is the most desirable strategy, it is usually not possible because of our insufficient ability to determine the primary underlying pain mechanisms in each individual. In order to move towards more mechanistically targeted treatment strategies, multiple aspects of the clinical pain condition (e.g. pain symptoms, sensory signs) needs to be systematically evaluated. Clinical evaluation should also include pain-related psychosocial variables associated with persistent pain so that these can be addressed in the pain management design.

References

1. Leung J, Moseley A, Fereday S, Jones T, Fairbairn T, Wyndham S. The prevalence and characteristics of shoulder pain after traumatic brain injury. Clin Rehabil. 2007;21(2):171–181.
2. Lew HL, Otis JD, Tun C, Kerns RD, Clark ME, Cifu DX. Prevalence of chronic pain, posttraumatic stress disorder, and persistent postconcussive symptoms in OIF/OEF veterans: polytrauma clinical triad. J Rehabil Res Dev. 2009;46(6):697–702.
3. Siddall PJ, McClelland JM, Rutkowski SB, Cousins MJ. A longitudinal study of the prevalence and characteristics of pain in the first 5 years following spinal cord injury. Pain. 2003;103(3):249–257.
4. Bryce TN, Biering-Sørensen F, Finnerup NB, et al. International spinal cord injury pain classification: part I. Background and description. Spinal Cord. 2012a;50(6):413–417.
5. Roosink M, Renzenbrink GJ, Geurts AC, Ijzerman MJ.Towards a mechanism-based view on post-stroke shoulder pain: theoretical considerations and clinical implications. NeuroRehabilitation. 2012;30(2):153–165.
6. Cruz-Almeida Y, Martinez-Arizala A, Widerström-Noga EG. Chronicity of pain associated with spinal cord injury: A longitudinal analysis. J Rehabil Res Dev. 2005;42(5):585–594.
7. Warms CA, Turner JA, Marshall HM, Cardenas DD. Treatments for chronic pain associated with spinal cord injuries: many are tried, few are helpful. Clin J Pain. 2002;18(3):154–163.
8. Widerström-Noga EG, Turk DC. Types and effectiveness of treatments used by people with chronic pain associated with spinal cord injuries: influence of pain and psychosocial characteristics. Spinal Cord. 2003;41(11):600–609.
9. Cardenas DD, Jensen MP. Treatments for chronic pain in persons with spinal cord injury: A survey study. J Spinal Cord Med. 2006;29(2):109–117.
10. Klit H, Finnerup NB, Overvad K, Andersen G, Jensen TS. Pain following stroke: a population-based follow-up study. PLoS One. 2011;6(11):e27607.
11. Naess H, Lunde L, Brogger J, Waje-Andreassen U. Post-stroke pain on long-term follow-up: the Bergen stroke study. J Neurol. 2010;257(9):1446–1452.
12. Douglas C, Wollin JA, Windsor C. Illness and demographic correlates of chronic pain among a community-based

sample of people with multiple sclerosis. Arch Phys Med Rehabil. 2008;89(10):1923–1932.
13. Levendoglu F, Ogun CO, Ozerbil O, Ogun TC, Ugurlu H. Gabapentin is a first line drug for the treatment of neuropathic pain in spinal cord injury. Spine. 2004;29(7):743–751.
14. Siddall PJ, Cousins MJ, Otte A, Griesing T, Chambers R, Murphy TK. Pregabalin in central neuropathic pain associated with spinal cord injury: a placebo-controlled trial. Neurology. 2006;7(10):1792–1800.
15. Rintala DH, Holmes SA, Courtade D, Fiess RN, Tastard LV, Loubser PG. Comparison of the effectiveness of amitriptyline and gabapentin on chronic neuropathic pain in persons with spinal cord injury. Arch Phys Med Rehabil. 2007;88(12):1547–1560.
16. Vranken JH, Dijkgraaf MG, Kruis MR, van der Vegt MH, Hollmann MW, Heesen M. Pregabalin in patients with central neuropathic pain: a randomized, double-blind, placebo-controlled trial of a flexible-dose regimen. Pain. 2008;136(1–2):150–157.
17. Norrbrink C, Lundeberg T. Tramadol in neuropathic pain after spinal cord injury: a randomized, double-blind, placebo-controlled trial. Clin J Pain. 2009;25(3):177-184.
18. Cardenas DD, Nieshoff EC, Suda K, et al. A randomized trial of pregabalin in patients with neuropathic pain due to spinal cord injury. Neurology. 2013;80(6):533–539.
19. Siddall PJ. Management of neuropathic pain following spinal cord injury: now and in the future. Spinal Cord. 2009;47(5):352–359.
20. Finnerup NB, Sorensen L, Biering-Sorensen F, Johannesen IL, Jensen T S. Segmental hypersensitivity and spinothalamic function in spinal cord injury pain. Exp Neurol. 2007a;207(1):139–149.
21. Baastrup C, Finnerup NB. Pharmacological management of neuropathic pain following spinal cord injury. CNS Drugs. 2008;22(6):455–475.
22. Vassend O, Quale AJ, Roise O, Schanke AK. Predicting the long-term impact of acquired severe injuries on functional health status: the role of optimism, emotional distress and pain. Spinal Cord. 2011;49(12):1193–1197.
23. Hoffman JM, Bombardier CH, Graves DE, Kalpakjian CZ, Krause JS. A longitudinal study of depression from 1 to 5 years after spinal cord injury. Arch Phys Med Rehabil. 2011;92(3):411–418.
24. Widerström-Noga EG, Cruz-Almeida Y, Felix ER, Adcock JP. Relationship between pain characteristics and pain adaptation type in persons with SCI. J Rehabil Res Dev. 2009;46(1):43–56.
25. Jensen MP, Kuehn CM, Amtmann D, Cardenas DD. Symptom burden in persons with spinal cord injury. Arch Phys Med Rehabil. 2007a;88(5):638–645.
26. Nicholson PK, Nicholas MK, Middleton J. Spinal cord injury-related pain in rehabilitation: A cross-sectional study of relationships with cognitions, mood and physical function. Eur J Pain. 2008;13(5):511–517.
27. Hirsh AT, Bockow TB, Jensen MP.Catastrophizing, pain, and pain interference in individuals with disabilities. Am J Phys Med Rehabil. 2011;90(9):713–722.
28. Kennedy P, Lude P, Taylor N. Quality of life, social participation, appraisals and coping post spinal cord injury: a review of four community samples. Spinal Cord. 2006;44(2):95–105.
29. Richards JS, Meredith RL, Nepomuceno C, Fine PR, Bennett G. Psycho-social aspects of chronic pain in spinal cord injury. Pain. 1980;8(3):355–366.
30. Summers JD, Rapoff MA, Varghese G, Porter K, Palmer RE. Psychosocial factors in chronic spinal cord injury pain. Pain. 1991;47(2):183–189.
31. Michalski D, Liebig S, Thomae E, Hinz A, Bergh FT. Pain in patients with multiple sclerosis: a complex assessment including quantitative and qualitative measurements provides for a disease-related biopsychosocial pain model. J Pain Res. 2011;4:219–225.
32. Middleton J, Tran Y, Craig A. Relationship between quality of life and self-efficacy in persons with spinal cord injuries. Arch Phys Med Rehabil. 2007;88(12):1643–1648.

33. Wollaars MM, Post MW, Brand N. Spinal cord injury pain: the influence of psychologic factors and impact on quality of life. Clin J Pain. 2007;23(5):383–391.

34. Kemp BJ, Bateham AL, Mulroy SJ, Thompson L, Adkins RH, Kahan JS. Effects of reduction in shoulder pain on quality of life and community activities among people living long-term with SCI paraplegia: a randomized control trial. J Spinal Cord Med. 2011;34(3):278–284.

35. IASP Task Force on Taxonomy Part III: Pain Terms, "A Current List with Definitions and Notes on Usage" (pp 209–214) Classification of Chronic Pain, Second Edition, edited by H. Merskey and N. Bogduk, IASP Press, Seattle, ©1994.

36. Waring WP 3rd, Biering-Sorensen F, Burns S, et al. 2009 review and revisions of the international standards for the neurological classification of spinal cord injury. J Spinal Cord Med. 2010;33(4):346–352.

37. Zeilig G, Rivel M, Weingarden H, Gaidoukov E, Defrin R. Hemiplegic shoulder pain: evidence of a neuropathic origin. Pain. 2013;154(2):263–271.

38. Boivie, J. Central pain. In McMahon, SB, Koltzenburg M (eds) Wall and Melzack's Text Book of Pain, Elsevier, London, 2003, pp.1057–1074.

39. Wasner G. Central pain syndromes. Curr Pain Headache Rep. 2010;14(6):489–496.

40. Treede RD, Jensen TS, Campbell JN, et al. Neuropathic pain: redefinition and a grading system for clinical and research purposes. Neurology. 2008;70(18):1630–1635.

41. Woolf CJ. Central sensitization: implications for the diagnosis and treatment of pain. Pain. 2011;152(3 Suppl):S2–15.

42. Woolf CJ, Salter MW. Neuronal plasticity: increasing the gain in pain. Science. 2000;288(5472):1765–1769.

43. Alm M, Saraste H, Norrbrink C. Shoulder pain in persons with thoracic spinal cord injury: prevalence and characteristics. J Rehabil Med. 2008;40(4):277–283.

44. Boivie J. Chapter 48 Central post-stroke pain. Handb Clin Neurol. 2006;81:715–730.

45. Latremoliere A, Woolf CJ. Central sensitization: a generator of pain hypersensitivity by central neural plasticity. J Pain. 2009;10(9):895–926.

46. Finnerup NB, Jensen TS. Spinal cord injury pain—mechanisms and treatment. Eur J Neurol. 2004;11(2):73–82.

47. Yezierski RP. Pain following spinal cord injury: pathophysiology and central mechanisms. Prog Brain Res. 2000;129:429–449.

48. von Hehn CA, Baron R, Woolf CJ. Deconstructing the neuropathic pain phenotype to reveal neural mechanisms. Neuron. 2012;73(4):638–652.

49. Backonja M, Woolf CJ. Future directions in neuropathic pain therapy: closing the translational loop. Oncologist. 2010;Suppl 2:24–29.

50. Yezierski RP. Spinal cord injury pain: spinal and supraspinal mechanisms. J Rehabil Res Dev. 2009;46(1):95–107.

51. Hulsebosch CE, Hains BC, Crown ED, Carlton SM. Mechanisms of chronic central neuropathic pain after spinal cord injury. Brain Res Rev. 2009;60(1):202–213.

52. Finnerup NB, Baastrup C. Spinal cord injury pain: mechanisms and management. Curr Pain Headache Rep. 2012;16(3):207–216.

53. Gwak YS, Kang J, Unabia GC, Hulsebosch CE. Spatial and temporal activation of spinal glial cells: Role of gliopathy in central neuropathic pain following spinal cord injury in rats. Exp Neurol. 2012;234(2):362–372.

54. Gwak YS, Hulsebosch CE. GABA and central neuropathic pain following spinal cord injury. Neuropharmacology. 2011a;60(5):799–808.

55. Gwak YS, Hulsebosch CE. Neuronal hyperexcitability: a substrate for central neuropathic pain after spinal cord injury. Curr Pain Headache Rep. 2011b;15(3):215–222.

56. Costigan M, Scholz J, Woolf CJ. Neuropathic pain: a maladaptive response of the nervous system to damage. Annu Rev Neurosci. 2009;32:1–32.

57. Knerlich-Lukoschus F, von d R-B, Lucius R, Mehdorn HM, Held-Feindt J. Spatiotemporal CCR1, CCL3(MIP-1alpha), CXCR4, CXCL12(SDF-1alpha) expression patterns in a rat spinal cord injury model of posttraumatic neuropathic pain. J Neurosurg Spine. 2011a;14(5);583–597.

58. Geng SJ, Liao FF, Dang WH, et al. Contribution of the spinal cord BDNF to the development of neuropathic pain by activation of the NR2B-containing NMDA receptors in rats with spinal nerve ligation. Exp Neurol. 2010;222(2):256–266.

59. Knerlich-Lukoschus F, Noack M, von der Ropp-Brenner B, Lucius R, Mehdorn HM, Held-Feindt J. Spinal cord injuries induce changes in CB1 cannabinoid receptor and C-C chemokine expression in brain areas underlying circuitry of chronic pain conditions. J Neurotrauma. 2011b;28(4):619–634.

60. Boroujerdi A, Zeng J, Sharp K, Kim D, Steward O, Luo ZD. Calcium channel alpha-2-delta-1 protein upregulation in dorsal spinal cord mediates spinal cord injury-induced neuropathic pain states. Pain. 2011;152(3):649–655.

61. Hasbargen T, Ahmed MM, Miranpuri G, Li L, Kahle KT, Resnick D, Sun D. Role of NKCC1 and KCC2 in the development of chronic neuropathic pain following spinal cord injury. Ann N Y Acad Sci. 2010;1198:168–172.

62. Meisner JG, Marsh AD, Marsh DR. Loss of GABAergic interneurons in laminae I-III of the spinal cord dorsal horn contributes to reduced GABAergic tone and neuropathic pain after spinal cord injury. J Neurotrauma. 2010;27(4):729–737.

63. Sandhir R, Gregory E, He YY, Berman NE. Upregulation of inflammatory mediators in a model of chronic pain after spinal cord injury. Neurochem Res. 2011;36(5):856–862.

64. Carlton SM, Du J, Tan HY, et al. Peripheral and central sensitization in remote spinal cord regions contribute to central neuropathic pain after spinal cord injury. Pain. 2009;147(1–3):265–276.

65. Widerström-Noga EG, Felix ER, Cruz-Almeida Y, Turk DC. Psychosocial subgroups in persons with spinal cord injuries and chronic pain. Arch Phys Med Rehabil. 2007;88(12):1628–1635.

66. Cruz-Almeida Y, Alameda G, Widerström-Noga EG. Differentiation between pain-related interference and interference caused by the functional impairments of spinal cord injury. Spinal Cord. 2009;47(5):390–395.

67. Felix ER, Cruz-Almeida Y, Widerström-Noga EG. Chronic pain after spinal cord injury: what characteristics make some pains more disturbing than others? J Rehabil Res Dev. 2007;44(5):703–715.

68. Widerström-Noga EG, Turk DC. Exacerbation of chronic pain following spinal cord injury. J.Neurotrauma 2004;21(10):1384–1395.

69. Jensen MP, Ehde DM, Gertz KJ, et al. Effects of self-hypnosis training and cognitive restructuring on daily pain intensity and catastrophizing in individuals with multiple sclerosis and chronic pain. Int J Clin Exp Hypn. 2011;59(1):45–63.

70. Widerström-Noga E, Biering-Sorensen F, Bryce T, et al. The international spinal cord injury pain basic data set. Spinal Cord. 2008;46(12):818–823.

71. Widerström-Noga EG, Biering-Sørensen F, Bryce T, Cardenas DD, Finnerup NB, Jensen MP, Richards JS, Siddall PJ. The International Spinal Cord Injury Pain Basic Data Set (version 2.0). Spinal Cord. 2014;52(4):282–286.

72. Bryce TN, Biering-Sørensen F, Finnerup NB, et al. International Spinal Cord Injury Pain (ISCIP) Classification: Part 2. Initial validation using vignettes. Spinal Cord. 2012b;50(6):404–412.

73. Wasner G, Deuschl G. Pains in Parkinson disease—many syndromes under one umbrella. Nat Rev Neurol. 2012;8(5):284–294.

74. 4 Jensen MP, Turner JA, Romano JM, Fisher LD. Comparative reliability and validity of chronic pain measures. Pain. 1999;83:157–162.

75. Kerns RD, Turk DC, Rudy TE. The West Haven-Yale Multidimensional Pain Inventory (WHYMPI). Pain. 1985;23:345–356.

76. Bouhassira D, Attal N, Fermanian J, et al. Development and validation of the Neuropathic Pain Symptom Inventory. Pain. 2004;108(3):248–257.

77. Attal N, Fermanian C, Fermanian J, Lanteri-Minet M, Alchaar H, Bouhassira D. Comparison of pain syndromes associated with nervous or somatic lesions and development of a new neuropathic pain diagnostic questionnaire (DN4). Pain. 2005;114(1–2):29–36.

78. Attal N, Fermanian C, Fermanian J, Lanteri-Minet M, Alchaar H, Bouhassira D. Neuropathic pain: are there distinct subtypes depending on the aetiology or anatomical lesion? Pain. 2008;138(2):343–353.

79. Galer BS, Jensen MP. Development and preliminary validation of a pain measure specific to neuropathic pain: the Neuropathic Pain Scale. Neurology. 1997;48(2):332–338.

80. Fishbain DA, Lewis JE, Cutler R, Cole B, Rosomoff HL, Rosomoff RS. Can the neuropathic pain scale discriminate between non-neuropathic and neuropathic pain? Pain Med. 2008;9(2):149–160.

81. Geber C, Klein T, Azad S, et al. Test-retest and interobserver reliability of quantitative sensory testing according to the protocol of the German Research Network on Neuropathic Pain (DFNS): a multi-centre study. Pain. 2011;152(3):548–556.

82. Felix ER, Widerström-Noga EG. Reliability and validity of quantitative sensory testing in persons with spinal cord injury and neuropathic pain. J Rehabil Res Dev. 2009;46(1):69–83.

83. Baron R, Förster M, Binder A. Subgrouping of patients with neuropathic pain according to pain-related sensory abnormalities: a first step to a stratified treatment approach. Lancet Neurol. 2012;11(11):999–1005.

84. Rolke R, Baron R, Maier C, et al. Quantitative sensory testing in the German Research Network on Neuropathic Pain (DFNS): standardized protocol and reference values. Pain. 2006;123(3):231–243.

85. Maier C, Baron R, Tolle TR, et al. Quantitative sensory testing in the German Research Network on Neuropathic Pain (DFNS): somatosensory abnormalities in 1236 patients with different neuropathic pain syndromes. Pain. 2010;150(3):439–450.

86. Eide PK, Jorum E, Stenehjem AE. Somatosensory findings in patients with spinal cord injury and central dysaesthesia pain. J Neurol Neurosurg Psychiatry. 1996;60(4):411–415.

87. Finnerup NB, Johannesen IL, Fuglsang-Frederiksen A, Bach FW, Jensen TS. Sensory function in spinal cord injury patients with and without central pain. Brain. 2003;126(Pt 1):57–70.

88. Hall BJ, Lally JE, Vukmanic EV, et al: Spinal cord injuries containing asymmetrical damage in the ventrolateral funiculus is associated with a higher incidence of at-level allodynia. J Pain. 2010;11(9):864–875.

89. Milhorat TH, Kotzen RM, Mu HT, Capocelli AL Jr, Milhorat RH. Dysesthetic pain in patients with syringomyelia. Neurosurgery. 1996;38(5):940–946.

90. Finnerup NB, Otto M, Jensen TS, Sindrup SH. An evidence-based algorithm for the treatment of neuropathic pain. Med Gen Med. 2007b;9(2):36.

91. Beric A, Dimitrijevic MR, Lindblom U. Central dysesthesia syndrome in spinal cord injury patients. Pain. 1988;34(2):109–116.

92. Wasner G, Lee BB, Engel S, McLachlan E. Residual spinothalamic tract pathways predict development of central pain after spinal cord injury. Brain. 2008;131(Pt 9):2387–2400.

93. Cruz-Almeida Y, Felix ER, Martinez-Arizala A, Widerström-Noga EG. Decreased spinothalamic and dorsal column medial lemniscus-mediated function is associated with neuropathic pain after spinal cord injury. J Neurotrauma. 2012;29(17):2706–2715.

94. Hong JH, Choi BY, Chang CH, et al. The prevalence of central post-stroke pain according to the integrity of the spino-thalamo-cortical pathway. Eur Neurol. 2012;67(1):12–17.

95. Hari AR, Wydenkeller S, Dokladal P, Halder P. Enhanced recovery of human spinothalamic function is associated with central neuropathic pain after SCI. Exp Neurol. 2009;216(2):428–430.

96. Zeilig G, Enosh S, Rubin-Asher D, Lehr B, Defrin R. The nature and course of sensory changes following spinal cord injury: predictive properties and implications on the mechanism of central pain. Brain. 2012;135(Pt 2):418–430.

97. Finnerup NB, Norrbrink C, Trok K, Piehl F, Johannesen IL, Sørensen JC, Jensen TS, Werhagen L.Phenotypes and predictors of pain following traumatic spinal cord injury: a prospective study. J Pain. 2014;15(1):40–48.

98. Crown ED, Gwak YS, Ye Z, et al. Calcium/calmodulin dependent kinase II contributes to persistent central neuropathic pain following spinal cord injury. Pain. 2012;153(3):710–721.

99. Densmore VS, Kalous A, Keast JR, Osborne PB. Above-level mechanical hyperalgesia in rats develops after incomplete spinal cord injury but not after cord transection, and is reversed by amitriptyline, morphine and gabapentin. Pain. 2010;151(1):184–193.

100. Baumgärtner U, Greffrath W, Treede RD.Contact heat and cold, mechanical, electrical and chemical stimuli to elicit small fiber-evoked potentials: merits and limitations for basic science and clinical use. Neurophysiol Clin. 2012;42(5):267–280.

101. Cruccu G, Aminoff MJ, Curio G, et al. Recommendations for the clinical use of somatosensory-evoked potentials. Clin Neurophysiol. 2008;119(8):1705–1719.

102. Wydenkeller S, Maurizio S, Dietz V, Halder P. Neuropathic pain in spinal cord injury: significance of clinical and electrophysiological measures. Eur J Neurosci. 2009;30(1):91–99.

103. Kramer JL, Taylor P, Haefeli J, et al. Test-retest reliability of contact heat-evoked potentials from cervical dermatomes. J Clin Neurophysiol. 2012a;29(1):70–75.

104. Ulrich A, Haefeli J, Blum J, Min K, Curt A. Improved diagnosis of spinal cord disorders with contact heat evoked potentials. Neurology. 2013;80(15):1393–1399.

105. Kramer JL, Haefeli J, Curt A, Steeves JD. Increased baseline temperature improves the acquisition of contact heat evoked potentials after spinal cord injury. Clin Neurophysiol. 2012b;123(3):582–589.

106. Kumru H, Soler D, Vidal J, et al. The effects of transcranial direct current stimulation with visual illusion in neuropathic pain due to spinal cord injury: an evoked potentials and quantitative thermal testing study. Eur J Pain. 2013;17(1):55–66.

107. Turk DC. Biopsychosocial perspective on chronic pain. In: Gatchel R, Turk DC, editors. Psychological approaches to chronic pain management: a clinician's handbook. New York: Guilford Press; 1996. p. 3–33.

108. Bowsher D. Central pain following spinal and supraspinal lesions. Spinal Cord.1999;37:235–238.

109. Grasso MG, Clemenzi A, Tonini A, et al. Pain in multiple sclerosis: a clinical and instrumental approach. Mult Scler. 2008;14(4):506–513.

110. Jensen MP, Moore MR, Bockow TB, Ehde DM, Engel JM. Psychosocial factors and adjustment to chronic pain in persons with physical disabilities: a systematic review. Arch Phys Med Rehabil. 2011;92(1):146–160.

111. Cleeland CS, Ryan KM. Pain assessment: global use of the Brief Pain Inventory. Ann Acad Med Singapore. 1994;23(2):129–138.

112. Bryce TN, Budh CN, Cardenas DD, et al. Outcome measures for pain after spinal cord injury: an evaluation of reliability and validity. J Spinal Cord Med. 2007;30:421–440.

113. Banks, SM, Kerns RD. Explaining high rates of depression in chronic pain: a diathesis-stress framework. Psychol Bull. 1996;119:95–110.

114. Hammell KW, Miller WC, Forwell SJ, Forman BE, Jacobsen BA. Fatigue and spinal cord injury: a qualitative analysis. Spinal Cord. 2009;47(1):44–49.

115. Turk DC, Rudy TE. Towards a comprehensive assessment of chronic pain patients. Behav Res Ther. 1987;25(4):237–49.

116. Widerström-Noga EG, Duncan R, Felipe-Cuervo E, Turk DC. Assessment of the impact of pain and impairments associated with spinal cord injuries. Arch Phys Med Rehabil. 2002;**83**(3): 395–404.

117. Romano JM, Turner JA, Jensen MP, et al. Chronic pain patient-spouse behavioral interactions predict patient disability. Pain 1995;**63**(3):353–360.

118. Stroud MW, Turner JA, Jensen MP, Cardenas DD. Partner responses to pain behaviors are associated with depression and activity interference among persons with chronic pain and spinal cord injury. J.Pain 2006;**7**(2):91–99.

119. Cano A, Weisberg JN, Gallagher RM. Marital satisfaction and pain severity mediate the association between negative spouse responses to pain and depressive symptoms in a chronic pain patient sample. Pain Med. 2000;**1**(1):35–43.

120. Widerström-Noga EG, Duncan R, Turk DC. Psychosocial profiles of people with pain associated with spinal cord injury: identification and comparison with other chronic pain syndromes. Clin J Pain. 2004;**20**(4):261–271.

121. Hanley MA, Raichle K, Jensen M, Cardenas DD. Pain catastrophizing and beliefs predict changes in pain interference and psychological functioning in persons with spinal cord injury. J.Pain 2008;**9**(9):863–871.

122. Boschen KA, Tonack M, Gargaro J. Long-term adjustment and community reintegration following spinal cord injury. Int J Rehabil Res. 2003;**26**(3):157–164.

123. Norrbrink BC, Kowalski J, Lundeberg T. A comprehensive pain management programme comprising educational, cognitive and behavioural interventions for neuropathic pain following spinal cord injury. J.Rehabil.Med. 2006;**38**(3):172–180.

124. Jensen MP, Turner JA, Romano JM. Changes after multidisciplinary pain treatment in patient pain beliefs and coping are associated with concurrent changes in patient functioning. Pain. 2007b;**131**(1–2):38–47.

125. Teasell RW, Mehta S, Aubut JA, et al. A systematic review of pharmacologic treatments of pain after spinal cord injury. Arch.Phys. Med Rehabil. 2010;**91**(5):816–831.

126. Jensen MP, Gammaitoni AR, Bolognese JA, et al. The pain quality response profile of pregabalin in the treatment of neuropathic pain. Clin J Pain. 2012;**28**(8):683–686.

127. Falah M, Madsen C, Holbech JV, Sindrup SH. A randomized, placebo-controlled trial of levetiracetam in central pain in multiple sclerosis. Eur J Pain. 2012;**16**(6):860–869.

128. Attal N, Cruccu G, Baron R, et al.; European Federation of Neurological Societies. EFNS guidelines on the pharmacological treatment of neuropathic pain: 2010 revision. Eur J Neurol. 2010;**17**(9):1113-e88.

129. Dickenson AH, Matthews EA, Suzuki R. Neurobiology of neuropathic pain: mode of action of anticonvulsants. Eur J Pain 2002;**6** Suppl A:51–60.

130. Guan Y, Ding X, Cheng Y, et al. Efficacy of pregabalin for peripheral neuropathic pain: results of an 8-week, flexible-dose, double-blind, placebo-controlled study conducted in China. Clin Ther. 2011;**33**(2):159–166.

131. Satoh J, Yagihashi S, Baba M, et al. Efficacy and safety of pregabalin for treating neuropathic pain associated with diabetic peripheral neuropathy: a 14 week, randomized, double-blind, placebo-controlled trial. Diabet Med. 2011;**28**(1):109–116.

132. Backonja M, Beydoun A, Edwards KR, et al. Gabapentin for the symptomatic treatment of painful neuropathy in patients with diabetes mellitus: a randomized controlled trial. JAMA 1998;**280**(21):1831–1836.

133. Rowbotham M, Harden N, Stacey B, Bernstein P, Magnus-Miller L. Gabapentin for the treatment of postherpetic neuralgia: a randomized controlled trial. JAMA 1998;**280**(21):1837–1842.

134. Kim JS, Bashford G, Murphy TK, Martin A, Dror V, Cheung R. Safety and efficacy of pregabalin in patients with central post-stroke pain. Pain. 2011;**152**(5):1018–1023.

135. Finnerup NB, Grydehøj J, Bing J, et al. Levetiracetam in spinal cord injury pain: a randomized controlled trial. Spinal Cord. 2009;**47**(12):861–867.

136. Jungehulsing GJ, Israel H, Safar N, et al. Levetiracetam in patients with central neuropathic post-stroke pain—a randomized, double-blind, placebo-controlled trial. Eur J Neurol. 2013;**20**(2):331–337.

137. Amr YM. Multi-day low dose ketamine infusion as adjuvant to oral gabapentin in spinal cord injury related chronic pain: a prospective, randomized, double blind trial. Pain Physician. 2010;**13**(3):245–249.

138. Eide PK, Stubhaug A, Stenehjem AE. Central dysesthesia pain after traumatic spinal cord injury is dependent on N-methyl-D-aspartate receptor activation. Neurosurgery. 1995;**37**(6):1080–1087.

139. Sindrup SH, Jensen TS. Efficacy of pharmacological treatments of neuropathic pain: an update and effect related to mechanism of drug action. Pain. 1999;**83**(3):389–400.

140. Dharmshaktu P, Tayal V, Kalra BS. Efficacy of antidepressants as analgesics: a review. J Clin Pharmacol. 2012;**52**(1):6–17.

141. Ansari A. The efficacy of newer antidepressants in the treatment of chronic pain: a review of current literature. Harv.Rev.Psychiatry 2000;**7**(5):257–277.

142. Cardenas DD, Warms CA, Turner JA, Marshall H, Brooke MM, Loeser JD. Efficacy of amitriptyline for relief of pain in spinal cord injury: results of a randomized controlled trial. Pain. 2002;**96**(3):365–373.

143. Vranken JH, Hollmann MW, van der Vegt MH, et al. Duloxetine in patients with central neuropathic pain caused by spinal cord injury or stroke: a randomized, double-blind, placebo-controlled trial. Pain. 2011;**152**(2):267–273.

144. Loubser PG, Donovan WH. Diagnostic spinal anaesthesia in chronic spinal cord injury pain. Paraplegia 1991;**29**(1):25–36.

145. Attal N, Gaude V, Brasseur L, et al. Intravenous lidocaine in central pain: a double-blind, placebo-controlled, psychophysical study. Neurology 2000;**54**(3):564–574.

146. Attal N, Guirimand F, Brasseur L, Gaude V, Chauvin M, Bouhassira D. Effects of IV morphine in central pain: a randomized placebo-controlled study. Neurology. 2002;**58**(4):554–563.

147. Barrera-Chacon JM, Mendez-Suarez JL, Jáuregui-Abrisqueta ML, Palazon R, Barbara-Bataller E, García-Obrero I. Oxycodone improves pain control and quality of life in anticonvulsant-pretreated spinal cord-injured patients with neuropathic pain. Spinal Cord. 2011;**49**(1):36–42.

148. Siddall PJ, Molloy AR, Walker S, Mather LE, Rutkowski SB, Cousins MJ. The efficacy of intrathecal morphine and clonidine in the treatment of pain after spinal cord injury. Anesth Analg. 2000;**91**(6):1493–1498.

149. Svendsen KB, Jensen TS, Bach FW. Does the cannabinoid dronabinol reduce central pain in multiple sclerosis? Randomized double blind placebo controlled crossover trial. BMJ. 2004;**329**(7460):253.

150. Rog DJ, Nurmikko TJ, Friede T, Young CA. Randomized, controlled trial of cannabis-based medicine in central pain in multiple sclerosis. Neurology. 2005;**65**(6):812–819.

151. Rog DJ, Nurmikko TJ, Young CA. Oromucosal delta9-tetrahydrocannabinol/cannabidiol for neuropathic pain associated with multiple sclerosis: an uncontrolled, open-label, 2-year extension trial. Clin Ther. 2007;**29**(9):2068–2079.

152. Rintala DH, Fiess RN, Tan G, Holmes SA, Bruel BM. Effect of dronabinol on central neuropathic pain after spinal cord injury: a pilot study. Am.J.Phys.Med.Rehabil. 2010;**89**(10):840–848.

153. Falci S, Best L, Bayles R, Lammertse D, Starnes C. Dorsal root entry zone microcoagulation for spinal cord injury-related central pain: operative intramedullary electrophysiological guidance and clinical outcome. J Neurosurg. 2002 Sep;**97**(2 Suppl):193–200.

154. Cioni B, Meglio M, Pentimalli L, Visocchi M. Spinal cord stimulation in the treatment of paraplegic pain. J Neurosurg. 1995;**82**(1):35–39.

155. Owen SL, Green AL, Stein JF, Aziz TZ. Deep brain stimulation for the alleviation of post-stroke neuropathic pain. Pain. 2006;120(1–2):202–206.

156. Boccard SG, Pereira EA, Moir L, Aziz TZ, Green AL. Long-term outcomes of deep brain stimulation for neuropathic pain. Neurosurgery. 2013;72(2):221–230.

157. Previnaire JG, Nguyen JP, Perrouin-Verbe B, Fattal C. Chronic neuropathic pain in spinal cord injury: efficiency of deep brain and motor cortex stimulation therapies for neuropathic pain in spinal cord injury patients. Ann.Phys.Rehabil.Med 2009;52(2):188–193.

158. Tan G, Rintala DH, Jensen MP, et al. Efficacy of cranial electrotherapy stimulation for neuropathic pain following spinal cord injury: a multi-site randomized controlled trial with a secondary 6-month open-label phase.J Spinal Cord Med. 2011;34(3):285–296.

159. Soler MD, Kumru H, Pelayo R, et al. Effectiveness of transcranial direct current stimulation and visual illusion on neuropathic pain in spinal cord injury. Brain. 2010;133(9):2565–2577.

160. Norrbrink BC, Lundeberg T. Non-pharmacological pain-relieving therapies in individuals with spinal cord injury: a patient perspective. Complement Ther.Med. 2004;12(4):189–197.

161. Norrbrink C, Lundeberg T. Acupuncture and massage therapy for neuropathic pain following spinal cord injury: an exploratory study. Acupunct Med. 2011;29(2):108–115.

162. Norrbrink C. Transcutaneous electrical nerve stimulation for treatment of spinal cord injury neuropathic pain. J Rehabil Res Dev. 2009;46(1):85–93.

163. Nayak S, Shiflett SC, Schoenberger NE, et al. Is acupuncture effective in treating chronic pain after spinal cord injury? Arch.Phys. Med Rehabil. 2001;82(11):1578–1586.

164. Rapson LM, Wells N, Pepper J, Majid N, Boon H. Acupuncture as a promising treatment for below-level central neuropathic pain: a retrospective study. J Spinal Cord.Med 2003;26(1):21–26.

165. Lee JA, Park SW, Hwang PW, et al. Acupuncture for shoulder pain after stroke: a systematic review. J Altern Complement Med. 2012;18(9):818–823.

166. Norrbrink C, Lindberg T, Wahman K, Bjerkefors A. Effects of an exercise programme on musculoskeletal and neuropathic pain after spinal cord injury—results from a seated double-poling ergometer study. Spinal Cord. 2012 Jun;50(6):457–461.

167. Mulroy SJ, Thompson L, Kemp B, et al.; Physical Therapy Clinical Research Network (PTClinResNet). Strengthening and optimal movements for painful shoulders (STOMPS) in chronic spinal cord injury: a randomized controlled trial. Phys Ther. 2011;91(3):305–324.

168. Molton IR, Graham C, Stoelb BL, Jensen MP. Current psychological approaches to the management of chronic pain. Curr.Opin. Anaesthesiol. 2007;20(5):485–489.

169. Heutink M, Post MW, Bongers-Janssen HM, et al. The CONECSI trial: results of a randomized controlled trial of a multidisciplinary cognitive behavioral program for coping with chronic neuropathic pain after spinal cord injury. Pain. 2012;153(1):120–128.

170. Jensen MP, Barber J, Romano JM, Molton IR, Raichle KA, Osborne TL, Engel JM, Stoelb BL, Kraft GH, Patterson DR. A comparison of self-hypnosis versus progressive muscle relaxation in patients with multiple sclerosis and chronic pain. Int J Clin Exp Hypn. 2009;57(2):198–221.

CHAPTER 26

The impact of fatigue on neurorehabilitation

Killian Welch and Gillian Mead

Introduction

Though difficult to define, and abstract in conceptualization, fatigue is an experience familiar to all. Consequently, it is not itself pathological but is experienced to an extreme and disabling degree in many neurological conditions. In chronic fatigue syndrome (CFS) extreme fatigue is the central feature of condition, and the physiological changes and behaviours associated with it probably contribute to the pervasiveness of symptoms and chronicity of the problem. These physiological changes and behaviours probably also contribute to fatigue in other conditions. These often represent potentially remediable factors, and consequently are important to identify and address. An individualized formulation is crucial to achieving this, a principle that will guide the structure of this chapter. First, we will consider how factors innate to neurological conditions and those secondary to them can contribute to fatigue. Then, we will discuss how understanding of these factors can be synthesized in the formulation to guide treatment. This chapter will focus on the commonest neurological conditions in which fatigue is prominent; multiple sclerosis (MS), stroke, Parkinson's disease (PD), and traumatic brain injury (TBI). The same principles are applicable to fatigue in other neurological conditions.

General issues

What is fatigue?

The distinction between 'normal' and 'pathological' fatigue is unavoidably arbitrary. Non-pathological fatigue would be the experience of being tired after exercise, with energy restored after rest [1]. Definitions of pathological fatigue vary, but that of the MS Council is a good example, namely: 'a subjective lack of physical and/or mental energy that is perceived by the individual or caregiver to interfere with usual and desired activities' [2]. The subjectivity of fatigue is emphasized in this definition, which is consistent with description of (post-stroke) fatigue as 'weariness unrelated to previous exertion levels and usually not ameliorated by rest' [3]. Other definitions, such as Staub and Bogousslavsky's, emphasize the subjective need for greater effort, which does seem to be a core feature of the fatigue experience in all contexts [4].

Although attempts have been made to separate physical and mental fatigue, this is often neither feasible nor useful. Others favour dividing fatigue in to 'central' and 'peripheral' components. Chaudhuri and Behan for example, define central fatigue as 'the failure to initiate and/or sustain attentional tasks and physical activities requiring self-motivation (as opposed to external stimulation)', whereas peripheral fatigue is regarded as primarily physical or muscular in nature [5]. Central fatigue would be exemplified by the perception that more effort is required to undertake a task than is normal in the absence of any overt physical disability (i.e. a sensory symptom), whilst peripheral fatigue might be characterized by the objective documentation that voluntary power declines during a task or on repetition of that task (i.e. a motor sign) [6]. Notwithstanding that neurophysiological testing is crucial in distinguishing the level of involvement of the motor system, in practice the usefulness even of this more considered distinction can be questionable [7]. Perceived levels of central and peripheral fatigue covary, and even in myasthenia gravis, that exemplar of 'peripheral fatigue', reports of mental fatigue are common [8].

Fatigue is dissociable from sleepiness, although there is overlapping symptomatology [9]. Sleepiness is a physiological phenomenon, depending on previous sleep and occurring at regular intervals following a circadian rhythm [10] By contrast, fatigue describes persistent physical or mental exhaustion, not necessarily accompanied by sleepiness, and which sleep cannot alleviate. A patient may have both, and they are associated with common factors, for example the release of proinflammatory cytokines [11]. Apathy, even harder to distinguish from fatigue, is a feeling of indifference; fatigued patients generally retain an interest in their hobbies and interests, they just do not have the energy to undertake them.

How to measure a subjective concept

Peripheral fatigue, as an acute tendency for force generating capacity to diminish during sustained effort, can be fairly easily described and quantified. It is attributed to mechanisms such as the failure of neuro-muscular transmission, metabolic disturbances, defects of muscle membranes, or peripheral circulatory failure [5]. Central fatigue is subjective, warranting intervention when a patient endorses the symptom, its importance, and desire for treatment. Many attempts have been made to quantify it. Mead et al. identified over 50 scales used to assess fatigue post stroke [12], some of the more commonly encountered being summarized in Table 26.1. Others have taken a different approach to assessing fatigue. For example, in stroke a semi-structured interview has been used, and 'caseness' defined as fatigue present most days for >50% of waking hours which interferes with everyday activities [13]. This approach has also been used to define CFS. It is clear,

Table 26.1 Commonly used scales to assess fatigue

	Items	Score range	Dimension	Advantages	Disadvantages
Fatigue Severity Scale (FSS)	9	1–7 (Likert-type)	Modality, severity, frequency, impact on life	Valid and reliable, Shown to differentiate from depression, most widely used	Sensitivity to change questionable
Fatigue Impact Scale	40	0–4 (Likert-type)	Physical, cognitive, psychosocial impact	Valid and reliable Used in many conditions	Long
Modified Fatigue Impact Scale	21	0–4 (Likert-type)	Cognitive, psychosocial, physical impact	Valid and reliable Used in many conditions	Designed specifically to assess the impact of fatigue on everyday life
Visual Analogue Scale	1	0–100 (mm)	Depends on question	Valid, simple, quick Used in many conditions	Reliability questioned

Kos D, et al, Neurorehabil Neural Repair 22, pp. 91–100, copyright © 2008. Reprinted by permission of SAGE Publications.

however, that all cut-offs for 'caseness' are arbitrary, and as all assessments rely on subjective reporting they do not differentiate inability to generate or maintain the required effort/force from disinclination to do so [6].

Attempts have been made to objectively quantify 'central' fatigue. In 'cognitive' fatigue, likely best conceptualized as one component of it, these have generally measured performance on tasks requiring sustained attention. Meaningful associations between subjective reports of fatigue and neuropsychological measures have been elusive, however [14]. This is perhaps unsurprising given the lack of an association between cognitive complaints and performance on neuropsychological assessment [15]. Though a recent study in MS did report an association between subjective fatigue and performance when executive demands were very high [16], and a stroke study related fatigue to attentional and executive impairment [17], objective measures of central fatigue are currently of little clinical utility.

Epidemiology

Community studies report a prevalence of debilitating fatigue lasting at least 6 months of around 5% [18]. Greater fatigue is weakly associated with increasing age, female gender and, possibly, lower socio-economic status [19, 20]. The prevalence of fatigue in neurological conditions is increased beyond what would be expected solely on the basis of age and disability, being estimated to affect 30–80% of patients (see Table 26.2) [21]. Patients also often report a qualitative difference in their experience of fatigue after acquiring a neurologic illness, describing it as 'overwhelming' and 'mind-numbing' [22, 23].

Impact of fatigue

Forty percent of MS and one-third of PD patients report fatigue as their most disabling symptom [24, 25]. Fatigue imposes significant socioeconomic consequences, including loss of work hours and may be the most important factor in loss of employment [26, 27].

Aetiology and associations

A combination of biological, psychological, and social factors contribute to fatigue in all patients. Though the relative contribution of each varies between diagnosis and patient, failure to consider each sphere can lead to suboptimal treatment in all. Obvious examples are failure to consider depression in an individual who has prominent fatigue following a stroke, or overlooking medication side effects in a patient with CFS. Psychosocial issues, including unhelpful health beliefs, are particularly important to identify in neurological disease, as these may be the most modifiable maintaining factors. Though divisions are fluid, in this section potential contributions to fatigue will be separated into 'primary' and 'secondary' factors. The former are directly attributable to the neurological disease process, while the latter are physiological, psychological, or behavioural changes occurring as direct or indirect consequences. CFS is an example of a condition in which extreme fatigue exists in the absence of overt neurological pathology, but the presence of immunological and endocrine abnormalities is well established. This demonstrates both the arbitrary separation between 'primary' and 'secondary' factors and the potentially profound impact that the latter can have. Effective treatment for CFS suggests what may improve fatigue in other conditions.

Table 26.2 Estimated prevalence of fatigue in selected neurological illness

Population	Estimated prevalence (%)
Multiple sclerosis	38–83
Stroke	36–77
Parkinson's disease	28–58
Traumatic brain injury	45–73
Myasthenia gravis	27–91
Motor neurone disease	44–83

Caseness is variably defined as scores above an arbitrary cut off on a fatigue rating scale or fatigue present for >50% of waking hours and interfering with everyday activities.

Modified from Kluger et al. [21].

Primary factors

Direct brain pathology

Neurological disorders are due to abnormalities of the structure or function of the nervous system. Those associated with fatigue affect diverse brain regions, however, and fatigue is also prominent in medical and psychiatric conditions, in which brain structural abnormalities are subtle or absent. Consequently, fatigue is unlikely to be localized to a discrete brain region.

Early structural magnetic resonance imaging (MRI) studies of MS did not find any correlation between subjective fatigue and lesion load or brain atrophy, although recently associations between fatigue and volume loss have been reported [28], with atrophy in the striatum, thalamus, frontal cortex, and parietal cortex particularly highlighted [29, 30]. In a 2009 cross-sectional study post-stroke fatigue was more common in stroke than transient ischaemic attack (TIA) patients, suggesting at least some post stroke fatigue might be attributable to brain damage [31]. Systematic review found no association between fatigue and white matter lesions or brain atrophy, however, although some studies did report an association with infratentorial or basal ganglia stroke [32]. No TBI studies examine correlations between structural abnormalities with fatigue, but clinical markers of injury severity do not predict fatigue [33]. A study in patients who had had penetrating TBI found that fatigue was associated with ventromedal prefrontal cortex damage [34]. Reduced grey matter volume is reported in CFS [35], with increased prefrontal cortex volume following treatment with cognitive behavioural therapy (CBT) [36]. In summary, when structural abnormalities are identified they implicate involvement of frontal and subcortical brain regions in fatigue.

As fatigue likely involves distributed brain regions, functional imaging may provide greater insights in to its mechanisms. These approaches generally support the concept that fatigue is associated with dysfunction of cortical–subcortical circuitry, particularly circuits involved in attention and executive function. In MS there is decreased regional glucose metabolism in the frontal cortex and basal ganglia of fatigued patients [37]; in TBI brain activity is increased in the middle frontal lobe, basal ganglia, and anterior cingulate during a speeded cognitive task [38]; in PD decreases in frontal lobe perfusion are greater in patients with fatigue than those without (which was associated with executive function impairments) [39]; and CFS patients had differing patterns of activation of prefrontal cortical regions compared to healthy controls [40]. Functional imaging studies of fatigued stroke patients have not been undertaken, but post-stroke fatigue has been related to attentional and executive impairment [17].

In summary, convergent data across neurological conditions suggest dysfunction in the striatal-thalamic-frontal system is important in fatigue. These impairments may necessitate higher levels of mental effort for complex tasks, which increases subjective fatigue. In conditions with damaged brain structure (e.g. MS, TBI) recruitment of expanded pools of cortical neurons likely reflects brain plasticity unmasking latent pathways. Though adaptive, it may be energy intensive, excessive use of neuronal pools resulting in fatigue [41]. In CFS disruption again seems present but likely arises through different routes, which may include mechanisms such as sustained abnormalities of attentional focus.

Inflammation and endocrine factors

Inflammation is associated with fatigue, as evident from the lethargy of acute infections. This is mediated by pro-inflammatory cytokines, which act on the brain to result in drowsiness, loss of appetite, decreased activity and withdrawal from social interaction [42]. The association between treatment with interferon-α (IFN-α) and fatigue (which is dissociable from depression) is well recognized [43]. As inflammatory degenerative disorders, elevated cytokines are particularly relevant to fatigue in MS and systemic lupus erythematosus (SLE). Cytokines are however also elevated post-stroke and TBI [44, 45], in CFS [46], and even in PD [47], and depression [48], likely also contributing to fatigue in these conditions.

Alterations in the hypothalamic-pituitary-adrenal (HPA) axis are among the most replicated findings in CFS, mild hypocortisolaemia being consistently reported and attributed to enhanced negative feedback in the HPA axis [49]. This contrasts with the increased HPA axis activity and raised cortisol levels seen in depression [50] Whereas hormonal changes are relatively subtle in MS and CFS, in TBI, (and obviously pituitary stroke), they can be gross and necessitate replacement treatment. In TBI these abnormalities are not restricted to the acute phase, with as many as 25% of long-term survivors showing one or more pituitary hormone deficiencies [51]. As well as hypocortisolaemia and hypothyroidism being obvious causes of fatigue, an association with lowered growth and sex hormone levels following TBI has been reported [52, 53].

Secondary factors

Other medical problems

The possibility of additional medical pathology must be remembered. There should be blood screens for common hematologic and metabolic conditions and thyroid dysfunction. Recommended investigations to aid diagnosis of CFS, exclude other conditions and 'red flags' for alternative diagnostic explanations are shown in Table 26.3. In MS vitamin D deficiency is common. Though an association with fatigue was not found in MS it has been in the general population; consequently, assessment of 25-hydroxy vitamin D levels may be considered [54]. Infections can worsen fatigue and should be excluded [55]. An MS exacerbation may present as fatigue prior to clinical manifestation [56].

Medication side effects

Medications frequently causing fatigue include antispasticity agents (e.g. baclofen or tizanidine), narcotic analgesics, sedative hypnotic or anticonvulsant agents, sedative antidepressants or anxiolytics, and antihypertensive medication [57]. Patients often report increased fatigue with IFN therapy, though fatigue often improves with time on interferon [58]. Pretreating with nonsteroidal anti-inflammatory may improve IFN-associated fatigue [57]. Hypertension or hypotension secondary to excessive antihypertensive use may be associated with post stroke fatigue, though whether there is a causal relationship is uncertain [59].

Mobility issues and environment

In stroke, TBI and MS ambulation can be compromised by spasticity and weakness. Gait can be inefficient, requiring excessive energy expenditure that quickly fatigues the patient [60]. This will reduce physical activity causing physical deconditioning. The

Table 26.3 Investigations to aid in diagnosis of CFS and to exclude other illness

All patients

Full blood count (FBC)

Urea, electrolytes, and creatinine (U&Es)

Liver function tests, including albumin (LFTs)

Thyroid function tests (TFTs)

Glucose random

Erythrocyte sedimentation rate (ESR)

C-reactive protein (CRP)

Calcium

Creatine kinase*

Ferritin*

Urinalysis

When indicated by history or examination

Antimitochondrial antibodies (AMA) if minor alterations in LFTs

Antinuclear antibody test (ANA)

Cytomegalovirus CMV)

Coeliac serology if diarrhoea/altered bowel habit, weight loss or history of autoimmune disorders and in patients with a family history of coeliac disease)

Epstein–Barr virus (EBV)

Extractable nuclear antigens (ENA)

Human immunodeficiency virus (HIV)

Hepatitis B and C

Lyme serology

Serology for chronic bacterial infections

Toxoplasma

Electrocardiogram (ECG) if any cardiological symptoms)

Features suggesting alternative diagnoses

Substantive unexplained weight loss

Objective neurological signs

Symptoms or signs of inflammatory arthritis or connective tissue disease

Symptoms or signs of cardiorespiratory disease

Symptoms of sleep apnoea

Clinically significant lymphadenopathy

In the all patients section, all investigations from those with asterisks would also be routinely done in neurology patients.

Contains public sector information licensed under the Open Government Licence v2.0. [154].

oxygen cost of breathing is increased in PD patients, meaning they require more energy simply to breath [61]. Energy loss with tremors and dyskinesias has also been demonstrated [62].

Hyperthermia contributes to fatigue during exercise in healthy people [63], but the strong association between heat and symptom exacerbation (Uhthoff's phenomenon) is a particular characteristic of MS. It affects 60–80% of MS patients and is attributed to increased body temperature inducing conduction block in vulnerable axons [64]. Deconditioning can result through avoidance of exercise/activity to prevent symptom exacerbation [65].

Psychiatric conditions

Fatigue is a core feature of depression, present in around 25% of people with neurological disorder [66]. Depression severity correlates with fatigue severity [67], and should never be dismissed as simply 'an appropriate reaction to a serious illness'. Indeed rather than being 'secondary' to neurological conditions its aetiology is often not clearly separable from the neurological disease process itself. A positive correlation has also been reported between anxiety and subjective fatigue [68].

Identification of depression in neurological conditions is complicated by many symptoms (e.g. fatigue, reduced attention and concentration, disturbed sleep) being features of the diseases themselves. Consequently greater emphasis should be placed on cognitive than somatic symptoms, the presence of guilt, worthlessness, hopelessness, and suicidality strongly suggesting depression. The pattern of fatigue observed in depression is rather different from that in neurological conditions. Fatigue in depression tends to be worst in the morning, improve as the day goes on, and not be relieved by sleep; MS fatigue, by contrast, is best in the morning, worsens as the day goes on, and rest gives some relief. Substance misuse is strongly associated with fatigue and should always be considered.

Sleep disorders

In neurological disorders fatigue has a consistent relationship with broken sleep. Correlations with daytime sleepiness however, though present in TBI and PD, are surprisingly weak in MS [69–71]. Nonetheless, patients reporting daytime sleepiness should be screened for potential sleep disorders, including obstructive sleep apnoea, narcolepsy and restless leg syndrome/periodic limb movement disorder. The latter is particularly common in MS [72], while sleep-disordered breathing is a particular issue after stroke [73], and various sleep disorders are core features of PD [74]. Initial insomnia in the absence of obvious medical cause suggests anxiety, while early morning waking with inability to get back to sleep is more characteristic of depression. Other disease-associated problems such as pain, spasticity and nocturnal micturition also impact on sleep and require specific interventions.

Pain

Pain is common and can be difficult to treat. Robust correlations between pain and fatigue are reported in various neurological conditions [75, 76]. It is speculated that pain may contribute to fatigue through a reduction in central motor drive [77]. If associated with activity it will encourage activity avoidance.

Poor nutrition

As 50–80% of in-hospital stroke patients have one or more eating difficulties related to neurologic deficits, it is unsurprising that 50% of stroke inpatients are malnourished [78] Westergren reported that 6 months post-stroke poorer nutritional status was closely related to a lack of energy [79]. Effects are likely bidirectional, giving rise to a vicious circle.

Deconditioning

Deconditioning is a complex physiological process in which the lack of use of the body's cardiovascular, neuromuscular, biomechanical, and musculoskeletal systems leads to a decrease in their functional capacity, and the body's efficiency [80]. This reduces the capacity for exercise and increase the perception of effort required for a given level of activity. Though evidence of significantly reduced physical fitness in CFS compared to sedentary controls is conflicting, a recent systematic review concluded that there was reduced physiological exercise capacity in CFS and that deconditioning is a perpetuating factor [81]. Though other factors likely contribute too, some evidence for the presence of deconditioning is provided by the proven efficacy of graded exercise programmes in reducing symptoms of CFS [82]. Neurological conditions are associated with substantial reductions in activity, and deconditioning has been reported in MS, stroke, TBI, and in PD [83–86].

Beliefs about activity/cognitive style

Cognitive factors believed to contribute to the maintenance of CFS include a tendency to focus on fatigue and perceive it as a negative experience (which consequently amplifies its perception) and beliefs of having a very limited ability to be active (leading to very low levels of activity) [87]. In CFS a strong belief in a physical cause of the illness, a strong focus on bodily sensations, and a poor sense of control over symptoms contribute to fatigue severity and functional impairment [88]. The importance of fear of symptom exacerbation in CFS was elegantly demonstrated in a cycling task. It was a more important determinant of distance travelled than physical symptoms, physical disability, mood, and other illness perceptions [89].

It is likely that similar cognitions and attentional biases magnify fatigue in some with neurological disorders. Beliefs about the dangers of activity may be expected in MS, given that elevated body temperature or prolonged exertion exacerbates symptoms [57]. Though unstudied, it is likely that after a catastrophic event such as stroke fears of provoking a further stroke inhibit engagement with exercise in some patients. It has been reported in MS that a sense of control (often referred to as self-efficacy), reduces feelings of fatigue, whereas focusing on bodily sensations aggravates it [90]. MS patients who catastrophize about experiencing symptoms (expecting the worst possible outcome), who are embarrassed about symptoms, or who believe symptoms are always a sign of physical damage are more likely to be fatigued [91]. A systematic review incorporating studies in cancer, CFS, MS, fibromyalgia, and healthy individuals confirmed a significant association between catastrophizing and fatigue [92]. Other cognitive styles also influence fatigue and activity levels. For example, a qualitative study examining what determined whether people resumed previously valued activities after stroke identified 'all-or-nothing' thinking as a barrier [93]. 'All-or-nothing behaviour', that is, overdoing things when feeling better then needing to rest for prolonged periods to recover, is associated with fatigue in MS [91].

Pre-injury factors and response to stressors

Personality is assumed to influence vulnerability to CFS, but cross-sectional studies confound state and trait effects. A prospective study did, however, report that higher emotional instability (an individual's tendency to experience psychological distress) and self-reported stress were risk factors for the condition [94]. Acute physical or psychological stress might trigger the onset of CFS, it being shown that severe stressful events or difficulties are more common in the period prior to onset of the illness than in population controls [95].

Having a severe neurological disorder is a significant stressor, and dispositional differences in response to stress must contribute to fatigue in at least some patients. Though prospective studies are lacking, cross-sectional data reports higher emotional instability is associated with greater fatigue in MS and cancer [96, 97]. An association between fatigue and perceived stress has also been reported [98].

Pre-stroke fatigue may increases the risk of post-stroke fatigue, but studies are retrospective and consequently susceptible to recall bias [99]. The picture is further complicated by fatigue itself being a risk factor for stroke [99].

Treatment

The multifactorial nature of fatigue is captured by a biopsychosocial formulation, which facilitates an individualized understanding of maintaining factors and guides multidisciplinary management. A model formulation is depicted in Figure 26.1. Unfortunately the evidence base for the treatment of fatigue in neurological conditions is poor. Most research on fatigue treatment has been in CFS and MS, so evidence will often be extrapolated from these conditions. The absence of overt neurological pathology in CFS means this must be done with caution. As discussed earlier, however, there is considerable overlap between biological, psychological, and behavioural findings in fatigued individuals across diagnoses, which provides some justification. 'Secondary' factors certainly contribute substantially to fatigue in neurological conditions, and being generally more modifiable than the disease process itself are important treatment targets.

Review treatment of the neurological condition and directly related problems

Though fatigue is a side effect of some immunomodulatory agents used to treat MS, disease modifying drugs can actually reduce fatigue. This is reported even with IFN-β, but the effect with glatiramer acetate is significantly greater [100]. A cross-sectional case-controlled study suggested natalizumab may have greatest effect [101].

PD drugs are implicated both in exacerbating and reducing fatigue. Pramiprexole has been associated with increased subjective fatigue in several randomized controlled trials (RCTs) [102], while carbidopa–levodopa reduced muscle fatigue in experimental studies [103]. Assessing subjective fatigue is further complicated in PD by whether the patient is in an 'on' or 'off' sate. Stroke and TBI do not currently have 'direct' treatments, but some symptomatic or secondary prevention interventions are associated with fatigue.

Identify and treat medical comorbidity and full medication review

Comorbid medical conditions are common in neurological disorders, and are almost universally associated with fatigue.

Sleep and nutrition

Sleep

Specific sleep disorders (discussed under 'Primary factors') should be identified and treated. Sleep phase disorders are addressed by entraining a regular sleep–wake cycle, and melatonin and/or light treatment may assist. CBT has good evidence in treating insomnia in the non-neurological population, with positive studies in TBI and MS [104, 105]. Though hypnotics and sedative antidepressants can be helpful, the high incidence of side effects (falls, hallucinations, sedation, cognitive deficits, bowel, and bladder problems, etc.) necessitates caution. Personal experience suggests trazodone and mirtazepine as sedative antidepressants associated with fewest problems, and if they must be used short-acting hypnotics (used short term) are preferable to long-acting ones.

First line treatment of periodic limb movement disorder (PLMD) is with dopamine agonists or Levodopa [106], and marked relief with ropinirole or pramipexole is reported in post-stroke restless leg syndrome (RLS) [107] Though significant depression must be treated, remember that antidepressants can aggravate RLS and PLMD [73]. Deep brain stimulation has been recommended for the treatment of insomnia in advanced PD [108].

Nutrition

All patients should be supported in having a balanced, healthy diet. Even skipping breakfast has been associated with fatigue [109]. In MS, RCTs report adherence to a low fat, low cholesterol diet supplemented with olive oil capsules significantly reduce fatigue [110], but vitamin D or omega-3-fatty acids do not [111, 112].

Carnitine contributes to cellular energy metabolism, and deficiency may reduce energy production through impaired fatty acid oxidation. An RCT of fatigued elderly individuals without current significant medical morbidity found 4 g a day of acetyl L-carnitine for 180 days reduced physical and mental fatigue compared to placebo [113]. In an open label randomized study in CFS acetylcarnitine and propionylcarnitine both reduced fatigue, though improvement was reduced with combined treatment [114]. A Cochrane review identified one active-comparator, cross-over randomized trial which found no difference between acetyl L-carnitine 2 g daily and amantadine 200 mg daily on MS fatigue; an open-label study showing reduced fatigue with levocarnitine did not meet inclusion criteria [115]. Despite reported benefit in various medical conditions, the impact of carnitine on fatigue has not been examined in other neurological conditions.

Physical aids and interventions

Physical aids

Use of orthoses or functional electrical stimulators can improve gait mechanics, promote energy conservation, and improve the safety of walking [57], but evidence they reduce fatigue is lacking.

Temperature control

Given the association between heat stress and MS symptom deterioration, simple strategies to minimize heat exposure, such as performing work or exercise during the early morning or late evening when it is cooler, seem sensible. Observational studies report benefit from simple cooling strategies such as cold showers, applying ice packs, and drinking cold beverages [65]. Precooling, essentially immersing the lower limbs in cool water, was shown to have some benefit in terms of walk performance and fatigue ratings [116]. In an RCT, cooling garments demonstrated subjective reductions in fatigue in thermally sensitive MS patients, though blinding of patients was not achieved [108]. Anecdotal evidence suggests 4-aminopyridine limits worsening of MS symptoms during heat exposure or exercise [65].

Treatment of psychiatric conditions

Treatment of depression and anxiety in neurological disease is discussed in Chapter 28. If insomnia is a major problem sedative antidepressants may be preferable, whereas energizing antidepressants, (such as selective serotonin reuptake inhibitors), may be first choice if fatigue is prominent but initial insomnia not a major issue [117]. Unfortunately, and likely reflecting the multifactorial nature of fatigue, cancer research shows that antidepressant

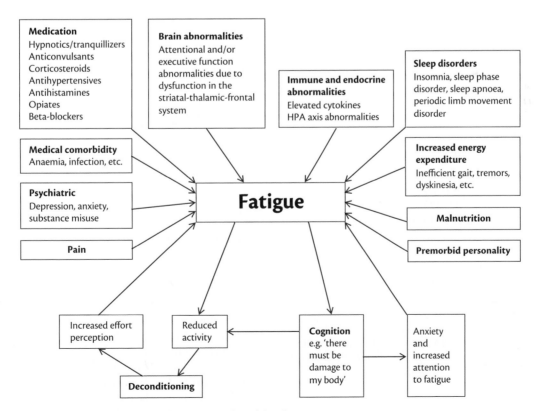

Fig. 26.1 Formulation-based approach to understanding fatigue in neurological disorders.

treatment may not improve fatigue even when it treats depression [118]. There is no evidence antidepressants improve fatigue in the absence of depression [119].

Exercise and energy conservation strategies

Exercise

Exercise improves exercise tolerance and reduces fatigue in healthy individuals as well as those with long-term conditions [120]. Benefit is however not limited to the physical dimension of fatigue, as exercise also improves mood, reduces anxiety and fear [121], and improves cognitive performance [122]. These benefits are likely consequent to associated physiological and anatomical changes, such as increased production of growth factors, increased efficiency of the cerebral vascular system, enhanced hippocampal neurogenesis, and regulation of the immune and endocrine systems [1]. Understanding of how this occurs is fast increasing, a recent study showing voluntary wheel-running induced gene expression in the mouse hippocampus [122]. As well as addressing deconditioning through these overtly neurobiological mechanisms, exercise may also influence effort perception.

Andreason et al. categorized exercise interventions as endurance training (ET), resistance training (RT), combined training (CT), and 'other' training modalities (OT) [123]. In general ET, or aerobic exercise, is most consistently beneficial. Walking is especially recommended, but swimming or cycling may also be appropriate [124]. Exercise programmes must be properly planned, gradually building levels of activity to promote increasing stamina and prevent unhelpful 'boom–bust cycles' occurring. This means regular exercise sessions start from a level that does not result in postexertional malaise, with the length and frequency of the exercise sessions progressively increasing. The CFS literature shows that, compared with a symptom-contingent approach, a time-contingent approach leads to greater improvements in fatigue and physical functioning [124]. A measurement (time, distance walked, etc.) rather than symptom experience should determine whether a session ends, this likely underpinning the superiority of graded exercise over adaptive pacing [82] Though patients may be anxious about undertaking an exercise programme, there is no reason why graded exercise carried out under appropriate professional supervision should be harmful. Research on the efficacy of exercise-based interventions in specific conditions are considered next.

Chronic fatigue syndrome

A 2011 meta-analysis of five RCTs supported the efficacy of graded exercise in the treatment of CFS [125]. Since this study the results of the PACE trial, the largest ($n = 640$) and most important trial of graded exercise therapy (GET), CBT, and adaptive pacing in CFS have been published. It reported that CBT and GET both had an odds ratio for trial recovery compared to standard care or adaptive pacing of around 3.5, and concluded they 'can safely be added to specialist medical care to moderately improve outcomes for CFS' [82]. Concerns about the safety of GET are not evidence based [126]. The underlying principle of gradually increasing activity may be applicable to cognitive activity too, implying CFS sufferers should be encouraged to undertake gradually more challenging intellectual tasks, starting from a tolerable level [124].

Multiple sclerosis

A 2011 systematic review reported exercise therapy has the potential for positive effect on MS fatigue [123]. Ten studies (seven

of which were RCTs, total 239 patients) examined the effect of endurance training, with some demonstrating a substantial effect. Findings were heterogeneous, with larger studies recruiting people fatigued at the start of the study more likely to show an effect. Analogous to concerns about a 'boom–bust' cycle in CFS, intensive training activities undertaken to exhaustion can reduce the effectiveness of treatment.

Stroke

Exercise post-stroke does lead to improvements in physical fitness [127]. Though data demonstrating an association between post-stroke fatigue and physical fitness are limited [128], extrapolating from data in other conditions one would expect associated improvements in fatigue. A randomized trial of 83 patients >4 months post-stroke demonstrated that 12 weeks of cognitive therapy augmented with graded activity training led to greater reductions in post-stroke fatigue than cognitive therapy alone [129].

Other conditions

As in the general population, in PD fatigue is significantly (negatively) associated with physical activity [130]. Aerobic conditioning programmes do increase fitness in PD [85], though an RCT of a weekly community gym-based exercise programme found no benefit on fatigue [131]. In contrast, semi-supervised home treadmill training was safe and associated with a significant reduction in fatigue [132]. While fitness training may improve cardiorespiratory fitness after traumatic brain injury [133], no trials examine impact on fatigue.

Energy conservation

The PACE trial clarified the superiority of graded exercise to pacing, the latter being no more effective than standard medical care [82, 116]. This is likely because pacing encourages adaptation to illness, whereas CBT and GET encourage gradual increases in activity with the aim of ameliorating the illness. This being said it is certainly possible to combine interventions aiming to increase activity and fitness with guidance on how to organise activities so they match energy levels, incorporate regular rest periods and adapt daily living activities to minimize unnecessary utilization of energy. A systematic review reported that in the short-term energy conservation strategies can reduce fatigue in MS [134]; there is also evidence in post-stoke fatigue [135]. Some benefit may derive from feelings of control and self-efficacy.

Address cognitions

The role of cognitive processes (e.g. excessive focus on bodily symptoms, fear of fatigue and catastrophization), in perpetuation of fatigue were discussed previously. It is, however, impossible to isolate cognitive and behavioural interventions. Even a purely exercise-based intervention will involve activity despite feeling fatigued, challenging beliefs such as 'activity is dangerous' [87]. This may partly explain why graded exercise performed as well as CBT in the PACE trial.

Chronic fatigue syndrome

While acknowledging the above, the efficacy of CBT in CFS is established; a 2011 meta-analysis of 16 RCTs reported that CBT and GET were equally effective, but the former may be better when patients have comorbid anxiety and depressive symptoms [125]. As described in the PACE trial, the aim of CBT is to address fears of engaging in activity/avoidance of activity which interact with physiological processes to perpetuate fatigue. Therapeutic strategies include examining the evidence underpinning beliefs and using behavioural experiments to test out fears. A baseline of activity and rest and a regular sleep pattern are established, and then gradual increases in both physical and mental activity collaboratively planned. Patients are also helped to address social and emotional problems through problem solving.

Multiple sclerosis

An RCT of 72 fatigued MS patients reported that though fatigue decreased with both interventions, reductions were greater with CBT than relaxation therapy (effect size 3.0 vs. 1.8) [136]. CBT combined explanation of the cognitive behavioural model of fatigue, activity scheduling, sleep hygiene, and changing unhelpful cognitions about fatigue. Changing perceptions of fatigue (e.g. perceiving it as more controllable, as time limited and as having less serious consequences) mediated decreases in fatigue [137]. An Internet-based version of this intervention with telephone support also resulted in significant reductions in fatigue [138], as did mindfulness training (compared to usual care) in an RCT of 150 patients [139]. Mindfulness aims to reduce stress through teaching a nonjudgmental awareness of moment-to-moment experience.

Stroke

As discussed Zedlitz et al. reported that, though CBT alone had beneficial effects, reductions in post-stroke fatigue were greater when cognitive therapy was augmented with graded activity training [129]. The cognitive component was delivered in small groups and emphasised pacing, improved planning of activities and relaxation, with rather less focus on challenging unhelpful cognitions than CBT in the CFS and MS trials. These results need replication, but do emphasize the importance of exercise/graded activity accompanying any cognitive intervention for post-stroke fatigue. A small uncontrolled pilot study has since suggested mindfulness-informed CBT was associated with a reduction in post-stroke fatigue [140].

Other conditions

No studies have examined the efficacy of cognitive interventions for fatigue in PD or moderate/severe TBI.

Multidisciplinary rehabilitation

Multidisciplinary rehabilitation aims to reduce symptoms, increase independence and maximise participation in society [141]. It is generally coordinated by a specialist doctor, delivered by a team of different therapists, and not protocolized, being tailored to individual needs and goals.

Several uncontrolled studies suggested multidisciplinary rehabilitation is beneficial in CFS [142]. Though impact on fatigue was not a specific focus in Khan et al.'s Cochrane review of the efficacy of multidisciplinary rehabilitation in MS, the review does summarize outcomes on this measure [141]. On the basis of two positive RCTs of outpatient rehabilitation they report there is limited evidence that high intensity programmes can provide short-term benefit in fatigue, and insufficient evidence that a lower intensity programme can reduce fatigue. A home based intervention had no impact on fatigue compared to standard care, and the only study comparing inpatient rehabilitation to standard care was negative. Though benefits of multidisciplinary rehabilitation have been reported in other neurological conditions, specific effects on fatigue have not been examined.

The potentially modest impact of multidisciplinary rehabilitation on fatigue in MS is initially surprising, as it likely includes elements of exercise treatment and cognitive interventions known to have good effect. This may reflect however that it is the delivery of evidence based interventions directed at specific areas of need that is important rather than simply access to a variety of professionals [143].

Medication

Drugs such as antidepressants have proven benefit in treating secondary conditions common in neurological disease which contribute to fatigue. This section will focus on drugs used specifically to treat fatigue.

Amantadine

A 2009 Cochrane review of amantadine in MS reported that though five RCTs met the criteria for inclusion, overall their quality was poor [144]. They reported small and inconsistent improvements in fatigue. Nonetheless, though unlicensed it is a commonly used treatment for MS fatigue, the standard dose being 100–200 mg morning and early afternoon [117]. It is generally well tolerated but side effects can include hallucinations, vivid dreams, nausea, hyperactivity, anxiety, insomnia, constipation, and rash. Its effects on fatigue in stroke, TBI, and PD are unreported.

Modafinil

Modafinil is a non-amphetamine-like drug approved for the management of narcolepsy and used for daytime fatigue in other conditions. Three RCTs examined the effect of Modafinil 200–400 mg on MS fatigue. The smallest showed a significant reduction in fatigue compared to placebo, apparent within three hours [145]; the others reported only a trend towards greater fatigue reduction ($p = 0.07$) [146] or no change [147]. Modafinil is generally well tolerated, but serious, life-threatening skin reactions, psychiatric adverse reactions (such as suicidal thoughts, depression, psychotic episodes) and cardiovascular adverse reactions (e.g. hypertension) have been reported [117]. A small non-placebo controlled study in stroke patients showed modafinil decreased fatigue severity in patients with brainstem and thalamic strokes (as well as MS patients), but not cortical infarctions [148]. Two small RCTs examined the impact of modafinil on PD fatigue. Though both did not report significant change on any of the fatigue severity scales used, one did report improvement in clinical global impression of fatigue [149]; no safety concerns were raised. A single-centre cross-over RCT in patients with (predominantly moderate or severe) TBI found that it improved daytime sleepiness, but not fatigue [150]. Though numerous studies fail to demonstrate greater effects on fatigue than (generally pronounced) placebo effects, modafinil is generally the first-line (unlicensed) pharmacological treatment for fatigue in neurological disease.

Other pharmacological agents

Two RCTs in MS did not separate effects of pemoline from placebo [117]; this, together with potential for liver toxicity, mean it is rarely used. Prokarin is a proprietary blend of histamine and caffeine, administered as a cream. A single small MS RCT suggested it reduced fatigue compared to placebo [151]. A single small RCT reported that methylphenidate 10 mg three times a day significantly reduced fatigue in PD and was well tolerated

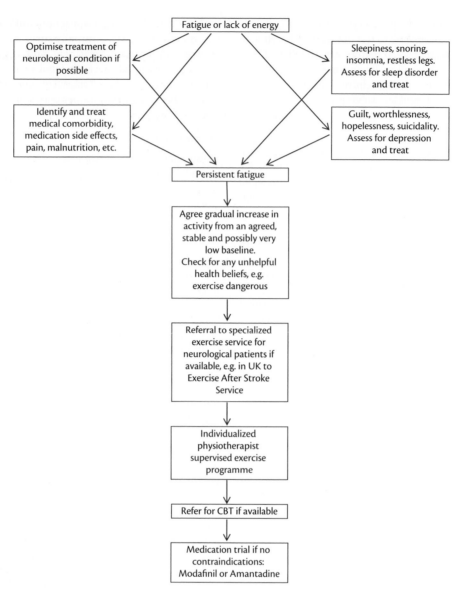

Fig. 26.2 Treatment of fatigue in neurological conditions.

[152]. It has not been evaluated in other neurological conditions. Lack of replication of this study, together with the fact it is a controlled drug, may worsen motor function and quality of life in PD, has a potential for abuse, and can cause insomnia, hypertension, and anorexia, have limited its use. An unreplicated randomized placebo-controlled crossover trial showed benefit from aspirin, daily dosage of 1300 mg, on MS-related fatigue [153].

A pragmatic approach to treating fatigue in neurological conditions

A treatment plan is detailed in Figure 26.2. Exercise has the best evidence and should be encouraged in all patients. Ideally, individually tailored programmes would be provided, such as the Exercise After Stroke programme delivered in some UK leisure centres. If not available, but mobility is reasonable, regular walks starting from a modest base are a good option. If there seem to be barriers/reservations about exercise, clinicians must explore what these are and correct any misunderstandings about the perceived dangers of activity/exercise. CBT has reasonable evidence, but availability is limited. Additionally, many neurological conditions are associated with significant cognitive impairment, which likely reduces the benefit of CBT. Though evidence for pharmacological treatments is weak, amantadine and modafanil are commonly used. Carnitine may hold some promise, but further trials are needed.

References

1. Harrington M. Neurobiological studies of fatigue. Prog Neurobiol. 2012;**99**:93–105
2. Mohr DC, Dick LP, Russo D, et al. The psychosocial impact of multiple sclerosis: Exploring the patients perspective, Health Psychology. 1999;**18**:376–382.
3. de Groot MH, Phillips SJ, Eskes GA. Fatigue associated with stroke and other neurologic conditions: implications for stroke rehabilitation. Arch Phys Med Rehabil. 2003;**84**:1714–1720.
4. Staub F, Bogousslavsky J. Fatigue after stroke: a major but neglected issue. Cerebrovasc Dis. 2001;**12**:75–81.
5. Chaudhuri A, Behan PO. Fatigue in neurological disorders. Lancet. 2004;**363**:978–988.

6. Vucic S, Burke D, Kiernan MC. Fatigue in multiple sclerosis: mechanisms and management. Clin Neurophysiol. 2010;**121**:809–817.

7. Gerber LH. Some unresolved issues for the study of fatigue: the way forward. PM R. 2010;**2**:466–468.

8. Paul RH, Cohen RA, Goldstein JM, Gilchrist JM. Fatigue and its impact on patients with myasthenia gravis. Muscle Nerve. 2000;**23**:1402–1406.

9. Neu D, Mairesse O, Hoffmann G, et al. Do sleepyand tiredgo together? Rasch analysis of the relationships between sleepiness, fatigue and nonrestorative sleep complaints in a nonclinical population sample. Neuroepidemiology. 2010;**35**:1–11.

10. Borbély AA. A two process model of sleep regulation. Hum Neurobiol. 1982;**1**:195–204.

11. Rohleder N, Aringer M, Boentert M. Role of interleukin-6 in stress, sleep, and fatigue. Ann N Y Acad Sci. 2012;**1261**:88–96.

12. Mead G, Lynch J, Greig C, Young A, Lewis S, Sharpe M. Evaluation of fatigue scales in stroke patients. Stroke. 2007;**38**:2090–2095.

13. Lynch J, Mead G, Greig C, Young A, Lewis S, Sharpe M. Fatigue after stroke: the development and evaluation of a case definition. J Psychosom Res. 2007;**63**:539–544.

14. Bailey A, Channon S, Beaumont J. The relationship between subjective fatigue and cognitive fatigue in advanced multiple sclerosis. Multiple Sclerosis. 2007;**13**:73–80.

15. Duits A, Munnecom T, van Heugten C, van Oostenbrugge RJ. Cognitive complaints in the early phase after stroke are not indicative of cognitive impairment. J Neurol. Neurosurg Psychiatry. 2008;**79**:143–146.

16. Holtzer R, Foley F. The relationship between subjective reports of fatigue and executive control in multiple sclerosis. J Neurol Sci. 2009;**281**:46–50.

17. Radman N, Staub F, Aboulafia-Brakha T, Berney A, Bogousslavsky J, Annoni J. Poststroke fatigue following minor infarcts A prospective study. Neurology. 2012;**79**:1422–1427.

18. Jason LA, Jordan KM, Richman JA, et al. A community-based study of prolonged fatigue and chronic fatigue. J Health Psychol. 1999;**4**:9–26.

19. Pawlikowska T, Chalder T, Hirsch S, Wallace P, Wright D, Wessely S. Population based study of fatigue and psychological distress. Br Med J. 1994;**308**:763–766.

20. Bültmann U, Kant I, Kasl SV, Beurskens AJ, van den Brandt, Piet A. Fatigue and psychological distress in the working population: psychometrics, prevalence, and correlates. J Psychosom Res. 2002;**52**:445–452.

21. Kluger BM, Krupp LB, Enoka RM. Fatigue and fatigability in neurologic illnesses Proposal for a unified taxonomy. Neurology. 2013;**80**:409–416.

22. Brown R, Dittner A, Findley L, Wessely S. The Parkinson fatigue scale. Parkinsonism Relat Disord. 2005;**11**:49–55.

23. Flinn NA, Stube JE. Post-stroke fatigue: qualitative study of three focus groups. Occupat Ther Int. 2010;**17**:81–91.

24. Friedman J, Friedman H. Fatigue in Parkinsons disease. Neurology. 1993;**43**:2016–2018.

25. Bakshi R. Fatigue associated with multiple sclerosis: diagnosis, impact and management. Multiple Sclerosis. 2003;**9**:219–227.

26. Smith MM, Arnett PA. Factors related to employment status changes in individuals with multiple sclerosis. Multiple Sclerosis. 2005;**11**:602–609.

27. Zesiewicz T, Patel-Larson A, Hauser R, Sullivan K. Social security disability insurance SSDI. in Parkinsons disease. Disabil Rehabil. 2007;**29**:1934–1936.

28. Marrie RA, Fisher E, Miller DM, Lee J, Rudick RA. Association of fatigue and brain atrophy in multiple sclerosis. J Neurol Sci. 2005;**228**:161–166.

29. Niepel G, Tench CR, Evangelou N. Deep gray matter and fatigue in MS. J Neurol. 2006;**253**:896–902.

30. Calabrese M, Rinaldi F, Grossi P, et al. Basal ganglia and frontal/parietal cortical atrophy is associated with fatigue in relapsing—remitting multiple sclerosis. Multiple Sclerosis. 2010;**16**:1220–1228.

31. Winward C, Sackley C, Metha Z, Rothwell PM. A population-based study of the prevalence of fatigue after transient ischemic attack and minor stroke. Stroke. 2009;**40**:757–761.

32. Kutlubaev M, Duncan F, Mead G. Biological correlates of post-stroke fatigue: a systematic review. Acta Neurol Scand. 2012;**125**:219–227.

33. Cantor JB, Ashman T, Gordon W, et al. Fatigue after traumatic brain injury and its impact on participation and quality of life. J Head Trauma Rehabil. 2008;**23**:41–51.

34. Pardini M, Krueger F, Raymont V, Grafman J. Ventromedial prefrontal cortex modulates fatigue after penetrating traumatic brain injury. Neurology. 2010;**74**:749–754.

35. de Lange FP, Kalkman JS, Bleijenberg G, Hagoort P, van der Meer, Jos WM, Toni I. Gray matter volume reduction in the chronic fatigue syndrome. Neuroimage. 2005; **26**:777–781.

36. de Lange FP, Koers A, Kalkman JS, et al. Increase in prefrontal cortical volume following cognitive behavioural therapy in patients with chronic fatigue syndrome. Brain. 2008;**131**:2172–2180.

37. Roelcke U, Kappos L, Lechner-Scott J, et al. Reduced glucose metabolism in the frontal cortex and basal ganglia of multiple sclerosis patients with fatigue A 18F-fluorodeoxyglucose positron emission tomography study. Neurology. 1997;**48**:1566–1571.

38. Kohl AD, Wylie G, Genova H, Hillary F, Deluca J. The neural correlates of cognitive fatigue in traumatic brain injury using functional MRI. Brain Injury. 2009;**23**:420–432.

39. Abe K, Takanashi M, Yanagihara T. Fatigue in patients with Parkinsons disease. Behav Neurol. 2000;**12**:103–106.

40. Caseras X, Mataix-Cols D, Giampietro V, et al. Probing the working memory system in chronic fatigue syndrome: a functional magnetic resonance imaging study using the n-back task. Psychosom Med. 2006;**68**:947–955.

41. Lapierre Y, Hum S. Treating fatigue. Int MS J. 2007;**14**:64–71.

42. Norheim KB, Jonsson G, Omdal R. Biological mechanisms of chronic fatigue. Rheumatology. 2011;**50**:1009–1018.

43. Capuron L, Gumnick JF, Musselman DL, et al. Neurobehavioral effects of interferon-α in cancer patients: phenomenology and paroxetine responsiveness of symptom dimensions. 2002;**26**:643–652.

44. Spalletta G, Bossu P, Ciaramella A, Bria P, Caltagirone C, Robinson R. The etiology of poststroke depression: a review of the literature and a new hypothesis involving inflammatory cytokines. Mol Psychiatry. 2006;**11**:984–991.

45. Mannix RC, Whalen MJ. Traumatic brain injury, microglia, and Beta amyloid, Int J Alzh Dis. 2012: 608732. doi: 10.1155/2012/608732.

46. Patarca R. Cytokines and chronic fatigue syndrome. Ann N Y Acad Sci. 2001;**933**:185–200.

47. Menza M, DeFronzo Dobkin R, Marin H, et al. The role of inflammatory cytokines in cognition and other non-motor symptoms of Parkinsons disease. Psychosomatics. 2010;**51**:474–479.

48. Dowlati Y, Herrmann N, Swardfager W, et al. A meta-analysis of cytokines in major depression. Biol Psychiatry. 2010;**67**:446–457.

49. Christley Y, Duffy T, Everall IP, Martin CR. The neuropsychiatric and neuropsychological features of chronic fatigue syndrome: revisiting the enigma. Curr Psychiatry Rep. 2013;**15**:1–9.

50. Hinkelmann K, Moritz S, Botzenhardt J, et al. Changes in cortisol secretion during antidepressive treatment and cognitive improvement in patients with major depression: A longitudinal study. Psychoneuroendocrinology. 2012;**37**:685–692.

51. Behan L, Phillips J, Thompson C, Agha A. Neuroendocrine disorders after traumatic brain injury, J Neurol Neurosurg Psychiatry. 2008;**79**:753–759.

52. Kelly DF, McArthur DL, Levin H, et al. Neurobehavioral and quality of life changes associated with growth hormone insufficiency after complicated mild, moderate, or severe traumatic brain injury. J Neurotrauma. 2006;**23**:928–942.

53. Agha A, Thompson CJ. High risk of hypogonadism after traumatic brain injury: clinical implications. Pituitary. 2005;**8**:245–249.

54. Knippenberg S, Bol Y, Damoiseaux J, Hupperts R, Smolders J. Vitamin D status in patients with MS is negatively correlated

55. with depression, but not with fatigue. Acta Neurol Scand. 2011;**124**:171–175.
55. Forwell SJ, Brunham S, Tremlett H, Morrison W, Oger J. Primary and nonprimary fatigue in multiple sclerosis. Int J MS Care. 2008;**10**:14–20.
56. Rosenberg JH, Shafor R. Fatigue in multiple sclerosis: a rational approach to evaluation and treatment. Curr Neurol Neurosci Rep. 2005;**5**:140–146.
57. Frohman TC, Castro W, Shah A, et al. Symptomatic therapy in multiple sclerosis. Ther Adv Neurol Disorders. 2011;**4**:83–98.
58. Hadjimichael O, Vollmer T, Oleen-Burkey M. Fatigue characteristics in multiple sclerosis: the North American Research Committee on Multiple Sclerosis NARCOMS. survey. Health Qual Life Outcomes. 2008;**6**:100.
59. Harbison J, Walsh S, Kenny R. Hypertension and daytime hypotension found on ambulatory blood pressure is associated with fatigue following stroke and TIA. Q J Med. 2009;**102**:109–115.
60. Huisinga JM, Filipi ML, Schmid KK, Stergiou N. Is there a relationship between fatigue questionnaires and gait mechanics in persons with multiple sclerosis? Arch Phys Med Rehabil. 2011;**92**:1594–1601.
61. Tzelepis GE, McCool FD, Friedman JH, Hoppin FG. Respiratory muscle dysfunction in Parkinsons disease. Am J Respir Crit Care Med. 1988;**138**:266–271.
62. Friedman JH. Fatigue in Parkinsons disease patients. Curr Treatm Options Neurol. 2009;**11**:186–190.
63. Nybo L. Hyperthermia and fatigue. J Appl Physiol. 2008;**104**:871–878.
64. Flensner G, Ek A, Söderhamn O, Landtblom A. Sensitivity to heat in MS patients: a factor strongly influencing symptomology-an explorative survey. BMC Neurol. 2011;**11**:27.
65. Davis SL, Wilson TE, White AT, Frohman EM. Thermoregulation in multiple sclerosis. J Appl Physiol. 2010;**109**:1531–1537.
66. Carson AJ, Ringbauer B, MacKenzie L, Warlow C, Sharpe M. Neurological disease, emotional disorder, and disability: they are related: a study of 300 consecutive new referrals to a neurology outpatient department. J Neurol Neurosurg Psychiatry. 2000;**68**:202–206.
67. Patrick E, Christodoulou C, Krupp L. Longitudinal correlates of fatigue in multiple sclerosis. Multiple Sclerosis. 2009;**15**:258–261.
68. Ziino C, Ponsford J. Measurement and prediction of subjective fatigue following traumatic brain injury. J Int Neuropsychol Soc. 2005;**11**:416–425.
69. Valko P, Waldvogel D, Weller M, Bassetti C, Held U, Baumann C. Fatigue and excessive daytime sleepiness in idiopathic Parkinsons disease differently correlate with motor symptoms, depression and dopaminergic treatment. Eur J Neurol. 2010;**17**:1428–1436.
70. Ponsford JL, Ziino C, Parcell DL, et al. Fatigue and sleep disturbance following traumatic brain injury—their nature, causes, and potential treatments. J Head Trauma Rehabil. 2012;**27**:224–233.
71. Mills RJ, Young CA. The relationship between fatigue and other clinical features of multiple sclerosis. Multiple Sclerosis J. 2011;**17**:604–612.
72. Kaminska M, Kimoff R, Schwartzman K, Trojan D. Sleep disorders and fatigue in multiple sclerosis: evidence for association and interaction. J Neurol Sci. 2011;**302**:7–13.
73. Hermann DM, Bassetti CL. Sleep-related breathing and sleep-wake disturbances in ischemic stroke. Neurology. 2009;**73**:1313–1322.
74. Diederich NJ, McIntyre DJ. Sleep disorders in Parkinsons disease: Many causes, few therapeutic options. J Neurol Sci. 2012;**314**:12–19.
75. Englander J, Bushnik T, Oggins J, Katznelson L. Fatigue after traumatic brain injury: association with neuroendocrine, sleep, depression and other factors. Brain Injury. 2010;**24**:1379–1388.
76. Naess H, Lunde L, Brogger J, Waje-Andreassen U. Post-stroke pain on long-term follow-up: the Bergen stroke study. J Neurol. 2010;**257**:1446–1452.
77. Mastaglia FL. The relationship between muscle pain and fatigue. Neuromusc Disord. 2012;**22**:S178–180.

78. Finestone HM, Greene-Finestone LS, Wilson ES, Teasell RW. Prolonged length of stay and reduced functional improvement rate in malnourished stroke rehabilitation patients. Arch Phys Med Rehabil. 1996;**77**:340–345.
79. Westergren A. Nutrition and its relation to mealtime preparation, eating, fatigue and mood among stroke survivors after discharge from hospital-a pilot study. Open Nurs J. 2008;**2**:15.
80. Clark LV, White PD. The role of deconditioning and therapeutic exercise in chronic fatigue syndrome CFS). J Mental Health. 2005;**14**:237–252.
81. Nijs J, Aelbrecht S, Meeus M, Van Oosterwijck J, Zinzen E, Clarys P. Tired of being inactive: a systematic literature review of physical activity, physiological exercise capacity and muscle strength in patients with chronic fatigue syndrome. Disabil Rehabil. 2011;**33**:1493–1500.
82. White P, Goldsmith K, Johnson A, et al. Comparison of adaptive pacing therapy, cognitive behaviour therapy, graded exercise therapy, and specialist medical care for chronic fatigue syndrome (PACE): a randomised trial. Lancet. 2011;**377**:823–836.
83. Saunders DH, Greig CA, Young A, Mead GE. Physical fitness training for stroke patients. Stroke. 2004;**35**:2235.
84. Sandroff BM, Sosnoff JJ, Motl RW. Physical fitness, walking performance, and gait in multiple sclerosis. J Neurol Sci. 2013;**328**:70–76.
85. Morris ME, Martin CL, Schenkman ML. Striding out with Parkinson disease: evidence-based physical therapy for gait disorders. Phys Ther. 2010;**90**:280–288.
86. Mossberg KA, Ayala D, Baker T, Heard J, Masel B. Aerobic capacity after traumatic brain injury: comparison with a nondisabled cohort. Arch Phys Med Rehabil. 2007;**88**:315–320.
87. Knoop H, Prins JB, Moss-Morris R, Bleijenberg G. The central role of cognitive processes in the perpetuation of chronic fatigue syndrome. J Psychosom Res. 2010;**68**:489–494.
88. Prins JB, van der Meer JWM, Bleijenberg G. Chronic fatigue syndrome. Lancet. 2006;**367**:346–355.
89. Silver A, Haeney M, Vijayadurai P, Wilks D, Pattrick M, Main C. The role of fear of physical movement and activity in chronic fatigue syndrome. J Psychosom Res. 2002;**52**:485–493.
90. Kos D, Kerckhofs E, Nagels G, D'hooghe M, Ilsbroukx S. Origin of fatigue in multiple sclerosis: review of the literature. Neurorehabil Neural Repair. 2008;**22**:91–100.
91. Skerrett TN, Moss-Morris R. Fatigue and social impairment in multiple sclerosis: the role of patients cognitive and behavioral responses to their symptoms. J Psychosom Res. 2006;**61**:587–593.
92. Lukkahatai N, Saligan LN. Association of catastrophizing and fatigue: A systematic review. J Psychosom Res. 2013;**74**:100–109.
93. Robison J, Wiles R, Ellis-Hill C, McPherson K, Hyndman D, Ashburn A. Resuming previously valued activities post-stroke: who or what helps? Disabil Rehabil. 2009;**31**:1555–1566.
94. Kato K, Sullivan PF, Evengard B, Pedersen NL. Premorbid predictors of chronic fatigue. Arch Gen Psychiatry. 2006;**63**:1267–1272.
95. Hatcher S, House A. Life events, difficulties and dilemmas in the onset of chronic fatigue syndrome: a case-control study. Psychol Med. 2003;**33**:1185–1192.
96. Merkelbach S, König J, Sittinger H. Personality traits in multiple sclerosis MS. patients with and without fatigue experience. Acta Neurol Scand. 2003;**107**:195–201.
97. Shun SC, Hsiao FH, Lai YH, Liang JT, Yeh KH, Huang J. Personality trait and quality of life in colorectal cancer survivors. Oncology Nursing Forum. 2011. **38**:E211–218.
98. Trojan DA, Arnold D, Collet J, et al. Fatigue in multiple sclerosis: association with disease-related, behavioural and psychosocial factors. Multiple Sclerosis. 2007;**13**:985–995.
99. Lerdal A, Bakken LN, Kouwenhoven SE, et al. Poststroke fatigue: A review. J Pain Symptom Manage. 2009;**38**:928–949.
100. Metz L, Patten S, Archibald C, et al. The effect of immunomodulatory treatment on multiple sclerosis fatigue. J Neurol Neurosurg Psychiatry. 2004;**75**:1045–1047.

101. Yildiz M, Tettenborn B, Putzki N. Multiple sclerosis-associated fatigue during disease-modifying treatment with natalizumab, interferon-beta and glatiramer acetate. Eur Neurol. 2011;**65**:231–232.

102. Pinter M, Pogarell O, Oertel W. Efficacy, safety, and tolerance of the non-ergoline dopamine agonist pramipexole in the treatment of advanced Parkinsons disease: a double blind, placebo controlled, randomised, multicentre study. J Neurol Neurosurg Psychiatry. 1999;**66**:436–441.

103. Friedman JH. Fatigue: a common comorbidity in Parkinsons disease. In: Pfeiffer RF, Bodis-Wollner I (eds) Parkinsons Disease and Nonmotor Dysfunction. Springer, New York, 2013, pp. 391–400.

104. Ouellet M, Morin CM. Efficacy of cognitive-behavioral therapy for insomnia associated with traumatic brain injury: a single-case experimental design. Arch Phys Med Rehabil. 2007;**88**:1581–1592.

105. Baron KG, Corden M, Jin L, Mohr DC. Impact of psychotherapy on insomnia symptoms in patients with depression and multiple sclerosis. J Behav Med. 2011;**34**:92–101.

106. Aurora RN, Kristo DA, Bista SR, et al. The treatment of restless legs syndrome and periodic limb movement disorder in adults—an update for 2012: practice parameters with an evidence-based systematic review and meta-analyses: an American Academy of Sleep Medicine clinical practice guideline. Sleep. 2012;**35**:1039–1062.

107. Lee S, Kim J, Song I, An J, Kim Y, Lee K. Poststroke restless legs syndrome and lesion location: anatomical considerations. Movement Disorders. 2009;**24**:77–84.

108. Mayer G, Jennum P, Riemann D, Dauvilliers Y. Insomnia in central neurologic diseases: Occurrence and management. Sleep Med Rev. 2011;**15**:369–378.

109. Tanaka M, Mizuno K, Fukuda S, Shigihara Y, Watanabe Y. Relationships between dietary habits and the prevalence of fatigue in medical students. Nutrition. 2008;**24**:985–989.

110. Weinstock-Guttman B, Baier M, Park Y, Feichter J, et al. Low fat dietary intervention with omega-3 fatty acid supplementation in multiple sclerosis patients, Prostaglandins. leukotrienes and essential fatty acids. 2005;**73**:397–404.

111. Kampman MT, Steffensen LH, Mellgren SI, Jørgensen L. Effect of vitamin D3 supplementation on relapses, disease progression, and measures of function in persons with multiple sclerosis: exploratory outcomes from a double-blind randomised controlled trial. Multiple Sclerosis J. 2012;**18**:1144–1151.

112. Torkildsen O, Wergeland S, Bakke S, et al. Omega-3 Fatty Acid Treatment in Multiple Sclerosis (OFAMS Study): a randomized, double-blind, placebo-controlled trial. Arch Neurol Archneurol. 201269:1044–1051.

113. Malaguarnera M, Gargante MP, Cristaldi E, et al. Acetyl L-carnitine ALC. treatment in elderly patients with fatigue. Arch Gerontol Geriatr. 2008;**46**:181–190.

114. Vermeulen RC, Scholte HR. Exploratory open label, randomized study of acetyl- and propionylcarnitine in chronic fatigue syndrome. Psychosom Med. 2004;**66**:276–282.

115. Tejani AM, Wasdell M, Spiwak R, Rowell G, Nathwani S. Carnitine for fatigue in multiple sclerosis. Cochrane Database Syst Rev. 2012;**5** Art. No.: CD007280. DOI: 10.1002/14651858.CD007280.pub3.

116. White A, Wilson T, Davis S, Petajan J. Effect of precooling on physical performance in multiple sclerosis. Multiple Sclerosis. 2000;**6**:176–180.

117. Amato MP, Portaccio E. Management options in multiple sclerosis-associated fatigue. Expert Opin Pharmacother. 2012;**13**:207–216.

118. Morrow GR, Shelke AR, Roscoe JA, Hickok JT, Mustian K. Management of cancer-related fatigue. Cancer Invest. 2005;**23**:229–239.

119. Choi-Kwon S, Choi J, Kwon SU, Kang D, Kim JS. Fluoxetine is not effective in the treatment of poststroke fatigue: a double-blind, placebo-controlled study. Cerebrovasc Dis. 2006;**23**:103–108.

120. Mock V, Frangakis C, Davidson NE, et al. Exercise manages fatigue during breast cancer treatment: a randomized controlled trial. Psycho-Oncology. 2005;**14**:464–477.

121. Dimeo FC, Thomas F, Raabe-Menssen C, Pröpper F, Mathias M. Effect of aerobic exercise and relaxation training on fatigue and physical performance of cancer patients after surgery. A randomised controlled trial. Supportive Care in Cancer. 2004;**12**:774–779.

122. Kohman RA, Rodriguez-Zas SL, Southey BR, Kelley KW, Dantzer R, Rhodes JS. Voluntary wheel running reverses age-induced changes in hippocampal gene expression. PloS One. 2011;**6**:e22654.

123. Andreasen A, Stenager E, Dalgas U. The effect of exercise therapy on fatigue in multiple sclerosis. Multiple Sclerosis J. 2011;**17**:1041–1054.

124. Van Cauwenbergh D, De Kooning M, Ickmans K, Nijs J. How to exercise people with chronic fatigue syndrome: evidence-based practice guidelines. Eur J Clin Invest. 2012;**42**:1136–1144.

125. Castell BD, Kazantzis N, Moss-Morris RE. Cognitive behavioral therapy and graded exercise for chronic fatigue syndrome: a meta-analysis. Clin Psychol Sci Pract. 2011;**18**:311–324.

126. Smith C, Wessely S. Unity of opposites? Chronic fatigue syndrome and the challenge of divergent perspectives in guideline development. J Neurol Neurosurg Psychiatry. 2012;doi:10.1136/jnnp-2012-303208.

127. Brazzelli M, Saunders D, Greig C, Mead G. Physical fitness training for stroke patients. Cochrane Database of Systematic Reviews 2011;CD003316.

128. Duncan F, Kutlubaev MA, Dennis MS, Greig C, Mead GE. Fatigue after stroke: a systematic review of associations with impaired physical fitness. Int J Stroke. 2012;**7**:157–162.

129. Zedlitz AM, Rietveld TC, Geurts AC, Fasotti L. Cognitive and graded activity training can alleviate persistent fatigue after stroke a randomized, controlled trial. Stroke. 2012;**43**:1046–1051.

130. Elbers R, van Wegen EE, Rochester L, et al. Is impact of fatigue an independent factor associated with physical activity in patients with idiopathic Parkinsons disease? Movement Disorders. 2009;**24**:1512–1518.

131. Winward C, Sackley C, Meek C, et al. Weekly exercise does not improve fatigue levels in Parkinsons disease. Movement Disorders. 2012;**27**:143–146.

132. Canning CG, Allen NE, Dean CM, Goh L, Fung VS. Home-based treadmill training for individuals with Parkinsons disease: a randomized controlled pilot trial. Clin Rehabil. 2012;**26**:817–826.

133. Hassett L, Moseley A, Tate R, Harmer A. Fitness training for cardiorespiratory conditioning after traumatic brain injury. Cochrane Database of Systematic Reviews 2008;CD006123.

134. Blikman LJ, Huisstede B, Kooijmans H, Stam HJ, Bussmann JB, van Meeteren J. Effectiveness of energy-conservation treatment in reducing fatigue in Multiple Sclerosis: a systematic review and meta-analysis. Arch Phys Med Rehabil. 2013;**94**:1360–1376.

135. Clarke A, Barker-Collo SL, Feigin VL. Poststroke fatigue: does group education make a difference? A randomized pilot trial. Top Stroke Rehabil. 2012;**19**:32–39.

136. van Kessel K, Moss-Morris R, Willoughby E, Chalder T, Johnson MH, Robinson E. A randomized controlled trial of cognitive behavior therapy for multiple sclerosis fatigue. Psychosom Med. 2008;**70**:205–213.

137. Knoop H, van Kessel K, Moss-Morris R. Which cognitions and behaviours mediate the positive effect of cognitive behavioural therapy on fatigue in patients with multiple sclerosis? Psychol Med. 2012;**42**:205.

138. Moss-Morris R, McCrone P, Yardley L, van Kessel K, Wills G, Dennison L. A pilot randomised controlled trial of an Internet-based cognitive behavioural therapy self-management programme MS Invigor8 for multiple sclerosis fatigue. Behav Res Ther. 2012;**42**:205–213.

139. Grossman P, Kappos L, Gensicke H, et al. MS quality of life, depression, and fatigue improve after mindfulness training. A randomized trial. Neurology. 2010;**75**:1141–1149.

140. Hofer H, Holtforth MG, Lüthy F, Frischknecht E, Znoj H, Müri RM. The potential of a mindfulness-enhanced, integrative neuro-psychotherapy program for treating fatigue following stroke: a preliminary study. Mindfulness. 2012;1–8.

141. Khan F, Turner-Stokes L, Ng L, Kilpatrick T, Amatya B. Multidisciplinary rehabilitation for adults with multiple sclerosis. Cochrane Database Syst Rev. 2011;CD006036. DOI: 10.1002/14651858.CD006036.pub2.

142. Vos-Vromans DC, Smeets RJ, Rijnders LJ, et al. Cognitive behavioural therapy versus multidisciplinary rehabilitation treatment for patients with chronic fatigue syndrome: study protocol for a randomised controlled trial (FatiGo). Trials. 2012;**13**:71.

143. Ravnborg M. Rehabilitation therapy in MS; a short-term, expensive, placebo. Multiple Sclerosis J. 2012;**18**:1377–1378.

144. Pucci E, Branãs P, D'Amico R, Giuliani G, Solari A, Taus C. Amantadine for fatigue in multiple sclerosis Cochrane Database Syst Rev. 2009;DOI:0.1002/14651858. CD002818.pub2

145. Lange R, Volkmer M, Heesen C, Liepert J. Modafinil effects in multiple sclerosis patients with fatigue. J Neurol. 2009;**256**:645–650.

146. Möller F, Poettgen J, Broemel F, Neuhaus A, Daumer M, Heesen C. HAGIL (Hamburg Vigil Study): a randomized placebo-controlled double-blind study with modafinil for treatment of fatigue in patients with multiple sclerosis. Multiple Sclerosis J. 2011;**17**:1002–1009.

147. Stankoff B, Waubant E, Confavreux C, et al. Modafinil for fatigue in MS A randomized placebo-controlled double-blind study. Neurology. 2005;**64**:1139–1143.

148. Brioschi A, Gramigna S, Werth E, et al. Effect of modafinil on subjective fatigue in multiple sclerosis and stroke patients. Eur Neurol. 2009;**62**:243–249.

149. Seppi K, Weintraub D, Coelho M, et al. The Movement Disorder Society Evidence-Based Medicine Review Update: Treatments for the non-motor symptoms of Parkinsons disease. Movement Disorders. 2011;**26**:S42–80.

150. Jha A, Weintraub A, Allshouse A, et al. A randomized trial of modafinil for the treatment of fatigue and excessive daytime sleepiness in individuals with chronic traumatic brain injury. J Head Trauma Rehabil. 2008;**23**:52–63.

151. Gillson G, Richards T, Smith R, Wright J. A double-blind pilot study of the effect of Prokarin™ on fatigue in multiple sclerosis. Multiple Sclerosis. 2002;**8**:30–35.

152. Mendonça DA, Menezes K, Jog MS. Methylphenidate improves fatigue scores in Parkinson disease: a randomized controlled trial. Movement Disorders. 2007;**22**:2070–2076.

153. Wingerchuk D, Benarroch E, O'Brien P, et al. A randomized controlled crossover trial of aspirin for fatigue in multiple sclerosis. Neurology. 2005;**64**:1267–1269.

154. The Scottish Government. Scottish Good Practice Statement on ME-CFS: Quick Reference Clinical Guide Scottish Government, Edinburgh, 2010.

CHAPTER 27

Neuropalliative rehabilitation—managing neurological disability in the context of a deteriorating illness

Gail Eva, Jo Bayly, and Diane Playford

Introduction: the relevance of rehabilitation in palliative care

On the face of it, the concepts of rehabilitation and palliative care may seem paradoxical. Rehabilitation is generally viewed as future-directed and goal-oriented, aiming to increase function and social participation. Palliative care, on the other hand, is seen to deal in loss—of independence, of social roles, and, ultimately, of a future. There is, however, strong alignment between the objectives of rehabilitation, and those of palliative care. According to Wade and de Jong [1], rehabilitation is a process of assessment and goal-setting, with interventions directed towards maximizing well-being and participation in order to achieve adaptation to disability and to minimize carer stress. The World Health Organization [2] defines palliative care as an approach that improves quality of life of patients and their families through assessment and treatment of physical, psychosocial and spiritual problems. Dame Cicely Saunders, a pioneer of the hospice movement in the United Kingdom, describes it thus: [palliative care will] 'not only help you to die peacefully, but also to live until you die' [3: p. xxiii].

In both rehabilitation and palliative care, the importance of a holistic approach is emphasized, that is, one which attends to physical, psychological, and social dimensions. Palliative rehabilitation enables people to be as active and independent as possible within the constraints of a deteriorating illness, taking a realistic approach to patient goals. It supports adaptation to disability and coming to terms with changed circumstances, striving to respond rapidly to changes in abilities, goals, and needs. It uses the expertise of a multidisciplinary team with effective coordination of care to ensure consistency in approach. It is accepting of uncertainty and loss, anticipating deterioration and allowing time for relevant issues to be addressed with patients and those close to them [4].

In short, it is a coordinated, team effort aimed at enabling people to participate to as full an extent as possible in all aspects of their daily lives. Crucially, this is as much about a patient's psychological resources as it is about their physical capacity.

Taking account of what patients say is important to them towards the end of life, it is evident that that palliative rehabilitation has a great deal to offer. A number of research studies [5–8] show that patients want their symptoms to be well managed, their care to be well coordinated, and to avoid the inappropriate prolongation of dying. They wish to be able to maintain a sense of control, achievement, and self-worth, and to relieve the burden upon others. Strengthening relationships with loved ones is particularly important, as is the opportunity to say goodbye and bring closure. Rehabilitation makes an important contribution in all of these domains. According to the National Council for Palliative Care [9], palliative rehabilitation provides strategies and support to help people to adapt to illness and disability, and to be able to acknowledge approaching death. It enables people to perceive some control in their lives, and to maintain a sense of self as worthwhile and competent. It opens up possibilities for pleasurable activities and provides the means to be engaged in these.

Palliative care has its origins in the care of cancer patients, and while many of the principles of good palliative care are relevant to any illness, there are differences between the needs of people with cancer and those with neurological conditions [10]. Disease trajectories in neurological conditions are less predictable with a longer time-course. They are characterized by periods of relapse and remission rather than steady decline. Patients may have multiple disabilities with cognitive, behavioural and communication problems in addition to physical deficits [11, 12]. A further, important consideration is that people with long-term neurological conditions, such as multiple sclerosis (MS) or Parkinson's disease, are likely to have extensive experience of managing life with a disability [13]. This expertise must be recognized and respected, and incorporated into all aspects of care and rehabilitation [14, 15].

The delivery of neuropalliative rehabilitation

While there is an increasing recognition of the need for palliative care provision for people with deteriorating, life-limiting neurological conditions, there is very little in the way of clinical guidelines or research that specifically addresses the provision and structure of neuropalliative rehabilitation. In palliative cancer care, four categories of rehabilitation have proved useful and could provide a framework in neurology: preventative, restorative, supportive, palliative, as set out in Table 27.1 [16].

It is important to recognize that patients do not fit into neat categories, and that several approaches will be appropriate simultaneously. For example, preventative, supportive, and palliative rehabilitation could be used to help a person with late-stage MS to manage fatigue: education on pacing and gentle exercise, supportive strategies to set and achieve reasonable, desirable goals, underpinned by the recognition that the patient's priorities will be shaped by their understanding of their prognosis.

It is not uncommon to find palliative care used as a synonym for end-of-life care, with the implication that palliative care is only appropriate when the end stages of illness are reached. In fact, the opposite is true, and the World Health Organization [2] emphasizes the importance of its implementation early on in the disease trajectory. Living with a deteriorating condition frequently entails managing significant disability, and early rehabilitation can prevent deconditioning as well as help people to understand and cope with the fact that they are not going to return to their previous level of function.

Patients report palliative care needs from diagnosis. In a study of stroke patients newly admitted to hospital, Burton et al. [17] found that 66% had concerns about dependence and disability, around 50% reported fatigue, pain, anxiety, and concerns about family, while 25% were worried about death and dying. A palliative approach at this stage can be valuable in giving patients the opportunity to ask difficult questions about their prognosis, to express and discuss their fears, and to acknowledge the difficulty of living with an uncertain, unpredictable future.

This support needs to be available within the context of whatever services are most appropriate for the patient's circumstances at the time, and specialist teams will need to work closely together to make sure that it is provided. Patients with long-term neurological conditions (LTNCs), characterized by extended periods of stable disability, will need preventative and restorative rehabilitation

from neurology experts just as much as they need supportive and palliative approaches. Sykes [18] cautions against patients being corralled into specialist palliative care services because generalist clinicians are not confident enough to raise end-of-life issues. The problem for service providers is that it is not a question of 'either restorative or palliative rehabilitation', it is a case of 'both ... and', and running these two seemingly incongruous approaches alongside each other is not straightforward. In the following sections we discuss the coordination of care between services, and the 'living with dying' paradox that neuropalliative rehabilitation needs to embrace.

Service delivery and teamwork

Delivering services for people with LTNCs requires collaboration between three specialties: neurology, palliative care, and rehabilitation. Turner-Stokes and colleagues [11] provide guidance about how this interdisciplinary working can be achieved and managed, setting out the conditions under which people with LTNCs should be referred to each of the specialties. Anyone with a suspected LTNC should be seen by a specialist neurological service for investigation and diagnosis, and, where an LTNC is confirmed, for on-going management including disease-modifying treatment and advice on self-management. Rehabilitation services will be required where a person develops significant disability that impacts on their independence or their ability to participate in their current environment. Where a person has a limited lifespan, distressing symptoms such as pain, fatigue, and breathlessness, and when they need help with end-of-life care-planning, access to palliative care services will be required.

Co-ordinating care across specialties is tricky, and there are a number of barriers to be aware of—and to overcome [18, 19]. Neurological and rehabilitation services might be reluctant to refer to palliative care if they perceive these services to be predominantly concerned with the needs of cancer patients. As previously noted, the longer-term, less predictable course of LTNCs might not fit well with usual palliative care service configuration, which is characterized by concentrated efforts over short periods [20]. However, if palliative care services do not routinely receive referrals for patients with LTNCs, opportunities to develop properly resourced and skilled services—including appropriate rehabilitation—are limited.

Rehabilitation is delivered by multidisciplinary teams, and as we have seen, there are likely to be several teams involved. The provision of skilled, appropriate, and timely rehabilitation therefore depends on good teamwork both within and across teams. With several professional groups contributing to a rehabilitation plan, there is a need to be clear about role overlap and role boundaries. Different professions contribute in unique but complementary ways to patient care: each has a particular perspective delivering a service—different things that are observed, different narratives of health and illness, different ways of responding to problems. Blurring professional roles and sharing expertise can result in creative and effective solutions to problems, but it can also be a source of misunderstanding, confusion, tension and rivalry [4]. To maximize the former and avoid the latter, it is useful to ensure clarity about four particular aspects: first, identifying who needs to be involved (including the patient and family) and establishing mechanisms for good communication; second, ensuring that

Table 27.1 Categories of rehabilitation in palliative care

Preventative	Information and education focused, aiming to reduce the impact and severity of potential disabilities.
Restorative	Provided in anticipation of patients returning to their pre-illness level of function without long-term effects. It is delivered in both acute and longer-term phases, across in-patient and domiciliary settings as patients return to valued roles.
Supportive	Accepts that improvement is unlikely and supports patients and their families to identify and maximize their physical, functional, psychological, and social resources. The focus is on adaptation to changed circumstance rather than restoration.
Palliative	Aims to limit the impact of advancing disease and acknowledges the reality of dying, helping patients and families to adjust to this. Symptom management, comfort, and opportunities for social interaction with close family and friends become paramount.

the primary objectives to be achieved are understood by everyone, and the plan of action is agreed; third, setting out the contribution of each individual to achieving the objectives, that is identifying which member of the team has the expertise to deal with which particular problem; and finally, agreeing the process that will be used for review and revision.

The paradox: affirming life, preparing for death

We have seen that the aim of palliative rehabilitation is to help people to live as actively as they can, making the most of the abilities and resources available to them, while at the same time acknowledging death and enabling people to do the things they need and wish to do in order to put their lives in order. In a study of occupational therapists' approaches to working with people with life-limiting illness, Bye [21: p. 9] quotes a respondent's description that perfectly illustrates the balancing process this requires:

> One minute you seem to be helping them to fight death off and another moment you are helping them to accept death . . . You are putting things in place to say go ahead, live, get on, get going, and at the same time you are saying to them, well no you can't do this, you really have to appreciate that fact now . . . You are doing it all at the same time. You are saying get up, get going, and slow up and accept death all at once, which is really contrasting.

Although these two orientations are in tension, they are not mutually exclusive; both need to be central to the provision of neuropalliative rehabilitation.

Content of neuropalliative rehabilitation

Neuropalliative rehabilitation follows the same process that would be used in other conditions. As shown in Figure 27.1, there is an iterative, cyclical process of assessment, problem identification, goal setting, interventions (either implementing these directly or signposting elsewhere), review, and discharge [4, 9, 13].

This generic process needs to be underpinned by specific palliative care skills which include a number of elements. Working in the context of a rapidly changing condition requires a flexible, responsive approach to planning. Families and carers are as central to the

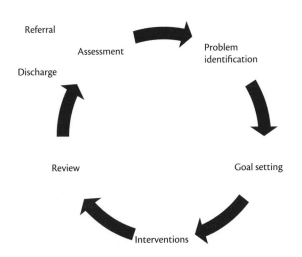

Fig. 27.1 Neuropalliative rehabilitation process.

process as patients, and it is important that they receive adequate and appropriate support. Health professionals need to understand that while deterioration is inevitable, the extent to which patients wish to acknowledge this will vary, and rehabilitation will need to be paced to take account of this. Patients and their families will be seeking information, and it can be challenging to provide this in the context of uncertainty. Effective communication depends on health professionals being comfortable discussing dying and the existential concerns that patients have.

Assessment strategies in neuropalliative rehabilitation

Assessment in neuropalliative rehabilitation requires a holistic, biopsychosocial approach, taking account of how the disease and treatment affects the person physically, functionally, psychologically and socially. The domains that should be assessed are set out in Table 27.2.

Assessment can be carried out through low key observation and conversational approaches, or via structured, standardized assessment tools, or a mixture of both. Many palliative rehabilitation clinicians favour a low-key approach, which has the advantage that patients are not put through rigorous, formal functional assessments that further deplete limited energy supplies, and may quickly be out of date as the disease progresses [21]. There is also a notion that standardized assessments with checklists are a barrier to developing relationships with patients, and that they are not sufficiently individualized and patient-focused. While relationship-building and patient-centredness are important in the assessment process, there is evidence to suggest that patients' concerns are more reliably through systematic, structured assessment. Homsi and colleagues [22] studied 200 patients consecutively referred to a palliative medicine programme, and compared open-ended questions with a 48-item symptom checklist. The median number of symptoms found using systematic assessment was ten-fold higher than those volunteered through open questioning.

The assessment process has to balance the need for a sufficiently detailed analysis of patients' problems such that a treatment plan can be formulated, with patients' fatigue and stamina as well as the potential for the process to reinforce the patient's sense of their limitations. The purpose of the assessment should be apparent both to the clinician and to the patient, with clear explanations of what is being done, why, and how it will contribute to the management plan. Assessment should be relevant to the activities a person will be carrying out—there is little purpose in assessing independence in dressing when this is not something a person needs or wishes to do without help. Similarly, it is helpful to include carers and family members in assessments where appropriate and possible—for example, a shower assessment together with the carer who will be helping the patient with the activity. In the later stages of illness, it is likely that the focus of assessment will shift from the patient to the carer's abilities and the environment of care.

Measuring outcomes

In addition to informing patients' care plans, information collected in the course of the assessment process can be used to measure the outcomes of neuropalliative rehabilitation. Measuring outcomes can help to demonstrate that the interventions provided are effective. It can also guide the development of services, monitor the

Table 27.2 Assessment in neuropalliative rehabilitation

Mobility	Ability to walk or to mobilize in a wheelchair.
Activities of daily living	The impact of illness on carrying out daily occupations—activities that are necessary as well as those which are desired.
Symptoms	For example, fatigue and energy levels, muscle weakness, spasticity, pain, respiratory problems, neuromuscular function, mood, cognitive function.
Living space	The physical and social environment in which the patient lives or will be living.
Communication	Speech and communication difficulties.
Nutrition	Eating and nutrition.
Resources	The personal strengths and resources that the patient has available, as well as those afforded by families, carers, communities, and the environment.
Relationships	The patient's relationship with those who are or will be providing care, looking in particular at how this affects the way in which he or she is allowed or enabled to function by others.
Prognosis	The likely future course of the illness, taking account of the potential for improving or maintaining function and quality of life, and of the patient's a view of the future.
Orientation to rehabilitation	The patient's perception of the need for and willingness to engage with rehabilitation.

impact of service developments and changes to practice, and show patients and their families that they are making progress [23, 24]. Outcome domains relevant to palliative rehabilitation include participation, goal attainment, self-efficacy, physical function, management of specific symptoms (notably pain, fatigue, and breathlessness), acceptance, and quality of life.

Measuring the outcomes of palliative rehabilitation can be challenging. Rehabilitation is often one component of a range of interventions provided by a multiprofessional team and it can be difficult to separate out the specific contribution of the rehabilitation element; many rehabilitation outcome measures anticipate that functional gains will be made, which is often not the case in palliative care where patients are deteriorating. Murtagh and colleagues [10: p. 43] point out that in palliative care, a successful outcome is not successful treatment of disease, but the ability, ultimately, to enable a 'good' death—that is, one that is free from distressing symptoms with psychosocial and spiritual needs addressed.

Goal setting

Goal setting is a core component of rehabilitation. It is a process of negotiation and discussion where a patient and health professional(s) decide on what the patient wants to achieve, and agree how they will work together to accomplish these things within a specified time frame. Patients need to be involved in the goal-setting process to ensure that goals are meaningful and relevant to them [25]. Goal setting provides a structure for the assessment process, for planning interventions, for review, and for measuring outcomes. It is particularly relevant in neuropalliative

rehabilitation, where working towards meaningful goals can provide patients with a sense of progress, self-sufficiency, and control. In context of deterioration and uncertainty, goals that foster insight and understanding can be just as important as those that are aimed at functional improvement [4].

To help patients to think about their goals, the following sorts of questions can be useful. 'What are the things in life that are important to you?' 'What would like to be able to do? Are there things that *need* to be able to do? Are these different to the things you *want* to do?' 'What do you feel you want to be able to do on your own, and what are you comfortable having some help with?' The answers to these questions need to be weighed against the patient's physical, psychological, and social resources, as well as how they fit with family and organizational priorities. Tension can arise when—for example—a patient's stated desire to remain at home conflicts with an elderly spouse's abilities to provide care in a locality where professional carers are a scarce resource.

As well as listening carefully to the content of patients' stories about what matters to them, we also need to attend to what the person is telling us indirectly about who they are and what makes life meaningful for them. A patient with very limited mobility might say, 'I used to be able to go for long walks in the country and I'd like to be able to do that again'. Rather than dismiss this as impossible and unrealistic, we can discuss with the patient what they enjoyed about the activity—perhaps the pleasure of exploration, being with other people with similar interests, and a sense of themselves as an active, outdoor kind of person. Understanding what the activity represents to the patient can make it possible to identify alternatives that could achieve the same things—a wheelchair-accessible trail, perhaps, or a picnic in the countryside.

It can be helpful to talk through some of the assumptions that patients make about what is possible and not possible, and what it is essential to do every day. Having some help with routine tasks, for example, can mean that a person has more energy available to do something that is pleasurable rather than necessary.

There is an important distinction to be made between *hopes* and *goals* [26]. A goal is clear and specific; it is something that a person has control over, and can work toward achieving. A hope, by contrast, is an indication of something that a person would like, that they do not have complete control over: 'I hope the weather will be good for our picnic next week', or 'I'm looking forward to by nephew's wedding in September'. Hopes can help to maintain optimism and a view of oneself as engaged in activities and events, even as these become more and more difficult.

Rehabilitation staff can be concerned about being seen to support patients' aspirations when they feel these are unrealistic. While it is neither helpful nor appropriate to be falsely encouraging—'Yes of course you will get better!' when recovery is not anticipated—it is also not necessary to undermine the strategies that patients use to maintain a sense of themselves as competent, worthwhile individuals. Normal human perception and behaviour is characterized by a tendency towards 'positive illusions': mild distortions of reality in which we hold unrealistically positive views of the self, exaggerate perceptions of personal control, and are unrealistically optimistic [27–29]. Moreover, these positive illusions appear to have protective psychological effects, which contribute significantly to a person's ability to adjust to severely threatening events.

Taylor [27] contends that adjustment to illness centres around three themes: a search for meaning in the experience, an attempt to regain mastery over the event in particular and over life in general, and an effort to enhance self-esteem. Patients might plan to travel abroad, or have ideas about manufacturing their own aids and adaptations, or resuming previously enjoyed hobbies, or they might look forward to being able to walk again. Research with people with metastatic spinal cord compression has shown that while patients take steps towards achieving these things, they also avoid situations in which their abilities could be directly challenged [30]. In this regard, patients' orientation to disability incorporates two apparently inconsistent attitudes (see Figure 27.2). On one hand, there is an acknowledgement that something significant has changed and that, as a consequence, functional boundaries and limitations will need to be explored, new self-management skills learned, and useful information sought. On the other hand, patients avoid acknowledging problems, determined to hold on to a sense of themselves as competent, resourceful human beings. These two orientations are in conflict, and patients look for ways to manage this tension by revising their expectations (changing the goalposts), indefinitely deferring anticipated pleasures, and by avoiding situations in which their abilities might be put to the test. Patients 'twin-track'—running their acknowledgement of changed circumstances alongside a view of themselves as capable. This overly-optimistic view of self and of future events does not necessarily prevent them from making sensible, practical plans for the present, and it can help to support self-esteem and a sense that life is worth living.

Maximizing function, mobility, and independence

In the context of a deteriorating condition, responding to the patient's desire for independence needs some careful thought. It can be helpful to focus on activity and participation as a means to foster an independence of spirit rather than to achieve the mastery of particular tasks. Cardol et al. [31: p. 1002] propose that 'the most valuable outcomes of rehabilitation are . . . possibilities or 'feasibilities' rather than specific achievements. Enabling a disabled person to be as independent as possible within the

limitations imposed by impairment, and to exercise autonomy in everyday life, form the bedrock of rehabilitation practice'. Recognizing that a person's impairments may rule out independence in the sense of performing an activity entirely on one's own, we can make a distinction between physically doing the activity oneself—'executional autonomy'—and being able to control the manner in which the activity is performed—'decisional autonomy' [32]. In other words, a person might not be able to put on a shirt without help, but they can exercise control over their environment through choosing what they wish to wear and instructing the helper about the way the task should be done. In palliative care rehabilitation, where the potential for improving a patient's executional autonomy is limited by advancing disease, this notion has particular relevance.

Modifying the environment and providing aids, equipment and adaptations can be enormously helpful in enabling people to continue to manage their desired activities. A wheelchair and a ramp can make the difference between being housebound, and getting out to the local shops. An adjustable-height hospital bed and a hoist in a downstairs room can make it possible for someone who can no longer transfer independently to continue to live at home. There are, however, a couple of considerations when providing large items of equipment. It is important to pay attention to the patient's physical environment and to the consequences of turning a home into what can feel like a mini hospital. There is also the issue that decisions about providing about expensive permanent or semi-permanent adaptations can be difficult to make when a prognosis is uncertain, when resources are limited, and when it is not clear how much use the person will be able to make of it. Openness, honesty, and good communication skills are required, as is being clear with patients about the alternatives and the advantages and drawbacks. Discussions with colleagues in the multiprofessional team can be invaluable in helping to make these decisions.

Rehabilitation approaches to the management of common symptoms

There are a number of symptoms that can aggravate the disability resulting from a neurological condition and impact on patients'

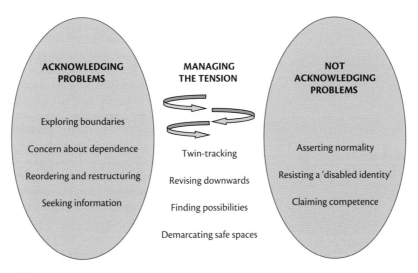

Fig. 27.2 Patients' response to disability.
Eva G, Paley J, Miller M, Wee B, Palliative Medicine (23), pp. 132–140, copyright © 2009 Reprinted by Permission of SAGE.

ability to participate in rehabilitation as well as to manage their daily activities. Rehabilitation approaches can contribute to their management. These are appropriate throughout a patient's disease trajectory, but careful attention to symptom management is particularly important around the initial diagnosis and at times of disease progression or following acute events.

Muscle weakness and deconditioning

Patients should be encouraged to remain physically active to minimize the onset of neuromuscular deconditioning. Low-intensity active exercises and movement therapies targeting large muscle groups may help maintain muscle power and exercise tolerance. While research into the potential benefits of exercise in advanced disease is limited, studies show that patients are willing to participate and do not appear to experience harm [33, 34]. Where independent low-intensity active exercise is not achievable due to the severity and nature of movement disorders, family members can be taught how to do active assisted and passive movements.

Equipment (such as a raised perching stool for kitchen activities, or a seat and rails in a bath or shower), mobility aids (for example, a walking frame), small aids (long-handled reachers and bottle openers, etc.), and adaptations (like a ramp in place of steps) can assist people to maintain their independence. However, as we discussed earlier, these should be introduced sensitively, attending to any psychological distress resulting from loss of independence, and understanding the significance and meaning to the person of increasing dependency. This is especially relevant for people diagnosed with rapidly progressive disease who may have had little time to adjust to the change in their function.

Breathlessness

Breathlessness is a multidimensional symptom incorporating physical, psychological, social, and environmental factors. It is responsive to non-pharmacological interventions delivered by a multiprofessional team [35]. Once potentially reversible causes have been excluded, rehabilitation interventions focus on directly or indirectly relieving the experience of breathlessness. Techniques that can be used to manage breathlessness are set out in Table 27.3.

Table 27.3 Techniques to alleviate the experience of breathlessness

Learning to use breathing techniques
Hand-held fan
Positioning and movement techniques
Exercise and physical activity
Learning to prioritize and pace activities
Mobility aids
Aids and adaptations to assist with daily activities
Modifying perceptions and negative beliefs
Acupressure/acupuncture
Non-invasive intermittent ventilation
Anxiety management
Distraction
Support for carers

Simon et al. [36] have identified five different patterns of episodic breathlessness in patients with advanced disease, examining the presence or absence of triggers, the predictability of the response, and the severity of the attack. Understanding the type of breathlessness can help clinicians to tailor specific management strategies.

Non-pharmacological breathlessness management services are increasingly being offered by specialist palliative care services and hospices. Interventions should be introduced early in anticipation of worsening breathlessness while the patient and carer have the motivation, physical and cognitive ability to integrate the strategies into daily routines. For patients with nocturnal hypoventilation and respiratory failure, referral to a ventilation service for non-invasive intermittent ventilation may improve sleep quality and daytime breathlessness [37, 38].

Fatigue

Like breathlessness, fatigue is a multifaceted symptom. Physical activity and exercise are the mainstays of rehabilitation management, combined with strategies to help patients to plan and pace their activities, cognitive therapy, treatment of underlying depression, and attention to risk factors such as poor nutrition and inactivity [39]. Teaching patients how to adapt movement patterns and postures can be helpful, such as sitting rather than standing to do a task. Energy conservation techniques equip patients and their carers with the skills to choose and balance desired activities or exercise with periods of recovery and rest. These strategies might be counterintuitive for patients whose past experience of healthy tiredness has taught them that rest is an effective remedy. Carers too can feel that they are being kind and supportive by encouraging the patient to be less active, without realising the adverse effects of deconditioning. Patients, carers, and other health professionals may need educating to understand that fatigue in the context of illness is different to ordinary tiredness, and that it needs to be actively managed.

Cough

In neuromuscular disease, varying restrictive lung disease patterns will develop according to the rate of disease progression and patterns of muscular weakness. In the palliative phase, alongside possible difficulties in swallowing and the presence of drooling, these can lead to recurrent chest infections, ineffective cough, and respiratory failure. It is important therefore that interventions to maximize respiratory capacity and assist cough are taught early to minimize and delay the onset of this respiratory insufficiency. Referral to specialist respiratory physiotherapy or ventilation intervention services for assessment will enable patients and carers to learn appropriate self-management techniques, such as breath stacking and manually assisted cough.

Some patients may require mechanically assisted cough devices such as lung volume recruitment bags or mechanical insufflator/exsufflators (cough assist machines). As the end of life approaches, palliative rehabilitation specialists can contribute to the support given to patients and families in making difficult decisions regarding on-going use of mechanical ventilation and cough assist devices.

Pain

Pain may be caused by the primary neurological condition or by comorbidities. Patients' perceptions of pain can guide treatment, and it can be helpful to find out whether patients can identify their own successful pain-relieving strategies, such as movement, positioning, relaxation, heat or cold, massage, or diversion [40]. Where pain is associated with movement, patients may become inactive. Carefully introduced and properly monitored exercise and movement therapy can help to encourage gentle activity, which, in turn, can prevent pain due to musculoskeletal immobility. These should be considered even when restoration of muscle function is not expected. Other non-pharmacological pain management interventions include transcutaneous electrical nerve stimulation (TENS), acupuncture and acupressure, soft tissue and massage therapies, mobility and other aids and equipment, and strategies to minimize the onset of pain when carrying out daily activities.

Speech and communication difficulties

Where it is likely that speech and communication will become impaired during the palliative phase, it is essential that referral to speech and language therapy services are made in good time. This allows interventions and strategies, including the use of augmented and alternative communication aids, to be established and adapted according to the needs and wishes of patients and carers as communication—and possibly also cognitive—abilities deteriorate. Enabling patients to continue to communicate for as long as possible is highly valued by both patients and carers. Where further deterioration is inevitable, families might need encouragement and support to discuss advanced care planning at a time when discussions are possible.

Swallowing

Difficulties in swallowing may occur long before the palliative phase and patients may have established support from their local speech and language therapy service. For other patients, swallowing problems may develop quickly, allowing little time for adjustment or accommodation and may herald the palliative phase of their disease. They may be associated with other symptoms such as drooling and cough and can be extremely distressing. Timely assessment is required to minimise the risk of aspiration pneumonia and reduced nutrition. Invasive procedures such as percutaneous endoscopic gastrostomy (PEG) and other enteral feeding devices are useful, but the risk of aspiration remains. In the palliative phase, sensitive negotiation and goal setting with patients and carers is needed, as autonomous choices balance known risks of aspiration against quality of life and on-going participation in family life and meal times.

The contrast between palliative rehabilitation in deteriorating vs stable neurological conditions

LTNCs are often divided into four groups:

1. Progressive conditions, for example, Parkinson's disease, motor neuron disease, and progressive MS.

2. Intermittent conditions, for example, epilepsy and relapsing remitting MS.

3. Single incident disorders, for example stroke, spinal cord injury, and traumatic brain injury.

4. Stable conditions, which have changing needs due to age, for example, post-polio syndrome and cerebral palsy.

The needs of people with progressive disease, where there is the possibility of serious disability and premature death, differ from those with single-incident disorder such as serious head injury, which results in profound disability. In the first group, the rehabilitation team will work with the patient in the early stages of the disease in the realm of preventative rehabilitation. After a relapse or in the early stages of progressive disease restorative rehabilitation may be provided in both in- and outpatient settings. As disability becomes more profound, supportive rehabilitation becomes the dominant model. Finally, where the person becomes severely disabled, palliative rehabilitation would be appropriate.

There is considerable evidence relating to the issues for people with slowly progressive disease such as MS. From the time of diagnosis the person with a progressive disease may have questions about death and dying and may need support around talking to their families about their prognosis and writing an advance directive. From diagnosis people can experience a sense of abandonment and isolation, which can continue for months or years [41]. Wollin [42] notes that feelings of disbelief and devastation are experienced not only by patients but also by their families, emphasizing the need for support for family relationships and not just individuals. These feelings of loss persist throughout the disease course. In MS, patients who have severe disability identify two significant areas of loss: the loss of personal independence and the loss of employment, which in turn lead to a loss of self-esteem, social contact, and income [43]. These multiple losses make adaptation and adjustment challenging, and cognitive behavioural therapy can be helpful in this regard. These feelings of loss, concern about death, and the need to adjust are traditionally the domain of palliative care but, where patients are well known to neurological services, the involvement of the neurological team may lead to better continuity of care.

As disease progresses, patients become less mobile and often become lost to follow up, particularly if they are admitted to nursing homes. These patients can experience pain, spasticity, fatigue, depression, pressure sores, and incontinence. While some neurological rehabilitation teams may have experience in the management of these problems, research evidence suggests that these symptoms are probably undermanaged in much of rehabilitation practice [44]. A dedicated MS palliative care service suggested that palliative care lead to improvements in five key symptoms: pain, nausea, vomiting, mouth problems, and sleeping difficulties; and also improved informal caregiver wellbeing.

These needs contrast with those following a single-incident disorder such as brain injury resulting in a low awareness state. In this context the main rehabilitation approaches used will be supportive and palliative rehabilitation, with an emphasis on enabling families to adjust to the 'ambiguous loss' associated with having a family member in a low awareness state, whether a persisting or permanent vegetative state (PVS) or a minimally conscious state. Kitzinger and Kitzinger [45] have outlined several key steps with regard to supporting families in a PVS. These include attention to appropriate decision-making processes in compliance with the Mental Capacity Act, good quality diagnosis care and information, regular patient review, and good palliative care.

Families, if they wish, should be supported to be actively engaged in the care programme of people with profound disabilities, and supported to undertake activities with their family member such as such as gentle massage, stretching, and stimulating activities (for example, listening to music). Families of patients with persistent disorders of consciousness should be offered counselling and support when they are ready to receive this, but family needs will change and so this support must be offered repeatedly.

Assisted dying—considerations for neuropalliative rehabilitation

Assisted dying remains a highly topical debate in palliative care. It is a complex subject and beyond the scope of this chapter to discuss in detail; however, there are aspects of the debate that have direct relevance for rehabilitation and it is therefore helpful for clinicians to have some understanding of the issues. Physician-assisted death is legal in certain parts of the world, for example in the Netherlands and the American state of Oregon. It is not currently legal in the UK despite several attempts in the last decade to introduce bills to Parliament to 'enable an adult who has capacity and who is suffering unbearably as a result of a terminal illness to receive medical assistance to die at his own considered and persistent request' [46: p. 179].

There is a fairly sizeable literature on patients' priorities and concerns at the end of life, but these focus mainly on the views of cancer patients and there is very little information specific to people with neurological conditions. What is apparent from this literature, however, and has relevance for rehabilitation at the end of life, is that disability and burden on others are both cited by patients as reasons for considering assisted suicide [47–49].

In a controversial report, the Commission on Assisted Dying [50] set out a case for allowing assisted dying in terminally ill adults. There are strong views on both sides of the debate, but the one aspect of the report that received unanimous support was the statement that comprehensive palliative care should be available to everyone living with life-threatening illness, at all times, and across all care settings. While one wants to avoid the naïve and simplistic view that given the proper care and facilities no-one would choose to die, it is vitally important to make sure that people reaching the end of life are able to live in a way that preserves their dignity and self worth.

This requires attention to be paid to an individual's impairment as well as to their physical environment and to social structures and attitudes. Disabled people giving evidence to the Commission expressed the concern that 'less politicized disabled people, or people who first develop an impairment later in life as a result of illness . . . might be more prone to adopt negative social perceptions about the status of disabled people in society', and that a sense of oneself as worthless and burdensome could influence judgements and decisions about whether life was worth living [50: p.291]. As we noted at the beginning of this chapter, rehabilitation in palliative care is concerned with enabling people to participate to as full an extent as possible in all aspects of their daily lives—making the most not only of their physical capacity, but also their psychological resources. Rehabilitation has an important part to play in supporting a person's perception of him or herself as a worthwhile individual with something to contribute to society, even in the late stages of illness.

Communication skills

Excellent communication skills underpin the delivery of neuropalliative rehabilitation. In addition to the basic good communication skills required in any healthcare context, there are two issues that have particular relevance in palliative care: being comfortable talking about death and dying, and being able to manage uncertainty.

Talking about dying

The National Service Framework for Long Term Conditions [51] emphasizes the importance of clinicians having the skills to address patients' fears and concerns about death. Patients are likely to have thoughts (and possibly fears) about the manner and timing of death, even if these are not voiced. For this reason, death and loss need to be on the agenda from the start, even when death is not imminent. People need to be given both the opportunity and the permission to ask questions, and clinicians need to find ways of making it clear to patients that they are comfortable having such conversations. Simply asking patients whether they have any fears or concerns about the future can be a way of doing this.

Managing uncertainty

Patients have many questions to which there are few straightforward answers: 'How quickly will I get worse?' 'Am I going to be able to walk again?' According to Murtagh et al. [10], 'The key to managing uncertainty is to acknowledge it—unacknowledged uncertainty causes problems; acknowledged uncertainty, carefully handled, can build trust'. The difficult bit is to maintain patients' trust and confidence in you—to recognize that this is not contingent on knowing all of the answers, but being willing to accept that sometimes there are no answers and to help patients and their families to face that and to manage the consequences. Some practical strategies for managing uncertainty are set out in Table 27.4.

Self-care strategies

For healthcare professionals, working with people who are reaching the ends of their lives is personally challenging. In this final section, we explore some of the factors that can contribute to stress in the workplace as well as some that counterbalance these, and we suggest some simple self-care strategies.

Sherman [52] proposes that job stressors fall into four categories: personal, interpersonal, health system, and professional.

Table 27.4 Strategies for managing uncertainty

For professionals	For patients
Recognize uncertainty, both one's own and that of other professionals.	Discover how much the patient wants to know.
Be honest with patients about uncertainty.	Discover how the patient feels about uncertainty.
Encourage open discussion of uncertainty among the multidisciplinary team.	Allow the patient to dictate the amount and pace of information.
	Avoid collusion with the patient or family.

Personal factors include our own previous life experiences of loss, illness, and death; the expectations we have of ourselves and of what we can deliver; and our attitudes and values—'good professionals can manage their emotions without it affecting their work', for example, or 'it is unprofessional to cry in the workplace'. *Interpersonal factors* relate both to interactions with patients and with colleagues. It is possible to become too invested in patients' problems without giving enough attention to personal replenishment [53]. Some patients can remind us powerfully of people we have known personally, making it hard to avoid over-identifying with their situation. Receiving inadequate emotional and practical support from colleagues can compound this. From a *health systems* perspective, the pressures inherent in the organizations in which we work can be stressful. Inadequate resources, poor coordination of care and bureaucracy can make it impossible to deliver what we would want for our patients, leading to feelings of frustration and powerlessness. The moral and ethical dilemmas that arise in palliative care can lead to *professional* dilemmas, particularly when patients' wishes conflict with codes of ethical conduct. For example, respecting a patient's autonomy and valuing the practice of goal setting can be difficult when that patient's stated goal is to end their life.

Signs of stress include: feelings of anxiety, guilt, anger, frustration, helplessness, self-doubt or insecurity; rumination; finding it difficult to take one's self away from the job (physically and mentally); conflict in teams; prolonged feelings of sadness and despair; over-investment in patients' problems, difficulty making decisions, and avoiding interactions with patients and their families. It is important to pay attention to feedback from others—it can sometimes be difficult to recognize or accept that we are stressed, and the observations of others can be helpful in this regard.

People who work in palliative care situations identify many rewards in their work which are valuable in counterbalancing some of these stressors. Vachon [53] highlights a number of ways in which doing a job that is meaningful and contributes to the good of society can be personally and professionally fulfilling. The opportunity to make a difference in people's lives at a very challenging time can engender a sense of being involved in something meaningful and important. The centrality of families and carers in the rehabilitation process makes it possible to work holistically and inclusively, experiencing reciprocity in relationships that are developed and receiving positive feedback where one's input has been helpful. Being instrumental in patients achieving their goals can provide families with good memories in difficult times. Contributing to patients being able to die where they chose, having put their affairs in order, enjoying warm relationships with those close to them can show us that death can be peaceful and well managed. The work can be intellectually stimulating, providing satisfaction in managing challenging ethical, practical, and professional situations well, and being part of a supportive network of colleagues who share the same ideals.

Stress is part of everyday life, and some amount of stress can be energizing and motivating. Attempting to eradicate stress altogether is likely to be both impossible and counter-productive. However, we do want to make sure that stress is well managed, and that we are controlling it, rather than the other way around. There are a number of things that we can do to manage and reduce stress [54]. These involve attending to both personal and environmental factors, gaining a clear understanding of ourselves and our work environment.

At a personal level, we need to understand our own resources, motivations, values, and limitations. We can use both behavioural and cognitive strategies to implement change where needed—doing things differently, as well as changing habits of thought and attitudes. Developing a level of self-awareness is important, particularly in understanding our personal philosophy of illness, suffering and death. Working with a mentor or clinical supervisor to do this can be beneficial. In terms of environmental factors, we need a realistic appraisal of external resources, identifying where they are plentiful and where they are limited. Having a clear understanding of what is expected of us, and what is reasonable and achievable within the resources available is extremely important. The New Economics Foundation [55] offers a set of simple, practical, evidence-based actions to promote well-being in everyday life. These are shown in Table 27.5.

Summary and conclusions

Patients tell us that what matters to them towards the end of life includes being able to maintain a sense of achievement and self-worth, and to enjoy their relationships with those close to them. The functional deterioration that patients experience and consequent loss of independence can cause psychological distress and social isolation. Although rehabilitation is traditionally thought of in terms of improvement and restoration, at the end of life it has a vital role to play in supporting people to adapt to changed circumstance and to limit the impact of advancing disease while acknowledging the reality of dying.

Excellent neuropalliative care requires a well-coordinated multi-professional team which brings together expertise in neurology, rehabilitation, and palliative care. The team needs to be able to manage the tension between supporting patients' goals and hopes while at the same time acknowledging the reality of death and dying openly, honestly and with sensitivity. This requires well-developed communication skills, and attention to the personal and professional challenges and rewards that working in this area entails.

Table 27.5 Five ways to well-being

Connect with people—family, friends, colleagues and patients. Building connections enriches daily life.
Be active. Find a physical activity that you enjoy and suits your level of ability. Exercise helps us to feel good.
Take notice. Be curious about your surroundings. Notice the things around you that are beautiful and unusual.
Keep learning. Try something new, set a challenge you will enjoy achieving.
Give. Do something nice for a friend or a stranger. Thank someone. Smile. Look out as well as in. Seeing yourself and your happiness as linked to a wider community can be incredibly rewarding.

References

1. Wade DT, de Jong BA. Recent advances in rehabilitation. Br Med J 2000;**320**:1385–1388.
2. World Health Organization. National Cancer Control Programmes: Policies and Managerial Guidelines, 2nd ed. WHO, Geneva, 2002.
3. Saunders C. Cicely Saunders: Selected Writings 1958–2004. Oxford University Press, Oxford, 2006.
4. Tookman AJ, Hopkins K, Scharpen-von-Heussen K. Rehabilitation in palliative medicine. In: Doyle D, Hanks G, Cherney N, Calman K (eds) Oxford Textbook of Palliative Medicine, 3rd edn. Oxford University Press, Oxford, 2004, pp. 1019–1033.
5. Aspinal F, Hughes R, Dunckley M, Addington-Hall. What is important to measure in the last months and weeks of life? A modified nominal group study. Int J Nurs Studies. 2006;**43**(4):393–403.
6. Heyland DK, Dodek P, Rocker G, et al, Canadian Researchers End-of-Life Care Network (CARENET). What matters most in end-of-life care: perceptions of seriously ill patients and their family members. CMAJ. 2006;**174**(5):627–633.
7. Steinhauser KE, Christakis NA, Clipp EC, McNeilly M, McIntyre L, Tulsky JA. Factors considered important at the end of life by patients, family, physicians, and other care providers. JAMA. 2000;**284**(19): 2476–2482.
8. Singer PA, Martin DK, Kelner M. Quality End-of-Life Care. Patients' Perspectives. JAMA. 1999;**281**(2): 163–168.
9. National Council for Palliative Care. Fulfilling Lives. Rehabilitation in Palliative Care. National Council for Palliative Care, London, 2000.
10. Murtagh FEM, Preston M, Higginson I. Patterns of dying: palliative care for non-malignant disease. Clin Med. 2004;**4**(1):39–44.
11. Turner-Stokes L, Sykes N, Silber E, on behalf of the Guideline Development Group. Long-term neurological conditions: management at the interface between neurology, rehabilitation and palliative care. Clin Med. 2008;**8**(2):186–191.
12. Department of Health. The National Service Framework for People with Long-term Neurological Conditions. Department of Health, London, 2005.
13. Barnes MP. Principles of neurological rehabilitation. J Neurol Neurosurg Psychiatry. 2003;**74**(Suppl IV):iv3–iv7.
14. Derksen J, Chochinov HM. Disability and end-of-life care: let the conversation begin. J Palliat Care. 2006;**22**(3):175–182.
15. Gill CJ. Disability, constructed vulnerability, and socially conscious palliative care. J Palliat Care. 2006;**22**(3):183–189.
16. Deitz JH. Rehabilitation Oncology. John Wiley & Sons Inc., New York, 1981.
17. Burton CR, Payne S, Addington-Hall J, Jones A. The palliative care needs of acute stroke patients: a prospective study of hospital admissions. Age Ageing. 2010;**39**:554–559.
18. Sykes N. Palliative care, neurology and rehabilitation: current levels of involvement. J Care Services Manage. 2008;**2**(2):194–202.
19. Turner-Stokes L, Sykes N, Silber E, Khatri A, Sutton L, Young. From diagnosis to death: exploring the interface between neurology, rehabilitation and palliative care in managing people with long-term neurological conditions. Clin Med. 2007;**7**(2):129–136.
20. Kristjanson LJ, Aoun SM, Yates P. Are supportive services meeting the needs of Australians with neurodegenerative disease and their families? J Palliat Care. 2006;**22**(3):151–157.
21. Bye R. When clients are dying: occupational therapists' perspectives. J Occupat Ther Res. 1998;**18**(1):3–24.
22. Homsi J, Walsh D, Rivera N, et al. Symptom evaluation in palliative medicine: patient report vs systematic assessment. Support Care Cancer. 2006;**14**:444–453.
23. Eva G. Measuring occupational therapy outcomes in cancer and palliative care. In: J Cooper (ed.) Occupational Therapy in Oncology and Palliative Care. John Wiley & Sons, Chichester, 2006, pp. 189–199.
24. Bausewein C, Daveson B, Benalia H, Simon ST, Higginson IJ. Outcome Measurement in Palliative Care: The Essentials. PRISMA, London. Available from http://www.csi.kcl.ac.uk/files/Guidance%20on%20Outcome%20Measurement%20in%20Palliative%20Care.pdf (accessed 19 August 2014).
25. Playford ED, Siegert R, Levack W, Freeman J. Areas of consensus and controversy about goal setting in rehabilitation: a conference report. Clin Rehabil. 2009;**23**:291–344.
26. Eva G. Goal setting. In: Nieland P, Simander R, Taylor J (eds) Physiotherapy in End of Life Care. Elsevier, Munich, 2013, pp. 39–41.
27. Taylor SE. Adjustment to threatening events: a theory of cognitive adaptation. Am Psychol. 1983;**38**(11):1161–1173.
28. Taylor SE, Brown JD. Illusion and well-being: a social psychological perspective on mental health. Psychol Bull. 1988;**103**(2):193–210.
29. Taylor SE, Kemeny ME, Reed GM, Bower JE, Gruenewald TL. Psychological resources, positive illusions, and health. Am Psychol. 2000;**55**(1):99–109.
30. Eva G, Paley J, Miller M, Wee B. Patients' constructions of disability in metastatic spinal cord compression. Palliat Med. 2009;**23**:132–140.
31. Cardol M, de Jong BA, Ward CD. On autonomy and participation in rehabilitation: a response. Disabil Rehabil. 2002;**24**(18):1001–1004.
32. Cardol M, de Jong BA, Ward CD. On autonomy and participation in rehabilitation. Disabil Rehabil., 2002;**24**(18):970–974.
33. Dal Bello-Haas V, Florence JM. Therapeutic exercise for people with amyotrophic lateral sclerosis or motor neuron disease. Cochrane Database Syst Rev. 2013;**5**:CD005229. DOI: 10.1002/14651858.CD005229.pub3.
34. Rietberg MB, Brooks D, Uitdehaag BMJ, Kwakkel G. Exercise therapy for multiple sclerosis. Cochrane Database Syst Rev 2004;**3**: CD003980. DOI: 10.1002/14651858.CD003980.pub2, 2004.
35. Booth S, Moffat C, Farquhar M, Higginson IJ, Burkin J. Developing a breathlessness intervention service for patients with palliative and supportive care needs, irrespective of diagnosis. J Palliat Care. 2011;**27**(1):28–36.
36. Simon ST, Higginson IJ, Benalia H, et al. Episodes of breathlessness: Types and patterns—a qualitative study exploring experiences of patients with advanced diseases. Palliat Med. 2013;**27**(6):524–532.
37. Shneerson J. Neuromuscular and skeletal diseases, and obstructive sleep apnoea. In: Amedzai SH, Baldwin D, Currow D (eds) Supportive Care in Respiratory Disease, 2nd edn. Oxford University Press, Oxford, 2012, pp. 215–234.
38. Royal College of Physicians, National Council for Palliative Care, British Society of Rehabilitation Medicine. Long-term neurological conditions: management at the interface between neurology, rehabilitation and palliative care. Concise Guidance to Good Practice series, No 10. RCP, London, 2008.
39. Lou JS, Weiss MD, Carter GT. Assessment and management of fatigue in neuromuscular disease. Am J Hospice Palliat Med. 2010;**27**(2):145–145.
40. Van den Broek J. Pain management. In: Nieland P, Simander R, Taylor J (eds) Physiotherapy in End of Life Care. Elsevier, Munich, 2013, pp. 47–61.
41. Johnson J. On receiving the diagnosis of multiple sclerosis: managing the transition. Multiple Sclerosis. 2003;**9**:82–88.
42. Wollin J, Yates PM, Kristjanson LJ. Supportive and palliative care needs identified by multiple sclerosis patients and their families. Int J Palliat Nurs. 2006;**12**:20–26.
43. Edmonds P, Vivat B, Burman R, Silber E, Higginson IJ. Loss and change: experiences of people severely affected by multiple sclerosis. Palliat Med. 2007;**21**(2):101–107.
44. Edmonds P, Hart S, Wei Gao, et al. Palliative care for people severely affected by multiple sclerosis: evaluation of a novel palliative care service. Multiple Sclerosis. 2010;**16**(5):627–636.
45. Kitzinger J, Kitzinger C. The 'window of opportunity' for death after severe brain injury: family experiences. Sociol Health Illness. 2013;**35**(7):1095–1112.
46. Harris D, Richard B, Phanna P. Assisted dying: the ongoing debate. Postgrad Med J., 2006;**82**:479–482.

47. Suarez-Almazor ME, Newman C, Hanson J, Bruera E. Attitudes of terminally ill cancer patients about euthanasia and assisted suicide: predominance of psychosocial determinants and beliefs over symptom distress and subsequent survival. Clin Oncol. 2002;**15**(20):2134–2141.

48. Filiberti A, Ripamonti C, Totis A, et al. Characteristics of terminal cancer patients who committed suicide during a home palliative care program. J Pain Sympt Manage. 2001;**22**(1): 544–553.

49. Emanuel EJ, Fairclough DL, Emanuel LL. Attitudes and desires related to euthanasia and physician-assisted suicide among terminally ill patients and their caregivers. JAMA. 2000**84**(19):2460–2468.

50. Commission on Assisted Dying. The Current Legal Status of Assisted Dying is Inadequate and Incoherent. Demos, London, 2011.

51. Department of Health. National Service Framework for Long Term Conditions. Department of Health, London, 2005.

52. Sherman DW. Nurses' stress and burnout: how to care for yourself when caring for patients and their families experiencing life-threatening illness. Am J Nurs., 2004;**104**(5):48–56.

53. Vachon MLS. The stress of professional caregivers. In: Doyle D, Hanks G, Cherney N, Calman K (eds) Oxford Textbook of Palliative Medicine, 3rd edn. Oxford University Press, Oxford, 2004, pp. 992–1004.

54. Schönleiter W P. Self-care for physiotherapists. In: Nieland P, Simander R, Taylor J (eds) Physiotherapy in End of Life Care. Elsevier, Munich, 2013, pp. 179–188.

55. Aked J, Marks N, Cordon C, Thompson S. Five Ways to Wellbeing. New Economics Foundation, London, Available from http://www.neweconomics.org/publications/entry/five-ways-to-well-being-the-evidence (accessed 19 August 2014).

CHAPTER 28

Recognition and management of functional (non-organic) symptoms after CNS damage

Lucia Ricciardi, Alan Carson, and Mark Edwards

Introduction

In clinical practice it is well known that some patients who have a recognized neurological disease or have experienced structural damage to the nervous system, may present with symptoms which are eventually unexplained by that disease or damage. These patients are often referred to as having 'functional overlay'. Functional overlay is relatively common: in a recent study [1] of over 3,000 consecutive outpatients presenting for the first time to neurological services, 12% of those with neurological disease or structural damage were also reported by their treating neurologist to have 'symptoms unexplained by disease'. There was no significant difference between different neurological diagnoses and the likelihood of patients having functional overlay, though some smaller studies have focused on particular causes of neurological disease and have reported some differences in the likelihood of functional overlay occurring in different disorders (e.g. a higher rate of somatoform disorders has been reported in those with Parkinson's disease as opposed to atypical parkinsonism and dementia [2, 3]).

In this chapter we consider the relevance of functional overlay to management of patients with central nervous system (CNS) damage. This task is rather difficult as few studies have explored in detail the diagnosis, pathophysiology and treatment of functional symptoms specifically in the setting of CNS damage. A major exception to this is the quite extensive study of patients who have an inexplicably catastrophic outcome after what appeared to be minor traumatic brain injury (mTBI), a phenomenon sometimes called post-concussional syndrome. We have therefore focused this chapter on this topic, while also drawing on evidence for the diagnosis, pathophysiology, and treatment of functional symptoms in a more general neurological setting.

Traumatic brain injury (TBI) is a common event, most commonly caused by road accidents, falls, sport injuries, and assaults, and can lead to death and disability. Approximately 80% of TBI are defined as 'mild' (mTBI) [4] and as such would intuitively not be expected to result in a poor outcome. However, poor, even catastrophic outcome is reported after such mTBI; such poor outcome may well be due to functional neurological symptoms, and this must be considered because it has a definite impact on management.

Although a universally accepted definition of mTBI is lacking, differing criteria including measures of Glasgow Coma Scale (GCS), duration of total loss of consciousness and duration of post-traumatic amnesia have been recommended and are widely used. Following comprehensive review of the scientific literature the World Health Organization (WHO) recommended the following definition [5]: 'Mild traumatic brain injury is an acute brain injury resulting from mechanical energy to the head from external force. Operational criteria for clinical identification include: (1). One or more of the following: confusion or disorientation, loss of consciousness for 30 minutes or less, post-traumatic amnesia for less than 24 hours, and/or other transient neurological abnormalities such as focal signs, seizure, and intracranial lesion not requiring surgery; AND (2). GCS score of 13–15 after 30 minutes post head injury or later upon presentation for health care. These manifestations of mTBI must not be due to drugs, alcohol, medications, caused by other injuries, or treatment for other injuries (e.g. systemic injuries, facial injuries, or intubation), caused by other problems (e.g. psychological trauma, language barrier, or coexisting medical conditions) or caused by penetrating craniocerebral injury'.

Acute symptoms of mTBI include: headache, dizziness, nausea, fatigue, vertigo, tinnitus, slurred speech, and poor concentration; these symptoms tend to recover within a matter of days or weeks after injury and most individuals (80–90%) report no apparent sequelae after 3 months. The prognosis of mTBI is therefore, in the majority of cases, excellent.

However 10–20% of patients with mTBI, (historically not very sympathetically termed the 'miserable minority' [6]) have persistent symptoms at one year after injury [7–9]. Many of these patients experience a chronic condition that is termed by many: 'post-concussion syndrome' (PCS), though for reasons outlined below this term is thought by some to be an inappropriate label for the condition. Patients with persistent symptoms after mTBI typically experience a combination of symptoms in physical (e.g. fatigue, headache), cognitive (e.g. concentration and memory deficit), and emotional (e.g. anxiety, irritability) domains [6, 10].

One important consideration that could explain some of the poor outcome at long-term follow-up of patients with mTBI is that patients who have mTBI are at risk due to lifestyle factors from other illness, including recurrent TBI. A high prevalence of alcohol abuse in those with head injury has long been recognized; one-third to two-thirds of patients with TBI are intoxicated at the time of injury, and approximately half of alcoholics have a history of TBI with loss of consciousness and/or hospitalization [11]. On this basis we could hypothesize that past personal and social life style might predispose to a more severe outcome following mTBI.

Following this line, a recent study has underlined once again the role of alcohol in head injury and has examined the subsequent risk of epilepsy. The findings are intriguing and suggest that the widely accepted association between mTBI and seizures may in fact be an artefact related to high rates of alcohol misuse in this population [12].

A second potential cause of poor outcome is that mTBI might trigger the onset of a functional neurological disorder, which has as its main symptoms those symptoms that are usually ascribed to 'PCS'. In support of this contention, there is no clear positive correlation between the severity of TBI and PCS development; on the contrary, moderate to severe injuries do not tend to cause PCS. This piece of evidence brings into question the use of the word 'concussion' to describe this syndrome: surely concussion would be expected to be most severe in those with moderate to severe TBI? Added to this is the finding that typical symptoms of 'PCS' are also seen in patients who have suffered (often minor) limb injuries where there is good evidence of there being *no* injury to the head. Such symptoms are also commonly seen in patients with chronic pain disorder, or even in healthy controls. These observations are part of the background against which there has been an ongoing debate as to whether 'PCS' is best considered a 'neurogenic' or a 'psychogenic' disorder, and also if for some patients it is a genuine entity at all or simply reflects deliberate generation of symptoms for financial gain.

A parallel debate has taken place with regard to functional neurological symptoms in general; fierce debates regarding terminology are underpinned by different levels of belief about the relevance of psychological factors in the triggering and maintenance of functional symptoms.

Historical background

The term PCS was used for the first time in 1834 in Grinker's neurology textbook. Between 1866 and 1882 Erichsen described in his publications what was defined as 'railway brain' or 'railway spine' as 'certain obscure injuries of the nervous system commonly met with as the results of shocks of the body received in collisions on railways' and he suggested that minor head and spine injuries might cause severe disabilities due to 'molecular disarrangement' in the nervous system. A number of contemporaneous medical authorities such as Wardsworth, Page, Strumpel, and Oppenheim debated the nature of this syndrome trying to clarify whether it was a 'functional' disorder (Page in 1883 used this term for the first time), an 'organic' brain damage or whether it reflected exaggeration of symptoms as a compensation law was approved in Europe at that time for personal injury.

In the 1880s Charcot defined a new distinct subcategory of hysteria, traumatic hysteria or hysteron-traumatism, in which minor body injury resulted in major physical and/or psychological disability. In particular, one of these 20 cases ('Le Log') developed typical symptoms of 'PCS' after what, by description, was a mild TBI. Charcot suggested that this disorder was caused by a combination of constitutional predilection to nervous degeneration and an 'agent provocateur' and that the physical trauma served as a trigger. In this view of an organic site of hysteria, Charcot integrated in a single concept the psyche and the soma as aetiological influences, a clear suggestion that the Cartesian separation of body and mind was inadequate with respect to disorders with 'psychosomatic' features. In the 1890s Friedman suggested a new nomenclature for the post-traumatic syndrome characterized by headache, dizziness, vasomotor instability, and intolerance to alcohol as 'the vasomotor symptom complex', and he proposed that it might be caused by deficit in intracranial circulation.

By the 1960s, two main theories were current. Miller supported the viewpoint of those who believed that PCS was a psychogenic disorder, magnified by the availability of financial compensation. This would appear to conflate ideas of involuntary psychogenic disorders with the production of physical symptoms deliberately for financial gain: malingering. Symonds supported the 'organicity' of the syndrome stating that 'it is questionable whether the effects of concussion, however slight, are ever completely reversible'.

Lishman, in recent years, suggested that both 'physiogenic' and 'psychogenic' factors are important in the genesis of PCS symptoms. From this point of view, organic factors are chiefly relevant in the earlier stages, whereas chronic symptoms are perpetuated by secondary 'neurotic' developments [13].

Recognition of functional symptoms in clinical practice

There has been a major shift in approach over the past 10–15 years with regard to such patients. The two main components of this shift in approach have been (1) an emphasis on making a diagnosis based on positive aspects of the history and physical signs rather considering the diagnosis of functional neurological symptoms as a diagnosis of exclusion, and (2) an acceptance that psychological factors, particularly childhood emotional trauma, may not be important for all patients who develop such symptoms, and certainly that the presence or absence of psychopathology should not unduly influence the diagnosis.

Regarding the importance of focusing on positive physical signs and investigation findings to support the diagnosis, rather than the presence of psychological distress, patients with functional movement disorders, including functional weakness, represent an important model since they have objective motor signs that are suitable for clinical and experimental measurement. Diagnosis in such patients relies on demonstrating an improvement/normalization of the movement disorder with distraction. There are various techniques that can be used depending on the symptom, including Hoover's sign for functional weakness (normalization of apparently weak hip extension by flexion of the contralateral hip) and change in frequency of functional tremor when the patient taps at a different frequency with the other hand. Sensory symptoms may break fundamental rules regarding anatomy (for example tubular visual field defects, where the size of the visual field defect is the same when assessed close to the patient and far away).

The commonest chronic symptoms after mTBI are sensory/cognitive, and thus are more difficult to diagnose as functional according to positive clinical criteria in comparison to motor signs, which can be directly observed. However, many of the chronic symptoms commonly reported in patients after mTBI are also reported by patients with functional neurological symptoms defined on positive clinical criteria. This especially applies to complaints of poor memory, which on neuropsychological testing is revealed to be related to poor attention and concentration.

There is a growing appreciation of the role of physical precipitating factors in the mechanism of functional neurological symptoms. Physical precipitants commonly include injury (typically limb injury), but also intercurrent illness, operations, drug reactions, etc. Such physical precipitants are reported in up to 80% of those with functional neurological symptoms. This clearly does not deny a role for psychological/emotional triggers, and indeed it is impossible to separate out the physical and psychological aspects of response to such physical triggers [14, 15]. This is in accordance with recent models of other functional somatic syndromes such as chronic fatigue syndrome and irritable bowel syndrome [16], which are typically preceded by a flu-like illness or an episode of infective diarrhoea, respectively. The common occurrence of physical precipitating factors triggering onset of functional neurological symptoms defined on positive clinical criteria clearly provides a plausible mechanistic link for the triggering of functional symptoms after mTBI.

Phenomenology of persistent symptoms seen after mTBI

In terms of prevalence of symptoms, headache and fatigue are the commonest symptoms at 6 months follow-up after mTBI [9, 17]. Other common symptoms are sleep disturbances, cognitive deficit (such as attention deficit and poor memory), speech deficit, dizziness, vision deficit (blurred vision, double vision), nausea, and vomiting [9]. Such symptoms are non-specific in nature and occur at similar rates after several other physical traumas. There is no evidence for their causality. In particular, currently available evidence does not support neuronal damage as the main underlying mechanism [5].

Headache is a cardinal feature and the most common symptom reported in PCS [18]. According to the International Classification of Headache Disorder, the onset of chronic post-traumatic headache attributed to mTBI should develop within 7 days after trauma [19]. It is still very controversial whether persistent headache after mTBI or neck trauma might be causally related to the traumatic event itself (for example as a triggered form of migraine) or if other causes such as functional basis, psychosocial expectation, compensation, or litigation are better explanations.

Cognitive deficits after mTBI that persist beyond 1 year are often proposed to reflect functional neurological symptoms [20, 21] or linked to secondary gain or malingering. It is important to note, however, that many patients with poor outcome after mTBI are receiving medication (often analgesics) and these too can have a direct effect on cognitive performance, as can coexistent mood problems. The most common complaint is that of memory and attention difficulties [22]. Recent studies have demonstrated that symptomatic patients with PCS after mTBI show cognitive sequelae such as reduced verbal fluency and working memory functioning compared to healthy controls and asymptomatic patients. However, the idea that mTBI can have sustained consequences, and that the subjectively experienced symptoms and difficulties in everyday situations might be related to objectively measurable parameters in neurocognitive function, is still matter of debate

and the majority of recent studies report a lack of evidence for this hypothesis [23–28] suggesting that the relationship between PCS and cognitive impairment is generally weak and that there are no mTBI-attributable cognitive deficits beyond 3 months after injury, although those patients with complicated mTBI, (ie with associated skull fractures or intracranial lesions) may have significant cognitive deficits [5].

When assessing cognitive symptoms after mTBI, traditional psychometric testing can be misleading. In addition, it is mandatory to perform tests of effort, which help to evaluate whether a patient's poor score on cognitive testing is likely to represent a false positive due to poor effort. Such tests cannot, however, distinguish between poor effort due to malingering and poor effort related to the underlying neurobiological mechanism behind functional neurological symptoms or factors such as low mood.

Efforts have been made to produce criteria for diagnosis of a specific functional cognitive disturbance after mTBI: cogniform disturbance or cogniform condition [29]. These criteria attempt to separate out causation (conversion disorder vs. facticious disorder vs. malingering) from the common symptoms that patients present with. They emphasize the need for effort testing, and the positive diagnostic use of identification of particular patterns of memory/cognitive disturbance (loss of remote autobiographical memory, inability to perform simple overlearned skills such as reading, writing, or simple maths) that are not commonly seen in those with even moderate brain injury. They also emphasize the positive diagnostic utility of incongruity between performance on cognitive tests and behaviour observed in a more natural setting.

Reports of speech and language deficits persisting one year after mTBI have described patterns of 'non credible speech and language deficit' including 'foreign accent syndrome', atypical dysarthria, stuttering, severe expressive aphasia, and speech apraxia. Foreign accent syndrome is a rare condition, which can follow a damage of right hemisphere, typically a cerebrovascular accident. It is characterized by changes in rhythm, prosody/intonation and phoneme production of speech in absence of other cognitive deficit such as aphasia. Recently, few cases of functional foreign accent syndrome have been reported after mTBI, in absence of structural CNS lesion [30, 31]. Cases of functional stuttering [32] have been reported after mTBI. Such cases were usually of sudden onset after mTBI in the absence of structural brain damage, and where the pattern of stuttering was inconsistent with the typical pattern of an organic stutter.

Non-epileptic seizures are events that resemble epileptic seizures but occur without epileptiform activity [33]. A small number of studies have investigated the concurrence of TBI and NES and have identified a prevalence of TBI ranging between 33–45% in samples of NES patients; in about 70% of these cases the injury was minimal (mTBI). These studies suggest mTBI as a comorbid factor in NES, and links mTBI to an increased prevalence of functional neurological symptoms. Patients with NES and TBI seem to be more likely to have psychiatric comorbidities such as mood disorders, anxiety, impulsive personality traits or disorders, and a history of abuse [34].

Treatment

There is very little specific data regarding management of functional symptoms that occur together with a neurological disease or structural damage. However, it seems highly likely that management of such symptoms can be informed by evidence (which itself is rather meagre) on how functional symtoms in general can be successfully managed. It is important to note that in patients with CNS damage, functional symptoms may in fact be the most treatable aspect of the disability the patient presents with. This underlines the importance of recognition and appropriate treatment of these symptoms.

Management of any condition is aided by successful communication of information about the diagnosis. This is likely to be of even greater importance in those with functional symptoms. Here, a sensitive and appropriate explanation can be a treatment in its own right. A lack of explanation is likely to increase attention towards symptoms and foster abnormal illness beliefs. In our own practice we concentrate on giving a diagnosis based on positive clinical signs (i.e. explaining what it is that is wrong) rather than explaining how the symptoms cannot be explained by the neurological disease/damage the patient has (i.e. explaining what the patient does not have). We feel it is important to give the symptoms a name, and we prefer the use of the word functional to describe symptoms, as it is relatively free of 'baggage' regarding the aetiology of the symptoms, and the term is acceptable to patients. We do not avoid discussing the possible relevance of psychological factors, but do so in a broad context, which accepts that many patients do not endorse such factors to be relevant. We emphasize reversibility of symptoms and discuss a broad rehabilitation approach to treatment. We suggest patients and their families look at online sources of information (such as the website www.neurosymptoms.org and the patient organization FND Hope).

There is some evidence to support the use of cognitive behavioural therapy (CBT) in those with functional symptoms. The main therapeutic techniques include the identification and adjustment of pathological automatic thoughts and proposing behavioural experiments to the patient, with the intent of disrupting the vicious cycle of the symptoms and their consequences [35–39]. Unfortunately, this technique is limited by the paucity of well-trained therapists and the lack of availability of it in some countries.

Two studies have also suggested the utility of psychodynamic psychotherapy for these patients; this is based on exploring past and early life experiences, relationships with parents, problematic emotions, and current life experiences [40, 41]. Such treatments may be facilitated in selected patients with the use of antidepressant or anxiolytic medications [42], and may be more effective for those with severe symptoms when given as part of inpatient multidisciplinary rehabilitation [43, 44].

More recently, promising results have been shown for specific forms of physiotherapy for those with functional motor symptoms [45]. In a retrospective cohort study Czarnecki et al. found that 1 week of intensive rehabilitation, based on 'motor reprogramming' techniques, was successful. Over 65% of patients reported that they were 'better' or 'much better' at discharge and at 2 years post-discharge [46]. Jordbru and coworkers [47] conducted a crossover, randomized study assessing the efficacy of 3 week inpatient rehabilitation programme on 60 patients with functional (psychogenic) gait disorders, compared to a waiting list control group. The programme consisted of physical activity within a cognitive behavioural framework. They showed an improvement in clinical scales assessing functional mobility and quality of life in over 70% of patients [47].

When specifically considering the management of PCS, current guidelines are available and suggest that all patients should be offered reassurance about the nature of their symptoms and advice on gradual return to normal activities after uncomplicated mTBI [48]. This advice includes efforts to normalize the presence of somatic symptoms after mTBI and to reassure patients and family that such symptoms do not reflect significant brain injury.

Recent systematic reviews have underlined the inconsistency of results and the lack of randomized clinical trials on the use of anti depressant drugs in mTBI patients; only one study found amitriptyline to substantially reduce headache after mTBI while sertraline was associated with significant improvement in depression, anger, aggression, functional disability, PCS, and cognition in mTBI patients [49].

Several studies have evaluated the efficacy of psychological treatments such as CBT, including three randomized controlled trials where authors showed some evidence that CBT may be effective in the treatment of persistent symptoms (beyond three months duration) after mTBI (for a review see [50]).

For those with severe complex symptoms after mTBI, a multidisciplinary approach combining physical and psychological treatment is often suggested as the most appropriate treatment, often taking place in an inpatient unit. Evidence in support of this approach for patients with persistent symptoms after mTBI is limited, though there is evidence in support of this approach for patients with chronic severe functional neurological symptoms in general.

Conclusions

It is well recognized that a percentage of patients with neurological disease and structural damage, including mTBI, develop functional symptoms. Efforts should be made to arrive at a positive diagnosis and to adopt a broad approach to explanation and treatment which does not solely focus on psychological factors. Such patients can be vulnerable to repeated investigations and unnecessary treatments. However, recovery can be aided by appropriate multidisciplinary intervention.

References

1. Stone J, Carson A, Duncan R, et al. Which neurological diseases are most likely to be associated with 'symptoms unexplained by organic disease'. J Neurol. 2012;**259**(1):33–38.
2. Onofrj M, Bonanni L, Manzoli L, Thomas A. Cohort study on somatoform disorders in Parkinson disease and dementia with Lewy bodies. Neurology. 2010;**74**(20):1598–1606.
3. Pareés I, Saifee TA, Kojovic M, et al. Functional (psychogenic) symptoms in Parkinson's disease. Mov Disord. 2013;**28**(12):1622–1627.
4. Kraus JF, Nourjah P. The epidemiology of mild, uncomplicated brain injury. J Trauma. 1988;**28**:1637–1643.
5. Carroll LJ, Cassidy JD, Holm L, Kraus J, Coronado VG. Methodological issues and research recommendations for mild traumatic brain injury: the WHO Collaborating Centre Task Force on Mild Traumatic Brain Injury. J Rehabil Med. 2004(43 Suppl):113–125.
6. Ruff RM, Camenzuli L, Mueller J. Miserable minority: emotional risk factors that influence the outcome of a mild traumatic brain injury. Brain Inj. 1996;**10**(8):551–565.
7. Iverson GL. Outcome from mild traumatic brain injury. Curr Opin Psychiatry. 2005;**18**(3):301–317.

8. Kraus J, Schaffer K, Ayers K, Stenehjem J, Shen H, Afifi AA. Physical complaints, medical service use, and social and employment changes following mild traumatic brain injury: a 6-month longitudinal study. J Head Trauma Rehabil. 2005;**20**(3):239–256.

9. Hou R, Moss-Morris R, Peveler R, Mogg K, Bradley BP, Belli A. When a minor head injury results in enduring symptoms: a prospective investigation of risk factors for postconcussional syndrome after mild traumatic brain injury. J Neurol Neurosurg Psychiatry. 2012;**83**(2):217–223.

10. Boake C, McCauley SR, Levin HS, et al. Diagnostic criteria for postconcussional syndrome after mild to moderate traumatic brain injury. J Neuropsychiatry Clin Neurosci. 2005;**17**(3):350–356.

11. Thornhill S, Teasdale GM, Murray GD, McEwen J, Roy CW, Penny KI. Disability in young people and adults one year after head injury: Prospective cohort study. Br Med J. 2000;**320**(7250):1631–1635.

12. Vaaramo K, Puljula J, Tetri S, et al. 5 Predictors of new-onset seizures: a 10-year follow-up of head trauma subjects with and without traumatic brain injury. J Neurol Neurosurg Psychiatry. 2014;**85**(6):598–602.

13. Lishman WA. Physiogenesis and psychogenesis in the 'post-concussional syndrome'. Br J Psychiatry. 1988;**153**:460–469.

14. Edwards MJ, Bhatia KP. Functional (psychogenic) movement disorders: merging mind and brain. Lancet Neurol. 2012;**11**(3):250–260

15. Stone J, Edwards MJ. How 'psychogenic' are psychogenic movement disorders? Mov Disord 2011;**26**:1787–1788.

16. Harrison NA, Brydon L, Walker C, et al. Neural origins of human sickness in interoceptive responses to inflammation. Biol Psychiatry. 2009;**66**(5):415–422.

17. Lannsjö M, af Geijerstam JL, Johansson U, Bring J, Borg J. Prevalence and structure of symptoms at 3 months after mild traumatic brain injury in a national cohort. Brain Inj. 2009;**23**(3):213–219.

18. Evans RW. The post concussion syndrome and the sequelae of mild head injury. In: Evans RW, ed Neurology and Trauma, 2nd edn. Oxford University Press, New York, 2006, pp. 95–128.

19. Headache Classification Committee of the International Headache Society (IHS). The International Classification of Headache Disorders, 3rd edition (beta version). Cephalalgia. 2013;**33**(9):629–808.

20. Greiffenstein FM, Baker JW. Comparison of premorbid and postinjury mmpi-2 profiles in late postconcussion claimants. Clin Neuropsychol. 2001;**15**(2):162–170.

21. Arciniegas DB, Anderson CA, Topkoff J, McAllister TW Mild traumatic brain injury: a neuropsychiatric approach to diagnosis, evaluation, and treatment. Neuropsychiatr Dis Treat. 2005;**1**(4):311–327.

22. Niogi SN, Mukherjee P, Ghajar J, et al. Structural dissociation of attentional control and memory in adults with and without mild traumatic brain injury. Brain. 2008;**131**(Pt 12):3209–3221.

23. Bohnen NI, Jolles J, Twijnstra A, Mellink R, Wijnen G. Late neurobehavioural symptoms after mild head injury. Brain Inj. 1995;**9**(1):27–33.

24. Sterr A., Herron K., Hayward C., Montaldi D. (2006). Are mild head injuries as mild as we think? Neurobehavioral concomitants of chronic post-concussion syndrome. BMC Neurol. **6**:7.

25. Chan RCK: Attention deficits in patients with persisting postconcussive complaints: a general deficit or specific component deficit? J Clin Exp Neuropsychol Neuropsychol Dev Cogn A. 2002;**24**:1081–1093.48

26. Kinnunen KM, Greenwood R, Powell JH, et al. White matter damage and cognitive impairment after traumatic brain injury. Brain. 2011;**134**:449–463.

27. Lange RT, Iverson GL, Franzen MDNeuropsychological functioning following complicated vs. uncomplicated mild traumatic brain injury. Brain Inj.. 2009;**23**:83–91.

28. Chen JK, Johnston KM, Frey S, Petrides M, Worsley K, Ptito A. Functional abnormalities in symptomatic concussed athletes: an fMRI study. Neuroimage. 2004;**22**:68–82.

29. Delis DC, Wetter SR. Cogniform disorder and cogniform condition: proposed diagnoses for excessive cognitive symptoms. Arch Clin Neuropsychol. 2007;**22**(5):589–604.

30. Cottingham ME, Boone KB. Non-credible language deficits following mild traumatic brain injury. Clin Neuropsychol. 2010;**24**(6):1006–1025.

31. Mahr G, Leith W. Psychogenic stuttering of adult onset. J Speech Hear Res. 1992;**35**(2):283–286.

32. Abudarham S, White A. 'Insuring' a correct differential diagnosis—a 'forensic' collaborative experience. Int J Lang Commun Disord. 2001;**36** Suppl:58–63.

33. Brown RJ, Syed TU, Benbadis S, LaFrance WC Jr, Reuber M. Psychogenic nonepileptic seizures. Epilepsy Behav. 2011;**22**(1):85–93.

34. Lafrance WC Jr, Deluca M, Machan JT, Fava JL. Traumatic brain injury and psychogenic nonepileptic seizures yield worse outcomes. Epilepsia. 2013;**54**(4):718–725.

35. Speckens AE, van Hemert AM, Spinhoven P, Hawton KE, Bolk JH, Rooijmans HG. Cognitive behavioural therapy for medically unexplained physical symptoms: a randomised controlled trial. Br Med J. 1995;**311**(7016):1328–1332.

36. LaFrance WC, Miller IW, Ryan CE, et al. Cognitive behavioral therapy for psychogenic nonepileptic seizures. Epilepsy Behav. 2009;**14**(4):591–596.

37. Goldstein LH, Chalder T, Chigwedere C, et al. Cognitive-behavioral therapy for psychogenic nonepileptic seizures: a pilot RCT. Neurology. 2010;**74**(24):1986–1994.

38. Sharpe M, Walker J, Williams C, et al Guided self-help for functional (psychogenic) symptoms: a randomized controlled efficacy trial. Neurology. 2011;**77**(6):564–572.

39. LaFrance WC Jr, Friedman JH. Cognitive behavioral therapy for psychogenic movement disorder. Mov Disord. 2009;**24**(12):1856–1857.

40. Hinson VK, Weinstein S, Bernard B, Leurgans SE, Goetz CG. Single-blind clinical trial of psychotherapy for treatment of psychogenic movement disorders. Parkinsonism Relat Disord. 2006;**12**(3):177–180.

41. Kompoliti K, Wilson B, Stebbins G, Bernard B, Hinson V. Immediate vs. delayed treatment of psychogenic movement disorders with short term psychodynamic psychotherapy: Randomized clinical trial. Parkinsonism & related disorders 2014;**20**(1):60–63.

42. Voon V, Lang AE. Antidepressant treatment outcomes of psychogenic movement disorder. J Clin Psychiatry. 2005;**66**(12):1529–1534.

43. Saifee TA, Kassavetis P, Pareés I, et al. Inpatient treatment of functional motor symptoms: a long-term follow-up study. J Neurol. 2012;**259**(9):1958–1963.

44. McCormack R, Moriarty J, Mellers JD, et al. Specialist inpatient treatment for severe motor conversion disorder: a retrospective comparative study. J Neurol Neurosurg Psychiatry. 2013;**85**(8):895–900

45. Nielsen G, Stone J, Edwards MJ. Physiotherapy for functional (psychogenic) motor symptoms: a systematic review. J Psychosom Res. 2013;**75**(2):93–102.

46. Czarnecki K, Thompson JM, Seime R, Geda YE, Duffy JR, Ahlskog JE. Functional movement disorders: successful treatment with a physical therapy rehabilitation protocol. Parkinsonism Relat Disord. 2012;**18**(3):247–251.

47. Jordbru AA, Smedstad LM, Klungsøyr O, Martinsen EW. Psychogenic gait disorder: A randomized controlled trial of physical rehabilitation with one-year follow-up. J Rehabil Med. 2014;**46**(2):181–187.

48. SIGN 130, Brain Injury Rehabilitation in Adults: A National Clinical Guideline. Healthcare Improvement Scotland, 2013.

49. Tyler GS, McNeely HE, Dick ML. Treatment of post-traumatic headache with amitriptyline. Headache. 1980;**20**(4):213–216

50. Al Sayegh A, Sandford D, Carson AJ. Psychological approaches to treatment of postconcussion syndrome: a systematic review. J Neurol Neurosurg Psychiatry. 2010;**81**(10):1128–1134.57

Technical concepts

sections

Technical concepts

CHAPTER 29

Promises and challenges of neurorehabilitation technology

William Rymer and Arun Jayaraman

Introduction

Over the last 20 years, there has been extraordinary growth in the development of rehabilitation technologies designed to enhance rehabilitation therapies. These include robotic systems for retraining upper and lower extremities (e.g. IMT Manus and Lokomat), as well as electrical stimulators reducing foot drop and shoulder subluxation, and wearable sensors to track actual performance. The motivation for the use of many of these technologies is simple to understand, since these devices serve to augment therapies delivered by the clinicians, increasing their reach, and they may also prove to be more cost effective as well, in some clinical settings.

To take the case of robotic locomotion therapies for example, such as those provided by the powered robotic gait trainer called the Lokomat® (a device designed and manufactured by Hocoma®), the intent was to improve and potentially to simplify locomotor gait training for patients with incomplete spinal cord injury, by providing a more intense dose of locomotor training while reducing the weight-bearing burden for the patient at the same time. It was shown earlier in a number of studies on animal models, for example, that locomotor training in which an animal is suspended above a treadmill so that the treadmill is allowed to promote 'passive' walking by moving the animal's legs, that even animals with complete spinal cord injury will often generate natural locomotor patterns within a relatively short period of time.

When the manual locomotor training approach was tested in humans, however, it has proved to be extremely laborious physically, in that several therapists were needed to move the limbs of a paralysed spinal cord subject by hand. Although this task was manageable initially when subjects were weak, in many cases the limbs developed progressively increasing spasticity, providing progressively larger and larger resistances to externally imposed motion. This barrier has proven difficult for therapists to manage. Furthermore, in order to do this training effectively, therapists need to sit low at the edge of a treadmill and to manually move the limbs of the patient to match the treadmill motion. This manual approach has proven to be physically demanding, a source of fatigue, and has even resulted in musculoskeletal and joint injuries to therapists. Furthermore, the approach also requires that there be many therapists involved, typically three or four for a single training session, to minimize therapist fatigue, making the economics of the training plan uncertain at best. (This is because insurance plans in many countries will cover only a single therapist for one training session.)

For all these reasons, engineers have been encouraged to develop alternate therapeutic devices that could substitute for the rather arduous human manual labour. In addition to serving as a substitute for such physical labour, gait-training devices such as the Lokomat® generate additional valuable information about patient impairment levels, as well as their response to locomotor therapy. This is because the robot sensors can register the amount of weight bearing that the patient can sustain, the tolerated gait speed, and the patterns of muscular activation, all measures of overall impairment levels.

Finally, the devices are also able to track precisely the amount of locomotor therapy that is actually delivered, such as the number of steps taken, the level of weight bearing utilized, the average gait speed, and the amount of time spent in training. As a consequence, such robotic devices have proven very popular, and there have been many advanced systems developed for upper and lower extremity training.

To date, however, the results of most of these robotic therapies have been surprisingly meager. In most published trials the responses of robotic training for either upper or lower extremity have been marginally better than those provided by an experienced therapist (e.g. Lo et al. [1] for upper extremity training in stroke survivors), and in some instances have even been somewhat worse [2], potentially for reasons relating to patient compliance and to the actual work performed.

Because of these inconsistent results, there has been an ongoing reassessment of the value of these robotic devices, both from the standpoint of the degree of clinical improvement that they generate, but also from the standpoint of their cost-benefit to the clinical service. Since these devices are uniformly rather expensive, it has become rather difficult to determine whether the investment required to purchase these devices is financially justifiable. For all these reasons, there are a number of legitimate concerns being raised now that require suitable answers.

1. Should robotic devices try to emulate the therapist?

   Many of these new robotic devices, especially robotic gait trainers, seek to emulate or to expand the capacity of the clinical therapist, so it would seem to be important to determine at the outset whether therapy performed without robots is effective. The answer, in brief, is not yet clear, and there are surprisingly few examples where the effects of non-robotic physical therapy have been carefully documented and shown to be positive.

In one recent publication summarizing the effects of locomotor treadmill training without robotic assistance, the effects of such training were inconclusive [3]. As a consequence, the notion that the robotic should emulate the therapist closely is unproven.

2. If robots are going to be used to augment the training offered by therapists, what are the appropriate control algorithms?

a. **Position control**—in early studies, locomotion robots were often configured as position control systems, imposing relatively rigid patterns of joint angular motion on the lower extremities during walking. This approach appeared to have considerable value in non-ambulatory weak patients, in that it preserved joint range of motion, and imposed controlled yet beneficial loading on bone and muscle. However, as soon as some degree of locomotor recovery emerged, these position-controlled robotic systems have proven to be of less of obvious value. This is because the subjects routinely begin to relax, allowing the gait trainer to do the work for them. In this way, a key ingredient for recovery, which is engagement and involves active subject participation, is at least partly lost, and the clinical outcomes routinely suffer.

b. **Impedance control**—here, the limbs are driven so that there is some freedom to move the robot within a spring-like force field, allowing more active subject participation, although the approach does not readily emulate the therapist's interactions with the patient. This impedance control has some inherent advantages, because it is less restrictive with regard to dictating limb motion, and it allows a degree of natural variability in the limb path.

On the other hand, it does not take account of the desired limb trajectory, in the way that an experienced therapist might seek to steer subject initiated voluntary limb motion, nudging limb movement progressively towards a more effective and safer movement pattern.

c. **Cooperative control**—here the robot most closely emulates the actions of the therapist in that the system provides assistance or guidance when there is some deviation from therapist-selected kinematic parameters, yet there is minimal intervention when the limb is moving appropriately. This approach appears to be the most promising, in that it allows the patient to expend effort constructively, to practise, and to learn key functional tasks en route to improving overall locomotor function.

One major remaining issue, however, is that we do not know how to define the movement 'error' precisely. For example, should endpoint motion follow a 'normal' hand path (in the case of the upper extremity) or should other norms be adopted?

Error reduction or error magnification for movement training?

In recent years there has been increasing interest in using control algorithms, in which the movement error revealed during voluntary motion by the patient is forcibly increased during training, either by moving the limb physically in a different direction using a robotic device (such as the IMT Manus system), or by distorting visual feedback displays to place the limb in a different position than actually visualized.

This approach has been actively explored during training with an upper extremity planar robot that can impose unusual types of force perturbations during voluntary limb motion to a target. (These perturbations include so-called 'negative viscosity', in which forces are applied in a direction orthogonal to the targeted limb motion with a magnitude that varies in proportion to the speed of such motion.)

The evidence so far is that this approach may expedite the rate of improvement, but may not necessarily achieve a substantially better long-term outcome, as measured in terms of movement accuracy or smoothness of voluntary motion, or in terms of functional clinical benefit (see [4]).

When should therapy be delivered?

There is ongoing debate about the optimal timing of physical or occupational therapy, as to whether the most effective time for therapy is early after a cerebral or spinal lesion, (within the first few weeks), or potentially later, or whether there is a difference in outcome.

There is little direct evidence to help us here, although there has been a recurring concern that early therapy may sometimes aggravate the severity of brain lesions. In animal models, for example, early therapy may very increase stroke lesion size. (Quite recently, findings from Martin Schwab's group in Zurich [5] have shown that in animal models, early exercise after a stroke may limit collateral sprouting from corticospinal fibres, potentially reducing efficacy of a rehabilitation treatment—in this case with NO-GO antibody.)

If the results of these animal studies can be generalized to human stroke or brain injury, it may be prudent to wait several weeks after a stroke before intensive therapy or drug treatments are initiated.

Next steps

It is our general thesis that training objectives for many robotic device applications in stroke and spinal cord injury are currently not well thought through, and as a consequence, failure to produce clinically significant benefits may be attributable to both unrealistic expectations about the impact of robotic therapies, and to the limitations of control algorithms used, rather than to any inherent limitation of robotic device design or performance itself.

One of the reasons for this claim is that the control model that is used for training by rehabilitation robots is that we are usually attempting to rapidly retrain an impaired limb motion to a movement path approximating a 'normal' movement trajectory. Unfortunately, this approach may not be realistic, and may ultimately be doomed to fail.

Furthermore, we also assume that the neural plasticity in other types of motor learning will help to restore the trajectory to a normal pattern. This idea is largely, if not completely, untested.

What movement trajectory should we be correcting to?

Many robotic systems correct the error in limb movement trajectory of the stroke or spinal cord injured patient toward a hypothetical idealized trajectory, related often to that displayed by a healthy control subject. Typically, a normal hand movement path, for example, in which an object is being picked up by the hand, involves essentially straight-line movement of the hand from its initial position toward the object, with the profile of hand velocity appearing to be a smooth, 'bell shaped ' velocity curve with low values for higher acceleration derivatives (i.e. approaching 'minimum jerk' properties). This type of linear movement profile appears to generate rather smooth movements routinely, although it remains unclear as to whether this smoothness is directly controlled by the nervous system, or whether it emerges naturally from the mechanical filtering properties of muscle and other tissues.

While the approach of emulating a straight-line movement is overtly rational (because we would certainly like to restore a movement trajectory toward the normal) at least in broad terms, it may not be the most effective. This is because generating the 'normal' hand trajectory may require that the stroke survivor retain the ability to program spatial and temporal features of muscle activation that are no longer within the subject's movement repertoire. Instead, it might be more helpful to target movement strategies that use some kind of progressive staging in modulating the movement path that is potentially more achievable, at least in the short term.

To illustrate, some years ago in our own research studies, (see [6]), we examined target-directed voluntary movement of the upper extremity in stroke survivors under two distinct conditions. In the first, we asked the subject to move in the horizontal plane to a displayed target above a table with no major support of arm weight provided. In this situation, in which shoulder and arm muscles were needed to support the weight of the limb, limb motion was overtly impaired, in that the range of voluntary hand movement was markedly reduced, and the hand trajectory was often rather irregular, often displaying a curved movement path.

We then supported the same subject's arm on a low friction surface, (here we used an air table), eliminating the need for the subject to oppose gravitational forces, and repeated the target acquisition sequence. Under these conditions, the hand movement trajectory improved radically, with many subjects now able to reach the targets throughout the available workspace. The hand trajectories were routinely much straighter and more accurate in the supported limb, although there were still some clear abnormalities in limb braking and target capture, presumably because of the abnormally low friction environment. (This low friction environment would not be experienced by many people in the course of daily living.)

Our premise in these studies was that while synergies (abnormal coupling between muscles acting to move the limb) were presumably a factor, other factors, such as a loss of the ability to predict the mechanical behaviour of the limb during relatively rapid motion apparently also contributed. This loss of the ability to plan for mechanical interactions between limb segments (or coupling torques) is sometimes described as an impairment or loss of an 'internal model' of the limb mechanics.

Suffice it to say that many features of abnormal motion do appear to be linked to an inability to predict how the limb kinematics will behave when the limb is moving rapidly over a low friction surface, whether or not there is a disruption of some internal model located within some part of the motor or premotor cerebral cortex.

Whether the motor impairments are due to loss of internal models, to abnormal synergies to reflex couplings, or to muscle weakness remains unclear. None the less, it is still likely that we are targeting unrealistic goals by asking stroke survivors to attempt to

---

Box 29.1 Promises of rehabilitation technologies

1. **Rehabilitation robotics** offers the promise that clinicians can expand their capacity to treat multiple patients effectively at the same time, while collecting detailed information about impairment level, and the response to therapy. Widespread use should allow low cost treatments to many patients.

2. **More advanced functional electrical stimulation (FES) applications** will potentially allow restoration of grip and arm motion in the paralysed upper extremity, and may even enable limited standing and walking in patients with complete spinal cord injury.

3. **FES** promises to maintain muscle mass in situation where voluntary motion is impaired, and it can help maintain skin integrity, bone mass and improve autonomic function, especially in patients with complete spinal cord injury.

4. **Virtual reality systems** are immersive, entertaining and will help patients practice their motor and sensory task, increasing the dose of relevant therapy.

Challenges of rehabilitation technologies

1. **Rehabilitation robots.** Although there were high expectations for the therapeutic impact and for the cost benefits that would accrue from the use of these systems, these expectations have not yet been fulfilled.

2. **FES.** Whereas more limited FES applications have been accepted, and are in widespread use (foot drop stimulators, shoulder pain therapies) more ambitious uses for grasp restoration or for standing have not found acceptance, because of the complexity of the technology and the need for operative placement.

3. **Virtual reality systems** are also in widespread use, but their use remains to be validated. This delay is linked, in part to the almost continuous change in the technology, coupled with uncertainty about the therapeutic benefit of many systems, especially the most advanced and costly version.

---

behave 'normally' by attempting to achieve straight-line smooth voluntary motion.

In short, we assert that a 'null' trajectory, such as that displayed during low friction minimal weight bearing settings may serve as a more manageable target for therapy training than current control strategies. We can then make an argument that trajectory estimated under zero load is the best indicator of the underlying limb trajectory, and that this should serve as a basis for a progressive path correction implemented as part of rehabilitation of the upper extremity and hand.

Conclusions

In the last 10–15 years, there has been an impressive growth in the numbers and kinds of advanced technologies available for treating patients with neurological disorders, including robotic trainers, electrical stimulation systems, virtual reality immersion trainers, and wearable sensors to track progress. Although enthusiasm for these technologies was initially very high, and expectations were that the systems would match or exceed the performance of therapists, these expectations have not been fully sustained, and technology-based therapies have proven to be only marginally more effective than advanced physical or occupational therapy, especially when this therapy is delivered by experienced clinicians.

Although it is now tempting to dismiss many of these new technologies as a fad, they bring to the clinic the ability to deliver precisely controlled interventions in a way that no therapist can readily emulate. Furthermore, they also bring the ability to quantify outcomes, as well as duration and intensity of therapy.

It is our belief that the limited efficacy shown so far may be related to the way these systems are used, rather than to any inherent flaws in their design or application. If more precise therapy models are utilized, we expect that therapeutic outcomes will be more substantial, especially if we apply these therapies earlier after the stroke or spinal cord injury.

This so-called 'window of opportunity' may well begin much earlier than we envision, and more importantly, may close within a relatively few weeks, essentially eliminating the potential value almost all rehabilitation trials that have been done to date (e.g. [1–4] and Box 29.1).

References

1. Lo AC, Guarino PD, Richards LG et al. Robot-assisted therapy for long-term upper-limb impairment after stroke. N Engl J Med. 2011;**365**(18):1749.
2. Hidler J, Nichols D, Pellucid M, et al. Multicenter randomized clinical trial evaluating the effectiveness of the Loomed in sub acute stroke. Neurorehabil Neural Repair. 2009;**23**(1):5–13.
3. Duncan PW, Sullivan KJ, Behrman AL, et al, LEAPS Investigative Team. Body-weight-supported treadmill rehabilitation after stroke. N Engl J Med.2011;**364**(21):2026–2036.
4. Abdollahi F, Case Lazarro ED, Listenberger M, et al. Error augmentation enhancing arm recovery in individuals with chronic stroke: a randomized crossover design. Neurorehabil Neural Repair. 2013;
5. Wahl AS, Omlor W, Rubio JC, Chen JL, Zheng H, Schröter A, Gullo M, Weinmann O, Kobayashi K, Helmchen F, Ommer B, Schwab ME. Neuronal repair. Asynchronous therapy restores motor control by rewiring of the rat corticospinal tract after stroke. *Science*. 2014;**344**(6189):1250–1255. doi: 10.1126/science.1253050.
6. Beer RF, Dewald JP, Rymer WZ. Deficits in the coordination of multijoint arm movements in patients with hemiparesis: evidence for disturbed control of limb dynamics. Exp Brain Res. 2000; **131**(3):305–319.

CHAPTER 30

Application of orthoses and neurostimulation in neurorehabilitation

Jacopo Carpaneto and Silvestro Micera

Introduction

In the next future, it is expected that the proportion of persons over 65 will increase by more than 70% in the industrialized countries, and by more than 200% worldwide. This age group is particularly prone to cerebrovascular accidents or neurodegenerative diseases. These trends pose significant challenges to the organization of health and social care services. At the same time, there is an increasing number of subjects (especially young subjects) suffering central nervous system injuries (spinal cord injury (SCI), or traumatic brain injury (TBI)) from a variety of new trend sports, and this creates a significant problem for our society.

In the last decades, new rehabilitation strategies based on electrical stimulation (ES), orthoses, and robotic devices have been proposed in order to overcame some limits of traditional rehabilitation techniques based on manual therapies (e.g. need for more therapist to manually assist patients during training, repetitive exercises, costs, quantitative assessment of motor recovery) [1, 2]. Different mechatronic systems such as passive and active foot orthoses, overground upper and lower limb trainers, body weight support systems, and exoskeleton have been developed [1–2]. The goal of this chapter is to summarize the main achievement in using ES or ES combined with orthosis in order to restore grasping and locomotor functions using different stimulation approaches.

Orthosis

Orthoses are non-surgical, wearable, and relatively low-cost devices applied externally to the upper or lower limb in order to restore or improve motor functions (e.g. grasping or walking) in subjects affected by different neuro-muscular disorders (e.g. SCI, stroke, TBI, multiple sclerosis, cerebral palsy, peripheral nerve injury). Orthoses can support movements, correct, and prevent injury in subjects both in acute and chronic conditions. Orthoses can be roughly classified as passive and active. Passive orthoses do not allow motion and they can be used for support purposes whereas active orthoses allow motion.

Upper limb orthoses [3] are mainly used in order to assist movements of weak muscles and allow functions with the main aims to increase range of motion (ROM), block undesired joints movements, enhance functions, and prevent contractures. This kind of orthoses can be classified as: clavicular and shoulder orthoses, arm orthoses, functional arm orthoses, and elbow orthoses.

Lower limb orthoses [1–2, 4–5] are mainly used to increase the quality and efficacy of walking, reducing or correcting abnormal gait patterns, and decreasing abnormal tone and posture. This kind of orthoses can be classified as: shoes orthosis, foot orthosis, ankle–foot orthosis, knee–ankle–foot orthosis, knee orthosis, and trunk hip–knee–ankle–foot orthosis.

In order to overcame one of the major limit of ES (i.e. fatigue, see next section), ES has been combined with orthoses obtaining systems called hybrid assistive systems (HAS) or hybrid orthotic systems (HOS) [6–7]. Some examples of these devices will be introduced and described in subsequent sections.

Electrical stimulation

ES is a widely used technique for artificially generating nerve and muscle activations in humans. A series of short electrical current pulses are applied between pairs of electrodes, which can be transcutaneous, percutaneous (through the skin), or implanted either directly onto the surface of the muscle (epimysial) or placed around the nerve (monopolar, bipolar, or multipolar cuffs). The stimulation pulses can be monophasic or charge-balanced biphasic (symmetric or asymmetric), with the latter providing optimal control of contraction force whilst minimizing tissue damage [8–9].

The current distribution generated between the anode and cathode changes the relative concentration of ions (e.g. potassium and sodium) resulting in hyperpolarization and depolarization of excitable cellular membranes. Action potentials can be generated in nerve axons once depolarization of their transmembrane potential exceeds –55 mV [10]. The volume of tissue surrounding the cathode, where nerve axons and fibre bundles can be activated, can be defined as an activation volume. Although ES can be used to directly activate muscle fibres [11], the excitation thresholds (and hence stimulation amplitudes) are typically significantly higher (>100) than the motoneurons that innervate the muscle. Thus most ES applications either target the motoneurons directly; or where their sub-branches innervate the target muscles (motor-points) [12]. During volitional activation of the muscles, the nerve (and hence muscle) fibres are activated asynchronously, allowing fine control of movement; with the larger (alpha) fibres recruited to provide stronger contractions. However, ES preferentially activates the larger (alpha) nerve fibres (and smaller fibres close to the electrode) synchronously, which can lead to loss of fine control and reduced fatigue resistance within the contracted muscle [8, 11, 13].

ES has been widely used for treatment of pain, muscle training, and functional restoration of movement. To obtain maximum functional benefit it is necessary for subjects to regularly use ES systems both clinically and at home [14]. Ideally, ES systems and their associated electrodes must therefore be able to selectively activate the target muscle, simple to configure, easy to set up (or don and doff), comfortable to use, and have an intuitive volitional control [8, 11, 13]. Different types of electrodes can be used to achieve ES [15]. In particular, surface stimulation, peripheral stimulation using invasive electrodes or spinal stimulation can be achieved.

It is possible to distinguish between functional electrical stimulation (FES) and therapeutic electrical stimulation (TES). In the first case, ES is used in order to elicit muscular contraction and to obtain functional activities (e.g. grasping or walking). In the second case, ES is used in order to improve impairments through therapeutic sessions (and not in a continuous way). A neuroprosthesis (NP) can be considered as a multichannel ES system, which is used to restore functional movements to muscles after damage to the nervous system [8, 11, 13]. Many NPs are used to help improve activities of daily living (e.g. grasping) or quality of life (e.g. bladder stimulation) [13]. The choice of electrode technology is based upon the required functionality for each subject. Most NP control systems generate predefined stimulation patterns in

response to user-defined interactions; with parameters temporally varying (e.g. amplitude vs. gait phase for locomotion) or parametrically varying (e.g. hand grasp). Finally, the main indications and contraindications of stimulations for patients affected by stroke and SCI are given in Table 30.1.

Walking neuroprostheses

The main goal of walking neuroprostheses (WNPs) is to enable individuals with lower extremity paralysis (i) to prevent of footdrop, (ii) to restore standing and transfer, and (iii) to restore gait functions.

Non-invasive WNPs

In the 1960s Liberson proposed the use of ES for hemiplegic footdrop (Figure 30.1A) [16]. This first prototype of WNP elicited dorsiflexion in a hemiplegic foot and synchronized the application of electrotherapy with the swing phase of gait. Several researchers developed similar systems [17] and Vodovnik's group in Ljubljana systematically investigated the use of FES for the restoration of gait [18]. These systems used surface electrodes over the tibialis anterior and over the common peroneal nerve and a heel switch, worn in the shoe of the paretic side, was used to turn on the stimulation when the foot was lifted off the ground and off at heel strike.

Standing can be obtained with surface ES of the quadriceps alone [19] even if better results have been obtained by also stimulating the hip extensor [20].

In 1983 Kralj proposed a closed-loop control of stimulation of the quadriceps muscle group and the peroneal nerves in three complete SCI patients [21]. These subjects were able to walk in parallel bars or with the aid of a roller walker for shorter distances.

Starting from these first studies, several systems have been developed thanks to the advances in ES technology (e.g. electrodes, electronics, control) obtaining more complex and efficient stimulation [11, 17].

The first lower limb surface ES system Food and Drug Administration (FDA) approved and commercially available was the Parastep developed by Sigmedics (www.sigmedics.com) and based upon work by Graupe [22]. It used 12 electrodes placed over the back, gluteals, and lower extremities and a walker with hand controls to regulate standing and sitting. Standing and walking for short distances is a very demanding task for patients with SCI at T4/T11 level, even using the Parastep [23–24]. Nevertheless, the Parastep has been used in approximately 400 patients for independent short-distance ambulation with positive physical and psychological benefits, making it an important option for thoracic-level traumatic paraplegics [25].

Other similar commercially available WNPs based on peroneal nerve stimulation are the WalkAide System (Innovative Neurotronics, Austin, TX www.walkaide.com), the Odstock O2CHS (Odstock Medical, Avon, MA), and the L300 NESS (www.bioness.com). Walkaide, developed at the University of Alberta, is a single-channel ES device attached to a molded cuff located below the knee. The timing and duration of the stimulation during walking is controlled by means of a tilt sensor and an accelerometer. The Odstock is a two-channel foot switch controlled stimulator. The timing of muscle activation can be adjusted so that a contraction can occur as weight is transferred on or off a footswitch or set to occur at other times in the gait cycle by adding a delay following a footswitch transition. The

Table 30.1 Indications and contraindications of ES for patients affected by stroke and SCI

Indications of ES	Contraindications of ES
Upper limb: • SCI patients C5–C6 levels (restoration of tetraplegic hand and arm function) • In some cases SCI patients C4 or higher level tetraplegia • Stroke patients with hemiplegia (enhancement of upper-limb function) Lower limb: • SCI patients with T4–T12 levels (restoration of paraplegic standing and stepping) • Stroke patients (treatment of ankle dorsiflexion weakness)	• Cardiac pacemakers or other implanted electrical stimulators • Peripheral vascular disease if possibility of causing thrombi to loosen • Hypertension or hypotension can affect autonomic responses • Obesity • Impaired sensation • Neoplastic tissue • Skin disease or cancer at area of stimulation • Cognitive issues affecting ability to provide feedback • Undiagnosed pain • Not over carotid sinus • Not over thoracic region • Not over phrenic nerve • Not over trunk if pregnant • Not over relatively superficial metal implants • Not transcerebrally at milliamp • Not through areas of broken or irritated skin

device is used as an orthotic aid, replacing conventional splinting and also as a training device assisting gait re-education. A similar peroneal nerve stimulator has been developed by Bioness (NESS L300), and it consists of a small unit attached to the upper calf. The device can be used to assist subjects during walking after stroke, SCI, multiple sclerosis, brain injury or tumour, and cerebral palsy.

These systems demonstrated a good acceptance and a long-term improvement in walking speed/skill in persons with different disabilities [26–32].

HAS mainly used orthoses in order to provide body weight support and allowing a reduction of stimulation during standing or gait stance phase. Examples of these devices consist in ES and orthotic components such as the Oswestry Parawalker orthosis [33], reciprocal gait orthosis [34], exoskeletal bracing [35–36], hip

(A)

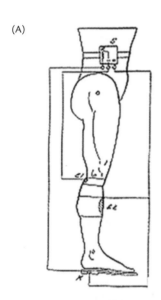

(B)

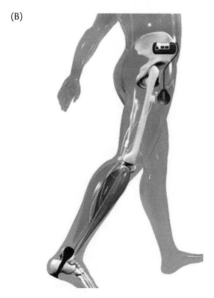

Fig. 30.1 (A) An approach for the stimulation of the quadriceps muscle group and the peroneal nerves; (B) the Actigate by Neurodan/Otto Bock.

Liberson WT, Holmquest HJ, Scot D, Dow M Functional electrotherapy: stimulation of the peroneal nerve synchronized with the swing phase of the gait of hemiplegic patients. Arch Phys Med Rehabil. 1961;42:101–105.

constraint orthosis [37], and very complex robotic orthosis (e.g. Lokomat [38]). Recently, a commercial knee–ankle–foot orthosis (Ottobock Sensor Walk) has been integrated with an ES system and a walker obtaining a walking rehabilitation system [39]. These devices have been tested in subjects with thoracic paraplegia allowing a reduction in muscle fatigue and an increase of walking speed.

In the last decades, multichannel stimulators and percutaneous and implanted electrodes have been developed and tested in order to overcome some of the main drawbacks of surface WNPs (i.e. reduced muscle selectivity, muscle fatigue, limited walking distance, fine control of joint trajectories).

Percutaneous WNPs

A more invasive approach in order to elicit spinal reflexes for ambulation is the use of percutaneous electrodes. This technique allows the direct activation and control of individual muscles. Researchers at the Cleveland Veterans Affairs (VA) Medical Center and Case Western Reserve University (CWRU; Cleveland OH) were able to synthetize complex activation of lower limb muscles using percutaneous electrodes [40]. Daly et al. [41], implanted 124 electrodes into the lower limb of 17 subjects. Good muscle response was found in 93% of electrodes also achieving gains in subject impairment and disability measures.

Implantable WNPs

CWRU/VA developed an implantable neuroprosthesis that can be used by SCI subjects for standing assisted transfer, and exercises [42]. This WNP consists of an eight-channel receiver–stimulator implanted in the anterior lower abdomen, epimysial and intramuscular electrodes, a wearable external control unit, a command ring (worn around the index finger), a transmitting coil, a charger, and a clinical programming station.

The epimysial electrodes were implanted bilaterally on the vastus lateralis for knee extension and on the gluteus maximus and the semimembranosus for hip extension, whereas intramuscular electrodes were implanted in the lumbar erector spinae for trunk support, with the main aim to provide postural support and power during the sit-to-stand and stand-to-sit transition. Twelve subjects with SCI at different levels (from C6 to T9) participated in a pilot study demonstrating that this kind of implantable WNP provides standing, allows the subject to perform some tasks in the environment, standing times range from 3 to >40 minutes, a limited swing-through walking with a walker, and less required assistance. User satisfaction was high.

An alternative to epimysial or intramuscular electrodes is represented by electrodes placed around or in the peripheral nerve. This approach allows the stimulation of target axons with a reduced surgery time, lower stimulation amplitudes, and better selectivity (recruitment of multiple muscles or independent motor unit pools) [43].

Nerve cuff electrodes, such as the CWRU spiral cuffs, have already been successfully used in chronic clinical applications. In one case study, a IST-16 system and four-contact spiral nerve-cuff electrodes were implanted in the distal branches of the femoral nerve innervating the quadriceps, obtaining good results in terms of cuff stability and selectivity and standing times [44–45]. Moreover, a flat interface nerve electrode (FINE), an evolution of the CWRU cuff electrodes, was recently placed intraoperatively around the tibial and/or common peroneal nerve, demonstrating the ability to selectively restore plantarflexion or dorsiflexion [43, 46].

Examples of commercial multichannel implantable peroneal nerve stimulator are the STIMuSTEP and the ActiGait (Neurodan/Otto Bock). The first device is a two-channel device able to produce dorsiflexion and inversion and eversion of the foot by means of the individual stimulation of the deep and superficial branches of the common peroneal nerve [47]. Power and control signals for stimulation are transmitted through the skin using radio telemetry from a transmitter unit worn externally over the implant, held in place by an elastic strap. The device is controlled using a foot switch placed in the users' shoe.

The Actigait (Figure 30.1B) consists of a nerve cuff with four tripolar electrodes placed around the common peroneal nerve, a control unit, a heel switch that triggers the initiation and termination of each stimulation sequence, and a clinical station [48]. Fifteen hemiplegic subjects participated in a study, with the main aim to evaluate the safety and performance of the device, obtaining improvement in walking speed and distance and good acceptance by patients [48].

Finally, a 'BIONic' foot drop stimulator has been developed and tested in one patient [49]. The device is based on a modified WalkAide system plus a BION, an injectable microstimulator that receives power and control information from an external transmitting coil (without the need for surgical implantation of wires) [50]. The results obtained demonstrated that BIONs were more selective in activating the ankle dorsiflexor muscles than surface stimulation of the common peroneal nerve, and produced a more balanced flexion of the ankle during walking [49].

Spinal WNPs

Spinal cord stimulation (epidural and intraspinal ES) are two new approaches that can be used to produce: (i) in case of epidural stimulation, rhythmic, locomotor-like movements in the legs, presumably due to the activation of afferent pathways; and (ii) in case of intraspinal stimulation an activation of spinal motoneurons and interneuron circuits [51–52]. Intraspinal ES was tested in the lumbosacral spinal cord of rats, cats, and frogs, evoking functional and complex movements of paralysed limbs [53–54]. On the other hand, hind limb stepping in partially and completely transected rats was obtained combining serotonergic agonism with epidural stimulation of the lumbar spinal cord (Figure 30.2) [55–56].

Recently, a 16-electrode array was implanted on the dura (L1–S1 cord segments) of a paraplegic subject (C7–T1 level) and epidural stimulation allowed some functional recovery (standing with assistance for some minutes and locomotor-like patterns) [57]. During this first case study, epidural stimulation showed to be able to reactivate previously silent spared neural circuits or promote plasticity.

While the results in animals have been very encouraging, several technical advancements (i.e. new electrodes, implantable stimulator, and control strategies) are necessary prior to any extensive translation in humans with SCI.

Main advantages and limits of the WNPs

ES systems for lower limbs, independently of the choice of electrodes (e.g. surface, percutaneous, or implantable), seem usable for standing and short distance walking, often in combination with orthoses and walkers. Some cons are related to insufficient selectivity, learning how to use the device properly, and donning and doffing procedures. In particular, these devices suffer from a risk from falling due to poor balance of the subjects, energy cost and fatigue, and slow speed of gait. Even if WNPs cannot be used today as a replacement for wheelchairs or as a mobility device, users appreciated the possibility to achieve standing and locomotion in small environments. Moreover, exercises and ambulation with a WNP allow a more positive health effect respect to the ambulation with only orthoses [8]. HAS seem able to improve balance and mobility even if with some disadvantages such as encumbrance and weight.

Grasping neuroprostheses

The main goal of grasping neuroprostheses (GNPs) is to enable individuals with upper extremity paralysis due to SCI and stroke (i) to use their hands in activities of daily living (ADL) and (ii) to perform therapeutic exercises.

Several GNPs have been developed in the past years using different approaches to achieve muscle recruitment.

Non-invasive GNPs

In the last decades, some NPs for the restoration of grasp functions have been developed, with surface electrodes, (e.g. Bionic Glove, Belgrade Grasping System, UNAFET 4, Compex II, and Bioness H200) [11, 58] (Figure 30.3). Despite some drawbacks and few clinical trials, GNPs demonstrated some clinical benefits to subjects [8, 13].

Starting from the pioneering work of Long in 1960 [59], the first devices consisted of a splint and they were able to provide capabilities of opening and closing the hand.

These prototypes were tested in quadriplegic patients [60] and in hemiplegic patients [61]. Following these preliminary studies and after technological improvement, the first commercial device has been developed: the NESS Handmaster (Ra'anana, Israel). The device was designed in order to be used by C5 tetraplegic patients as well as with hemiplegic (stroke) patients. It is based on five surface electrodes embedded into an orthosis and able to stimulate five muscles (flexor digitorum superficialis (FDS), extensor pollicis brevis (EPB), flexor pollicis longus (FPL), extensor digitorum communis (EDC), and thenar). Two functional grasps (i.e. key and palmar grips) and some exercise modes can be selected using an external switch on the control unit. This device has been used for small clinical trials in subjects with a cervical SCI between C4 and C6 [62] and subacute and chronic stroke [63–64].

More recently, this device (now known as the NESS H200 Hand Rehabilitation System (Bioness, Inc, Valencia, CA) has been used in a large clinical trials on chronic stroke patients [65] reporting as some beneficial effects on muscle hypertonia, pain, oedema, and passive ROM. These effects confirmed what obtained in previous studies with a small number of patients.

The Bionic Glove [66] is a fingerless glove with a forearm sleeve worn over surface electrodes that is placed over the finger flexors and extensors. Voluntary wrist movements (e.g. wrist extension for grasping and wrist flexion for release) can be used to control the ES and to produce opening and closing of the hand. Tested in subjects with C5–C7 SCI, it provided an improvement of the independence in these subjects [67].

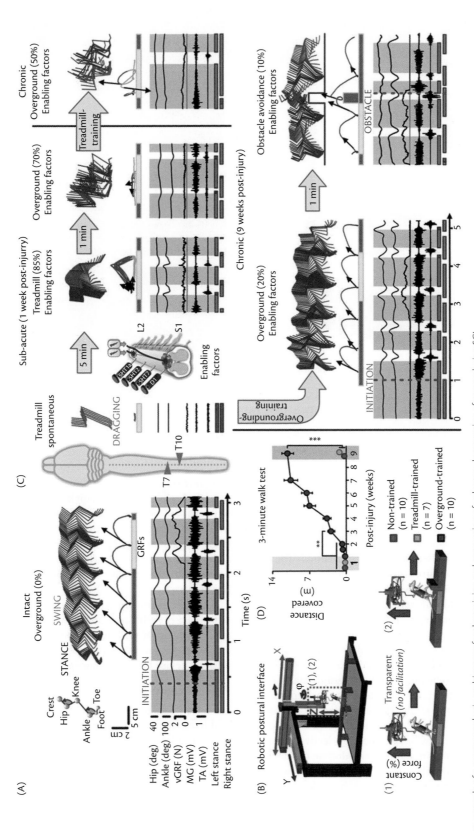

Fig. 30.2 An example of a neuroprosthetic multisystem for the training and restoration of voluntary locomotion after paralyzing SCI.

From van den Brand R, Heutschi J, Barraud Q, DiGiovanna J, Bartholdi K, Huerlimann M, Friedli L, Vollenweider I, Moraud EM, Duis S, Dominici N, Micera S, Musienko P, Courtine G. Restoring voluntary control of locomotion after paralyzing spinal cord injury. Science. 2012 Jun 1;336(6085):1182–5. Reprinted with permission from AAAS.

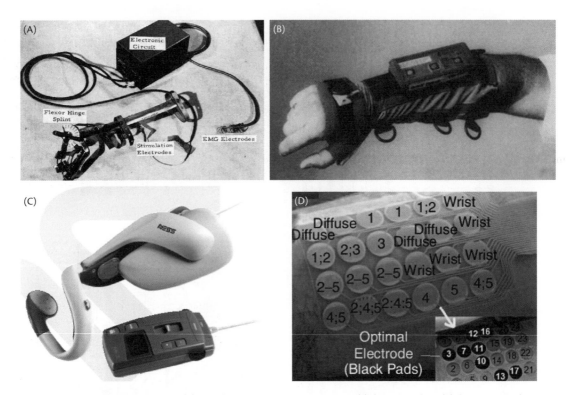

Fig. 30.3 Different examples of GNP to restore grasping: (A) one of the first non-invasive prototype; (B) the Bionic Glove; (C) the NESS H200 by Bioness; (D) a flexible transcutaneous electrode array.

(A) From Vodovnik, L.; Long, C.; Reswick, J.B.; Lippay, A.; Starbuck, D. Myo-Electric Control of Paralyzed Muscles. Biomedical Engineering, IEEE Transactions on. 1965; BME-12(3 and 4):169–72. (B) Reprinted from Archives of Physical Medicine and Rehabilitation, 80(3), Dejan Popović, Aleksandar Stojanović, Andjelka Pjanović, Slobodanka, Radosavljević, Mirjana Popović, Stevan Jović, Dragan Vulović, Clinical evaluation of the bionic glove, 299–304, Copyright (1999), with permission from Elsevier. (D) Reprinted from Artificial Organs, Ana Popović-Bijelić, Goran Bijelić, Nikola Jorgovanović, Dubravka Bojanić, Mirjana B. Popović, Dejan B. Popović, Multi-Field Surface Electrode for Selective Electrical Stimulation, 448–452, Copyright (2005), with permission from John Wiley & Sons Ltd.

The Belgrade Grasping System [68] (and its successor, the ActiGrips System), is a GNP that also allows reaching function. It has four stimulation channels (three to generate grasping function and one to stimulate the triceps brachii muscle and to allow elbow extension). The grasping function (i.e. hand opening and closing) is externally controlled through a push button. The subject's shoulder velocity, measured through a goniometer, was used to stimulate the triceps brachii muscle and to control the reaching function. The Belgrade Grasping System was tested in eight subjects with chronic tetraplegia and it resulted in an improvement in hand grasping activity [58]. Concerning its therapeutic efficiency, it was tested in 12 chronic tetraplegics with a complete sensory–motor lesion at C5/C6 level shoulder [58]. This GNP was marketed as ActiGrips System and it has been commercially available since 2003. Even if they provided interesting performance in terms of motor recruitment, all the above mentioned GNPs were characterized by common drawbacks such as: risk of generate undesired movements due to a limited muscle selectivity, muscle fatigue, difficulty in control, in donning and doffing the devices, and in the electrode positioning [69]. Despite these drawbacks, GNPs based on transcutaneous electrodes are by far least invasive and are therefore regularly used for therapeutic applications of ES (TES) [14, 68, 70–72].

More recently, arrays of small transcutaneous electrodes have been developed and positioned over the portion of the forearm in order to selectively activate finger muscles [70, 73–74]. Early transcutaneous electrode arrays were constructed with flexible straps with integrated isolated conductive rubber patches [75]. More recently flexible printed circuit boards with individual electrolyte soaked pads [76], as well as novel embroidered electrodes [77] have been used. The control of these arrays selecting the optimal electrode location and stimulation parameters can be done using an automatic algorithm [78]. The use of embroidered electrode technology can also improve muscle selectivity and practicability of this approach [69].

Finally, a non-invasive modular hybrid neuro-orthosis (OrthoJacket [79]) has been proposed for the restoration of hand and arm functions in high tetraplegic SCI subjects. OrthoJacket combines ES for the activation of paralysed muscles with an orthotic device for the mechanical stabilization.

Percutaneous GNPs

The advantages of the percutaneous electrode are the elimination of skin resistance and cutaneous pain issues, greater muscle selectivity, and lower stimulation currents. Percutaneous electrodes are particularly usefully in activating small, deep muscles, such as the intrinsic muscles of the hand.

Starting from a first clinical trial with percutaneous electrodes implanted in C6 tetraplegic patient [80], a 30 percutaneous electrodes GNP (FESMate) was developed in the 1980s [81]. The device was able to provide several stimulation patterns for several hand grasps and upper extremity motions. The FESMate was controlled by different commands (i.e. push button, head switches, voice, sip and puff, and shoulder motion). This system has been tested with subjects with cervical SCI (C4–C6) and hemiplegia to produce hand, forearm, elbow, and shoulder movements, but limited data are available in terms of clinical outcome of the experiments.

GNPs using implanted peripheral neural and muscular electrodes

The implantation of electrodes and stimulators that deliver current directly to the targeted nerves is still investigated in order to solve some of the main drawbacks of surface approach. Two very interesting approaches will be described here, showing their promising clinical achievements: (i) a fully implantable device (Freehand) and the (ii) use of cuff electrodes.

The Freehand is an implantable device developed with the main aim to restore lateral and palmar grasps in subjects with C5-C5 tetraplegia [82–83]. This implantable GNP is based on a fully implantable stimulator located in the subject's anterior chest. The stimulator is connected with eight epimysial or intramuscular electrodes implanted near motor points of hand and forearm muscles. The stimulator communicates with and external programmable control unit by means of a radiofrequency transmitting coil. An additional sensor detects contralateral shoulder movements and uses this signal to control the opening and closing of the hand. The system has been implanted in more than 250 tetraplegic patients (C5 and C6 level) [8]. From the results of a multicenter study with 51 C5 and C6 tetraplegic subjects [84] and other small studies [85–86], the Freehand was able to improve pinch force and grasp release abilities, resulting in a greater independency in performing ADLs. Patients expressed satisfaction [84] and the implant seemed very robust to failure (i.e. a survival rate of 98.7% considering 238 electrodes implanted for a time ranging from 3 years up to 16 years [87]). Despite these promising clinical results, the Freehand was not commercially available since 2011. A second version, not yet commercially available, has been recently developed (Figure 30.4) [88]. This new version increased the number of stimulation electrodes (i.e. from 8 to 12 allowing better upper limb functions such as forearm pronation and reaching by elbow extension) and it allows the recording of electromyography (EMG) from two muscles. One of the main improvements is the possibility to control the GNP with ispilateral muscles (i.e. wrist extension for grasp and wrist flexion for release) eliminating the need for contralateral shoulder movements. A recent study [88] in three C5/C6 SCI subjects obtained results similar to the first version (i.e. effective grasp and release function with high level of user satisfaction) [88]. Moreover, a case study with one stroke patient has been recently published and it demonstrated the effectiveness of the GNP with a resulting increase of the active range of finger extension, of the lateral pinch force, of the number of objects grasped and released, and of qualitative assessment scores [89].

A preliminary evaluation of nerve cuff electrodes in humans has been done intraoperatively in the ulnar and radial nerves of 21 human subjects [91]. The obtained results demonstrated the possibility to selectively and independently activate at least one muscle from one nerve. In a following study [92], nine spiral cuff electrodes were implanted in a chronic study (up to three years) in two subjects (C1 and C5 level respectively). A cuff electrode with four individually controllable stimulation sites was implanted in the radial nerve of both subjects and one received an additional

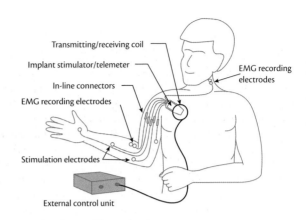

Fig. 30.4 The scheme of the Freehand system.
Kilgore KL, Hart RL, Montague FW, Bryden AM, Keith MW, Hoyen HA, Sams CJ, Peckham PH. An implanted myoelectrically-controlled neuroprosthesis for upper extremity function in spinal cord injury. Conf Proc IEEE Eng Med Biol Soc. 2006;1:1630–3.

cuff in the musculocutaneous nerve. The nerve conduction velocity, the threshold recruitment, the recruitment stability, and the recruitment selectivity were tested demonstrating that these electrodes were able to provide full and graded muscle contraction (similar to from muscle-based electrodes) in all target muscles without adverse changes in the nerve (recruitment properties or sensory effects).

Intraspinal GNPs

Starting from past experiments with animals [53–54], it seems that intraspinal ES may provide a means of artificially eliciting movements avoiding some disadvantages of conventional FES systems (i.e. recruitment of coordinated patterns of muscle contractions and reduction of fatigue due to a more physiological recruitment order). Recent experiments in monkeys [93–94] showed that using multisite intraspinal ES it is possible to restore coordinated activation of multiple muscles and control reaching and grasping movements. In Figure 30.5, an example of the potentials of this approach to restore grasping force is provided.

Main advantages and limits of GNPs

FES systems for upper limbs based on surface stimulation (i.e. Bionic Glove and NESS) seem able to restore some upper limb tasks (and in particular palmar grasp, hold, and release) even if the difficulties with donning and doffing, a reduced muscle stimulation selectivity, and control issues prevent a large clinical use of these devices [8, 11, 95]. The percutaneous approach (such as the NEC FESMate [96]) seems able to overcome some limits of surface electrodes (i.e. better selectivity, reduced pain, lower stimulation currents, reduced donning and doffing time) even if it is not suitable for long-term clinical use and it is afflicted by an increased risk of electrode breakage and infection. Finally, implantable systems (e.g. Freehand [83]) seem a solution that can be used in long-term clinical use thanks to a reduced risk of damage and infection, a low rate of failure [8, 11, 85], high selectivity of muscle stimulation, greater ADLs independence, better grasp, hold, and release, and high satisfaction. Of course, implantable systems require an additional surgery for the implantation of the GNP, a risk of tissue growth affecting the nerve, and high costs.

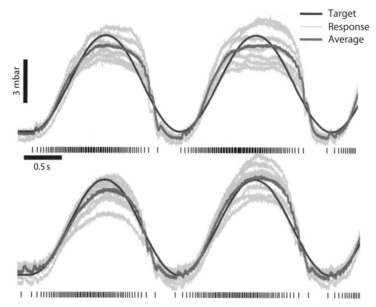

Fig. 30.5 Grip force achieved using two different encoding approaches for the intraspinal stimulation.
Zimmermann JB, Seki K, Jackson A. Reanimating the arm and hand with intraspinal microstimulation. J Neural Eng. 2011 Oct;8(5):054001.

Therapeutic electrical stimulation

ES of paralysed limbs can provide therapeutic benefits in SCI and post stroke patients [8, 13]. Exercises based on TES induce some positive physiological changes and in particular they can prevent osteoporosis, muscle atrophy, increase of body fat mass, and cardiovascular complications. Moreover, TES can promote/facilitate motor relearning and reduce spasticity and shoulder pain [13]. Exercises can be induced using body weight support devices or arm or leg cycle ergonomoters. Examples of arm or leg-cycle ergometers are the ERGYS (Therapeutic Alliances Inc., Fairborn, OH), the R300 (Restorative Therapies, Baltimore, MD), and the MotoMed (Reck-Technik, Betzenweiler, Germany). These systems combined stationary leg-cycle ergometer with surface ES to allow persons with little or no voluntary leg movement (e.g. SCI) to actively pedalling. Moreover, some of the above cited GNPs or WNPs or HAS can also be used not only to restore motor functions but also as a therapeutic systems. Finally, more sophisticated approaches for ES-based therapeutic exercises are based on robotic devices able to compensate arm or body weight [2]. One example combines a multichannel surface electrical stimulator applied to distal muscles in order to provide grasp and release movements of the hand, with a commercial robotic exoskeleton (ArmeoSpring, Hocoma AG) to provide gravity compensation of the shoulder and elbow [97]. A different system for the lower limb (RT600, Restorative Therapies, Baltimore, MD) combines two motorized footplates and a partial body weight support with the surface ES of leg and gluteal muscles in order to support stepping and standing.

Current challenges and future directions

Studies have shown that through regular use of ES, patients are able to help the recovery of some upper and lower limb function. However, despite much promise, ES-based neuroprostheses are limited by the tedious donning and doffing of stimulation electrodes and sensors, manual control parameter adjustment, fast onset of fatigue, physical therapist support. Clinicians often find the systems to be time consuming and overly complicated to use. Therefore, although ES technology has been used for decades and its benefits widely published, its use in the clinic is largely absent. To improve the situation it is necessary to increase the efficacy of the devices and their clinical usability. For example, non-invasive solutions have to provide an easy way for donning and doffing and for customizing the stimulation parameters. At the same time, more invasive solutions (based on peripheral or spinal stimulation) are still far from an extensive clear demonstration of clinical efficacy. Problems such as long-term usability and selectivity need to be addressed before an extensive clinical application could become possible.

Finally, hybrid solutions based on the synergistic use of ES and other approaches can be also envisaged in the future. For instance, new robotic-based training methodologies have emerged that promise to improve rehabilitation of patients who are unable to perform motor activities (walking, reaching, grasping). Examples of such patients are stroke survivors and SCI patients. Studies have shown that such robotic assistive devices can lead to very positive therapeutic outcomes. Despite the promise of robot-assisted therapy, a number of disadvantages limit its widespread use in the clinic. Such therapy mainly provides passive movements of limbs, which leads to low activity of muscles and metabolism. Moreover, robotic systems can lead to abnormal muscle activation patterns. Also, robotic gait trainers for rehabilitation generally lack actuated ankle joints. Such actuation is difficult to implement as application of high torque to the feet may be dangerous. Individual limitations of the robotic and ES therapies can be eliminated by combining the two modalities. Immediate advantages include promotion of normal muscle activation, the possibility for practice of normal patterns earlier during rehabilitation, reduced requirements on physical therapist support, and ankle/hand activation. The current studies show that there is interest in combined ES-robotic trainers, but that research and development are very much in the initial stages.

References

1. Díaz I, Gil JJ, Sánchez E. Lower-limb robotic rehabilitation: literature review and challenges. J Robotics. 2011;1–11: doi: 10.1155/2011/759764.

2. del-Ama AJ, Koutsou AD, Moreno JC, de-los-Reyes A, Gil-Agudo A, Pons JL. Review of hybrid exoskeletons to restore gait following spinal cord injury. J Rehabil Res Dev. 2012;49(4):497–514.

3. Tyson SF, Kent RM. The effect of upper limb orthotics after stroke: a systematic review. NeuroRehabilitation. 2011;28(1):29–36.

4. Ferris DP, Sawicki GS, Domingo A. Powered lower limb orthoses for gait rehabilitation. Top Spinal Cord Inj Rehabil. 2005;11(2):34–49.

5. Hasan SA, Hoque MZ. Lower limb orthoses: A review. J Chittagong Med Coll Teach Assoc. 2009 19(1):33–36.

6. Popovic D, Tomović R, Schwirtlich L. Hybrid assistive system—the motor neuroprosthesis. IEEE Trans Biomed Eng. 1989;36(7):729–737.

7. Popovic DB. Externally powered and controlled orthotics and prosthetics. The Biomedical Engineering Handbook. Joseph D. Bronzino, CRC Press, Boca Raton, FL, 2000, pp. 142/1–17.

8. Ragnarsson KT. Functional electrical stimulation after spinal cord injury: current use, therapeutic effects and future directions. Spinal Cord. 2008;46(4):255–274.

9. Keller T, Ellis MD, Dewald JP. Overcoming abnormal joint torque patterns in paretic upper extremities using triceps stimulation. Artif Organs. 2005;29(3):229–232.

10. Kandel ER, Schwartz JH, Jessell TM, Principles of Neural Science, Appleton & Lange, New York, 1991.

11. Peckham PH, Knutson JS. Functional electrical stimulation for neuromuscular applications. Annu Rev Biomed Eng. 2005;7:327–360.

12. Durand DM, Grill WM, Kirsch R. Electrical stimulation of the neuromuscular system. In: He B (ed.) Neural Engineering. Springer, Berlin, 2005, pp. 157–191.

13. Sheffler LR, Chae J. Neuromuscular electrical stimulation in neurorehabilitation. Muscle Nerve. 2007;35(5):562–590.

14. Alon G, Levitt SF, McCarthy PA. Functional electrical stimulation enhancement of upper extremity functional recovery during stroke rehabilitation: a pilot study. Neurorehabil Neural Repair 2007;21:207

15. Navarro X, Krueger TB, Lago N, Micera S, Stieglitz T, Dario P. A critical review of interfaces with the peripheral nervous system for the control of neuroprostheses and hybrid bionic systems. J Peripher Nerv Syst. 2005;10(3):229–258.

16. Liberson WT, Holmquest HJ, Scot D, Dow M Functional electrotherapy: stimulation of the peroneal nerve synchronized with the swing phase of the gait of hemiplegic patients. Arch Phys Med Rehabil. 1961;42:101–105.

17. Lyons GM, Sinkjaer T, Burridge JH, Wilcox DJ. A review of portable FES-based neural orthoses for the correction of drop foot. IEEE Trans Neural Syst Rehabil Eng. 2002;10(4):260–279.

18. Vodovnik L, Crochetiere WJ, Reswick JB. Control of a skeletal joint by electrical stimulation of antagonists. Med Biol Eng. 1967;5(2):97–109.

19. Bajd T, Kralj A, Sega J, Turk R, Benko H, Strojnik P. Use of a two-channel functional electrical stimulator to stand paraplegic patients. Phys Ther. 1981;61(4):526–527.

20. Kuzelicki J, Kamnik R, Bajd T, Obreza P, Benko H. Paraplegics standing up using multichannel FES and arm support. J Med Eng Technol. 2002;26(3):106–110.

21. Kralj A, Bajd T, Turk R, Krajnik J, Benko H. Gait restoration in paraplegic patients: a feasibility demonstration using multichannel surface electrode FES. J Rehabil R D. 1983;20(1):3–20.

22. Graupe D, Kohn K. Functional electrical stimulation for ambulation by paraplegics. Krieger, Malabar, FL, 1994.

23. Brissot R, Gallien P, Le Bot MP, et al. Clinical experience with functional electrical stimulation-assisted gait with Parastep in spinal cord-injured patients. Spine. 2000;25(4):501–508.

24. Jacobs PL, Johnson B, Mahoney ET. Physiologic responses to electrically assisted and frame-supported standing in persons with paraplegia. J Spinal Cord Med. 2003;26(4):384–389.

25. Graupe D, Kohn KH. Functional neuromuscular stimulator for short-distance ambulation by certain thoracic-level spinal-cord-injured paraplegics. Surg Neurol. 1998;50(3):202–207.

26. Wieler M, Stein RB, Ladouceur M, et al. Multicenter evaluation of electrical stimulation systems for walking. Arch Phys Med Rehabil 1999;80:495–500.

27. Taylor PN, Burridge JH, Dunkerley AL, et al. Clinical use of the Odstock dropped foot stimulator: its effect on the speed and effort of walking. Arch Phys Med Rehabil. 1999;80(12):1577–1583.

28. Hausdorff JM, Ring H. Effects of a new radio frequency-controlled neuroprosthesis on gait symmetry and rhythmicity in patients with chronic hemiparesis. Am J Phys Med Rehabil. 2008;87(1):4–13.

29. van Swigchem R, Vloothuis J, den Boer J, Weerdesteyn V, Geurts AC. Is transcutaneous peroneal stimulation beneficial to patients with chronic stroke using an ankle-foot orthosis? A within-subjects study of patients' satisfaction, walking speed and physical activity level. J Rehabil Med. 2010;42(2):117–121.

30. Damiano DL, Prosser LA, Curatalo LA, Alter KE. Muscle plasticity and ankle control after repetitive use of a functional electrical stimulation device for foot drop in cerebral palsy. Neurorehabil Neural Repair. 2013;27(3):200–207.

31. Everaert DG, Stein RB, Abrams GM, et al. Effect of a foot-drop stimulator and ankle-foot orthosis on walking performance after stroke: a multicenter randomized controlled trial. Neurorehabil Neural Repair. 2013;27(7):579–591.

32. Taylor P, Humphreys L, Swain I. The long-term cost-effectiveness of the use of Functional Electrical Stimulation for the correction of dropped foot due to upper motor neuron lesion. J Rehabil Med. 2013;45(2):154–160.

33. McClelland M, Andrews BJ, Patrick JH, Freeman PA, el Masri WS. Augmentation of the Oswestry Parawalker orthosis by means of surface electrical stimulation: gait analysis of three patients. Paraplegia. 1987;25(1):32–38.

34. Solomonow M, Baratta R, Hirokawa S, et al. The RGO Generation II: muscle stimulation powered orthosis as a practical walking system for thoracic paraplegics. Orthopedics. 1989;12(10):1309–1315.

35. Goldfarb M, Korkowski K, Harrold B, Durfee W. Preliminary evaluation of a controlled-brake orthosis for FES-aided gait. IEEE Trans Neural Syst Rehabil Eng. 2003;11(3):241–248.

36. Kobetic R, To CS, Schnellenberger JR, et al. Development of hybrid orthosis for standing, walking, and stair climbing after spinal cord injury. J Rehabil Res Dev. 2009;46(3):447–462.

37. Audu ML, To CS, Kobetic R, Triolo RJ. Gait evaluation of a novel hip constraint orthosis with implication for walking in paraplegia. IEEE Trans Neural Syst Rehabil Eng. 2010;18(6):610–618.

38. Jezernik S, Colombo G, Keller T, Frueh H, Morari M. Robotic orthosis lokomat: a rehabilitation and research tool. Neuromodulation. 2003;6(2):108–115.

39. Sharma N, Mushahwar V, Stein R. Dynamic optimization of FES and orthosis-based walking using simple models. IEEE Trans Neural Syst Rehabil Eng. 2013;22(1):114–126.

40. Kobetic R, Marsolais EB.Synthesis of Paraplegic Gait with Multichannel Functional Neuromuscular Stimulation. IEEE Trans Rehabil Eng. 1994;2:66–79.

41. Daly JJ, Kollar K, Debogorski AA, et al. Performance of an intramuscular electrode during functional neuromuscular stimulation for gait training post stroke. J Rehabil Res Dev. 2001;38(5):513–526.

42. Davis JA Jr, Triolo RJ, Uhlir J, et al. Preliminary performance of a surgically implanted neuroprosthesis for standing and transfers—where do we stand? J Rehabil Res Dev. 2001;38(6):609–617.

43. Schiefer MA, Freeberg M, Pinault GJ, et al. Selective activation of the human tibial and common peroneal nerves with a flat interface nerve electrode. J Neural Eng. 2013;10(5):056006.

44. Fisher LE, Miller ME, Bailey SN, et al. Standing after spinal cord injury with four-contact nerve-cuff electrodes for quadriceps stimulation. IEEE Trans Neural Syst Rehabil Eng. 2008;16(5):473–478.

45. Fisher LE, Tyler DJ, Anderson JS, Triolo RJ. Chronic stability and selectivity of four-contact spiral nerve-cuff electrodes in stimulating the human femoral nerve. J Neural Eng. 2009;6(4):046010.

46. Schiefer MA, Polasek KH, Triolo RJ, Pinault GC, Tyler DJ. Selective stimulation of the human femoral nerve with a flat interface nerve electrode. J Neural Eng. 2010;7(2):26006.

47. Kenney L, Bultstra G, Buschman R, et al. An implantable two channel drop foot stimulator: initial clinical results. Artif Organs. 2002;26(3):267–270.

48. Burridge JH, Haugland M, Larsen B, et al. Phase II trial to evaluate the ActiGait implanted drop-foot stimulator in established hemiplegia. J Rehabil Med. 2007;39(3):212–218.

49. Weber DJ, Stein RB, Chan KM, et al. BIONic WalkAide for correcting foot drop. IEEE Trans Neural Syst Rehabil Eng. 2005;13(2):242–246.

50. Loeb GE, Zamin CJ, Schulman JH, Troyk PR. Injectable microstimulator for functional electrical stimulation. Med Biol Eng Comput. 1991;29(6):NS13–19.

51. Bamford JA, Mushahwar VK. Intraspinal microstimulation for the recovery of function following spinal cord injury. Prog Brain Res. 2011;194:227–239.

52. Tator CH, Minassian K, Mushahwar VK. Spinal cord stimulation: therapeutic benefits and movement generation after spinal cord injury. Handb Clin Neurol. 2012;109:283–296.

53. Giszter SF, Mussa-Ivaldi FA, Bizzi E. Convergent force fields organized in the frog's spinal cord. J Neurosci. 1993;13(2):467–491.

54. Bamford JA, Putman CT, Mushahwar VK. Intraspinal microstimulation preferentially recruits fatigue-resistant muscle fibres and generates gradual force in rat. J Physiol. 2005;569(Pt 3):873–884.

55. Gerasimenko Y, Roy RR, Edgerton VR. Epidural stimulation: comparison of the spinal circuits that generate and control locomotion in rats, cats and humans. Exp Neurol. 2008;209(2):417–425.

56. van den Brand R, Heutschi J, Barraud Q, et al. Restoring voluntary control of locomotion after paralyzing spinal cord injury. Science. 2012;336(6085):1182–1185.

57. Harkema S, Gerasimenko Y, Hodes J, et al. Effect of epidural stimulation of the lumbosacral spinal cord on voluntary movement, standing, and assisted stepping after motor complete paraplegia: a case study. Lancet. 2011;377(9781):1938–1947.

58. Popovic MR, Popovic DB, Keller T. Neuroprostheses for grasping. Neurol Res. 2002;24(5):443–452.

59. Long C. An electrophysiologic splint for the hand. Arch Phys Med Rehabil. 1963;44:499–503.

60. Vodovnik L, Long C 2nd, Reswick JB, Lippay A, Starbuck D. Myo-electric control of paralyzed muscles. IEEE Trans Biomed Eng. 1965;12(3):169–172.

61. Merletti R, Acimovic R, Grobelnik S, Cvilak G. Electrophysiological orthosis for the upper extremity in hemiplegia: feasibility study. Arch Phys Med Rehabil. 1975;56:507.

62. Snoek GJ, IJzerman MJ, in 't Groen FA, Stoffers TS, Zilvold G. Use of the NESS handmaster to restore hand function in tetraplegia: clinical experiences in ten patients. Spinal Cord. 2000;38(4):244–249.

63. Alon G, McBride K, Ring H. Improving selected hand functions using a noninvasive neuroprosthesis in persons with chronic stroke. J Stroke Cerebrovasc Dis. 2002;11(2):99–106.

64. Ring H, Rosenthal N. Controlled study of neuroprosthetic functional electrical stimulation in sub-acute post-stroke rehabilitation. J Rehabil Med. 2005;37(1):32–36.

65. Meijer JW, Voerman GE, Santegoets KM, Geurts AC. Short-term effects and long-term use of a hybrid orthosis for neuromuscular electrical stimulation of the upper extremity in patients after chronic stroke. J Rehabil Med. 2009;41(3):157–161.

66. Prochazka A, Gauthier M, Wieler M, Kenwell Z. The bionic glove: an electrical stimulator garment that provides controlled grasp and hand opening in quadriplegia. Arch Phys Med Rehabil. 1997;78(6):608–614.

67. Popovic D, Stojanovic A, Pjanovic A, eet al. Clinical evaluation of the bionic glove. Arch Phys Med Rehabil. 1999;80(3):299–304.

68. Popovic DB, Popovic MB, Stojanovic A, Pjanovic A, Radosavljevic S, Vulovic D. Clinical evaluation of the Belgrade grasping system. Proceedings of the Vth Vienna Workshop on FES. Vienna, 1998, pp. 247–250.

69. Micera S, Keller T, Lawrence M, Morari M, Popovic DB. Wearable neural prostheses. Restoration of sensory-motor function by transcutaneous electrical stimulation. IEEE Eng Med Biol Mag. 2010;29(3):64–69.

70. Popovic MB, Popovic DB, Sinkjaer T, Stefanovic A, Schwirtlich L. Clinical evaluation of Functional Electrical Therapy in acute hemiplegic subjects. J Rehabil Res Dev. 2003;40(5):443–453.

71. Popovic MB, Popovic DB, Schwirtlich L, Sinkjaer T. Functional electrical therapy (FET): clinical trial in chronic hemiplegic subjects. Neuromodulation. 2004;7(2):133–140.

72. Mangold S, Keller T, Curt A, Dietz V. Transcutaneous functional electrical stimulation for grasping in subjects with cervical spinal cord injury. Spinal Cord. 2005;43:1–13.

73. Malešević NM, Popovic Maneski LZ, Ilic V, et al. A multi-pad electrode based functional electrical stimulation system for restoration of grasp. J Neuroeng Rehabil. 2012;9:66.

74. Westerveld AJ, Schouten AC, Veltink PH, van der Kooij H. Selectivity and resolution of surface electrical stimulation for grasp and release. IEEE Trans Neural Syst Rehabil Eng. 2012;20(1):94–101.

75. Nathan RH. The isometric action of the forearm muscles. J Biomech Eng. 1992;114(2):162–169.

76. Popovic-Bijelic A, Bijelic G, Jorgovanovic N, Bojanic D, Popovic MB, Popovic DB. Multi-field surface electrode for selective electrical stimulation. Artif Organs. 2005;29(6):448–452.

77. Lawrence M, Gross GP, Lang M, Kuhn A, Keller T, Morari M. Assessment of finger forces and wrist torques for functional grasp using new multichannel textile neuroprostheses. Artif Organs. 2008;32(8):634–638.

78. Popovic DB, Popovic MB. Automatic determination of the optimal shape of a surface electrode: selective stimulation. J Neurosci Methods. 2009;178(1):174–181.

79. Schill O, Wiegand R, Schmitz B, et al. OrthoJacket: an active FES-hybrid orthosis for the paralysed upper extremity. Biomed Tech (Berl). 2011;56(1):35–44.

80. Peckham PH, Marsolais EB, Mortimer JT. Restoration of key grip and release in the C6 tetraplegic patient through functional electrical stimulation. J Hand Surg Am. 1980;5(5):462–469.

81. Handa Y, Hoshimiya N. Functional electrical stimulation for the control of the upper extremities. Med Prog Technol. 1987;12(1–2):51–63.

82. Keith MW, Peckham PH, Thrope GB, Buckett JR, Stroh KC, Menger V. Functional neuromuscular stimulation neuroprostheses for the tetraplegic hand. Clin Orthop Relat Res. 1988;(233):25–33.

83. Keith MW, Peckham PH, Thrope GB, et al. Implantable functional neuromuscular stimulation in the tetraplegic hand. J Hand Surg Am. 1989;14(3):524–530.

84. Peckham PH, Keith MW, Kilgore KL, et al. Efficacy of an implanted neuroprosthesis for restoring hand grasp in tetraplegia: a multicenter study. Arch Phys Med Rehabil. 2001;82(10):1380–1388.

85. Taylor P, Esnouf J, Hobby J. The functional impact of the Freehand System on tetraplegic hand function. Clinical Results. Spinal Cord. 2002;40(11):560–566.

86. Wuolle KS, Bryden AM, Peckham PH, Murray PK, Keith M. Satisfaction with upper-extremity surgery in individuals with tetraplegia. Arch Phys Med Rehabil. 2003;84(8):1145–1149.

87. Kilgore KL, Peckham PH, Keith MW, et al. Durability of implanted electrodes and leads in an upper-limb neuroprosthesis. J Rehabil Res Dev. 2003;40(6):457–468.

88. Kilgore KL, Hoyen HA, Bryden AM, Hart RL, Keith MW, Peckham PH. An implanted upper-extremity neuroprosthesis using myoelectric control. J Hand Surg Am. 2008;33(4):539–550.

89. Knutson JS, Chae J, Hart RL, et al. Implanted neuroprosthesis for assisting arm and hand function after stroke: a case study. J Rehabil Res Dev. 2012;**49**(10):1505–1516.

90. Kilgore KL, Hart RL, Montague FW, et al. An implanted myoelectrically-controlled neuroprosthesis for upper extremity function in spinal cord injury. Conf Proc IEEE Eng Med Biol Soc. 2006;**1**:1630–1633.

91. Polasek KH, Hoyen HA, Keith MW, Tyler DJ. Human nerve stimulation thresholds and selectivity using a multi-contact nerve cuff electrode. IEEE Trans Neural Syst Rehabil Eng. 2007;**15**(1):76–82.

92. Polasek KH, Hoyen HA, Keith MW, Kirsch RF, Tyler DJ. Stimulation stability and selectivity of chronically implanted multi-contact nerve cuff electrodes in the human upper extremity. IEEE Trans Neural Syst Rehabil Eng. 2009;**17**(5):428–437.

93. Moritz CT, Lucas TH, Perlmutter SI, Fetz EE. Forelimb movements and muscle responses evoked by microstimulation of cervical spinal cord in sedated monkeys. J Neurophysiol. 2007;**97**(1):110–120.

94. Zimmermann JB, Seki K, Jackson A. Reanimating the arm and hand with intraspinal microstimulation. J Neural Eng. 2011;**8**(5):054001.

95. Alon G, McBride K, Ring H. Improving selected hand functions using a noninvasive neuroprosthesis in persons with chronic stroke. J Stroke Cerebrovasc Dis. 2002;**11**(2):99–106.

96. Popovic MR, Popovic DB, Keller T. Neuroprostheses for grasping. Neurol Res. 2002;**24**(5):443–452.

97. Crema A, McNaught A, Albisser U, Bolliger M, Micera S, Curt A, et al. A hybrid tool for reaching and grasping rehabilitation: The ArmeoFES. Proc IEEE EMBS. 2011;3047–3050.

CHAPTER 31

Technology to enhance arm and hand function

Arthur Prochazka

Introduction

According to the Centres for Disease Control and Prevention, in 2010 there were 8.3 million stroke survivors in the US [1]. Nearly a million individuals in North America live with spinal cord injury (SCI), half of whom have tetraplegia [2]. Up to 60% of these people find it hard or impossible to perform activities of daily life (ADLs) because of poor upper limb (UL) function [3]. The main deficits are poor control of the proximal muscles, difficulty extending the elbow and wrist, difficulty in grasping (and particularly in releasing objects), and in about 30% of cases, significant to severe spastic hypertonus. Spastic hypertonus develops in 20–30% of stroke survivors 6 to 18 months post-stroke [4–7]. Spastic hypertonus is associated with reduced range of motion (ROM), pain, and contractures [8, 9]. Several studies have shown that spasticity can impede ADLs [5, 6, 10].

Based on the International Classification of Functioning and Disability [11], meaningful recovery of UL function should be viewed as the ability to incorporate the paretic limb in home and community activities and therefore to enhance participation. Examples include the ability to hold and cut food, open a jar or medicine bottle, and sign a cheque. Hand function, including dextrous manipulation, is at the top of the 'wish-list' of stroke survivors and individuals with tetraplegia due to SCI [12, 13]. In fact, a recent questionnaire survey of 220 stroke survivors found that the most important outcome was the ability to use the paretic arm in meaningful ways [13, 14]. One person said 'It is a big deal to be able to use your arm again. I think most of the doctors think it is not. It is a big deal to be able to use your arm again psychologically as well as physically' [13: p. 1217]. This underscores the meaningfulness of arm and hand recovery from the person's perspective.

Before considering the technology that has been developed to restore UL function, it is important to understand the time-course of spontaneous recovery and current treatment strategies.

Spontaneous recovery of hand function after stroke and SCI

For a year or more after a stroke or SCI, arm and hand function spontaneously recover, initially quickly, then levelling off. The extent to which a person regains useful function in ADLs depends on the severity of the injury [15, 16]. It has been suggested that after a stroke 'no emergence of arm synergies at 4 weeks is associated with poor outcome at 6 months' [17]. Full recovery of UL function occurs in only about 12% of stroke survivors [17]. Spontaneous recovery, particularly in the first few weeks, provides a shifting baseline that must be taken into account when comparing the efficacy of treatments, for example in randomized controlled trials (RCTs). This is a serious obstacle in some cases. For example, a recent study showed that in order to provide sufficient statistical power when comparing treatments in the acute or subacute period after SCI, the sample size required can be completely prohibitive, given the relatively small number of similar cases likely to be encountered in large cities, or even in whole countries [2].

Brief summary of conventional rehabilitation techniques

Duration

The duration of inpatient rehabilitation varies widely from country to country. For stroke survivors in the US, this decreased from 20 to 12 days between 1994 and 2001, with up to 61% of patients not receiving any follow-up therapy [18]. This has forced therapists to focus more on compensatory strategies than on restoring function. On discharge, patients are provided with passive aids such as ankle and knee braces or splints, arm slings, and canes. Some patients continue exercising after discharge, but a survey of stroke participants in our programme revealed that after a few months, the only exercise they did with any consistency was passive stretching, largely to relieve hypertonus.

Two treatment regimes based on neurophysiological principles, the Bobath technique, which aims to restore normal coordination, and proprioceptive neuromuscular facilitation, which uses stretching to restore ROM, have been widely used since the 1960s, with strong adherents in each camp [19–24]. An RCT that compared these two methods concluded that there were no substantial difference between them in improving ADLs [25].

Exercise

According to the American Heart Association, 'physical activity remains a cornerstone in the current armamentarium for risk factor management for the prevention and treatment of stroke and cardiovascular disease' [26]. Most rehabilitation clinics have a range of passive exercise devices for hand and arm function, such as therapy putty, skateboards, incline boards, stacking cones, ring trees, and peg boards. Hand exercises are occasionally performed with spring-loaded splints, or splints that transfer wrist extensor torque to finger extensors. Higher-functioning patients are taught ROM exercises of the arm and hand, passive stretching to reduce hypertonus, squeezing a ball, and other exercises. There is evidence that the more physiotherapy of this type that patients receive, the better the motor outcome [27].

Compensatory strategies

It has long been generally accepted by therapists that in severely disabled stroke survivors, therapy should be restricted to minimizing contractures and pain [28] and teaching compensatory methods, for example tying shoelaces with one hand, or using simple assistive devices, such as a universal cuff, to hold tools and utensils [29]. Compensatory strategies may, however, inhibit spontaneous functional recovery. For example, stroke survivors often lean forward from the hip to position the more affected hand to grasp or stabilize objects. It has been argued that once compensatory strategies become habitual, they lead to 'learned non-use,' a form of motor neglect [30]. Thus, while compensatory strategies are useful and empowering, they may reduce the motivation of patients, therapists, and medical device companies to pursue new therapies, exercise regimes, or technologies.

Cost

As will become apparent, cost and reimbursement are crucial factors in the adoption of new treatments and technologies. For this reason, approximate costs are given in what follows, to provide the reader with a basis for comparison between the various methods and devices discussed. The costs are based on North American data and are provided in US dollars. Costs in other developed countries are broadly similar, though of course with some local variance. In some cases the costs are absorbed by government healthcare agencies or insurance companies. When individuals do not have this financial support, the cost of devices and treatments can be prohibitive.

Constraint-induced movement therapy (CIMT)

Originally called forced-use training [31], CIMT has been adopted by rehabilitation institutes around the world to treat stroke survivors. Movements of the less-affected UL are constrained for 6–7 hours for 2 weeks, forcing the more affected UL to be used in intensive practice of tasks relevant to the subject [3, 32]. The Stroke Rehabilitation Evidence-Based Review (SREBR) endorses this approach: 'Exposure to stimulating and complex environments and involvement in tasks or activities that are meaningful to the individual with stroke serves to increase cortical reorganization and enhance functional recovery' [33–35]. Other features of CIMT are 'shaping' (gradually increasing the difficulty of tasks) and a 'transfer package:' a behavioural contract specifying post-treatment activities. An important limitation of CIMT is that subjects must have at least 20° of voluntary wrist extension and 10° voluntary finger extension [32]. This excludes 85–90% of people with hemiparetic hands [33, 36]. There is disagreement on whether the strategy of preventing the less-affected arm from taking part in intensive exercise therapy is beneficial or not. Numerous papers have appeared in the last few years that favour bilateral training [37–41].

The CIMT course offered at the Taub therapy clinic at the University of Alabama in Birmingham costs around $6K. Pressure for reimbursement has risen as a result of a multi-centre trial confirming that CIMT produces clinically relevant improvements in arm function [42]. Less intensive protocols have been suggested, such as *modified* CIMT (mCIMT) [43–45], comprising CIMT for 30 min, three times a week and wearing a mitt on the less-affected hand for 5 hours a day, for 5 days a week. The efficacy of mCIMT is yet to be confirmed in RCTs.

In an effort to provide standardized UL exercises at minimal cost to stroke survivors, a group at the University of British Columbia developed the graded repetitive arm supplementary programme (GRASP: [46]). It is self-administered during rehabilitation in an in-patient setting, with follow-up at home. It has three difficulty levels chosen according to the UL Fugl-Meyer assessment of function. The participant receives an exercise book containsing instructions for each exercise, and a kit containing inexpensive equipment (e.g. ball, bean bag, towel, paper clips). Repetitive exercises including strengthening, range of motion and fine motor skills are designed to improve ADLs. GRASP is recommended by the Canadian Stroke Best Practice Guidelines (www.strokebestpractices.ca) and has been adopted by over 100 sites in several countries.

Tendon transfer surgery

It is important when evaluating novel devices that enhance UL function, to be aware of the existing medical alternatives. One of these is surgically to shift the tendon of a muscle that remains under voluntary control from its original attachment to a new one, to replace the action of a paralysed muscle [47]. A recent survey found that 70% of tetraplegic people who had received tendon transfers were satisfied with the results, 77% reported a positive impact on their lives, 68% reported improvements in ADLs, 66% reported improved independence, and 69% reported improvement in occupation [48]. Tendon transfers are only available in specialized centres. Less than half of the 137 tetraplegic people recently surveyed had ever been told about this option and only 9% had had the procedure [12]. Nearly 80% said they would be willing to spend 2–3 months being less independent while recovering from surgery, ultimately to become more independent. Tendon transfers carry the risk of infection and involve several months of recovery during which motor function is actually reduced. The movements that are restored may not be as natural as anticipated, and although in principle, tendon transfers are reversible, this involves more surgery. Because abnormal connective tissue growth and changes in muscle and tendon will have occurred, the anatomical relationship will not be completely restored. This can be a disincentive to people hoping for a 'cure'.

Mechanical splints and exoskeletal devices

Numerous passive and powered mechanical devices in the form of articulated splints and supports that act as exoskeletons have been developed and tested over the years. Notable recent devices include the ReWalk (ReWalk Robotics: www.rewalk.com) [49] and the Ekso Bionic Suit (www.eksobionics.com) for ambulation and the *Saebo*Flex for hand grasp and release (www.saebo.com). The *Saebo*Flex (Figure 31.1) is a spring-loaded, passive device that holds the wrist and fingers in extension. The user grasps an object by voluntarily flexing the fingers. The springs assist in re-opening the hand to release the object. Another spring-loaded splint, the MossRehab 'RELEAS' (www.mossrehab.com/

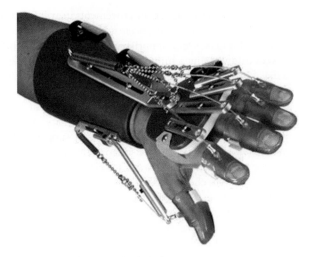

Fig. 31.1 The Saeboflex spring-loaded splint.

Therapeutic-Modalities-Tools/releas.html) recently came onto the market at a cost of ~$200. Powered orthoses for hand grasp and release have also entered clinical trials [50].

Therapeutic and functional electrical stimulation

Weak or paralysed muscles can be activated by trains of electrical pulses applied either with surface stimulators and electrodes or with implanted stimulators and leads. In both cases it is the nerves innervating the muscles that are activated [51]. Muscles denervated as a result of peripheral nerve injury or the destruction of spinal motoneurons cannot be activated in this way. Therapeutic electrical stimulation (TES) refers to cyclical stimulation to increase muscle strength. Functional electrical stimulation (FES) refers to voluntarily triggered stimulation to assist in functional tasks. Studies have shown that TES can reduce hypertonus and improve motor function. Surface FES stimulators for foot-drop

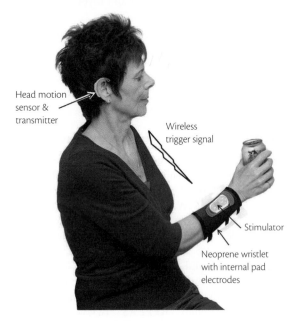

Head motion sensor & transmitter

Wireless trigger signal

Stimulator

Neoprene wristlet with internal pad electrodes

Fig. 31.2 The Rehabtronics wireless-triggered hand stimulator.

have been commercially available in Europe since the late 1970s [52], and more recently in North America [53, 54].

In the late 1970s a therapeutic programme for hand function involving daily FES-assisted biofeedback exercises was initiated at the Rancho Los Amigos Rehabilitation Hospital in Los Angeles [55–57]. The FES devices comprised hinged splints containing surface electrodes and stimulators activated by push-button. The first commercial hand stimulator was the Automove, which detects weak voluntary electromyographic (EMG) activity of muscles associated with weak voluntary contractions, and then stimulates these same muscles to augment the contractions [58]. Improvements in subsequent unassisted voluntary function have been reported [59–63]. In the 1990s, two designs of surface hand stimulators were developed for people with tetraplegia, the Handmaster [64] and the Bionic Glove [65]. The Handmaster was subsequently commercialized as the Bioness H200 [65, 66]. It comprises a hinged splint containing moistened pad electrodes, and a stimulator triggered by push-button. It costs about US$7,000. The Bionic Glove, an FES garment triggered by wrist movements was shown to provide functional and therapeutic benefits to people with tetraplegia [67]; however, it did not survive the commercialization process.

Stroke survivors have difficulty flexing and extending the wrist, so alternative methods of triggering these devices voluntarily have been developed. Accelerometers built into small earpieces are used to detect toothclicks or head nods. Radiofrequency signals are then transmitted to the FES garment [68]. A wristlet based on the head-nod method is being developed by Rehabtronics Inc. (www.rehabtronics.com) (Figure 31.2). This will cost about $2,000 and is scheduled for commercial release in 2015.

Implanted devices for enhancing UL function

A fully implanted UL FES device developed at Case Western Reserve University [69, 70] was approved by the Food and Drug Administration in 1997 and marketed by Neurocontrol as the 'Freehand System.' About 200 of these devices were implanted in people with C4–C5 tetraplegia. An external control unit wirelessly activated an implanted stimulator that delivered pulse trains to muscles in the forearm to elicit different hand movements. Shoulder or wrist movements were used to select the movements. Though many recipients benefited, the Freehand System was withdrawn from the market in 2002 [71]. An improved multichannel version of the device that is controlled myoelectrically (by EMG signals picked up with electrodes implanted in muscles still under voluntary control) has recently been implanted in several individuals with tetraplegia [72, 73]. The device has also been implanted in a person with stroke, though interestingly, myoelectric control was unsuccessful in this case study [74]. Other novel implantable devices for UL function include the Finetech STIMuGRIP [75] and an implantable system called the Stimulus Router that requires only the leads to be implanted, with pulse trains coupled through the skin from a wireless-triggered wristlet stimulator [76].

Virtual reality (VR) training and computer gaming

A recent meta-study concluded that 'VR and video game applications are novel and potentially useful technologies that can be combined with conventional rehabilitation for upper arm improvement after stroke' [77]. In 1992 a glove instrumented with sensors was developed to enable VR games for rehabilitation purposes [78]. Actuators in the palm of the glove provided resistance to finger and thumb flexion according to the virtual object grasped, enhancing the experience [79]. Affordable VR devices from the computer gaming world have recently been adapted for motor rehabilitation, most notably the Nintendo Wii [80–84]. The Wii allows users to play computer games with a hand-held motion sensor. It was not designed for rehabilitation and it lacks dextrous tasks requiring grasp/release, pronation/supination, wrist flexion/extension, pinch-grip/ release, and picking up and transferring objects. The resistance to movement presented by real objects in tasks of daily life is also lacking. In spite of these shortcomings, a recent study suggests that VR games played on the Wii provide a safe, feasible, and potentially effective alternative to facilitate rehabilitation therapy and promote motor recovery after stroke [85]. The Wii has been embraced by rehabilitation clinics around the world, showing the need for affordable in-home devices that make exercise therapy enjoyable and thereby increase adherence.

Robotic UL exercise training

Over the last 20 years, powered robotic systems have been developed for UL rehabilitation. The simplest of these are servo motors that impose repetitive, continuous passive movements on limbs [86, 87]. In some cases attachments are provided that mimic objects found in ADLs (PrimusRS: btetech.com; E-Link: www.biometric-sltd.com). The MIT-Manus rehabilitation robot provides arm supports and applies planar forces that assist or resist voluntary motion during target-tracking on a monitor [88, 89]. In an important recent study of 127 chronic stroke participants, in those who did 36 hours of MIT-Manus robot-assisted exercise over 12 weeks, UL function improved by about the same amount as in those who received equivalent therapist-supervised intensive training and in those who received usual care [90]. In their discussion of this disappointing outcome, the authors noted that their participants received an unexpectedly large amount of additional rehabilitation, possibly reflecting self-selection of highly motivated people or better access to rehabilitative services in the Veterans Administration system within which the study was conducted. Another factor was the inclusion of severely impaired participants: the mean baseline Fugl-Meyer score was 20 (out of a full range of 66). Functional outcomes of intensive exercise therapy in individuals with low levels of motor function are generally lower than in those with moderate to mild impairment at baseline (see later).

The KINARM, developed by Dr Steven Scott at Queens University, Kingston, Canada, is another example of a planar robotic device that supports the arm [91]. So far, it has been used mainly for assessing individual joint contributions to UL movement. The Motorika ReoGo is a floor-mounted telescopic servo, which applies forces in three dimensions to the UL [92]. It has been deployed in at least one large chain of rehabilitation hospitals in the USA. The most recent device of this type is the multi-degree-of-freedom ARMin arm robot, commercialized by Hocoma, the makers of the Lokomat® gait-training robot [93]. This device has an exoskeleton structure that enables the training of movements in 3-D space, as well as grasp and release of an instrumented gripper. It detects voluntary effort and assists when needed. It incorporates computer games to motivate the users.

Training with rehabilitation robots does not necessarily improve scores on ADL tests [90, 94, 95]. A recent meta-analysis [35] concludes: 'Sensorimotor training with robotic devices improves functional and motor outcomes of the shoulder and elbow, however, it does not improve functional and motor outcomes of the wrist and hand.' This could be partly due to the fact that the existing devices do not exercise dextrous hand movements. Another factor that has only recently been recognized is the tendency of clients whose movements are assisted by robots, to take advantage of the assistance and progressively reduce their own effort [96]. This has been termed 'slacking.' Unfortunately it has also been shown that it is the client's own effort that is the key to functional improvement with exercise training [97], The aforementioned robotic systems cost from $60K to $150K and require dedicated personnel within a clinical setting. A simpler robot, the 'Hand Mentor,' comprises a powered wrist splint. This device exercises hand and wrist only. In a recent small-scale RCT ($n = 17$) of the Hand Mentor, the rating of mood increased more in a group that used the device in addition to repetitive task practice than in a group receiving repetitive task practice only. Other outcome measures were similar in the two groups [98].

In spite of the large amount of effort and expense involved in developing these robotic rehabilitation systems in the last two decades, actual deployment in clinics or in patients' homes has so far been limited, presumably because of complexity, cost, and the fact that dose-equivalent non-robotic therapy may be equally effective. Research on the use of rehabilitation robotic-based technologies for improving UL function and use after stroke remains in its infancy and with a considerable gap between clinic-based and home-based programmes. A recent review of rehabilitation robotics concluded with the following recommendation: 'To maximize efficacy for a large clinical population, the authors propose that future task-oriented robots need to incorporate yet-to-be developed adaptive task presentation algorithms that emphasize acquisition of fine motor coordination skills while minimizing compensatory movements' [99].

Passive exercise devices incorporating computer gaming

Given the large cost of robotic devices and the realization that what may count most in rehabilitation is the client's own efforts to move rather than external assistance [98], there is an increased interest in passive devices that promote UL exercise. Simple devices that support the weight of the arm either with slings or articulated arms attached to wheelchairs have been used in rehabilitation clinics for many years. The most sophisticated of these devices, which incorporates computer gaming to improve motivation, is the Hocoma ArmeoSpring [100]. This device is a spring-loaded, articulated arm support, developed from the Therapy Wilmington Robotic Exoskeleton (T-WREX) [101]. It is primarily suitable for ROM exercises. It is provided with an instrumented gripper, enabling grasp and release to be detected and incorporated into the games. It costs over $60K and is therefore only suitable for clinics. In a recent study [102], 23 chronic hemiparetic patients completed 36 1-hour sessions using the ArmeoSpring. Improvements of between 2 and 10% were reported in a variety of outcome measures, including functional tests such as the Fugl-Meyer Arm (FMA) test and the Wolf Motor Function test [103]. In another study, 12 tetraplegic

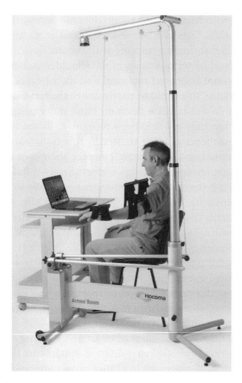

Fig. 31.3 The Armeo® Booom.

participants performed ArmeoSpring training with one of their affected arms for a total of 15 hours spread over 5 weeks. This was additional to conventional occupational and physical therapy. There were few functional benefits in the limbs receiving the training compared with the limbs that did not [104]. However, in a subgroup of participants with partial hand function at baseline, there was a significantly larger increase in one of the functional outcome measures in the treated limbs.

A related device, the ArmeoBoom, comprises an overhead crane that supports the forearm with a sling that can move up and down, providing partial weight support (Figure 31.3). A motion sensing device at the top of the frame tracks the position of the hand. The device provides ROM exercises in a computer gaming environment, but like the Wii, it lacks dextrous tasks such as grasp–release, pinch–grip and pronation–supination. It costs around $16K, and so could conceivably be provided for in-home use on a rental basis. In a study on eight sub-acute stroke participants, EMG patterns of UL muscles were compared during elbow and shoulder joint excursions with and without gravity compensation provided by a precursor of the ArmeoSpring [105]. Arm movement excursions were facilitated without impairing motor control. In another study on a related device, seven chronic stroke participants received 18 half-hour sessions over 6 weeks of reach training with computer games [106]. There was a median increase of 3 points in the FMA after training and a significantly increased work area of the hemiparetic arm, as indicated by the normalized area of circles drawn by the participants.

A gaming workstation designed for motor rehabilitation, the 'ReJoyce' (Rehabilitation Joystick for Computerized Exercise), enables clients to perform task-oriented, intensive arm and hand exercises in the guise of computer games [107–109]. It was designed to provide tasks that mimic a variety of common ADLs, including

those requiring dextrous manipulation: grasping, moving and releasing objects having weight and resistance to movement, bimanual rotation of a steering wheel, pouring fluid from a can, holding a jar and twisting its lid, pinch-gripping and lifting small objects, sliding and pinch-gripping coins on a surface (Figure 31.4). The client is presented with a choice of 10 games and a slider to set an initial difficulty level. The difficulty levels of games are incremented upon successful completions of each stage of a game. The ReJoyce has been used independently by clients in clinics or at home. It has also been used for in-home telerehabilitation (see next section), whereby the choice and difficulty of games are controlled remotely over the Internet by a tele-coach, along with two-way audiovisual communication with the client.

The use of technology for in-home exercise therapy

In developed countries only 5–10% of chronic stroke survivors attend outpatient therapy sessions on a regular basis. There is therefore an urgent need to improve adherence to in-home exercise programmes to improve health status, cognitive function, participation and quality of life. To address this need, early supported discharge (ESD) programmes have been, or are being, implemented in several countries [110, 111]. They involve home visits, typically 1 hour/day for 6–8 weeks by one or more allied health professionals. A recent meta-study, [110] came to the conclusion that stroke patients with mild to moderate disability receiving ESD can attain similar or superior functional outcomes compared to in-patient rehabilitation at a cost lower than usual care (http://ebrsr.com/evidence-review/7-outpatient-stroke-rehabilitation).

Telerehabilitation has been proposed as a means of delivering continuing outpatient therapy in a more convenient and affordable way [112]. According to a recent analysis by the Alberta Health Services, 2 hours of travel by therapists are allocated to each ESD home visit. Given that the home visit itself lasts about an hour, this means that two-thirds of the time, and therefore two-thirds of the cost, is taken up by travel. During the 1-hour visit, 20–25 min are dedicated to UL exercises, 20–25 min to cognitive/perceptual therapy, and 10–15 min to mobility. All of these functions could, in principle, be performed on devices such as the ReJoyce in the home, supervised over the Internet by tele-coaches, thus eliminating the travel component. Several clients can be supervised simultaneously by one tele-coach, further reducing costs.

So far, telerehabilitation has focused mainly on psychological, cognitive, and vocational rehabilitation. However, various pilot studies of tele-supervised training for motor function have taken place over the last decade [79, 113–116]. Recent studies involving the home-use of ReJoyce systems in stroke and SCI subjects have shown that in-home exercises with telerehabilitation and FES produced improvements in UL motor function exceeding the minimal clinically important difference [107, 117–119]. Participants who had the largest increases in Action Research Arm Test (ARAT) scores were those whose baseline scores were in the mid-range. This is in line with previous work showing that the initial severity of a stroke determines the extent of recovery [120].

There are numerous barriers to the widespread adoption of telerehabilitation by healthcare providers and reimbursement agencies [121]. These include cost, an insufficient evidence base, lack of reimbursement, laws regulating telerehabilitation, professional

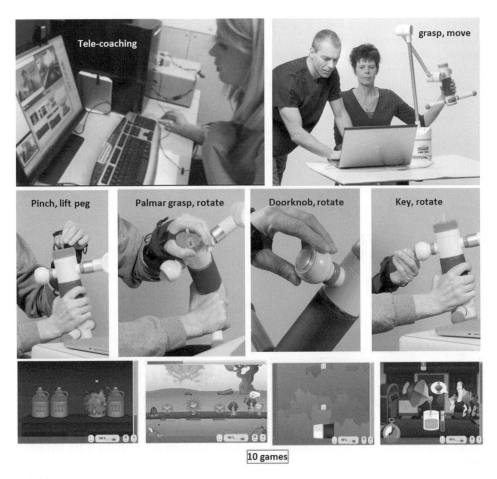

Fig. 31.4 The ReJoyce telerehabilitation system.

Outcome evaluation

Numerous tests of upper extremity function have been developed over the years. To quote from a recent review article [122] 'The most frequently cited UL performance measures include the ARAT [123, 124], Box and Blocks Test (BB) [125], Chedoke Arm and Hand Activity Inventory (CAHAI) [126], Jebsen–Taylor Hand Function Test (JTT) [127], Nine-Hole Peg Test [128], and the Wolf Motor Function Test (WMFT) [103]. The most frequently cited self-reporting measures include the Stroke Impact Scale (SIS) [129] and the Motor Activity Log (MAL) [130].' The ARAT and the BB test have recently been identified as having the strongest relationship to clinical utility [131].

Recently, attempts have been made to develop entirely quantitative UL performance measures. These include the Toronto Rehabilitation Hand function test, which was shown to have a moderate to strong construct validity in assessing unilateral hand motor function in persons with tetraplegia [132]. The KinArm allows the quantification of numerous movement parameters

during visual reaching tasks [133]. This may provide a better resolution of sensorimotor impairment than standard clinical tests. It also allows position sense to be quantified [134]. The ReJoyce system incorporates an automated hand function test, which takes about 5 minutes to complete, and proceeds with automated screen prompts. It provides an overall score that correlates well with the ARAT and Fugl-Meyer arm and hand function tests [135]. It also provides scores related to individual variables such as grasp strength, whole-arm ROM, pronation–supination, pinch-grip, and dexterity. It can be performed in the clinic or remotely. Once a client has done the test, the system automatically suggests games and difficulty levels that match the client's abilities.

Satisfaction/dissatisfaction with therapy and assistive devices

A problem that has increasingly concerned researchers, healthcare providers, health policy analysts, insurers, and equipment manufacturers, is the difficulty of relating the outcomes of the standard UL tests to real-world needs, most notably independence, employment, community participation, and quality of life. There are questionnaires that provide some insight into these factors from the client's point of view, for example, the Psychosocial Impact of Assistive Devices Scale [136], the Functional Independence Measure (FIM) [137], the Spinal Cord Independence Measure (SCIM) [138] and the Stroke Impact

Scale. These instruments are used to varying degrees to make decisions on the level of home-care needed by individuals. They are also used by insurers and government healthcare agencies to decide on which treatments and devices to reimburse. This is often a make-or-break factor in whether a given treatment or device survives clinically and commercially or not. Unfortunately, at this stage, there are no satisfactory quantitative means of measuring the impact of an intervention on the aforementioned list of real-world needs. Activity monitoring with the use of accelerometers has been proposed, but unfortunately simple accelerometry does not distinguish between movements that are relevant (e.g. job-related manipulation of objects) and those that are not (e.g. arm movements during walking, whole-body accelerations while travelling in a car and so on). Some progress is being made in this respect with the use of multiple sensors, enabling hand opening and closing to be detected specifically [139]. Even so, it will be challenging to distinguish between motor events that relate to the items in the list and those that do not.

Guidelines for selecting UL rehabilitation technologies

Many factors are involved in the choice of methods and devices for UL rehabilitation. Costs must be carefully weighed against the anticipated benefits. Low-cost, structured, conventional exercise programmes, exemplified by the GRASP protocol, are being increasingly adopted in both the clinic and outpatient settings, but because the exercises tend to be repetitive and uninteresting, adherence can be a problem. Wearable, spring-loaded splints are of relatively low cost and may improve motor function during rehabilitation. In principle, they could also be useful as aids to daily living, but their current appearance and bulk may be a barrier for some potential users. FES splints such as the Bioness H200 are increasingly being used in rehabilitation clinics, and FES wristlets currently under development may enable outpatient usage in ADLs as well. Implantable FES devices hold promise, but they are relatively costly and still in the experimental stage. VR exercise therapy has grown rapidly in recent years with the advent of low-cost gaming devices such as the Nintendo Wii and the Xbox Kinect. These devices were not developed for rehabilitation and they do not involve dextrous tasks, nor interaction with real-life objects. They are mainly useful for improving whole-arm ROM. The gaming aspect of VR training is now recognized as a key factor in motivating clients and maintaining their adherence to exercises. Various robotic UL rehabilitation devices incorporating VR gaming have been developed over the last 25 years. They are expensive and therefore they are only found in well-funded clinics. It is still unclear whether they offer significant advantages over conventional occupational therapy. With the growing realization that the client's own efforts rather than external assistance are the key to functional improvement, attention has turned to simpler, less costly, passive devices that use VR gaming. Another growing trend is to extend the period of time that clients perform outpatient exercise therapy with the use of such devices in the home. Internet-based tele-coaching has the potential to maximize the efficacy and duration of in-home exercise therapy, but various barriers must be overcome before this becomes mainstream.

Conclusion

In this chapter we reviewed some of the UL disabilities following stroke and SCI. Conventional approaches to treatment were discussed, and current and emerging technologies that may enhance function, such as active mechanical orthoses and FES devices, were described. Surface FES systems that augment simple hand grasp–release are increasingly seen as useful adjuncts to therapy, particularly in the subacute stages of recovery after stroke or SCI. Their long-term use in ADLs is less common, but with the advent of convenient, low-cost systems that can be voluntarily triggered and used independently in the outpatient setting, this mode of usage may expand in the coming years. Exercise therapy has been identified as being crucial in maximizing the functional outcomes after stroke and SCI. Numerous technological approaches have been proposed to improve adherence to exercise programmes, including computer gaming with purpose-designed rehabilitation robots as well as passive devices. Tele-supervised in-home rehabilitation is still in its early stages, but will probably become an important part of rehabilitation in the future. The costs/benefits ratio will no doubt determine the eventual success or failure of the various technological approaches discussed.

Acknowledgements

This work was supported by the Canadian Institutes for Health Research.

Disclosure of conflict of interest

The author of this chapter has a financial interest in Rehabtronics Inc., manufacturer of the hand stimulator shown in Figure 31.2 and the ReJoyce System shown in Figure 31.4.

References

1. Fang J, Shaw K, George M. Prevalence of Stroke—United States, 2006–2010. Morbidity and Mortality Weekly Report (MMWR). 2012;**61**(20):379–382.
2. Fawcett JW, Curt A, Steeves JD, et al. Guidelines for the conduct of clinical trials for spinal cord injury as developed by the ICCP panel: spontaneous recovery after spinal cord injury and statistical power needed for therapeutic clinical trials. Spinal Cord. 2007;**45**:190–205.
3. Van Der Lee JH, Wagenaar RC, Lankhorst GJ, Vogelaar TW, Deville WL, Bouter LM. Forced use of the upper extremity in chronic stroke patients: results from a single-blind randomized clinical trial. Stroke. 1999;**30**:2369–2375.
4. Kong KH, Lee J, Chua KS. Occurrence and temporal evolution of upper limb spasticity in stroke patients admitted to a rehabilitation unit. Arch Phys Med Rehabil. 2012;**93**:143–148.
5. Sommerfeld DK, Eek EU, Svensson AK, Holmqvist LW, Von Arbin MH. Spasticity after stroke: its occurrence and association with motor impairments and activity limitations. Stroke. 2004;**35**:134–139.
6. Lundstrom E, Terent A, Borg J. Prevalence of disabling spasticity 1 year after first-ever stroke. Eur J Neurol. 2008;**15**:533–539.
7. Watkins CL, Leathley MJ, Gregson JM, Moore AP, Smith TL, Sharma AK. Prevalence of spasticity post stroke. Clin Rehabil. 2002;**16**:515–522.
8. Rizzo MA, Hadjimichael OC, Preiningerova J, Vollmer TL. Prevalence and treatment of spasticity reported by multiple sclerosis patients. Mult Scler. 2004;**10**:589–595.
9. Gracies JM. Pathophysiology of spastic paresis. II: Emergence of muscle overactivity. Muscle Nerve. 2005;**31**:552–571.

10. Welmer AK, Von Arbin M, Widen Holmqvist L, Sommerfeld DK. Spasticity and its association with functioning and health-related quality of life 18 months after stroke. Cerebrovasc Dis. 2006;**21**:247–253.

11. WHO. International Classification of Functioning, Disability and Health (ICF) [Online]. World Health Organization. 2013. Available: http://www.who.int/classifications/icf/en/ (accessed 20 August 2014).

12. Anderson KD, Friden J, Lieber RL. Acceptable benefits and risks associated with surgically improving arm function in individuals living with cervical spinal cord injury. Spinal Cord. 2009;**47**:334–338.

13. Barker RN, Brauer SG. Upper limb recovery after stroke: the stroke survivors' perspective. Disabil Rehabil. 2005;**27**:1213–1223.

14. Barker RN, Gill TJ, Brauer SG. Factors contributing to upper limb recovery after stroke: a survey of stroke survivors in Queensland Australia. Disabil Rehabil. 2007;**29**:981–989.

15. Fugl-Meyer AR, Jaasko L, Leyman I, Olsson S, Steglind S. The post-stroke hemiplegic patient. 1. a method for evaluation of physical performance. Scand J Rehabil Med. 1975;**7**:13–31.

16. Nakayama H, Jorgensen HS, Raaschou HO, Olsen TS. Recovery of upper extremity function in stroke patients: the Copenhagen Stroke Study. Arch Phys Med Rehabil. 1994b;**75**:394–398.

17. Kwakkel G, Kollen BJ, Van Der Grond J, Prevo AJ. Probability of regaining dexterity in the flaccid upper limb: impact of severity of paresis and time since onset in acute stroke. Stroke. 2003;**34**:2181–2186.

18. Wolf SL, Winstein CJ, Miller JP, Blanton S, Clark PC, Nichols-Larsen D. Looking in the Rear View Mirror When Conversing With Back Seat Drivers: The EXCITE Trial Revisited. Neurorehabil Neural Repair. 2007;**21**:379–387.

19. Bobath B. Treatment of adult hemiplegia. Physiotherapy. 1977;**63**:310–313.

20. Bobath B. The application of physiological principles to stroke rehabilitation. Practitioner. 1979;**223**:793–794.

21. Bobath K, Bobath B. Spastic paralysis treatment of by the use of reflex inhibition. Br J Phys Med. 1950;**13**:121–127.

22. Voss DE, Knott M. Patterns of motion for proprioceptive neuromuscular facilitation. Br J Phys Med. 1954;**17**:191–198.

23. Barraclough R. Methods of proprioceptive neuromuscular facilitation; as applied to the re-education of the hemiplegic patient. Physiotherapy. 1958;**44**:252–257.

24. Knutsson E. Proprioceptive neuromuscular facilitation. Scand J Rehabil Med Suppl. 1980;**7**:106–112.

25. Dickstein R, Hocherman S, Pillar T, Shaham R. Stroke rehabilitation. Three exercise therapy approaches. Phys Ther. 1986;**66**:1233–1238.

26. Gordon NF, Gulanick M, Costa F, et al. Physical activity and exercise recommendations for stroke survivors: an American Heart Association scientific statement from the Council on Clinical Cardiology, Subcommittee on Exercise, Cardiac Rehabilitation, and Prevention; the Council on Cardiovascular Nursing; the Council on Nutrition, Physical Activity, and Metabolism; and the Stroke Council. Circulation. 2004;**109**:2031–2041.

27. Sunderland A, Tinson DJ, Bradley EL, Fletcher D, Langton Hewer R, Wade DT. Enhanced physical therapy improves recovery of arm function after stroke. A randomised controlled trial. J Neurol Neurosurg Psychiatry. 1992;**55**:530–535.

28. Barreca S. Management of the Post Stroke Hemiplegic Arm and Hand: Treatment Recommendations of the 2001 Consensus Panel. Heart and Stroke Foundation of Ontario, 2001.

29. Nakayama H, Jorgensen HS, Raaschou HO, Olsen TS. Compensation in recovery of upper extremity function after stroke: the Copenhagen Stroke Study. Arch Phys Med Rehabil. 1994a;**75**:852–857.

30. Taub E, Crago JE, Burgio LD, et al. An operant approach to rehabilitation medicine: overcoming learned nonuse by shaping. J Exp Anal Behav. 1994;**61**:281–293.

31. Wolf SL, Lecraw DE, Barton LA, Jann BB. Forced use of hemiplegic upper extremities to reverse the effect of learned nonuse among chronic stroke and head-injured patients. Exp Neurol. 1989;**104**:125–132.

32. Taub E, Uswatte G, King DK, Morris D, Crago JE, Chatterjee A. A placebo-controlled trial of constraint-induced movement therapy for upper extremity after stroke. Stroke. 2006;**37**:1045–1049.

33. Boake C, Noser EA, Ro T, et al. Constraint-induced movement therapy during early stroke rehabilitation. Neurorehabil Neural Repair. 2007;**21**:14–24.

34. Van Peppen RP, Kwakkel G, Wood-Dauphinee S, Hendriks HJ, Van Der Wees PJ, Dekker J. The impact of physical therapy on functional outcomes after stroke: what's the evidence? Clin Rehabil. 2004;**18**:833–862.

35. Foley N, Mehta S, Jutai J, Staines E, Teasell R. Upper Extremity Interventions. Evidence-based review of stroke rehabilitation. 2013;**10**: 1–163. [Online]. Canadian Stroke Network: ebrsr.com. Available from http://ebrsr.com/sites/default/files/Module-10-upper-extremity_FINAL_16ed.pdf (accessed 30 September 2014).

36. Dobkin BH. Confounders in rehabilitation trials of task-oriented training: lessons from the designs of the EXCITE and SCILT multicenter trials. Neurorehabil Neural Repair. 2007;**21**: 3–13.

37. Van Delden AE, Peper CE, Beek PJ, Kwakkel G. Unilateral versus bilateral upper limb exercise therapy after stroke: a systematic review. J Rehabil Med. 2012;**44**:106–117.

38. Whitall J, Waller SM, Sorkin JD, et al. Bilateral and unilateral arm training improve motor function through differing neuroplastic mechanisms: a single-blinded randomized controlled trial. Neurorehabil Neural Repair. 2011;**25**:118–129.

39. Chan MK, Tong RK, Chung KY. Bilateral upper limb training with functional electric stimulation in patients with chronic stroke. Neurorehabil Neural Repair. 2009;**23**:357–365.

40. McCombe Waller S, Whitall J. Bilateral arm training: why and who benefits? NeuroRehabilitation. 2008;**23**:29–41.

41. Summers JJ, Kagerer FA, Garry MI, Hiraga CY, Loftus A, Cauraugh JH. Bilateral and unilateral movement training on upper limb function in chronic stroke patients: A TMS study. J Neurol Sci. 2007;**252**:76–82.

42. Wolf SL, Winstein CJ, Miller JP, et al. Effect of constraint-induced movement therapy on upper extremity function 3 to 9 months after stroke: the EXCITE randomized clinical trial. JAMA. 2006;**296**:2095–2104.

43. Page, S. J., Sisto, S. A., Levine, P., Johnston, M. V, Hughes, M. 2001. Modified constraint induced therapy: a randomized feasibility and efficacy study. J Rehabil Res Dev, **38**: 583–590.

44. Page SJ, Levine P. Modified constraint-induced therapy extension: using remote technologies to improve function. Arch Phys Med Rehabil. 2007a;**88**:922–927.

45. Page SJ, Levine P. Modified constraint-induced therapy in patients with chronic stroke exhibiting minimal movement ability in the affected arm. Phys Ther. 2007b;**87**:872–878.

46. Harris JE, Eng JJ, Miller WC, Dawson AS. A self-administered Graded Repetitive Arm Supplemntary Program (GRASP) improves arm function during inpatient stroke rehabilitation: a multi-site randomized controlled trial. Stroke. 2009;**40**:2123–2128.

47. Freehafer AA, Kelly CM, Peckham PH. Tendon transfer for the restoration of upper limb function after a cervical spinal cord injury. J Hand Surg. 1984;**9**:887–893.

48. Wuolle KS, Bryden AM, Peckham PH, Murray PK, Keith M. Satisfaction with upper-extremity surgery in individuals with tetraplegia. Arch Phys Med Rehabil. 2003;**84**:1145–1149.

49. Esquenazi A, Talaty M, Packel A, Saulino M. The ReWalk powered exoskeleton to restore ambulatory function to individuals with thoracic-level motor-complete spinal cord injury. Am J Phys Med Rehabil. 2012;**91**:911–921.

50. Allington J, Spencer SJ, Klein J, Buell M, Reinkensmeyer DJ, Bobrow J. Supinator Extender (SUE): a pneumatically actuated robot for

forearm/wrist rehabilitation after stroke. Conf Proc IEEE Eng Med Biol Soc. 2011;**2011**:1579–1582.

51. Stein RB, Prochazka A. Impaired motor function: functional electrical stimulation.. In: Lozano AM, Gildenberg PL, Tasker RR (eds) Textbook of Stereotactic and Functional Neurosurgery. Springer, Berlin, 2009, pp. 3047–3060.

52. Vodovnik L, Bajd T, Kralj A, Gracanin F, Strojnik P. Functional electrical stimulation for control of locomotor systems. CRC Crit Rev Bioeng. 1981;**6**:63–131.

53. Taylor P, Burridge J, Dunkerley A, et al. Clinical audit of 5 years provision of the Odstock dropped foot stimulator. Artif Organs. 1999;**23**:440–442.

54. Stein RB, Chong S, Everaert DG, et al. A multicenter trial of a footdrop stimulator controlled by a tilt sensor. Neurorehabil Neural Repair. 2006;**20**:371–379.

55. Baker L, Yeh C, Wilson D, Waters RL. Electrical stimulation of wrist and fingers for hemiplegic patients. Phys Ther. 1979;**59**:1495–1499.

56. Taylor PN, Burridge J, Swain ID. Electrical stimulation to improve hand function and sensation following chronic stroke. In: Proceedings of the 5th International Workshop on FES. Vienna, Austria 1995, pp. 359–362.

57. Waters R, Bowman B, Baker L, Benton L, Meadows P. Treatment of hemiplegic upper extremity using electrical stimulation and biofeedback training. In: Popovic DJ (ed.) Advances in External Control of Human Extremities. Yugoslav Committee for Electronics and Automation, Belgrade,1981, pp. 251–266.

58. Hansen GVO. EMG-controlled functional electrical stimulation of the paretic hand. Scand J Rehabil Med. 1979;**11**:189–193.

59. Heckmann J, Mokrusch T, Kroeckel A, Warnke S, Von Stockert T, Neundoerfer B. Electromyogram-triggered neuromuscular stimulation for improving the arm function of acute stroke survivors: a randomized pilot study. Eur J Phys Med Rehabil. 1997;**7**:138–141.

60. Francisco G, Chae J, Chawla H, et al. Electromyogram-triggered neuromuscular stimulation for improving the arm function of acute stroke survivors: a randomized pilot study. Arch Phys Med Rehabil. 1998;**79**:570–575.

61. Cauraugh JH, Kim S. Two coupled motor recovery protocols are better than one: electromyogram-triggered neuromuscular stimulation and bilateral movements. Stroke. 2002;**33**:1589–1594.

62. Chae J. Neuromuscular electrical stimulation for motor relearning in hemiparesis. Phys Med Rehabil Clin N Am. 2003;**14**:S93–109.

63. De Kroon JR, Ijzerman MJ, Chae J, Lankhorst GJ, Zilvold G. Relation between stimulation characteristics and clinical outcome in studies using electrical stimulation to improve motor control of the upper extremity in stroke. J Rehabil Med. 2005;**37**:65–74.

64. Nathan RH. US Patent #5,330,516. Device for generating hand function. US Patent Office: 15 claims, 6 drawing sheets. 1994.

65. Prochazka A, Gauthier M, Wieler M, Kenwell Z. The bionic glove: an electrical stimulator garment that provides controlled grasp and hand opening in quadriplegia. Arch Phys Med Rehabil. 1997;**78**:608–614.

66. Weingarden HP, Zeilig G, Heruti R, et al. Hybrid functional electrical stimulation orthosis system for the upper limb: effects on spasticity in chronic stable hemiplegia. Am J Phys Med Rehabil. 1998;**77**:276–281.

67. Popovic D, Stojanovic A, Pjanovic A, et al. Clinical evaluation of the bionic glove. Arch Phys Med Rehabil. 1999;**80**:299–304.

68. Prochazka A. Method and Apparatus for controlling a device or process with vibrations generated by tooth clicks. USA, 6,961,623 patent application. 2005.

69. Keith MW, Peckham PH, Thrope GB, et al. Implantable functional neuromuscular stimulation in the tetraplegic hand. J Hand Surg. 1989;**14**:524–530.

70. Peckham PH, Keith MW, Kilgore KL, et al., Implantable Neuroprosthesis Research Group. Efficacy of an implanted neuro-prosthesis for restoring hand grasp in tetraplegia: a multicenter study. Arch Phys Med Rehabil. 2001;**82**:1380–1388.

71. Hall SW. Commercializing neuroprostheses: The business of putting the brain back in business. BA Molecular Biology Thesis, Princeton University, 2003. Available from http://portal.bm.technion.ac.il/Labs/niel/Public%20Data/Publications/Hall_Thesis.pdf (accessed 30 September 2014).

72. Hart RL, Bhadra N, Montague FW, Kilgore KL, Peckham PH. Design and testing of an advanced implantable neuroprosthesis with myoelectric control. IEEE Trans Neural Syst Rehabil Eng. 2011;**19**:45–53.

73. Kilgore KL, Hart RL, Montague FW, et al. An implanted myoelectrically-controlled neuroprosthesis for upper extremity function in spinal cord injury. Conf Proc IEEE Eng Med Biol Soc. 2006;**1**:1630–1633.

74. Knutson JS, Chae J, Hart RL, et al. Implanted neuroprosthesis for assisting arm and hand function after stroke: a case study. J Rehabil Res Dev. 2012;**49**:1505–1516.

75. Spensley J. STIMuGRIP(R); a new Hand Control Implant. Conf Proc IEEE Eng Med Biol Soc. 2007;**1**:513.

76. Gan LS, Ravid E, Kowalczewski JA, Olson JL, Morhart M, Prochazka A. First permanent implant of nerve stimulation leads activated by surface electrodes, enabling hand grasp and release: the stimulus router neuroprosthesis. Neurorehabil Neural Repair. 2012;**26**:335–343.

77. Saposnik G, Levin M. Virtual reality in stroke rehabilita-tion: a meta-analysis and implications for clinicians. Stroke. 2011;**42**:1380–1386.

78. Burdea G, Langrana N, Roskos E, Silver D, Zhuang J. A portable dextrous master with force feedback Presence. 1992;**1**: 18–28.

79. Popescu VG, Burdea GC, Bouzit M, Hentz VR. A virtual-reality-based telerehabilitation system with force feedback. IEEE Trans Inf Technol Biomed. 2000;**4**:45–51.

80. Allen D. You're never too old for a Wii. Nurs Older People. 2007;**19**:8.

81. Cowley AD, Minnaar G. New generation computer games: Watch out for Wii shoulder. Br Med J. 2008;**336**:110.

82. Deutsch JE, Borbely M, Filler J, Huhn K, Guarrera-Bowlby P. Use of a low-cost, commercially available gaming console (Wii) for rehabilitation of an adolescent with cerebral palsy. Phys Ther. 2008;**88**:1196–1207.

83. Graves LE, Ridgers ND, Stratton G. The contribution of upper limb and total body movement to adolescents' energy expenditure whilst playing Nintendo Wii. Eur J Appl Physiol. 2008;**104**:617–623.

84. Robinson RJ, Barron DA, Grainger AJ, Venkatesh R. Wii knee. Emerg Radiol. 2008;**15**:255–257.

85. Saposnik G, Teasell R, Mamdani M, et al. Effectiveness of virtual reality using Wii gaming technology in stroke rehabilitation: a pilot randomized clinical trial and proof of principle. Stroke. 2010;**41**:1477–1484.

86. Dirette D, Hinojosa J. Effects of continuous passive motion on the edematous hands of two persons with flaccid hemiplegia. Am J Occupat Ther. 1994;**48**:403–409.

87. Salter RB. History of rest and motion and the scientific basis for early continuous passive motion. Hand Clin. 1996;**12**:1–11.

88. Aisen ML, Krebs HI, Hogan N, Mcdowell F, Volpe BT. The effect of robot-assisted therapy and rehabilitative training on motor recovery following stroke. Arch Neurol. 1997;**54**:443–446.

89. Hogan N, Krebs HI, Rohrer B, et al. Motions or muscles? Some behavioral factors underlying robotic assistance of motor recovery. J Rehabil Res Dev. 2006;**43**:605–618.

90. Lo AC, Guarino PD, Richards LG, et al. Robot-assisted therapy for long-term upper-limb impairment after stroke. N Engl J Med. 2010;**362**:1772–1783.

91. Dukelow SP, Herter TM, Bagg SD, Scott SH. The independence of deficits in position sense and visually guided reaching following stroke. J Neuroeng Rehabil. 2012;**9**:72.

92. Bovolenta, F, Sale P, Dall'armi V, Clerici P, Franceschini M. Robot-aided therapy for upper limbs in patients with stroke-related

lesions. Brief report of a clinical experience. J Neuroeng Rehabil. 2011;**8**:18.

93. Nef T, Riener R. Three-Dimensional Multi-Degree-of-Freedom Arm Therapy Robot (ARMin). In: Dietz V, Nef T, Rymer WZ (eds) Neurorehabilitation Technology. Springer, London, 2012, pp. 141–157.

94. Prange GB, Jannink MJ, Groothuis-Oudshoorn CG, Hermens HJ, Ijzerman MJ. Systematic review of the effect of robot-aided therapy on recovery of the hemiparetic arm after stroke. J Rehabil Res Dev. 2006;**43**:171–184.

95. Kwakkel G, Kollen BJ, Krebs HI. Effects of robot-assisted therapy on upper limb recovery after stroke: a systematic review. Neurorehabil Neural Repair. 2008;**22**:111–121.

96. Reinkensmeyer DJ, Akoner O, Ferris DP, Gordon KE. Slacking by the human motor system: Computational models and implications for robotic orthoses. Conf Proc IEEE Eng Med Biol Soc. 2009;**1**:2129–2132.

97. Kahn LE, Lum PS, Rymer WZ, Reinkensmeyer DJ. Robot-assisted movement training for the stroke-impaired arm: Does it matter what the robot does? J Rehabil Res Dev. 2006;**43**:619–630.

98. Kutner NG, Zhang R, Butler AJ, Wolf SL, Alberts JL. Quality-of-life change associated with robotic-assisted therapy to improve hand motor function in patients with subacute stroke: a randomized clinical trial. Phys Ther. 2010;**90**:493–504.

99. Schweighofer N, Choi Y, Winstein C, Gordon J. Task-oriented rehabilitation robotics. Am J Phys Med Rehabil. 2012;**91**:S270–279.

100. Reinkensmeyer D.. Functional assisted gaming for upper-extremity therapy after stroke: background, evaluation, and future directions of the spring orthosis approach.. In: Dietz V, Nef T, Rymer WZ (eds) Neurorehabilitation Technology. Springer, London, 2012, pp. 327–341.

101. Sanchez RJ, Liu J, Rao S, et al. Automating arm movement training following severe stroke: functional exercises with quantitative feedback in a gravity-reduced environment. IEEE Trans Neural Syst Rehabil Eng. 2006;**14**:378–389.

102. Colomer C, Baldovi A, Torrome S, et al. Efficacy of Armeo(R) Spring during the chronic phase of stroke. Study in mild to moderate cases of hemiparesis. Neurologia. 2013;**28**:261–267.

103. Wolf SL, Catlin PA, Ellis M, Archer AL, Morgan B, Piacentino A. Assessing Wolf motor function test as outcome measure for research in patients after stroke. Stroke. 2001;**32**:1635–1639.

104. Zariffa J, Kapadia N, Kramer JL, et al. Feasibility and efficacy of upper limb robotic rehabilitation in a subacute cervical spinal cord injury population. Spinal Cord. 2012;**50**:220–226.

105. Prange GB, Jannink MJ, Stienen AH, Van Der Kooij H, Ijzerman MJ, Hermens HJ. Influence of gravity compensation on muscle activation patterns during different temporal phases of arm movements of stroke patients. Neurorehabil Neural Repair. 2009;**23**:478–485.

106. Krabben T, Prange GB, Molier BI, et al. S. Influence of gravity compensation training on synergistic movement patterns of the upper extremity after stroke, a pilot study. J Neuroeng Rehabil. 2012;**9**:44.

107. Kowalczewski J, Chong SL, Galea M, Prochazka A. In-Home Tele-Rehabilitation Improves Tetraplegic Hand Function. Neurorehabil Neural Repair. 2011;**25**:412–422.

108. Kowalczewski J, Prochazka A. Technology improves upper extremity rehabilitation. Prog Brain Res. 2011a;**192**:147–159.

109. Lange BS, Requejo P, Flynn SM, et al. The potential of virtual reality and gaming to assist successful aging with disability. Phys Med Rehabil Clin N Am. 2010;**21**:339–356.

110. Teasell R, Foley N, Bhogal SK, Speechley M. Outpatient Stroke Rehabilitation. Evidence-based review of stroke rehabilitation. 7: 1-41, 2013 [Online]. Canadian Stroke Network: ebrsr.com. Available: http://ebrsr.com/sites/default/files/Chapter7_Outpatients_FINAL_16ed.pdf (accessed)

111. Fisher RJ. Implementing early supported discharge in stroke care. Nat Rev Neurol. 2011;**8**:176.

112. Winters JM. Telerehabilitation research: emerging opportunities. Annu Rev Biomed Eng. 2002;**4**:287–320.

113. Heuser A, Kourtev H, Winter S, et al. Telerehabilitation using the Rutgers Master II glove following carpal tunnel release surgery: proof-of-concept. IEEE Trans Neural Syst Rehabil Eng. 2007;**15**:43–49.

114. Piron L, Turolla A, Agostini M, et al. Assessment and treatment of the upper limb by means of virtual reality in post-stroke patients. Stud Health Technol Inform. 2009;**145**:55–62.

115. Langan J, Delave K, Phillips L, Pangilinan P, Brown SH. Home-based telerehabilitation shows improved upper limb function in adults with chronic stroke: A pilot study. J Rehabil Med. 2013;**45**:217–220.

116. Reinkensmeyer DJ, Pang CT, Nessler JA, Painter CC. Web-based telerehabilitation for the upper extremity after stroke. IEEE Trans Neural Syst Rehabil Eng. 2002;**10**:102–108.

117. Kowalczewski J, Prochazka A. Technology improves upper extremity rehabilitation. In: Green AM, Chapman CE, Kalaska JF, Lepore F (eds.) Enhancing Performance for Action and Perception. Elsevier, Amsterdam, 2011b, pp. 147–159.

118. Kowalczewski J, Gritsenko V, Ashworth N, Ellaway P, Prochazka A. Upper-extremity functional electric stimulation-assisted exercises on a workstation in the subacute phase of stroke recovery. Arch Phys Med Rehabil. 2007;**88**:833–839.

119. Buick A, Unterschultz L, Kowalczewski J, Carson RG, Prochazka A. Use of accelerometers and MEPs to assess corticospinal excitability following novel combined therapy in chronic stroke. In: Society for Neuroscience, 42nd AGM, New Orleans, 2012, p. 276.20.

120. Wade DT, Hewer RL. Functional abilities after stroke: measurement, natural history and prognosis. J Neurol Neurosurg Psychiatry. 1987;**50**:177–182.

121. Cohn ER. Telerehabilitation in 2012: policy and infrastructure challenges to ubiquitous deployment across the United States. In: RESNA Annual Conference—2012, Baltimore, MD. Available from http://www.rerctr.pitt.edu/Graphics/Poster/RERC_TR_0119_12.png (accessed 30 September 2014).

122. Lang CE, Bland MD, Bailey RR, Schaefer SY, Birkenmeier RL. Assessment of upper extremity impairment, function, and activity after stroke: foundations for clinical decision making. J Hand Ther. 2013;**26**:104–114;quiz 115.

123. Lang CE, Wagner JM, Dromerick AW, Edwards DF. Measurement of upper-extremity function early after stroke: properties of the action research arm test. Arch Phys Med Rehabil. 2006;**87**:1605–1610.

124. Lyle RC. A performance test for assessment of upper limb function in physical rehabilitation treatment and research. Int J Rehabil Res. 1981;**4**:483–492.

125. Mathiowetz V, Volland G, Kashman N, Weber K. Adult norms for the Box and Block Test of manual dexterity. Am J Occup Ther. 1985;**39**:386–391.

126. Barreca S, Gowland CK, Stratford P, et al. Development of the Chedoke Arm and Hand Activity Inventory: theoretical constructs, item generation, and selection. Top Stroke Rehabil. 2004;**11**:31–42.

127. Jebsen RH, Taylor N, Trieschmann RB, Trotter MJHLA. An objective and standardized test of hand function. Arch. Physical Med. Rehab. 1969;**50**:311–319.

128. Heller A, Wade DT, Wood VA, Sunderland A, Hewer RL, Ward E. Arm function after stroke: measurement and recovery over the first three months. J Neurol Neurosurg Psychiatry. 1987;**50**:714–719.

129. Duncan PW, Wallace D, Lai SM, Johnson D, Embretson S, Laster LJ. The stroke impact scale version 2.0. Evaluation of reliability, validity, and sensitivity to change. Stroke. 1999;**30**:2131–2140.

130. Uswatte G, Taub E, Morris D, Vignolo M, Mcculloch K. Reliability and validity of the upper-extremity Motor Activity Log-14 for measuring real-world arm use. Stroke. 2005;**36**:2493–2496.

131. Connell LA, Tyson SF. Clinical reality of measuring upper-limb ability in neurologic conditions: a systematic review. Arch Phys Med Rehabil. 2012;**93**:221–228.

132. Kapadia N, Zivanovic V, Verrier M, Popovic MR. Toronto rehabilitation institute-hand function test: assessment of gross

motor function in individuals with spinal cord injury. Top Spinal Cord Inj Rehabil. 2012;**18**:167–186.

133. Coderre AM, Zeid AA, Dukelow SP, et al. Assessment of upper-limb sensorimotor function of subacute stroke patients using visually guided reaching. Neurorehabil Neural Repair. 2010;**24**:528–541.

134. Dukelow SP, Herter TM, Moore KD, et al. Quantitative assessment of limb position sense following stroke. Neurorehabil Neural Repair. 2010;**24**:178–187.

135. Prochazka A, Kowalczewski J. A fully-automated, quantitative test of upper limb function J Motor Behav. 2015;**47** in press.

136. Jutai J, Day H. Psychosocial Impact of Assistive Devices Scale (PIADS). Technology and Disability 2002;**14**:107–111

137. Dodds T, Martin D, Stolov W, Deyo R. A validation of the functional independence measurement and its performance among rehabilitation inpatients. Arch Phys Med Rehabil. 1993;**74**:531–536.

138. Itzkovich M, Gelernter I, Biering-Sorensen F, et al. The Spinal Cord Independence Measure (SCIM) version III: reliability and validity in a multi-center international study. Disabil Rehabil. 2007;**29**:1926–1933.

139. Friedman N, Bachman M, Reinkensmeyer DJ. Device and method for providing hand rehabilitation and assessment of hand function, filed May 25, 2012. USA patent application US **13**/481,685. 2013.

CHAPTER 32

Technology to enhance locomotor function

Rüdiger Rupp, Daniel Schließmann,
Christian Schuld, and Norbert Weidner

Introduction

The loss of mobility due to sensorimotor dysfunction of the lower extremities has devastating effects on the quality of life of affected individuals and their ability to remain independent in the community. This in particular applies to patients with neurological gait disorders of the central nervous system (CNS) like stroke, Parkinson's disease (PD), multiple sclerosis (MS), or spinal cord injury (SCI). Stroke is one of the most prevalent neurological conditions worldwide (1.1 million first strokes per year in Europe) and the leading cause for persistent disabilities in adults [1]. Moreover, the burden of stroke is high and is likely to increase in future decades [2]. A stroke is typically followed by a hemiparesis, which frequently affects walking function. In stroke rehabilitation gait restoration has high priority, since mobility is a key prerequisite for independence. Hemiparesis, in combination with the unsteadiness to walk, promotes reduced motor activities, resulting in further gait deterioration, acceleration of cardiovascular diseases, and musculoskeletal abnormalities. Therefore, the ultimate aim of gait rehabilitation is to provide patients an efficient and safe walking ability. Another patient group with severe restrictions of walking function are PD patients. More than 1 million people in the United States suffer from PD, which affects approximately 1 in 100 Americans older than 60 years [3]. In most patients the first symptoms appear in the age between 50 and 60, and 5–10% of the affected persons are younger than 40 [4]. Gait is one of the most affected motor characteristics of this disorder, although symptoms of PD vary. The gait pattern in PD is characterized by small shuffling steps and a general slowness of movement (bradykinesia). Patients with PD have difficulties initiating steps, but also stopping. MS affects approximately 400,000 people in the United States and 2.5 million worldwide [5]. More than 200 people are diagnosed with MS each week in the United States. MS typically begins between 20 and 40 years of age and is the leading cause of non-traumatic disability in young adults. Gait disturbances are among the most prevalent disabilities in MS, which are related to paresis, drop foot, spasticity, loss of balance, sensory ataxia, and fatigue.

In the US an estimated number of 250,000 (Europe: 330,000) people suffer from SCI with 11,000 new injuries per year [6], of which 40% are tetraplegic. Though the SCI has a traumatic origin in the majority of patients (45%), during the last decade the percentage of non-traumatic patients is constantly growing. This contributed to a trend seen in industrial countries that the number of incomplete lesions increases, which nowadays constitute approx. 60–70% of the overall population.

Compensation versus restoration

In the rehabilitation of gait disorders two main concepts—namely compensation and restoration—are applied. Compensation means that lost motor functions are substituted by other, preserved functions or by assistive technology. Restoration means that a weak or lost function is recovered by training. Compensation is the preferred approach in the rehabilitation of individuals with severe CNS injuries, such as motor and sensory complete SCI. Adaptive equipment and/or neuroprostheses based on functional electrical stimulation (FES) are employed as compensatory strategies [7] to perform functional activities and to increase the level of independence in individuals with persistent handicap. Therapeutic strategies emphasizing on compensation in the rehabilitation of gait include [8]:

1. Gait training using compensatory movement strategies, for example, compensate for restriction in plantar dorsiflexion by increased hip flexion or trunk movements.

2. Strengthening innervated musculature with preserved voluntary control, emphasizing muscles required to perform compensatory movements.

3. Adaptive equipment like knee–ankle–foot orthoses, reciprocing gait orthosis and/or FES splints mainly for correction of drop foot.

4. Providing appropriate equipment to enhance activity and participation. Examples are wheelchairs, walkers or canes.

In contrast to compensation a restorative rehabilitation approach aims to reinstall a normal movement pattern and to avoid compensatory movements at the same time. Over the last two decades restorative strategies have gained high acceptance among therapists due to scientific findings about the intrinsic capacity of the CNS for use-dependent neuroplasticity and reorganisation. Restorative therapies are typically applied to individuals with a high potential for neurological recovery, for example, motor incomplete SCI

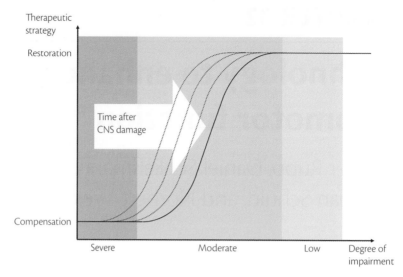

Fig. 32.1 Dependency of the therapeutic strategy and the degree of the impairment.

usually in the subacute stage after CNS injury. The therapeutic strategies emphasizing restoration in rehabilitation after CNS injury include [8]:

1. Locomotor training involving body weight-supported step training on a treadmill and/or overground. Stepping assistance can be provided manually or using robotic gait orthosis. In some cases, these strategies are combined with mechanical orthoses and/or strengthening of innervated musculature.

2. Conventional gait training involving practice of static and dynamic standing balance, stepping, and walking. Like in locomotor training these strategies are combined with mechanical orthosis and/or strengthening of innervated musculature.

3. Functional electrical stimulation therapy for neuromuscular re-education and functional training emphasizing on normal movement patterns.

At this point, there is no evidence regarding the optimal timing and combination of compensation-based therapies in relation to restoration-based approaches for patients with spared sensorimotor function. Based on clinical experience, the more sensorimotor function is preserved the more and earlier restorative strategies should be employed. Training should be balanced towards compensation in cases with little remaining voluntary movement (Figure 32.1). In patients with little or maximal impairment the choice of compensation versus restoration is rather easy, whereas in persons with moderate impairments the boundaries of compensation and restoration become indistinct. In other instances, compensatory strategies support restorative efforts: Compensatory walking aids like braces may improve the knee or ankle joint stability and thus allow a person with substantially preserved voluntary motor function to take part in a restorative gait therapy. In any case, technology plays an important role in the implementation of both strategies in the clinical as well as the domestic environment.

The aim of this chapter is to provide an overview of the established and most recent technology to promote locomotion either by restorative or a compensatory means and to provide insights to limitations of current technology together with challenges and opportunities of future developments.

Clinical evidence of restorative gait therapies

After extensive animal research demonstrated the feasibility and success of task specific locomotor training approaches, the concept of body weight supported treadmill training (BWSTT) was introduced into the clinical setting. The key component of BWSTT is the support of the patient's body weight by a harness in combination with a static (counterweights) or dynamic (springs and/or active drives) weight reduction system. The latter has the advantage to compensate for the moment of inertia caused by the counterweights at higher gait speeds, when fast vertical shifts of the body centre occur. In case of weak muscles or spasticity the stepping movements, and under certain circumstances also the trunk, are manually assisted by up to three therapists.

Over the last 15 years BWSTT has been established as a standard therapy in the gait rehabilitation of patients with stroke [9], incomplete SCI [10], and MS [11]. PD patients receive treadmill training to improve their hypokinesia-induced gait impairment [12]. Besides positive effects related to walking speed and endurance, normalization of the muscular activation pattern, and improved capability for weight bearing reductions in spasticity and increases in cardiopulmonary efficiency have also been shown following BWSTT [13]. It has to be noted that most of these studies included subjects in the subacute or chronic stage. A randomized, controlled multicentre clinical trial comparing 12 weeks of manual-assisted BWSTT with conventional overground gait training in acute subjects (incomplete SCI patients within 8 weeks post trauma) did not find differences in walking speed and distance nor the locomotor subscore of the Functional Independence Measure [14] between the two groups 6 months after study inclusion [15]. Interestingly, both treatment groups showed much better outcomes compared to a historic control group. The authors discuss that both the treadmill and the conventional gait training group received a much higher therapy intensity and duration than those usually applied in clinical routine [16].

Neurobiological basis for an effective locomotor training

It has been proposed for more than 250 years that activity patterns for locomotion originate from segmental spinal circuits. But it was the work of Sherrington [17] and Brown [18] in the beginning of the 20th century that truly moved this field forward. In these studies, they found that, with appropriate sensory stimuli from the periphery, spinalized cats generated patterned movements that mimicked those exhibited during swing and stance phases of locomotion. What they originally termed 'the intrinsic factor' has now become known as the central pattern generator (CPG). The CPG is a cluster of neuronal networks in the CNS, including the spinal cord, that can generate basic rhythmical motor patterns. These networks play an important role in tasks such as chewing and breathing and are also involved in the generation of the flexion and extension patterns during walking [19]. Recent clinical studies confirm older observations showing that in humans the pattern generator networks for walking are located in the lower thoracic and upper lumbar spinal cord comparable to findings obtained in several animal species [20, 21].

The imagination of the CPG being something like the 'sinoatrial node of the spinal cord' is completely wrong. This neuronal network needs sufficient input from supraspinal respectively cortical neurons to receive some sort of pushing signal for generation of a walking pattern [22]. Additionally, afferent feedback from the periphery is necessary to continuously adapt the weighting of pre-programmed patterns, so called movement primitives [23], to the actual environmental conditions [24]. In this context, some stimuli seem to be more efficient in activating the CPG than others. It has been shown in complete SCI subjects that the physiological movement of the hip joint, in particular the extension at the end of the stance phase, and the appropriate gait-phase related loading of the foot soles are the key trigger sources of the spinal gait pattern generator [25]. Based on the findings about the functionality of the locomotor pattern generators additional experiments with spinalized cats and rats have been performed, which proofed that the CPG can be trained by appropriate paradigms and that herewith a better functional outcome can be achieved [26]. The reason for these improvements is the live-long ability of the CNS for reorganization of neural connections, so called neuroplasticity [27]. This ability for adaptation and learning is not only present in the brain, but also in the spinal cord. A recent experiment in cats applied a sequential dual-lesion paradigm consisting of: (1) an initially unilateral hemisection of the spinal cord at a level well rostral to the CPG located in the lumbosacral segments, resulting in an incomplete paralysis of the hindlimbs; and (2) a complete injury 3 weeks later two segments caudal to the first level. The main idea of this paradigm is that if intrinsic changes occurred within the spinal cord itself during locomotor recovery after the initial hemisection, these changes could probably be retained and expressed very early after a second, and complete, spinalization a few segments below. Directly after the hemisection the cats showed an altered gait pattern at both hindlimbs, which normalized by gait training in the next 3 weeks. Immediately after complete spinalization cats showed normal hindlimb locomotion without any pharmacological stimulation. This indicates that the incomplete spinal injury had induced plastic changes within the spinal circuitry below the level of lesion, such that the CPG was already primed to re-express locomotion after the complete SCI [28].

Principles of motor learning

The fundamental concept of restoration of motor functions is based on the assumption that practice of respective movements induces plastic changes in the altered CNS representing the structural correlate of motor learning. Moreover, the frequency and duration of practice correlates with the level of motor performance. Thus, repetition represents the key factor for successful motor learning. Although this may be the most effective way to improve short term performance during the training session, it is not sufficient for retaining motor skills over time. A set of factors—called principles of motor learning—have been identified that contribute to the long-term retention of a newly acquired skill (Table 32.1) [29]. Among them are the degree of active participation and motivation of the patient, an appropriate intrinsic and extrinsic feedback, the adaptation of the complexity of the movement task, and contextual interference, in which variability and diversification of the movement tasks are explicit components of the gait training.

Overview of effective treadmill training parameters

Although the general framework of the principles of motor learning is well known, it does not translate into detailed recommendations for practitioners to perform BWSTT. A systematic evaluation of BWSTT variables in stroke patients revealed that a faster walking speed with body weight support ranging from 35–50% lead to the most physiological gait pattern [30]. The most effective afferent stimuli for activation of the CPG have been identified by studying the muscular activation patterns in individuals with complete SCI during systematic variation of the degree of hip extension and of foot loading [25]. It was shown that hip extension initiated swing phase and that a sufficient degree of foot loading is necessary to elicit a CPG efferent output. Based on these results it can be concluded that the degree of body weight support should be adjusted to the minimal amount of support with the caveat that joint overloading (like hyperextension of the knee) needs to be avoided. A poorly documented detail in studies using BWSTT is the use of handrails and details on the mechanical design of the weight support system, in particular the design of the attachment point(s) of the overhead suspension. With only one attachment point, which does not restrict rotational movements, the individual to be trained on the treadmill may have a hard time to stabilize in the transversal plane, in particular with higher degrees of body weight support. In those cases handrail use is mandatory to achieve a physiological gait pattern. In case a patient shows improvements during the rehabilitation process, based on practical experience it is advisable to first increase treadmill speed until a normal walking speed is reached followed by a stepwise decrease of body weight support until full weight bearing is achieved [31, 32].

Patient-related variables have a strong impact on the therapy success. Starting task-specific training early on after CNS injury seems to yield better rehabilitative outcomes [33, 34]. SCI patients with an initially incomplete lesion and preserved sensory and some motor function caudal to the level of lesion will most likely develop a relevant walking function [35]. However, tetraplegic SCI patients compared to paraplegics need higher muscle forces in the lower extremities for an ambulatory function [36].

Table 32.1 The principles of motor learning

Principle of motor learning	Explanation
Task specifity	'Walking can only be learned by walking'. To improve a specific skill, the respective movement task or a closely related needs to be practised.
Active participation	Active participation of the patient forms the basis for initiation of neuronal plastic changes. Motivation and eagerness strongly influence the therapy outcome.
Repetition	For transfer of short-term adaptations in motor control into sustained movement patterns, the movement task has to be repeated often.
Adaptation of the complexity ('Shaping')	The difficulty of a movement task has to be chosen according to the functional status of the patient. A too simple movement task is boring and thus does not challenge the patient, a too complex, not executable task is overloading the patient and is therefore frustrating.
Feedback	Inherent as well as augmented feedback of the motor performance forms an essential component of a therapy for normalization of pathological movement patterns.
Variability 'contextual interference'	Whereas repetition of the same movement task leads to an increased performance of the trained movement, the introduction of variability enhances the learning process and retention. Diversification increases the active participation of a patient.
Distributed practice	In general, shorter, distributed sessions with intermittent pause periods seem to be more effective than longer block sessions ('massed practice').
Generalization	Improved motor skills in an artificial environment, e.g. treadmill or locomotion robot do not necessarily lead to enhanced skills in a natural environment. Dedicated therapeutic interventions are needed to transfer training skills to daily-life activities.

Locomotion robots for automated gait training

Technical specifications of robotic locomotion systems

After the benefits of treadmill therapy were proven, 10 years ago the first steps were undertaken towards automation of BWSTT with the development of motor-driven gait orthoses [37] or specialized locomotion training devices [38]. The main aim of these developments was to free therapists from the exhausting work of manually assisting the stepping movements and to perform a therapy in a more standardized fashion (Figure 32.2). The active components of the robots consist mainly of electric motors or pneumatically driven actuators in combination with spindles, gears, or bowden cables. Pneumatic actuators have the advantage of inherent lower stiffness, which reduces the risk of injuries. However, if they are used in highly dynamic configuration, they consume a high amount of compressed air and need sophisticated controllers to compensate their nonlinearities. Within the class of active devices there are technically more simple devices, which are

mainly based on an end-effector approach, and complex devices, in which several degrees of freedom (DOF) of several joints are actively driven independently.

The end-effector based systems use footplates to guide the movements of the foot in space. Examples of machines based on the end-effector approach for the lower extremity is the Gait Trainer (RehaHesse, Berlin, Germany) and the more sophisticated G-EO (Reha Technology, Olten, Switzerland) [38, 39]. Their main advantage is their easy setup, since no technical joint axes of the device have to be aligned with the axes of the anatomical joints. Furthermore, they only use one or two drives per extremity to generate a two-dimensional planar motion. With the G-EO device walking and stair climbing/ascending can be trained in the same therapy session without adaption of the machine (Figure 32.3). However, in end-effector devices the movements originate from the most distal segment of the extremity and therefore—though the kinematic movement pattern looks similar to the physiological situation—the kinetics of the generated movements may not be perfectly physiological. However, this seems to be crucial for the success of the therapy [25]. Additionally, in end-effector based robots only information about forces and/or position of the most distal part of the extremity is available, which may be too unspecific for control of a physiological kinetic and kinematic movement trajectory. For separation of the complex movement task of a physiological, reciprocal gait pattern into single, less complex subtasks the degree of support has to be separately adjustable for each joint. A physiological movement of all joints of an extremity can only be achieved by the use of active drives, which support the movements of the main DOF of a dedicated joint. Additionally, an individualized setup of a joint and movement phase related resistance is only possible with actively driven exoskeletons.

Actuated exoskeletons normally operate in conjunction with a system for partial body weight unloading and a moving treadmill. Examples for actively driven exoskeletons are the well-established Lokomat, the LOPES, and ALEX devices [40–42]. Because active components including their controllers form the most expensive parts of a robotic device, usually a compromise between costs and functionality in terms of generating a perfect physiological trajectory in three dimensions has to be made. Therefore robotic locomotion training machines are mainly generating movements in the sagittal plane, whereas movements in the frontal or transversal plane are not supported or even restricted. However, many patients have weak leg abductor and adductor muscles and practitioners often wish to have the possibility for robotic training of these muscle groups, which are highly relevant for a physiological walking pattern. A general challenge of the application of exoskeletons is their proper adjustment and alignment to the anatomical constraints of the different types of joints. Due to their mechanical complexity exoskeletons are often time consuming in their initial setup and in everyday applications.

Though actively driven exoskeletons represent the state of the art of robotics technology they still leave room for improvement [43]. Most of the systems are operating in a position control mode, which means that the actively driven joints follow predefined reference trajectories. Hence, the position-controlled robot does not integrate the patient's residual capabilities and support is provided even during gait phases, where the voluntary force of the patient would be sufficient for a physiological movement. In this condition the robotic device does not help, but hinders a patient

(A) 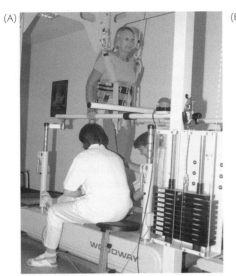 (B)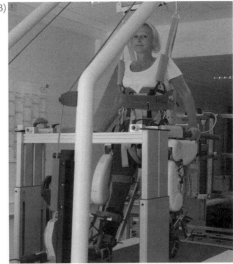

Fig. 32.2 Comparison between manually assisted (a) and automated (b) treadmill training.

to perform a given motor task. To overcome this limitation several, more compliant control concepts were introduced—first of all the impedance control concept [44]. In a pure impedance control scheme the current position of the robot is virtually coupled to a reference position by a simulated spring and damper assembly with adjustable stiffness and damping values. With reduced spring stiffness, patients can participate more actively and experience more movement variability. However, they can also lead to unfavourable movement patterns and become more and more

affected by the inertia of the robot as impedance is reduced. Therefore, an adaptive impedance control scheme in the sense of 'assist-as-needed' should be implemented into the active devices to challenge the patient as much as possible and to provide support, when and where it is needed [45]. Special focus should be put on the fact that a physiological movement does not consist of a highly reproductive movement pattern, but contains some inherent variability. Therefore, robotic devices should also incorporate a control scheme that allows for small deviations from the reference trajectory and enables patients to improve their gait patterns on a trial-and-error basis. A pilot study incorporating this control scheme shows promising results [46]. Nevertheless, until now none of these prototypically implemented, highly sophisticated control concepts have found their way into routine clinical applications. Though the underlying reasons can only be speculated, it seems that due to the need for individual, regular tuning of the control algorithms and their limited robustness these systems can only be handled by highly experienced technicians, who are normally not present in a clinical environment.

Clinical evidence in effectiveness of robotic locomotion therapy

With the support of locomotion robots the maximum time per therapy session is only determined by the training capacity of the patient and no longer by the physical constraints of the therapists. Furthermore, a reproducible gait pattern independent of environmental conditions can be achieved [40]. Despite robotic therapeutic devices became a clinical routine rehabilitative therapy over the years, the question regarding their efficacy compared to conventional treatment has still to be answered. Due to the well known advances of industrial robots regarding higher precision, higher reproducibility and product quality and faster production time therapists and patients tend to rate robotic therapies as being more effective than manual therapies. In contrast to this assumption, results of randomized controlled trials comparing robot-assisted therapy with conventional gait training including BWSTT do not indicate a general superiority of robotic training. Based on this evidence it was suggested to completely

Fig. 32.3 The end-effector based G-EO training robot supporting users in practising walking and stair climbing.
With kind permission of Reha Technology AG, Olten, Switzerland.

disestablish robotic therapies in clinical routines [47]. Although study participants and training regimes varied to a large degree, studies focusing on non-ambulatory subjects found advantages of robot-aided gait training [34, 48, 49]. Studies on ambulatory subjects found conventional gait training consisting of postural tasks, overground walking, speed tasks, symmetry of lower limb movements, stair climbing, and BWSTT to be more effective [50, 51]. Taken together, these results suggest that, at this point, robot-aided treadmill training is most effective for severely affected, non-ambulatory patients, whereas it is less effective in already ambulatory patients.

Why do robots not lead to a superior outcome in patients with minor gait disorders despite their ability to generate highly reproducible stepping patterns over a prolonged training session? Apparently, in non-ambulatory patients the training intensity in respect to the number of repetitions seems to be important for improvement, whereas in ambulatory patients other factors contributing to an enhanced locomotor performance (Table 32.1) become more relevant [52]. A clear disadvantage of the robotic devices currently used in clinical routine is the lack of an assist-as-needed control scheme, which does not sufficiently challenge the patient. Device developers have to keep in mind that during training the task has to be repeated, not the movement. In conclusion, the principles of motor learning (Table 32.1) have to be implemented more consequently into robotic devices to improve the effectiveness of robotic locomotion therapies in ambulatory patients. An appropriate feedback functionality and control algorithms allowing for deviations from the uniform walking pattern might be key components for an improved therapy. It has to be emphasized that a robot alone does not represent a stand-alone tool, which promotes gait rehabilitation through all stages of rehabilitation. Moreover, its full potential can only be utilized if robotic tools are embedded in a comprehensive gait therapy concept [50, 53].

Extended possibilities of technology for enhancement of locomotion

Up to now, locomotion robots have proved their feasibility and safety after many therapy sessions. They clearly help to reduce physical workload in therapists engaged in the gait rehabilitation process. So far, the developmental process of robotic locomotion devices has been mainly guided by the scope of perfectly mimicking the motor behaviour of a human therapist. However, robotic locomotion devices, even at their current stage of implementation and with all their technological limitations, can go beyond this scope and may open up novel areas of applications. Further enhancement of gait rehabilitation outcomes may be achieved by (1) transferring robotic training devices in application fields, which are currently insufficiently covered by therapists (e.g. home-based training), and (2) extending the therapeutic options by utilizing the multidimensional sensors of a robot.

Robots for home-based locomotion therapy

Due to increasing economical restrictions in the health care system the length of primary rehabilitation is continuously getting shorter [54]. With the help of robotic locomotion devices the sufficient intensity of task-oriented gait training can be sustained in the clinical setting. However, a dramatic reduction of the quantity

and quality of the training occurs after discharge from primary rehabilitation. Although systematic experimental investigations are missing, results from previous clinical studies with comparable patient populations suggest that a long-term, mid-intensity locomotion training over several months seems to be more effective than the application of training protocols with high intensity for only a few weeks [37, 55]. This fact underlines the need for technically advanced locomotion therapy systems for home use, but so far only a few of them exist. A simple transfer of the existing robotic devices to the patients' homes is not possible since most of them are restricted to the application in a clinical or outpatient setting due to their size, weight and price. Furthermore, all of the devices have to be operated by experienced therapists.

The main technical challenges of a home-based locomotion therapy device are safety issues and its self-operation by the user. An appropriate method to minimize the risk of injuries is to put the user in a safe training position, like a semi-recumbent position of the body as implemented for the 'MoreGait' (**M**otorized **o**rthosis for home **Re**habilitation of **Gait**) device. This locomotion robot consists of a special seat in combination with an inclined backrest, two pneumatically driven exoskeletons to assist movements of the legs (actively driven knee and ankle joint, positively driven hip joint) and a special apparatus (stimulative shoe, Video 32.1) to generate a physiological foot loading pattern without the need for verticalization of the user (Figure 32.4).

The therapeutic functionality of the novel device is based on highly dynamic leg movements (up to 30 double steps per minute) combined with a physiological, gait phase related loading of the foot soles and an adaptive feedback of the joint-specific deviations from the reference trajectory. From a neurobiological point of view it represents a device that aims at the enhancement of neural plasticity at different levels of the CNS: First, it generates the key sensory stimuli necessary for activation of the CPG at the spinal level [25] and second, provides external feedback about the performance of the movements to compensate for the loss of sensation and/or proprioception and to enhance relearning at a supraspinal level (Figure 32.5).

To assess the feasibility and efficacy of this device a baseline-study with 25 chronic motor incomplete individuals with SCI, who were already ambulatory (Walking Index for Spinal Cord Injury (WISCI) II [56] ≥ 5) at study onset, was conducted. After 8 weeks of daily, up to 45-min long therapy sessions at home, the gait speed and endurance improved approximately 50% compared to

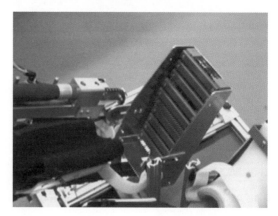

📹 **Video 32.1** The 'MoreGait'-device and its stimulative shoe in operation.

baseline. Additionally, the mean WISCI II increased by 4 points [57]. These improvements are in the range of those achieved with stationary, treadmill-based locomotion robots [37]. Interestingly, there was an almost linear increase in gait speed and endurance over the 8 weeks of therapy, indicating that a prolonged therapy beyond 8 weeks might lead to even better outcomes.

The feasibility study showed that it is possible to generate highly dynamic leg movements including a physiological sensory stimulation of the foot sole in a safe manner with a compact and transportable robotic locomotion training device. Due to the dedicated safety concept of the machine during 1,100 training sessions only one therapy related adverse event occurred [58].

Real-time feedback of gait parameters

In contrast to therapists, robots, with their integrated angular and torque sensors, are capable of continuously measuring kinematic and kinetic parameters of several joints simultaneously. It was successfully demonstrated that this feature allows highly reliable measurements of maximal voluntary isometric muscle force of lower extremities [59]. Therefore, these parameters may

be used for documentation and guidance of the rehabilitation process. More importantly, real-time analysis of acquired sensor data and direct feedback of selected parameters to users brings new perspectives to gait rehabilitation [60]. Besides impaired motor function patients with relevant neurological disease conditions suffer frequently from concomitant sensory deficits, in particular proprioceptive sensory dysfunction (altered position/vibration sense), with resulting gait ataxia. Even patients with substantial motor functions are in most instances unable to compensate the lack of proprioception through vague visual (mirror) or auditory feedback (therapist instructions), or through physical guidance of impaired extremities. In addition, feedback provided by therapists may vary over time and between therapists. The principle of instrumented, augmented feedback, in which impaired proprioception is substituted by providing additional external information, may help to overcome these problems [61]. The overall goal of feedback is to promote relevant, persistent and transferable improvements in gait function. For feedback training, parameters of instrumental gait analysis may be used, among them joint angles, ground reaction forces, joint moments,

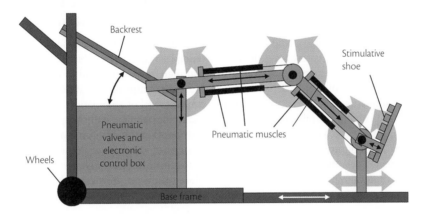

Fig. 32.4 Overview of the 'MoreGait' concept for robotic locomotion training at home (black arrows mark adjustable parts for adaption to the individual user, light grey arrows indicate actively driven parts).

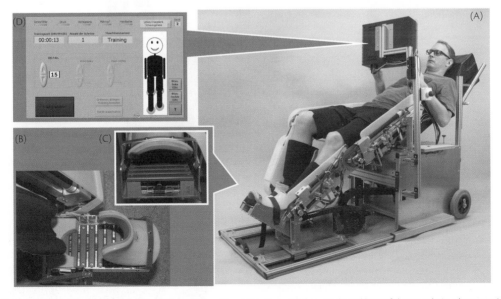

Fig. 32.5 A subject during training in the 'MoreGait'-device (A), top (B) and front (C) view of the medio-lateral bars of the stimulative shoe, user interface, and feedback screen (D).

time-distance parameter, symmetry indices, or muscular activation patterns. The feedback modality may be either visual (graphical or numeric deviations from the physiological gait pattern), auditory, tactile, or multimodal [62].

A promising approach is to use implicit 'visual feedback distortion' to influence the gait pattern. Following this concept a gait variable (e.g. step length on one side while walking on a treadmill) is visually fed back to the user and gradually distorted over time. In healthy subjects a systematic modulation of step length away from symmetry could be achieved without explicit knowledge of the manipulation [63]. Studies examining the role of the focus of attention in healthy subjects have consistently demonstrated that instructions inducing an external focus (directed at the movement effect) are more effective than those promoting an internal focus (directed at the body movements) [64]. However, patients with sensory-motor impairments may not always benefit from feedback in the same way healthy subjects do, as they often comprehend how to influence a pathological movement, but are physically not able to [62]. Therefore, in patients with more severe impairment it may be advisable to start with less complex feedback of the movement performance of a single joint. As soon as the performance improves, the quality of the feedback provided will be gradually shifted towards the success of the movement task. The latter seems to facilitate automaticity in motor control, which is the ability to walk without continuously thinking about its low-level details, and to promote the energy-efficiency of movements.

A very sophisticated implementation of feedback is virtual reality. Virtual reality is increasingly used in combination with robotic devices, which combine elements for motor and cognitive training and have a high motivational aspect (Figure 32.6). Feedback methods can turn a rather monotonous exercise into an exciting and comfortable one, which results in a higher willingness to participate in a training, and thereby in a higher training intensity and potentially in a better motor performance [65, 66].

Additionally, it has been shown that besides motor skills also physical performance and cognitive function may improve in PD during complex challenging conditions, such as obstacle stepping in a virtual environment [42, 67].

Despite the tremendous technical progress made over the last few years the overall evidence supporting additional feedback training strategies is rather limited [68, 69]. In particular, information about long-term carry over effects of feedback training is missing. Few studies select their feedback strategies and paradigms implemented in locomotion robots according to the principles and concepts of motor learning (Table 32.1). For example, feedback, which is continuously provided, does not support but rather blocks the learning process [70, 71]. Moreover, the information content of the feedback has to be carefully adapted to the cognitive capacity of the patient, since the performance of a movement task is decreasing during mental stress. Nevertheless, feedback-based rehabilitation strategies represent a very promising and emerging field in gait rehabilitation of patients with predominantly sensory dysfunction.

Technology for substitution of locomotor function

In patients with persistent sensorimotor impairments restorative therapies might not be able to induce relevant neuroplastic changes and thereby may not lead to relevant functional improvements. In this case compensatory strategies are applied to achieve an independent level of ambulation. In a compensatory approach assistive technology traditionally plays an important role and is meant to assist people with different levels of impairments in their ambulatory function in various ways. Wheelchairs, scooters, walkers, braces, and canes are examples of assistive devices for enhancement of mobility. More people use assistive technologies related to mobility (6.4 million) than any other general type of assistive technology [72].

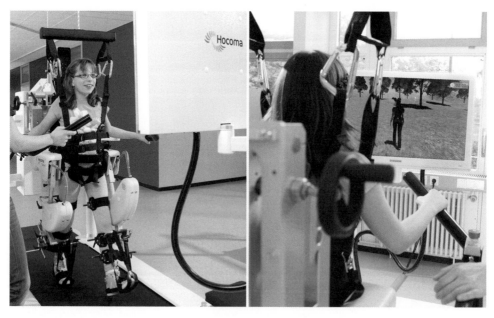

Fig. 32.6 Driven gait orthosis 'LokomatPro' with pediatric module and virtual reality.
With kind permission of Hocoma AG, Volketswil, Switzerland and SRH Hospital Neckargemünd, Germany.

Manual and electric wheelchair technology

In patients with severe restrictions of voluntary motor function the wheelchair represents the most effective assistive device for enhancement of mobility of otherwise immobile individuals. For many people with disabilities a wheelchair is more than an assistive device in particular in developing countries [73]. It is the means by which they achieve inclusion and increases access to opportunities for education, employment, and participation within the home environment and the community. A manual wheelchair is designed for people who have enough upper-body, arm, and hand strength to self-propel the wheels of the chair. Users of manual wheelchairs must have sufficient balance and posture to sit upright in the wheelchair because there is not much back support. In addition to providing mobility, an appropriate wheelchair supports cardiopulmonary fitness, physical health and quality of life.

From a technological viewpoint an ideal manual wheelchair has to fulfil several prerequisites to be safe, comfortable and efficient. The design criteria of a manual wheelchair strongly depend on its intended use and the level of activity of the end user (Figure 32.7). While it may be sufficient to have a heavy folding frame wheelchair for pure indoor use in persons with low activity level, a lightweight rigid frame wheelchair is the best choice for outdoor use in persons with a higher activity level. The latter can be handled by the users themselves for transportation in a car. A crucial factor for safety and comfort is the proper adjustment of the seating position. In long-term wheelchair users it is extremely important to find the correct position for optimal propulsion in order to avoid shoulder complications [74].

If wheelchairs are intended to be used over an extended period of time, it is advisable to use them in combination with seat cushions to avoid pressure sores. Seat cushions are available in a variety of designs from simple foam cushions to complex pressurized, self-adjusting air cushions. The selection of the cushion mainly depends on the individual risk to develop pressure sores.

If wheelchair users do not have enough upper extremity strength or trunk stability to operate a manual wheelchair in any environment, an electrical drive for supporting the manual propelling movements can be added. Some of the commercially available systems (e.g. e-motion, Abler, Albstadt, Germany) are completely integrated in a wheel and can easily replace the wheels of a conventional manual wheelchair. They measure the manual effort by integrated torque sensors, thereby detecting the navigational intent of the user.

Depending on the environmental conditions the system autonomously controls the levels of additionally applied torque or may even decelerate the wheelchair in downhill conditions. Power-assisted manual wheelchairs help to maintain a certain level of physical activity in combination with a prolonged period of mobility.

Electric wheelchairs are intended to be used by people who need support for their upper body and who are unable to move a manual chair with their arms and hands. A power chair has a more supportive seat and often a headrest for people who aren't able to hold themselves upright. The traditional control interface of an electrical wheelchair is a joystick mounted at the distal end of the armrest. Several adapters like hand rests are used to allow control in persons, in whom almost no voluntary hand and finger movements are preserved. More sophisticated control options including chin control, suck-and-puff control, eye-movement control, or even brain control, are available to enable steering an electrical wheelchair by individuals with severe motor impairments.

Motor-driven exoskeletons for independent overground walking

Driven by the recent technological progress leading to higher capacities of rechargeable batteries, to miniaturized electronics and higher efficiency of electrical drives complex exoskeletons for overground walking have matured to a premarket stage over the last few years (Video 32.2). In 2012, a female with complete SCI successfully finished the London Marathon in 16 days with one of the two most sophisticated systems (Figure 32.8). Currently, it cannot be determined whether any of these systems will be accepted by the intended users as personal assistance systems and will successfully survive on the market. Before broader application, the inherent problem of minimizing the risk of falls and injuries has to be solved properly. Quantitative data on adverse events, negative health effects and the reliability and robustness of the devices during everyday use in the community have yet to be obtained [75, 76]. The preservation, or even gain, of independence are crucial factors influencing the end user acceptance. Another significant obstacle for successful market introduction is the price of the devices ranging currently from 50,000 to 80,000€. Potential users of active exoskeletons have to fulfil certain physical requirements. Sufficient voluntary trunk stability to shift the body centre of mass from one leg to the other and

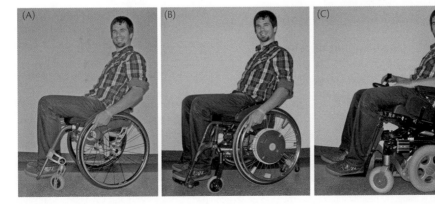

Fig. 32.7 Wheelchairs with different levels of support to the user: (A) light-weight rigid frame manual wheelchair, (B) manual wheelchair equipped with power assisted wheels, and (C) electric wheelchair with joystick control.

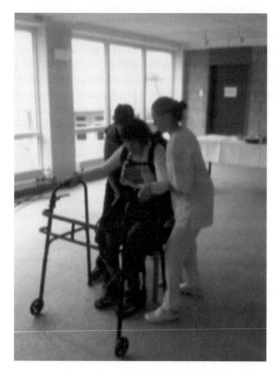

📹 **Video 32.2** An individual with a motor incomplete SCI sitting up and walking with the Ekso (Ekso Bionics, Richmond, CA, USA) exoskeleton.

unrestricted arm movements for handling of crutches to obtain additional body stability and to control the user interface of the device are mandatory. Hence, only paraplegic individuals will be able to operate such a device. Contraindications are restricted joint mobility, severe spasticity, and autonomous dysfunctions (e.g. autonomic dysreflexia and hypotension due to venous pooling during verticalization). Taken these facts together, it is presumed that no more than 10% of individuals with SCI, the main target group of manufacturers of exoskeletons, will profit from such a device. Therefore, for the majority of end users with SCI exoskeletons at their current stage are not a serious alternative to the wheelchair as a relatively inexpensive, efficient, and socially accepted assistive mobility device.

Future developments and challenges

Task-oriented gait therapies either conventional or with robotic support demonstrated to be efficient components of a restorative gait rehabilitation programme. After their first commercial availability robotic training devices have been increasingly integrated into clinical routine over the last decade. In industrialized countries there is another reason why robotic locomotion devices will become an integral component of gait rehabilitation—demography. The population is constantly getting older due to a longer life expectancy, in combination with a declining birth rate. As a consequence, qualified therapists will become sparse paralleled by an increasing demand for such therapies in the aging population.

The tremendous progress of hard- and software technology allowed for the implementation of sophisticated robotic training devices with several degrees of freedom of actively driven joints, multiple kinematic and kinetic sensors, and sophisticated methods for virtual reality [77, 78]. Their combined application with CNS excitation modulating therapies like spinal cord stimulation [79], transcranial direct current stimulation [80], or repetitive transcranial magnetic stimulation [81–83] holds promise for outcome improvements beyond the currently achievable extent.

Despite the technological advances to promote mobility and ambulation a number of issues have to be addressed in the future.

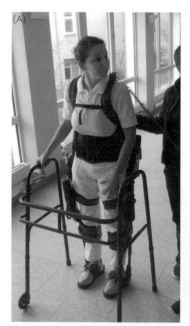 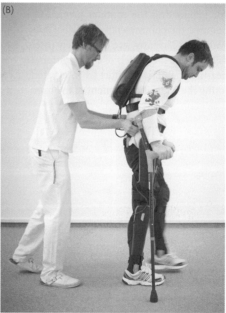

Fig. 32.8 Exoskeletons for overground walking: (A) healthy subject with the Ekso exoskeleton (Ekso Bionics, Richmond, CA, USA) and (B) individual with complete thoracic SCI with the ReWalk exoskeleton.
Argo Medical, Yokneam Ilit, Israel, with kind permission of the Trauma Center Murnau, Germany.

The efficacy of robotic-assisted gait rehabilitation has to be further improved by a consequent application of principles of motor learning and their consistent implementation into robotic controllers [84]. Complex exoskeletons allow for systematic investigation and identification of technical components and therapeutic approaches most effective for gait restoration. Certainly, they help to enhance our understanding about motor control and learning, which in turn will promote the optimization of current robotic devices and the development and integration of novel technologies. In the future, robotic locomotion training devices will evolve as true patient-cooperative systems. A major milestone into this direction has been achieved recently with the non-invasive detection of the level of participation directly from brain signals [85].

Early clinical predictors are needed to determine which patients will most likely recover a relevant ambulatory function with a restorative approach. For example, it is quite challenging to decide whether patients with sensorimotor complete SCI in the acute and early subacute phase will undergo rehabilitative therapies aiming for restoration rather than compensation, or vice versa.

Systematic investigations are needed to identify the influence of therapy parameters like speed, degree of body weight support, duration, and repetition of the therapy sessions on the outcome. In particular, dose–outcome relationships in different patient groups with different degrees of impairment need to be determined. Eventually, a true personalized, evidence-based gait rehabilitation may become reality.

There is a high demand for innovative solutions to translate skills trained in artificial environments such as a treadmill to overground locomotion and activities of daily living. First proof of principle studies successfully employed such devices in animal experiments. However, the challenging translation into the clinical arena has yet to be accomplished [86].

After all, it is important to keep in mind that the outcome of all restorative therapies is determined by the degree of spared CNS tissue in respective neurological disease entities. This raises the fundamental question: how much more functional recovery can be gained with an optimal restorative protocol beyond the level achieved by currently administered conventional rehabilitative protocols? Even the most advanced rehabilitative approach will—depending on the severity of the CNS lesion—only promote a limited recovery.

At this point neuroregenerative therapies aiming for axon regrowth and remyelination are urgently needed. Animal studies have identified numerous such interventions, which have been shown to promote structural and functional recovery in CNS disease and trauma. Although, their successful clinical translation has not been achieved yet, recent animal studies clearly demonstrated a superior outcome of these neuroregenerative interventions when combined with task-oriented rehabilitative therapies. These studies generate new questions regarding the appropriate timing of a regenerative intervention in relation to neurorehabilitative therapies [87, 88].

Although a higher degree of neurological recovery by clinical introduction of novel neuroprotective or -regenerative therapies can be expected, it is likely that motor impairments of different degree will persist after severe CNS damage. To promote ambulation in these cases an ideal technical walking aid would detect the movement intent of the user and reanimate the paralysed muscles. Research on such neuroprostheses for restoration of walking on the basis of FES started almost 50 years ago. However, they never made their way out of the lab [89], because end users have to fulfil a lot of prerequisites and muscle fatigue occurs quickly due to non-physiological activation of nerves and muscles. The limitations of purely FES-based lower extremity neuroprostheses may be overcome by the combination of FES, either applied non-invasively with surface electrodes, or by implanted stimulators and active orthosis [90]. In cases, where some motor functions are preserved, scalable, modular hybrid neuroprostheses need to be developed that can be adapted to the individual handicap and needs of potential end users [91]. Current exoskeletons mostly use electrical actuators with gearboxes, which are too heavy and bulky to be worn under clothes. Novel actuators based on materials shortening in the presence of electrical fields, such as dielectric elastomers and ferroelectric polymers, offer new possibilities in terms of power efficiency and miniaturization. If the high voltages needed for their operation can be safely handled or if the force-generating capabilities of carbon nanotubes or nanowires can be transferred from the microscopic to the macroscopic level, artificial muscles made from these novel materials will allow for the realization of agile, lightweight, and wearable exoskeletons [92–94]. Alternative concepts like fuel-powered artificial muscles may solve the problem of energy storage and supply [95].

It is well known from prosthetics that the implementation of an intuitive control of an assistive device is highly relevant for the users' acceptance [96]. Most recent advances in brain–computer interfaces may effectively allow for the detection of the movement intent of the end user from recordings of multiple brain neurons [97]. Whether the same performance can be achieved non-invasively by electroencephalographic detection of muscle synergies needs to be shown in future studies [98, 99]. To gain practical relevance brain–computer interfaces have to prove their usability in the end users' home environment, without the need for daily calibration and tuning of the decoding algorithms by technical experts [100].

For real embodiment of a compensatory assistive locomotion device tactile and spatial information obtained by pressure and inertial sensors needs to be fed back to the user. A recently performed evaluation of a somatosensory prosthesis in Rhesus macaque monkeys, using intracortical microstimulation, shows that the performance on a tactile task is equivalent whether stimuli are delivered to the native finger or to a prosthetic finger [101].

Conclusion

Technology plays an important role in compensatory and restorative neurorehabilitative approaches. In hardly any other domain than in the rehabilitation of neurological patients did the scientific findings about the intrinsic plasticity of the CNS induce a critical appraisal of established therapy concepts. In the meantime, task-specific therapies, in particular BWSTT, have become an inherent component of gait rehabilitation programmes for neurological patients. The availability of locomotion robots overcame the physical restrictions of manually assisted training. However, there is no clear evidence for a superiority of the robotic training. This seems to be associated with the lack of implementation of principles of motor learning into robotic devices. Nevertheless, locomotion robots open new therapeutic opportunities. Among them are the continuation of intensive locomotion training in the home environment and increase of the effectiveness of the training by using real-time feedback of movement variables, up to virtual reality based methods.

It has to be emphasized that a locomotion robot cannot represent a complete gait rehabilitation programme. Such tools have to be embedded into a multifaceted, comprehensive therapy concept.

Beyond their therapeutic possibilities complex exoskeletons are impressive research tools that allow for systematic investigations of effective therapy parameters and thereby help to enhance our understanding about motor control and learning.

Whether exoskeletons at their current stage will challenge established and accepted mobility tools such as the wheelchair in individuals suffering from severe sensorimotor impairment has to be demonstrated. The continuing technological progress will enhance compensatory assistive locomotion devices by implementation of highly effective electrochemical actuators and somatosensory feedback. However, more clinical trials are needed to provide an objective basis, whether technology driven innovations in the field of neurorehabilitation are capable to outperform conventional rehab approaches. The close dialogue between neuroscientists, engineers, physicians, therapists, patients, and health care service providers will be a prerequisite to ensure a steady progress in the future.

References

1. Warlow C, van Gijn J, Dennis M, et al. Stroke: Practical management, 3rd edn. Blackwell Publishing, Oxford, 2008.
2. Feigin VL, Lawes CM, Bennett DA, Barker-Collo SL, Parag V. Worldwide stroke incidence and early case fatality reported in 56 population-based studies: a systematic review. Lancet Neurol. 2009;8(4):355–369.
3. Fritsch T, Smyth KA, Wallendal MS, Hyde T, Leo G, Geldmacher DS. Parkinson disease: research update and clinical management. South Med J. 2012;105(12):650–656.
4. Trenkwalder C, Schwarz J, Gebhard J, et al. Starnberg trial on epidemiology of Parkinsonism and hypertension in the elderly. Prevalence of Parkinson's disease and related disorders assessed by a door-to-door survey of inhabitants older than 65 years. Arch Neurol. 1995;52(10):1017–1022.
5. Tullman MJ. Overview of the epidemiology, diagnosis, and disease progression associated with multiple sclerosis. Am J Manag Care. 2013;19(2 Suppl):S15–20.
6. Wyndaele M, Wyndaele JJ. Incidence, prevalence and epidemiology of spinal cord injury: what learns a worldwide literature survey? Spinal Cord. 2006;44(9):523–529.
7. Taylor P, Humphreys L, Swain I. The long-term cost-effectiveness of the use of functional electrical stimulation for the correction of dropped foot due to upper motor neuron lesion. J Rehabil Med. 2013;45(2):154–160.
8. Somers MF. Compensation and restoration in rehabilitation after spinal cord injury: A review of the evidence. Top Spinal Cord Inj Rehabil. 2011;16(Suppl. 1):65.
9. Hesse S, Bertelt C, Jahnke MT, et al. Treadmill training with partial body weight support compared with physiotherapy in nonambulatory hemiparetic patients. Stroke. 1995;26(6):976–981.
10. Dietz V. Locomotor training in paraplegic patients. Annals of neurology. 1995;38(6):965.
11. Swinnen E, Beckwee D, Pinte D, Meeusen R, Baeyens JP, Kerckhofs E. Treadmill training in multiple sclerosis: can body weight support or robot assistance provide added value? A systematic review. Mult Scler Int. 2012;2012:240274.
12. Mehrholz J, Friis R, Kugler J, Twork S, Storch A, Pohl M. Treadmill training for patients with Parkinson's disease. Cochrane Database Syst Rev. 2010(1):CD007830.
13. Hicks AL, Ginis KA. Treadmill training after spinal cord injury: it's not just about the walking. J Rehabil Res Dev. 2008;45(2):241–248.
14. Hall KM, Cohen ME, Wright J, Call M, Werner P. Characteristics of the Functional Independence Measure in traumatic spinal cord injury. Arch Phys Med Rehabil. 1999;80(11):1471–1476.
15. Dobkin B, Apple D, Barbeau H, et al. Weight-supported treadmill vs over-ground training for walking after acute incomplete SCI. Neurology. 2006;66(4):484–493.
16. Wolpaw JR. Treadmill training after spinal cord injury: good but not better. Neurology. 2006;66(4):466–467.
17. Sherrington CS. Flexion-reflex of the limb, crossed extension-reflex, and reflex stepping and standing. J Physiol. 1910;40(1–2):28–121.
18. Brown TG. The intrinsic factors in the act of progression in the mammal. Proc R Soc Lond B Biol Sci. 1911;84:308–319.
19. Grillner S, Zangger P. How detailed is the central pattern generation for locomotion? Brain research. 1975;88(2):367–371.
20. Dimitrijevic MR, Gerasimenko Y, Pinter MM. Evidence for a spinal central pattern generator in humans. Ann N Y Acad Sci. 1998;860:360–376.
21. Harkema S, Gerasimenko Y, Hodes J, et al. Effect of epidural stimulation of the lumbosacral spinal cord on voluntary movement, standing, and assisted stepping after motor complete paraplegia: a case study. Lancet. 2011;377(9781):1938–1947.
22. Singh A, Balasubramanian S, Murray M, Lemay M, Houle J. Role of spared pathways in locomotor recovery after body-weight-supported treadmill training in contused rats. J Neurotrauma. 2011;28(12):2405–2416.
23. Lacquaniti F, Ivanenko YP, Zago M. Patterned control of human locomotion. J Physiol. [2012;590(Pt 10):2189–2199.
24. Pearson KG. Neural adaptation in the generation of rhythmic behavior. Annu Rev Physiol. 2000;62:723–753.
25. Dietz V, Muller R, Colombo G. Locomotor activity in spinal man: significance of afferent input from joint and load receptors. Brain. 2002;125(Pt 12):2626–2634.
26. Edgerton VR, Courtine G, Gerasimenko YP, et al. Training locomotor networks. Brain Res Rev. 2008;57(1):241–254.
27. Wolpaw JR. The education and re-education of the spinal cord. Progr Brain Res. 2006;157:261–280.
28. Rossignol S, Frigon A. Recovery of locomotion after spinal cord injury: some facts and mechanisms. Annu Rev Neurosci. 2011;34:413–440.
29. Krakauer JW. Motor learning: its relevance to stroke recovery and neurorehabilitation. Curr Opin Neurol. 2006;19(1):84–90.
30. Chen G, Patten C. Treadmill training with harness support: selection of parameters for individuals with poststroke hemiparesis. J Rehabil Res Dev. 2006;43(4):485–498.
31. Chen G, Patten C, Kothari DH, Zajac FE. Gait deviations associated with post-stroke hemiparesis: improvement during treadmill walking using weight support, speed, support stiffness, and handrail hold. Gait Posture. 2005;22(1):57–62.
32. Hesse S, Werner C, Paul T, Bardeleben A, Chaler J. Influence of walking speed on lower limb muscle activity and energy consumption during treadmill walking of hemiparetic patients. Arch Phys Med Rehabil. 2001;82(11):1547–1550.
33. Van Peppen RP, Kwakkel G, Wood-Dauphinee S, Hendriks HJ, Van der Wees PJ, Dekker J. The impact of physical therapy on functional outcomes after stroke: what's the evidence? Clin Rehabil. 2004;18(8):833–862.
34. Mayr A, Kofler M, Quirbach E, Matzak H, Frohlich K, Saltuari L. Prospective, blinded, randomized crossover study of gait rehabilitation in stroke patients using the Lokomat gait orthosis. Neurorehabil Neural Repair. 2007;21(4):307–314.
35. Curt A, Van Hedel HJ, Klaus D, Dietz V. Recovery from a spinal cord injury: significance of compensation, neural plasticity, and repair. J Neurotrauma. 2008;25(6):677–685.
36. Wirz M, van Hedel HJ, Rupp R, Curt A, Dietz V. Muscle force and gait performance: relationships after spinal cord injury. Arch Phys Med Rehabil. 2006;87(9):1218–1222.

37. Wirz M, Zemon DH, Rupp R, et al. Effectiveness of automated locomotor training in patients with chronic incomplete spinal cord injury: a multicenter trial. Arch Phys Med Rehabil. 2005;86(4):672–680.

38. Hesse S, Werner C, Uhlenbrock D, von Frankenberg S, Bardeleben A, Brandl-Hesse B. An electromechanical gait trainer for restoration of gait in hemiparetic stroke patients: preliminary results. Neurorehabil Neural Repair. 2001;15(1):39–50.

39. Hesse S, Tomelleri C, Bardeleben A, Werner C, Waldner A. Robot-assisted practice of gait and stair climbing in nonambulatory stroke patients. J Rehabil Res Dev. 2012;49(4):613–622.

40. Colombo G, Wirz M, Dietz V. Driven gait orthosis for improvement of locomotor training in paraplegic patients. Spinal Cord. 2001;39(5):252–255.

41. Winfree KN, Stegall P, Agrawal SK. Design of a minimally constraining, passively supported gait training exoskeleton: ALEX II. IEEE Int Conf Rehabil Robot. 2011;2011:5975499.

42. van der Kooij H, Veneman J, Ekkelenkamp R. Design of a compliantly actuated exo-skeleton for an impedance controlled gait trainer robot. Conf Proc IEEE Eng Med Biol Soc. 2006;1:189–193.

43. Huang VS, Krakauer JW. Robotic neurorehabilitation: a computational motor learning perspective. J Neuroeng Rehabil. 2009;6:5.

44. Riener R, Lunenburger L, Jezernik S, Anderschitz M, Colombo G, Dietz V. Patient-cooperative strategies for robot-aided treadmill training: first experimental results. IEEE Trans Neural Syst Rehabil Eng. 2005;13(3):380–394.

45. Hussain S, Xie SQ, Jamwal PK. Adaptive Impedance Control of a Robotic Orthosis for Gait Rehabilitation. IEEE Trans Syst Man Cybern B Cybern. 2013;17(2):442–451.

46. Schuck A, Labruyere R, Vallery H, Riener R, Duschau-Wicke A. Feasibility and effects of patient-cooperative robot-aided gait training applied in a 4-week pilot trial. J Neuroeng Rehabil. 2012;9:31.

47. Dobkin BH, Duncan PW. Should body weight-supported treadmill training and robotic-assistive steppers for locomotor training trot back to the starting gate? Neurorehabil Neural Repair. 2012;26(4):308–317.

48. Husemann B, Muller F, Krewer C, Heller S, Koenig E. Effects of locomotion training with assistance of a robot-driven gait orthosis in hemiparetic patients after stroke: a randomized controlled pilot study. Stroke. 2007;38(2):349–354.

49. Schwartz I, Sajin A, Fisher I, et al. The effectiveness of locomotor therapy using robotic-assisted gait training in subacute stroke patients: a randomized controlled trial. PM R. 2009;1(6):516–523.

50. Hidler J, Nichols D, Pelliccio M, et al. Multicenter randomized clinical trial evaluating the effectiveness of the Lokomat in subacute stroke. Neurorehabil Neural Repair. 2009;23(1):5–13.

51. Hornby TG, Campbell DD, Kahn JH, Demott T, Moore JL, Roth HR. Enhanced gait-related improvements after therapist-versus robotic-assisted locomotor training in subjects with chronic stroke: a randomized controlled study. Stroke. 2008;39(6):1786–1792.

52. Hornby TG, Reinkensmeyer DJ, Chen D. Manually-assisted versus robotic-assisted body weight-supported treadmill training in spinal cord injury: what is the role of each? PM R. 2010;2(3):214–221.

53. van Hedel HJ. Weight-supported treadmill versus over-ground training after spinal cord injury: from a physical therapist's point of view. Phys Ther. 2006;86(10):1444–1445; author reply 5–7.

54. NSCISC. The 2006 Annual Statistical Report for the Model Spinal Cord Injury Care System. National SCI Statistical Center, 2006, Available from https://www.nscisc.uab.edu/PublicDocuments/reports/pdf/NSCIC%20Annual%202006.pdf (accessed 20 August 2014).

55. Hicks AL, Adams MM, Martin Ginis K, et al. Long-term body-weight-supported treadmill training and subsequent follow-up in persons with chronic SCI: effects on functional walking ability and measures of subjective well-being. Spinal Cord. 2005;43(5):291–298.

56. Dittuno PL, Ditunno JF, Jr. Walking index for spinal cord injury (WISCI II): scale revision. Spinal Cord. 2001;39(12):654–656.

57. Rupp R, Plewa H, Schuld C, et al. Ein motorisiertes Exoskelett zur automatisierten Lokomotionstherapie im häuslichen Umfeld—Ergebnisse einer Pilotstudie mit inkomplett Querschnittgelähmten. Neurologie & Rehabilitation. 2011;17(1):13–20.

58. Rupp R, Plewa H, Schuld C, Gerner HJ, Hofer EP, Knestel M. MotionTherapy@Home—First results of a clinical study with a novel robotic device for automated locomotion therapy at home. Biomedizinische Technik Biomedical engineering. 2011;56(1):11–21.

59. Bolliger M, Banz R, Dietz V, Lunenburger L. Standardized voluntary force measurement in a lower extremity rehabilitation robot. J Neuroeng Rehabil. 2008;5:23.

60. Lunenburger L, Colombo G, Riener R. Biofeedback for robotic gait rehabilitation. J Neuroeng Rehabil. 2007;4:1.

61. Hunt MA. Movement retraining using real-time feedback of performance. J Vis Exp. 2013(71):e50182.

62. Sigrist R, Rauter G, Riener R, Wolf P. Augmented visual, auditory, haptic, and multimodal feedback in motor learning: a review. Psychon Bull Rev. 2013;20(1):21–53.

63. Kim SJ, Krebs HI. Effects of implicit visual feedback distortion on human gait. Experimental brain research. 2012;218(3):495–502.

64. Wulf G, Shea C, Lewthwaite R. Motor skill learning and performance: a review of influential factors. Med Educ. 2010 Jan;44(1):75–84.

65. Schuler T, Brutsch K, Muller R, van Hedel UJ, Meyer-Heim A. Virtual realities as motivational tools for robotic assisted gait training in children: A surface electromyography study. NeuroRehabilitation. 2011;28(4):401–411.

66. Lewek MD, Feasel J, Wentz E, Brooks FP, Jr., Whitton MC. Use of visual and proprioceptive feedback to improve gait speed and spatiotemporal symmetry following chronic stroke: a case series. Phys Ther. 2012;92(5):748–756.

67. Mirelman A, Maidan I, Herman T, Deutsch JE, Giladi N, Hausdorff JM. Virtual reality for gait training: can it induce motor learning to enhance complex walking and reduce fall risk in patients with Parkinson's disease? J Gerontol A Biol Sci Med Sci. 2011;66(2):234–240.

68. Laver KE, George S, Thomas S, Deutsch JE, Crotty M. Virtual reality for stroke rehabilitation. Cochrane Database Syst Rev. 2011;9:CD008349.

69. Tate JJ, Milner CE. Real-time kinematic, temporospatial, and kinetic biofeedback during gait retraining in patients: a systematic review. Phys Ther. 2010;90(8):1123–1134.

70. Ikegami T, Hirashima M, Osu R, Nozaki D. Intermittent visual feedback can boost motor learning of rhythmic movements: evidence for error feedback beyond cycles. J Neurosci. 2012;32(2):653–657.

71. Schmidt RA, Lee TD. Motor Control and Learning; A Behavioral Emphasis, 4th edn. USA Human Kinetics, Champaign, IL, 2005.

72. Scherer MJ. The change in emphasis from people to person: introduction to the special issue on assistive technology. Disabil Rehabil. 2002;24(1–3):1–4.

73. WHO. Guidelines on the Provision of Manual Wheelchairs in Less Resourced Settings. World Health Organization, Geneva, 2008.

74. Akbar M, Balean G, Brunner M, et al. Prevalence of rotator cuff tear in paraplegic patients compared with controls. J Bone Joint Surg Am. 2010;92(1):23–30.

75. Esquenazi A, Talaty M, Packel A, Saulino M. The ReWalk powered exoskeleton to restore ambulatory function to individuals with thoracic-level motor-complete spinal cord injury. Am J Phys Med Rehabil. 2012;91(11):911–921.

76. Zeilig G, Weingarden H, Zwecker M, Dudkiewicz I, Bloch A, Esquenazi A. Safety and tolerance of the ReWalk exoskeleton suit for ambulation by people with complete spinal cord injury: a pilot study. J Spinal Cord Med. 2012;35(2):96–101.

77. Reinkensmeyer DJ, Boninger ML. Technologies and combination therapies for enhancing movement training for people with a disability. J Neuroeng Rehabil. 2012;9:17.

78. Adamovich SV, Fluet GG, Tunik E, Merians AS. Sensorimotor training in virtual reality: a review. NeuroRehabilitation. 2009;**25**(1):29–44.

79. Minassian K, Hofstoetter U, Tansey K, Mayr W. Neuromodulation of lower limb motor control in restorative neurology. Clin Neurol Neurosurg. 2012;**114**(5):489–497.

80. Danzl MM, Chelette KC, Lee K, Lykins D, Sawaki L. Brain stimulation paired with novel locomotor training with robotic gait orthosis in chronic stroke: A feasibility study. NeuroRehabilitation. 2013;**33**(1):67–76.

81. Wang RY, Tseng HY, Liao KK, Wang CJ, Lai KL, Yang YR. rTMS combined with task-oriented training to improve symmetry of interhemispheric corticomotor excitability and gait performance after stroke: a randomized trial. Neurorehabil Neural Repair. 2012;**26**(3):222–230.

82. Yang YR, Tseng CY, Chiou SY, et al. Combination of rTMS and treadmill training modulates corticomotor inhibition and improves walking in Parkinson disease: a randomized trial. Neurorehabil Neural Repair. 2013;**27**(1):79–86.

83. Benito J, Kumru H, Murillo N, et al. Motor and gait improvement in patients with incomplete spinal cord injury induced by high-frequency repetitive transcranial magnetic stimulation. Topics in spinal cord injury rehabilitation. 2012;**18**(2):106–112.

84. Marchal-Crespo L, Reinkensmeyer DJ. Review of control strategies for robotic movement training after neurologic injury. J Neuroeng Rehabil. 2009;**6**:20.

85. Wagner J, Solis-Escalante T, Grieshofer P, Neuper C, Muller-Putz G, Scherer R. Level of participation in robotic-assisted treadmill walking modulates midline sensorimotor EEG rhythms in able-bodied subjects. Neuroimage. 2012;**63**(3):1203–1211.

86. Dominici N, Keller U, Vallery H, et al. Versatile robotic interface to evaluate, enable and train locomotion and balance after neuromotor disorders. Nat Med. 2012;**18**(7):1142–1147.

87. Wang D, Ichiyama RM, Zhao R, Andrews MR, Fawcett JW. Chondroitinase combined with rehabilitation promotes recovery of forelimb function in rats with chronic spinal cord injury. J Neurosci. 2011;**31**(25):9332–9344.

88. Zhao RR, Andrews MR, Wang D, et al. Combination treatment with anti-Nogo-A and chondroitinase ABC is more effective than single treatments at enhancing functional recovery after spinal cord injury. Eur J Neurosci. 2013;**38**(6):2946–2961.

89. Marsolais EB, Kobetic R. Development of a practical electrical stimulation system for restoring gait in the paralyzed patient. Clin Orthop Relat Res. 1988;**233**:64–74.

90. Bulea TC, Kobetic R, Audu ML, Schnellenberger JR, Triolo RJ. Finite state control of a variable impedance hybrid neuroprosthesis for locomotion after paralysis. IEEE Trans Neural Syst Rehabil Eng. 2013;**21**(1):141–151.

91. del-Ama AJ, Koutsou AD, Moreno JC, de-los-Reyes A, Gil-Agudo A, Pons JL. Review of hybrid exoskeletons to restore gait following spinal cord injury. J Rehabil Res Dev. 2012;**49**(4):497–514.

92. Madden JD. Mobile robots: motor challenges and materials solutions. Science. [Review]. 2007 Nov 16;**318**(5853):1094–1097.

93. Carpi F, Kornbluh R, Sommer-Larsen P, Alici G. Electroactive polymer actuators as artificial muscles: are they ready for bioinspired applications? Bioinspir Biomim. 2011;**6**(4):045006.

94. Foroughi J, Spinks GM, Wallace GG, et al. Torsional carbon nanotube artificial muscles. Science. 2011;**334**(6055):494–497.

95. Ebron VH, Yang Z, Seyer DJ, Kozlov ME, Oh J, Xie H, et al. Fuel-powered artificial muscles. Science. 2006;**311**(5767):1580–1583.

96. Schultz AE, Kuiken TA. Neural interfaces for control of upper limb prostheses: the state of the art and future possibilities. PM R. 2011;**3**(1):55–67.

97. Collinger JL, Wodlinger B, Downey JE, et al. High-performance neuroprosthetic control by an individual with tetraplegia. Lancet. 2013;**381**(9866):557–564.

98. Alessandro C, Delis I, Nori F, Panzeri S, Berret B. Muscle synergies in neuroscience and robotics: from input-space to task-space perspectives. Front Comput Neurosci. 2013;**7**:43.

99. Contreras-Vidal J, Presacco A, Agashe H, Paek A. Restoration of whole body movement: toward a noninvasive brain-machine interface system. IEEE Pulse. [Review]. 2012;**3**(1):34–37.

100. Courtine G, Micera S, DiGiovanna J, Millan Jdel R. Brain-machine interface: closer to therapeutic reality? Lancet. [Comment]. 2013;**381**(9866):515–517.

101. Berg JA, Dammann JF, 3rd, Tenore FV, Tabot GA, Boback JL, Manfredi LR, et al. Behavioral demonstration of a somatosensory neuroprosthesis. IEEE Trans Neural Syst Rehabil Eng. 2013;**21**(3):500–507.

CHAPTER 33

Enhancing independent community access and participation: services, technologies, and policies

Luc Noreau, Geoffrey Edwards,
Normand Boucher, Francois Routhier,
Claude Vincent, Hubert Gascon, and
Patrick Fougeyrollas

Introduction: community access

The prevalence of disability is currently estimated to be about 15% worldwide with significant variations across countries [1]. This figure will increase over time due to various factors, including the ageing of the population, particularly in developing countries. However, as Stephen Hawking said, 'Disability need not be an obstacle to success' [1]. Individual accomplishment in the life of persons with disabilities (PWD) has much to do with: (1) effective participation in valued life activities, (2) achievement of culturally and developmentally appropriate social roles, (3) contribution to various aspects of community life, and (4) full citizenship. The UN Convention on the Rights of Persons with Disabilities [2] enshrines the right to full and effective participation, including rights to accessibility, to live independently and be included in the community, and to participate in political, public and cultural life, recreation and sports. The Convention also emphasizes that various types of environmental factors hinder or facilitate full and effective participation in society of PWD on an equal basis with others. This paradigm stems from a shift in the conceptualisation of disability, from individual responsibility for disabling situations (e.g. impairments causing disadvantages in social and economic life) to a person–environment interactive process, such as depicted in contemporary disability models, including the International Classification of Functioning, Disability and Health [3] and the Disability Creation Process [4].

While rehabilitation, which aims to develop mental and physical capabilities, has the potential to facilitate independent and community living of PWD, in many cases access to services and technologies that meet their needs in the community is essential to ensure effective participation. Overall, efforts to provide better community access have led to limited success and a substantial number of PWD continue to face environmental barriers to their participation as equal members of society. An optimal analysis of factors that could enhance participation requires the use of a taxonomy of environmental dimensions (e.g. physical, technological and social). Initial thinking regarding community access often focuses on physical access as defined by architectural and physical elements in the environment (ramps, kerb cuts, etc.). However, this is only one aspect of a comprehensive vision of the environmental dimensions influencing participation [5]. Other environmental dimensions and community services that influence participation, include home care and support, primary health care, transportation, social and family support, education and job training, and technologies to enhance mobility, communication and home adaptation [1, 6, 7]. In some instances, social policies and programmes that regulate such dimensions vary from country to country.

An in-depth analysis of the influence of environmental factors on participation might well consider a three-level approach to the environmental dimension [4, 8, 9], corresponding to elements in the person's immediate environment (microsystem), the community where the person lives (mesosystem) and the societal dimension of the living environment (macrolevel). The aim of this chapter is to identify and describe critical elements in the environment that could contribute to optimal participation and to indicate how a favourable environment could facilitate participation. The main aspects considered are access to services and technology, as well as social policies. Since there are important variations in environmental and cultural issues across societies, this chapter focuses mainly on issues related to developed countries. Furthermore, many of the issues related to community access apply to PWD in general and not specifically to those with neurological impairments.

Services

Primary health care

Disability may be associated with a wide range of medical conditions, some of which result in poor health and substantial health care needs. Indeed, PWD may have complex and continuing health care needs related to their primary medical condition or associated impairments [10], making the management of health care challenging. While specialised health care is sometimes necessary to treat complex conditions, in terms of primary health care, the needs of PWD require services similar to those of the general population. Such care is an essential component of the provision of services along the continuum of health care from promotion to curative and rehabilitative care [11].

In concrete terms, access to primary health care that facilitates community access is a key issue for PWD as, overall, they are more vulnerable health-wise than persons without disabilities [12]. They report significantly greater prevalence and more frequent medical conditions including pain and fatigue [13], which can affect physical functioning and community participation. For example, severe bowel dysfunction is associated with barriers to personal relationships, feelings about self, and home life [14] while satisfaction with participation is consistently associated with a lower level of fatigue, pain, depression, stress, and anxiety [15]. In persons with neurological conditions (e.g. spinal cord injury), medical conditions such as bone density problems, depression, and sexual and reproductive health also need to be considered [16].

Important milestones such as the UN Convention and the Americans with Disabilities Act reinforced the right of PWD to get effective access to the highest standards of health care, without discrimination. However, PWD are often excluded from general health care [17] due to various constraints that can lead to dissatisfaction with services they do receive [18, 19]. Because of chronic medical conditions, there is a higher rate of primary health care utilization among PWD [20], even though access to health care is sometimes seen as a fight or an ongoing challenge on the continuum of health care [21]. Having access to health care, even on a limited basis, does not mean that needs are satisfied as unmet needs in PWD can be three times higher than in the general population [22].

There are various causes and constraints that increase unmet needs in PWD and some are related to limited access to primary health care. Major barriers are associated with physical inaccessibility, poor communication by service providers, funding issues, and a lack of knowledge and expertise regarding disability. Physical accessibility of facilities and equipment can be an issue: for example, offices and clinics often do not have accessible examination tables and scales [23]. While building entrances are usually accessible, the interiors (narrow doorways, cluttered exam rooms, inaccessible bathrooms) may not be accessible to wheelchair users [24]. Reports suggest that clinic administrators' significant lack of knowledge regarding accessible medical equipment and disability regulations could partly explain why medical practices lack such equipment [25, 26].

While inadequate communication between patients and physicians can be a barrier that limits access to health care in the general population, PWD also encounter barriers that place them at increased risk of experiencing ineffective patient–physician communication [27]. For example, they are more likely to think that service providers do not treat them equally to persons without disabilities for aspects such as listening to them, explaining treatment or involving them in treatment decisions. Some barriers are more structural and involve a lack of alternative means of communication such as large print or Braille materials and sign language interpreters for persons with sensory disabilities [28]. Overall, accessible communication means providing content in formats that are usable and understandable by persons with specific disabilities (vision, hearing, speech) or with limited ability to read or understand [29]. It also means ensuring a proper level of health literacy to facilitate decision-making and treatment instructions and follow-up. A lack of training for health care providers regarding how to care for PWD can also have a negative impact on health care coordination or quality [19, 28, 30]. This in turn can lead to a focus on people's disabilities rather than possible secondary complications or health problems, thus undermining primary health care.

Health care is funded through different sources depending on the jurisdiction and services required (government budgets, public or private health insurance, out-of-pocket expenses). Affordability of services is a major issue even without disabilities, but PWD are more likely to experience a lack of affordable health care, even in developed countries [1]. This leads to postponing efforts to seek health care or not buying needed medications because they are too costly [20]. Furthermore, since PWD have lower rates of employment, they are less likely to be able to afford private health insurance or may be excluded from such insurance because of pre-existing conditions. Access to insurance is critical as uninsured PWD report more problems getting needed care or medications than their insured counterparts [31].

This combination of physical, social, and economic barriers makes it difficult for many PWD to have access to and receive the quality health care they need, which affects their potential to be active in society and achieve full citizenship. There are various service models that foster integrative approaches or minimise barriers to accessing health care in PWD [32, 33]. The World Report on Disability [1] suggested 'reasonable accommodations' focusing on changes in health care facilities, including structural modifications, use of universal design features, and alternative approaches to presenting health information. To enhance 'disability knowledge' among health care providers, dissemination of information to practitioners should be encouraged through initiatives such as the 'Actionable Nuggets' project [34] aimed at providing primary care physicians with concise, but concrete, information on major issues related to the health of people with spinal cord injury. Moreover, encouraging the use of disability models is critical in ensuring that health care providers have a better understanding of the concept of functioning and participation as a crucial component of the definition of health that goes beyond disease and medical complications [35].

Community support programmes

Persons with disabilities want to live in the community of their choice. To do so they may need residential resources, home care services, family support, and transportation. No serious discussion about the social participation of PWD can take place without including the services they need to live, as independently as possible, in a regular home environment.

Table 33.1 Categories of home care services

Physical help	Includes all the services required daily to meet basic needs: personal hygiene, dressing, moving about and eating within the home
Domestic help	Includes all regular or occasional services to look after household tasks everyone has to perform in the home, such as doing laundry, preparing meals, washing dishes, going grocery shopping, and maintaining the home inside and out
Help within the community	Includes all services required to compensate for disabling situations vis-à-vis the social demands of daily life in an ordinary home environment. Examples include budget, correspondence, administrative procedures, and social services. Excluded are services related to recreation, transportation, community action and involvement, which are complementary to home care services but could require personal or human support and accompaniment
Health care	Includes all specialized nursing and paramedical services provided in the home

Home care services mean all the services required by PWD and provided in their home, with the aim of compensating for their functional disabilities and disabling situations in the daily life activities they need to perform to live in their regular home environment, with due respect for their personal choices. Home care services are generally divided into four categories [40]: physical help, domestic help, help within the community, and health care (Table 33.1).

Access to home care services within the framework of a person-centred or independent living model is an approach increasingly used to enable PWD to live and participate in the community. The Independent Living Movement has played an important role in keeping PWD, especially those with motor disabilities, in the community by advocating the principles of control over one's life and the services needed to carry out activities of daily living [36, 37]. This movement originated in the United States and then, in the late 1980s and 1990s, developed in Europe, especially in the Scandinavian countries [38, 39]. The importance of this phenomenon is confirmed in the majority of post-industrial societies [40]. Generally, service recipients from the Independent Living Movement include persons with very severe physical disabilities, but this formula is also offered to persons with intellectual disabilities and mental health problems [39, 41, 42]. It takes different forms and has different names depending on the context, such as direct payments, personal assistance, personal budget, etc.

Defining a person's needs with regard to home care services should be an empowering experience and cannot be dissociated from the reality of where the person chooses to live, what support the family needs, and transportation for the person to fulfil expected social roles.

This requires a person-centred needs assessment. The main objective of this assessment is to pinpoint the exact tasks the person wants to perform, in which he/she encounters disabling situations or difficulties, even with technical aids or human support. The assessment should cover any need which the person

thinks must be met to enable him/her to live at home as comfortably as possible in his/her own opinion. Having established the list of needs for home care services, the next step is to detail the tasks and qualifications of the staff needed to address them as well as how often and for how long the services are needed. The ultimate aim is to make it possible for PWD to buy and personally manage some or all of the home care services they need.

Different types of formulas have been developed and experiences with direct allocation have varied in different countries but they have all encountered difficulties with implementation [38, 39]. Some observers of the Independent Living Movement insist on assessing the impact of these formulas on the overall environment of PWD, with regard to their ability to act, and the impact on the community as a whole, with regard to development of partnerships with other grassroots organizations [38, 43, 44]. Problems noted include aspects related to difficulties recruiting and training workers and working conditions, or needs assessment, and the paternalistic control of professionals [39, 45–47]. In response to some of these difficulties, some American Independent Living centres have created training programmes for community workers in collaboration with various states. 'Most of these efforts are designed to establish a set of core standards and training programs for personal assistant services workers across the continuum of services and community-based settings' [37]. This formula is very important for many PWD since it allows them to remain active in their community while keeping some control over decisions that affect them with regard to personal services.

Support for families

Since the early 1980s, when policies to foster the integration of PWD were adopted, nearly an entire generation of children, adolescents, and young adults with disabilities have lived with their families, regardless of the origin, type, or severity of the disabilities. In addition, the declining number of births per family, which reduces the number of people who can support the family as a unit, the increasing number of divorces, and geographic mobility as well as the changing demographics of parenting are other changes that have an impact on families, including its structure, access to family support, and the availability of mothers or other family caregivers. Disability policies must consider all these realities. Support for families appears to be a critical element in the process of integrating children with disabilities in ordinary living environments.

A major contribution of research focusing on the impact of disabilities on families is the development of the concept that the family is a system in itself, consisting of four subsystems (marital, parental, fraternal, and extended) that are constantly interacting and are influenced by its structural characteristics, life cycle and functions [48]. This concept underscores the interdependence of the individuals who make up the family system. When one of them has a disability, all of them are affected and feel the effects. The family system must adapt to and cope with a situation where the unexpected high level of care and support needed is a burden on family caregivers, whose health and well-being can be jeopardised if they do not receive outside support.

In many instances, there are not enough family resources to support the family's 'natural' resilience in overcoming difficult situations. Heiman [49] stresses the importance of the social network and support provided by service networks. Different support strategies may be considered. Tétreault et al. [50] proposed a typology of these strategies based on the needs of families. It consists of four categories: (1) support (informational; for accompaniment and help with decision-making; judicial–legal; financial; educational; psychosocial; for assistance in daily life; for recreation, sports, and social activities; for transportation; etc.); (2) respite; (3) child minding (child caring); and (4) emergency support (accommodation, financial, caretaking, etc.). When determining which strategies to choose, the characteristics and needs expressed by the families in interaction with the individual characteristics of the child with disabilities must all be taken into account.

From the viewpoint of interventions focusing on assisted resilience [51], support strategies act as protective factors that strengthen the family's resilience and help it respond positively to the challenges involved in meeting the specific needs of the child with disabilities. Growing out of the study of the positive adaptation of children to traumatic events and chronic adversity [52], the work on resilience expanded from looking at individual resilience to studying family, collective, and societal resilience [53]. McCubbin and McCubbin [54] were the first to examine family resilience by looking at the different characteristics that help families resist disruption in the face of change and adapt to crisis situations. Studying resilience helps to understand not only why some families manage to survive traumatic events and adversity, but also how they manage to grow and emerge stronger from the ordeal [55]. The concept of resilience is of great interest for family support services, especially with the emergence of the concept of 'assisted resilience' as distinct from natural resilience, which refers to the individual's and family's own strengths and abilities [53]. Assisted resilience interventions are characterized by: (1) focus on and development of the potential of individuals or families at risk; (2) identification of existing resources in the individual's or family's circle; and (3) implementation of prevention programmes and of a maieutic approach for intervention strategy.

For families of children with disabilities, managing to cope with a situation that could become chronically difficult is conditioned by the interaction between the characteristics of the child, his/her family and the environment. Neither the population of children with disabilities nor families are homogeneous. The nature and severity of the impairment (cognitive, motor, sensory, communication) and its impact on the day-to-day functioning of the child, as well as the presence of physical or mental health or behaviour problems are all characteristics that make each situation different. This heterogeneity, combined with age and gender, results in needs of varying types and intensity. In addition, socioeconomic level, schooling, family size and structure, access to an informal network of significant persons, proximity of services, personal and family resources are all characteristics that make families different from each other. They have an effect on family resilience and on parents' availability and ability to fulfil their parental role in a way that fosters the optimal development of their child. Support for families is essential if the implementation of current disability policies is to be a success.

Employment and education

In the field of education, one sees the same trend towards integration in a regular school environment of PWD, be they children, adolescents or adults, instead of within a specialised structure. This is undoubtedly one of the most important and critical changes in practice in the past forty years towards true participation in community life. There is increasing discussion about inclusive education, as opposed to an emphasis on inclusive pedagogy. An inclusive approach, however, is still driven by differing trends and tensions that sometimes make it difficult to address individual differences [56]. This move towards inclusivity is even more important when it involves returning to work or returning to the community after a trauma. The scientific community is particularly interested in this latter dimension, given the great complexity of the process where a range of social and psychosocial variables influence the return to community living [57–60]. This educational and employment issue has been widely addressed in recent years from the standpoint of social and community participation, which is marked by transitions, that is, critical moments in the life cycle of individuals. Many factors influence youth transitions [62] from secondary to post-secondary education and then to the workforce (Table 33.2). The presence of a disability makes these transitions even more complex.

The last 15 years have seen an increased focus on the transition from adolescence to young adulthood [61], especially in the US and the UK. Part of the trend in both countries is driven by laws that require transition planning to be part of youth education programming, starting at age 14. Under US law, educators are asked to provide annual statements of transition services, including

Table 33.2 Factors influencing youth transition

Internal organizational characteristics of the school (including administrative and teaching staff)	Peer influence
Scholastic participation	Behaviour problems and psychological health
Participation in the social life of the school	Financing for post-secondary education
Cognitive ability	Experience in the first year of post-secondary studies
Parental socioeconomic status	Competence (problem solving and other skills)
Family and community social and cultural capital (family time, time available to invest in cultural activities)	Coop study programmes that provide opportunities for work and study
Family history (separation, death, divorce, child custody, parental role and attitude toward the child's studies)	Volunteer work
Balance expectations between work, education, and family responsibilities	First work experience
Personal, scholastic, and professional aspirations (of both the youth and the parents)	Study–work combination
Career planning	Unemployment experience; quality and length of work

if appropriate, a statement of the interagency responsibilities or linkages necessary to meet each child's specific needs. In Canada there are so-called 'mixed' programmes to facilitate the transition from youth to adulthood. Little is known, however, about the effectiveness of such programmes [59].

Moreover, in professional settings, especially related to rehabilitation, concerns about transition are emerging while in the research field, especially in Anglo-Saxon countries, studies have shown the importance of such factors for years. Compared to youth without disabilities, youth with disabilities are half as likely to participate in post-secondary education. Rates of unemployment and under-employment in youth with disabilities are cause for concern (over 55% and 75% for youth with moderate or severe disabilities, respectively). Transition to adulthood for young adults with cerebral palsy and other disabilities is a difficult and sometimes delayed process. The transition from adolescence to adulthood has been examined by trying to establish a profile of the health and needs of groups of people with different diagnoses (cerebral palsy, spina bifida, and traumatic brain injury). It appears that the transition to post-secondary education and the workforce varies depending on the diagnosis and its characteristics [62].

Summary of personal and community service accessibility issues for people with disabilities

Accessibility to social, communal, and medical support services is revealed to be complex and problematic across the range of disabilities encountered, and this despite the enactment of laws designed to ensure full access and participation as a basic human right. Part of the difficulty is that the personal, communal, and societal levels are so intertwined it is difficult to develop robust practical programmes that simultaneously address all three levels. However, recognition that there are three levels to deal with is an important tool for moving forward in the provision of more effective services. In the area of assistive technologies, on the other hand, most technologies have been traditionally aimed at the personal level. It is only in the past few years that the range of technologies has broadened. It is of great interest and relevance, therefore, to examine the current developments of assistive technologies, as a complement to our understanding of the accessibility of support services.

Technologies

Writing a section on technologies designed to support either the rehabilitation process or the ongoing challenges of living with disabilities has never been more challenging than it is today. The last few years have seen a burgeoning not just of new technologies but of entirely new categories of technology, and there are no signs that the rate of evolution is slowing down. If anything, it is accelerating. There is a need to find some kind of order in this rapidly changing area.

To provide a useful structure, the most recent version of the Disability Creation Process developed by Fougeyrollas et al. [63] was used. This has the additional advantage of framing the technology within its social context as part of a broader process of supporting greater access to community services, as outlined in the remainder of this chapter. Compared to the International Classification of Functioning, Disability and Health, the model promulgated by the World Health Organization, which relates the biological conditions of impairment to the activities, social participation, and inclusion of PWD within the larger community, the Disability Creation Process model gives the environment a more central place.

As previously described, the micro-, meso-, and macroscales correspond to the personal level, the community level and the societal level of activities, respectively. This provides a useful basis for situating the rapidly changing landscape of technologies, and we adopt this framework in the following discussion.

Microscale, personal technologies

The microscale concerns personal technologies that are under the immediate purview of the user, which may be adopted, modified or exchanged without the need to comply with any formal regulations. Microlevel technologies therefore correspond to most 'assistive devices' designed to meet the individual needs of people living with disability, and include individualized technologies for assisting those with sensory and cognitive deficits and for improving mobility, such as wheelchairs and navigational aids. A typical example of a microlevel technology is a wheelchair.

Meso-scale, communal technologies

The meso-scale concerns technologies which cannot be easily picked up and carried and whose use is generally regulated by regional statutes. These include traditional technologies such as home adaptations, domotics, environmental care systems, and adaptations to public and private vehicles. They also include new technologies such as the so-called 'smart environments'. A good example of meso-level technology is the adaptation of a vehicle to support drivers with disabilities; such adaptations must be approved by regional governments.

Macroscale, societal technologies

Macroscale technologies are primarily large, networked infrastructures, which must be supported and regulated at the national and international levels. These include the Internet and communication and information technologies that harness the Internet and operate at societal levels such as social networks. They also include large-scale infrastructure adaptations such as those being considered for the development of so-called 'smart cities'. The infrastucture used to support a technology such as Twitter is a macro-scale technology; however, the device used to access Twitter may be a microscale technology. Hence the technologies involved in each of these levels are relatively different, although there is some blurring of the lines at the boundaries between them.

The macrolevel of technology is a maturing arena for new technologies that has not been widely studied or even acknowledged in the rehabilitation community. However, technological innovation on this scale is on the rise and, especially via the smart cities research focus, we are likely to see a growing number of enabling infrastructure-based technologies specifically geared to supporting PWD in the coming years. Furthermore, although most 'smart' technologies are still experimental, they are also developing rapidly, driven by strong market pressure. As a result, the 'technology landscape' may look very different in a decade than it does today.

The Disability Creation Process model includes, like the International Classification of Functioning, Disability and Health, an explicit acknowledgement of the role played by daily activities and social roles, and many technologies have been developed to support these needs. However, even these activities and roles are changing in the broader context of today's knowledge economy, and technologies on different scales may serve to support those needs. Where relevant, we indicate the relationships between technologies, activities/roles and personal factors, such as capabilities and identity issues, in order to better situate their role within the broader dimensions of this section.

Personal, microscale technologies

Assistive devices

Populations that present neurological deficits include adults with spinal cord injury [64, 65], traumatic brain injury [66, 67], stroke [68], and adults with neurovisual deficits [69]. Three types of assistive devices are particularly common in clinical programs for these populations: assistive technologies for cognition, visual aids, and electronic aids for daily living.

A popular assistive technologies for cognition (ATC) tool is the personal digital assistant [66], which is a small hand-held computer, also known as palmtop, hand-held PC, hand-held and, more recently, tablet and smartphone, used to help compensate for behavioural memory deficits, which is the most common complaint among individuals with acquired brain injury (Figure 33.1). Behavioural memory deficits involve working and prospective memory, attention and executive functions, as these are engaged in the performance of everyday activities, such as taking medications, planning and organizing schedules, keeping appointments, performing multi-step tasks, and dealing with distractions [66]. Another commonly used ATC is television-assisted prompting, which issues reminders that help to achieve task completion [67]. There is also the planning and execution assistant and trainer [70], which is a new device that helps users stay focused and on task despite surprises and distractions. It is a hand-held electronic calendar and address book that features automatic cueing to start and

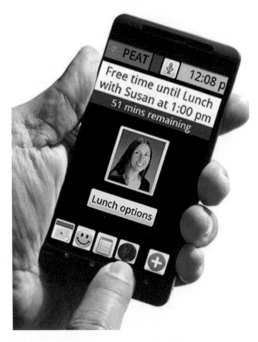

Fig. 33.1 The Planning and Execution Trainer (PEAT).
Source: Brain Aid http://brainaid.com/

stop daily activities and has a built-in telephone, fax, and Internet. Finally, the assistive technology support process completes the list of ATCs. This support, with the use of sensors placed in the home, encourages the completion of a task that has already been started or issues reminders about tasks required in a specific location or after specific actions [68].

Regarding assistive technologies for neurovisual deficits, many have been tested. Various types of eyewear may assist in reducing falls; prisms and telescopic lenses may improve visual attention and minimize the impact of visual field deficits. Technologies to improve computer use, way finding, and home safety may also enhance user functionality [69].

Electronic aids for daily living (EADLs) are used by individuals who struggle with manipulation tasks and mobility. Those—also known as environmental control units or environmental control systems—are assistive technology interventions prescribed by rehabilitation professionals to increase autonomy and hence improve quality of life. Electronic aids enable users to independently operate electronic devices, such as telephones, door openers, bed positions, lights, computers, and personal entertainment systems, through alternative access within the home or workplace [64, 65]. EADLs, while not technically 'smart devices', may be viewed as a first step in that direction [71].

Scientific evidence in support of the links between the use of ATCs, visual aids and EADLs on the one hand, and social participation on the other, remains to be established. Larger study samples are required to ensure generalizability. Furthermore, participants need to use identical technologies (same brand and model) in a wide variety of environments and social contexts to achieve more robust assessments. For example, it is necessary to observe a group of subjects taking on a variety of social roles, assuming responsibilities and participating in the social life of the community, both with and without their assistive devices. Finally, it is important to note that ATCs, visual aids and EADLs are evolving far too rapidly to permit adequate and full testing of any one device. As a result, there are many studies that are 'non experimental', that is, do not include any form of direct intervention, control group or randomised controlled trial for the target population. Instead, these studies focus on user perceptions and clinical recommendations. Questionnaire-based surveys and qualitative methods [65, 68] are preferred for assessing reported use and perceptions. Efforts to evaluate specific devices tend to adopt an exploratory approach based on small group interventions without a control group [66] or sometimes they may adopt a cross-sectional design with a control group [64]. One study used a randomized controlled crossover design [67]; main outcomes showed a significant advantage for prospective memory prompting (72% completion) compared to no prompting (43% completion) and higher task completion with television-assisted prompting for researcher-assigned experimental tasks (81%) compared to self-selected preferred (68%) or not preferred (68%) tasks. Overall, more studies of actual use are required to assess the real value of these technologies for increasing social participation among populations with neurological impairments.

Communication devices

The use of communication aids has been assessed more specifically for people with cerebral palsy [72, 73] or for post-traumatic brain injury and post-coma patients presenting a minimum of conscious functioning [74, 75]. Two types of assistive technology are used in clinical settings: alternative augmentative communication (AAC) devices and communication devices for a minimally conscious state.

AAC devices encompass communication methods used to supplement or replace speech or writing for those with impairments in the production or comprehension of spoken or written language. AAC is used by people with a wide range of speech and language impairments, including congenital impairments such as cerebral palsy and acquired conditions such as amyotrophic lateral sclerosis and Parkinson's disease. AAC can be a permanent addition to a person's communication programme or a temporary aid [76, 77]. The two most important elements appreciated by people who rely on AAC are: (1) saying exactly what they want to say, and (2) saying it as fast as they can. AAC devices have evolved dramatically over the past 30 years. Originally little more than printed tables of symbols to which the user pointed to communicate different messages, later versions exploited dedicated voice synthesizers. Modern AAC services are provided by portable computers, tablets and smart phones, and use a range of voice synthesizers (Figure 33.2).

Regarding communication devices for the minimally conscious state, the technology offers writing opportunities to persons emerging from a minimally conscious state who are affected by extensive motor disabilities. These are based on specific arrangements of optic, tilt, or pressure microswitches (linked to preferred environmental stimuli) and eyelid, toe and finger responses [74, 75]. For writing, the use of optic sensors and scanning keyboard emulators for persons with pervasive motor disabilities and lack of head control can help manage basic writing [72].

Concerning the scientific evidence in support of these technologies, there is very little compared to that available for ATCs and EADLs. Interview-based surveys [92] and reports of clinical expertise [77] are the primary means of reporting on these technologies. Specific product assessments, on the other hand, rely on exploratory intervention strategies in small groups without a control group [72, 74, 75].

Many different AAC technologies are commercially marketed and they evolve rapidly. As with other assistive technologies, this makes it difficult to assess their impact on social participation. An effective study would need to observe a group of individuals using the same technology in different settings and contexts, without undue effort, with and without their aids. Such studies are difficult to organize because they require a lot of resources and are intrusive in the lives of participants (require monitoring 24 hours a day). Furthermore, AAC devices and communication devices for the minimally conscious must be individually programmed and require many hours of training. As a result, studies involving large groups are extremely difficult to organise, let alone publish. Most studies present strategy choices rather than attempting to measure effects [77]. Furthermore, keeping up with new products poses additional challenges, especially for technologies that support brain injury or stroke. Factors affecting the integration of aided communication in everyday life contexts are complex. For many adults, the lack of key supports, including the availability of communication partners, restricts the contexts in and extent to which aided communication is used.

Mobility devices

Within the set of all possible assistive devices for PWD, mobility devices such as wheelchairs (manual or powered), scooters, walkers, and rollators are the most heavily used [78]. Many populations with neural deficits, people with spinal cord injury [79], acquired brain trauma [80], multiple sclerosis [81], cerebral palsy [82], and Parkinson's disease [83] are subject to use them. For example, among those with spinal cord injury, for whom functional mobility is considered one of the aspects that most affects their social participation [84], the wheelchair provides the most common and effective solution to enhanced mobility. Indeed, 82% of people with spinal cord injury possessed at least one wheelchair, and 60% of these depend totally on their wheelchair for moving around [85].

Many positive impacts result from the use of mobility devices on populations with neural impairments as well as other groups. Indeed, mobility devices have positive effects on activity and participation within daily activities of various populations [86], in particular people with spinal cord injury or who have suffered a stroke. Overall, powered wheelchairs and scooters improve independence in mobility, and increase mobility-related participation in everyday activities [87] as well as having measurable positive impacts on overall mobility [88, 89], quality of life, pain and discomfort [89]. Wheelchair use, whether manual or powered, also facilitates the ability to perform social roles and participate in the community [90] among patients recovering from neural impairments [91, 92]. Furthermore, the impacts of assistive devices on the users' informal caregivers [93] shows how mobility devices contribute to reducing some of the physical and emotional burden, but can also increasing caregiver injury, anxiety about user injury, accessibility issues, and social stigma. A few studies have signalled some negative impacts, particularly for the use of manual wheelchairs among people with spinal cord injury. Injuries due to excessive use and acute injuries are among the issues commonly reported [94, 95]. Furthermore, wheelchairs themselves may be perceived as a limiting factor to full social participation [96] and increase dependence on others [91]. For children and adolescents, benefits of mobility devices have also shown that independent powered mobility is associated with developmental, cognitive, and psychosocial skills such as spatial cognition, independence, and

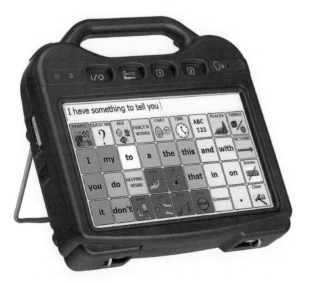

Fig. 33.2 Alternative augmentative communication (AAC).
Source: University of Colorado www.ucdenver.edu.

emotion [97]. Powered mobility decreases perceived levels of stress of parents with children with cerebral palsy at the time of wheelchair delivery, and increases satisfaction with their child's social and play skills, their ability to go where desired, sleep and wake patterns, and belief that the general public accepts their child [98]. For the same population, powered mobility also increased parents' positive perceptions of their child's social skills, increased the number of mobility activities during play, and may have positively impacted the quality of play for the children [99]. There exist few studies that examine the specific benefits of scooters, walkers and rollators as compared to wheelchairs. Despite this, it seems reasonable to assume that similar effects and impacts can be observed throughout populations with neurological disorders.

During the past ten years, mobility technologies have evolved beyond these more conventional devices and new mobility technologies have emerged. For example, the iBOT is an advanced powered wheelchair that allows a user to rise to the same height as a standing person while remaining supported on the two rear wheels (Figure 33.3). This device hence allows an individual to perform a variety of activities that were difficult or impossible with conventional mobility devices, such as holding an eye-level conversation, using up or down ramps, traversing outdoor surfaces such as grass and dirt trails, and climbing curbs. One problem with this device is it is nonetheless awkward to use in constrained spaces such as bathrooms [100]. Users with people with spinal cord injury report improved employment satisfaction [101], while users with a range of neurological impairments report better independent functional mobility skills in a community environment [102], greater access to work and outdoor environments, enhanced community access and improved social interaction [103]. Unfortunately, production and sales of the device ceased in 2009 due to its high cost and weak market share. Another advanced device, the TopChair, combines powered wheels and caterpillar tracks so as to enhance

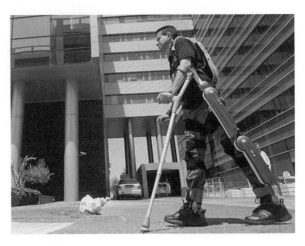

Fig. 33.4 Exoskeletons.
Source: www.internetmedicine.com

user autonomy in both indoor and outdoor environments. Its most appreciated capability is the ability to climb or descend staircases [104].

Finally, a mobility enhancement device that has been viewed by many as a long term solution to mobility needs for PWD is the exoskeleton [105, 106], also called a power suit or muscle suit (Figure 33.4). At least one has been commercially available for several years, albeit with rudimentary capability and at a very high cost [106]. The development of exoskeleton capability has, however, taken a lot longer than originally expected and results today are still far from mature. Several suits have been successfully deployed in the laboratory under limited conditions and for short durations. Separate development efforts are underway for upper body and lower body exoskeletons, the needs of each are somewhat different. Exoskeleton devices are aimed at several applications, of which mobility devices for PWD are but one possible use. Other uses include for soldiers, for caregivers, construction, hazardous work environments, etc. Although costs for robotic components have dropped dramatically in recent years, the complex nature of these devices means that commercial availability of products at prices comparable to even high end wheelchairs or other mobility devices is unlikely for many years yet to come.

Communal, mesoscale technologies

Motor vehicle adaptation—private and public

Transportation via either personal or public vehicles is absolutely essential to ensure success in carrying out day-to-day activities as well as for full participation in community life in contemporary society. Among individuals who have disabilities in general and spinal cord injuries in particular [96, 107], transportation has been shown to be a significant barrier to community participation. In order to overcome the limitations that prevent the use of a motor vehicle, many types of adaptation have been developed. For personal automobiles, the most important modifications concern the primary controls (steering, accelerator, and brakes)—for example, mechanical hand controls that do not require gripping to operate (e.g. right-angle pull/push and rotate/push operations), a steering spinner (such as using knobs or balls) or zero-effort steering device, and a parking brake extension or reduced-effort brakes [108, 109] (Figure 33.5). In addition, several systems may need to be moved into more accessible locations (e.g. the

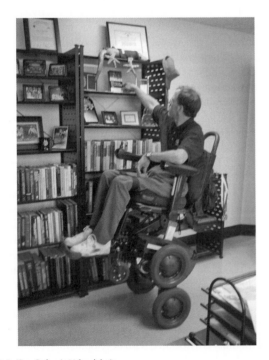

Fig. 33.3 iBot Robotic Wheelchair.
Source: Hizook www.hizook.com.

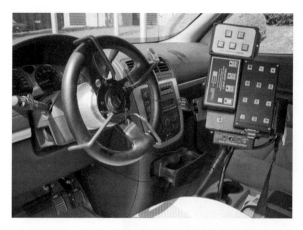

Fig. 33.5 Adaptation of the primary controls of a vehicle.
Constance-Lethbridge Rehabilitation Centre (http://www.constance-lethbridge.qc.ca/)

accelerator and dashboard controls). Other common modifications include the implementation of automated doors (opening and closing), and the lowering of the floor (such as in a van) [108]. Of course, many modern vehicles already come equipped with characteristics which facilitate use that may be considered 'universal'—(e.g. an automatic transmission shifter without a thumb button, power steering, a collision warning system, power brakes, and automated doors) [110]. Vehicle access is also an important consideration, especially for wheelchair users—common adaptations include the installation of a semi- or fully automated ramp or lift (Figure 33.6) or use of a grasp enhancer [109]. Finally, seat adaptations may also be required for a safe and effective driving experience, including the possibility to use the wheelchair itself as the driver's seat when suitably clamped in place [111]. In addition to these physical transformations, most states require evaluation by a competent specialist of the driving capabilities of the potential user [108, 111, 112]. The costs of these adaptations can range up to about $90,000, although limited modifications can be sometimes made for a few hundred dollars [111, 112].

For public transport (bus, metro, paratransit van, etc.), adaptations may include the installation of a ramp or lift, or the use of designs that eliminate steps, include a lowered floor, or eliminate the gap between platform and vehicle (Figure 33.6). For both public

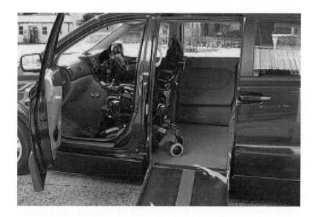

Fig. 33.6 Adapted vehicle with automated ramp.
Motor Equipment News (www.motorequipmentnews.co.nz) http://motorequipmentnews.co.nz/articles/passionate-brothers-making-difference-disabled-drivers

and private vehicles, wheelchair tiedowns that limit wheelchair motion are an important feature [108, 113]. Each country has its own legislative and regulating authority for these adaptations—most will have to meet safety norms.

Home adaptation and automation (smart homes)

It is important to highlight the differences between assistive devices (micro-scale technology) and smart homes (meso-scale technology). First, the latter, in comparison to most assistive technologies, cannot be easily picked up and carried and their use is generally regulated by regional statutes. For example, assistive devices like EADLs (e.g. a switch on a wheelchair that can be activated by a person to turn on different electronic devices) or stand-alone devices (e.g. radio passive infrared receiver and voice receiver) are single devices [114]. However, when technology refers to a simply connected system (e.g. a warden call button or a community alarm) or a more complex system linked to an external infrastructure (e.g. a domestic device that interacts with a city-based infrastructure to support telecare services), it is more than a simple assistive device. We call such complex systems 'smart homes' because of their dependence on external infrastructures and also because these systems may react to the individual and perform a range of supportive actions (Figure 33.7).

Smart homes include automation of domestic features, security features, multimedia and telecare services [115]. There can be many levels of 'ambient intelligence' in different smart homes [71] and different systems have been proposed. Aldridge [116] proposes five levels: (1) homes with intelligent objects; (2) homes with intelligent, communicating objects; (3) connected homes; (4) learning homes; and (5) attentive homes. Mann and Milton [117] propose eight levels, which to some extent go further than Aldridge's levels to what might be called a sixth, proactive level. For example, attentive homes will assess individuals' lifestyle trends based on an analysis of their daily activities and then issue 'prompts or verbal feedback' to help people succeed in undertaking daily activities effectively and safely [117].

There is little real evidence of the application of smart home technology to support neurological conditions specifically; rather, these are developments that support wide ranges of disability, including those with neurological impairments. It is nonetheless possible to point to examples of smart homes in automation and security features [114]. In the UK, for example, many residential projects involving smart homes have been tested. Some include a bath monitor, cooker monitor and voice feedback system [118]. Another includes a communal kitchen area for a range of residents and has technology demonstrator sites in England, including the iHouse, with a number of scenarios to support cognitive and sensory impairments [119].

These initiatives offer a full range of automation and safety features that are intended for a mixed population of wheelchair users, brain injury victims and people with sensory impairments [119]. In telecare services, there is a wide variety of devices that are commonly used with people with neurological diagnoses, namely pendant alarms, fall detectors, bed occupancy sensors, pull cords, movement sensors, smoke/heat/flood detectors and carbon monoxide monitors, automated lighting, location sensors, activity sensors, well-being monitors, and medication reminder systems [114].

One promising set of technologies for smart homes involves the use of tele-operated robotic arms that are located in the home but

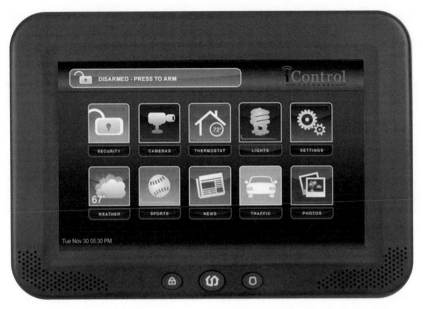

Fig. 33.7 Smart home device.
Source: Forbes http://blogs-images.forbes.com/amywestervelt/files/2012/03/iControl.jpg.

are remotely operated by a caregiver. The use of such tele-operated arms has been studied for assisting a person to rise from bed, wash, dress, eat, and fetch needed items [120]. These systems could help people with both motor and cognitive impairments. Smart homes with high levels of ambient intelligence can also schedule and organise household repairs, food and service deliveries [117].

No evidence yet exists concerning the impact of smart homes on social participation; these developments are complex to build and not enough have been implemented to support extensive impact studies. Instead, the scientific literature reports on project ideas and plans, technical prototypes, and the strengths and limitations of different smart home components. One common element can be found in most of these papers, however; even if different people have a similar diagnostic profile and present similar cognitive or motor limitations, each person has different needs in terms of home automation, personal safety, communication preferences, and telecare services. Hence, smart homes must be able to adapt to context, or must be designed around the specific needs of each client (e.g. use or not of specific assistive technologies, prompts, and reminders, what caregivers are able to provide by way of additional services, what can be monitored at a distance, and which tasks are amenable to automated or tele-operated strategies) [121]. Furthermore, both the type and quality of telecare services may raise ethical questions around privacy issues [122]. The most pressing objections against telecare are concerned with depersonalising care, increasing the isolation of patients, and using technology to achieve cost savings rather than health gains.

Societal, macro-scale technologies

Regional infrastructures for smart cities

Smart homes will need to rely on a variety of regional infrastructures in order to function effectively [123]. In addition, these infrastructures will support the development of smart environments other than those found in residences and private vehicles.

These infrastructures must also be developed with users with disabilities in mind. Otherwise, they risk becoming another barrier to inclusion [123].

Research concerned with identifying responsive infrastructures and determining their structure is still embryonic, although some progress has been made in the past five years. Smart homes will require both location-based and object-based local infrastructures [124] in order to support context-aware functionality [125]. Disability-specific ontologies are suggested [123, 124] to anchor data representation schemes. This is an important point as the development of such ontologies requires the collaboration of individuals involved in rehabilitation or disability studies on the one hand, and computer specialists and researchers on the other. Furthermore, the disability-specific ontologies will need to interface with geospatial ontologies to support location-based service provision within the context of enhanced mobility.

Data including information on public buildings (location, accessibility, services provided), events, accessible city routes, information on public transport, and relevant navigational data will need to be provided via these infrastructures [126] (Figure 33.8). Furthermore, combined with information concerning public transport routes, it could be important to develop reliable and robust pedestrian support infrastructures [71], which have somewhat different needs than those used to support vehicle movements, whether public or private.

The infrastructures provided need to accommodate dynamic changes in the locations of individuals and, as a result, changing configurations for service provision [127] and must also track service provision across micro-, meso-, and macro-scales [128]. In addition to semantic (ontology) approaches, multi-agent-based architectures are expected to play a major role [129]. So-called smart garments are also expected to play an intermediate role between the home-based individual and the city-based infrastructure [130].

Applications to be supported include transportation and navigation services [131], telecare and monitoring [128], tele-operation

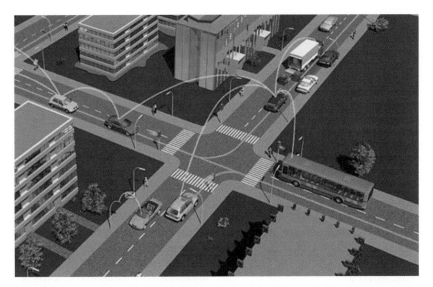

Fig. 33.8 Intelligent transportation system.
Source: http://technologynewhere.wordpress.com/2010/05/12/intelligent-transportation-system/ Technologynewhere blog on wordpress

of robotic devices [120], services for remote ordering and delivery [117], adapted learning [132], and informational [133] environments. Within the framework of so-called 'caring cities', specific infrastructures to support the use of technologies by the homeless are also called for. There is a relationship between the homeless and disability; many of the homeless struggle with issues of disability [134] and inadequate health care responses. Issues that are more specific to homeless populations that should be addressed via appropriate infrastructures include the need to develop mutual protection arrangements and the need to replace defective or stolen devices. Access to learning infrastructures is also important [132].

Social networking and the Internet

Another constellation of service provision at the macro-scale is access to and use of social networking and other Internet-based services (Figure 33.9). Access is an issue; as the Internet has become more complex and multimodal, accessibility for the disabled has declined [133], particularly due to a lack of recognition among designers of Internet services of the need to incorporate flexible features that increase accessibility.

Nonetheless, despite the difficulties, social networking in particular, but also other services provided by the Internet (see Table 33.3), has already proven to be an effective tool for a range of disabilities.

More negative aspects of the Internet experience include the unconscious prevalence of conventional able-bodied ideas even when disability is acknowledged [145], the presence of multimedia files that are often inaccessible (no subtitles, garbled sound, etc. [133]), and the dangers that sexual predators represent for children [135]. In addition, many users with disabilities are quite computer-savvy but are unable to fully exploit the medium because there are significant barriers. This is particularly true for people with visual impairments [146].

Although there is much room for development, there is growing evidence of the value of social networking and other Internet services. On the other hand, large-scale infrastructures are not validated through specific studies of use but rather through a

maturing understanding of the most relevant architectures, which will also take time to develop.

Summary of technologies accessibility issues for people with disabilities

The whole field of technology aids for PWD has grown rapidly over recent years, and emphasis is shifting from personal aids (microsystem), towards home aids (mesolevel), and even large-scale infrastructures (macrolevel). However, the impacts of these technologies are becoming harder to measure given the rate of deployment of new technologies and the emergence of new classes of technology for which reliable assessment procedures are still lacking. Technologies that address the specific needs of persons with neurological deficits are also increasingly becoming available. The ultimate efficacy of all these technologies depends at least as strongly on social and economic policies in support of PWD, towards which we now turn our attention.

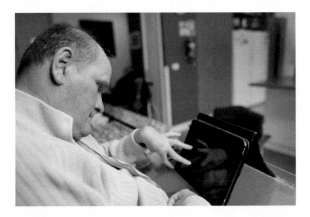

Fig. 33.9 Social networking and the internet.
Source: Gary Radler gary@garyradlerphoto.com
Website: http://www.garyradler.com/Stock/Portraits-of-People-with-a-3/i-TJ2qSnj/A

Table 33.3 Social networking and the Internet increasing access to community

Interrupting patterns of isolation and loneliness [135]	Increased autonomy [136]
Finding a job [137, 138]	Greater control over complex communication situations [139]
Disability networking [140]	Accessing news services [138]
Online dating [138]	Accessing online learning environments [141]
Self and group advocacy [140]	Accessing useful information, such as concerning sexuality [142]
Benefits of anonymity [hence reduced stigmatisation] and disinhibition [135, 143]	Participating in group discussions [e.g. via blogging [144]], accessing tools that enhance independent living [e.g. apps [138]]

Social policies and disability

Trying to define the complex relationship that has developed between disability and public policy is a challenge, particularly when dealing with certain national traditions and practices. These policies, which are the result of interventions by public agencies, have been deployed in different ways and in different sectors over the past four decades with the aim of helping PWD participate in community activities. They are complex and generally agreed to be fragmented [147, 148], since they take different forms as they endeavour to meet individual and collective needs, improve health and well-being, compensate for losses and damages incurred, and redistribute wealth to achieve equality. With respect to disability, they include responding with specific measures to the needs of PWD, as is the case with home care, home adaptations, and adapted transport (the so-called 'disability policy'), while in other cases responses are delivered through general interventions targeting the population as a whole.

For the majority of developed countries, the organisational structures of the policies inherited from the 1970s were reformed in the early 2000s. From measures aimed at supporting specialized institutions, an approach focusing on human rights to eliminate obstacles to social participation now dominates the political landscape. In this process, the role of policy is reaffirmed as an essential factor in keeping persons with disabilities in the community.

Stemming from this, an approach targeting personal compensation for additional costs incurred as a result of having disabilities or impairments or experiencing disability situations is implemented in a way that separates income-related issues from additional costs. The logic behind compensation for costs is mostly applied without regard to individual income and underscores collective responsibility for the social consequences of disability (PWD generally have reduced incomes). This approach is the subject of more and more discussions across different revisions of income security measures [148, 149].

The dimensions related to the issue of income and income replacement in the event of an accident takes us into a very complex realm where insurance provisions co-exist alongside social assistance and solidarity that often vary depending on the causes of the accident. In the current situation of economic instability, the welfare state is slowly being transformed into a hybrid system connecting the state and civil society and in which the roles of the different stakeholders such as community organisations, charities, foundations and, to a lesser extent, family caregivers, in responding to these needs are becoming blurred. In this process, we should stress the importance given to the progressive accessibility of the built environment and public transport [150, 151]. All these elements that help to redefine the system reflect both a need to modulate the way things are done and a reaffirmation of their essential role in supporting PWD in their participation in regular activities in the community.

In contrast with earlier assistance policies, contemporary societies are characterized by active national and regional policies and diversified disability support programmes. On the other hand, in the context of public budget constraints and reduction of the size of the state, OCDE countries tend increasingly to transfer responsibilities from the central state to regional and local authorities [152].

The situation is rendered still more complex by the tendency of different states to each have a unique historically-based welfare organization for income security and disability support programmes. One way to understand eligibility to those programmes is to distinguish between specific access on the basis of work status, work accidents, and disability insured causes such as traffic accidents, from access to disability programmes that flow from social security measures available for all citizens. However, this complex network of situations means both access to income security and to specific forms of compensation are generally inequitable across different populations, especially for PWD.

Recently, there has been a shift towards offering direct payments rather than access to services, which are in any case diminishing because of cost-cutting practices. This shift appears on the surface to align with the Independent Living ideology—in particular, it attributes a broader interpretation of the role of the personal budget to cover the needs of PWD. In principle, the individual is provided with increased freedom of choice and controls who provides the disability support. Generally these programmes favour a transfer of public resources towards less costly services from social economy organizations and private agencies.

Direct payment and personal budget management are valuable solutions in apparent fit with values of the disability rights movement but they do not suit the abilities and choices of every PWD. Moreover, such a policy could reduce collective responsibility and may exacerbate redistribution problems for vulnerable citizens.

Summary of social policies issues for people with disabilities

There is no modern example of a really equitable universal disability insurance policy in developed countries. Such a system would make a distinction between basic income security for all citizens, high enough to cover basic needs and prevent the fall into poverty; and universal insurance for disability-related additional costs whatever the causes of disability, work situation, and household status.

Discussion and conclusion

The issue of enhancing community access and promoting full participation of PWD in society is still highly challenging in spite of significant improvements over the last few decades at all levels.

The increasing importance of the social model of disability and the efforts of advocates of the disability movement have led to the passing of new laws or conventions based on human rights principles that mandate the reduction of barriers to full participation. These, in turn, have led to changes in how services are organized and delivered, in the ranges of health care and technologies being promoted and what they are called upon to do, and in the social and disability policies in play at national, international, and regional levels.

Service delivery is still, however, fragmentary and inadequate overall at addressing the range of support services required to ensure full participation. Many gaps still exist—there are significant inadequacies in the ability to deliver health care to PWD, to support families and for young or adult PWD to get an education and find work, not to mention participate more fully in leisure activities. Different countries have different strategies for dealing with this—none are currently fully successful. One of the key insights to emerge in recent years is the role of resiliency in handling the challenges posed by disability, whether at the level of the individual, the family, or the community. As a result, there has been a partial shift in service delivery towards enhancing resiliency rather than only offering direct support.

In counterpoint to the problems of service delivery, however, we are currently in the middle of a major technological revolution. Technological aids are broadening from devices that assist individuals to more environmentally engaged technologies that offer support for homes and households, as well as global infrastructures that operate at macroscopic levels, providing adapted or 'smart' services for both individuals and communities—smarter and more caring cities, for example, and Internet-enhanced communications environments. On the other hand, these technological innovations are occurring so quickly that adequate testing and assessment of their support for PWD is weak and largely ineffectual—new technologies replace older ones faster than they can be evaluated. Furthermore, earlier experiences with personal assistive devices showed that although these devices can enhance the lives of PWD, their benefits are often overestimated by the developers. The issue of ensuring adequate testing remains problematical as a result.

Finally, socioeconomic policies in relation to disability are shifting in a number of important ways. There is a growing recognition of the need to separate the provisions of social security for all citizens, which include insurance for basic costs associated with disability, from the additional and endemic costs of engaging in full participation while living with disability, costs which can be both individual but also societal. An example of the latter is the lower income typical for PWD—hence compensation for disability needs to incorporate awareness of systemic income disparities that also affect PWD. Another recent change among developed countries has been to offer more direct payment programmes in lieu of access to services, which allows PWD a choice among different service providers. The approach emphasizes the increasing autonomy available to PWD as a result of the changes under way, a net gain if nothing compromising emerges. There are fears, however, that direct payment schemes may abrogate responsibility on the part of government towards the need to construct social and physical environments that are less disabling. The call for physical environments that meet the requirements of universal design offers an example of the pressure on states to ensure full participation and citizenship.

An interesting observation that may be made is that, although developments in service provision, policy-making, and technological development are necessarily inter-related, the impacts of changes in any one area on the others are often poorly understood—for example, how does a successful new technology change service provision or policy-making? What is the relationship between the realization of the role of resiliency in service provision and the development of smart environments?

Overall, we may observe an emerging 'disability economy', driven by both social and technological innovation, but the exact form it will take is still evolving and is difficult to affirm. An important challenge to ensure social change, however, is rooted in the fact that a fundamental shift needs to occur in culture, not just the culture of disability but, in a more expansive way, the culture of 'ability'. Universal design is not aimed at designing

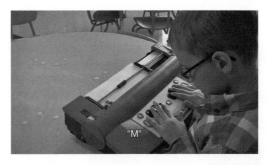

Video 33.1. Assistive Technology in Action - Meet Mason (related to section 2.1.1 Assistive Devices): In this video, you'll meet Mason, a young boy with vision loss who, with the help of assistive technologies, is able to learn reading and writing in the same classroom as his sighted peers.
(Source: http://www.youtube.com/watch?annotation_id=annotation_761049&feature=iv& src_vid=bYKUx OdUAao&v=xMHuWGUEu2M)
This video is credited by the Family Center on Technology and Disability(www.fctd.info/)

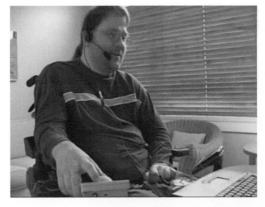

Video 33.2. Wireless Technologies for People with Disabilities (related to section 2.1.1 Assistive Devices): This video presents a number of assistive technologies that have been developed over the past years for persons with significant physical disabilities to help them with their activities of daily living. Stand-alone devices, as well as solutions that make use of commercially available technologies such as personal computers have given people more control over their home environments.
(Source: https://www.youtube.com/watch?v=J0qllstWw-M)
This video is credited and produced by The Neil Squire Society(www.neilsquire.ca/)

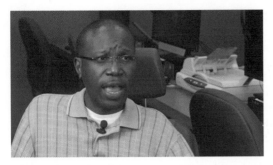

Video 33.3. FAU Assistive Technology Lab (related to section 2.1.1 Assistive Devices): This video gives a brief introduction to the many types of assistive technology, like Electronic aids for daily living (EADLs).

(Source:http://www.youtube.com/watch?v=wphcu2MuWX4)

This video is credited by the Florida Atlantic University (www.osd.fau.edu/)

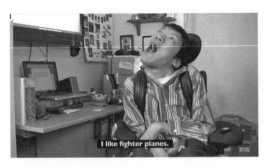

Video 33.4. Assistive Technology in Action - Meet Jared (related to section 2.1.1 Assistive Devices): In this video, you'll meet Jared, a young man with cerebral palsy who controls his computer using a sip and puff switch. That computer access allows Jared to run a business creating dynamic graphics and websites.

(Source: https://www.youtube.com/watch?v=bYKUxOdUAao)

This video is credited by the Family Center on Technology and Disability (www.fctd.info/)

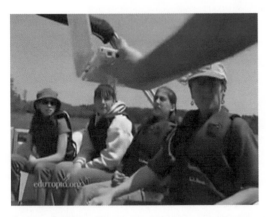

Video 33.5. Assistive Technology: Enabling Dreams (related to section 2.1.2Communication Devices): This video shows the use by disabled students of alternative augmentative communication (AAC) devices. From voice-activated software to customized laptops, tech is changing the way disabled students communicate, learn, and play.

(Source: http://www.youtube.com/watch?v=rXxdxck8Gic)

This video is credited by Edutopia (www.Edutopia.org)

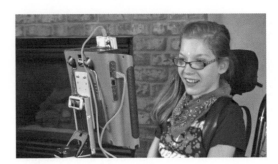

Video 33.6. Assistive Technology in Action - Meet Elle (related to section 2.1.2Communication Devices): In this video you'll meet Elle, a young woman with cerebral palsy who with the help of assistive technologies, is able to communicate with family, friends, and teachers. We invite you to view and share this video with your colleagues and the families you serve.

(Source: http://www.youtube.com/watch?v=p46F0IbYEUA)

This video is credited by the Family Center on Technology and Disability (www.fctd.info/)

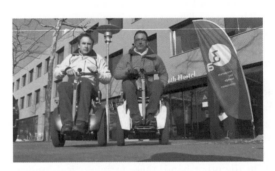

Video 33.7. Go everywhere with GENNY 2.0 (related to section 2.1.3Mobility Devices): This video shows how mobility devices can improve daily mobility for persons with disabilities.

(Source: http://www.youtube.com/watch?v=p46F0IbYEUA)

This video is credited by Genny Mobility (www.gennymobility.com/)

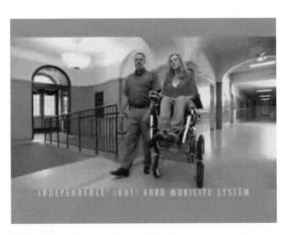

Video 33.8. iBot Robotic Wheel chair Commercial(related to section 2.1.3 Mobility Devices): This video portrays how mobility devices can improve daily mobility for persons with disabilities.

(Source: http://www.youtube.com/watch?v=O7otewMk9pc)

This video is credited by DEKA research (www.dekaresearch.com)

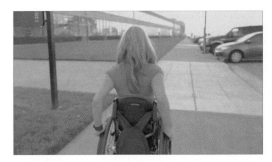

Video 33.9. Tamara Mena ~ Ekso test pilot: Believe (related to section 2.1.3 Mobility Devices): This video portrays how mobility devices can improve daily mobility for persons with disabilities.
(Source:http://spectrum.ieee.org/biomedical/bionics/goodbye-wheelchair-hello-exoskeleton)
This video is credited by Spectrum IEEE (www.spectrum.ieee.org/)

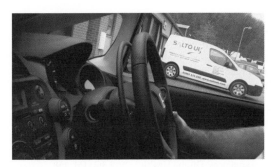

Video 33.12. Autoadapt K5 Gas under-ring - Bewick Mobility (related to section 2.2.1 Motor Vehicle Adaptation): This video shows how a car can be adapted to allow persons with disabilities to drive.
(Source: http://www.youtube.com/watch?v=nB08tJYMksg)
This video is credited by AutoAdapt (www.autoadapt.com/en/)

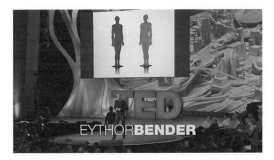

Video 33.10. Eythor Bender: Human exoskeletons - for war and healing (related to section 2.1.3 Mobility Devices): This video shows how mobility devices can improve daily mobility for persons with disabilities.
(Source: http://www.ted.com/talks/eythor_bender_demos_human_exoskeletons)

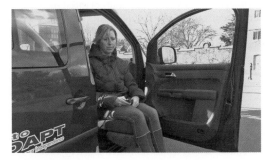

Video 33.11. TurnyEvo car seat lift (related to section 2.2.1 Motor Vehicle Adaptation): This video shows how a car can be adapted to allow persons with disabilities to drive.
(Source: http://www.youtube.com/watch?v=zvOPtV6aSTI)
This video is credited by AutoAdapt (www.autoadapt.com/en/)

environments for PWD; it is aimed at designing environments for people with all forms and levels of ability. One of largest inhibitors to this is the attitudes and understanding of the common citizen—the social representations that people maintain of each other. And social representations do not change quickly. It may take another generation before we see the true shape of the new economy.

Acknowledgements

The authors are greatly indebted of the generous contribution of Mr David Fiset, research coordinator at CIRRIS, for supporting the preparation of the manuscript and to Ms Bernadette Wilson for the English translation.

References

1. World Health Organization. World Report on Disability. World Health Organization (WHO), Geneva, 2011.
2. United Nations. Convention on the Rights of Persons with Disabilities. United Nations (UN), New York, 2006.
3. World Health Organization. International Classification of Functioning, Disability and Health (ICF). World Health Organization (WHO), Geneva, 2001.
4. Fougeyrollas P, Beauregard L. Disability: an interactive person-environment social creation. In: Albrecht G, Bury M. (eds) Handbook of Disability Studies. SAGE Publications, Inc., Thousand Oaks, CA, 2001, pp. 171–195.
5. Felicetti T. Barriers to community access: It's about more than curb cuts. The Case Manager. 2005;16(1):70–72.
6. Office des personnes handicapées du Québec. À part entière, pour un véritable exercice du droit à l'égalité des personnes handicapées. In: Office des personnes handicapées du Québec (OPHQ). Gouvernement du Québec, Drummondville, 2009.
7. The Commission on Accreditation of Rehabilitation Facilities. Medical Rehabilitation: Standards Manual. The Commission on Accreditation of Rehabilitation Facilities (CARF), Tucson, AZ, 2003.
8. Bronfenbrenner U. The ecology of human development. Harvard University Press, Cambridge MA, 1979.
9. Whiteneck G, Fougeyrollas P, Gerhart KA. Elaborating the model of disablement. In: Fuhrer MJ(ed.) Assessing Medical Rehabilitation Practices: The Promise of Outcomes Research. Paul H. Brookes Publishing Co., Baltimore, MD, 1997, pp. 91–102.

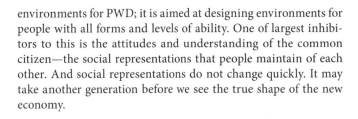

10. Iezzoni LI, O'Day BL. More than ramps: a guide to improving health care quality and access for people with disabilities. Oxford University Press, Oxford, 2006.

11. World Health Organization. The world health report 2008: primary health care now more than ever. World Health Organization (WHO), Geneva, 2008.

12. Bowers B, Esmond S, Lutz B, Jacobson N. Improving Primary Care for Persons with Disabilities: The nature of expertise. Disabil Soc. 2003;18(4):443–455.

13. Patterson BJ, Doucette WR, Lindgren SD, Chrischilles EA. Living with disability: Patterns of health problems and symptom mediation of health consequences. Disabil Health J. 2012;5(3):151–158.

14. Roach M, Frost F, Creasey G. Social and personal consequences of acquired bowel dysfunction for persons with spinal cord injury. J Spinal Cord Med. 2000;23(4):263–269.

15. Yorkston KM, Bamer A, Johnson K, Amtmann D. Satisfaction with participation in multiple sclerosis and spinal cord injury. Disabil Rehabil. 2012;34(9):747–753.

16. McColl MA, Aiken A, McColl A, Sakakibara B, Smith K. Primary care of people with spinal cord injury: Scoping review. Can Fam Physician. 2012;58(11):1207–1216.

17. Stein MA, Stein PJ, Weiss D, Lang R. Health care and the UN disability rights convention. Lancet. 2009;374(9704):1796–1798.

18. Fouts BS, Andersen E, Hagglund K. Disability and satisfaction with access to health care. J Epidemiol Community Health. 2000;54(10):770–771.

19. Iezzoni LI, Long-Bellil LM. Training physicians about caring for persons with disabilities: 'Nothing about us without us!'. Disabil Health J. 2012;5:136–139.

20. Gulley SP, Altman BM. Disability in two health care systems: access, quality, satisfaction, and physician contacts among working-age Canadians and Americans with disabilities. Disabil Health J. 2008;1:196–208.

21. Guilcher SJT, Craven BC, Lemieux-Charles L, Casciaro T, McColl MA, Jaglal SB. Secondary health conditions and spinal cord injury: an uphill battle in the journey of care. Disabil Rehabil. 2013;35(11):894–906.

22. McColl MA, Jarzynowska A, Shortt SED. Unmet health care needs of people with disabilities: population level evidence. Disabil Soc. 2010;25(2):205–218.

23. Scheer J, Kroll T, Neri MT, Beatty P. Access barriers for persons with disabilities: the consumer's perspective. J Disabil Policy Studies. 2003;13(4):221–230.

24. Mudrick NR, Breslin ML, Liang M, Yee S. Physical accessibility in primary health care settings: Results from California on-site reviews. Disabil Health J. 2012;5(3):159–167.

25. Pharr J. Accessible medical equipment for patients with disabilities in primary care clinics: Why is it lacking? Disabil Health J. 2013;6(2):124–132.

26. Pharr J, Chino M. Predicting barriers to primary care for patients with disabilities: A mixed methods study of practice administrators. Disabil Health J. 2013;6(2):116–123.

27. Smith DL. Disparities in patient-physician communication for persons with a disability from the 2006 Medical Expenditure Panel Survey (MEPS). Disabil Health J 2009;2(206–215).

28. Morrison EH, George V, Mosqueda L. Primary care for adults with physical disabilities: perceptions from consumer and provider focus groups. Fam Med. 2008;40(9):645–651.

29. Story MF, Kailes JI, Donald CM. The ADA in action at health care facilities. Disabil Health J. 2010;3(4):245–252.

30. Kroll T, Neri M. Experiences with care co-ordination among people with cerebral palsy, multiple sclerosis, or spinal cord injury. Disabil Rehabil. 2003;25(19):1106–1114.

31. Iezzoni LI, Frakt AB, Pizer SD. Uninsured persons with disability confront substantial barriers to health care services. Disabil Health J. 2011;4(4):238–244.

32. Carmona R, Giannini M, Bergmark B, Cabe J. The Surgeon General's Call to Action to Improve the Health and Wellness of Persons with Disabilities: historical review, rationale, and implications 5 years after publication. Disabil Health J. 2010;3(4):229–232.

33. McColl MA, Shortt S, Godwin M, et al. Models for Integrating Rehabilitation and Primary Care: A Scoping Study. Arch Phys Med Rehabil. 2009;90(9):1523–1531.

34. Actionable Nuggets. Welcome to ACTIONABLE NUGGETS web-based support. Kingston, Ontario: Actionable Nuggets; 2013. Available from: http://www.actionnuggets.ca/ (accesswed 20 August 2014).

35. Madden R, Ferreira M, Einfeld S, et al. New directions in health care and disability: the need for a shared understanding of human functioning. Aust N Z J Public Health. 2012;36(5):458–461.

36. DeJong G. Independent living: from social movement to analytic paradigm. Arch Phys Med Rehabil. 1979;60(10):435–446.

37. Stone R, Newcomer R. Advances and issues in personal care. Clin Geriatr Med. 2009;25(1):35–45.

38. Lord J, Hutchison P. Individualised support and funding: building blocks for capacity building and inclusion. Disabil Soc. 2003;18(1):71–86.

39. Waterplas L, Samoy E. L'allocation personnalisée: le cas de la Suède, du Royaume-Uni, Des Pays-Bas et de la Belgique. Revue Française des affaires sociales. 2005;59 (2):61–101.

40. Boucher N. Le dispositif de soutien à domicile des personnes ayant des incapacités, un facteur d'exclusion? In: Gagnon É, Pelchat Y, Édouard E (eds) Politiques d'intégration, rapports d'exclusion Action publique et justice sociale. Presses de l'Université du Québec, Québec, 2008, pp. 331–348.

41. Ridley J, Jones LYN. Direct what? The untapped potential of direct payments to mental health service users. Disabil Soc. 2003;18(5):643–658.

42. Spandler H, Vick N. Opportunities for independent living using direct payments in mental health. Health Social Care Community. 2006;14(2):107–115.

43. Hutchison P, Pedlar A, Dunn P, Lord J, Arai S. Canadian Independent Living Centres: impact on the community. Int J Rehabil Res. 2000;23(11):61–74.

44. Stainton T, Boyce S. 'I have got my life back': users' experience of direct payments. Disabil Soc. 2004;19(5):443–454.

45. Carmichael A, Brown L. The future challenge for direct payments. Disabil Soc. 2002;17(7):797–808.

46. Duffy S. Individual budgets: transforming the allocation of resources for care. J Integrated Care. 2005;13(1):8–16.

47. Pearson C. Keeping the cash under control: whats the problem with direct payments in Scotland? Disabil Soc. 2004;19(1):3–14.

48. Turnbull AP, Turnbull HR, Erwin E, Soodak L. Families, professionals, and exceptionality. Merrill/Prentice Hall, Englewood Cliffs, NJ, 1986.

49. Heiman T. Parents of Children with disabilities: resilience, coping, and future expectations. J Dev Phys Disabil. 2002;14(2):159–171.

50. Tétreault S, Blais-Michaud S, Marier Deschênes P, Beaupré P, Gascon H, Boucher N, Carrière M. How to support families of children with disabilities? An exploratory study of social support services. Child & Family Social Work. 2014;19 :272–281.

51. Jourdan-Ionescu C. Intervention écosystémique individualisée axée sur la résilience. Revue québecoise de psychologie. 2001; 22(1): 163–183.

52. Rutter M. Psychsocial resilience and protective mechanisms. Am J Orthopsychiatry. 1987;57(3):316–331.

53. Ionescu S. Traité de resilience assistée. Presses Universitaires de France, Paris, 2011.

54. McCubbin HI, McCubbin MA. Typologies of resilient families: emerging roles of social class and ethnicity. Family Relations. 1988;37(3):247–254.

55. Patterson JM. Understanding family resilience. J Clin Psychol. 2002;58(3):233–246.

56. Norwich B. Education, inclusion and individual differences: recognising and resolving dilemmas. Br J Educ Studies. 2002; 50(4):482–502.

57. Boschen KA, Tonack M, Gargaro J. Long-term adjustment and community reintegration following spinal cord injury. Int J Rehabil Res. 2003;26(3):157–164.

58. Charlifue S, Gerhart K. Community integration in spinal cord injury of long duration. NeuroRehabilitation. 2004;19(2):91–101.

59. King GA, Baldwin PJ, Currie M, Evans J. Planning successful transitions from school to adult roles for youth with disabilities. Children's Health Care. 2005;34(3):193–216.

60. Krause JS. Years to employment after spinal cord injury. Arch Phys Med Rehabil. 2003;84(9):1282–1289.

61. Neubert D. The role of assessment in the transition to adult life process for students with disabilities. Exceptionality. 2003;11(2):63–75.

62. Stewart D, Law M, Jaffer S. Transition to adulthood for youth with complex needs and their families. CanChild Centre for Childhood Disability Research, Ontario, 2005.

63. Fougeyrollas P. La funambule, le fil et la toile: transformations réciproques du sens du handicap. Presses de l'Université Laval, Québec, 2010. 338 p.

64. Rigby P, Ryan SE, Campbell KA. Electronic aids to daily living and quality of life for persons with tetraplegia. Disabil Rehabil Assistive Technol. 2011;6(3):260–267.

65. Verdonck MC, Chard G, Nolan M. Electronic aids to daily living: be able to do what you want. Disabil Rehabil Assistive Technol. 2011;6(3):268–281.

66. Gentry T, Wallace J, Kvarfordt C, Lynch KB. Personal digital assistants as cognitive aids for individuals with severe traumatic brain injury: A community-based trial. Brain Inj. 2008;22(1):19–24.

67. Lemoncello R, Sohlberg MM, Fickas S, Prideaux J. A randomised controlled crossover trial evaluating Television Assisted Prompting (TAP) for adults with acquired brain injury. Neuropsychol Rehabil. 2011;21(6):825–846.

68. Lindqvist E, Borell L. The match between experienced difficulties in everyday activities after stroke and assistive technology for cognitive support. Technol Disabil. 2010;22(3):89–98.

69. Copolillo A, Ivanoff SD. Assistive technology and home modification for people with neurovisual deficits. NeuroRehabilitation. 2011;28(3):211–220.

70. Levinson R. The Planning and Execution Assistant and Trainer (PEAT). J Head Trauma Rehabil. 1997;12(2):85–91.

71. Mann WC. Smart technology for aging, disability, and independence: The state of the science. Wiley-Interscience, New York, 2005.

72. Lancioni G, Singh N, O'Reilly M, et al. Using an optic sensor and a scanning keyboard emulator to facilitate writing by persons with pervasive motor disabilities. J Dev Phys Disabil. 2007;19(6):593–603.

73. Matter B, Feinberg M, Schomer K, Harniss M, Brown P, Johnson K. Information needs of people with spinal cord injuries. J Spinal Cord Med. 2009; 32(5):545–554.

74. Lancioni GE, O'Reilly MF, Singh NN, Oliva D, Buonocunto F, Belardinelli MO. Technology-assisted writing opportunities for a man emerged from a minimally conscious state and affected by extensive motor disabilities. Dev Neurorehabil. 2011;14(2):123–127.

75. Lancioni GE, Singh NN, O'Reilly MF, et al. Promoting adaptive behavior in persons with acquired brain injury, extensive motor and communication disabilities, and consciousness disorders. Res Dev Disabil. 2012;33(6):1964–1974.

76. Smith MM, Connolly I. Roles of aided communication: perspectives of adults who use AAC. Disabil Rehabil Assistive Technol. 2008; 3(5):260–273.

77. Wallace T, Bradshaw A. Technologies and strategies for people with communication problems following brain injury or stroke. NeuroRehabilitation. 2011;28(3):199–209.

78. LaPlante MP, Kaye HS. Demographics and trends in wheeled mobility equipment use and accessibility in the community. Assistive Technol. 2010;22(1):3–17.

79. Cooper RA, Cooper R. Quality-of-life technology for people with spinal cord injuries. Phys Med Rehabil Clin N Am. 2010; 21(1):1–13.

80. Hillier SL, Sharpe MH, Metzer J. Outcomes 5 years post-traumatic brain injury (with further reference to neurophysical impairment and disability). Brain Inj. 1997;11(9):661–675.

81. Souza A, Kelleher A, Cooper R, Cooper RA, Iezzoni LI, Collins DM. Multiple sclerosis and mobility-related assistive technology: systematic review of literature. J Rehabil Res Dev. 2010;47:213–223.

82. Rodby-Bousquet E, Hagglund G. Use of manual and powered wheelchair in children with cerebral palsy: a cross-sectional study. BMC Pediatr. 2010;10(1):59–66.

83. Mutch W, Dingwall-Fordyce I, Downie AW, Paterson JG, Roy SK. Parkinson's disease in a Scottish city. Br Med J. 1986; 292 534–536.

84. Noreau L, Fougeyrollas P. Long-term consequences of spinal cord injury on social participation: the occurrence of handicap situations. Disabil Rehabil. 2000;22(4):170–180.

85. Post MW, van Asbeck FW, van Dijk AJ, Schrijvers AJ. Services for spinal cord injured: availability and satisfaction. Nature Publishing Group, London, 1997.

86. Salminen AL, Brandt A, Samuelsson K, Töytäri O, Malmivaara A. Mobility devices to promote activity and participation: a systematic review. J Rehabil Med. 2009; 41(9):697–706.

87. Löfqvist C, Pettersson C, Iwarsson S, Brandt A. Mobility and mobility-related participation outcomes of powered wheelchair and scooter interventions after 4-months and 1-year use. Disabil Rehabil Assistive Technol. 2012; 7(3):211–218.

88. Auger C, Demers L, Gélinas I, Miller WC, Jutai JW, Noreau L. Life-space mobility of middle-aged and older adults at various stages of usage of power mobility devices. Arch Phys Med Rehabil. 2010; 91(5):765–773.

89. Davies A, De Souza LH, Frank AO. Changes in the quality of life in severely disabled people following provision of powered indoor/outdoor chairs. Disabil Rehabil. 2003;25(6):286–290.

90. Rousseau-Harrison K, Rochette A, Routhier F, Dessureault D, Thibault F, Côté O. Impact of wheelchair acquisition on social participation. Disabil Rehabil Assistive Technol. 2009;4(5):344–352.

91. Barker DJ, Reid D, Cott C. The experience of senior stroke survivors: factors in community participation among wheelchair users. Can J Occup Ther. 2006;73(1):18–25.

92. Rousseau-Harrison K, Rochette A, Routhier F, Dessureault D, Thibault F, Côté O. Perceived impacts of a first wheelchair on social participation. Disabil Rehabil Assistive Technol. 2012;7(1):37–44.

93. Mortenson WB, Demers L, Fuhrer M, J,, Jutai JW, Lenker J, DeRuyter F. How assistive technology use by individuals with disabilities impacts their caregivers: a systematic review of the research evidence. Am J Phys Med Rehabil 2012;91:984–998.

94. Seitz AL, McClure PW, Finucane S, Boardman Iii ND, Michener LA. Mechanisms of rotator cuff tendinopathy: Intrinsic, extrinsic, or both? Clin Biomech. 2011;26(1):1–12.

95. Yang J, Boninger ML, Leath JD, Fitzgerald SG, Dyson-Hudson TA, Chang MW. Carpal tunnel syndrome in manual wheelchair users with spinal cord injury: a cross-sectional multicenter study. Am J Phys Med Rehabil. 2009;88(1007–1016).

96. Chaves ES, Boninger ML, Cooper R, Fitzgerald SG, Gray DB, Cooper RA. Assessing the influence of wheelchair technology on perception of participation in spinal cord injury. Arch Phys Med Rehabil. 2004;85(11):1854–1858.

97. Nisbet PD. Assessment and training of children for powered mobility in the UK. Technol Disabil. 2002;14(4):173–182.

98. Tefft D, Guerette P, Furumasu J. The impact of early powered mobility on parental stress, negative emotions, and family social interactions. Phys Occupat Ther Pediatr. 2011;31(1):4–15.

99. Guerette P, Furumasu J, Tefft D. The positive effects of early powered mobility on children's psychosocial and play skills. Assist Technol. 2013; 25(1):39–48.

100. Cooper RA, Boninger ML, Cooper R, et al. Use of the Independence 3000 IBOT Transporter at home and in the community. J Spinal Cord Med. 2003; 26(1):79–85.

101. Cooper RA, Boninger ML, Cooper R, Fitzgerald SG, Kellerher A. Preliminary assessment of a prototype advanced mobility device in the work environment of veterans with spinal cord injury. NeuroRehabilitation. 2004; 19(2):161–170.

102. Uustal H, Minkel JL. Study of the independence IBOT 3000 mobility system: An innovative power mobility device, during use in community environments. Arch Phys Med Rehabil. 2004;**85**(12):2002–2010.

103. Arthanat S, Desmarais JM, Eikelberg P. Consumer perspectives on the usability and value of the iBOT® wheelchair: findings from a case series. Disabil Rehabil Assistive Technol. 2012; **7**(2):153–167.

104. Laffont I, Guillon B, Fermanian C, et al. Evaluation of a stair-climbing power wheelchair in 25 people with tetraplegia. Arch Phys Med Rehabil. 2008;**89**(10):1958–1964.

105. Esquenazi A, Talaty M, Packel A, Saulino M. The ReWalk powered exoskeleton to restore ambulatory function to individuals with thoracic-level motor-complete spinal cord injury. Am J Phys Med Rehabil. 2012; **91**(11):911–921.

106. Quintero HA, Farris RJ, Goldfarb M, editors. Control and implementation of a powered lower limb orthosis to aid walking in paraplegic individuals. Rehabilitation Robotics (ICORR), 2011 IEEE International Conference,2011 June 29–July 1.

107. Silver J, Ljungberg I, Libin A, Groah S. Barriers for individuals with spinal cord injury returning to the community: A preliminary classification. Disabil Health J. 2012; **5**(3):190–196.

108. Babirad J. Chapter 21. Driver evaluation and vehicle modification. In: Olson DA, DeRuyter F (eds). Clinician's Guide to Assistive Technology. St Louis, Mosby, 2002, pp. 351–376.

109. Nead R. Chapter 2—Driver retraining and adaptive equipment. In: Schultheis MT, DeLuca J, Chute DL (eds). Handbook for the Assessment of Driving Capacity. Elsevier, Oxford, 2009, pp. 21–34.

110. Ellis RD, Talbot GL. Chapter 16. Universal design and the automobile. In: Pellerito JM (ed.). Driver Rehabilitation and Community Mobility. Mosby, St Louis, 2006, pp. 345–355.

111. van Roosmalen L, Paquin GJ, Steinfeld AM. Quality of life technology: the state of personal transportation. Phys Med Rehabil Clin N Am. 2010; **21**(1):111–125.

112. Hunter-Zaworski K, Nead R. Chapter 21—Transportation, driving, and community access. In: Sisto SA, Druin E, Sliwinski MM (eds) Spinal Cord Injuries Management and Rehabilitation. Elsevier, Oxford, 2009, pp. 495–518.

113. RESNA. Section 20: Wheelchair seating systems for use in motor vehicles-draft. In: American National Standards Institute (ANSI)/ Rehabilitation Engineering Society of North America (RESNA), editor. RESNA WC-4. Arlington, VA, 2009.

114. Dewsbury G, Linskell J. Smart home technology for safety and functional independence: The UK experience. NeuroRehabilitation. 2011;**28**(3):249–260.

115. Bierhoff I, van Berlo A, Abascal J, et al. Chapter 3. Smart home environment. In: Roe PRW (ed.) Towards an Inclusive Future Impact and Wider Potential of Information and Communication Technologies. COST, Brussels, 2007,p p. 110–156.

116. Aldrich F. Smart homes: past, present and future. In: Harper R(ed.) Inside the Smart Home: Springer, London, 2003,p p. 17–39.

117. Mann WC, Milton BR. Home automation and smart homes to support independence. In: Mann WC (ed.) Smart Technology for Aging, Disability, and Independence. John Wiley & Sons Inc., New York, 2005, pp. 32–66.

118. Orpwood R. The Gloucester smart house. J Dementia Care. 2001; **9**:28–31.

119. Martin S, Beamish E. Evaluation of Ardkeen Supported Living Option. Belfast: Social Research Centre, University of Ulster, 2008.

120. Helal A, Abdulrazak B. TeCaRob: Tele-care using telepresence and robotic technology for assisting people with special needs. Int J ARM. 2006;7(3):46–53.

121. Swann J. Equipment and adaptations for helping stroke survivors. NursResidential Care. 2006;8(3):126–129.

122. Sorell T, Draper H. Telecare, surveillance, and the Welfare State. Am J Bioethics. 2012;**12**(9):36–44.

123. Kadouche R, Abdulrazak B, Giroux S, Mokhtari M. Disability centered approach in smart space management. Int J Smart Home. 2009;**3**(2):13–26.

124. Wongpatikaseree K, Ikeda, M, Buranarach M, Supnithi T, Lim AO, Tan Y. (eds) Activity recognition using context-aware infrastructure ontology in smart home domain. Seventh International Conference on Knowledge, Information and Creativity Support Systems (KICSS), 2012.

125. Doukas C, Metsis V, Becker E, Le Z, Makedon F, Maglogiannis I. Digital cities of the future: Extending @home assistive technologies for the elderly and the disabled. Telematics and Informatics. 2011;**28**(3):176–190.

126. Macagnano E, (ed). Intelligent urban environments: towards e-inclusion of the disabled and the aged in the design of a sustainable city of the future. A South African example. 5th International Conference on Urban Regeneration and Sustainability: Sustainable City, 2008 24–26 September, Skiathos, Greece.

127. Lim S, Chung L, Han O, Kim J-H. (eds) An interactive cyber-physical system (CPS) for people with disability and frail elderly people. 5th International Conference on Ubiquitous Information Management and Communication (ICUIMC '11), 2011, New York, NY, USA.

128. LeRouge C, Gaynor, M, Chien-Ching L, Ma AJ. Multi-level technical infrastructure for diabetes chronic care management in China. 43rd Hawaii International Conference on System Sciences (HICSS), 2010, pp. 1–10.

129. Cook DJ, Youngblood GM, Jain G. Algorithms for Smart Spaces. The Engineering Handbook of Smart Technology for Aging, Disability, and Independence: John Wiley & Sons Inc., New York, 2008, pp. 767–783.

130. Park S, Jayaraman S. Smart textiles: a platform for sensing and personalized mobile information-processing. J Textile Institute. 2003;**94**(3–4):87–98.

131. Helal AA, Mokhtari M, Abdulrazak B. The engineering handbook of smart technology for aging, disability, and independence: John Wiley & Sons, Computer Engineering Series, 2008. Available from http://ca.wiley.com/WileyCDA/WileyTitle/productCd-0471711551.html (accessed 30 September 2014).

132. Campin S. Brisbane—towards a learning city and a city of learning communities. International Conference on Engaging Communities, 14–17 August, Brisbane, Australia, 2005.

133. Ellis K, Kent, M. Disability and New Media. Taylor & Francis, London, 2010.

134. Bessey M, Kelly S. The Impact of Technology on the Homeless. 2011. Available from http://superawesomegood.com/wp-content/uploads/2012/02/ImpactofTechnologyontheHomeless.pdf (accessed 20 August 2014).

135. Christopherson KM. The positive and negative implications of anonymity in Internet social interactions: 'On the internet, nobody knows you're a dog'. Computers in Human Behavior. 2007; **23**(6):3038–3056.

136. Grimaldi C, Goette T. The Internet and the independence of individuals with disabilities. Internet Research. 1999;9(4):272–280.

137. Carey AC, Potts BB, Bryen DN, Shankar J. Networking towards employment: experiences of people who use augmentative and alternative communication. Research and Practice for Persons with Severe Disabilities. 2004;**29**(1):40–52.

138. Ritchie H, Blanck P. The promise of the Internet for disability: a study of on-line services and web site accessibility at Centers for Independent Living. Behavioral Sciences & the Law. 2003; **21**(1):5–26.

139. Benford P, Standen P. The internet: a comfortable communication medium for people with Asperger syndrome (AS) and high functioning autism (HFA)? J Assist Technol. 2009; **3**(2):44–53.

140. Zubal-Ruggieri R. Making links, making connections: internet resources for self-advocates and people with developmental disabilities. Intellectual and Developmental Disabilities. 2007; **45**(3):209–215.

141. Tosh D, Werdmuller B. Creation of a learning landscape: weblogging and social networking in the context of e-portfolios. 2004. Available from: http://benwerd.com/wp-content/uploads/2012/07/learning-landscape.pdf (accessed 20 August 2014).

142. Ahmed OH, Sullivan SJ, Schneiders AG, Mccrory P. iSupport: do social networking sites have a role to play in concussion awareness? Disabil Rehabil. 2010; **32**(22):1877–1883.

143. Suler J. The online disinhibition effect. CyberPsychology & Behavior. 2004;7:321–326.
144. McClimens A, Gordon F. People with intellectual disabilities as bloggers: What's social capital got to do with it anyway? J Intellect Disabil. 2009;13(1):19–30.
145. Stendal K, Balandin S, Molka-Danielsen J. Virtual worlds: A new opportunity for people with lifelong disability? J Intellect Dev Disabil. 2011;36(1):80–83.
146. Hollier SE. The Disability Divide: A study into the impact of computing and internet-related technologies on people who are blind or vision impaired. PhD Thesis, Curtin University of Technology, Perth, Autralia, 2007. Available from http://digitalcommons.ilr.cornell.edu/gladnetcollect/340/?utm_source=digitalcommons.ilr.cornell.edu%2Fgladnetcollect%2F340&utm_medium=PDF&utm_campaign=PDFCoverPages (accessed 30 September 2014).
147. McColl M, Jongbloed L. Disability and social policy in Canada. Jongbloed M-aML, editor. Captus University Publications, Toronto, 2006.
148. Prince MJ. Absent citizens: Disability politics and policy in Canada: Cambridge University Press, Cambridge, 2009.
149. Grover C, Piggott L. Disability and social (in)security: emotions, contradictions of 'inclusion' and employment and support allowance. Social Policy and Society. 2013;12(03):369–380.
150. Bromley RDF, Matthews DL, Thomas CJ. City centre accessibility for wheelchair users: The consumer perspective and the planning implications. Cities. 2007;24(3):229–241.
151. Imrie R. Disability and discourses of mobility and movement. Env Planning A. 2000;32(9):1641–1656.
152. Cohu S, Lequet-Slama D, Velche D. Les politiques en faveur des personnes handicapées dans cinq pays européens. Grandes tendances. Revue française des affaires sociales. 2005;2(2):9–33.

CHAPTER 34

Virtual reality for neurorehabilitation

Robert Riener

Introduction

What is virtual reality?

The term 'virtual reality' (VR) was popularized in the late 1980s by Jaron Lanier, one of the pioneers of the field. At the same time, also the term 'artificial reality' came up. The Encyclopaedia Britannica describes VR as 'the use of computer modelling and simulation that enables a person to interact with an artificial three-dimensional (3D) visual or other sensory environment' [1]. Furthermore, it states that 'VR applications immerse the user in a computer-generated environment that simulates reality through the use of interactive devices, which send and receive information and are worn as goggles, headsets, gloves, or body suits' [1]. For example, a user wearing a head-mounted display with a stereoscopic projection system can view animated images of a virtual environment. The immersion is enhanced by the use of motion sensors that pick up the user's movements and adjust the view on the visual display in real-time accordingly; the user can even pick up and manipulate virtual objects that she or he sees through the visual display, and also wearing data gloves that are equipped with joint angular position sensors, or even with force-feedback modules that provide the sensation of touch [1]. Thus, VR usually refers to a technology designed to provide interaction between user and artificially generated environments. This interaction is supposed to be more natural, direct, or real than pure simulation technologies delivering only numerical or simple graphical outcomes.

There are further terms, especially applied in the area of rehabilitation, that refer to VR applications, such as 'feedback', 'biofeedback' and 'augmented feedback'. Feedback allows patients to evaluate their movement success as well as detect potential movement errors [2, 3]. Concepts that are mostly being deployed are, for example, verbal feedback and mirrors placed in front of the patients, giving visual and/or acoustic feedback [4]. Other approaches include biofeedback—processes that monitor a patient's performance using physiological measurements [5]. With the advent of modern media technologies, also the technology of 'augmented feedback' has nowadays become increasingly popular [6, 7]. Augmented feedback can be defined as 'the provision of supplementary sensory information (visual, auditory, or haptic) brought by technological means, which would not normally be present in the usual environment' [8]. A good overview of VR technologies applied to medicine has been presented by Riener and Harders [9]. That source serves as a basis for some of the chapters and text passages of this article.

Principle of virtual reality

Main components

VR comprises two main components: the user environment and the virtual environment (Figure 34.1) [9]. While the user interacts with the VR system, the two environments communicate and exchange information through a barrier called interface. The interface can be considered as a translator between the user and the VR system. When the user applies input actions (e.g. motion, force generation, speech, etc.), the interface translates these actions into digital signals, which can be processed and interpreted by the system. On the other hand, the system's computed reactions are also translated by the interface into physical quantities, which the user can perceive through the use of different display and actuator technologies (e.g. images, sounds, feeling of touch, etc.). Finally, the user interprets this information and reacts to the system accordingly.

Importance of multi-modality

In VR applications, the exchange of different physical quantities between the user and the virtual environment occurs via different channels, also called modalities. Such modalities can be sound, vision, or touch. Communicating with multiple modalities is called multimodal interaction. Multimodal interaction allows several types of modalities to be simultaneously exchanged between the user and the virtual environment. The goal of applying multimodal interaction is to provide a complete and realistic image of the situation, to give redundant information (e.g. for safety reasons), to increase the quality of presence, and to provide a more intensive stimulation of the human neurophysiological system, when applied to rehabilitation.

Problems of the use of VR

Increasing use of VR also turned up some problems due to the technology. Sometimes users experience so-called cybersickness [10, 9] with symptoms of nausea, dizziness, eye-strain, headache, disorientation, or vomiting. Of course, the level of sickness depends on the susceptibility of the user. Symptoms can appear during the exposure to the VR and last for hours after the exposure. Technical issues may be main origins for cybersickness. For example, a 15 ms lag in a head-mounted display can already induce cybersickness in the user.

Rationale for the use of virtual reality in rehabilitation

Rehabilitation has the goal to restore previously lost movement capabilities, to learn compensatory movements or to treat

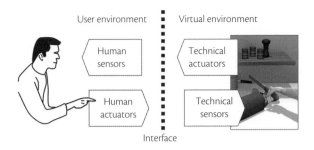

Fig. 34.1 Bidirectional exchange of information in VR systems.
Riener R, Harders M. Virtual reality in medicine. Springer; 2012. [9]).

cognitive and psychological deficits that enable subjects to cope with daily life and, thus, increase quality of life [9]. VR technologies in rehabilitation are thereby mostly employed in physiotherapy, occupational therapy, and psychotherapy. Applications in physiotherapy and occupational therapy usually consist of methods to recover limb functionality after disease or accident. In psychotherapy, VR is mostly used to treat phobias or stress diseases or trauma. VR technologies can also be applied to provide feedback as assistance during activities of daily living (ADL).

The three key concepts of physiological rehabilitation are *repetition* of the movement that needs to be rehabilitated, *active participation* of the patient, and *performance feedback*. Movement repetition is important both for motor learning and the corresponding cortical changes [11]. Active participation in gait training was shown to increase therapy outcome [12]. The same is true for the rehabilitation of the upper extremities, when stroke patients are forced to use their paretic arm due to constraint induced movement therapy (CIMT) [13]. The repeated practice must also be linked to incremental success at some task or goal. In the intact nervous system, this is achieved by trial and error practice, with feedback about the performance success provided by the senses (e.g. vision, audition, proprioception).

VR is a powerful tool to motivate the participants to active participation, while providing augmented performance feedback. VR in rehabilitation provides motivating training that can be superior to training in a real situation [7]. It was shown that increased motivation and active participation can lead to increased efficiency and advancements of motor learning in neurorehabilitation [14, 15]. Enriched environments, highly functional and task-oriented practice environments were shown to be necessary for motor re-learning and recovery after stroke [15].

There are different factors influencing the motivation of a subject using VR technologies. First, the VR task should show functionally meaningful reactions to the motor performance of the patient to increase motivation [16]. Another factor influencing the motivation is the kind of reward provided in order to keep the patient always engaged and interested [17, 18]. Last but not least, motivation can also be affected by the difficulty level of the VR exercise. Best results have been obtained when the difficulty is adapted to the motor and cognitive capabilities of the patient [19, 20, 21, 22].

Besides the aspects of improving active participation through motivation, VR allows testing of different methods of motor training, types of feedback provided, and different practice schedules for comparative effectiveness in improving motor function in patients. VR technology does not replace the real environment, but it provides a convenient tool for manipulating these factors, setting up automatic training schedules and for training, testing, and recording participants' motor responses. The VR environment settings, choice of tasks, and level of difficulty can be easily and gradually adjusted to the human subject with respect to motor abilities, cognitive abilities, interests, age, etc.

Another advantage for using VR technologies in neurorehabilitation is that it automatically provides context specific instructions. Just by seeing the virtual environment can stimulate and invite the patient to get active just by intuition, without any further oral explanations given by the therapist. For instance, a virtual path in the nature, with a virtual ball lying on the ground, may stimulate the user to walk to the ball and shoot it away; or a table with a virtual bottle and an empty glass invites the subject to grasp the bottle and fill the glass. Furthermore, VR can be a good solution for training of dangerous tasks, which may be too difficult to train for in the real setting, such as special gait-related tasks (risk of falling) or use of edgy and sharp tools for different manipulative tasks (risk of arm/face injuries).

Technical prerequisites

Recording technologies

A human operator presents actions to the VR system in various forms, for instance, as positions and movements, forces and torques, speech and sounds as well as physiological quantities (see Figure 34.2, Table 34.1), which need to be measured by recording technologies and fed as input modality into the virtual environment [9]. The choice of method or device to measure such information depends on the physical properties of the information to be transferred and the range of the signal to be measured.

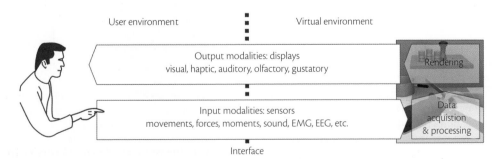

Fig. 34.2 Multimodal, bidirectional interaction between the user and the virtual environment.
Riener R, Harders M. Virtual reality in medicine. Springer; 2012. [9]).

Table 34.1 Examples of different input modalities and recording technologies, see also [9]

Physiological function	Information transferred	Physical quantities	Measurement device examples
Voice, speech	Sound, acoustics, words, commands	Sound pressure, frequency	Microphone
Muscle activities, segmental kinematics and kinetics	Posture and body motion; mechanical load	Position, velocity, angle, acceleration; force, moment	Joystick, goniometer, accelerometer
Physiological functions	Cardiovascular state, thoughts, well-being	Heart rate, temperature, electrophysiological quantities	Thermometer, electromyogram (EMG), electroencephalogram (EEG), pulse oximeter

Recording of positions and movements

For many VR applications it is required to measure positions and movements of body segments or objects used by the human operator [9]. Measurement of positions and movements can be based on resistive, capacitive, inductive, ultrasound, or optical sensing principles. The position and movement measuring systems can be classified into three categories depending on structure and design. These are desktop systems, body-mounted systems, and contact-free systems. Desktop systems are designed for being used on a desk. Such devices are standard computer mice or game joysticks. More complex joystick-type devices exist that allow rendering of several degrees of freedom, for example in spatial (3D) range. Body-mounted sensing systems are usually used to measure the posture or movement of the human. The equipment needs to be attached to the body of the subject (Figure 34.3). Examples are goniometers, gyroscopes, accelerometers, and inclinometers in order to measure angles, velocity, or acceleration, respectively. Inertial sensors, such as accelerometers and gyroscopes, are used to measure motion and orientation. Inertial sensors are widely applied in head-mounted displays to track the angular motion of the user's head. Goniometers are used to measure joint angles. Many versions are based on resistive measurement principles using potentiometers. Contact-free systems (remote systems) can capture the position and motion of the body in space without mechanical contacts between the subject and the sensing unit [23]. This type of sensing system is often preferable since it gives a large scope and the users are normally not encumbered by wires and bulky components. Several systems are based on optical, acoustic, or magnetic measuring principles [24]. Most common are passive optical systems, commercially available by companies such as Qualysis AB, Gothenburg, Sweden, or Vicon Motion Systems Limited, Oxford, UK. Eye-tracking systems are used to detect and record the positions and movements of one or both eyes of the viewer while looking at any real or virtual object, for example on a screen [25].

Recording of forces and torques

Sensing user interaction forces and torques is important, especially for force feedback controllers implemented in haptic devices and robots. Forces and torques are usually measured by resistive (strain gauges), piecoelectric, capacitive, and optical methods. They can be recorded by desktop systems (e.g. joysticks or computer mice with force feedback), lab-mounted systems (e.g. ground reaction platforms, instrumented holds, and bars) or by body-mounted systems (e.g. pressure-measuring insoles).

Recording of sound

There is a large variety of sound and speech recording systems available. They differ from each other in terms of their setup (mounted on a desk, a wall, or the user's head), their connection (with wires or wireless), the number of recording channels (mono, stereo, or array of microphones) [26], and the processing technology (e.g. sound detections or speech analysis) [27].

Recording of physiological signals

Physiological signals, representing activities of the peripheral and autonomous nervous system, can also be used as input modality for VR systems, for example, to detect if the user of any VR scenarios gets emotionally involved or even stressed. Measurable quantities are, for example, muscle activity, faze, pupil size, nerve signals, cardiovascular signals (heart rate, blood pressure), metabolic signals (blood gas concentration), respiration variables, body temperature, and skin conductance [28, 29].

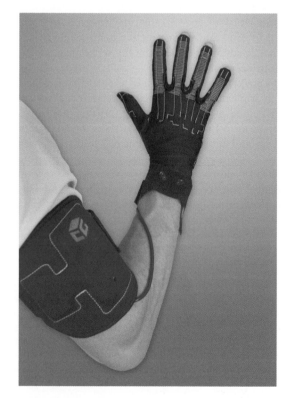

Fig. 34.3 CyberGlove III, including 18 to 20 sensors.
With kind permission of CyblerGlove Systems LLC.

Display technologies

Visual displays

Various hardwares exist for the visual display of computer-generated images. Presentation of 2D pictures can be performed by simple computer monitors or projection systems. For stereo rendering of graphical information different methods have been developed to present the correct stereo image to the respective eye [9].

One method is to encode the images for the respective eyes via light polarization. Filters are employed to distinctly polarize the left- and right-eye stereo image. Users apply glasses with corresponding polarization filters, thus, letting only the appropriately polarized images pass each filter. This display strategy can be implemented by using two projectors equipped with rotated linear polarizers. The rendered images are projected simultaneously onto the same surface. Passive stereo glasses are worn, which contain matching rotated linear polarizers. Instead of polarization, also different colours (red/green, blue/green or only slightly shifted colours) can be used to distinguish the right and left image. Furthermore, stereoscopic images can be generated by head-mounted displays, or autostereoscopic screens, which do not require any glasses worn by the user.

There different levels of immersion are encountered with the use of different graphical display systems. The simplest solutions are desktop systems, based on standard computer screens. A straightforward extension of desktop VR is the enlargement of the display area. This widens the provided field of view, thus, increasing the sense of immersion. Moreover, additional users can participate in the viewing of the presented VR content [30]. The most immersive graphical display systems are those, where the user is placed inside of a virtual world, while blocking out cues from the real environment in order to obtain a sense of presence—the feeling of actually being in the simulated environment. Two key examples in this category are cave-like setups and head-mounted displays. In the former a user stands inside a small room, whose walls are used as projection surfaces. The virtual world is displayed on the latter via rear-projection [31]. In the second immersive display type, a head-mounted setup is worn, which houses small screens in front of the eyes [32]. By tracking head movements of a user, the views of the virtual world are updated according to the changes in viewing position and orientation. However, head-mounted displays are often too heavy and uncomfortable for prolonged usage.

Auditory displays

There are many different techniques for generating sound in a virtual environment with the purpose of providing a realistic impression or to provide instructions or warnings. Auditory signals can be generated by headphones or loudspeakers. Headphones are the simplest solution for displaying sound to the VR user. They are often used together with head-mounted displays. Headphones can produce stereo sound and they can suppress noise from the surrounding environment. However, as in the most common devices the characteristics of the sound are independent of the user's position and orientation, the user may perceive the sound as unrealistic when moving the head.

Sound can also be displayed by loudspeakers. They are often used together with a screen or projector. Compared to headphones, loudspeakers can be used by multiple users, and the user does not have to wear equipment covering the ears. Alternatively to the use of a single speaker to produce mono sound, numerous speakers can be used to produce different qualities of stereo sound (e.g. 2 speakers for stereo sound, 6 or more speakers for surround sound, 64 or more speakers for a method based on the wave field synthesis)

Haptic displays

The term haptics originates from the 19th century, where it was used mainly in relation to psychophysics research. It is derived from the Greek word *haptikos*, which means 'able to touch/grasp'. Today it is used to describe all tactile, kinaesthetic, and proprioceptive perceptions of the human body. An important aspect to note about haptics is that it involves both a passive receptive and an active explorative component, thus, requiring bidirectional input and output. Tactile perception is related to the sense of touch, which includes the feeling of pressure, vibration, temperature, and pain. The tactile cues are perceived by a variety of receptors located under the surface of the human skin. Each receptor responds to different stimuli. For example, mechanoreceptors sense pressure and vibration, thermoreceptors detect changes in skin temperature, and nociceptors sense pain.

Many haptic devices have been built to date, as research devices but also as commercially available products. The majority incorporate only the force feedback component of touch, thus, providing mainly kinaesthetic and proprioceptive sensations [33]. The most famous of these interfaces is the PHANToM device from SensAble Technologies (Figure 34.4A). Originally developed at Massachusetts Institute of Technology, it can now be found in many research labs concerned with haptics. The device can provide haptic interaction only for a single point (usually in the form of a pen or finger gimbal), but has a large range of motion and a wide range of uses. While the PHANToM is based on a series kinematic structure, other haptic displays have parallel kinematic structures. Prominent examples of parallel robots are the hexapod with six degrees of freedom, the Delta robot, and parallel mechanisms based on the pantograph principle.

The CyberGrasp, Cyber-Glove Systems LLC (Figure 34.4B) with its 22 sensors is another haptic device, which is based on a wearable concept. Actuators attached to each finger allow the user to grip and feel a virtual object with four fingers. Furthermore it can be attached to the Cyber-Grasp exoskeleton. Another wearable device is the exoskeleton MAHI of Sledd and O'Malley [34], which provides force feedback mainly to the palm of the user as well as the elbow (Figure 34.4C). It can be used in combination with the cyberglove to add haptic feeback to the fingers.

Only a few solutions support tactile feedback, which is harder to generate as the biological process of tactile receptors are not fully understood [33], and as there are bigger design challenges to meet the spatial and temporal requirements of tactile perception. Tactile displays can be used to provide tactile perception to the finger tips (Figure 34.4D).

Rendering technologies

Rendering in computer graphics

Typical elements required for graphical rendering are sources of light, objects in the environment, and the camera (or eye) viewing the scene. Moreover, physical processes (e.g. light reflection and image formation in the camera) are also essential components. These basic ingredients can be found in most standard rendering approaches and softwares. However, in some specialized cases

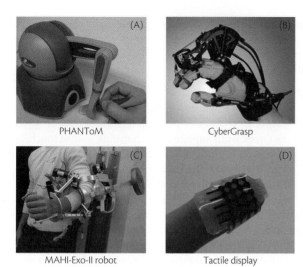

Fig. 34.4 Variety of different haptic display devices: (A) PHANToM, (B) CyberGrasp, (C) MAHI Exoskeleton, and (D) tactile display. (A) With kind permission of SMS Lab, ETH Zurich, Switzerland, (B) with kind permission of CyberGlove Systems LLC; (C) with kind permission of Rice University and Marcia O'Malley; (D) with kind permission of Ig-Mo Koo.

(e.g. in volume rendering), different image creation paradigms are followed [36]. The real physics underlying the mentioned processes are complex, therefore, often simplifications are made, especially if real-time performance is required. This becomes visible as a trade-off between the levels of photorealism and interactivity. More information can be found in Riener and Harders [9]. Graphical rendering algorithms are available in contemporary graphics libraries, such as the so-called 'Open Graphics Library' (OpenGL)—a widespread, platform-independent, cross-language application programming interface for creating 3D depictions of graphical objects.

Auditory rendering

Due to the development of high-capacity computer technology, sound is not any more restricted to simple replay of prerecorded samples. Sound has made its way towards VR, where rendering of sound is used for creating virtual auditory environments analogous to graphics rendering [37]. There are two major principles to render the acoustic information to the virtual environment. The first principle is to display prerecorded sound samples. The sound samples are usually static and non-parameterized. To simulate different virtual situations, often a large number of sound samples are required. These different sound samples may be played simultaneously or one after the other depending on the user activity and interaction with the virtual scenario. This principle is commonly used to render the background scenario in virtual environments by adding for example, twittering birds, rushing waters, passing cars, a human audience, machine noise, or music. The second principle of sound rendering is either based on real-time synthesizing of sound sources as they are generated by the physical properties of the sound emitting components and materials, or on modulating the sound signals as they appear in the vicinity of the ear of the listener [38].

Haptic rendering

Haptic rendering refers to the process of creating haptic impressions or force feedback from a virtual environment through haptic displays. The process consists of two main steps: collision detection and contact force computation. Collision detection is a process to detect the intersection occurring between the user (in the virtual environment) and the virtual object the user is interacting with. As soon as the interacting body part of the user (e.g. the user's fingertip, object hold and moved by the hand, foot, toe) penetrates the virtual object (e.g. a wall, surface of a desk, a static object), a collision between the user and the object takes place, which implies that the user touches the virtual object. Haptic devices must then render reaction forces that prevent the user from penetrating too deep into the virtual object. The rendered force should resemble the contact force when touching an equivalent object in a real scenario. Some basic haptic rendering techniques for rigid objects of simple geometry are presented in Riener and Harders [9].

Generation of virtual environments

Unlimited number of both fictional and genuine virtual environments can be applied in VR aided rehabilitation. Virtual environments can either be static or include dynamic elements such as changing weather and time conditions, altering topography, or even procedurally growing flora [39]. These characteristics, in combination with pleasant or unpleasant background music and other acoustic stimuli, can hence be used to influence the level of arousal and valence of patients affecting their emotional experience [40, 41].

There are various elements involved in the generation of virtual environments, including navigation, interaction, autonomy, and scripting. The generation of virtual environments can be made more efficient by modelling certain characteristics of different user types using the environment [42]. For example, users of a virtual shopping mall might interact very differently to the environment and each other than users of a flight simulator environment [42]. Virtual environments generated with high fidelity should, in addition, have an interesting story that causes users to suspend disbelief and get immersed in the environment. Artificial intelligence is an important part of making realistic interactions in virtual environments. For example, a virtual tour of a historical site can be made more interesting by augmenting it with a virtual guide, who has the knowledge structure of the virtual site, but is also given a 'personality' so that the virtual guide can emulate a real guide [43].

A particular type of virtual environments are encountered in serious games, which are games designed for purposes other than entertainment, such as to educate or to train [44]. In a literature survey on the impact of computer games and serious games, it was found that knowledge acquisition/content understanding was a frequent outcome of games, suggesting that games might have a beneficial effect [45].

Reeve presents an introduction to narrative-based serious games [46]. According to Reeve, serious games have clear objectives for player achievement that are transferable to spaces outside the game world; they are rarely ends in themselves but mechanisms to improve skills in other domains. Within serious games, the role of the narrative becomes more pronounced because of the requirement to deliver specific learning outcomes. Reeve categorized the types of narratives in games as follows [46]: (i) in *linear traditional* games the users must successfully complete a stage before receiving the next episode of the game; (ii) in *branching narrative* games every decision made in the game has a unique set of consequences, which reflects real life; (iii) games with *parallel paths* have the game content predefined but the user can sequence the material in a manner of his or her choosing, rather like connecting assorted lengths of a pipe; (iv) In a *dynamic narrative* structure the game is without declared goals, but is an open-ended experience that develops a continuing story through the behaviour and interactions of characters and forces within the milieu.

McQuiggan et al. [47] developed a narrative-centred learning environment called Crystal Island, which was a serious game for studying eighth-grade microbiology, and compared it to traditional instructional approaches. Although the learning gain in students was less than the traditional approach, the narrative-centred game had motivational benefits with regards to self-efficacy, presence, interest, and perception of control [47].

In serious games, storytelling can be used as a tool for motivation, for example by using storytelling as a reward [48]. Storytelling can also be used to give serious games a specific form that is easy to understand [48]. When game scenes of serious games fit within an overall narrative, learner interest is maintained [44]. McDaniel et al. [49] provide a conceptualization of the nature and function of storytelling in serious games.

In an early work on the desirable characteristics of games, Malone [50] lists *variable difficulty* as one of the desirable features. According to Malone, good computer games should be playable at different difficulty levels, which can be chosen automatically by the game according to how well the player does, or can be chosen by the player [50]. The first idea, that the game chooses a difficulty level based on how well the player performs, is similar to the idea in flow theory of matching task challenge to user skill in order to sustain user motivation for a task [51]. The idea of automatically adjusting difficulty level of games has been very influential in shaping the design of serious games over the last two decades. For example, different parts of a complex serious game can be individually adapted to match user performance. A more sophisticated machine learning approach is to have game agents learn from their experience and adapt themselves in real-time based on user performance [52]. In another approach, game parameters and behaviours of computer-controlled opponents can be adapted in real-time according to the proficiency of the player in the game [53]. In an educational game, adaptation rules can be designed to examine learner performance and adapt a specific game scenario based on how well the learner is doing [54].

In any game, rewards and scores are important components. They give feedback to the user in an attempt to both demonstrate correct versus incorrect answers, but can also act as a motivating entity [55]. There has been some debate about the role of rewards in affecting intrinsic motivation—the inherent tendency to seek out novelty and challenges in games and not work towards rewards [56]. While some researchers opine that rewards negatively affect intrinsic motivation [57], others argue that there is no such negative effect [58]. Nonetheless, rewards remain a key part of games, and are often related to the concept of *scores*, which are points awarded to users based on how well they perform in a game. Score motivates game play by rewarding behaviour and providing a gauge of performance, enabling comparison and competition [59]. The presence of *high score lists* in games has been argued to encourage user participation [60].

Virtual-reality supported physiotherapy
Virtual-reality supported ankle rehabilitation
At Rutgers University, Burdea and colleagues developed the VR-supported haptic device called 'Rutgers Ankle' [61]. The system consists of a hexapod platform as a haptic interface that provides forces in 6 degrees of freedom to the patient's foot, in response to his or her movement performance in a game-like VR exercise (Figure 34.5). The patient is treated in a sitting posture, with the foot attached via a footplate to the hexapod device. Two exercise games have been developed. In the first one, the patient uses the foot to steer a virtual airplane through a virtual sky. As the plane moves forward, a series of open square hoops are presented on the screen. The goal is for the participant to manoeuvre the plane through the hoops without hitting the sides. This is done by mapping the ankle movement to the flight path, where for instance ankle dorsiflexion can cause the nose of the plane to point upward, elevation can cause the plane to go toward the left, etc. The difficulty level can be adjusted by changing the number and placement of hoops, airplane speed, and the amount of resistance provided by the haptic interface. A second game calls for the participant to pilot a virtual speedboat over the ocean while avoiding buoys, again by moving the ankle up and down or in and out. A recent addition to these games is that the user can experience task-related haptic effects such as a jolt when a buoy or hoop is hit, or to change the environmental conditions by adding turbulence to the air or water implemented by generating a low-frequency side-to-side vibration of the platform. The Rutgers Ankle system has been validated on patients with orthopaedic disorders, which showed that the VR-based training had a positive effect in task accuracy (defined as the number of hoops entered versus the missed ones), ankle range of motion, ankle torque production, one leg stance time, and stair descent time.

A recent study by Mirelman et al. [62] compared robotic intervention using the Rutgers Ankle system for patients exercising with and without an attached VR system. The researchers did not only compare standard neurological tests for both groups, but also investigated the distance walked and the steps taken in everyday life using an accelerometer based system. The group that received

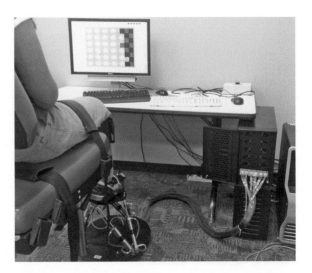

Fig. 34.5 VR application in ankle rehabilitation using the Rutgers Ankle.
Copyright Rutgers Tele-Rehabilitation Institute. Reprinted by permission.

VR-augmented training showed greater changes in walking velocity, distance, and number of steps taken.

Virtual-reality supported gait rehabilitation

Gait rehabilitation is applied for patients with paralysed lower extremities due to lesions of the central or peripheral nervous system (e.g. after stroke or spinal cord injury) [9]. The goals of the therapy are to restore motor function and improve movement coordination, to learn new motion strategies and to prevent secondary complications such as muscle atrophy, osteoporosis, and spasticity, in order to improve quality of life, and finally get back to normal daily activities and participation in the society.

Treadmill training

Treadmill training is part of a rehabilitation programme administered to patients with neurological gait disorders in order to improve walking capabilities. Some clinical research groups are using VR systems that are coupled to standard commercially available treadmills used in rehabilitation. Baram and Miller studied the effects of VR on the walking abilities of multiple sclerosis patients [63]. Their study included 16 patients. They found an average short-term improvement of 24% increase in walking speed compared to baseline after exercising with VR.

Using a treadmill mounted on a 6 degree of freedom motion platform with a coupled VR system, Fung et al. could not only investigate walking, but also turning movements [64]. They showed that gait performance (i.e. gait speed), could be increased in stroke patients, when providing auditory and visual feedback during treadmill training [64].

Jaffe et al. have used VR technology to train obstacle avoidance during walking in chronic post-stroke patients [65]. Virtual obstacles were displayed in a head-mounted display together with a video image of the patient's legs. They compared real world and virtual world obstacle avoidance training. Patients who received VR training showed significantly greater improvements in fast paced velocity than patients who trained with real objects. Improvements in obstacle clearance and step length of the non-paretic side were also higher in the VR group, but not significantly.

Similarly, Chuang et al. [66] compared training with and without VR in coronary artery bypass graft patients, and found that patients training with VR achieved significantly better cardiopulmonary improvement. Yang et al. [67] also compared treadmill training with and without VR in stroke patients, and found improvements in walking speed, community walking time and self-reported walking ability in the VR group.

While most approaches use treadmills in combination with monitors or other display devices to render the virtual environments in front of the patient, others project the visual contexts (e.g. obstacles) directly onto the instrumented treadmills. This allows training foot positioning relative to environmental properties [68]. Such devices are likewise used to allow functional gait rehabilitation in elderly people or improve gait adaptability in people with stroke [69]. Further investigations of the effects of VR training on gait biomechanics with individuals post-stroke were performed by Deutsch et al. [70] and Mirelman et al. [62].

Treatment of Parkinson's disease

One of the primary symptoms of Parkinson's disease is hypokinesia, that is, difficulty in the initiation and continuation of motions, in particular during ambulation. These symptoms tend to worsen as the disease progresses. Although the symptoms can be mitigated by drugs such as L-dopa, these drugs can become less effective over time and may produce unwanted side effects, such as chorea and athetotic movements. Thus, a complementary method to treat hypokinetic gait in Parkinson's disease could offer patients a way to delay or reduce drug use while still maintaining or even improving gait function. Such an alternative method is based on an interesting phenomenon associated with patients with Parkinson's disease termed kinesia paradoxa. Patients with Parkinson's disease, who are unable to ambulate, or even unable to initiate a step on open ground are, paradoxically, able to step over objects placed in their path with little difficulty. Weghorst and colleagues have conducted a number of studies to ascertain, whether VR technology provides a way to take advantage of this phenomenon and facilitate walking in Parkinson's disease patients by presenting virtual objects overlaid on the natural world [71]. Several other technologies have been developed and applied to assist Parkinson patients during daily life activities (see later).

Robot-assisted gait training

Several devices for robot-assisted gait training have been developed over the last decades and were shown to cause significant improvement of gait function in patients suffering from stroke or spinal cord injury [72]. Robots for treadmill walking typically consist of a body weight support system, an actuated exoskeletal mechanism in combination with a treadmill or an actuated end-effector based mechanism in order to drive the limbs of the patient. Examples are the Lokomat [73, 74], which uses actuators in hips and knees to automate treadmill walking, the WalkTrainer [75], the Bowden cable-driven LOPES robot [76], and the Autoambulator.

Robot-aided VR exercises have been used to increase the motivation and physical engagement of children with cerebral palsy [77, 78, 79, 80]. VR exercises have also been used to motivate subjects suffering from stroke [81]. The study of Mirelman et al. [62] investigated the effects of VR training compared with a robot alone. In the following section, the principles of VR in gait rehabilitation will be explained with the example of the Lokomat gait orthosis.

Gait rehabilitation with the Lokomat

The Lokomat gait orthosis was developed in the Spinal Cord Injury Center at the University Hospital Balgrist Zurich, for improvement and automation of neurorehabilitative treadmill training [73, 74]. It consists of two actuated leg orthoses, which are strapped to the patient's legs. On each orthosis, two motors, one at the hip joint and one at the knee joint, guide the patient's legs along a physiological walking pattern. The orthosis is synchronized with the belt speed of a treadmill. Together with the body weight support system, the orthosis allows even non-ambulatory patients to perform walking movements.

Therapists and physicians can choose the optimal training scenario and set the VR and game parameters in such way that patient-specific motor deficits are addressed in the best way. For example, in a project with cerebral palsy children, the motor function training aims to increase the maximal force output of hip and knee flexors/extensors, to exercise and improve maximum joint range of motion, speed adaptation during walking, translation of visual input into motor output (eye/head coordination) and initiation/termination of gait. Four training scenarios of daily living were implemented as virtual tasks that address the above-mentioned training goals [79]. For muscle strengthening and to increase the range of motion, the patients waded through deep snow in a virtual world or kicked a virtual soccer ball. In order to exercise the starting and stopping of gait and the increase and decrease of walking speed, the patients have to walk within a street traffic scenario, where they have to cross a street at a traffic light. Patients exercise gait-eye coordination (translation of visual input into motor output) and leg motion coordination in the street traffic scenario and in an obstacle course (Table 34.2).

Studies in healthy subjects showed that VR enabled healthy subjects to perform more accurate movements during obstacle stepping [82]. Subjects were given auditory, visual and haptic feedback on their foot clearance and the distance to obstacles they had to overstep. Performance was measured as foot clearance over the obstacle and the number of obstacles hit. This study showed that subjects had higher performance with auditory feedback than with visual feedback. Additionally, the authors showed that 3D vision did not improve performance compared to 2D visions. In patients, a study by Bruetsch et al. showed that VR had the potential to increase active participation of children with cerebral palsy compared to gait therapy alone [77]. Participation was thereby quantified by electromyography (EMG) measurements.

If sound is used, it should be properly timed with a visual or haptic event. In order to create a realistic impression, the sound should not be delayed more than 20 ms after the occurrence of the visual or haptic event. An example is the collision of the foot with a virtual obstacle. When the foot impacts the virtual wall, the graphical and haptic displays show the foot contact with the wall with a minimal time shift to the acoustics.

The Lokomat system can also serve as a haptic display that renders the force interaction between the user's foot and a virtual object [79, 82] (Figure 34.6). As the Lokomat was not built to be used as a haptic display, it only has motors at the hip and knee joints, whereas the ankle joint cannot be actuated. Therefore, contact forces on the toes cannot be displayed directly. Nevertheless, it is possible to produce a quasi-realistic haptic perception by tricking the tactile system with synchronized visual and acoustic cues into believing the interaction would happen at the toes. Impedance control is normally used to display haptic objects in the virtual environment. Typical sampling times for haptic rendering lie in the range of 500–1000 Hz. Below 500 Hz, the rendering of stiff objects may become unstable. The haptic rendering has been directly included within the Lokomat control architecture. An impedance controller computes a corrective force from the difference between desired and real position. It implements a spring-damper system

as an internal impedance model. The reaction force is computed from the stiffness of the spring-damper system. Computation of the contact forces can be done by impulse based methods or by penalty based methods. An impulsive force is applied on contact of the foot with the object and pushes the foot out of the virtual object. Thereby, the position of the foot in Cartesian space must be computed as a function of hip and knee angles and length of shank and thigh. When shank length is known, estimation of the length of thigh and foot can be done, using the method of Winter [83]. Then, during contact with the object, the desired haptic interaction forces can be computed. In penalty based methods, the interaction force will be computed depending upon the penetration depth and/or the penetration velocity [82]. Additional friction terms can help creating a realistic feeling.

Virtual-reality supported arm rehabilitation

Arm rehabilitation is applied for patients with paralysed upper extremities due to lesions of the central or peripheral nervous system (e.g. after stroke or spinal cord injury) [9]. The goals of the therapy are to restore motor function and improve movement coordination, to learn new motion strategies (compensatory movements, trick movements), and to prevent secondary complications such as muscle atrophy, osteoporosis, and spasticity, in order to improve quality of life, and finally get back to normal daily activities and participation in the society.

Arm therapy systems

Chen et al. [84] and Duff et al. [85] developed VR systems where arm kinematics are tracked with cameras and reflective markers. In both cases, the patient performs reaching motions that are shown on the screen. In the case of Duff et al. [85], different auditory cues are also used to give feedback about the movement. King et al. [86] developed a similar system, but combined the optical tracking with an 'arm skate' system for tracking on a table. Subramanian et al. [2] were able to show that such exercise with VR and optical tracking can lead to a slight improvement in arm function over conventional physical exercise, possibly due to better feedback. Mumford et al. [87] also used cameras to track a cylinder that was grasped by the user and moved along a horizontal display. Augmented feedback was given to reinforce speed, trajectory and placement.

Alamri et al. [88] developed a system for arm impairment diagnosis and rehabilitation based on a data glove and visual display. Tasks include arranging blocks, moving a cup, working out with a dumbbell and others. Similarly, Merians et al. [89] developed a hand training system based on a CyberGlove and a simple 3D representation of the hand. Connelly et al. [90] were able to show slightly, though not significantly, greater improvement when training with a glove in VR compared to normal training.

An adaptive virtual scenario was developed by Cameirão et al. [19]. The arm was again tracked using cameras and markers, and data gloves allow finger tracking. The virtual environment consists of several different tasks, and a personalized training module allows difficulty to be adapted to the individual patient.

In contrast to the above groups, who applied camera tracking systems or wearable data gloves, Fong et al. [91] used a touch screen to simulate an automated teller machine for patients with acquired brain injury. The goal of their system was to train both

Table 34.2 Therapy goals of a virtual scenario used with cerebral palsy patients

	Soccer	Obstacle	Traffic	Snow
Muscle strength		+		+
Range of motion	+	+		
Walking speed	+		+	
Limb coordination	+	+		
Cognition	+		+	

cognitive ability (using the machine) and motor ability. Similarly, Lewis et al. [92] developed a system where the forearm and wrist are secured in a fibreglass cast mounted on a load cell. The application of forces and torques to the cell controls the movement of a submarine shown on the display.

There are several groups that have shown that augmented feedback exercises promote recovery in patients suffering from stroke [93, 94] and lead to smoother arm movements [95].

Robot-aided arm rehabilitation

The advantages of robotic arm training are that the therapist can get assisted, e.g. relieved from the weight of the patient's arm, the training can get longer and more intensive (up to 20 times more movement repetitions per training session), and the movements can be measured and used for therapy assessment. Furthermore, by adding special VR technologies the training can get much more entertaining and motivating. Implementation of task-oriented games can support to learn activities of daily life. Examples of arm therapy robots are the MIT-Manus [96], which allows training movements in the horizontal plane (Figure 34.7A), the T-WREX (commercialized as Armeo®Spring, Hocoma AG, Switzerland) [97], a passive gravity-balancing orthosis allowing arm movements in 5 degrees-of-freedom (Figure 34.7B), the Bi-Manu-Track [98], a single joint actuator that allows training of distal arm functions, the Gentle/s system, an endeffector-based robot that is based on the Haptic Master with 4 active and 2 passive degrees-of-freedom [99], the first bimanual training robot MIME [100], several passive

systems based on the PHANToM haptic device [101], the ADAPT, a robot for training with different tools [102], ARMin [103], which is a device with 7 active degrees of freedom (Figure 34.8) and several hand master systems, to support finger movements, such as the Rutgers Master [104].

One of the key elements for a successful rehabilitation is the motivation of the patient. It is also known that task-orientated training improves motor recovery in patients [105]. Audiovisual displays can ideally be used to present tasks and instructions to the patient [89, 106–108]. Therefore, most systems are connected to a visual display with a virtual environment, where the robot acts as an input device for playing games and performing tasks (Figure 34.7, and Figure 34.9). The movement can be represented by a virtual avatar, by projecting a real camera image to the virtual world or by mapping the subject's movement to any other object (e.g. virtual ball or virtual car). During motor training also cognitive tasks can be exercised.

One of the first robot-aided VR training system was developed by Adamovich and coworkers [106, 109]. It allows training of different exercises of the hand within a virtual environment. The hand movements were recorded by a CyberGlove device (CyberGlove Systems, San Jose, CA, USA), whereas finger forces were applied with a RutgersMaster [104]. In this way, the range of motion could be trained for each finger independently. A graphical bar on the screen serves to display the amount of flexion force of each finger, which encourages the patient to flex and extend the fingers as much as possible. Another exercise enabled to train fast hand closing speeds. This was implemented by a motivating

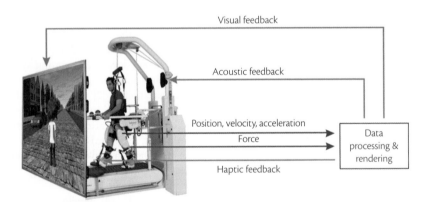

Fig. 34.6 The Lokomat VR setup.

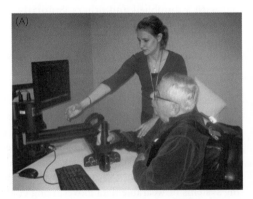
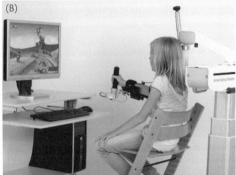

Fig. 34.7 Examples of arm rehabilitation robots applied in combination with VR displays: (A) MIT Manus; (B) Armeo®Spring Pediatric, Hocoma AG, Switzerland. (A) By courtesy of H. I. Krebs; (B) picture: Hocoma, Switzerland.

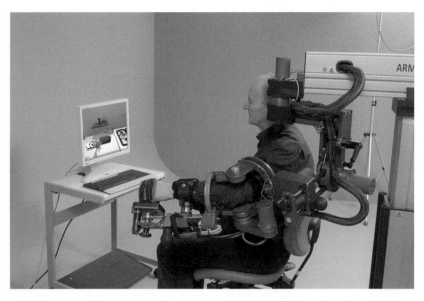

Fig. 34.8 ARMin IV with 7 degrees of freedom.

butterfly game, where the task of the user is to wink the hand faster than a predetermined threshold in order to chase away the butterfly from the virtual hand.

Several studies have also attempted to explicitly improve patient motivation in robot-aided rehabilitation using elements such as difficulty adaptation, short- and long-term goals, music, and other elements [110, 111].

Virtual reality applications with ARMin

ARMin was developed at ETH Zurich in collaboration with University Hospital Balgrist Zurich. The newest version of the device consists of 7 active degrees of freedom and allows the training of functional movements (Figure 34.8). The exoskeleton is attached to the patients arm with two cuffs, one on the upper and one on the lower arm [103]. ARMin is connected to a virtual environment to provide visual and auditory feedback. The system has two computers, a control system with the real-time operating system Matlab xPC-Target and a host computer with the graphical user interface. The API of xPC is used to poll the needed data from the control system. For graphical rendering the GIANTS game engine, Coin3D, later also UNITY were used.

There are currently three different modes used for training, such as mobilization mode, simple games, and ADL tasks. In the mobilization mode the therapist is able to teach and repeat movements. The therapist determines the choice of joints to be moved as well as the range of motion and speed of the movement. The movement taught by the therapist is smoothened and then stored by the robot. A position controller repeats the stored trajectory, while the patient can remain completely passive. The joint angles of the robot are mapped to a virtual hand of the avatar on the screen (Figure 34.9). The goal of this mode is to foster blood circulation, reduce spasticity in the hemiparetic arm, prevent joint contractures, train muscle strength, etc.

To train joint movements simple games have been implemented. In the ball game the patient controls a virtual bar to catch a ball. The joint to be involved and the range of motion are selected by the therapist. The handle can be moved in one, two,

or three dimensions, depending on the motor skills of the patient and the training preferences of the therapist. Furthermore, difficulty level, amount of support, and ball behaviour are adjustable to the patients' needs. The robot supports the patient with an as-much-as-needed control strategy. In another game, coordination can be trained by moving a ball through the randomly generated labyrinth. Again, the workspace is adjustable by the therapist and then mapped to the plane representing the labyrinth. The walls are haptically rendered with a penalty-based approach. To train coordination, the force applied against the walls must not exceed a given threshold. Otherwise, the patient has to restart from the beginning of the labyrinth. Additionally, appealing sound is given as a reward, when the end of the labyrinth has been reached.

A third mode enables the training of ADL tasks (Figure 34.9) [112]. The patient has to perform functional movements with the whole arm to achieve the tasks and train activities he or she can use in daily life. Realistic tasks have been implemented according to a

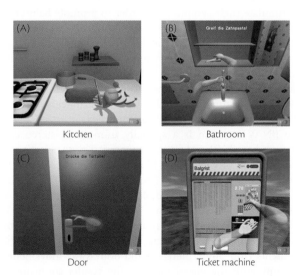

Fig. 34.9 Activities of daily living (ADL) tasks that can be trained with ARMin.

list defined by several criteria (e.g. importance in daily life, feasib-lility with ARMin). Besides the visual feedback, auditory feedback is applied to maximally involve the patient in the virtual world. Furthermore, perception when interacting with objects is mim-icked by sound feedback. As the third modality, haptic feedback has been implemented to support the patient (e.g. haptic table) or to enhance the level of realism by adding friction and weight to objects. To simplify collision detection, only the end-effector posi-tion (representing the hand), is considered for haptic interaction. Virtual objects are rendered as cylinders or cuboids. To calculate the haptic feedback each object is modeled by a spring-damper system. When a collision occurs the calculated force is applied at the endeffector by the controller. While the visual and audi-tory feedback use a sampling rate of 60 Hz, the haptic feedback is rendered with 1 kHz. During the rehabilitation of patients it is important that the training is linked to the real world in order to maximize the transfer to daily life. Realistic behaviour of objects is provided by the physics and collision detection engine of GIANTS. Instead of 3D-vision lighting and shadow effects help to perceive visual depth in the virtual world. Important in reha-bilitation therapy is the adaptability of the virtual world to the skills of the patient. Therefore, the avatar hand can be moved by the therapist to a position, where the patient can reach all objects needed within the range of movement available to him or her. The ADL training system has been evaluated with healthy subjects and stroke patients [112]. Besides using the visual feedback to present the task and arm movement it was also used to display the virtual tunnel of the patient-cooperative control strategy (Figure 34.7B).

Further virtual reality applications

Balance training

One of the first reports about the use of VR for balance training has been provided by Jacobson et al. [113]. The authors describe a VR system for balance training of subjects with vestibular disorders, which they call the Balance Near Automatic Virtual Environment (BNAVE).

Subjects with peripheral vestibular disorders frequently suffer from disequilibrium during standing and walking, and visual blurring during head movements. They are often treated in ves-tibular rehabilitation programmes by exposure to situations that stimulate their symptoms in order to promote habituation. Typically, patients are taken through a gradually changing type of exposure that progressively adds situations and positions pro-voking and increasing their symptoms (e.g. dizziness, motion sickness, loss of balance). Due to habituation, the symptoms get weaker during the course of the treatment. VR technologies can support such training, as large immersive visual fields can be cre-ated and changed rapidly to suit patient needs.

The BNAVE system is a spatially immersive, stereoscopic, projection-based VR system that encompasses a subject's entire horizontal field of view, and a large portion of the vertical field of view, when looking forward (viewing angle is 200° in the hori-zontal and 95° in the vertical direction). The validity of the sys-tem's immersion was tested in a pilot study. Both normal and vestibular-impaired subjects responded to the visual stimuli provided by the BNAVE system with substantial greater head movements (100–300% increase) and body sway movements in synchrony with the visual motion. The results confirmed the robust effect of the visual stimuli provided by the system on pos-tural responses.

VR training has been used successfully to rehabilitate func-tional balance and mobility also in both traumatic brain injury (TBI) survivors and healthy elderly subjects [114]. In another study, an experimental group that received VR therapy in addi-tion to conventional physical therapy improved in balance more than the control group that received only physical therapy [115].

VR exercises have also been used to improve dynamic balance control in a short-sitting position of three wheelchair users, fol-lowing spinal cord and head injuries [116]. The patients showed increased motivation to perform a centre-of-pressure-controlled video game-based exercise and increased dynamic short-sitting balance. The patients exhibited increases in practice volume and attention span during training with the game-based tool. In addition, they demonstrated substantial improvements in dynamic balance control. These observations indicate that a video-game-based exercise approach can have a substantial posi-tive effect by improving dynamic short-sitting balance.

Back training

Recently, a commercial product, called Valedo®Motion (Hocoma AG, Volketswil, Switzerland), came out that can be used for functional low back pain therapy, through a motivating exercise environment. The system uses two lightweight orientation sen-sors to record small movements from the patient's lumbar spine, and provides real-time augmented performance feedback to help the patient improve their movement awareness. Various exercises have been designed to help improve the patient's mobilization, proprioception, stabilization and balance. The use of real-time visual feedback using VR technology not only helps to improve patient's compliance and motivation, but also supports therapists by providing direct assessments of trunk movement quality.

Cognitive training

Psychophysiological stimulation to increase engagement and motivation

VR exercises such as arm training can only be effective if the par-ticipant is motivated to exercise and is appropriately challenged. Particularly motivation has been shown to have a major influence on the rehabilitation outcome [9, 12, 14, 117]. While it is impos-sible to measure motivation itself while a person is immersed in VR, we can assume that certain psychological states (high engage-ment, appropriately balanced workload) can ensure high motiva-tion. For example, it is desirable to control cognitive workload since research in healthy subjects has shown that motor learning decreases in the presence of distracting cognitive tasks that pre-sent cognitively overchallenging situations [118, 119]. On the other hand, tasks without cognitive workload may be considered bor-ing, thus, decreasing the motivation to exercise.

Cognitive workload can be unobtrusively measured in VR with the use of so-called psychophysiological measurements (record-ings of the body's response to psychological states). Originally used for workload recognition in applications such as flight simu-lation, they were extensively investigated for both upper extrem-ity [120, 121] and lower extremity [29, 122] rehabilitation within the FP7 European project MIMICS. The project demonstrated the possibility of classifying workload using psychophysiological measurements and using them to adapt task difficulty. The dem-onstrated systems essentially consisted of two feedback loops: a 'fast' feedback loop to provide physical assistance during each motion and a 'slow' feedback loop to adapt difficulty every few minutes (Figure 34.10). Since then, several other studies have proposed alternative methods of recognizing cognitive workload from psychophysiological measurements applied in rehabilitation [123–125], but it is not yet clear what approach would be optimal with regard to accuracy, robustness and patient comfort.

Quantifying cognitive load during the training can be achieved by evaluation of physiological quantities such as electrocardiogram (ECG), galvanic skin response (GSR), breathing frequency, and skin temperature [29]. This is possible, as all psychological quantities as behavioural, social, and emotional aspects are reflected in physiological signals of the body [126]. Using autoadaptive linear classification methods [122], these physiological signals can be processed to determine the cognitive load in real time. By adapting the training environment and task difficulty of the virtual environment, it is possible to control the physiological and psychological state of subjects during gait and arm rehabilitation in a closed loop fashion.

Training of cognitive function after brain damage

Mild cognitive impairment and memory impairment

There is a lot of potential in using VR technology for memory training of persons with mild cognitive impairments (MCI). Guo et al. [127] developed a virtual kitchen and tested it with persons with MCI and found a high acceptability rate. In a study by Kizony et al. [128], a virtual supermarket environment was used to train executive functions for persons with MCI, resulting in an improvement in executive functions. VR can also be used for memory training in healthy elderly individuals. In a study done to test the effect of VR-aided memory training (VRMT) on memory in healthy elderly persons, it was found that the experimental group using VRMT showed significantly better improvement in memory tests than the control group who underwent face-to-face training [129].

Dementia and Alzheimer's disease

In a feasibility study on the application of VR, Flynn et al. [130] developed a virtual environment of a park and tested it with persons with dementia. They found that persons with dementia could feel present in the environment and interact with objects, thus,

justifying the use of virtual reality to train cognitive functions that persons. Exergaming, (i.e. the combination of games and exercise), can be another way to achieve cognitive stimulation in dementia, which can lead to improvements in cognitive functions and also motor performance, as shown in a study done by Colombo et al. [131]. In older adults with questionable dementia, VR-based memory training was able to improve objective memory performance [132].

Impairment in spatial orientation and navigational skills is one of the major symptoms of Alzheimer's disease (AD) [133], and can be a threat to both individual and public safety [134]. Tests with tasks performed in virtual environments are a cost-effective way of assessing navigational skills in persons with AD [134]. VR also offers the opportunity to rehabilitate spatial orientation in persons with AD, in a cost-effective manner [135]. Bouchard et al. [136] present a set of specific guidelines for designing and implementing effective serious games targeting persons with AD, including choosing right in-game challenges, designing appropriate interaction mechanisms, providing dynamic difficulty adjustments, and producing effective visual and auditory assets to maximize cognitive training. The application of serious games to rehabilitate persons with AD is still at a nascent stage and, therefore, such guidelines can be useful for future researchers.

Traumatic brain injury

VR has been found to be a valid tool to assess memory and learning in individuals with traumatic brain injuries (TBI) [137]. In a study performed to train executive functions in people with TBI, training in a virtual supermarket was compared to training with conventional occupational therapy [138]. It was found that transfer to daily functions in the real world is better in the case of virtual training than conventional therapy [138]. A 4-week intervention that consisted of non-immersive VR exercises resulted in improvement in verbal and visual learning tasks in persons with TBI [139]. In an online VR based training, patients with TBI showed an increase in working memory and attention levels from pre- to post-training [140].

Attention deficit hyperactivity disorder

Virtual environments are a promising method for rehabilitation of attention deficit hyperactivity disorders (ADHD). Rizzo et al. [141] have developed a head-mounted display based VR scenario called the Virtual Classroom designed for the assessment and possible rehabilitation of attention processes. Cho et al. [142] found in a study that immersive VR with cognitive training can improve the attention span of children and adolescents with behavioural problems and help them learn to focus on tasks.

Autistic spectrum disorder

Bauminger et al. [143] did a study to evaluate the effectiveness of a 3-week intervention using a cooperation enforcing virtual environment called StoryTable, which was used to facilitate collaboration and positive social interaction for 6 children, aged 8–10 years, with autistic spectrum disorder (ASD). In the StoryTable, users could manipulate objects and characters within the context of a specific story background setting. Many different scenarios (or backgrounds) were made available, each having different characters, which children could use to create and narrate stories. The intervention resulted in an increase in positive social behaviours and decrease in stereotypic, repetitive behaviours in the children [143].

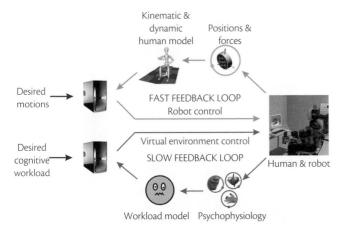

Fig. 34.10 Adding a psychophysiological 'slow' feedback loop to rehabilitation in order to complement 'fast' robot control.

In another work, Herrera et al. [144] developed a VR-based learning environment, where a shopping activity was recreated. Within this learning environment, the tool 'I am going to act as if . . .' aimed at facilitating the understanding of imagination in people with ASD. An intervention with two children with ASD using this VR-based learning environment resulted in improved functional use of objects and improved imagination understanding [144].

Phobias

There are different areas of psychotherapy in which the application of VR can prove to be an effective tool [9]. Wiederhold and Wiederhold [145] were one of the first who recognized the potential of VR as a tool in psychotherapy, in order to treat patients suffering from different phobias. Examples are acrophobia (fear of height), aviatophobia (fear of flying, see Figure 34.11), fear of driving, social phobias, claustrophobia (fear of small spaces), or agoraphobia (fear of large spaces). Comprehensive reviews were presented by Krijn et al. [146] and Brahnam and Jain [147].

Post-traumatic stress disorder

Persons with post-traumatic stress disorders (PTSD) show symptoms of fear, helplessness, insomnia, after having been exposed to an extreme stressor or traumatic event. PTSD is characterized by three distinct types of symptoms: (1) they re-experience the event again and again in their imagination, (2) they try to avoid reminders of the event, and (3) they are hyper-aroused for at least 1 month after the traumatic event [148]. VR-graded exposure therapy is employed at the point when exposure therapy would normally be introduced. According to Rothbaum et al. [149], VR-graded exposure therapy has several advantages over conventional exposure approaches. First, the technology of VR allows to introduce a shared experience between the therapist and participant that is practically impossible without VR. For example, it is almost impossible to bring the clinician to the traumatic scenery that caused the disorder, and share all the PTSD patient's imagined scenes. Second, VR extends the range of options available to a clinician by allowing the opportunity to expose to situations that are difficult, expensive and/or time-consuming in real life. For instance, using a virtual airplane the therapist can expose the patient to the airport and spend time on a virtual airplane taking off, flying in smooth and turbulent weather, and landing, repeatedly, without leaving the office, all within the typical therapy hour. Third, in a VR setting, the therapist can titrate the situation, thus, creating the perfect exposure for the patient. For example, the patient can experience a certain situation in an airplane, with all features, except one (e.g. excluding turbulence) until the patient is ready to confront herself or himself with turbulence in the frame of the therapy. Fourth, VR-graded exposure therapy augments the patient's imaginative capacities with visual, auditory, olfactory, and even haptic computer-generated experiences (i.e. in more modalities than in conventional therapy). In this way, VR provides a rich sensory and evocative therapeutic environment that may be particularly helpful for patients who are reluctant to recall feared memories, have difficulty to emotionally engage in the traumatic memory, or are not very good at imagining situations [149]. Rizzo et al. [150] developed a VR-graded exposure therapy for veterans from the Iraq and Afghanistan wars and found that out of 20 treatment completers, 16 no longer met PTSD criteria at post-treatment. A survivor of the World Trade Center attack of 11 September 2001 was exposed over a course of six 1-hour VR-graded exposure therapy sessions, to virtual planes flying over the World Trade Center, jets crashing into the World Trade Center, etc. After the therapy, he successfully reduced acute PTSD symptoms [151]. In another study, VR-graded exposure therapy could reduce the difficulties reported with PTSD patient at the Naval Medical Center, San Diego [152]. In a randomized, controlled trial of VR-graded exposure therapy versus 'treatment as usual' with active duty military personnel suffering from combat-related PTSD, it was found that 7 out of 10 participants improved at least by 30% in the VR group, whereas only 1 out of the 9 returning participants showed similar improvement in the treatment as usual group [153].

Virtual-reality supported assistance

Gait assistance

Systems that assist gait are almost exclusively based on augmented rather than virtual reality, providing visual and auditory cues to assist walking in daily life. They are most commonly used with Parkinson's disease patients, who exhibit hypokinesia or so-called gait freezing events. When such an event is detected, the wearable augmented reality system provides a cue that remains until the freezing has been corrected by the user [154–156].

Similar systems are also used by multiple sclerosis and cerebral palsy patients, where the goal is to stabilize gait by providing appropriate feedback. In the example application of Baram and Miller (2007) and Baram and Lenger (2012), a sound generator provides a tick each time the user takes a step [157, 158]. The user is instructed to adjust gait so as to produce a balanced rhythmic auditory cue. Additionally, visual feedback is provided

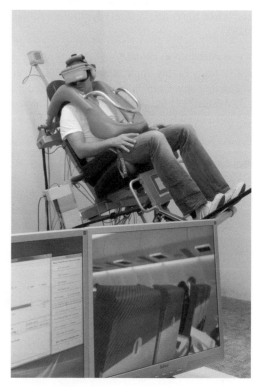

Fig. 34.11 Simulator for the treatment of aviatophobia (fear of flying). Courtesy of Prof. A. Mühlberger, University of Würzburg, Germany.

by a head-mounted display that shows an image of transverse lines which respond dynamically to the user's motion, much like a real floor fixed in space. Either one or both types of feedback together can be used to establish an improved gait pattern and faster walking speed.

Assistance for people with visual or auditory impairments

Systems that support visually and hearing impaired people in daily life collect information from the real environment and display it via other senses such as hearing and touching [159]. As such, they are again examples of augmented rather than virtual reality.

Most devices for the visually impaired are navigation systems, which record the environment using cameras or distance sensors, then provide feedback to the user [160–162]. They are based on positioning methods, radio frequency identification tags, or computer vision [163]. More expensive solutions make use of sensors built into the environment while cheaper ones are built into clothing [164] or mobile phones [165]. Feedback is most commonly provided via auditory displays. Two such examples are the NAVIG [161] and AudioNav [165] systems, where different sensing technologies are fused to sense the position in the environment and head orientation using Global Positioning System, camera, compass, accelerometer, and inclinometer signals attached to the user's body or head. Spatially rendered semantic audio information is used to guide the user and mediate the location of recognized objects.

Alternatively, devices for the visually impaired can also provide haptic feedback. One such example is an instrumented handle that supplements conventional white canes using haptic-augmented feedback. Pulses of a spinning wheel mimic the impact with a distant obstacle and vibrotactile feedback informs about distances to objects. As the implemented infrared and ultrasonic range sensors can also detect obstacles in the far distance and above head level, the safety of the user is increased [160].

Devices for the hearing impaired record sound, and then provide information to the user via visual displays such as head-mounted displays or mobile phones. While it can be difficult to interpret rich audio information, such as human speech, with such devices, some implementations do exist and have shown promising results [166, 167].

Wheelchair assistance

Webster et al. [168] examined whether the use of a computer-assisted therapy (CAT) system in combination with a wheelchair simulator device would be effective in improving real world performance on a wheelchair obstacle course in a group of patients with stroke and unilateral neglect syndrome. In addition, they examined, whether this training influenced the number of falls experienced by participants during their inpatient hospital stay. Forty patients (38 men, 2 women) with right hemisphere stroke participated. All patients were right-handed and showed evidence of unilateral neglect, defined as specific scores on two standard tests of neglect, the Random Letter Cancellation Test and the Rey–Osterrieth Complex Figure test. The patients who had received the VR-CAT training made fewer errors, and hit significantly fewer ($p \leq 0.0001$) obstacles with the left side of their wheelchair during the real world wheelchair obstacle course test than did participants in the control group, who had not received

this training (1.3 vs. 5.1 collisions). In addition, participants in the VR-trained group sustained significantly fewer falls ($p \leq 0.02$) than those in the control group (2 of 19 patients in CAT group; 8 of 19 in the control group). The virtual performance tests, conducted on participants in the CAT group, showed improved performance after the training for both the video tracking and VR wheelchair obstacle test, indicating that a learning effect had occurred in the virtual world.

Discussion

Relevance of VR for increase of motivation

VR is a powerful tool to motivate the participants to active participation, while providing augmented performance feedback. VR in rehabilitation provides motivating training that can be superior to training in a real situation [7, 169]. It was shown that increased motivation [14] and active participation [15] can lead to increased efficiency and advancements of motor learning in neurorehabilitation. Enriched environments, highly functional and task-oriented practice environments were shown to be necessary for motor re-learning and recovery after stroke [15]. Additionally, VR can be utilized to test different methods of motor training, types of feedback provided, and different practice schedules for comparative effectiveness in improving motor function in patients. VR technology provides a convenient mechanism for manipulating these factors, setting up automatic training schedules and for training, testing, and recording participants' motor responses.

Through game-like characteristics, VR technology can increase the overall motivation of patients during therapy [2, 170]. One game element that has been addressed quite extensively and has shown to be important is the possibility to adjust the level of difficulty of a VR exercise to the capabilities of patients [19–22]. In addition, studies have shown that VR exercises should show functionally meaningful reactions to the motor performance of the patient to increase motivation [16]. The same study did not find any differences in engagement between VR exercises that differed in providing explicit task goals, frequent performance feedback or competitive training. The authors argued that this could be due to differing preferences and expectations of participating subjects towards the VR exercises. Other game mechanics that have been proposed to encourage motivation are reward systems, variable content, and intuitive tasks [17, 18].

Relevance of VR-based feedback for motor learning

Robotic assistance can reduce a patients' effort to actively participate during training. This has been shown for both upper- and lower-extremity therapy [171, 172]. The primary cause for this effect can be attributed to the passive guidance the robot provides during training [171]. Such continuous guidance preserves desired movement kinematics, reducing actual movement errors. The absence of errors eventually leads to a reduction of effort and, thus, negatively affects the overall effectiveness of the training [173]. Therefore, VR-based feedback of movement is an important factor for motor learning, since it allows patients to evaluate their movement success as well as detect potential movement errors [3, 94]. Conventional concepts that are mostly being deployed are, for example, verbal feedback and mirrors placed in front of the patients, in order to give visual and/or acoustic feedback [4]. However, more and more computer-assisted feedback methods are currently entering the clinical sites, such as audiovisual bio-feedback and VR technologies [5].

One can distinguish two different types of VR-based feedback. First, feedback as being used in assistive devices has the primary goal to inform or warn the user about different environmental or body-related situations, such as high joint loads, battery depletion, obstacles, etc. The number of signals and the amount of information are usually limited to avoid confusion of the user and the persons in her or his vicinity. Consequently, signals are displayed in a time-discrete way, only when needed, and not in a continuous manner. In contrast, in therapeutic applications, the feedback signal contains a rather rich amount of information about the kind and quality of the movement performed usually displayed in a continuous or quasi-continuous manner. This is required to shape the movement and the underlying neuronal and muscular activity in a continuous way, resulting in a satisfactory gait or arm function that holds on in the long run.

Relevance of complexity

The complexity of rehabilitation systems often depends on the level of impairment of patients. If the level of impairment and required functionality of the rehabilitation system is low, inexpensive options often suffice. An example is augmenting a simple glove with Xbox instead of expensive custom-made gloves for finger training in post-stroke patients [174]. Gesture recognition systems are another way of providing inexpensive and immersive virtual reality-based rehabilitation for mildly impaired patients. A prominent example of such a device is Microsoft's Kinect (http://www.microsoft.com/en-us/kinectforwindows/), which has been used to make several interactive and motivating VR-based rehabilitation systems [175, 176].

Another wireless controller is Nintendo's Wii (http://www.nintendo.com/wii), which has also been successfully applied to rehabilitation. In a pilot randomized clinical trial with stroke patients, Saposnik et al. [177] used the Wii in conjunction with publicly available sports and cooking virtual reality environments. They found that, compared to recreational training, the group of stroke patients using the Wii showed significant improvement in standard motor function tests [177]. Wii has been a popular off-the-shelf activity-promoting device used in other studies such as in balance rehabilitation in patients with acquired brain injury [178], in complementing traditional rehabilitation [179], in cerebral palsy rehabilitation [180], and in movement therapy to promote upper-extremity function post-stroke [181].

Popular video games are increasingly being rediscovered and used in rehabilitation. For example, a 3D version of the popular game Tetris® (http://www.tetris.com/) was used to evaluate flexible thinking in deaf and hard of hearing children, and it was found that practising 3D spatial rotations did indeed improve flexible thinking [182]. Tetris has found another use in early PTSD therapy, when the symptoms of the disorder are not full blown. In a pilot study [183], participants underwent simulated post-traumatic stress by watching a film consisting of scenes of injury and death. The experimental group, who played Tetris®, had a reduced frequency of flashback of the traumatic scenes as compared to the control group that did no task [183]. Tetris has also found use in cognitive rehabilitation for increasing reaction time and a positive sense of well-being among elderly persons [184]. Playing simple arcade video games like Pacman and Donkey Kong

were also found to enhance reaction time among elderly persons [185, 186] but not cognition. Therefore, more complex games would be required to train other cognitive functions like executive control and memory processes.

On the other end of the spectrum are more sophisticated rehabilitation systems which are required in the case of more severely impaired patients, or in disorders for which simple games do not suffice. An example of a high-end system is an immersive virtual environment, consisting of computers, real-time graphics, visual displays, body tracking sensors, and specialized interface devices that serve to immerse a participant in a computer-generated simulated world that changes in a natural way with head and body motion [187]. The capacity of VR technology to create controllable, multisensory, interactive 3D stimulus environments, within which a person can become immersed and interact, offers clinical assessment and intervention options that are not possible using simple games or traditional neuropsychological methods [187]. This is relevant for cases in which the nature of the disorder under therapy often precludes the use of simple computer games, for example full-fledged PTSD. PTSD is often encountered in veterans who are returning from combat, which is enormously stressful from a physical, emotional, cognitive, and psychological perspective [188]. Therefore, PTSD therapy must reflect that intensity [188], which can be achieved with immersive VR, and which is not possible with simple games or traditional neuropsychological methods. Additionally, persons undergoing immersive VR therapy can practise in a controlled environment and can measure their success in real-time through feedback [189]. Numerous researchers have used immersive VR systems for PTSD therapy with positive results [150–153].

For severely motor-impaired patients who cannot support themselves during therapy, for example stroke patients who have an impaired limb, sophisticated systems take the form of robot-assisted therapy. A robot can support the patient's impaired limb, making therapy less demanding both for the patients and the human therapist [190]. Additionally, robotic devices can also implement novel forms of mechanical manipulation that are impossible for therapists to emulate, which may ultimately enhance movement recovery of patients [190]. Robot-assisted rehabilitation can be extended by adding immersive VR with head-mounted display and haptic feedback so that patients can feel and manipulate objects in a large 3D workspace. Haptic devices can also be used as standalone rehabilitation interfaces, by providing different kinds of adjustable haptic forces like assistance and friction that can be changed in magnitude according to the level of disorder of the patient [191]. Another complex immersive VR environment, which can be used for rehabilitation is a 'cave' consisting of a room whose walls, ceiling and floor surround a viewer with projected images on a virtual reality environment [31].

Looking at the landscape of rehabilitation systems, one can conclude that although off-the-shelf games and hardware can be, and indeed are, used for rehabilitation, their applicability is restricted to mild disorders. When the severity of the disorder is high, sophisticated, custom-built VR environments and hardware are more appropriate.

Clinical relevance and evidence

Abovementioned applications and results indicate that patients' motor and cognitive functions can be improved through the use of VR technologies. Plenty of single case studies and some larger randomized clinical trials have been performed showing specific beneficial effects in many therapeutic and assistive areas. Increased engagement and motivation, improved performance, and often also positive physiotherapeutic outcomes were observed. Such studies include VR-aided treatment of single joints using haptic input devices, gait training studies performed on a treadmill with or without robotic support, arm therapy studies applying kinematic input devices or robotic support. Positive effects have been observed also when VR is applied for balance or back training. Additionally, VR technology has been used for the training of cognitive function, for example to increase motivation and engagement, to treat patients with mild cognitive impairments, dementia, TBI, ADHD, or ASD. In the area of psychotherapy, VR has been applied not only to the treatment of many different phobias such as aviatophobia, claustrophobia, and social phobias, but also to the treatment of eating disorders and PTSD.

There is a subgroup of applications, where feedback of information as provided by a display device of a VR system serves mainly to deliver an assistive function in the patient's home or work environment or during leisure. This can help elderly or patients with motor or sensory impairments to better cope with the challenges of daily life. Any additional therapeutic effect in these applications is, however, not excluded, but even desired.

Abovementioned studies show that sensory-motor or cognitive functions of patients can be improved through the application of VR technology. A systematic review performed by Henderson et al. [192] provides some evidence that movement training with immersive VR yields functional improvements in the upper extremities of stroke patients. In contrast, Laver et al. [193] published another systematic review, based on the selection of 19 younger studies, where they concluded that the effect of interactive games shows only limited improvements of arm and gait function in stroke patients. However, several studies are still ongoing and, so far, it is not at all clear, which kind of feedback and intensity must be applied at which phase after the stroke to obtain the maximum outcome.

Limitations of current systems

Rizzo et al. [194] came to the conclusion that the field of VR rehabilitation is still in an early phase. While weaknesses in areas of interface and display technologies are apparent, they do not threaten the viability of the field. They further concluded, that VR-technology in rehabilitation will continue to grow, gain further mainstream acceptance and eventually have a significant, positive impact on rehabilitation sciences [194]. Similarly, Adamovic et al. [195] concluded that VR-technology may be an 'optimal tool for designing therapies that target neuroplastic mechanisms in the nervous system', since it allows training in complex environments that might not be possible in the real world. They, however, point out, that the full potential of VR in rehabilitation will only emerge after research has identified the effect of various sensory-motor manipulations on neural processes [195].

Thus, the limitations of current systems can be discussed from two points of views: first, from the effect on the human user, and second, from the usability of the technology. With respect to the effects on the human user, it is not fully understood which technical features cause which motivational and therapeutic effect. Technical features to be distinguished concern the complexity of the displayed information, such as the displayed dimension (2D/3D), bandwidth and ranges, kind of rendered information, quality of the signals, kind of virtual environment, number of objects, story and game elements etc. The features implemented can have different effects on the user's perception, experienced presence, engagement, and eventually, on the therapeutic outcome.

Usability of the technology refers to the complexity of the technical components, and includes aspects such as weight and size, donning and doffing time, comfort, adjustability, adaptability, and immersion. Usability and price of the technology affect, eventually, the acceptance by the wearer and the clinician who is working with the technology. It is clear, that current VR systems are not optimal with respect to both effect on the human user and usability of the technology.

Outlook

So far, neither individual patient characteristics, nor the perspectives of the clinician, and the dynamics between the individual, clinician, and the technology are taken into account when prescribing the right amount and modality of motor or cognitive training features. However, not much is known so far about the exact mechanisms that may lead to a meaningful outcome for the *individual* subject. The different features of the VR technology have different effects on individuals. It is always only a special choice of specific adjustments and choices of VR features that may have an effect on an individual subject with his or her specific clinical properties.

Future studies will analyse further clinical data of large randomized clinical trials, in order to find clusters of responders (in contrast to non-responders) that show a significant rehabilitation outcome as a function of specific VR features and modalities. This may lead to novel individualized VR-enhanced training concepts that, for the first time, take into account single-patient perspective and clinical expertise to maximize the rehabilitation outcome of that individual patient.

In a later step this may lead to novel diagnostic tests providing predictors or markers that will allow screening and classifying of patients into different groups. Depending on the group, only specific technical modalities may be required to treat the individual. In this way, specific individualized technologies and training paradigms may be applied in a more effective way.

Further developments will yield novel technical systems that will be easier to don and doff, more comfortable to wear, provide a much better immersion, and will have no or only little technical artefacts and physiological side effects, such as cybersickness. This will increase the acceptance of the technology, if the therapeutic effect is significant, and the price tolerable.

Conclusion

VR is a powerful tool to motivate the participants to actively participate, while it provides augmented performance feedback. VR-enhanced rehabilitation settings can provide a highly motivating training that can be superior to training in a real situation. Increased motivation and active participation can lead to increased efficiency and advancements of motor learning in neurorehabilitation.

Several applications exist showing that patients' motor and cognitive functions can be improved through the use of VR technologies. Plenty of single case studies and some larger randomized clinical trials have been performed showing specific beneficial effects in many therapeutic and assistive areas. Increased engagement and motivation, improved performance, and often also positive physiotherapeutic outcomes were observed.

Despite the many technological achievements and positive results in many therapeutic and assistive applications, not much is known so far about the exact mechanisms that may lead to a meaningful outcome for the individual subject. Therefore, randomized clinical trials will have to find clusters of responders that show a significant rehabilitation outcome as a function of specific VR features and modalities. This may lead to novel individualized VR-enhanced training concepts that will take into account single patient perspective and clinical expertise to maximize the rehabilitation outcome of individual patients.

Acknowledgements

Special thanks go to Aniket Nagle, Domen Novak, Roland Sigrist, and Lukas Zimmerli who contributed to the writing and editing of this book chapter.

References

1. Britannica E. 'Virtual Reality (VR)'; 2011. Encyclopædia Britannica Online. Available from: http://www.britannica.com/EBchecked/topic/630181/virtual-reality (accessed 21 August 2014).
2. Subramanian S, Knaut L, Beaudoin C, McFadyen B, Feldman A, Levin M. Virtual reality environments for post-stroke arm rehabilitation. J Neuroeng Rehabil. 2007;4(1):20.
3. van Vliet PM, Wulf G. Extrinsic feedback for motor learning after stroke: What is the evidence? Disabil Rehabil. 2006;28(13):831–840.
4. Dobkin BH. The Clinical Science of Neurologic Rehabilitation, 2nd edn. Oxford University Press, New York, 2003.
5. Horowitz S. Biofeedback applications: a survey of clinical research. Altern Comp Ther. 2006;12(6):275–281.
6. Chiviacowsky S, Wulf G. Feedback after good trials enhances learning. Res Q Exerc Sport. 2007;78:40–47.
7. Holden MK. Virtual environments for motor rehabilitation: review. Cyberpsychol Behav. 2005;8(3):187–211.
8. Didier JP. Learning and teaching: two processes to bear in mind when rethinking physical medicine and rehabilitation. In: Rethinking physical and rehabilitation medicine. Collection de L'Académie Européenne de Médecine de Réadaptation. Springer, Paris, 2010, pp. 3–17.
9. Riener R, Harders M. Virtual reality in medicine. Springer, Berlin, 2012.
10. Kim YY, Kim EN, Park MJ, Park KS, Ko HD, Kim HT. The application of biosignal feedback for reducing cybersickness from exposure to a virtual environment. Presence: Teleoperators and Virtual Environments. 2008;17(1):1–16.
11. Kwakkel G, Wagenaar RC, Koelman TW, Lankhorst GJ, Koetsier JC. Effects of intensity of rehabilitation after stroke. A research synthesis. Stroke. 1997;28(8):1550–1556.
12. Liebermann DG, Buchman AS, Franks IM. Enhancement of motor rehabilitation through the use of information technologies. Clin Biomech. 2006;21(1):8–20.
13. Bonaiuti D, Rebasti L, Sioli P. The constraint induced movement therapy: a systematic review of randomised controlled trials on the adult stroke patients. Eur J Phys Rehabil Med. 2007;43(2):139–146.
14. Loureiro R, Amirabdollahian F, Cootes S, Stokes E, Harwin W. Using haptics technology to deliver motivational therapies in stroke patients: Concepts and initial pilot studies. Proceedings of Eurohaptics 2001, Birmingham, UK. 2001, p. 6.
15. Johnson MJ. Recent trends in robot-assisted therapy environments to improve real-life functional performance after stroke. J Neuroeng Rehabil. 2006;3:29.
16. Zimmerli L, Jacky M, Lünenburger L, Riener R, Bolliger M. Increasing patient engagement during virtual reality–based motor rehabilitation. Arch Phys Med Rehabil. 2013;.
17. Lövquist E, Dreifaldt U. The design of a haptic exercise for post-stroke arm rehabilitation. In: Proceedings of the 6th International Conference on Disability, Virtual Reality & Associated Technologies. Esbjerg, Denmark: Citeseer, 2006, pp. 18–20.
18. Pareto L, Broeren J, Goude D, Rydmark M. Virtual reality, haptics and post-stroke rehabilitation in practical therapy. In: Proceedings of the 7th International Conference on Disability, Virtual Reality & Associated Technologies, with ArtAbilitation. Maia, Portugal, 2008, pp. 245–252.
19. Cameirão MS, Badia BS, Oller ED, Verschure PFMJ. Neurorehabilitation using the virtual reality based Rehabilitation Gaming System: methodology, design, psychometrics, usability and validation. J Neuroeng Rehabil. 2010;7(1):1–14.
20. Reid D. A model of playfulness and flow in virtual reality interactions. Presence: Teleoperators and Virtual Environments. 2004;13(4):451–462.
21. Riva G, Castelnuovo G, Mantovani F. Transformation of flow in rehabilitation: The role of advanced communication technologies. Behav Res Methods. 2006;38(2):237–244.
22. Zimmerli L, Krewer C, Gassert R, et al. Validation of a mechanism to balance exercise difficulty in robot-assisted upper-extremity rehabilitation after stroke. J Neuroeng Rehabil. 2012;9(1):1–13.
23. Patel S, Park H, Bonato P, et al. A review of wearable sensors and systems with application in rehabilitation. J Neuroeng Rehabil. 2012;9(12):1–17.
24. Zhou H, Hu H. Human motion tracking for rehabilitation—A survey. Biomed Signal Proc Control. 2008;3(1):1–18.
25. Barea R, Boquete L, Mazo M, López E. System for assisted mobility using eye movements based on electrooculography. IEEE Trans Neural Syst Rehabil Eng. 2002;10(4):209–218.
26. Ballou G. Handbook for sound engineers. Focal Press, Burlington MA, 2005.
27. Benzeghiba M, De Mori R, Deroo O, et al. Automatic speech recognition and speech variability: A review. Speech Communication. 2007;49(10–11):763–786. Intrinsic Speech Variations.
28. Andreassi JL. Psychophysiology: Human Behavior and Physiological Response, 5th edn. Lawrence Erlbaum Associates, Inc., Mahwah, NJ, 2007.
29. Koenig A, Omlin X, Zimmerli L, et al. Psychological state estimation from physiological recordings during robot assisted gait rehabilitation. J Rehabil Res Dev. 2011;48(4):367–386.
30. Krueger W, Froehlich B. The responsive workbench. computer graphics and applications, iEEE. 1994;14(3):12–15.
31. Cruz-Neira C, Sandin DJ, DeFanti TA, Kenyon RV, Hart JC. The CAVE: audio visual experience automatic virtual environment. Communications of the ACM. 1992;35(6):64–72.
32. Sutherland IE. A head-mounted three dimensional display. In: Proceedings of the December 9-11, 1968, fall joint computer conference, part I. AFIPS '68 (Fall, part I). ACM; New York, NY, 1968, pp. 757–764.
33. Coles TR, Meglan D, John NW. The role of haptics in medical training simulators: a survey of the state of the art. IEEE Trans Haptics. 2011;4(1):51–66.
34. Sledd A. Performance enhancement of a haptic arm exoskeleton. haptic interfaces for virtual environment and teleoperator systems. Haptics'06, Arlington, VA, USA, 14th Symposium on Haptics. 2006, pp. 375–381.
35. Koo IM, Jung K, Koo JC, Nam JD, Lee YK, Choi HR. Development of soft-actuator-based wearable tactile display. IEEE Trans Robotics. 2008;24(3):549–558.

36. Kaufman A, Mueller K. Overview of volume rendering. In: Hansen CD, Johnson CR, editors. The Visualization Handbook. Academic Press, London, 2005, pp. 127–174.

37. Funkhouser T. Sounds Good to Me! Computational Sound for Graphics, Virtual Reality, and Interactive Systems. SIGGRAPH 2002, San Antonio, TX. 2002.

38. Wand M, Strasser W. A real-time sound rendering algorithm for complex scenes. Technical Note, University of Tübingen, WSI-2003-5, ISSN 0946-3852 2003.

39. Zimmerli L, Verschure P. Delivering environmental presence through procedural virtual environments. In: Presence 2007: The 10th Annual International Workshop on Presence, Foment de les Arts Decoratives (FAD), Barcelona, Spain 2007, pp. 335–338.

40. Bernardi L, Porta C, Sleight P. Cardiovascular, cerebrovascular, and respiratory changes induced by different types of music in musicians and non-musicians: the importance of silence. Heart. 2006;**92**(4):445–452.

41. Bradley MM, Lang PJ. Affective reactions to acoustic stimuli. Psychophysiology. 2000 **2**;37:204–215.

42. Tanney S, Schwartz P, Yen S, Shen L, Furness T. A design method for virtual environments using narrative and pattern languages. Technical Report R-98-13, Human Interface Technology Lab, University of Washington, 1998.

43. Ibanez J, Aylett R,Ruiz-Rodarte R. Storytelling in virtual environments from a virtual guide perspective. Virtual Reality. 2003;**7**(1):30–42.

44. Johnson WL, Vilhjálmsson, Marsella S. Serious games for language learning: How much game, how much AI? In: AIED (Artificial Intelligence in Education: Supporting Learning through Intelligent and Socially Informed Technology). Proceedings of the 2005 conference on Artificial Intelligence in Education: Supporting Learning through Intelligent and Socially Informed Technology vol. 125; 2005, pp. 306–313.

45. Connolly TM, Boyle EA, MacArthur E, Hainey T, Boyle JM. A systematic literature review of empirical evidence on computer games and serious games. Computers Educ. 2012;**59**(2):661–686.

46. Reeve C. Narrative-based serious games. In: Petrovic O, Brand A (eds) Serious Games on the Move. Springer, Vienna, 2009, pp. 73–89.

47. McQuiggan S, Rowe J, Lee S, Lester J. Story-based learning: the impact of narrative on learning experiences and outcomes. In: Woolf B, Aïmeur E, Nkambou R, Lajoie S (eds) Intelligent Tutoring Systems. vol. 5091 of Lecture Notes in Computer Science. Springer, Berlin, Heidelberg, 2008, pp. 530–539.

48. Bopp MM. Storytelling and motivation in serious games. Research Report of the Enhanced Learning Experience and Knowledge Transfer Project (ELEKTRA), available from http://cordis.europa.eu/project/rcn/80640_en.html accessed 29 September 2014.

49. McDaniel R, Fiore SM, Nicholson D. Serious storytelling: Narrative considerations for serious games researchers and developers. Serious Game Design and Development: Technologies for Training and Learning. 2010;13–30.

50. Malone TW. What makes things fun to learn? Heuristics for designing instructional computer games. In: Proceedings of the 3rd ACM SIGSMALL symposium and the first SIGPC symposium on Small systems. ACM, 1980, pp. 162–169.

51. Csikszentmihalyi M. Beyond boredom and anxiety. Jossey-Bass, San Francisco, 2000.

52. Mehta M, Ram A. Runtime Behavior adaptation for real-time interactive games. IEEE Trans Computat Intellig AI Games. 2009;**1**(3):187–199.

53. Tan CH, Tan KC, Tay A. Dynamic game difficulty scaling using adaptive behavior-based AI. IEEE Trans Computat Intellig AI Games. 2011;**3**(4):289–301.

54. Peirce N, Conlan O, Wade V. Adaptive educational games: providing non-invasive personalised learning experiences. In: Second IEEE International Conference on Digital Games and Intelligent Toys Based Education, DIGITEL 2008, Banff, AB, Canada, pp. 28–35.

55. Vogel JJ, Greenwood-Ericksen A, Cannon-Bowers J, Bowers CA. Using virtual reality with and without gaming attributes for academic achievement. J Res Technol Educ. 2006;**39**(1):105–118.

56. Ryan RM, Deci EL. Self-determination theory and the facilitation of intrinsic motivation, social development, and well-being. Am Psychol. 2000;**55**(1):68–78.

57. Deci EL, Koestner R, Ryan RM. A meta-analytic review of experiments examining the effects of extrinsic rewards on intrinsic motivation. Psychol Bull. 1999;**125**(6):627–668.

58. Cameron J, Pierce WD. Reinforcement, reward, and intrinsic motivation: a meta-analysis. Rev Educ Res. 1994;**64**(3):363–423.

59. Toups Z, Kerne A, Hamilton W. Motivating play through score. In: ACM Computer Human Interaction 2009 Workshop on Engagement by Design, 2009, CHI 2009, Boston, MA, USA, pp. 4–9.

60. King D, Delfabbro P, Griffiths M. Video game structural characteristics: a new psychological taxonomy. Int J Ment Health Addiction. 2010;**8**(1):90–106.

61. Girone M, Burdea G, Bouzit M, Popescu V, Deutsch JE. Orthopedic rehabilitation using the 'Rutgers ankle' interface. Medicine Meets Virtual Reality. 2000;**70**:89–95.

62. Mirelman A, Bonato P, Deutsch J. Comparative study randomized controlled trial research support. Stroke. 2009;**40**(1):169–174.

63. Baram Y, Miller A. Virtual reality cues for improvement of gait in patients with multiple sclerosis. Neurology. 2006;**66**(2):178–181.

64. Fung J, Richards CL, Malouin F, McFadyen BJ, Lamontagne A. A treadmill and motion coupled virtual reality system for gait training post-stroke. Cyberpsychol Behav. 2006;**9**(2):157–162.

65. Jaffe DL, Brown DA, Pierson-Carey CD, Buckley EL, Lew HL. Stepping over obstacles to improve walking in individuals with poststroke hemiplegia. J Rehabil Res Dev. 2004;**41**(3):283–292.

66. Chuang TY, Sung WH, Lin CY. Application of a virtual reality–enhanced exercise protocol in patients after coronary bypass. Arch Phys Med Rehabil. 2005;**86**(10):1929–1932.

67. Yang YR, Tsai MP, Chuang TY, Sung WH, Wang RY. Virtual reality-based training improves community ambulation in individuals with stroke: A randomized controlled trial. Gait Posture. 2008;**28**(2):201–206.

68. van Ooijen M, Roerdink M, Trekop M, Visschedijk J, Janssen T, Beek P. Functional gait rehabilitation in elderly people following a fall-related hip fracture using a treadmill with visual context: design of a randomized controlled trial. BMC Geriatr. 2013;**13**(1):34.

69. Heeren J, van Ooijen M, Janssen T, et al. C-mill therapy improves gait adaptability in the chronic phase after stroke. In: 7th World Congress for NeuroRehabilitation. vol. 26. Melbourne, Australia, 2012, p. 76.

70. Deutsch J, Paserchia C, Vecchione C, et al. Improved gait and elevation speed of individuals post-stroke after lower extremity training in virtual environments. J Neurol Phys Ther. 2004;**28**(4):185–186.

71. Weghorst S. Augmented reality and Parkinson's disease. Comm ACM. 1997;**40**(8):47–48.

72. Husemann B, Muller F, Krewer C, Heller S, Koenig E. Effects of locomotion training with assistance of a robot-driven gait orthosis in hemiparetic patients after stroke: a randomized controlled pilot study. Stroke. 2007;**38**(2):349–354.

73. Colombo G, Joerg M, Schreier R, Dietz V. Treadmill training of paraplegic patients using a robotic orthosis. J Rehabil Res Dev. 2000;**37**(6):693–700.

74. Riener R, Lünenburger L, Maier IC, Colombo G, Dietz V. Locomotor training in subjects with sensori-motor deficits: an overview of the robotic gait orthosis Lokomat. J Healthcare Eng. 2010;**1**(2):197–216.

75. Stauffer Y, Allemand Y, Bouri M, et al. The WalkTrainer–a new generation of walking reeducation device combining orthoses

and muscle stimulation. IEEE Trans Neural Syst Rehabil Eng. 2009;**17**(1):38–45.

76. Veneman JF, Kruidhof R, Hekman EE, Ekkelenkamp R, Van Asseldonk EH, van der Kooij H. Design and evaluation of the LOPES exoskeleton robot for interactive gait rehabilitation. IEEE Trans Neural Syst Rehabil Eng. 2007;**15**(3):379–386.

77. Brütsch K, Schuler T, Koenig A, et al. Influence of virtual reality soccer game on walking performance in robotic assisted gait training for children. J Neuroeng Rehabil. 2010;**7**(1):15.

78. Brütsch K, Koenig A, Zimmerli L, et al. Virtual reality for enhancement of robot-assisted gait training in children with neurological gait disorders. J Rehabil Med. 2011;**43**(6):493–499.

79. Koenig A, Wellner M, Koneke S, Meyer-Heim A, Lunenburger L, Riener R. Virtual gait training for children with cerebral palsy using the Lokomat gait orthosis. Studies Health Technol Informat. 2008;**132**:204–209.

80. Patritti B, Sicari M, Deming L, et al. Enhancing robotic gait training via augmented feedback. In: Engineering in Medicine and Biology Society (EMBC), Annual International Conference of the IEEE, 2010, Buenos Aires, Argentina, pp. 2271–2274.

81. Zimmerli L, Duschau-Wicke A, Riener R, Mayr A, Lünenburger L. Virtual reality and gait rehabilitation: Augmented feedback for the Lokomat. In: International Conference on Virtual Rehabilitation, Haifa, Israel, 2009, pp. 150–153.

82. Wellner M, Schaufelberger A, von Zitzewitz J, Riener R. Evaluation of visual and auditory feedback in virtual obstacle walking. Presence: Teleoperators and Virtual Environments. 2008;**17**(5):512–524.

83. Winter DA. Biomechanics and Motor Control of Human Movement, 3rd edn. John Wiley & Sons Inc., Hoboken, NJ, 1990.

84. Chen Y, Duff M, Lehrer N, et al. A novel adaptive mixed reality system for stroke rehabilitation: principles, proof of concept, and preliminary application in 2 patients. Top Stroke Rehabil. 2011;**18**(3):212–230.

85. Duff M, Chen Y, Attygalle S, et al. An adaptive mixed reality training system for stroke rehabilitation. IEEE Trans Neural Syst Rehabil Eng. 2010;**18**(5):531–541.

86. King M, Hale L, Pekkari A, Persson M, Gregorsson M, Nilsson M. An affordable, computerised, table-based exercise system for stroke survivors. Disabil Rehabil Assist Technol. 2010;**5**(4):288–293. PMID: 20302419.

87. Mumford N, Duckworth J, Thomas PR, Shum D, Williams G, Wilson PH. Upper limb virtual rehabilitation for traumatic brain injury: Initial evaluation of the elements system. Brain Inj. 2010;**24**(5):780–791. PMID: 20353283.

88. Alamri A, Eid M, Iglesias R, Shirmohammadi S, El-Saddik A. Haptic virtual rehabilitation exercises for poststroke diagnosis. IEEE Trans Instrument Measurement. 2008;**57**(9):1876–1884.

89. Merians AS, Poizner H, Boian R, Burdea G, Adamovich S. Sensorimotor training in a virtual reality environment: does it improve functional recovery poststroke? Neurorehabil Neural Repair. 2006;**20**(2):252–267.

90. Connelly L, Jia Y, Toro ML, Stoykov ME, Kenyon RV, Kamper DG. A Pneumatic glove and immersive virtual reality environment for hand rehabilitative training after stroke. IEEE Trans Neural Syst Rehabil Eng. 2010;**18**(5):551–559.

91. Fong K, Chow K, Chan B, et al. Usability of a virtual reality environment simulating an automated teller machine for assessing and training persons with acquired brain injury. J Neuroeng Rehabil. 2010;**7**(1):1–9.

92. Lewis GN, Woods C, Rosie JA, Mcpherson KM. Virtual reality games for rehabilitation of people with stroke: perspectives from the users. Disabil Rehabil Assist Technol. 2011;**6**(5):453–463. PMID: 21495917.

93. Piron L, Tonin P, Atzori AM, et al. The augmented-feedback rehabilitation technique facilitates the arm motor recovery in patients after a recent stroke. Studies Health Technol Informat. 2003;p. 265–267.

94. Subramanian SK, Massie CL, Malcolm MP, Levin MF. Does provision of extrinsic feedback result in improved motor learning in the upper limb poststroke? A Systematic review of the evidence. Neurorehabil Neural Repair. 2010;**24**(2):113–124.

95. Huang H, Ingalls T, Olson L, Ganley K, Rikakis T, He J. Interactive multimodal biofeedback for task-oriented neural rehabilitation. In: 27th Annual International Conference of the Engineering in Medicine and Biology Society. IEEE-EMBS 2005. Shanghai, 2005, pp. 2547–2550.

96. Krebs HI, Hogan N, Volpe BT, Aisen ML, Edelstein L, Diels C. Overview of clinical trials with MIT-MANUS: a robot-aided neuro-rehabilitation facility. Technol Health Care. 1999;**7**(6):419–423.

97. Housman SJ, Le V, Rahman T, Sanchez RJ, Reinkensmeyer DJ. Arm-training with T-WREX after chronic stroke: preliminary results of a randomized controlled trial. In: IEEE International Conference on Rehabilitation Robotics (ICORR), Noordwijk, The Netherlands, 2007,p p. 562–568.

98. Hesse S, Werner C, Pohl M, Rueckriem S, Mehrholz J, Lingnau ML. Computerized arm training improves the motor control of the severely affected arm after stroke. Stroke. 2005;**36**:1960–1966.

99. Harwin W, Loureiro R, Amirabdollahian F, et al. The GENTLE/S project: A new method of delivering neuro-rehabilitation. Assistive Technology—Added Value to the Quality of Life AAATE. 2001;**1**:36–41.

100. Lum P, Burgar C, Van der Loos M, Shor P, Majmundar M, Yap R. MIME robotic device for upper-limb neurorehabilitation in subacute stroke subjects: A follow-up study. J Rehabil Res Dev. 2006;**43**(5):631–642.

101. Broeren J, Rydmark M, Björkdahl A, Sunnerhagen KS. Assessment and training in a 3-dimensional virtual environment with haptics: a report on 5 cases of motor rehabilitation in the chronic stage after stroke. Neurorehabil Neural Repair. 2007;**21**(2):180–189.

102. Choi Y, Gordon J, Park H, Schweighofer N. Feasibility of the adaptive and automatic presentation of tasks (ADAPT) system for rehabilitation of upper extremity function post-stroke. J Neuroeng Rehabil. 2011;**8**(1):1–12.

103. Nef T, Guidali M, Riener R. ARMin III—arm therapy exoskeleton with an ergonomic shoulder actuation. Appl Bionics Biomech. 2009;**6**(2):127–142.

104. Bouzit M, Burdea G, Popescu G, Boian R. The Rutgers Master II-new design force-feedback glove. IEEE/ASME Trans Mechatronics. 2002;**7**(2):256–263.

105. Bayona NA, Bitensky J, Salter K, Teasell R. The role of task-specific training in rehabilitation therapies. Top Stroke Rehabil. 2005;**12**(3):58–65.

106. Adamovich SV, Merians AS, Boian R, et al. A virtual reality-based exercise system for hand rehabilitation post-stroke. Presence: Teleoperators and Virtual Environments. 2005;**14**(2):161–174.

107. Broeren J, Claesson L, Goude D, Rydmark M, Sunnerhagen KS. Virtual rehabilitation in an activity centre for community-dwelling persons with stroke. Cerebrovasc Dis. 2008;**26**(3):289–296.

108. Podobnik J, Munih M, Cinkelj J. HARMiS—Hand and arm rehabilitation system. In: Proceedings of 7th International Conference on Disability, Virtual Reality & Associated Technologies, Maia and Porto, Portugal, 2008, pp. 237–244.

109. Boian R, Sharma A, Han C, et al. Virtual reality-based post-stroke hand rehabilitation. In: Proceedings of Medicine Meets Virtual Reality. vol. 85. Newport Beach CA, IOS Press, 2002, pp. 64–70.

110. Colombo R, Pisano F, Delconte C, Micera CMC S, Dario P, Minuco G. Design strategies to improve patient motivation during robot-aided rehabilitation. J Neuro-eng PMCID. 2007;**4**(3):12.

111. Mihelj M, Novak D, Milavec M, Ziherl J, Olenšek A, Munih M. Virtual rehabilitation environment using principles of intrinsic motivation and game design. Presence: Teleoperators and Virtual Environments. 2012;**21**(1):1–15.

112. Guidali M, Duschau-Wicke A, Broggi S, Klamroth-Marganska V, Nef T, Riener R. A robotic system to train activities of daily living in a virtual environment. Med Biol Eng Computing. 2011;49(10):1213–1223.

113. Jacobson J, Redfern M, Furman J, et al. Balance NAVE: a virtual reality facility for research and rehabilitation of balance disorders. Proceedings of the ACM Symposium on Virtual Reality Software and Technology, Banff, AB, Canada, 2001, pp. 103–109.

114. Bisson E, Contant B, Sveistrup H, Lajoie Y. Functional balance and dual-task reaction times in older adults are improved by virtual reality and biofeedback training. Cyberpsychol Behav. 2007;10(1):16–23.

115. Kim JH, Jang SH, Kim CS, Jung JH, You JH. Use of virtual reality to enhance balance and ambulation in chronic stroke: a double-blind, randomized controlled study. Am J Phys Med Rehabil. 2009;88(9):693–701.

116. Betker AL, Desai A, Nett C, Kapadia N, Szturm T. Game-based exercises for dynamic short-sitting balance rehabilitation of people with chronic spinal cord and traumatic brain injuries. Phys Ther. 2007;87(10):1389–1398.

117. Robertson IH, Murre JMJ. Rehabilitation of brain damage: brain plasticity and prinicples of guided recovery. Psychol Bull. 1999;125(32):544–575.

118. Redding GM, Rader SD, Lucas DR. Cognitive load and prism adaptation. J Motor Behav. 1992;24(3):238–246.

119. Taylor JA, Thoroughman KA. Motor adaptation scaled by the difficulty of a secondary cognitive task. PLoS One. 2008;3(6):e2485.

120. Novak D, Ziherl J, Olensek A, et al. Psychophysiological responses to robotic rehabilitation tasks in stroke. IEEE Trans Neural Syst Rehabil Eng. 2010;18(4):351–361.

121. Novak D, Mihelj M, Ziherl J, Olensek A, Munih M. Psychophysiological measurements in a biocooperative feedback loop for upper extremity rehabilitation. IEEE Trans Neural Syst Rehabil Eng. 2011;19(4):400–410.

122. Koenig A, Novak D, Omlin X, et al. Real-time closed-loop control of cognitive load in neurological patients during robot-assisted gait training. IEEE Trans Neural Syst Rehabil Eng. 2011;19(4):453–464.

123. Badesa FJ, Morales R, Garcia-Aracil N, Sabater JM, Perez-Vidal C, Fernandez E. Multimodal interfaces to improve therapeutic outcomes in robot-assisted rehabilitation. IEEE Trans Syst Man Cybernet Part C: Appl Rev. 2012;42(6):1152–1158.

124. Guerrero CR, Marinero JCF, Turiel JP, Muñoz V. Using 'human state aware' robots to enhance physical human–robot interaction in a cooperative scenario. Computer Methods Programs Biomed. 2013;112(2):250–259.

125. Shirzad N, Van der Loos HFM. Adaptation of Task Difficulty in Rehabilitation Exercises Based on the User's Motor Performance and Physiological Responses. In: IEEE International Conference on Rehabilitation Robotics (ICORR). Seattle, Washington, USA, 2013, pp. 1–6. Available from http://ieeexplore.ieee.org/xpl/articleDetails.jsp?arnumber=6650429&refinements%3D4269248155%26punumber%3D6636282%26sortType%3Dasc_p_Sequence%26filter%3DAND%28p_IS_Number%3A6650332%29 (accessed 29 September 2014).

126. Hugdahl K. Psychophysiology: The mind-body Perspective. Harvard University Press, Cambridge MA, 1995.

127. Guo WH, Lim SYE, Fok SC, Chan GYC. Virtual reality for memory rehabilitation. Int J Computer Appl Technol. 2004;21(1/2):32–37.

128. Kizony R, Korman M, Sinoff G, Klinger N E Josman. Using a virtual supermarket as a tool for training executive functions in people with mild cognitive impairment. In: Proceedings of the 9th International Conference on Disability, Virtual Reality & Associated Technologies. Laval, France, 2012..

129. Optale G, Urgesi C, Busato V, et al. Controlling memory impairment in elderly adults using virtual reality memory training: a randomized controlled pilot study. Neurorehabil Neural Repair. 2010;24(4):348–357.

130. Flynn D, van Schaik P, Blackman T, Femcott C, Hobbs B, Calderon C. Developing a virtual reality-based methodology for

131. people with dementia: A feasibility study. Cyberpsychol Behav. 2003;6(6):591–611.

131. Colombo M, Marelli E, Vaccaro R, et al. Virtual reality for persons with dementia: An exergaming experience. Gerontechnology. 2012;11(2):402–405.

132. Man DWK, Chung JCC, Lee GYY. Evaluation of a virtual reality-based memory training programme for Hong Kong Chinese older adults with questionable dementia: a pilot study. Int J Geriatr Psychiatry. 2012;27(5):513–520.

133. Miller B, Ikonte C, Ponton M, et al. A study of the Lund-Manchester research criteria for frontotemporal dementia. Clinical and single-photon emission CT correlations. Neurology. 1997;48(4):937–941.

134. Cushman LA, Stein K, Duffy CJ. Detecting navigational deficits in cognitive aging and Alzheimer disease using virtual reality. Neurology. 2008;71(12):888–895.

135. Rizzo AA, Buckwalter JG, Neumann U, et al. The virtual reality mental rotation spatial skills project. Cyberpsychol Behav. 1998;1(2):113–119.

136. Bouchard B, Imbeault F, Bouzouane A, Menelas BA. Developing serious games specifically adapted to people suffering from Alzheimer. In: Ma M, Oliveira M, Hauge J, Duin H, Thoben KD (eds) Serious Games Development and Applications. vol. 7528 of Lecture Notes in Computer Science. Springer, Berlin Heidelberg, 2012, pp. 243–254.

137. Matheis RJ, Schultheis MT, Tiersky LA, DeLuca J, Millis SR, Rizzo A. Is learning and memory different in a virtual environment? Clin Neuropsychol. 2007;21(1):146–161.

138. Jacoby M, Averbuch S, Sacher Y, Katz N, Weiss PL, Kizony R. Effectiveness of executive functions training within a virtual supermarket for adults with traumatic brain injury: a pilot study. IEEE Trans Neural Syst Rehabil Eng. 2013;21(2):182–190.

139. Grealy MA, Johnson DA, Rushton SK. Improving cognitive function after brain injury: The use of exercise and virtual reality. Arch Phys Med Rehabil. 1999;80(6):661–667.

140. Gamito P, Oliveira J, Pacheco J, et al. Traumatic brain injury memory training: a virtual reality online solution. Int J Disabil Hum Dev. 2011;10(4):309–312.

141. Rizzo A, Buckwalter J, Bowerly T, et al. The virtual classroom: A Virtual Reality Environment for the assessment and rehabilitation of attention deficits. Cyberpsychol Behav. 2000;3(3):483–499.

142. Cho B, Ku J, Jang D, et al. The effect of virtual reality cognitive training for attention enhancement. Cyberpsychol Behav. 2002;5(2):129–137.

143. Bauminger N, Goren-Bar D, Gal E, et al. Enhancing social communication in high-functioning children with autism through a co-located interface. In: IEEE 9th Workshop on Multimedia Signal Processing (MMSP), Chania, Crete, Greece, 2007, pp. 18–21.

144. Herrera G, Alcantud F, Jordan R, Blanquer A, Labajo G, De Pablo C. Development of symbolic play through the use of virtual reality tools in children with autistic spectrum disorders: Two case studies. Autism. 2008;12(2):143–157.

145. Wiederhold BK, Wiederhold MD. A review of virtual reality as a psychotherapeutic tool. Cyberpsychol Behav. 1998;1(1):45–52.

146. Krijn M, Emmelkamp P, Olafsson R, Biemond R. Virtual reality exposure therapy of anxiety disorders: A review. Clin Psychol Rev. 2004;24(3):259–281.

147. Brahnam S, Jain LC. Advanced computational intelligence paradigms in healthcare 6: Virtual Reality in Psychotherapy, Rehabilitation, and Assessment.. vol. Studies in Computational Intelligence 337. Springer, Berlin, 2011.

148. Yehuda R. Post-traumatic stress disorder. N Engl J Med. 2002;346(2):108–114. PMID: 11784878.

149. Rothbaum BO, Rizzo A, Difede J. Virtual reality exposure therapy for combat-related posttraumatic stress disorder. Ann N Y Acad Sci. 2010;1208(1):126–132.

150. Rizzo A, Newman B, Parsons T, et al. Development and clinical results from the virtual Iraq exposure therapy application for PTSD. In: International Conference on Virtual Rehabilitation, Haifa, Israel, 2009, pp. 8–15.

151. Difede J, Hoffman HG. Virtual reality exposure therapy for World Trade Center post-traumatic stress disorder: A case report. Cyberpsychol Behav. 2002;**5**(6):529–535.

152. Wood DP, Murphy J, Center K, et al. Combat-related post-traumatic stress disorder: A case report using virtual reality exposure therapy with physiological monitoring. Cyberpsychol Behav. 2006;**10**(2):309–315.

153. McLay RN, Wood DP, Webb-Murphy JA, et al. A randomized, controlled trial of virtual reality-graded exposure therapy for post-traumatic stress disorder in active duty service members with combat-related post-traumatic stress disorder. Cyberpsychol Behav Social Netw. 2011;**14**(4):223–229.

154. Bächlin M, Plotnik M, Roggen D, Giladi N, Hausdorff J, Tröster G. A wearable system to assist walking of Parkinson s disease patients. Methods Inf Med. 2010;**49**(1):88–95.

155. Baram Y, Aharon-Peretz J, Simionovici Y, Ron L. Walking on virtual tiles. Neural Proc Lett. 2002;**16**(3):227–233.

156. Espay AJ, Baram Y, Dwivedi AK, et al. At-home training with closed-loop augmented-reality cueing device for improving gait in patients with Parkinson disease. J Rehabil Res Dev. 2010;**47**(6):573–581.

157. Baram Y, Miller A. Auditory feedback control for improvement of gait in patients with multiple sclerosis. J Neurol Sci. 2007;**254**(1):90–94.

158. Baram Y, Lenger R. Gait improvement in patients with cerebral palsy by visual and auditory feedback. Neuromodulation: Technol Neural Interf. 2012;**15**(1):48–52.

159. Ong SK, Shen Y, Zhang J, Nee AY. Augmented reality in assistive technology and rehabilitation engineering. In: Fuhrt B, (ed.) Handbook of Augmented Reality. Springer, Berlin, 2011, pp. 603–630.

160. Gallo S, Chapuis D, Santos-Carreras L, et al. Augmented white cane with multimodal haptic feedback. In: 3rd IEEE RAS and EMBS International Conference on Biomedical Robotics and Biomechatronics (BioRob), Tokyo, Japan, 2010, pp. 149–155.

161. Katz BG, Kammoun S, Parseihian G, et al. NAVIG: augmented reality guidance system for the visually impaired. Virtual Reality. 2012;**16**(4):253–269.

162. Walker BN, Lindsay J. Navigation performance with a virtual auditory display: effects of beacon sound, capture radius, and practice. human factors. J Hum Factors Ergon Soc. 2006;**48**(2):265–278.

163. Zhang J, Ong S, Nee A. Navigation systems for individuals with visual impairment: A survey. In: Proceedings of the 2nd International Convention on Rehabilitation Engineering & Assistive Technology. Singapore Therapeutic, Assistive & Rehabilitative Technologies (START) Centre, 2008, pp. 159–162.

164. Zhang J, Lip CW, Ong SK, Nee AY. Development of a shoe-mounted assistive user interface for navigation. Int J Sensor Netw. 2011;**9**(1):3–12.

165. Fallah N. AudioNav: a mixed reality navigation system for individuals who are visually impaired. ACM SIGACCESS Accessibility and Computing. 2010;(96):24–27.

166. Moustakas K, Tzovaras D, Dybkjær L, Bernsen NO. A modality replacement framework for the communication between blind and hearing impaired people. In: Stephanidis C (ed.) Universal Access in Human–Computer Interaction. Applications and Services. Springer, Berlin, 2009, pp. 226–235.

167. Konya Y, Siio I. A caption presentation system for the hearing impaired people attending theatrical performances. In: Nijholt A, Romão T, Reidsma D (eds) Advances in Computer Entertainment. Springer, Berlin, 2012, pp. 274–286.

168. Webster J, McFarland P, Rapport L, Morrill B, Roades L, Abadee P. Computer-assisted training for improving wheelchair mobility in unilateral neglect patients. Arch Phys Med Rehabil. 2001;**82**(6):769–775.

169. Sveistrup H. Motor rehabilitation using virtual reality. J Neuroeng Rehabil. 2004;**1**(1):10.

170. Keshner E. Virtual reality and physical rehabilitation: a new toy or a new research and rehabilitation tool? J Neuroeng Rehabil. 2004;**1**(1):8.

171. Israel JF, Campbell DD, Kahn JH, Hornby TG. Metabolic costs and muscle activity patterns during robotic-and therapist-assisted treadmill walking in individuals with incomplete spinal cord injury. Phys Ther. 2006;**86**(11):1466–1478.

172. Wolbrecht ET, Chan V, Reinkensmeyer DJ, Bobrow JE. Optimizing compliant, model-based robotic assistance to promote neurorehabilitation. IEEE Trans Neural Syst Rehabil Eng. 2008;**16**(3):286–297.

173. Secoli R, Milot MH, Rosati G, Reinkensmeyer DJ. Effect of visual distraction and auditory feedback on patient effort during robot-assisted movement training after stroke. J Neuroeng Rehabil. 2011;**8**(1):1–10.

174. Morrow K, Docan C, Burdea G, Merians A. Low-cost virtual rehabilitation of the hand for patients post-stroke. In: 2006 International Workshop on Virtual Rehabilitation. IEEE, New York, NY, 2006, pp. 6–10.

175. Chang YJ, Chen SF, Huang JD. A Kinect-based system for physical rehabilitation: A pilot study for young adults with motor disabilities. Res Dev Disabil. 2011;**32**(6):2566–2570.

176. Huang JD. Kinerehab: a kinect-based system for physical rehabilitation: a pilot study for young adults with motor disabilities. In: The Proceedings of the 13th International ACM SIGACCESS Conference on Computers and Accessibility. ACM, Dundee, UK, 2011, pp. 319–320.

177. Saposnik G, Teasell R, Mamdani M, et al. Effectiveness of virtual reality using Wii gaming technology in stroke rehabilitation a pilot randomized clinical trial and proof of principle. Stroke. 2010;**41**(7):1477–1484.

178. Gil-Gómez JA, Lloréns R, Alcañiz M, Colomer C. Effectiveness of a Wii balance board-based system (eBaViR) for balance rehabilitation: a pilot randomized clinical trial in patients with acquired brain injury. J Neuroeng Rehabil. 2011;**8**(1):30.

179. Taylor MJ, McCormick D, Impson R, Shawis T, Griffin M. Activity promoting gaming systems in exercise and rehabilitation. J Rehabil Res Dev. 2011;**48**(10):1171–1186.

180. Deutsch JE, Borbely M, Filler J, Huhn K, Guarrera-Bowlby P. Use of a low-cost, commercially available gaming console (Wii) for rehabilitation of an adolescent with cerebral palsy. Phys Ther. 2008;**88**(10):1196–1207.

181. Mouawad MR, Doust CG, Max MD, McNulty PA. Wii-based movement therapy to promote improved upper extremity function post-stroke: a pilot study. J Rehabil Med. 2011;**43**(6):527–533.

182. Passig D, Eden S. Improving flexible thinking in deaf and hard of hearing children with virtual reality technology. Am Ann Deaf. 2000;**145**(3):286–291.

183. Holmes EA, James EL, Coode-Bate T, Deeprose C. Can playing the computer game 'Tetris' reduce the build-up of flash-backs for trauma? A proposal from cognitive science. PloS One. 2009;**4**(1):e4153.

184. Goldstein J, Cajko L, Oosterbroek M, Michielsen M, Van Houten O, Salverda F. Video games and the elderly. Soc Behav Personal. 1997;**25**(4):345–352.

185. Clark JE, Lanphear AK, Riddick CC. The effects of videogame playing on the response selection processing of elderly adults. J Gerontol. 1987;**42**(1):82–85.

186. Dustman RE, Emmerson RY, Steinhaus LA, Shearer DE, Dustman TJ. The effects of videogame playing on neuropsychological performance of elderly individuals. J Gerontol. 1992;**47**(3):P168–P171.

187. Rizzo A, Reger G, Gahm G, Difede J, Rothbaum BO. Virtual reality exposure therapy for combat-related PTSD. In: LeDoux JE, Keane T,

Shiromani P (eds) Post-Traumatic Stress Disorder. Springer, Berlin, 2009, pp. 375–399.

188. Rizzo A, Morie JF, Williams J, Pair J, Buckwalter JG. Human emotional state and its relevance for military VR training. DTIC Document, The Proceedings of the 11th International Conference on Human Computer Interaction, HCI International 2005, Las Vegas, USA, 2005.

189. Broeren J, Rydmark M, Sunnerhagen KS. Virtual reality and haptics as a training device for movement rehabilitation after stroke: a single-case study. Arch Phys Med Rehabil. 2004;85(8):1247–1250.

190. Kahn LE, Lum PS, Rymer WZ, Reinkensmeyer DJ. Robot-assisted movement training for the stroke-impaired arm: Does it matter what the robot does? J Rehabil Res Dev. 2006;43(5):619.

191. Takahashi Y, Terada T, Inoue K, et al. Haptic device system for upper limb motor and cognitive function rehabilitation: grip movement comparison between normal subjects and stroke patients. In: IEEE International Conference on Rehabilitation Robotics (ICORR). IEEE, Noordwijk, The Netherlands, 2007, pp. 736–741.

192. Henderson A, Korner-Bitensky N, Levin M. Virtual reality in stroke rehabilitation: a systematic review of its effectiveness for upper limb motor recovery. Top Stroke Rehabil. 2007;14(2):52–61.

193. Laver K, George S, Thomas S, Deutsch JE, Crotty M. Virtual reality for stroke rehabilitation. Stroke. 2012;43(2):e20–e21.

194. Rizzo A, Kim GJ. A SWOT analysis of the field of virtual reality rehabilitation and therapy. Presence: Teleoperators and Virtual Environments. 2005;14(2):119–146.

195. Adamovich SV, Fluet GG, Tunik E, Merians AS. Sensorimotor training in virtual reality: a review. Neurorehabilitation. 2009;25(1):29–44.

Index

Note: page numbers in *italics* refer to figures and tables.

spinal cord injury 51–2
see also ageing
electrical enabling motor control
   (eEmc) 135–6
   application in motor paralysis 144
   effect on bladder function 142–3
electrical epidural stimulation 73
electrical stimulation (ES) 363–4
   indications and contraindications *364*
   therapeutic 370
   transcranial 174
   in upper limb rehabilitation 376
   see also neuroprostheses; transcranial direct
      current stimulation
electric wheelchairs 393
electroejaculation 306
electroencephalography (EEG) 161–2
   small fibre evoked potentials 319
   studies after stroke 165
electromagnetic neuromodulation
   (emEmc) 137–9
electromyography (EMG)
   in documentation of progress 212, *213*
   EMG exhaustion phenomenon 69–71
   in subject-specific modelling 219
electronic aids for daily living (EADLs) 404
electrophysiological assessment, spinal
   neuronal function 67–8
Emara, T.H. *181*
embryonic stem cells (ESCs) 149–50, *153*
   GRNOPC1, trials in acute spinal cord
      injury 156
   transplantation in Parkinson's disease 152
emotional dysregulation, cognitive
   rehabilitation 268
enabling motor control (Emc)
   electrical stimulation 135–6, 142–3, 144
   electromagnetic stimulation 137–9
   pharmacological stimulation 136–7
   synergism with sensorimotor training 140
   transcutaneous electrical
      stimulation *139*–40
end-effector based robotic locomotor
   systems 388, *389*
end of life issues
   assisted dying 348
   oral feeding problems 279
endothelin-1 injection, as a model of ischemic
   stroke 130
enemas 300
energy conservation strategies 334, 346
energy demands, hemiparetic gait 214–15
Engel, G.L. 8
enteral nutrition 278
environmental factors 4
   age-related 48
environmental qualifiers, ICF 5
ephedrine, in orthostatic hypotension 103
epidural stimulation, spinal walking
   neuroprostheses 366
epilepsy
   altered neurogenesis 150–1
   sexual dysfunction 289
   see also antiepileptic drugs
epimysial electrodes 365
epinephrine (adrenaline) 91
   in bradycardia 102
EPOS study 29
erectile dysfunction 100
   in multiple system atrophy (MSA) 289

in Parkinson's disease 289
   treatment 304–5, 306
   see also sexual dysfunction
erection, physiology of 288
Erichsen, J.E. 353
Ericsson, K.A. 255
error-based adaptation 56, *57*
errorless learning 263
erythropoeitin, in orthostatic hypotension 103
Escorpizo, R. and Stucki, G. 6
e-therapy, in aphasia 258
EuroQol 19, 20
Eva, G. 341–9
evidence-based practice v
   therapies for elderly patients 51
evidence levels 43–4
EXCITE (Extremity Constraint Induced
   Therapy Evaluation) trial 41, 59, 60,
   240–1
executive function deficits, cognitive
   rehabilitation 267–8
exercise
   benefits of 334, 347
   conventional techniques 374
exercise-induced fever 105
exercise programmes, effect on chronic
   pain 322
exercise progression *239*
exercise variety *239*
exoskeleton devices 388–9, *406*
   future developments 395, 396
   for independent walking 393–4
   in virtual reality training 421, *422*
exposure therapy, use of virtual reality 430
eye-tracking systems 420

F
faecal impaction 107–8
faecal incontinence 107
   prevention of 291
   see also bowel dysfunction
fainting (syncope) 95
falls 48
   risk assessment 51
families
   contribution to rehabilitation 50
   support services 401–2
fatigue
   aetiology and associations 329
      direct brain pathology 330
      inflammation and endocrine factors 330
      secondary factors 330–2
   definitions of 328
   epidemiology 329
   formulation-based approach *333*
   impact of 329
   investigation of *331*
   management of 346
   measurement of 328–9
   in peripheral nerve disorders 225
   treatment 332
      cognitive factors 334–5
      exercise and energy conservation
         strategies 334
      medication 335–6
      multidisciplinary rehabilitation 335
      nutrition 333
      physical aids 333
      pragmatic approach *336*
      of psychiatric conditions 333–4

sleep disorders 332–3
   temperature control 333
feasibility studies 41
feedback training strategies 391–2, 418
   game-based training 423
   virtual reality training 419, 431–2
fertility, after spinal cord injury 291
fertility support 292
FESMate device 368–9
fesoterodine, in detrusor overactivity 293
fetal progenitor cells 149
   transplantation in Parkinson's disease 152
fetal striatal allografts, use in Huntington's
   disease 153
fibroblasts, conversion in functional
   neurons 151–2
Finetech–Brindley bladder stimulation
   system *294*, 297
Fish, J. 267
fixed proportional recovery, stroke 31–2
FLAME (Fluoexetine for Motor Recovery after
   Acute Ischemic Stroke) trial 197, 201
flat interface nerve electrodes (FINEs) 365–6
flexor reflex activity, and spasticity 77
fludrocortisone, in orthostatic
   hypotension 103
fluid intake
   in management of urinary incontinence 298
   in orthostatic hypotension 102
flunarizine, combination with cortical
   stimulation *186*
fluoxetine
   effect on practice-dependent plasticity 199,
      200
   in stroke patients 199, 201, *203*
   in premature ejaculation 306
Flynn, D. 429
Fong, K. 425–6
food consistency 275, 278
foot drop, ankle–foot orthoses *231*
force feedback controllers, virtual reality
   systems 420
foreign accent syndrome 354
Fougeyrollas, P. 399–413
fractional anisotropy (FA) 162, *169*
Franz, S. 112–120
Freehand system *369*, 376
Fregni, F. 179, *184*, *185*
frontal opercular infarction *276*
Fugl–Meyer (FM) scores
   change in the sensitive period after
      stroke 57, *58*
   improvements after stroke
      predictability 31
      recovery of dexterity 30
functional assessment, in clinical trials 38
   standardization of 40
functional baseline definition 36
functional connectivity analysis 167
functional electrical stimulation (FES) 83,
   230, 364
   in gait disturbance 386, 395
   in orthostatic hypotension 104
   promises and challenges *361*
   in upper limb rehabilitation 376, 380
functional imaging
   assessment of network connectivity 167
   evolution of cerebral reorganization after
      stroke 163
   in fatigue 330